Roenigk's Dermatologic Surgery

Current Techniques in
Procedural Dermatology

Third Edition

Roenigk's Dermatologic Surgery

Current Techniques in Procedural Dermatology

Third Edition

Edited by

Randall K. Roenigk
Mayo Clinic
Rochester, Minnesota, U.S.A.

John Louis Ratz
Center for Dermatology and Skin Cancer
Tampa, Florida, U.S.A.

Henry H. Roenigk, Jr.
Arizona Advanced Dermatology
Scottsdale, Arizona, U.S.A.

informa
healthcare

New York   London

Informa Healthcare USA, Inc.
270 Madison Avenue
New York, NY 10016

© 2007 by Informa Healthcare USA, Inc.
Informa Healthcare is an Informa business

No claim to original U.S. Government works
Printed in the United States of America on acid-free paper
10 9 8 7 6 5 4 3 2 1

International Standard Book Number-10: 0-8493-3718-6 (Hardcover)
International Standard Book Number-13: 978-0-8493-3718-5 (Hardcover)

Visit the Informa Web site at
www.informa.com

and the Informa Healthcare Web site at
www.informahealthcare.com

DEDICATION

To those who learn from this book and are happy with their success practicing dermatologic surgery

To the patients who entrust us with their care and benefit from a physician's dedication to life-long learning

To institutions such as Cleveland Clinic, Mayo Clinic, Northwestern University, and others that provided training for our authors

To professional colleagues with whom we have interacted over the years teaching courses, working with professional societies, educating the public and who appreciate our efforts on behalf of the specialty

To support staff at our institutions and private practices without whom we could not do what we do

And to our wives Julie, Kathie, and Shirley, along with our children, who put up with many extra hours away from them to see patients, write, teach, and do research. Without your support we would not be able to succeed at work and our lives would be incomplete.

The first edition of this textbook was published in 1988 and at that time, we felt we were helping to define a growing subspecialty in dermatology—dermatologic surgery. We asked a prominent plastic surgeon and an otolaryngologist to write forewords for the book. Both acknowledged the dermatologist's expertise in some surgical procedures but reminded us that collaboration across specialties was important. We continued that theme in the second edition published in 1996. In both editions, we mentioned the experience of Dr. Jacques Joseph who was dismissed from Wolff's Clinic in 1896 for performing a cosmetic procedure. His example serves as a reminder that change is not easy, and agents of change are often ostracized.

Fred Mohs, a general surgeon from Madison Wisconsin, published his first paper on chemosurgery in 1941. At that time, Dr. Mohs was not highly regarded by the surgical community. When I came to Mayo, I heard comments from general surgeons, such as "we hoped the Mohs procedure would die when Dr. Mohs died!" It takes time and perseverance, but good ideas with real value normally prevail to become the standard of care. It turns out Dr. Mohs had two good ideas: a better method to completely check the margins of a specimen and, since he used zinc chloride paste to fix the tissue and did not close the wounds, we learned a great deal about second intention wound healing.

General surgeons and other surgical specialties ignored Mohs' procedure because they did not want to read the pathology, and it was not practical to perform this procedure in a traditional operating room. In the late 1960s, some bold dermatologists who were willing to practice outside the normal bounds of dermatology began to expand their skills in surgery. This included novel procedures such as hair transplantation, dermabrasion, and laser, among others. Since dermatologists were learning surgery and are trained during their residency in the clinical and pathology diagnosis of skin cancer, the Mohs procedure was a natural fit. The efficiency of this practice was helped because dermatologists routinely practice in a clinic, not an operating room, and frozen section technology became readily available in the 1970s. As a result, a dermatologist could operate on three or four patients at one time in the clinic using local anesthesia, get a frozen section in about one hour, and read the histology before taking additional tissue. In those days, most wounds were left to heal by second intention. It did not take long before dermatologists realized that they could close surgical defects after Mohs surgery for skin cancer, so the wound healed better and faster. Thus was born oncologic and reconstructive dermatologic surgery, two of the three major areas that make up the body of knowledge of our subspecialty.

Since the first edition of *Roenigk's Dermatologic Surgery* in 1988 and the second edition in 1996, the reconstructive skills of dermatologic surgeons have expanded considerably. Dermatologic surgeons now repair most of their defects, including many that would have been referred to other surgeons in the past. We do these procedures with better skill because of the number of cases we perform. Based on Medicare data, dermatologists perform more skin lesion excisions, Mohs surgery for skin cancer, primary repairs, and skin flaps than any other medical specialty. Because dermatologic surgeons today routinely perform these procedures on an outpatient basis instead of a hospital operating room, the cost of care has greatly reduced while quality and access have also improved. As a result, the reconstructive surgery section of our book has been greatly expanded in this edition.

All population and demographic studies tell us that skin cancer will continue to increase because of the aging of the baby boomers. At the same time, even more patients are looking for ways to avoid the signs of aging. Combine patient demand with the surgical skills learned through removing cancer along with the dermatologist's appreciation for the appearance of the skin, and the third major area—cosmetic dermatologic surgery—becomes a logical extension of our subspecialty and ever-expanding body of knowledge. This edition of *Roenigk's Dermatologic Surgery* has added new chapters on technology used for cosmetic procedures, such as lasers and light sources as well as minimally invasive procedures such as soft tissue augmentation, ambulatory phlebectomy, and Botox®. We have greatly expanded our cosmetic dermatologic surgery section while also maintaining a balance, since many older procedures still have value, having withstood the test of time.

In the 1970s, several societies were founded to promote education in dermatologic surgery, including the American Society for Dermatologic Surgery and the American College of Mohs Micrographic Surgery and Cutaneous Oncology, among others. A peer-review journal, now named *Dermatologic Surgery*, was started, which currently enjoys the seventh highest impact factor among 35 peer-reviewed dermatology journals. It became clear that residents must learn dermatologic surgery as part of their dermatology training. The American Board of Dermatology and the Residency Review Committee for Dermatology recognized this change in practice and adopted new program requirements for dermatology training and reorganized the certifying exam in dermatology, adding a section on surgery. It also became clear that fellowship training beyond the residency was an important way for some residents to gain added skills. Most of these fellowships were established by the American College of Mohs Micrographic Surgery and Cutaneous Oncology, but in 2003, the Accreditation Council for Graduate Medical Education approved the adoption of a new subspecialty of dermatology—procedural dermatology.

The Residency Review Committee now accredits 35 fellowships in this subspecialty while the American Board of Dermatology is considering a subspecialty-certifying exam in procedural dermatology. Regardless of when a dermatologist was a resident or how much surgery was taught in their training program, it is incumbent on all physicians to maintain their skills and engage in lifelong learning.

Population demographics and the increasing cost of health care have supported the growth of dermatologic surgery over the past 40 years because we provide ready access to cost-effective, high-quality outpatient care for skin disease and the signs of aging, which was heretofore unavailable. Our mission as editors of the Third Edition of *Roenigk's Dermatologic Surgery: Current Techniques in Procedural Dermatology* has been to provide one source for the most up-to-date yet comprehensive information that broadly describes what is currently accepted as state of the art in dermatologic surgery. Reading this text is an important way for dermatologists who perform surgery to maintain or improve their surgical skills. We hope that the pages of this book become wrinkled and the binding cracked with regular use.

Randall K. Roenigk, MD
John Louis Ratz, MD
Henry H. Roenigk, Jr., MD

Contents

PART V: CUTANEOUS RECONSTRUCTION

PART VI: COSMETIC DERMATOLOGIC SURGERY

Contributors

Eric Adelman Health Policy and Practice, American Academy of Dermatology, Schaumburg, Illinois, U.S.A.

Tina S. Alster Department of Dermatology, Georgetown University Medical Center, Washington, D.C., U.S.A.

Mathew M. Avram Division of Dermatology, University of California, Los Angeles, California, U.S.A.

Philip Bailin Division of Dermatologic Surgery, Department of Dermatology, Cleveland Clinic Foundation, Cleveland, Ohio, U.S.A.

Kenneth Beer Palm Beach Esthetic Center, West Palm Beach, Florida and Department of Dermatology, University of Miami, Miami, Florida, U.S.A.

Wilma F. Bergfeld Department of Dermatology and Pathology, Cleveland Clinic Foundation, Cleveland, Ohio, U.S.A.

Steven C. Bernstein University of Montreal, Montreal, Quebec, Canada

Melissa A. Bogle Laser and Cosmetic Surgery Center of Houston, Houston, Texas, U.S.A.

Paul H. Bowman The Bowman Institute for Dermatologic Surgery, Tampa, Florida, U.S.A.

Jerry D. Brewer Mayo Clinic, Rochester, Minnesota, U.S.A.

David G. Brodland Departments of Dermatology and Otolaryngology, University of Pittsburgh Medical Center, Pittsburgh, Pennsylvania, U.S.A.

Harold J. Brody Emery University School of Medicine, Atlanta, Georgia, U.S.A.

Marc D. Brown Department of Dermatology, University of Rochester Medical Center, Rochester, New York, U.S.A.

Alastair Carruthers Department of Dermatology, University of British Columbia, Vancouver, British Columbia, Canada

Jean Carruthers Department of Ophthalmology, University of British Columbia, Vancouver, British Columbia, Canada

Misty D. Caudell University of South Florida College of Medicine, Tampa, Florida, U.S.A.

Roger I. Ceilley University of Iowa, Iowa City, Iowa, U.S.A.

Elbert H. Chen Department of Dermatology, Columbia University, New York, New York, U.S.A.

Nor Chiao M.D. Anderson Cancer Center, University of Texas, Houston, Texas, U.S.A.

Holly L. F. Christman University of California, San Francisco, California, U.S.A.

Joel L. Cohen AboutSkin Dermatology and DermSurgery and Department of Dermatology, University of Colorado, Boulder, Colorado, U.S.A.

Brett Coldiron Health Policy and Practice, American Academy of Dermatology, Schaumburg, Illinois, U.S.A.

William P. Coleman III Tulane University School of Medicine, New Orleans, Louisiana, U.S.A.

Michael E. Contreras Department of Dermatology, University of New Mexico, Albuquerque, New Mexico, U.S.A.

Jennifer Z. Cooper Department of Dermatology, University of Rochester Medical Center, Rochester, New York, U.S.A.

Daniel C. Dapprich Mayo Clinic, Rochester, Minnesota, U.S.A.

Terence M. Davidson University of California, School of Medicine, San Diego, California, U.S.A.

Jeffrey S. Dover SkinCare Physicians, Chestnut Hill, Massachusetts, U.S.A.

Zoe Diana Draelos Department of Dermatology, Wake Forest University School of Medicine, Winston-Salem, North Carolina, U.S.A.

Raymond G. Dufresne, Jr. Department of Dermatology, Brown Medical School, Brown University, Providence, Rhode Island, U.S.A.

Dirk M. Elston Department of Dermatology, Geisinger Medical Center, Danville, Pennsylvania, U.S.A.

Michael J. Fazio Department of Dermatology, Skin Cancer Surgery Center, University of California Davis, Sacramento, California, U.S.A.

Neil A. Fenske University of South Florida College of Medicine, Tampa, Florida, U.S.A.

Edgar F. Fincher Moy-Fincher Medical Group, Los Angeles, California, and Stanford University Medical Center, Stanford, California, U.S.A.

Frederick Fish Department of Dermatology, University of Minnesota, Minneapolis, Minnesota, U.S.A.

James E. Fitzpatrick Department of Dermatopathology, University of Colorado Health Sciences Center, Denver, Colorado, U.S.A.

Oren Friedman Department of Otorhinolaryngology, Mayo Clinic, Rochester, Minnesota, U.S.A.

Robert J. Friedman Department of Dermatology, New York University School of Medicine, New York, New York, U.S.A.

Trephina Galloway   Division of Dermatologic Surgery, Department of Dermatology, Cleveland Clinic Foundation, Cleveland, Ohio, U.S.A.

Hayes B. Gladstone   Stanford University, Stanford, California, U.S.A.

Hugh M. Gloster, Jr.   University of Cincinnati, Cincinnati, Ohio, U.S.A.

Jeffry A. Goldes   Associated Dermatology of Helena, Helena, Montana, U.S.A.

Loren E. Golitz   Department of Dermatopathology, University of Colorado Health Sciences Center, Denver, Colorado, U.S.A.

William J. Grabski   Brooke Army Medical Center, Fort Sam Houston, Houston, Texas, U.S.A.

Donald J. Grande   Department of Dermatology, Boston University School of Medicine, Stoneham, Massachusetts, U.S.A.

Hubert T. Greenway   Scripps Clinic and Research Foundation, La Jolla, California, U.S.A.

Roy C. Grekin   University of California, San Francisco, California, U.S.A.

C. William Hanke   Laser and Skin Surgery Center of Indiana, Carmel, Indiana, U.S.A.

Ali Hendi   Department of Dermatology, Mayo Clinic, Jacksonville, Florida, U.S.A.

William B. Henghold   The Skin Cancer Center of Northwest Florida, Pensacola, Florida, U.S.A.

Whitney A. High   Department of Dermatopathology, University of Colorado Health Sciences Center, Denver, Colorado, U.S.A.

Harry J. Hurley   West Chester, Pennsylvania, U.S.A.

Michael S. Kaminer   SkinCare Physicians, Chestnut Hill, Massachusetts, U.S.A.

Grace F. Kao   Department of Pathology and Laboratory Medicine, Baltimore VA Medical Center, Baltimore, Maryland, and George Washington University, Washington, D.C., U.S.A.

Wynn H. Kao   Department of Dermatology, University of Puerto Rico Medical Center, San Juan, Puerto Rico

Arielle N. B. Kauvar   New York Laser and Skin Care and New York University School of Medicine, New York, New York, and SUNY Downstate Medical Center, Brooklyn, New York, U.S.A.

Jefferson J. Kaye   The Ochsner Clinic, New Orleans, Louisiana, U.S.A.

Malcolm S. Ke   Department of Dermatology, University Hospitals of Cleveland, Case Western Reserve University, Orange Village, Ohio, U.S.A.

Tatiana Khrom   SUNY Downstate Medical Center, Brooklyn, New York, U.S.A.

Glenn Kolansky   Advanced Dermatology Surgery Center, Tinton Falls, New Jersey, U.S.A.

Christopher B. Kruse   Advanced Dermatology Surgery Center, Tinton Falls, New Jersey, U.S.A.

Emanuel G. Kuflik   Department of Medicine, New Jersey Medical School, Newark, New Jersey, U.S.A.

Jeff Lander   Department of Dermatology, University of Minnesota, Minneapolis, Minnesota, U.S.A.

Joshua E. Lane   Section of Dermatology, Department of Medicine, The Medical College of Georgia, Augusta, Georgia, U.S.A.

Robert C. Langdon   Shoreline Dermatology, Guilford, Connecticut, U.S.A.

Gary P. Lask   Division of Dermatology, University of California, Los Angeles, California, U.S.A.

Hann Lee   The Division of Dermatology and the Section of Plastic Surgery, The Keck School of Medicine University of Southern California, Los Angeles, California, U.S.A.

Peter K. Lee   Department of Dermatology, University of Minnesota, Minneapolis, Minnesota, U.S.A.

Barry Leshin   The Skin Surgery Center, Winston-Salem, North Carolina, U.S.A.

Yong Li   The Division of Dermatology and the Section of Plastic Surgery, The Keck School of Medicine University of Southern California, Los Angeles, California, U.S.A.

P. Lillis   University of Colorado Health Sciences Center, Denver, Colorado, U.S.A.

Katherine K. Lim   Mayo Clinic, Scottsdale, Arizona, U.S.A.

Clifford Warren Lober   University of South Florida College of Medicine, Tampa, Florida, U.S.A.

Wesley Low   University of California, School of Medicine, San Diego, California, U.S.A.

Leslie C. Lucchina   Department of Dermatology, Brigham and Women's Hospital and Harvard Medical School, Boston, Massachusetts, U.S.A.

Deborah F. MacFarlane   M.D. Anderson Cancer Center, University of Texas, Houston, Texas, U.S.A.

Diego E. Marra   Department of Dermatology, Brigham and Women's Hospital, Harvard Medical School, and Mohs Surgery Center, Dana Farber Cancer Institute, Boston, Massachusetts, U.S.A.

Elizabeth I. McBurney   Department of Dermatology, Louisiana State University, New Orleans, Louisiana, U.S.A.

Terri McGillis   Department of Dermatologic Surgery, Cleveland Clinic Foundation, Cleveland, Ohio, U.S.A.

Jon G. Meine   Department of Dermatologic Surgery, Cleveland Clinic Foundation, Cleveland, Ohio, U.S.A.

J. Ramsey Mellette, Jr. University of Colorado Health Sciences Center, Denver, Colorado, U.S.A.

Jeffrey L. Melton Department of Dermatology, University of Illinois at Chicago, Chicago, Illinois, U.S.A.

Allison J. Moosally Department of Dermatologic Surgery, Cleveland Clinic Foundation, Cleveland, Ohio, U.S.A.

Greg S. Morganroth University of California, San Francisco, California and Stanford University, Stanford, California, U.S.A.

Ronald L. Moy Department of Skin Cancer and Dermatologic Surgery, UCLA School of Medicine, Los Angeles, California, U.S.A.

Rhoda S. Narins Dermatology Surgery and Laser Center of New York, White Plains, New York and Department of Dermatology, New York University Medical Center, New York, New York, U.S.A.

Tri H. Nguyen Department of Dermatology and Otorhinolaryngology, University of Texas M.D. Anderson Cancer Center, Houston, Texas, U.S.A.

Suzanne M. Olbricht Department of Dermatology, Lahey Clinic, Burlington, Massachusetts and Department of Dermatology, Harvard Medical School, Boston, Massachusetts, U.S.A.

David S. Orentreich Mt. Sinai School of Medicine, New York, New York, U.S.A.

Norman Orentreich New York University School of Medicine, New York, New York, U.S.A.

Clark C. Otley Mayo Clinic, Rochester, Minnesota, U.S.A.

R. Steven Padilla Department of Dermatology, University of New Mexico, Albuquerque, New Mexico, U.S.A.

Clifford S. Perlis Fox Chase Cancer Center, Philadelphia, Pennsylvania, U.S.A.

P. Kim Phillips Mayo Clinic, Rochester, Minnesota, U.S.A.

Tania Phillips The Division of Dermatology and the Section of Plastic Surgery, The Keck School of Medicine University of Southern California, Los Angeles, California, U.S.A.

Kevin S. Pinski American Institute-Dermatology, Chicago, Illinois, U.S.A.

Christine Poblete-Lopez Department of Dermatology, Cleveland Clinic Foundation, Cleveland, Ohio, U.S.A.

Sheldon V. Pollack University of Toronto, Toronto, Ontario, Canada

Steven Proper University of Florida School of Medicine, Tampa, Florida, U.S.A.

Divya Railan Colby Skincare, San Jose, California, U.S.A.

Henry W. Randle Mayo Clinic, Jacksonville, Florida, U.S.A.

Désirée Ratner Department of Dermatology, Columbia University, New York, New York, U.S.A.

John Louis Ratz Center for Dermatology and Skin Cancer, Tampa, Florida, U.S.A.

Saadia Lakhany Raza Department of Dermatology, Emory University, Atlanta, Georgia, U.S.A.

Darrell S. Rigel Department of Dermatology, New York University School of Medicine, New York, New York, U.S.A.

June K. Robinson Department of Dermatology, Northwestern University Feinberg School of Medicine, Chicago, Illinois, U.S.A.

Henry H. Roenigk, Jr. Arizona Advanced Dermatology, Scottsdale, Arizona, U.S.A.

Randall K. Roenigk Mayo Clinic, Rochester, Minnesota, U.S.A.

Thom W. Rooke Mayo Clinic, Rochester, Minnesota, U.S.A.

Nathan Rosen McGill University, Montreal, Quebec, Canada

Timothy J. Rosio Anew Skin™ Dermatology, Folsom-Auburn, California, U.S.A.

Richard M. Rubenstein Dermal and Subcutaneous Tumors, Wellington Regional Medical Center, Wellington, Florida, U.S.A.

Adam I. Rubin University of Pennsylvania, Philadelphia, Pennsylvania, U.S.A.

Vernell St. John Health Policy and Practice, American Academy of Dermatology, Schaumburg, Illinois, U.S.A.

Stuart J. Salasche University of Arizona Health Sciences Center, Tucson, Arizona, U.S.A.

Richard K. Scher College of Physicians and Surgeons, Columbia University, New York, New York, U.S.A.

Bryan C. Schultz Loyola University Stritch School of Medicine, Maywood, Illinois, U.S.A.

Robert A. Schwartz New Jersey Medical School, Newark, New Jersey, U.S.A.

Kevin Spohr Dermal and Subcutaneous Tumors, Wellington Regional Medical Center, Wellington, Florida, U.S.A.

Thomas Stasko Vanderbilt University Medical Center, Nashville, Tennessee, U.S.A.

J. Barton Sterling Spring Lake, New Jersey, U.S.A.

Dow B. Stough Department of Dermatology, University of Arkansas for Medical Sciences, Little Rock, Arkansas, U.S.A.

Sharon Thornton Division of Dermatologic Surgery, Department of Dermatology, Cleveland Clinic Foundation, Cleveland, Ohio, U.S.A.

Christopher Tignanelli University of Medicine and Dentistry of New Jersey, New Jersey Medical School, Newark, New Jersey, U.S.A.

Rochelle Torgerson Mayo Clinic, Rochester, Minnesota, U.S.A.

Abel Torres   Loma Linda University School of Medicine, Loma Linda, California, U.S.A.

Thomas A. Victor   Department of Pathology and Laboratory Medicine, Evanston Northwestern Healthcare, Evanston, Illinois, U.S.A.

Allison T. Vidimos   Department of Dermatology, Cleveland Clinic Foundation, Cleveland, Ohio, U.S.A.

Richard F. Wagner, Jr.   University of Texas Medical Branch, Galveston, Texas, U.S.A.

Tom Wang   Department of Otolaryngology, Oregon Health Science Center, Portland, Oregon, U.S.A.

Melanie Warycha   Department of Dermatology, New York University School of Medicine, New York, New York, U.S.A.

Carl V. Washington   Department of Dermatology, Emory University, Atlanta, Georgia, U.S.A.

Robert A. Weiss   Department of Dermatology, Johns Hopkins University School of Medicine, and MD Laser Skin and Vein Institute, Baltimore, Maryland, U.S.A.

Ronald G. Wheeland   University of Arizona College of Medicine, Tucson, Arizona, U.S.A.

Duane C. Whitaker   University of Arizona, Tucson, Arizona, U.S.A.

Andrea Willey   Department of Dermatology, University of Minnesota, Minneapolis, Minnesota, U.S.A.

Gregory J. Wilmoth   Mayo Clinic, Rochester, Minnesota, U.S.A.

Dana Wolfe   University of California, School of Medicine, San Diego, California, U.S.A.

David T. Woodley   The Division of Dermatology and the Section of Plastic Surgery, The Keck School of Medicine University of Southern California, Los Angeles, California, U.S.A.

Randall J. Yetman   Cleveland Clinic Foundation, Cleveland, Ohio, U.S.A.

Mark J. Zalla   Dermatology Associates of Northern Kentucky, Florence, Kentucky, and Department of Dermatology, University of Cincinnati, Cincinnati, Ohio, U.S.A.

Priya Zeikus   Department of Dermatology, Brown Medical School, Brown University, Providence, Rhode Island, U.S.A.

John A. Zitelli   Shadyside Medical Center, Pittsburgh, Pennsylvania, U.S.A.

1

Surgical Preparation, Facilities, and Monitoring

Diego E. Marra
Department of Dermatology, Brigham and Women's Hospital, Harvard Medical School, and Mohs Surgery Center, Dana Farber Cancer Institute, Boston, Massachusetts, U.S.A.

Edgar F. Fincher
Moy-Fincher Medical Group, Los Angeles, California, and Stanford University Medical Center, Stanford, California, U.S.A.

Ronald L. Moy
Department of Skin Cancer and Dermatologic Surgery, UCLA School of Medicine, Los Angeles, California, U.S.A.

INTRODUCTION

To deliver the highest level of surgical care to the patient in the office setting, there must be adequate preparation prior to surgery. The steps include proper preparation of the skin, appropriate instrument selection and care, and an adequate facility for the procedure as well as to meet any unexpected needs.

SURGICAL PREPARATION OF THE SKIN

The goal of surgical preparation is twofold. The surgeon must do everything possible to decrease the chance of wound contamination and subsequent infection, which may lead to complications secondary to the infection. In addition, adequate antisepsis is essential to prevent infection transfer to office personnel, medical equipment, and other patients.

Bacteriology

It is impossible to sterilize the skin completely. Ten to twenty percent of the resident flora is found in the deeper layers of the skin, primarily within the pilosebaceous units. Most of the resident flora, however, is in the superficial layers of the skin. The normal flora varies considerably with the anatomic site. Approximately 90% of the resident aerobic bacteria is *Staphylococcus epidermidis*. Additional strains include *Staphylococcus aureus*, micrococci, diphtheroids, streptococci, and some gram-negative bacilli. The skin may also contain several transient and pathogenic microorganisms. These are the bacteria usually involved in wound infection and, fortunately, are easily removed by adequate surgical preparation. The single most commonly found organism in wound infections is *S. aureus*. Staphylococci and, to a lesser degree, streptococci are the most common offenders in outpatient surgery. In the hospital setting, the majority of pathogens in surgical wounds are gram-negative bacteria. These include *Escherichia coli, Pseudomonas aeruginosa, Klebsiella, Enterobacter,* and *Proteus* species. This difference between the hospital and the private office reflects cross-contamination in the hospital environment.

Antiseptic Agents

An ideal antiseptic agent should rapidly destroy all microorganisms without any risk of toxicity, irritation, or allergenicity. No one antiseptic agent satisfies all of these criteria, but some come closer than others (Table 1).

Soaps

Ordinary soaps have very little antibacterial effect. However, their mechanical emulsifying action removes a large portion of the superficial transient and pathogenic bacteria. Thus, an adequate scrub with a soap or detergent, preferably combined with the killing power of an antiseptic, is the first and most important step in prepping the skin.

Chlorhexidine

Chlorhexidine gluconate is a biguanide agent that is very effective against a wide range of gram-positive and gram-negative bacteria. Chlorhexidine produces rapid bacterial destruction and binds with the protein of the stratum corneum to leave some degree of residual action. It is not damaging to the skin and is not absorbed through it. There is no evidence of systemic toxicity. It also appears to be more resistant to contamination than many of the other antiseptic agents. Chlorhexidine has been shown to be safe for use on the oral mucosa, but the sudsing base can be irritating to the conjunctiva, so it should be kept away from the eyes. It can also be toxic to the middle ear. Therefore, it should not be placed into the auditory canal. This precaution applies to many other antiseptic agents. At the present time, chlorhexidine appears to be the agent of choice for a surgical scrub.

Iodophors

Pure iodine is a rapidly acting, powerful antiseptic agent. However, it tends to be unstable and is irritating to the skin.

Table 1   Antiseptic Scrubs

Type	Composition	Spectrum	Onset	Sustained Activity	Comments
Alcohol	Isopropyl/ethyl alcohol	Gram +	Fast	None	No killing of spores, antibacterial only; 70% more effective than 90%
Iodophor	Iodine + surfactant (betadine)	Gram +, gram −	Moderate	Up to 1 hr (longer acting than plain iodine)	Must be dry to be effective tissue damaging; inactivated by blood, serum; may be absorbed through skin
Hexachlorophene	Polychlorinated biphenyl (Phisohex)	Gram +	Slow–must remain in contact with skin >3 min	Yes	Teratogen, not sporicidal–do not use in pregnant women; CNS toxic–do not use in infants
Chlorohexadine	Biguanide (Hibiclens)	Gram +, gram −	Fast	Yes	Do not use near eyes or ears. Use betadine instead
Benzalkonium	Quaternary ammonium detergent (Zephiran)	Gram +, gram −	Slow	None	Prone to contamination

Most of the problems associated with elemental iodine have been addressed by the development of iodophors, which are a combination of iodine and a polymer. The water soluble complex slowly releases free iodine. The lower concentration of iodine is less irritating to the skin and, although less effective than iodine, is still an excellent antiseptic. Povidone-iodine is one of the most popular iodophor complexes. This aqueous solution may be applied as a final skin prep. A detergent base may be added (betadine surgical scrub) to produce a sudsing antiseptic preoperative scrub. These agents have a wide range of antibacterial activity, including the destruction of some bacterial spores.

The iodophors may occasionally cause skin reactions in iodine-sensitive individuals. Although it is of little risk in cutaneous surgery, iodine toxicity can result from absorption when iodophors are applied to large areas of denuded skin. Aqueous iodine preparations should not be used as wound cleansers because the iodine may have a denaturing effect on the exposed tissues.

Alcohols

Alcohols are good antiseptics, but their full effectiveness is not often achieved in the usual clinical application. Seventy percent ethyl alcohol can destroy 90% of cutaneous bacteria within two minutes if constant alcohol moisture is maintained during that time period. However, a single wipe with an ethyl alcohol-soaked swab produces a reduction of only 75% of the cutaneous bacteria. This reduction is predominantly mechanical and not bactericidal, and relies on alcohol as an organic solvent to remove oil and debris containing large numbers of bacteria. Alcohol should not be applied to an open wound because, like iodine, it denatures and damages tissue protein. Isopropyl alcohol is somewhat less irritating to the tissues than ethyl alcohol. It can cause some degree of vasodilatation, which may enhance the bleeding of small needle puncture sites. Because they are flammable, alcohol-based products should not be used in the presence of electrosurgical equipment.

Benzalkonium Chloride

Quaternary ammonium compounds are cationic agents and are easily inactivated by anionic compounds such as soaps, detergents, blood, and other organic materials. Benzalkonium chloride destroys many gram-positive and some gram-negative bacteria and fungi. However, it is now seldom used because it lacks effectiveness against *Mycobacterium tuberculosis, P. aeruginosa,* spores, and many viruses. In fact, the product may become contaminated by some of these organisms.

Hair Removal

Shaving should be avoided if possible. It has been shown that shaving traumatizes the skin and promotes bacterial growth, which results in an increased incidence of wound infections. If hair must be removed, it is preferable to clip away only the hair that interferes with surgery. Small areas may be cut satisfactorily using scissors. Electric clippers are convenient, but small spicules of hair should be removed carefully to avoid their introduction into the surgical site.

Marking Proposed Incision Lines

Most skin surgery is facilitated by drawing proposed incision lines on the skin prior to the actual incision. Traction and contraction often cause tissue distortion, and deviation from the proposed incision can thus be avoided. The proposed incision lines should be marked prior to injection of local anesthesia. The patient should be sitting up or standing so as to account for gravitational effects on relaxed skin tension lines. The use of dots instead of lines reduces the smudging and allows for more precision in the marking. There are a number of types of surgical markers available. Standard markers use gentian violet and are nontoxic. Preoperative prepping with alcohol will rub off the gentian violet, but Betadine and Hibiclens may not. There have been no reported cases of tattooing.

Draping

Most office procedures are performed using disposable drapes. These are impermeable to moisture. Cotton drapes, in contrast, are supple, porous, and more comfortable for the patient. If a fenestrated paper drape is used, it should be laminated with a layer of plastic between two sheets of paper. Nonlaminated paper drapes are chemically treated to resist moisture. Pure plastic drapes are available with an adhesive margin around the fenestration. This keeps the drape stable and is particularly useful when one is working in anatomic concavities.

Preparation of the Surgeon

The surgeon must also be prepared to enter the now sterile surgical environment in an antiseptic manner. Because gloves are occasionally punctured or defective, and because bacteria multiply rapidly in the warm, moist environment inside gloves, there should be minimal bacteria present on the hands prior to placing on sterile surgical gloves. Standard surgical scrubs are used for hospital operating rooms; however, studies show that a brief scrub with effective agents may be just as effective. Regular washing with an antiseptic detergent, such as chlorhexidine gluconate, before and between cases should result in a very low degree of bacterial contamination of the hand, in part because of its residual antibacterial effect.

Masks clearly help protect the staff from splashes of blood or other fluids (such as injected anesthesia, irrigation, etc.). However, whether masks provide protection to the patient is less clear. According to Ritter, there appears to be no difference in the total number of airborne bacterial pathogens in surgical rooms whether face masks are worn or not. A comparison by Caliendo of infection rates between lacerations repaired by physicians with ($n = 47$) and without ($n = 44$) face masks revealed no statistically significant difference. In fact, the single wound infection observed in that study occurred in a patient treated by a mask-wearing physician. On the basis of these data and his own report showing no change in the incidence of hospital operating room wound infections after discontinuing the use of face masks for a six-month time period, Orr concluded that the use of face masks may not serve any purpose vis-à-vis patient protection. It should be noted, however, that talking and coughing or sneezing may propel significant amounts of bacteria up to 1 and 3 m away, respectively, and as Belkin points out, masks significantly decrease such flow.

Clothing should be specific for the operating room. Street clothes should not be worn, as such clothing not only can bring microorganisms into the surgical area, but can also become contaminated by blood or other fluids; therefore, street clothes can transfer contamination to other areas at work or at home. It should be noted, however, that, as Belkin points out, specific surgical attire has not been shown to decrease infection rates, although this has not been extensively studied.

PREPARATION AND STERILIZATION OF SURGICAL INSTRUMENTS

Instrument Cleaning

After instruments have been used, they should be rinsed with warm water to remove debris. If they are soaked, it is best to add a detergent to the water. A detergent used for cleaning instruments should be of neutral pH. Acid detergents will break down the stainless steel surface and result in a black stain. Basic detergents leave a brown, rust-like deposit on the instrument. This appears after autoclaving and may interfere with the operation of the instrument since it is usually retained in the joint areas. All tissue and foreign materials must be carefully removed from the instruments. This material may be removed manually by scrubbing with a stiff plastic brush, or by means of an ultrasonic cleaner. If using the latter, the instruments are placed in ultrasonic cleaner fluid, which consists of water and a neutral pH detergent. Sonic waves are produced and are transformed in the fluid to mechanical energy, which dislodges foreign material from instrument surfaces. The ultrasonic cleaner removes only surface debris; it is not a disinfecting or sterilizing process. After the instruments have been removed from the ultrasonic cleaner and rinsed, they should be dried. Ultrasonic cleaning can remove lubrication in hinged areas. To restore this lubrication, instruments should be placed in instrument oil. This restores lubrication but may leave a greasy film on the surface, and some physicians prefer to use instrument oil only when necessary. Other oils, silicone spray, or grease should be avoided because they tend to bake when autoclaved and stiffen rather than lubricate the joints. Before the instruments are packed, they should be inspected to make sure they are in proper working order. Scissor blades can be tested for sharpness by cutting a piece of tissue paper. The cut should be smooth and without resistance. The tips of forceps and hemostats should be aligned. The opposing surfaces of needle holders should meet completely and be able to grasp 6–0 nylon suture securely from any angle. Many instrument manufacturers will sharpen and repair instruments at a very reasonable cost.

Sterilization

Most methods of sterilization efficiently destroy vegetative forms of bacteria. However, it is imperative in the sterilization of surgical instruments to use a method that will adequately destroy bacterial spores as well.

Steam Autoclave

Steam at 100°C destroys vegetative bacterial forms, but not spores. By increasing the pressure above ambient levels, the steam autoclave reaches a temperature of 121°C. When this environment is maintained for more than 15 minutes, all microorganisms are destroyed. The recommended cycle times for most autoclaves are somewhat longer. The 15-minutes exposure time begins when steam has penetrated all areas. This may require an additional 5 to 15 minutes, depending on the size of the surgical pack. The main disadvantage of steam sterilization is the gradual dulling of sharp edges, although this is less of a problem with high quality instruments. The steam autoclave may be used for the sterilization of most surgical materials including metal, cloth, paper, glassware, and heat-resistant plastics. Steam autoclaves are best operated with distilled water.

Chemiclave

The chemiclave is very similar to the steam autoclave but with lower humidity, usually less than 15%. The low humidity reduces damage to sharp surgical edges. Instruments are drier at the end of the autoclave cycle. However, instead of distilled water, the chemiclave uses a special chemical solution that contains formaldehyde, methylethyl ketone, acetone, and a mixture of several alcohols. Use of this system requires close adherence to protocol to prevent environmental contamination.

Dry Heat

Dry heat autoclaves are small, modified ovens. These units are inexpensive, and, due to the absence of moisture, there is no problem with corrosion or dulling. Dry heat sterilization requires high temperatures and prolonged exposure times. The usual instrument-packing materials (cloth, paper, or plastic) cannot be used for dry heat sterilization due to the high temperatures. The instruments must be placed in special containers or sterilized in metal trays or foil packs.

Gas Sterilization

Gas sterilization is an effective alternative for instruments and materials that cannot be exposed to heat. This process requires elaborate equipment and prolonged exposure times. Because it relies on the use of ethylene oxide gas, a known carcinogen, mutagen, and neurotoxin, this sterilization method is restricted to large institutional settings. Dermatologic surgeons may need to make arrangements for access to such a facility for sterilization of specialized equipment such as a dermabrasion handpiece or dermatome. It is important to remember that ethylene oxide penetrates porous materials and aeration is necessary prior to use: 24 hours for paper and thin rubber; 96 hours for plastics; and 7 days for polyvinyl chloride and items of plastic or rubber sealed in plastic.

Chemical (Cold Tray) Sterilization

A variety of disinfectant solutions or germicides are available. Most are a combination of ingredients such as a low concentration of alcohol, a detergent, an antirust additive, and a quaternary ammonium compound antiseptic. These antiseptic agents are easily inactivated and contaminated and are not effective against *M. tuberculosis, Pseudomonas,* or bacterial spores. Glutaraldehyde preparations are the only agents that are reliable for use as cold sterilizing agents. Glutaraldehyde reaches its maximum antibacterial effect when it is buffered to a pH of 8.5. However, it is relatively unstable at this pH and tends to polymerize over a period of weeks. Therefore, activated glutaraldehyde must be renewed frequently. Unbuffered glutaraldehyde antiseptics are also available, and although they are more stable, studies indicate that the unbuffered forms are less effective. Glutaraldehydes, however, are not without problems. First, although vegetative forms of bacteria are adequately destroyed within a few minutes, several hours are required to destroy spores. Second, if contamination occurs or a contaminated instrument is replaced in the solution, 8 to 10 hours must elapse before any instrument in that solution can be considered sterile. Third, because glutaraldehyde can be irritating to the skin and mucosal surfaces, it should be rinsed from the instruments with sterile water prior to use, potentially introducing an additional contamination factor. In short, chemical sterilization should not be performed on instruments used for incisional surgery.

Instrument Packing
Cloth

The traditional instrument pack material used in hospitals is cloth, but this is not as frequently used in the private office. Cloth must be laundered and, due to its permeability, the instrument storage time is significantly reduced. To be an effective barrier, the cloth wrapping material should be a tight-weave 270-thread count Pima cotton fabric.

Paper

Disposable paper packs are far more convenient than cloth for use in the private office. Crepe paper wraps are available for use as a wrap similar to cloth. Paper envelopes are easier to use. The most convenient choice is a paper/transparent pack that is self-sealing. The transparent side of the pack allows one to see the contents. A built-in heat-sensitive indicator on the paper surface changes color when it has been exposed to the autoclave cycle. It is important to remember this indicator shows that the pack has been exposed to heat but does not guarantee the adequacy of the sterilization process. For this purpose, special autoclave monitors are available. These are inserted into the packs to check periodically on the thoroughness of sterilization.

Open Containers and Solutions

Some prefer to autoclave instruments unpacked in metal trays. After the sterile trays are removed, the instruments are removed as needed from them. Another variation is to remove the freshly sterilized instruments from the autoclave tray and transfer them to a germicide holding solution. Both of these techniques introduce all the possibilities of storage contamination associated with cold sterilization, and should be avoided if possible.

All surgical instruments should be compartmentalized into separate packs or containers so that the container is violated only once for a particular procedure (Fig. 1).

Instrument Storage

After instruments have been autoclaved, they should be stored in a manner that will maintain sterility. Prior to autoclaving, the date should be written on packs for later reference. Storage time will vary depending upon the packing material used (Table 2). Well-sealed paper/transparent pouches have the longest storage time—up to 12 months. Instruments must be stored away from moisture. Any wet surgical pack must be considered contaminated. Packs should be subjected to limited handling. Handling traumatizes the paper surfaces and may result in breaks in the barrier. An instrument pack filing system should be devised so the office assistant does not have to search through several packs to find the desired item.

Surgical Tray Setup

In preparation for surgery, the surgical instruments must be arranged on a sterile tray. This is usually done by placing a sterile barrier drape over a tray such as the Mayo stand (Fig. 2). A disposable barrier drape consists of a layer of polyethylene film laminated between two layers of paper. Instruments should be packed such that, when the pouch is opened a short distance above die tray, the instruments fall out handle-first onto the tray. This avoids damage to the delicate instrument tips as well as preventing puncture of the barrier drape. The instruments are then arranged neatly on the tray with transfer forceps (Fig. 3). Suture material and scalpel blades may be added last.

SURGICAL FACILITY

Not all offices have space available for a room devoted exclusively to surgical procedures. The largest examination room available should be equipped for minor surgical procedures. The physician who performs only limited minor surgical procedures will not require a fully equipped suite; however, those with a larger surgical practice will require most of the recommended items and perhaps two or three similar surgical rooms.

Surgical Suite

A separate room should be reserved for surgical procedures. The surgical suite will usually contain more equipment than

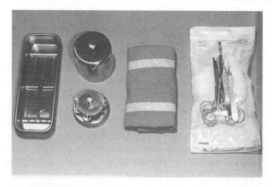

Figure 1 Surgical instruments compartmentalized to avoid contamination.

Table 2 Instrument Packing and Storage

Method	Advantages	Disadvantages	Safe storage time
Commercially packaged, pre-sterilized, disposable items	Fast and simple	Expensive	Sterile until opened or damaged
Sealed paper transparent pouches	Fast packing and opening; excellent barrier; instruments are visible	Moderately expensive	12 months
Nonwoven synthetic fabric	Disposable; tear resistant	Expensive; moisture retention	3–4 months
Paper wrap	Inexpensive	Tears and punctures easily	3–8 weeks
Muslin wrap	Most economical; lies flat and becomes sterile field drape	Must be laundered; produces lint; short shelf life	3–4 weeks; 6–12 months if immediately sealed in plastic after sterilization
Disinfectant holding solution	Minimal materials required; fast	Unreliable; prone to contamination; skin irritation	Must be replaced and instruments resterilized every 2 weeks or more often

an examination room. Minimizing the patient volume in this room will decrease the chance of damage to delicate and expensive items. The room should be at least 160 square feet. For major procedures 250 square feet is recommended. It is possible to do surgery in a much smaller room, but space will be tight and there will be insufficient room for ancillary and emergency equipment (Fig. 4). A hard-surfaced floor is easiest to keep clean; however, floor contamination is rarely a problem in dermatologic surgery. Although explosive anesthetic agents are no longer used, laws in some states require a conductive, hard-surfaced floor for licensed operating rooms. The walls should be covered with a washable material. The ceilings in most offices are constructed of standard suspended acoustic ceiling material. Acoustic tile is satisfactory for office surgery, but not adequate to meet the requirements for a licensed facility. That may require a ceiling of solid, nonporous material, which is easier to clean and is possibly more sanitary.

There should be ample counter space with a large, laboratory-style sink (licensing may require the sink to be near, but outside, the operating room) (Fig. 5). There should be adequate cabinet space, while overhead cabinet storage is recommended. The entry doors should be oversized to allow easy passage of a wheel-chair or stretcher cart. The operating room should be situated so there is room for additional storage nearby. Laboratory and sterilizing areas should also be in close proximity.

Lighting

The basic room lighting should be fluorescent. Three to four ceiling modules containing four 48-inch fluorescent lights each should provide adequate basic room light for 160 square feet or less. Ceiling or wall-mounted lights are preferred because they do not use valuable floor space and are usually more flexible in their range of coverage (Fig. 6). Single-point source, spotlight-type lights should be avoided. Harsh shadows are produced and make surgical visualization difficult. Single-point lights, such as head-mounted lights, are useful for supplemental lighting; The primary surgical light should come from multiple points or from a large reflector to produce shadowless light. Halogen lights produce a high-intensity natural light with minimal heat production. All surgery lights should have a transparent, protective safety shield to minimize the hazards associated with bulb failure. The light head should be periodically cleaned and inspected to make sure there are no loose or defective parts. Once the surgeon is gloved, the assistant can manipulate the light into the optimal position. Many surgery lights have accessory handles that can be sterilized and attached to the light for manipulation by the gloved surgeon. The sterilized handles should be cuffed to prevent contamination.

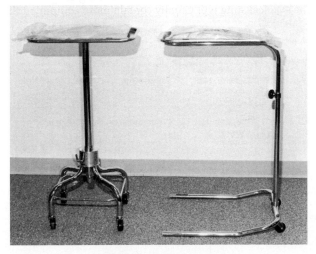

Figure 2 The Mayo stand.

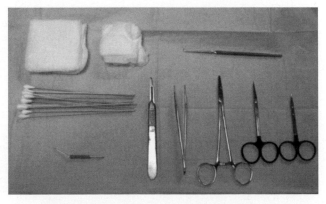

Figure 3 Proper arrangement of instruments on a tray.

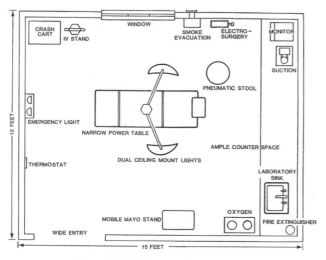

Figure 4 Ideal set-up of surgical suite.

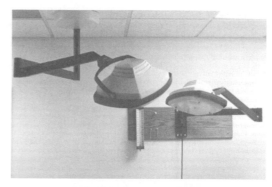

Figure 6 Wall-mounted lights.

Atmosphere

Hospital operating rooms often have laminar flow air systems to minimize contamination, and such a system may be required for accreditation. However, there is little evidence to indicate that these systems alter the rate of infection. Most postoperative infections do not arise from contamination from the inanimate environment. They are usually due to contamination from the patient, surgeon, surgical material, or breaks in sterile technique. The room should have good temperature control. Preferably, the operating room should have its own temperature-regulating system. The temperature of the room may rise considerably during long procedures performed under warm surgical lights. A sound system providing soothing music serves to distract the patient and minimizes the awareness of strange noises produced during surgery.

Surgical Table

Next to adequate lighting, a good surgical table is one of the most important features of the operating room. The ease of surgery will be greatly facilitated by an adaptable table that allows proper positioning. A full-power table is highly recommended. However, for those who wish to have a licensed operating room, some codes require the operating table to be ungrounded and have no electrical connection.

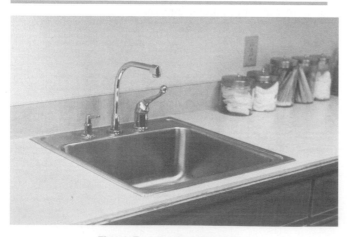

Figure 5 Laboratory-style sink.

This is not a significant hazard for outpatient cutaneous surgery. A wide table may increase patient comfort but may be less convenient for the surgeon working on midline structures. The table should be relatively thin, particularly at the head end. This allows the surgeon to put his or her legs under the table while seated and working in the head and neck region. The table should adapt to several positions. A well-contoured table may be comfortable for the patient lying supine but may not accommodate the patient in the prone or lateral position. The table should be adjustable for Trendelenburg and proctoscopic positions. Side rails are a useful option for attaching armboards or surgical trays.

Surgical Stool

Some procedures are best performed with the surgeon seated. A good surgical stool should be on rollers and have pneumatic height adjustment. The height adjustment is usually hand-controlled but a foot adjustment is a convenience for the gloved surgeon. Some stools are available with an extended backrest, which can provide valuable arm support.

Surgical Stands

A surgical tray attached to a power table is inflexible and may present problems. It is better to have an independent table that may be moved about the surgical field. The most common choice is a Mayo table or stand. A Mayo table is recommended because it rests on four casters and can be easily shifted with the surgeon's foot. The traditional Mayo stand is constructed with two casters and one or two legs and is not as stable. The advantages of the Mayo stand is the ease of placement directly over the patient.

Electrosurgical Equipment

A wide variety of electrosurgical equipment is available. The surgeon must tailor the equipment to the procedures performed. Most simple office procedures require coagulation and electrodesiccation. Dermatologic surgeons involved in advanced micrographic and reconstructive procedures, however, may not benefit from a higher degree of coagulation or the ability to generate cutting current. Sterile sheaths are available to cover electrosurgical handpieces; alternatively, autoclaveable units may be purchased and packed with each surgical setup. When extensive electrosurgery, particularly cutting current, is used in the course of a procedure, a large amount of smoke and a disagreeable odor are produced. This plume is not only offensive to patients, but is potentially infectious. Therefore, a smoke evacuation

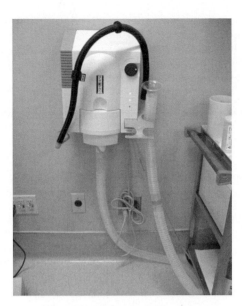

Figure 7 Smoke evacuation system.

system should be a standard equipment in any surgical suite (Fig. 7).

Emergency Equipment

Fire Extinguisher

An often overlooked hazard in the operating room is fire. This is a particular risk with laser surgery, but combustible items may also be easily ignited with electrosurgery. Many of the fire extinguishers supplied with medical offices dispense a fire-retardant powder. This may be effective but is not recommended for spraying in the region of a surgical wound. A gas fire extinguisher should be available.

Resuscitation Equipment

Every office should be equipped with a crash cart or emergency kit to store drugs and equipment for cardiopulmonary resuscitation (Fig. 8). All offices should be equipped with devices that permit medical personnel to

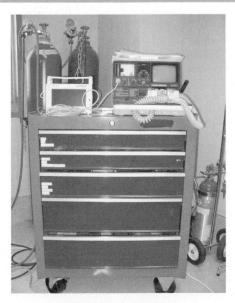

Figure 8 Crash cart.

provide mouth-to-mouth resuscitation without risk of contamination. Such masks equipped with one-way valves should be available to all of the treatment areas. Surgeons, particularly those involved in advanced procedures and especially those working in accredited facilities, should maintain current their advanced cardiac life support certification.

Oxygen

An oxygen system is recommended for use in patients with respiratory distress. The physician should be familiar with the indications and contraindications of oxygen administration.

Suction

Suction equipment is a useful addition to any operating room. It may be necessary in some emergencies and also for fluid aspiration during some procedures. For nonemergency suction use, an electrical pump-type suction unit is recommended. Venturi suction attachments are available for use with oxygen tanks. These are satisfactory when a brief period of suction is required for emergency procedures. However, these attachments require a high oxygen flow and deplete the oxygen supply rapidly.

Defibrillator

Although not a common item in private offices, a defibrillator with a cardiac monitor is a useful addition to the office in which advanced surgical procedures are performed, particularly on elderly patients.

Monitoring Equipment

In addition to a cardiac monitor combined with a defibrillator, other forms of patient status should be considered in a complete surgical facility. Such monitoring devices are mandatory for patients who undergo some form of conscious sedation, particularly intravenous sedation, and are standard equipment in accredited surgical facilities. A digital pulse oximeter provides continuous monitoring of the pulse rate as well as the oxygen saturation level. This allows the physician to readily identify the patient who has significant respiratory depression that interferes with adequate blood oxygenation. Pulse oximeters are useful in all patients, but may be somewhat unreliable in patients with severe chronic obstructive pulmonary disease or significant peripheral vascular disease. Continuous blood pressure monitoring is essential for sedated patients. An automatic blood pressure monitoring device is highly recommended. For any of these monitoring devices, it is recommended to have a machine that prints out a hard copy record of the data. Otherwise, the information should be carefully charted on a flow sheet at regular intervals.

Wheelchair

Some patients may need assistance exiting the surgery suite. An office wheelchair may prove valuable in such an occurrence.

Back-Up Equipment

The surgeon should be adequately prepared to deal with power failures should they occur during the course of a surgical procedure. Emergency lights are available that have a continuous charging battery system. When a failure to the charging system is detected, the lights are automatically activated. These units will provide adequate ambient lighting for the room. An auxiliary source of power should be available for the operation of electrosurgical equipment, power surgical table, and surgical lights. A 600-watt generator will run all of these devices adequately. Storage battery back-up systems with similar outputs are available and may be necessary when the use of a generator is not feasible. A back-up should be available for any mechanical equipment necessary for the completion of a surgical procedure.

Individual Protective Equipment

Because of increasing concerns about physician and employee exposure to contagious diseases, such as human immunodeficiency virus and the hepatitis viruses, special attention needs to be directed at protecting the medical care worker. Universal precautions dictate that surgical gloves be worn for all potential contact with bodily fluids. Employees should also wear gloves when handling and sorting used instruments. Strong consideration should be given to the use of masks and eye protection for nearly all surgical procedures. There is clear evidence that the smoke plume generated by lasers and electrosurgical units may harbor viable viral particles. Standard surgical masks are designed to prevent droplet transmission from physician to patient, and offer little protection against potentially infectious plumes. This emphasizes the importance of utilizing an adequate smoke evacuation system during such procedures.

Accreditation

In the 1970s, a trend toward office-based surgery led to the creation of a specialty-specific accrediting body charged with developing standards and ensuring compliance with office-based surgery protocols. Since then, it has become possible for advanced dermatologic surgeons to establish their own accredited ambulatory surgical facilities. Accreditation may be obtained through the Accreditation Association for Ambulatory Health Care (AAAHC), the Joint Commission of Accreditation of Hospitals (JCAHO), the Institute for Medical Quality (IMQ), or Medicare. The laws for state licensing vary and may be different from requirements of the national agencies. It is now possible to hire consultants to streamline the process of accreditation, an option that is particularly appealing for those contemplating designing and building their own surgical facility.

While this is undoubtedly a major undertaking and requires significant commitment of time and capital, there are countless reasons in favor of pursuing accreditation. First, and most importantly, such a setting maximizes patient comfort and safety. Second, it provides the surgeon with an ideal environment that is at once customized to the surgeon's preferences and capable of meeting any eventuality that may be encountered in the course of advanced surgical procedures. Third, procedures performed in such facilities, while meeting hospital-level standards, offer significant cost savings to patients and third-party payors when compared with hospital-based facilities. Fourth, Medicare reimburses accredited ambulatory surgical facilities. Finally, and perhaps of greatest significance to the field, accreditation validates and legitimizes the dermatologic surgeon's unique training, skills, and expertise vis-a-vis other surgical specialties. As such, accreditation should be, if not sought, then at least strongly considered by any physician for whom dermatologic surgery encompasses a major component of clinical practice.

BIBLIOGRAPHY

Surgical Preparation of the Skin

Alexander JW, Fischer JE, Boyajian M, Palmquist J, Morris MJ. The influence of hair-removal methods on wound infections. Arch Surg. 1983; 118(3):347–352.

Butcher HR, Ballinger WF, Gravens DL, et al. Hexachlorophene concentrations in the blood of operating room personnel. Arch Surg 1973; 107:70–74.

Chlorhexidine and other antiseptics. Med Lett Drugs Ther. 1976; 18(21):85–86.

Contaminated povidone-iodine solution. Northeastern United States. MMWR 1980; 29:553–555.

Cruse PJE, Foord R. The epidemiology of wound infection. A ten year prospective study of 62,939 wounds. Surg Clin North Am 1980; 60:27–40.

Dharan S, Pittet D. Environmental controls in operating theatres. J Hosp Infect 2002; 51(2):79–84.

Dixon RE, Kaslow RA, Mackel DC, et al. Aqueous quarternary ammonium antiseptics and disinfectants: use and misuse. JAMA 1976; 236:2415–2417.

Evans CA, Smith WM, Johnston EA, Giblett ER. Bacterial flora of the normal human skin. J Invest Dermatol 1950; 15:305–324.

Kaul AF, Jewett F. Agents and techniques for disinfection of the skin. Surg Gynecol Obstet 1981; 152:677–685.

Kimbrough RD. Review of recent evidence of toxic effects of hexachlorophene. Pediatrics 1973; 51:391–394.

Rodeheaver G, Bellamy W, Kody M, et al. Bactericidal activity and toxicity of iodine-containing solutions in wounds. Arch Surg 1982; 117:181–186.

Rosenberg A, Alatary SD, Peterson AF. Safety and efficacy of the antiseptic chlorhexidine gluconate. Surg Gynecol Obstet 1976; 143:789–792.

Roth RR, James WD. Microbiology of the skin: resident flora, ecology, infection. J Am Acad Dermatol 1989; 20(3):367–390. Review.

Sebben JE. Avoiding infection in office surgery. J Dermatol Surg Oncol 1982; 8:455–458.

Seropian R, Reynolds BM. Wound infections after preoperative depilatory versus razor preparation. Am J Surg 1971; 121:251–254.

Simmons BP. Guidelines for hospital environmental control. Infect Control 1982; 2:131–137.

Simmons BP. Guidelines for prevention of surgical wound infections. Infect Control 1982; 3:187–196.

Strachan C. Antibiotic prophylaxis in "clean" surgical procedures. World J Surg 1982; 6:273–280.

Whitaker DC, Grande DJ, Johnson SS. Wound infection rate in dermatologic surgery. J Dermatol Surg Oncol 1988; 14(5):525–528.

Preparation and Sterilization of Surgical Instruments

Association of Perioperative Registered Nurses. Recommended practices for cleaning and caring for surgical instruments and powered equipment. AORN J 2002; 75(3):627–630, 633–636, 638 passim.

Allen KW, Humphreys H, Sims-Williams RF. Sterilization of instruments in general practice: what does it entail? Public Health 1997; 111(2):115–117.

Altemeier WA, Burke JF, Pruitt BA, Sandusky WR. American College of Surgeons Manual on Control of Infection in Surgical Patients. Philadelphia: J.B. Lippincott, 1976.

Association for Advancement of Medical Instrumentation Sterilization Committee. Good Hosptial Practice: Ethylene Oxide Gas-Ventilation Recommendations and Safe Use. AAMI. 1981.

Belkin NL. The evolution of the surgical mask: filtering efficiency versus effectiveness. Infect Control Hosp Epidemiol 1997; 18(1):49–57.

Belkin NL. Use of scrubs and related apparel in health care facilities. Am J Infect Control 1997; 25(5):401–404.

Bond WW, Favero MS, Petersen NJ, et al. Inactivation of hepatitis B virus by intermediate-to-high level disinfectant chemicals. J Clin Microbiol 1982; 18:535–538.

Caputo RA, Odlaug TE. Sterilization with ethylene oxide and other gases. In: Lawrence CA, Block SS, eds. Disinfection, Sterilization, and Preservation. Philadelphia: Lea & Febiger, 1983:47–64.

Caliendo JE. Surgical masks during laceration repair. JACEP 1976; 5(4):278–279.

Doust BC, Lyon AB. Face masks in infection of the respiratory tract. JAMA 1918; 71:1216–1219.

Gorman SP, Scott EM, Russell AD. A review: antimicrobial activity, uses and mechanism of action of glutaraldehyde. J Appl Bacteriol 1980; 48:161–190.

Kuhn R. Care and handling of surgical instruments. Part II. Med Product Sales 1982; 13:84–86.

Mallison GF, Standard PG. Safe storage times for sterile packs. Hospitals 1974; 48:77–80.

Orr NW. Is a mask necessary in the operating theatre? Ann R Coll Surg Engl 1981; 63(6):390–392.

Pepper RE. Comparison of the activities and stabilities of alkaline glutaraldehyde sterilizing solutions. Infect Control 1980; 1:90–92.

Perkins JJ. Principles and Methods of Sterilization in Health Sciences. Springfield, IL: Charles C Thomas, 1980:154–167, 286–311.

Ritter MA, Eitzen H, French ML, Hart JB. The operating room environment as affected by people and the surgical face mask. Clin Orthop Relat Res 1975(111):147–150.

Rutala WA, Weber DJ. New disinfection and sterilization methods. Emerg Infect Dis 2001; 7(2):348–353.

Sebben JE. Sterilization and care of surgical instruments and supplies. J Am Acad Dermatol 1984; 11:381–392.

Simmons BP. Guidelines for hospital environmental control. Infect Control 1981; 2:133–146.

Surgical Facility

Accreditation Association for Ambulatory Health Care. AAAHC Guidebook for Office Based Surgery Accreditation. 2004.

American National Standard for the Safe Use of Lasers: ANSI Z126.1, New York: American National Standards Institute, Inc., 1980.

Davey WP. Quality improvement and management in a dermatology office. Arch Dermatol 1997; 133(11):1385–1387.

Elliott RA. Organization and efficient function of office surgery. In: Schultz RC, ed. Outpatient Surgery. Philadelphia: Lea & Febiger, 1979:52–75.

Elliott RA. The design and management of an aesthetic surgeon's office and surgery suite. In: Regnault P, Daniel R, eds. Aesthetic Plastic Surgery: Principles and Techniques. Boston: Little, Brown 1984.

Elliott RA, Hoehn JG. The office surgery suite. Clin Plast Surg 1983; 10:225–246.

Kesheimer K, Davey WP. Continuous quality improvement in a dermatologic surgery office. Arch Dermatol 2000; 136(11):1400–1403.

Maloney M. The surgical suite. In: Grekin RC, ed. The Dermatologic Surgical Suite, Design and materials. New York: Churchill Livingstone, 1991.

Mallison GFL. The inanimate environment. In: Bennett JV, Brachman PS, eds. Hospital Infections Boston: Little, Brown, 1979: 81–92.

Morello DC, Colon GA, Fredricks S, Iverson RE, Singer R. Patient safety in accredited office surgical facilities. Plast Reconstr Surg 1997; 99(6):1496–1500.

Pawlson LG, Torda P, Roski J, O'Kane ME. The role of accreditation in an era of market-driven accountability. Am J Manag Care 2005; 11(5):290–293.

Sebben JE. Fire hazards and electrosurgery. J Dermatol Surg Oncol 1990; 16:421–424.

Taylor D, Iqbal Y. How to clear accreditation hurdles. Outpatient Surg Mag 2001; 2:32–39.

Tobin HA. Designing the facility. In: Lee KJ, Stewart C, eds. Ambulatory Surgery and Office Procedures in Head and Neck Surgery. Orlando, FL: Grune & Stratton, 1986: 303–314.

Tobin HA. Office surgery: the surgical suite. J Dermatol Surg Oncol 1988; 14(3):247–255.

Watson AB, Loughman J. The surgical diathermy: principles of operation and safe use. Anesth Intensive Care 1978; 6: 310–321.

2

Instrumentation

Saadia Lakhany Raza and Carl V. Washington
Department of Dermatology, Emory University, Atlanta, Georgia, U.S.A.

INTRODUCTION

It is an exciting time in dermatologic surgery as the field continues to expand through the innovation and advancement of new techniques and procedures. It has become imperative for the dermatologic surgeon to become familiar with the wide variety of instruments available, as well as their many uses in order to effectively and efficiently perform specific procedures. In this chapter, the array of surgical instruments available to the dermatologic surgeon will be covered. The purpose of this review is not to be exhaustive, but rather to focus on those options most commonly utilized, and those most critical to the practice of dermatologic surgery.

BLADE HANDLES

Traditionally the #3 Bard-Parker standard blade handle has been the most widely used by cutaneous surgeons (Fig. 1). Its wide body fits comfortably in the palm and has an area large enough to provide a secure grip. This handle accommodates all blades No. 15 and lower. The weighted design of this instrument helps to stabilize the entire unit during the incision, so when properly used, the force needed to cut is counterbalanced by the weight of the handle. It is available with and without calibrations, which are useful for measuring lesion sizes. Another Bard-Parker design is the #3 round knurled handle, which accepts the same blade array as the standard handle.

Other handles have been designed in order to create a more precise gripping surface and a better fit in the hand of the surgeon (Fig. 1). Thinner and lighter than the #3 handle, the #9 handle is held more like a pencil during the incision. The #7 handle is a much thinner, longer instrument, and is available with or without a textured gripping surface. The cylindrical or hexagonal Beaver handle is used in combination with the small Beaver blades. This is most useful for difficult-to-reach areas, which require more precise, delicate maneuvering.

Disposable blade handles with attached blades are available, but these are weighted differently than the standard #3 handle and are less desirable for fine surgical work.

BLADES

Many types of blades are available to the dermatologic surgeon. They are generally manufactured of either stainless steel or carbon steel. Carbon steel is stronger than stainless steel and allows for more precise cutting of loose tissue such as around the eyelid and the groin. However, stainless steel blades are more commonly used in dermatologic surgery, likely because these inexpensive blades are adequate for most procedures. Blades on disposable scalpels, as well as Beaver blades, are generally composed of stainless steel.

The main parts of the blade include the tip, the cutting edge, and the eye of the blade, where it attaches to the handle. The opening in the blade is the eye and its shape will determine which type of handle fits a given blade. Blades most commonly used in dermatologic surgery include the Nos. 15, 15c, 11, and 10 (Fig. 2).

The No. 15 blade is the workhorse of cutaneous surgeons. Its convex cutting edge, or belly, is the sharpest surface, and incisions should be initiated with this edge instead of the tip. A variation of the No. 15 blade is the No. 15c blade, which is distinguished by its overall compact size and a more acute angle of the tip. It is useful in smaller anatomic regions and areas with delicate skin such as that found in the ears, eyelids, lips, and genitalia. The No. 11 blade has a sharp, pointed tip, which is ideal for stab incisions and for removing fine sutures. Larger than the belly of the No. 15 blade, the wide, convex sharp edge of the No. 10 blade is most advantageous for large excisional surgeries, especially on thick tissue such as the back, and for sectioning tissue in preparation for examination during Mohs micrographic surgery.

The most commonly used Beaver blades are sizes 6400 and 6700; these are designed to be used in conjunction with the Beaver handles (Fig. 1). The 6400 blade has a rounded tip while the 6700 blade is similar in shape to the 15c blade.

The double edged–Gillette® Super Blade (Fig. 3) is a very thin and extremely sharp stainless steel blade. It can be broken in half to eliminate one sharp edge so that shave biopsies and tangential excisions can be performed easily and safely.

Another useful tool is the DermaBlade® by Personna Medical (Fig. 3), which has a long sharp stainless steel edge, much like the razor blade. Its advantage is the increased safety allowed by the flexible plastic cover, which encases the entire blade except the cutting edge. The blade can be flexed between the thumb and index finger to achieve a desirable angle to easily remove a protuberant or flat lesion.

While there are number of choices of blades and blade handles available, in the end it is the surgeon's personal preference and experience, which determine which one should be used.

PUNCH

One of the most important and widely utilized tools is the skin punch (trephine) developed by Edward Keyes in 1879. The original Keyes punch is designed with a metallic handle,

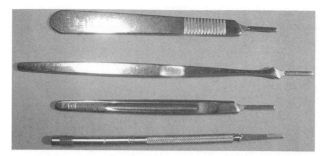

Figure 1 *Top to bottom*: #3, #7, #9, Beaver handle. (The Beaver handle has an attached 6400 Beaver blade.)

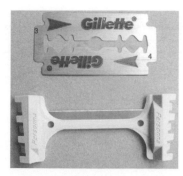

Figure 3 Gillette® Super Blade (*top*) and DermaBlade®.

a lumen with angled sides, and an annular cutting edge so that a larger area of epidermis than dermis is removed. Punch diameters range from 1–10 mm. The stainless steel blade has multiple uses including full thickness skin biopsies, and creation of both float grafts for depressed scars and donor grafts for hair transplantation. Also the 2–4 mm diameter punches can be used to remove cartilage plugs in order to allow granulation tissue to grow through the punch site when second-intention healing is the preferred mechanism for wound healing on the ear. The smaller Loo punch (Fig. 4) has less beveled edges and is better designed for creating floating punch grafts in order to improve the appearance of depressed scars. Both the Keyes and Loo punch blades will dull eventually with use and require maintenance. The skin punch is also available as a single use disposable instrument in a range of blade diameters and has the obvious advantage of an initial sharp edge.

SCISSORS

Scissors are divided into two main groups according to whether they have sharp or blunt tips. Additionally, they can be classified according to the length of the handle, as well as the characteristic of the blade (curved, straight, smooth, or serrated). The main function of sharp-tipped scissors tends to be precise cutting of tissue whereas blunt tips are preferred for minimizing unnecessary trauma during tissue dissection and undermining by pushing

nerves and vessels to the side rather than cutting through them. Both types of scissors are available with either straight or curved blades.

Most cutting scissors are manufactured from stainless steel, which will tend to become dull over time. It is imperative that cutting scissors be kept sharp enough to allow precise cutting and minimize crush injury to the tissue. Blade inserts made from tungsten carbide, which is stronger and more durable than stainless steel, are available. The inserts maintain a sharper edge and can help to minimize instrument turnover. However the inserts are expensive and will add to the cost of the scissors.

Cutting scissors commonly used include the iris, Stevens tenotomy, and Gradle scissors (Fig. 5). Iris scissors are short with pointed tips and are helpful in areas where the scalpel blade would not provide adequate control of tissue during cutting such as the loose tissue of eyelid or groin. Gradle scissors, with tapered tips, were originally designed for ophthalmologic use, and are ideal for resecting the delicate tissue in the periorbital and genital areas. The Stevens tenotomy scissors also have tapered ends and are similar to the Gradle scissors in their function.

Dissecting scissors include the Ragnell, Metzenbaum, and blunt-tipped Stevens tenotomy scissors (Fig. 6). Generally, the larger the dissection field, the larger the scissors that should be used to maximize efficiency. Scissors with larger handle-to-blade ratios allow for a more controlled dissection and require less effort in opening the jaw blades. The Metzenbaum and Ragnell scissors work similarly, but the thinner tips of the Ragnell scissors allow a more gentle dissection. In the more delicate periocular, periorbital, and genital areas, the blunt-tipped Stevens tenotomy scissors are preferable due to their overall smaller size, which provides better control of the tissue dissection.

With most of the scissor types described above, the super-cut feature is a relatively new option. These instruments

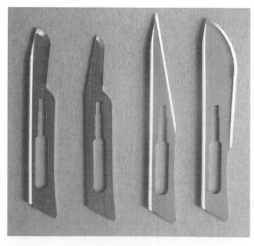

Figure 2 *Left to right*: 15, 15c, 11, 10 scalpel blades.

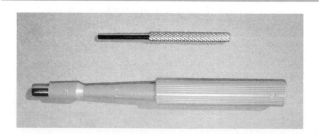

Figure 4 Loo punch (*top*), disposable punch tool (*bottom*).

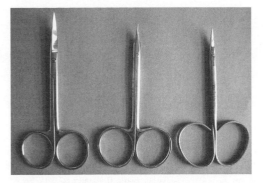

Figure 5 *Left to right*: Iris, Stevens tenotomy, Gradle scissors.

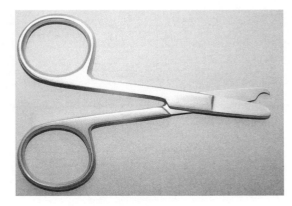

Figure 7 Littauer suture-cutting scissors.

are designed with a razor edge on one blade. The disadvantage is that they may tend to dull more quickly.

While not essential to all dermatologic surgeons, suture scissors are a useful addition to some (Fig. 7). When used exclusively for this purpose, these allow for less of the blunting of dissecting and cutting scissors, which tends to occur when these more expensive scissors are used to cut suture.

NEEDLE HOLDERS

Needle holders (Fig. 8) used in dermatologic surgery tend to be smaller and more delicate than those used in other types of procedures due to the fact that the needles and sutures used in dermatologic surgery are correspondingly smaller and more delicate. The Webster is a commonly used needle holder with its narrow jaws, which are available with either smooth or finely serrated surfaces. The serrated surface provides a better grip on the needle, but, however, can cause fraying of fine suture while tying knots and so generally the smooth surface is preferable.

For surgical procedures on thick tissue, such as on the back, the serrated heavy Halsey needle driver is a more appropriate tool, which can accommodate the larger needle and suture material generally required in these areas.

The Castroviejo, an alternative needle holder, is an even more delicate instrument designed for ultrafine surgery and needles. It is most useful for periorbital procedures. It is held much like a pencil, and so a left-handed surgeon can use it as easily as a right-handed one. It is available

with and without a lock–release mechanism, which requires some experience to use it proficiently.

FORCEPS

Forceps convert the surgeon's pincer grip into a much more controlled, delicate motion and have become essential in most dermatologic surgeries. A variety of forceps are available, but those used most commonly used in cutaneous procedures include the Adson, Bishop-Harmon, and jeweler's forceps (Fig. 9).

The Adson forceps are the most commonly used forceps and have wide serrated handles, which taper to long, narrow tips. Three or four fingers are placed on one side of the forceps and the thumb on the opposite handle. The Bishop-Harmon forceps is a smaller instrument designed for handling more delicate tissue such as the eyelid. Its handles have three holes on each side to facilitate a better grip and easier manipulation.

Additionally, forceps are designed with different tips to increase the efficiency of the instrument (Fig. 10). Choosing the appropriate tips will help to avoid crush injury while still maintaining stability of the tissue or suture. The widely used 2×1 teeth tips have two sharp points on one tip and a single point on the opposite tip; these are suitable for reconstruction because they allow for traction while minimizing tissue trauma. Serrated tips apply firm pressure and are

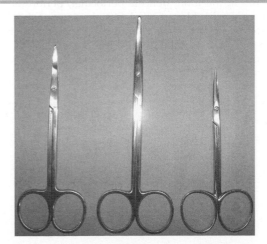

Figure 6 *Left to right*: Ragnell, Metzenbaum, and blunt-tipped Stevens tenotomy.

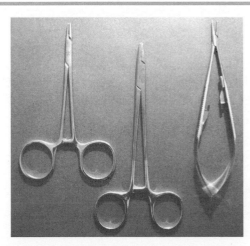

Figure 8 *Left to right*: Webster, Halsey, Castroviejo needle holders.

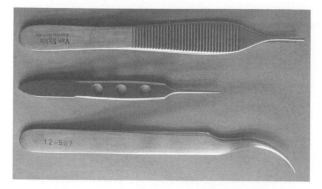

Figure 9   Adson, Bishop-Harmon, jeweler's forceps.

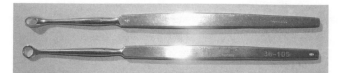

Figure 11   Fox (*top*) and Piffard (*bottom*) curettes.

useful for grasping a bleeding vessel or stabilizing tissue, which will be excised such as a cyst. The platform tips facilitate needle grasping during suturing.

Jeweler's forceps with very narrow tips are useful for removing suture which has become caught under skin.

In the end, the size of surgeon's hand, the intended function, as well as previous surgical experience will determine which forceps work most effectively for each surgeon.

CURETTES

Curettes have multiple functions in dermatologic surgery. The characteristic semisharp blade aids in distinguishing friable malignant tissue characteristic of certain types of skin cancers, which will scrape away with gentle pressure, leaving intact normal skin. This feature makes this a useful tool during electrodessication and curettage. In addition, for similar reasons, curettes are helpful prior to taking an initial stage during Mohs micrographic surgery. They may also be used to smooth out wound edges or to remove desiccation debris, where second-intention healing is a superior option for healing. This simple tool can also quickly remove small benign lesions, such as acrochordons and seborrheic keratoses.

The round Fox head and the oval head Piffard curettes (Fig. 11) are most commonly used in dermatologic surgery. Different curette sizes are available according to the diameter of the head. Generally, with a larger tumor or lesion, a curette with a larger head diameter should be used. Disposable curettes are available; however, the blade is sharper and so requires careful use in order to avoid excessive tissue damage.

SKIN HOOKS

Originally designed for tissue retraction and visualization, their ability to handle tissue with minimal trauma and crush injury have made skin hooks an essential instrument in cutaneous surgery. The Guthrie, sharp double-pronged

retractor and the single pronged Frazier hooks are most often used by dermatologic surgeons for retracting skin edges (Fig. 12). In addition, single pronged hooks are often substituted for forceps during placement of buried subcutaneous sutures, to minimize any crush injury, which could be induced by forceps.

STAPLES

Since 1908, surgical stapling has been used for wound closure and has continued to become more popular due to the increased efficiency and speed with which they can be placed. Disposable skin staples (Fig. 13) are generally made of stainless steel or titanium, and create less tissue strangulation than suturing. Staples are an ideal method of closure for noncosmetic areas such as the scalp and for large wounds on the extremities. They also can be used to secure skin grafts, particularly in larger wounds. Hemostats can be used to remove these staples; or, staple removers are widely available, which are designed to easily extract the staples.

ADDITIONAL INSTRUMENTS

A small hemostat such as the Halstead hemostat (Fig. 14), also known commonly as a mosquito clamp, is a thin instrument with long opposing jaws. It is available with either straight or curved tips. The hemostat can be used to secure and clamp substantial bleeding vessels during surgery, which are then cauterized or tied off. In addition, blades can be carefully removed from the blade handle with a hemostat.

Although not essential to a cutaneous surgical procedure, towel clamps can be used to organize the surgical tray and secure the operative field. Small Backhaus towel clamps (Fig. 15) are helpful for strategically placing towels around the surgical field in order to protect the patient while maintaining a clean field. Also, the larger Backhaus clamp can be used to anchor electrocautery wiring to the surgical tray.

Another instrument which was originally designed for ophthalmologic use, the chalazion clamp (Fig. 16) is also very helpful in cutaneous surgery to stabilize free margins such as the eyelid, earlobe, and lips. The clamp is

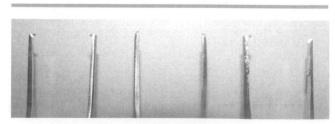

Figure 10   2 × 1 toothed, serrated and platform tips.

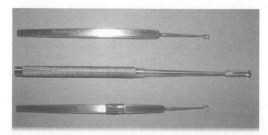

Figure 12   Guthrie (*top*), sharp double-pronged retractor (*middle*), Frazier hooks (*bottom*).

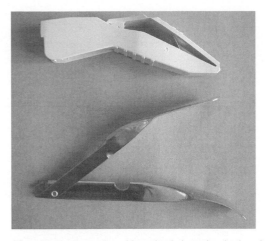

Figure 13 Disposable stapler with preloaded staples (*top*) and staple remover (*bottom*).

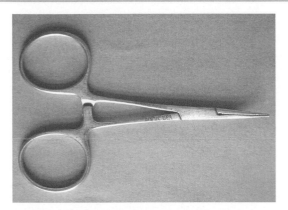

Figure 14 Halstead hemostat.

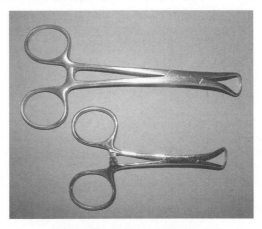

Figure 15 Backhaus towel clamps.

a modification of the traditional forceps with a smooth plate on one end and an oval ring on the opposing end. A thumb screw mechanism is used to secure the tissue between the ring and the plate. The circumferential pressure has the added benefit of providing some hemostasis to the involved tissue; however, care must be taken in order to avoid strangulating the tissue.

A periosteal elevator is a useful instrument for procedures, which require separating the periosteum from the

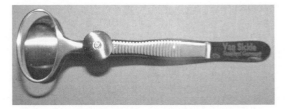

Figure 16 Chalazion clamp.

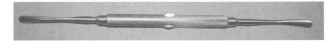

Figure 17 Freer periosteal elevator.

underlying bone. The Freer periosteal elevator (Fig. 17) is designed with two curved ends, one sharp and the other blunt. This instrument can also be used during biopsies or excisions, which require the nail avulsion. The blunt end is advanced under the nail plate and nail folds to separate the nail plate from the nail bed and hyponychium. Periosteal elevators can also be used to create a subcutaneous tunnel for suspension sutures or implant placement.

CONCLUSION

Given the array of instruments available, it is important to sample as many as possible and then to make informed decisions of which ones to incorporate into any procedure. In the end, it will be the experience and personal preference of each surgeon which will determine which instruments function most effectively in his or her hands.

BIBLIOGRAPHY

Bernstein G. Instrumentation for Mohs surgery. In: Mohs F, Mikhail GR, eds. Mohs Micrographic Surgery. Philadelphia: W.B. Saunders, 1991:61–76.

Bernstein G. The 15c scalpel blade. J Dermatol Surg Oncol 1987; 13:969.

Dimino-Emme L, Washington CV, Tran NT. Surgical instrumentation and wound closure materials. In: Ratz JL, Geronemus RG, Goldman MP, Maloney ME, Padilla RS, eds. Textbook of Dermatologic Surgery. Philadelphia: Lippincott-Raven, 1998:97–115.

Diwan R. Instruments for dermatologic surgery. In: Lask GP, Moy RL, eds. Principles and Techniques of Cutaneous Surgery. New York: McGraw-Hill, 1996:85–99.

Goldberg LH, Segal RJ. Surgical pearl: a flexible scalpel for shave excision of skin lesions. J Am Acad Dermatol 1996; 35:452–453.

Grabski WJ, Salasche SJ, Mulvaney MJ. Razor-blade surgery. J Dermatol Surg Oncol 16:1121–1126.

Hochberg J, Murray GF. Principles of operative surgery. In: Sabiston DC, Lyerly HK, eds. Textbook of Surgery: The Biological Basis of Modern Surgical Practice. Philadelphia: W.B. Saunders, 1997:253–263.

Keyes EL. The cutaneous punch. J Cutan Genitourin Dis 1887; 5:98–101.

Raza SL, Sengelmann RD. Instrumentation and sutures. In: Snow SN, Mikhail GR, eds. Mohs Micrographic Surgery. Wisconsin: University of Wisconsin Press, 2004:33–42.

Salache SJ, Winton GB, Adnot J. Surgical pearls. Dermatol Clin 1989; 7:75–110.

3

Closure Materials

Misty D. Caudell, Clifford Warren Lober, and Neil A. Fenske
University of South Florida College of Medicine, Tampa, Florida, U.S.A.

SUTURE

History

For thousands of years, we have been searching for an ideal suture material. Naturally occurring materials such as cotton, bark fiber, horsetails, and the mouthparts of pitcher ants have been used to close wounds. Innovative physicians tried violin strings, wooden sticks, and other devices for the same purpose. When synthetic materials such as nylon were developed for other purposes, surgeons adapted them to wound closure. It was not until the 1970s that synthetic polymers were developed specifically for use as suture materials on the basis of their physical, chemical, and biological properties.

Characteristics

Suture materials may be made of naturally occurring substances or synthetic polymers, monofilament or multifilament, dyed or undyed, and may be coated or uncoated. The chemical composition of a suture material may be either well determined (e.g., synthetic chemical polymers) or less specifically defined (e.g., surgical gut). Both the chemical composition and the physical construction of the suture determine the final properties of the suture material.

Several parameters are used to describe the physical characteristics of sutures (Table 1). Tensile strength is calculated by dividing the maximum load by the original cross-sectional area of suture material. Breaking strength is that load required to cause the suture material to rupture. Elasticity is the ability of a substance to undergo nonpermanent deformation, and plasticity refers to the ability of the material to stretch nonelastically without rupturing, or the ability of a substance to be permanently deformed without fracturing. Materials stretch elastically prior to undergoing plastic deformation. Memory is the ability of a substance to return to its original physical configuration following deformation.

Capillarity refers to the ability of suture material to conduct fluids. Multifilament and uncoated sutures tend to have a greater capillarity than monofilament and coated sutures. It has been clearly shown that multifilament and uncoated sutures tend to permit greater passage of bacteria into wounds and promote infection.

Sutures should elicit a minimal degree of tissue reactivity. Naturally occurring material is absorbed by phagocytosis and enzymatic degradation (e.g., surgical gut, rapidly or silk, very slowly). This tends to induce a greater degree of inflammatory response than synthetic polymers such as polyglycolic acid or polyglactin 910, which are degraded primarily by hydrolysis.

In addition to evaluating sutures on the basis of measurable physical characteristics, surgeons compare sutures on the basis of "performance characteristics." These subjectively evaluated parameters include pliability, ease of handling, visibility, and knot security. Knot security is the ability of a knot to hold without breaking or stretching and reflects the material's elasticity, plasticity, tensile strength, and memory.

Suture materials are available in different sizes. The number of zeros indicated on a suture package reflects the size of the enclosed suture material. As the number of zeros increases, the diameter of the suture material decreases. A 6–0 strand of nylon suture, for example, is narrower than a 4–0 strand of nylon suture. The designation in terms of zeros, however, does not correspond to an exact physical size but to a range of sizes allowed by the United States Pharmacopoeia to attain a given tensile strength. For this reason a strand of 4–0 polyglactin 910 is not necessarily the same diameter as a 4–0 strand of surgical gut. Suture materials are available in dyed and undyed forms. They are dyed to enhance visibility.

Suture materials have been arbitrarily designated by the United States Pharmacopoeia as either absorbable or nonabsorbable. An absorbable suture loses most of its tensile strength in the tissue 60 days following implantation. A nonabsorbable suture is resistant to enzymatic degradation and hydrolysis. Many of the so-called nonabsorable sutures are, in fact, physiologically absorbable. Silk, for example, which is a nonabsorbable suture according to the *United States Pharmacopoeia* definition, loses 50% tensile strength in two months to one year.

Basic Characteristics of Wound Healing

In order to understand what to expect of sutures, the basic physiology of wound healing must be understood. During the first four to six days after wounding, minimal wound strength is gained, and the surgical site is essentially dependent upon sutures to maintain closure. During the burst of fibroplasia and collagen production that begins between the fifth and sixth day after wounding, wound strength is rapidly gained. This increase in strength continues as remodeling of the wounded dermis progresses and plateaus after approximately 70 days. The maturation phase of wound healing continues for at least one year.

A surgical wound never attains the same cutaneous tensile strength of normal uncut skin. Two weeks after sutures

Table 1 Physical Characteristics of Sutures

Tensile strength	Maximum load divided by the original cross-sectional area of suture material
Breaking strength	Load required to cause suture material to rupture
Elasticity	The ability of a substance to undergo nonpermanent deformation
Plasticity	The ability of a material to stretch nonelastically without rupturing, or the ability to be permanently deformed without fracturing
Pliability	The ease with which a substance is bent
Memory	The ability of a substance to return to its original physical configuration following deformation
Capillarity	The ability of suture material to conduct fluids, higher with braided (or multifilament) sutures than with monofilament sutures
Tissue reactivity	Reactivity of tissue to suture; greater with naturally occurring materials (absorbed by phagocytosis and enzymatic degradation) than with synthetic polymers (degraded primarily by hydrolysis)
Performance characteristics	Subjective parameters which include pliability, ease of handling, visibility, and knot security
Knot strength	The ability of a knot to hold without breaking or stretching; reflects the material's elasticity, plasticity, tensile strength, and memory
Coefficient of friction	Reflects ease of passage of suture through tissue, with increasing coefficient indicating increased resistance; knot strength increases with increasing coefficient of friction
Absorbable suture	Suture that loses most tensile strength in the tissue 60 days following implantation
Nonabsorbable suture	Suture that is resistant to hydrolysis and enzymatic digestion

are implanted, surgical wounds have achieved only 3% to 5% of the original cutaneous strength, or approximately 7% of the ultimate tensile strength that the repaired wound will achieve. By the end of the third week, 20% of the final tensile strength is achieved, and by one month only 50% of ultimate wound strength (or 35% of the original strength) is attained. Wounds never gain more than 80% of the strength of intact unwounded skin.

All sutures are foreign bodies and thus produce an inflammatory response in the host dermis (Table 2). This inflammatory response peaks between the second and seventh day following implantation. Between the second and seventh day, there is an abundance of polymorphonuclear leukocytes, lymphocytes, and large monocytes. By the fourth day, there is an increasing number of mononuclear cells, macrophages, and fibroblasts. Between the third and eighth day, the epithelial cells deeply invade suture tracts and do not cease their migration until cells migrating from the needle entrance site meet cells advancing from the needle exit site (contact inhibition). In the case of absorbable sutures, the inflammatory cell reaction is noted to increase when absorption begins and persists until all of the foreign material is eliminated. In the case of nonabsorbable sutures, a comparatively acellular reaction persists, in which a fibrous capsule is laid down around the sutures at 10 to 16 days. In general, monofilament sutures produce less inflammatory response than multifilament sutures. Keep in mind that absorbable suture used in an area of infection or active inflammation may undergo a premature loss of function and thus compromise wound integrity.

Absorbable Sutures

Absorbable sutures (Tables 3 and 4) are placed into the subcutaneous tissue to eliminate dead space and into the dermis to minimize tissue tension during wound healing.

Absorbable sutures must be placed well into the dermis and subcutaneous tissue to facilitate their subsequent absorption by inflammation, enzymatic degradation, or hydrolysis. If absorbable sutures are placed too superficially, they may persist for a prolonged period of time and thus have an increased tendency to be transepidermally eliminated ("spit") from the wound. This can compromise the appearance of the scar. Absorbable sutures are not intended to be used too close to the skin surface. This slows absorption and increases the likelihood of epithelialization of the suture tunnels. This epithelialization can result in permanent suture tracts and cyst formation. Moreover, superficially placed dyed sutures may be visible through the skin, especially in light skinned individuals.

Surgical Gut

The first reference to catgut as an absorbable suture was by Galen of Pergamon, circa 150 AD. Although the origin of the name catgut is obscure, it has nothing to do with cats. It has been suggested that it was derived from the word "kit-gut," from "kit," an Arabian dancing master's fiddle that had strings made from sheep intestine.

Surgical gut sutures are derived from naturally occurring purified connective tissue (mostly collagen) of the submucosal layer of the small intestine of sheep and the serosal layer of the small intestine of cattle. Surgical gut is absorbed by proteolytic enzymatic degradation. As surgical gut sutures are derived from organic sources, there is no assurance of chemical uniformity among them. Manufacturing procedures may produce weak spots. This may cause uneven absorption and premature rupture of the sutures. Similarly, the physical parameters (e.g., width) of a given strand of surgical gut may vary.

In comparison with other absorbable suture materials presently available, surgical gut sutures tend to lose their

Table 2 Inflammatory Response to Suture in the Dermis

Day post-implantation	Host response
2–7	Abundance of polymorphonuclear leukocytes, lymphocytes, and monocytes
4	Increasing number of mononuclear cells, macrophages, and fibroblasts
3–8	Epithelial cells deeply invade suture tracts and do not cease their migration until cells migrating from the needle entrance site meet cells advancing from the needle exit site (contact inhibition)
Indefinite	For absorbable sutures, inflammatory cell reaction increases when absorption begins and persists until all foreign material is eliminated
	For nonabsorbable sutures, a comparatively acellular reaction persists, in which a fibrous capsule is laid down around the sutures at 10 to 16 days

Table 3 Characteristics of Absorbable Sutures

Suture type	Components	Degradation process and absorption	Type and construction	Strength retention post-implantation	Other
Surgical gut	Collagen from submucosal layer of the small intestine of sheep and the serosal layer of the small intestine of cattle	Enzymatic degradation and phagocytosis	Fast absorbing gut, essentially monofilament Plain surgical gut, undyed or dyed, essentially monofilament Chromic gut (treated with chromic salts), undyed or dyed, essentially monofilament	Nearly all tensile strength is lost at 1 week 40% at 1 week, no tensile strength at 2 weeks Coating delays physical absorption, actual retention of tensile strength beyond 14 days is negligible	Marked inflammatory response; absorbed rapidly in infected tissue; rinse briefly in tepid water before use; used for ophthalmic surgery, skin grafts, and in children when suture removal difficult
Polyglycolic acid (Dexon)	Synthetic homopolymer of glycolic acid, may be coated with a co-polymer of glycolide and epsilon-caprolactone (Polycaprolate)	Hydrolysis, degrades to glycolic acid, then absorbed and metabolized by the body, absorption is essentially complete between 60 and 90 days	Braided, coated (Dexon II) undyed or dyed Braided, uncoated (Dexon), undyed or dyed	65% at 2 weeks, 35% at 3 weeks	Good tensile strength, excellent knot security, coating minimizes tissue drag and facilitates handling
Polyglactin 910 (Vicryl)	Synthetic heteropolymer of glycolide (90%) and L-lactide (10%), coated with equal parts of a copolymer of glycolide and lactide (polyglactin 370) and calcium stearate	Hydrolysis, degrades to glycolic and lactic acids, then absorbed and metabolized by the body, absorption nearly complete by 70 days postimplantation (by 42 days for Vicryl Rapide)	Braided, coated (Vicryl Rapide), undyed Braided, Coated (VICRY), Undyed or Violet Braided, coated, with Triclosan (Vicryl Plus Antibacterial), Undyed or Violet	50% at 5 days, no tensile strength at 10–14 days 75% at 2 weeks, 50% at 3 weeks, 25% at 4 weeks, no tensile strength at 5 weeks	Mimics some characteristics of surgical gut with less tissue reactivity Excellent handling and knot security
Lactomer (Polysorb)	Synthetic heteropolymer of glycolide and L-lactide, coated with a mixture of a copolymer of caprolactone and glycolide, and calcium stearoyl lactylate	Hydrolysis, degrades to glycolic and lactic acids, then absorbed and metabolized by the body, absorption nearly complete by 70 days postimplantation	Braided, coated (Polysorb), undyed or violet	Tensile strength 140% U.S.P. minimal knot strength before implantation, 80% U.S.P. minimum knot security at 2 weeks, 30% U.S.P. minimum knot security at 3 weeks	Excellent handling and knot security
Polydioxanone (PDS)	Synthetic homopolymer of paradioxanone	Hydrolysis, less inflammatory response when compared with polyglactin 910; absorption complete at 180 days	Monofilament (PDS), undyed (Clear), blue or violet	70% at 2 weeks, 50% at 4 weeks, 25% at 6 weeks	Monofilament valuable when potential wound infection is a concern; major advantage is significant tensile strength retention; more difficult to handle than braided synthetics (high memory)

(Continued)

Table 3 Characteristics of Absorbable Sutures (*Continued*)

Suture type	Components	Degradation process and absorption	Type and construction	Strength retention post-implantation	Other
Polyglyconate (Maxon)	Synthetic copolymer of glycolic acid and trimethylene carbonate	Hydrolysis; absorption complete within 180 days	Monofilament (Maxon), undyed (Clear) or green	75% at 2 weeks, 50% at 4 weeks, 25% at 6 weeks	Monofilament valuable when potential wound infection is a concern; significant tensile strength retention; improved handling characteristics when compared with polydioxanone
Polyglecaprone 25 (Monocryl)	Synthetic copolymer of glycolide and epsilon-caprolactone	Hydrolysis; absorption complete at 90–120 days	Monofilament (Monocryl), undyed or violet	Dyed: 65% at 1 week, 30% at 2 weeks, no tensile strength at 4 weeks. Undyed: 50% at 1 week, 20% at 2 weeks, no tensile strength at 3 weeks	Minimal tissue reactivity, good choice for absorbable running intradermal, pliable, low memory
Glycomer 631 (Biosyn)	Synthetic polyester of glycolide (60%), dioxanone (14%), and trimethylene carbonate (26%)	Hydrolysis; absorption complete at 90–110 days	Monofilament (Biosyn), undyed or violet	75% U.S.P. minimum knot security at 2 weeks, 40% U.S.P. minimum knot security at 3 weeks	Minimal tissue reactivity, may be used as absorbable running intradermal, pliable, low memory, delayed absorption in comparison with polyglecaprone 25
Polyglytone 6211 (Caprosyn)	Synthetic polyester of glycolide, caprolactone, trimethylene carbonate, and lactide	Hydrolysis; absorption complete at 56 days	Monofilament (Caprosyn), undyed and uncoated	50–60% original knot strength at 5 days, 20–30% at 10 days, no tensile strength at 3 weeks	Similar loss of strength and mass as surgical gut sutures, but is easier to work with (lower drag forces) and is associated with fewer infections than surgical gut, greater pre-implantation strength than gut

Table 4 Tensile Strength Retention Post-Implantation

Fast Absorbing			
Gut	Chromic Gut	Vicryl	
	Dyed Monocryl		
Plain Surgical Gut		Dexon	PDS
Vicryl Rapide		Polysorb	Maxon
Undyed Monocryl		Biosyn	
Caprosyn			
Week 1	Week 2	Week 3	Week 4

Note: Number of days postimplantation when tensile strength is approximately 50% original implantation is noted.

strength rapidly. For this reason, surgical gut sutures may be inappropriate to use in patients predisposed to delayed wound healing (e.g., the elderly). Although absorption is markedly variable for the aforementioned reasons, approximately 60% of the tensile strength of surgical gut is lost one week following implantation into a wound, and effectively, no tensile strength remains in two weeks. Surgical gut is a foreign organic substance in human recipient tissue and elicits a markedly inflammatory response. Through this inflammatory response, surgical gut is broken down and absorbed. Surgical gut is absorbed more rapidly in infected tissue or in areas of active inflammation. Histologic examination of tissues sutured with surgical gut reveals striking inflammatory response within four days, peaking at day 9.

In an attempt to retard the absorption of surgical gut sutures, they may be treated with chromic salts. Although physical absorption is delayed, the actual retention of tensile strength beyond 14 days is negligible. Chromic gut sutures may persist beyond two weeks in the dermis, and a continuous inflammatory reaction persists until they are absorbed. Plain surgical gut can be heat treated to accelerate loss of tensile strength and absorption. This fast absorbing gut is not to be used internally, and is primarily used for surface (epidermal, superficial) sutures that are needed for only five to seven days (e.g., face), as nearly all of its original strength is lost within seven days of implantation. Compared with other suture materials used for surface sutures, fast absorbing gut elicits the most inflammation.

In contrast to most other sutures, which should be kept dry, surgical gut should be rinsed briefly in sterile tepid water before use to reduce tissue irritation. Surgical gut should not be pulled or stretched, as this may weaken the suture. As with all sutures, care should be taken to avoid grasping the suture with a needle driver (holder).

Although the use of surgical gut sutures has decreased during the last decades, there is one application for which surgical gut continues to be used. In procedures such as blepharoplasty, surgeons frequently choose to have sutures in place for only a few days. In this delicate area, where suture removal may be problematic, the use of "mild ophthalmic chromic gut" may be advantageous. The suture line is covered with tape and the sutures are rapidly absorbed. When the tape is removed a few days later, the sutures are generally removed simultaneously. Surgical gut sutures are also used for skin grafts and in children, when suture removal may be difficult.

Polyglycolic Acid

Polyglycolic acid (Dexon™, a product of Syneture became commercially available in 1971. It was originally manufactured by Davis & Geck and is now manufactured by Syneture. This braided absorbable synthetic homopolymer of glycolic acid (hydroacetic acid) provided for the first time a suture of uniform chemical composition. Glycolic acid initially reacts with itself to form the cyclic ester glycolide, which is subsequently converted to a high molecular weight linear chain polymer. This polymer is made into sutures when, in either its dyed or undyed form, it is crushed into small granules, melt-extruded through a mold to form fibers, heat-stretched, braided, restretched, and heat-treated again to make the braiding tight and more uniform. Polyglycolic acid suture is supplied in an uncoated (Dexon S) or a coated (Dexon II) form. The coating consists of a copolymer of glycolide and epsilon-caprolactone (Polycaprolate™, a product of Syneture), which is noncollagenous and nonantigenic. Coated polyglycolic acid suture is undyed (beige color) or dyed green, violet, or bicolored. Uncoated polyglycolic acid suture is either undyed (beige color) or dyed green to enhance visibility.

Since polyglycolic acid is not a naturally occurring organic substance, it elicits far less inflammatory response than surgical gut. It is absorbed primarily by hydrolysis rather than by a host inflammatory response. The polymer degrades to glycolic acid, which is then absorbed and metabolized by the body. Polyglycolic acid possesses good tensile strength and excellent knot security. According to the product description prepared by the manufacturer, two weeks after implantation into a wound approximately 65% of the initial tensile strength of polyglycolic acid sutures remains, and three weeks after implantation approximately 35% of the original tensile strength remains, for both coated and uncoated forms.

Many surgeons report noticeable tissue resistance to the passage of uncoated polyglycolic acid sutures. Thus is the genesis of the coated suture material that minimizes tissue drag and facilitates handling, in terms of ease of knot tying and passage through tissue.

Polyglactin 910 and Lactomer™ (A Product of Syneture)

With the appearance of polyglactin sutures (Vicryl™, a product of Ethicon) in 1974, surgeons were able to use a synthetic heteropolymer consisting of 90% glycolide and 10% L-lactide. More recently, Syneture, has developed Lactomer, a glycolide and lactide synthetic polyester suture (Polysorb™). Both of these glycolic acid/lactic acid copolymer sutures are braided, multifilament, coated, absorbable synthetic sutures. Lactide and glycolide are cyclic intermediates of lactide and glycolic acid that are more easily converted into fiber-forming polymers than are their parent free acids. The addition of lactic acid to the glycolic acid reduces crystallinity and increases pliability. In the manufacturing of polyglactin 910 sutures, the heteropolymer is melted in the presence of a catalyst, extruded into fibers, braided, heat-stretched to make the braiding tighter and more uniform and sterilized using ethylene oxide. Both polyglactin 910 and Lactomer are available undyed or dyed violet to enhance visibility. Polyglactin 910 and Lactomer are degraded by hydrolysis to glycolic and lactic acids, which are then absorbed and metabolized by the body. A coating is added to improve the overall handling properties of this multifilament braided suture. Polyglactin 910 (Vicryl) is coated with a mixture composed of equal parts of a copolymer of glycolide and lactide (polyglactin 370) and calcium stearate, and may be supplied in an antibacterial form, which is impregnated with triclosan (Vicryl plus Antibacterial™, a product of Ethicon). Lactomer (Polysorb) is coated with a mixture of a caprolactone and glycolide copolymer and calcium stearoyl lactylate.

It is important that absorbable suture material, when used for deep sutures, retain significant functional tensile strength for several weeks following implantation into a wound. Polyglactin 910 (Vicryl), Lactomer (Polysorb), and polyglycolic acid (Dexon) are braided synthetic absorbable sutures, which behave similarly in terms of retention of tensile strength. The residual tensile strength of a 4–0 suture of polyglactin 910 is consistently greater than that of polyglycolic acid when measured weekly. The difference in tensile strength between these two materials, however, should be of minimal clinical significance if wounds of the dermis and subcutaneous tissues are closed using appropriate surgical techniques that minimize wound tension. According to information supplied by the manufacturer, polyglactin 910 (Vicryl™) suture retained 75% of its original tensile strength at two weeks postimplantation, 25% of its original tensile strength at four weeks postimplantation, and essentially no tensile strength at five weeks postimplantation in rats. Lactomer (Polysorb™) shares a similar rate of loss of tensile strength.

Ideally, absorbable suture material should disappear as rapidly and completely as possible following its loss of functional tensile strength. Polyglactin 910 and Lactomer are absorbed more rapidly than is polyglycolic acid. In one study comparing the absorption of polyglactin 910 and polyglycolic acid, the absorption of polyglycan 910 began at approximately 40 days following its implantation into rats and was nearly complete by day 70. At 90 days, no polymer remained in the tissue. Although the absorption of polyglycolic acid was also noted to begin at approximately 40 days following its implantation, approximately half of the material remained in the tissue at 90 days, and "significant quantities" were present when the study was terminated at 120 days.

Vicryl Rapide (a product of Ethicon) is designed to lose strength rapidly and to mimic some characteristics of surgical gut, but with less tissue reactivity, because it is a synthetic absorbable suture degraded by hydrolysis rather than proteolysis. It is made of polyglactin 910 (the same polymer as Vicryl), but with a lower molecular weight. It is coated similarly to Vicryl. According to information supplied by the manufacturer, Vicryl Rapide retained 50% of its original tensile strength at five days postimplantation in rats, and no original tensile strength remained at 10 to 14 days postimplantation. In rats, absorption continues and is essentially complete by 42 days postimplantation. Vicryl Rapide is not intended to be used for deep closures, but only for superficial wound support required for 7 to 10 days (e.g., skin grafts, face).

Polydioxanone

In 1982, the synthetic homopolymer polydioxanone (PDS™, a product of Ethicon) became commercially available. This monofilament synthetic absorbable suture is prepared by polymerizing the monomer paradioxanone to a high molecular weight compound that can be melt extruded into a monofilament. The suture may be dyed using Drug and Cosmetic Violet No. 2 dye and thus be highly visible. Polydioxanone is particularly valuable when potential wound infection is a concern, because its monofilament construction prevents organisms from being entrapped by or traveling along the interstices of suture strands.

Polydioxanone is similar to polyglycolic acid (Dexon), polyglactin 910 (Vicryl), and Lactomer (Polysorb) in that it is degraded by hydrolysis rather than by phagocytosis and inflammation. When compared with polyglactin 910, a far less severe host inflammatory response is induced by polydioxanone.

A major advantage of polydioxanone suture is that it retains significant tensile strength for over a month. Polydioxanone retains 70% of its original tensile strength at two weeks postimplantation, 50% of its original tensile strength at four weeks postimplantation, and 25% of its original tensile strength at six weeks postimplantation. As surgical wounds attain only 3 to 5% of original skin tensile strength by two weeks following placement of sutures, this added suture tensile strength may be clinically significant in those wounds closed under some degree of tension. Polydioxanone is rapidly absorbed between 140 and 180 days postimplantation. At 140 days, approximately 80% of the polymer remains, and at 180 days, no significant material is present in the host tissue.

Polyglyconate

Polyglyconate (Maxon™, a product of Syneture) became commercially available in 1985. It was originally manufactured by Davis & Geck, and is now manufactured by Syneture. It is a synthetic monofilament absorbable polyglyconate suture composed of a copolymer of glycolic acid and trimethylene carbonate. It was developed to exhibit the synthetic monofilament advantages of polydioxanone (PDS), which are decreased risk of infection and prolonged tensile strength after implantation, but with improved handling properties. Some state that polyglyconate demonstrates superior handling when directly compared with polyglactin (Vicryl, Polysorb), as polyglyconate lacks memory, passes easily through tissue, and demonstrates superior strength. Animal studies indicate that polyglyconate retains 75% original tensile strength at two weeks postimplantation, 50% original tensile strength at four weeks postimplantation, and 25% at six weeks postimplantation (similar to polydioxanone). Absorption is essentially complete by 180 days.

Poliglecaprone 25

Poliglecaprone 25 (Monocryl™, a product of Ethicon) is a more recently developed synthetic absorbable monofilament suture composed of a copolymer of glycolide and epsilon-caprolactone. It is pliable and elicits minimal tissue reactivity (virtually inert in tissue). Because of its minimal reactivity, it may be utilized as a running intradermal suture, allowing prolonged superficial wound support without risk of railroad track deformity associated with prolonged use of nonabsorbable surface (epidermal, superficial) sutures. Moreover, it is not necessary to remove the suture, which can be difficult in some patients, with use of nonabsorbable running intradermal sutures. It is supplied in dyed and undyed forms. According to data supplied by the manufacturer, dyed poliglecaprone 25 retains 65% to 70% of its original tensile strength at one week after implantation and 30% to 40% at two weeks postimplantation. By four weeks postimplantation, essentially no tensile strength remains. Undyed poliglecaprone 25 retains 50% to 60% of its original tensile strength at one week after implantation and 20% to 30% at two weeks postimplantation. By three weeks postimplantation, undyed poliglecaprone has lost essentially all original tensile strength. Absorption for both is essentially complete at 91 to 119 days.

Glycomer 631

Glycomer 631 (Biosyn™, a product of Syneture) is a more recently developed synthetic absorbable monofilament suture composed of a polyester of glycolide (60%), dioxanone (14%), and trimethylene carbonate (26%). It elicits minimal tissue reactivity and exhibits physical characteristics, such as high flexibility and low memory, similar to poliglecaprone 25 (Monocryl). In comparison with poliglecaprone 25, glycomer 631 passes through tissue more easily, but knot security is slightly inferior. It is degraded by hydrolysis to glycolic acid, dioxanoic acid, propane diol, and carbon dioxide, which are then absorbed and metabolized by the body. According to data supplied by the manufacturer, although both products have similar total mass absorption profiles, Glycomer 631 (Biosyn) provides an additional week of wound support. Animal studies indicate that tensile strength is 70% of U.S.P. minimum knot strength at two weeks postimplantation and 40% U.S.P. minimum knot strength at three weeks postimplantation. According to the manufacturer, absorption of glycomer 631 is essentially complete between 90 and 110 days. A study of glycomer 631 in rats indicated that absorption was complete in three to six months (in comparison with absorption of poliglecaprone 25, which was completely absorbed by 90 days and polydioxanone, which was completely absorbed by six months); however, absorption in humans may be at a different rate.

Polyglytone 6211

Polyglytone 6211 (Caprosyn™, a product of Syneture) is a recently developed monofilament synthetic absorbable suture. It is a polyester of glycolide, caprolactone, trimethylene carbonate, and lactide. It is uncoated and undyed, and it is designed to lose tensile strength rapidly to mimic some characteristics of surgical gut. Absorption occurs via hydrolysis, yielding less inflammatory response than surgical gut.

Animal studies indicate that all original tensile strength is lost by 21 days after implantation and absorption is essentially complete by 56 days postimplantation. According to information provided by the manufacturer, knot strength decreases to 50% to 60% of original strength at five days postimplantation and to 20% to 30% at 10 days postimplantation. In one study comparing polyglytone 6211 and chromic gut sutures, polyglytone 6211 was easier to work with (as it is smooth and exhibits lower drag forces), was associated with fewer infections, and exhibited greater preimplantation strength. Both polyglytone 6211 and chromic gut sutures had no appreciable strength at three weeks postimplantation, and both demonstrated a similar loss of mass rate.

Nonabsorbable Sutures

Nonabsorbable sutures (Table 5) are typically used to oppose the skin surface. When used to oppose the skin surface, the sutures should be just tight enough to approximate, not strangulate, tissues. The wound edema that develops postoperatively increases the tension on the sutures and may cause them to "cut in" if they are firmly placed at the time of surgery.

Nonabsorbable sutures may be used as deep sutures ("buried" or "subcutaneous") to provide prolonged mechanical support for a healing wound (e.g., facelift). The use of nonabsorbable sutures in the deep tissues should not be viewed as an alternative to proper surgical techniques (e.g., proper planning of wound configuration, undermining, etc.) that minimize wound tension.

Silk

Silk has been used for centuries to close wounds. For the first half of this century, absorbable catgut and nonabsorbable silk were the standards for virtually all wound closures. Surgical silk is derived from the domesticated silkworm species Bombyx mori of the family Bombycidae, the larva of which spins silk to weave its cocoon. Silk sutures are processed to isolate the protein fibroin, remove the natural waxes and gums (sericin), dyed black, braided, and coated with wax or silicone to decrease tissue friction and reduce capillarity. Silk is a naturally occurring organic substance and induces a striking host inflammatory response, second only to surgical gut. It is degraded by phagotocytosis and the actions of enzymes. Like surgical gut and other organic materials, silk may vary in its exact chemical composition, and the diameter of each strand may be somewhat nonuniform.

An outstanding quality of silk is its ease of handling. Despite the development of numerous synthetic polymers, silk remains the standard by which all suture materials are judged with regard to ease of handling. Its ease of passage through tissue and pliability remain unsurpassed by any other material presently available. Unfortunately, its tensile strength is very low, and it exhibits high capillarity, which increases the risk of infection.

Although silk is classified as a nonabsorbable suture according to the United States Pharmacopoeia, it is, in fact, gradually absorbed. It loses approximately 50% of its strength in one year and has no significant tensile strength two years after implantation. In reality, it behaves as a very slowly absorbing suture material. Owing to its reactivity, it is rarely used for cutaneous closures, but is commonly used on mucosal surfaces and intertriginous areas because it is soft and pliable, thus resulting in minimal discomfort.

Nylon

In the 1930s and 1940s, numerous synthetic materials were developed for the clothing industry, the rubber industry, and other commercial ventures. Surgeons were quick to adapt these synthetic polymers as suture materials. Nylon, polyester, rayon, and other materials were tried. These synthetic polymers were uniform in composition and, as nonorganic materials, generally elicited less tissue reactivity than organic materials. They are available in either mono- or multifilament forms. Nylon suture is composed of long-chain aliphatic polymers of Nylon 6 or Nylon 6,6. Because of the elasticity of nylon suture, it is well suited for surface (epidermal, superficial) closure. Monofilament nylon (Ethilon™, a product of Ethicon; Dermalon™ and Monosof™, products of Syneture) has a great deal of memory, and its proclivity for knot slippage is well known. However, this shortcoming is easily conquered by increasing the number of knot throws and firmly setting knots. Multifilament braided nylon sutures (Nurolon™, a product of Ethicon; Surgilon™, a product of Syneture) exhibit decreased memory in comparison with monofilament nylon; however, they are also associated with a slightly higher infection rate because they are braided.

Like silk, some synthetic polymers are gradually absorbed by host tissues. In vivo, nylon loses tensile strength at a rate of approximately 15% to 20% per year by hydrolyzation.

Polypropylene

In 1970, polypropylene (Prolene™, a product of Ethicon; Surgipro™ II, a product of Syneture) was introduced as the first synthetic nonabsorbable material specifically developed for use as suture. Both Prolene and Surgipro II are monofilament synthetic sutures. Prolene is made of an isotactic crystalline stereoisomer of polypropylene (a synthetic linear polyolefin), containing few or no unsaturated bonds. Surgipro II is made of polypropylene and polyethylene.

Table 5 Characteristics of Nonabsorbable Sutures

Suture type	Components	Degradation process and absorption	Type and construction	Strength retention post-implantation	Other
Silk	Organic protein called fibroin, derived from larva of domesticated silk work Bombyx mori, with sericin gum removed	Phagocytosis and enzymatic degradation, gradual encapsulation by fibrous connective tissue	Braided, coated (wax or silicone), dyed (Black)	38% at 8 months, 50% at 1 year, no significant tensile strength at 2 years	Significant inflammatory tissue response, outstanding ease of handling, low tensile strength, high capillarity, good for mucosal surfaces
Nylon (Ethilon, Nurolon, Dermalon, Monosof, Surgilon)	Synthetic long-chain aliphatic polymer of Nylon 6 or Nylon 6,6	Hydrolysis, gradual encapsulation by fibrous connective tissue	Monofilament, undyed (Clear), black (Ethilon, Monosof), green (Ethilon), Blue (Dermalon) Braided, Uncoated (Nurolon); Braided, Coated with Silicone (SURGILON)	15–20% loss of tensile strength per year	Minimal inflammatory response, high tensile strength, high memory (decreased knot security), excellent elasticity, good for epidermal approximation
Polypropylene (Prolene, Surgipro II)	Synthetic polymer of polypropylene (Prolene) or polypropylene and polyethylene (Surgipro II)	Gradual encapsulation by fibrous connective tissue	Monofilament, undyed (Clear) or blue (Prolene, Surgipro II)	No significant change known to occur	Minimal inflammatory reaction, does not adhere to tissue (ideal as "pull-out" running intradermal suture), high plasticity, high memory, poor knot security
Polyester (Novafil, Vascufil)	Synthetic copolymer of polytetramethylene ether glycol and butylene terephthalate; Vascufil is coated with an absorbable polymer of ecaprolactone, glycolide and poloxamer 188 (Polytribolate)	Gradual encapsulation by fibrous connective tissue	Monofilament, undyed (Clear) or pigmented with Copper Phthalocyanine Blue (Novafil, Vascufil)	No significant change known to occur	Minimal inflammatory reaction, high plasticity and elasticity, excellent handling
Polyester (Mersilene, Ethibond Excel, Surgidac, Ti-cron)	Synthetic polyester composed of polyethylene terephthalate	Gradual encapsulation by fibrous connective tissue	Braided, uncoated (Mersilene), undyed or Green Braided, uncoated (Surgidac), undyed or green Braided, coated with polybutilate (Ethibond Excel), undyed or green Braided, coated with silicone (Ti-cron), undyed or blue	No significant change known to occur	Minimal tissue reactivity, last indefinitely once implanted, ideal for prosthetic implantations and cardiovascular surgery, good handling characteristics, high tensile strength
Hexafluoro-propylene-VDF (Pronova)	Synthetic polymer blend of poly (vinylidene fluoride) and poly (vinylidene fluoride-co-hexafluoro-propylene)	Gradual encapsulation by fibrous connective tissue	Monofilament, dyed blue (Pronova)	No significant change known to occur	Minimal tissue reactivity, lacks tissue adherence, possible choice for "pull-out" sutures

Polypropylene has tensile strength exceeding that of nylon, passes easily through tissue and induces a minimal host inflammatory response. It does not adhere to tissue and is therefore well suited as a "pull-out" running intradermal suture. It is either clear or dyed blue. Polypropylene is noted for its plasticity, which is advantageous during wound healing, as it will expand with tissue swelling to accommodate the wound. Disadvantages include high memory (more than nylon), poor knot security, and lack of elasticity.

Polybutester

In 1984, polybutester (Novafil™, a product of Syneture) was introduced as a synthetic monofilament suture. It is a copolymer of poly(glycol) tetraphthalate and poly(butylene) terephthalate. Polybutester suture passes easily through tissue and induces a minimal host inflammatory response. Its functional tensile strength is similar to that of nylon. It is not absorbed, nor is any significant change in strength retention known to occur in vivo.

Polybutester has a marked degree of plasticity and elasticity. It feels like a rubber band. At loads of only 25% of its knot breaking level, polybutester suture stretches to 50% of its total elongation capacity. Comparatively, nylon stretches to 25% of its total elongation capacity, and polyglycolic acid suture to 11% at similar loads. However, total elongation capacity for polybutester is similar to that of nylon. This plasticity enables the suture material to expand as the wound undergoes its edematous healing phase. Polybutester exhibits approximately twice the elasticity of nylon sutures. Its elasticity allows it to subsequently contract as the edematous phase of wound healing resolves.

Polyester

Polyester sutures (Mersilene™ and Ethibond Excel™, products of Ethicon; Ti-cron™ and Surgidac™, products of Syneture) are synthetic nonabsorbable braided multifilament sutures composed of polyethylene terephthalate. Because they elicit minimal tissue reactivity and last indefinitely once implanted, they are used for prosthetic implantations, facelifts, and cardiovascular surgery. They exhibit good handling characteristics and high tensile strength. Mersilene and Surgidac are uncoated, and therefore have a higher coefficient of friction when pulled through tissue. Ethibond is coated with polybutilate, which was the first synthetic coating developed specifically as a suture lubricant, and Ti-cron is coated with silicone.

Hexafluoropropylene-VDF

Hexafluoropropylene-VDF suture (Pronova, a product of Ethicon) is a newly developed monofilament suture made of a polymer blend of poly(vinylidene fluoride) and poly(vinylidene fluoride-co-hexafluoropropylene). This suture exhibits lack of adherence to tissues, similar to polypropylene (Prolene, Surgipro), which makes it a possible choice for "pull-out" sutures. Like polypropylene, it resists involvement in infection and elicits a minimal tissue inflammatory response. It is not absorbed, nor does it weaken after implantation. It is dyed blue.

STAPLES

Surgical staples are used because they permit rapid wound closure, reduce tissue trauma, elicit minimal inflammatory response, and are cost effective. In animal studies, undressed wounds closed with staples were less likely to become infected by surface contamination with *Staphylococcus aureus* than wounds closed with silk or nylon sutures.

The stapling guns presently available tend to evert wound edges and thus facilitate wound healing. Surgical staples may be particularly useful in hair-bearing areas such as scalps, for closing scalp reductions or closing donor sites following hair transplantation. Staples may additionally be used on the trunk and extremities and may be used to secure a split thickness skin graft to the recipient site.

On nonfacial skin, the results obtainable by staples are comparable to those one might expect using other nonabsorbable sutures. On facial areas, however, many believe that a more exact approximation of tissue and thus a better cosmetic result may be obtained using sutures rather than staples.

All staples, once inserted into the skin, make an incomplete rectangle; the top cross-limb lies on the skin surface parallel to the skin and perpendicular to the wound, the legs extend into the skin, and the pointed tips are bent inward and lie beneath the skin parallel to the top cross-limb. The depth of staple penetration is increased when more downward pressure is applied to the staple gun against the tissue. If the top cross-limb of the staple is too close to the wound, resulting in direct contrast with the wound, then permanent crosshatching may result.

Metal surgical staples are made of inert stainless steel. Ethicon, Autosuture™ (U.S. Surgical, Tyco Healthcare Group LP), and 3M market automatic disposable staplers with different features. Available options include rotatable heads that make them easier to use in hard-to-reach locations, regular or wide staple width, different height options, reloadable or non-reloadable, and number of staples per stapler (Fig. 1). Some may have a pre-cocked position of partial staple closure, which facilitates the placement of grafts by "hooking into" the graft tissue and opposing wound edges. This feature also facilitates wound edge eversion for linear and flap repairs.

SUTURE AND STAPLE REMOVAL

Many factors determine the cosmetic outcome for any wound. Crikelair's studies demonstrated that the size of the suture and needle used to insert it are relatively unimportant in terms of final cosmetic result. Sutures removed within seven days generally leave no skin marks, while in instances when it is necessary to leave sutures in place over

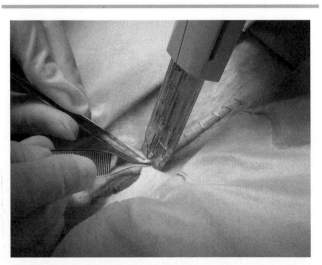

Figure 1 Surgical stapler. *Source:* PXW35 Proximate® Plus MD Skin Stapler. *Source:* Courtesy of Ethicon, Inc.

two weeks, persistent marks may result in "railroad track" appearance. This is understandable in view of the time course of wound healing and the host inflammatory response to sutures, as previously detailed.

It has been recommended by some that all sutures on the face, assuming a layered closure, be removed by the fifth day, if possible, with alternating sutures having been removed on the second to third day following placement. The same author suggests that sutures in the eyelids be completely removed by the second to third day, those in the extremities and anterior trunk at the sixth or seventh day, and those on the sole of the foot and back at 7 to 10 days. Others have suggested that sutures on the back and those placed in areas affected by a great deal of motion be left in place for two weeks or longer. These generalizations can only be used as guidelines. The proper time to remove sutures is determined by balancing cosmetic considerations, which dictate removal of sutures as rapidly as possible to avoid suture marks, functional considerations such as ensuring that the wound does not dehisce, and cost. These considerations will reflect the anatomy of the site involved, the degree of tension on the wound, the use of subcutaneous sutures, and the amount and direction of tension exerted by underlying muscles.

Because stainless steel staples cause minimal tissue reaction, some believe they may be left in place for longer periods of time than suture, which may prevent spreading of the scar.

TISSUE ADHESIVES

Tissue adhesives have been used since 1949, when cyanoacrylate adhesives were initially synthesized. The cyanoacrylate tissue adhesives are liquid monomers that, upon exposure to moisture from the skin, polymerize via an exothermic reaction to create strong bonds, which maintain tissue opposition. Butyl-cyanoacrylates (Indermil® Tissue Adhesive, marketed by U.S. Surgical and a trademark of Henkel Corporation, manufactured by Henkel Loctite (Ireland) Ltd.; Histoacryl™, a product of B. Braun) are somewhat brittle and exhibit poor tensile strength. Newer 2-octylcyanoacrylate exhibits greater tensile strength and flexibility. Octylcyanoacrylate was initially marketed as TraumaSeal by Tri-Point Medical, but is currently distributed as Dermabond Topical Skin Adhesive by Ethicon.

Tissue adhesives may be used for superficial approximation of traumatic lacerations and for surgical wounds under no or minimal static or dynamic tension (Fig. 2). They should be used in conjunction with deep dermal sutures that yield wounds with almost perfectly approximated edges before superficial closure. In these types of wounds, there is no increased dehiscence in comparison with wound edge approximation achieved with traditional suture. Studies have shown that tissue adhesives yield equivalent or superior cosmetic results in comparison with traditional superficial suture closures. They demonstrate equal or fewer wound infections, and cyanoacrylate has been demonstrated to have an antimicrobial effect. Although cyanoacrylate costs more than suture, wounds may be closed faster with tissue adhesive in comparison with suturing, with decreased chance of accidental needle stick injury. The time saved increases with increasing length of the closure. The major disadvantage of cyanoacrylate is reduced tensile strength (octylcyanoacrylate tensile strength is similar to 5–0 suture).

Tissue adhesives should not be used in patients who may exhibit delayed wound healing, or in patients who have

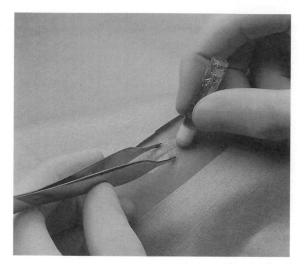

Figure 2   Application of tissue adhesive. *Source:* DERMABOND™ Topical Skin Adhesive. *Source:* Courtesy of Ethicon, Inc.

known allergies to cyanoacrylate or formaldehyde, as they are broken down to formaldehyde. Cyanoacrylate should not be used on mucosal surfaces, on skin regularly exposed to body fluids, or on skin with dense hair.

In addition to lacerations and linear closures, tissue adhesives may be useful to secure skin grafts (in combination with several cardinal sutures), closure of flaps and fragile skin (as they do not tear through tissues or strangulate them), and in patients who tend to heal with hypertrophic or keloid scarring.

When applying tissue adhesive, care should be taken to use minimal pressure, to minimize the chance of introducing the adhesive between the wound edges. It should be applied over the wound plus 5 to 10 mm on either side. A thin film should be applied, as a thick film or large droplet of adhesive may cause patient discomfort or the sensation of heat, as a result of the exothermic polymerization process. Dermabond Topical Skin Adhesive must be applied in three coats, High Viscosity Dermabond in two layers (information from manufacturer), and Indermil Tissue Adhesive in only one coat. Care should be taken to minimize runoff; the patient should be positioned so that the wound is parallel to the floor. The tissue adhesive should not come into contact with the eye. High Viscosity Dermabond was developed to minimize this risk when used near vital structures such as the eye, or to minimize runoff on curved structures such as the nose.

After application, once the adhesive has completely dried, a clean dressing may be applied, but no topical ointment or liquid should be applied directly to the cyanoacrylate. The patient should be instructed to avoid picking or scratching and to avoid placing tape directly over the adhesive, as these may cause premature detachment of the adhesive from the tissue. The adhesive may be wet briefly while showering, but prolonged water exposure (swimming, wet dressing, excessive perspiration) should be avoided. The tissue adhesive will gradually slough off in 5 to 10 days. If removal is desired before that time, acetone or petrolatum may facilitate its removal.

WOUND CLOSURE TAPES

Wound closure tapes may be used at the time of surgery over the suture line to provide an occlusive environment or to approximate wound edges under minimal tension. They may be used at the time of suture removal to decrease tension across the wound and to reinforce the wound. Many wound tapes are available (e.g., Steri-Strip, a product of 3M; Coverstrip, a product of Beirsdorf, Inc.), but few exhibit significant adhesiveness when used alone. Therefore, an adhesive such as tincture of benzoin or gum mastic must be used with these tapes to enhance their effectiveness. In comparison with tincture of benzoin, gum mastic (Mastisol™ Liquid Adhesive, a product of Ferndale Labs, Inc.) demonstrates superior adhesive qualities and decreased incidence of contact dermatitis.

SURGICAL NEEDLES

The ideal needle should cause minimal tissue trauma, which is achieved by being as narrow as possible while maintaining strength, being sharp enough to cut through tissue with minimal resistance, and resisting bending or breaking when pushed through tissue. Most surgical needles are made of stainless steel.

The needle is divided into the needle point, which extends from the extreme tip of the needle to the maximum cross-section of the body, the needle body, which is the portion which is grasped by the needle holder, and the needle eye, which may be either closed, French (split or spring), or swaged (eyeless) (Fig. 3). Virtually all sutures in use today are directly attached to the needles (swaged) rather than being threaded through a hole in the needle. This permits use of a smaller-diameter needle and thus less tissue trauma when sutures are placed. The needle body may be flattened to stabilize its security when grasped with the needle holder.

Needle size may be determined by several measurements (Fig. 4). Needle length is the curved distance measured along the needle from the point to the swage. Chord length specifies the distance between the extreme needle point to the swage, measured in a straight line. The diameter specifies the thickness of the needle itself. The radius refers to the distance from the body of the needle to the center of the circle created by the needle if the arc of the needle were extended to complete a full circle.

Needles are available in a variety of shapes including straight, half curved, ¼ circle, ⅜ circle, ½ circle, ⅝ circle, and

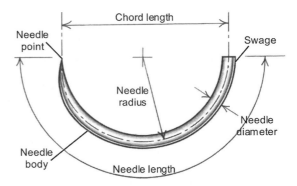

Figure 4 Anatomy of a needle. *Source*: Courtesy of Ethicon, Inc.

compound curved. The majority of needles used by dermatologic surgeons have an arc of 135 degrees (⅜ of a circle).

The terminology used to describe needles has developed in a haphazard fashion. One must determine which needles one prefers and learn the terminology of that particular manufacturer (Table 6; Fig. 5). Needle types suited to cutaneous surgery, common to most manufacturers, include the conventional cutting and reverse cutting needles (Fig. 6). The conventional cutting needle has a triangular point and body. The flat base of the triangle faces away from the wound and the apex of the triangle faces toward the wound (toward the center of the arc). This permits the suture to "ride" in the needle tract; if there is any tension on the wound, the suture will tend to "cut in" toward the wound edges. To avoid this difficulty, the reverse cutting needle was developed. Like the conventional needle, the reverse cutting needle has a triangular configuration but the apex of the triangle points away from the wound incision rather than toward it. This needle is particularly good for tough and difficult-to-penetrate tissues.

Reverse cutting needles currently available include the C (cutting, Syneture), FS (for skin, Ethicon), P (plastic,

Table 6 Needle Codes Applicable to Cutaneous Surgery

Code	Meaning	Cutting edge (if applicable)
Ethicon:		
CE	Cutting edge	
CFS	Conventional for skin	Conventional cutting
CP	Cutting point	
CPS	Conventional plastic surgery	Conventional cutting
CPX	Cutting point extra large	
FS	For skin	Reverse cutting
FSL	For skin large	Reverse cutting
FSLX	For skin extra large	Reverse cutting
OPS	Ocular plastic surgery	Side cutting (spatula)
P	Plastic	Reverse cutting, precision point
PC	Precision cosmetic	Conventional cutting
PS	Plastic surgery	Reverse cutting, precision point
PSL	Plastic surgery large	Reverse cutting, precision point
PSLX	Plastic surgery extra large	Reverse cutting, precision point
SFS	Spatulated for skin	Side cutting (spatula)
TE	Three eighths	
Syneture:		
C	Cutting	Reverse cutting
DX	DermaX	X cutting
HE	Plastic/ophthalmic surgery	Reverse cutting
P	Plastic	Reverse cutting, premium
PC	Plastic cutting	Conventional cutting

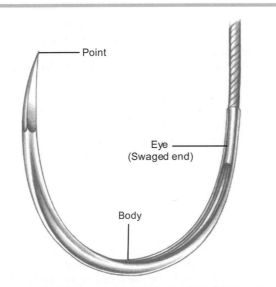

Figure 3 Needle components. *Source*: Courtesy of Ethicon, Inc.

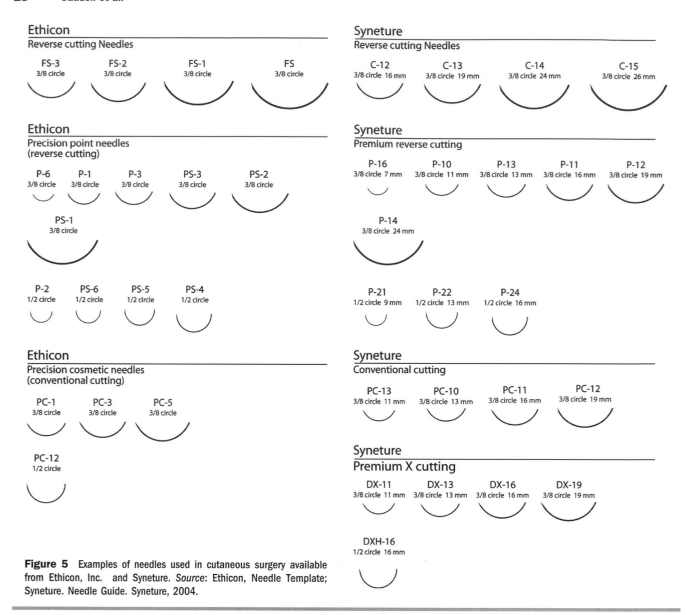

Figure 5 Examples of needles used in cutaneous surgery available from Ethicon, Inc. and Syneture. *Source*: Ethicon, Needle Template; Syneture. Needle Guide. Syneture, 2004.

Syneture and Ethicon), PS (plastic surgery, Ethicon). The "C" and "FS" needles are less finely honed than the "P" and "PS" needles, but are about half the price. For facial skin, the "P" or "PS" needles are recommended. Needle selection for nonfacial skin is per individual preference.

Conventional cutting needles currently available include the PC Prime™ needle (precision cosmetic, a product of Ethicon) and the "PC" needle (plastic cutting, a product of Syneture). The PC Prime needle has conventional cutting edges, a narrow point, a narrow diameter, and fine wire diameter. It has a flattened body for better stability when grasped with a needle driver and is superior for delicate surgery. The "PC" needle is finely honed and is a competitor of the PC Prime needle.

The DermaX™ ("DX," a product of Syneture) needle is a newly developed, uniquely shaped needle, which features four cutting surfaces (x-cutting). In cross-section, the tip is shaped like a diamond with concave sides, with cutting surfaces on the lateral aspects as well as on the superior and inferior surfaces (Fig. 7). It was designed specifically for

cosmetic surgery and delivers vertical and horizontal precision control, low tissue drag and easy penetration. According to the manufacturer, the needle shape facilitates depth placement and precision control during deep (subcuticular) approximation.

The number assigned to a suture (for example P-3 or DX-11), which appears on the package after the series designation, has different meaning for different manufactures. For needles manufactured by Ethicon, the numeric assignment is somewhat arbitrary, but as a general rule, the needle length increases as the numeric designation decreases (PS-1 is longer than PS-2). For needles manufactured by Syneture, the numeric designation usually increases with increasing needle length (but not always). For DermaX needles, the numeric designation refers to the length of the needle (in millimeters).

A word about needle holders is appropriate. The needle holder should be the appropriate size for the needle selected (a large needle should be held with a needle holder with larger heavier jaws, a small needle should be held with a

Conventional Cutting

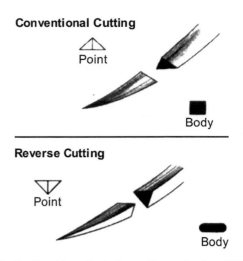

Reverse Cutting

Figure 6 Needle points and body shapes. *Source*: Courtesy of Ethicon, Inc.

Table 7 Average Retail Prices for Selected Sutures[a]

Suture type	Needle type			
	FS	P	PS	PC
Ethilon	$35.21	$86.35	$84.15	88.84[b]
Silk	$35.17	$77.09	$93.37	
Prolene, blue	$66.10[c]	$119.50	$117.55	$128.57
Monocryl		$112.34	$108.55	$99.06
PDS II	$80.00[c]	$129.40[c]	$129.40[c]	
Vicryl, undyed	$45.02[b]	$97.22	$99.23	$125.90[c]
Vicryl, violet	$55.96	$116.00[c]		
Vicryl Rapide		$127.60[c]	$128.40[c]	$142.50[c]
Plain gut	$60.70[c]	$94.00	$96.71	$125.60[c]
Chromic gut	$60.70[c]	$109.52	$95.25	

[a]Prices were obtained by web search on 12/29/04 for retail suture suppliers. Prices are for one box of 12 18" sutures.
[b]May be falsely low because no prices were available from the most expensive vendor, which was priced about 20–35% higher than the other two vendors sampled.
[c]May be falsely elevated because no prices were available from the least expensive vendors, which were priced about 20–35% lower than the other vendor sampled.
Abbreviations: FS, for skin (reverse cutting); P, plastic (reverse cutting, precision point); PS, plastic surgery (reverse cutting, precision point); PC, precision cosmetic (conventional cutting, finely honed).
Source: http://www.careexpress.com (Accessed December 2004); http://www.delasco.com/pcat/1/Surgery/Monocryl (Accessed December 2004); http://www.harrell-medical.com (Accessed December 2004).

fine-jawed needle holder). The needle should be grasped one-third to one-half the distance from the swaged end to the tip, as the swaged area is the weakest part of the needle.

CLOSURE MATERIAL SELECTION

When choosing closure material, one should consider the location of the wound, static and dynamic wound tension, presence of wound infection or fever (faster degradation possible) and cost of closure material. Select smallest diameter suture material that will achieve the closure objective, yet not compromise closure integrity. The size of absorbable suture should be guided by the expected tension (e.g., 3–0 or 4–0 if tension is present, 5–0 if no tension present). If wound tension is unavoidably high, then an absorbable suture with extended tensile strength, such as Maxon or PDS should be considered. If the wound is not under tension, then deep more conventional sutures without extended tensile strength retention such as Dexon II, Polysorb, Vicryl, or Biosyn may be considered. These absorbable sutures are more cost effective.

If fever or potential for infection is high, then deep sutures composed of synthetic monofilament are desirable, as braided sutures are associated with higher rates of infection and are more likely to be degraded rapidly in the presence of infection or fever.

For running intradermal sutures, polypropylene (Prolene, Surgipro), poliglecaprone 25 (Monocryl), or glycomer 631 (Biosyn) may be considered. They are comparably priced and all exhibit minimal tissue reactivity. Poliglecaprone 25 (Monocryl) and glycomer 631 (Biosyn) are absorbable, but polypropylene (Prolene, Surgipro), which is nonabsorbable, exhibits superior plasticity (Tables 7–9).

For surface approximation, the smallest suture appropriate for the area should be used (face 5–0 or 6–0, trunk 4–0, extremities 4–0 or 5–0, under tension 4–0). Nylon (Ethilon, Dermalon, Monosof) is ideal as it is relatively inexpensive, has good tensile strength, and exhibits excellent elasticity. If significant postoperative edema is expected, then polybutester (Novafil) may be considered, as it exhibits excellent plasticity and elasticity. Surface approximation of mucosal surfaces or intertriginous areas are best achieved with silk, which is soft and pliable and, therefore, more comfortable. For punch biopsies, shorter sutures (Look™, a product of Surgical Specialties Corporation) are available, providing significant cost savings.

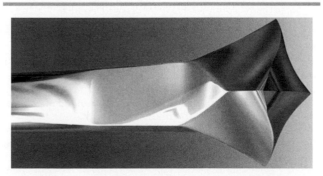

Figure 7 DermaX™ Needle. *Source*: Courtesy of Syneture.

Table 8 Example Retail Prices for Selected Sutures[a]

Suture type	Needle type		
	C or CE	P, PC, or PRE	DX
Dermalon	$57.49	$100.69	$118.29
Surgipro		$122.49	$118.29
Biosyn	$54.26	$144.73	$139.99
Maxon	$55.33	$118.03	
Polysorb	$46.86	$105.27	
Dexon II	$79.96		
Caprosyn		$99.77	

[a]Retail prices were obtained from Henry Schein, Inc. on 12/30/04. Prices are for one dozen 18" sutures.
Abbreviations: C, cutting (reverse cutting); P, plastic (reverse cutting, finely honed); PC, plastic cutting (conventional cutting, finely honed); DX, DermaX (X-cutting).

Table 9 Example Retail Prices for Staplers and Tissue Adhesives[a]

Dermabond Topical Skin Adhesive	$329.50
Dermabond, High Viscosity	$456.00[b]
3M DS & MS Precise Multi-Shot Disposable Skin Stapler (Arcuate)	$75.01
Reusable handle for use with 3M DS & MS Staplers	$222.00
3M PGX disposable, regular style (no additional handle required)	$112.29
3M precise staple remover	$36.00

[a]Prices were obtained by web search on 12/29/04 and 1/16/05 for retail suppliers. Prices are for 12 tubes of Dermabond™, 12 staplers with 15 staples, 12 stapler handles, and 12 staple removal kits.

[b]May be falsely elevated because no prices were available from the least expensive vendor.

Source: http://www.careexpress.com (Accessed December 2004); http://www.delasco.com/pcat/1/Surgery/Monocryl (Accessed December 2004); http://www.woundcare-products.com/products_001. cfm?C5561.

BIBLIOGRAPHY

Artandi C. A revolution in sutures. Surg Gynecol Obstet 1980; 150(2):235–236.

Aston SJ. The choice of suture material for skin closure. J Dermatol Surg 1976; 2(1):57–61.

Bennett RG. Selection of wound closure materials. J Am Acad Dermatol 1988; 18(4 Pt 1):619–637.

Blomstedt B, Osterberg B. Suture materials and wound infection. An experimental study. Acta Chir Scand 1978; 144(5):269–274.

Blondeel PN, Murphy JW, Debrosse D, et al. Closure of long surgical incisions with a new formulation of 2-octylcyanoacrylate tissue adhesive versus commercially available methods. Am J Surg 2004; 188(3):307–313.

Brandy DA. The quicklift: A modification of the S-lift. Cosmetic Dermatol 2004; 17(6):351–360.

Campbell JP, Swanson NA. The use of staples in dermatologic surgery. J Dermatol Surg Oncol 1982; 8(8):680–690.

Chu CC. Mechanical properties of suture materials: an important characterization. Ann Surg 1981; 193(3):365–371.

Craig PH, Williams JA, Davis KW, et al. A biologic comparison of polyglactin 910 and polyglycolic acid synthetic absorbable sutures. Surg Gynecol Obstet 1975; 41(1):1–10.

Craven NM, Telfer NR. An open study of tissue adhesive in full-thickness skin grafting. J Am Acad Dermatol 1999; 40(4):607–611.

Crikelair GF. Skin suture marks. Am J Surg 1958; 96(5):631–639.

Deutsch HL. Observations on a new absorbable suture material. J Dermatol Surg 1975; 1(4):49–51.

Eiferman RA, Snyder JW. Antibacterial effect of cyanoacrylate glue. Arch Ophthalmol 1983; 101(6):958–960.

Ethicon, Inc. Product information. In: Ethicon Wound Closure Manual. Ethicon, 2004, 88–109.

Ethicon, Inc. The surgical needle. In: Ethicon Wound Closure Manual Ethicon, 2004, 42–53.

Ethicon, Inc. The suture. In: Ethicon Wound Closure Manual. Ethicon, 2004, 10–40.

Ethicon, Inc. Topical skin adhesives. In: Ethicon Wound Closure Manual. Ethicon, 2004, 68.

Ethicon, Needle Template.

Freeman BS, Homsy CA, Fissette J, et al. An analysis of suture withdrawal stress. Surg Gynecol Obstet 1970; 131(3):441–448.

Fulton JE Jr., Saylan Z, Helton P, et al. The S-lift facelift featuring the U-suture and O-suture combined with skin resurfacing. Dermatol Surg 2001; 27(1):18–22.

Georgiade G, Riefkohl R, Serafin D, et al. Use of skin staples in plastic surgery. Ann Plast Surg 1980; 5(4):324–325.

Harris DR. Healing of the surgical wound, I. Basic considerations. J Am Acad Dermatol 1979; 1(3):197–207.

Harris DR. Healing of the surgical wound, II. Factors influencing repair and regeneration. J Am Acad Dermatol 1979; 1(3):208–215.

Hermann JB. Tensile strength and knot security of surgical suture materials. Am Surg 1971; 37(4):209–217.

Herrmann JB, Kelly RJ, Higgins GA. Polyglycolic acid sutures. Laboratory and clinical evaluation of a new absorbable suture material. Arch Surg 1970; 100(4):486–490.

Holt GR, Holt JE. Suture materials and techniques. Ear Nose Throat J 1981; 60(1):12–18.

Howes EL, Harvey SC. The strength of the healing wound in relation to the holding strength of the catgut suture. N Engl J Med 1929; 200:1285–1291.

Howes EL. Strength studies of polyglycolic acid versus catgut sutures of the same size. Surg Gynecol Obstet 1973; 137(1):15–20.

Howes EL. The immediate strength of the sutured wound. Surgery 1940; 7:24–31.

Howes EL. The strength of wounds sutured with catgut and silk. Surg Gynecol Obstet 1933; 57:309–311.

http://www.careexpress.com (Accessed December 2004).

http://www.delasco.com/pcat/1/Surgery/Monocryl (Accessed December 2004).

http://www.harrellmedical.com (Accessed December 2004).

http://www.syneture.com/products/sutures/absorbable/content_caprosyn.shtml (Accessed December 2004).

http://www.syneture.com/products/sutures/absorbable/body_caprosyn.shtml (Accessed December 2004).

http://www.syneture.com/products/sutures/absorbable/content_biosyn.shtml (Accessed December 2004).

http://www.syneture.com/products/sutures/absorbable/content_dexon2.shtml (Accessed December 2004).

http://www.syneture.com/products/sutures/absorbable/content_dexons.shtml (Accessed December 2004).

http://www.syneture.com/products/sutures/absorbable/content_maxon.shtml (Accessed December 2004).

http://www.syneture.com/products/sutures/absorbable/content_polysorb.shtml (Accessed December 2004).

http://www.syneture.com/products/sutures/absorbable/top_biosyn.shtml (Accessed December 2004).

http://www.syneture.com/products/sutures/absorbable/top_dexon2.shtml (Accessed December 2004).

http://www.syneture.com/products/sutures/absorbable/top_dexons.shtml (Accessed December 2004).

http://www.syneture.com/products/sutures/absorbable/top_maxon.shtml (Accessed December 2004).

http://www.syneture.com/products/sutures/absorbable/top_polysorb.shtml (Accessed December 2004).

http://www.syneture.com/products/sutures/non-absorbable/body_ticron.shtml (Accessed December 2004).

http://www.syneture.com/products/sutures/non-absorbable/body_surgidac.shtml (Accessed December 2004).

http://www.syneture.com/products/sutures/non-absorbable/body_surgipro.shtml (Accessed December 2004).

http://www.syneture.com/products/tissue_adhesives/index.shtml (Accessed December 2004).

http://www.syneture.com/specialties/plastic/dermax.shtml (Accessed December 2004).

http://www.woundcare-products.com/products_001.cfm?C561.

Jenkins HP, Hrdina LS, Ownes FM, et al. Absorption of surgical gut (catgut). Arch Surg 1942; 45:74–102.

Johnson A, Rodeheaver GT, Durand LS, et al. Automatic disposable stapling devices for wound closure. Ann Emerg Med 1981; 10(12):631–635.

Larena-Avellaneda A, Debus ES, Diener H, et al. Species-dependent premature degradation of absorbable suture materials caused by infection—impact on the choice of thread in vascular surgery. Vasa 2004; 33(3):165–169.

Laufer N, Merino M, Trietsch HG, et al. Macroscopic and histologic tissue reaction to polydioxanone, a new, synthetic, monofilament microsuture. J Reprod Med 1984; 29(5):307–310.

Lehman RA, Hayes GJ, Leonard F. Toxicity of alkyl 2-cyanoacrylates. II. Bacterial growth. Arch Surg 1966; 93(3):447–450.

Lerwick E. Studies on the efficacy and safety of polydioxanone monofilament absorbable suture. Surg Gynecol Obstet 1983; 156(1):51–55.

Lesesne CB. The postoperative use of wound adhesives. Gum mastic versus benzoin, USP. J Dermatol Surg Oncol 1992; 18(11):990.

Lober CW, Fenske NA. Suture materials for closing the skin and subcutaneous tissues. Aesthetic Plast Surg 1986; 10(4):245–247.

MacKinnon AE, Brown S. Skin closure with polyglycolic acid (DEXON). Postgrad Med J 1978; 54(632):384–385.

Mackenzie D. The history of sutures. Med Hist 1973; 17(2):158–168.

Madsen ET. An experimental and clinical evaluation of surgical suture materials. Surg Gynecol Obstet 1953; 97(1):73–80.

Molea G, Schonauer F, Bifulco G, et al. Comparative study on biocompatibility and absorption times of three absorbable monofilament suture materials (polydioxanone, poliglecaprone 25, glycomer 631). Br J Plast Surg 2000; 53(2):137–141.

Moy RL, Kaufman AJ. Clinical comparison of polyglactic acid (VICRYL) and polytrimethylene carbonate (MAXON) suture material. J Dermatol Surg Oncol 1991; 17(8):667–669.

Moy RL, Lee A, Zalka A. Commonly used suture materials in skin surgery. Am Fam Physician 1991; 44(6):2123–2128.

Moy RL, Quan MB. An evaluation of wound closure tapes. J Dermatol Surg Oncol 1990; 16(8):721–723.

Moy RL, Waldman B, Hein DW. A review of sutures and suturing techniques. J Dermatol Surg Oncol. 1992; 18(9):785–795.

Nilsson T. Mechanical properties of PROLENE and ETHILON sutures after three weeks in vivo. Scand J Plast Reconstr Surg 1982; 16(1):11–15.

Osterburg B, Blomstedt B. Effect of suture materials on bacterial survival in infected wounds. Acta Chir Scand 1979; 145:432–434.

Pineros-Fernandez A, Drake DB, Rodeheaver PA, et al. CAPROSYN, another major advance in synthetic monofilament absorbable suture. J Long Term Eff Med Implants 2004; 14(5):359–368.

Postlethwait RW, Smith BM. A new synthetic absorbable suture. Surg Gynecol Obstet 1975; 140(3):377–380.

Postlethwait RW, Willigan DA, Ulin AW. Human tissue reaction to sutures. Ann Surg 1975; 181(2):144–150.

Postlethwait RW. Long-term comparative study of nonabsorbable sutures. Ann Surg 1970; 171(6):892–898.

Postlethwait RW. Polyglycolic acid surgical suture. Arch Surg 1970; 101:489–494.

Quinn JV, Osmond MH, Yurack JA, et al. N-2-butylcyanoacrylate: risk of bacterial contamination with an appraisal of its antimicrobial effects. J Emerg Med 1995; 13(4):581–585.

Ray JA, Doddi N, Regula D, et al. Polydioxanone (PDS*), a novel monofilament synthetic absorbable suture. Surg Gynecol Obstet 1981; 153(4):497–507.

Rodeheaver GT, Beltran KA, Green CW, et al. Biomechanical and clinical performance of a new synthetic monofilament absorbable suture. J Long Term Eff Med Implants 1996; 6(3–4):181–198.

Rodeheaver GT, Borzelleca DC, Thacker JG, et al. Unique performance characteristics of NOVAFIL. Surg Gynecol Obstet 1987; 164(3):230–236.

Rodeheaver GT, Nesbit WS, Edlich RF. NOVAFIL. A dynamic suture for wound closure. Ann Surg 1986; 204(2):193–199.

Salthouse TN. Biologic response to sutures. Otolaryngol Head Neck Surg 1980; 88(6):658–664.

Singer AJ, Quinn JV, Clark RE, et al. Closure of lacerations and incisions with octylcyanoacrylate: a multi-center randomized trial. Surgery 2002; 131(3):270–276.

Singer AJ, Thode HC Jr. A review of the literature on octylcyanoacrylate tissue adhesive. Am J Surg 2004; 187(2):238–248.

Stillman RM, Bella FJ, Seligman SJ. Skin wound closure. The effect of various wound closure methods on susceptibility to infection. Arch Surg 1980; 115(5):674–675.

Swanson NA, Tromovitch TA. Suture materials, 1980s: properties, uses, and abuses. Int J Dermatol 1982; 21(7):373–378.

Syneture. Needle Guide. Syneture, 2004.

Van Winkle W Jr., Hastings JC. Considerations in the choice of suture material for various tissues. Surg Gynecol Obstet 1972; 135(1):113–126.

Varma S, Ferguson HL, Breen H, et al. Comparison of seven suture materials in infected wounds—an experimental study. J Surg Res 1974; 17(3):165–170.

Watts GT. Sutures for skin closure. Lancet 1975; 1(7906):581.

4

Medical Evaluation

Priya Zeikus and Raymond G. Dufresne, Jr.
Department of Dermatology, Brown Medical School, Brown University, Providence, Rhode Island, U.S.A.

INTRODUCTION

A detailed medical history and pertinent physical examination are important factors in the preoperative evaluation of the dermatologic surgery patient. This evaluation provides screening for the detection of diseases and other comorbidities that may affect surgical outcome. The evaluation thus allows the surgeon to appropriately plan the surgical procedure and anticipate potential complicating factors.

Many patients undergoing dermatologic surgery have pre-existing medical conditions. Most commonly these include diabetes, heart disease, clotting disorders, hypertension, and psychiatric or neurological illnesses. Careful consideration of patients' medical condition is critical in planning and preparing for the surgery. At times, coordination with the primary care physician who is managing the chronic health problems of the patient is important.

MEDICAL HISTORY

The evaluation of a patient's medical history and review of systems (ROS) is imperative prior to surgery (Table 1). The medical interview should include fundamental questions regarding past medical history, previous surgeries, current medications, medication allergies, pregnancy, tobacco, and alcohol use. The interview should inquire about chronic medical conditions particularly diabetes, heart disease, renal insufficiency, clotting disorders, and infectious diseases such as hepatitis B and C HIV. A history of herpes simplex virus is important when planning per oral surgery. Previous surgical history should also be elicited, including prior surgical complications such as bleeding, infection, or poor wound healing. Social history is important to plan for care in the perioperative period.

All medications, including over-the-counter and herbal medications should be documented. This review will uncover potential drug interactions and may elicit medical problems not detected in the ROS. Dietary supplements and herbal medications are not routinely self-reported by patients during the medical interview and may exacerbate bleeding in the perioperative period. Patients should be asked specifically about anticoagulant medications. Warfarin, enoxeparin, clopidogrel, persantine, heparin, aspirin, nonsteroidal inflammatory agents, and vitamin E are potential medications that can cause excessive bleeding during surgery. Table 2 lists these common anticoagulants and their mechanism of action.

PHYSICAL EXAMINATION

As dermatologic surgery is often a limited procedure and poses only minor risk to the patients, a focused physical exam is sufficient. However, the physical examination should be tailored to the nature and type of excision that is planned. The lesion should be closely examined for size, location, and relationship to potential danger areas or natural skin lines. Any evidence of facial asymmetry should be noted. Associated nerves and blood vessels in that anatomic region should be identified, as this will help aid in planning the surgical approach. The confirmation of local neurological function is also important prior to surgery. Examination should check for associated regional lymphadenopathy, if indicated. Photographing the skin lesion at the time of the physical examination captures an accurate description of the lesion and also serves as a reference for the future surgery.

The physical examination should include vital signs, assessment of the patient's functional status, mental status, affect, and overall appearance. on the basis of the ROS and nature of the procedure, the physical examination can be expanded as needed. Further laboratory evaluation or assistance from other consultants or the primary care physician may occasionally be needed.

LABORATORY TESTING

Routine laboratory testing prior to dermatologic surgeries is not usually indicated. Most dermatologic procedures are outpatient procedures with only local anesthesia, and the rates of preoperative morbidity and mortality with dermatologic surgeries are low. Most laboratory abnormalities can be predicted from a patient's physical examination and medical history. Moreover, laboratory anomalies, when discovered, rarely lead to changes in perioperative treatment. If patients have significant medical conditions, such as a bleeding disorder (or other conditions that could affect surgical outcome), appropriate laboratory testing and diagnostic studies are recommended.

AREAS OF SPECIAL CONCERN

Cardiovascular Disease

The initial history and physical examination should be attentive to cardiac disorders, including coronary artery disease (recent myocardial infarction, unstable angina), congestive heart failure, and presence of a pacemaker or

Table 1 Medical History

Current medications: specifically, anticoagulants and antiplatelet agents, herbal medications, over-the-counter medications
Medication allergies: allergies to antibiotics, topical antibiotics, latex, adhesives
Medical conditions:
 Cardiac disease: angina, heart failure, high blood pressure, artificial valves, defibrillators, pacemakers
 Hematologic disease: anticoagulants, bleeding disorders
 Diabetes mellitus: Type I or II, of control, insulin and/or other glycemic medications, renal or ocular disease
 Infectious disease: Hepatitis B, C, HIV/AIDS, Herpes simplex virus, Methicillin resistant Staph aureus
 Pregnancy: trimester of pregnancy, breastfeeding
 Renal disease: dialysis dependent, status post transplant
 Neurological and psychiatric disease: dementia, seizures, frequent fainting spells, anxiety, depression, obsessive compulsive disorder/body dysmorphic disorder
 Pulmonary: chronic obstructive pulmonary disease, asthma
 Liver disease: hepatitis, previous blood transfusion, illicit drug use, alcohol use
 Immunocompromised/immunosupressed: cancer, chemotherapy, transplant, immunosuppressive therapy
Previous surgeries/hospitalizations
Social history: alcohol, tobacco, recreational drug use
Family history: history of skin cancers, melanoma
Review of systems

implantable defibrillator device. The American College of Cardiology and American Heart Association have proposed a detailed algorithm that is based on the assessment of clinical history and symptoms, prior cardiac evaluation and treatment, functional capacity of the patient and the surgery specific risk. The overall cardiac risk estimated with dermatologic procedures is reportedly less than 1%. However, those patients with high cardiac risk factors such as acute myocardial infarction in the last seven days, unstable or severe angina, severe arrhythmias or severe valvular disease causing symptoms should have supplemental preoperative evaluation and testing by a cardiologist.

Table 2 Anticoagulant and Antiplatelet Agents

Medication	Mechanism of causing bleeding
Nonsteroidal anti-inflammatory drugs Ibuprofen Diclofenac	Inhibition of platelet cyclooxygnease pathway
Heparin	Binds to antithrombin and inhibits factors H, IX,X,XI, and XII
Warfarin	Inhibition of synthesis of vitamin K clotting factors, H, VII, IX, and X
Enoxeparin	Inhibition of coagulation factor X
Aspirin	Irreversibly blocks thromboxane A_2 synthesis by platelets
Clopidogrel	Inhibition of ADP-mediated platelet activation and aggregation
Dipyrimadole	Inhibition of platelet aggregation by inhibiting platelet phosphodiesterase
Herbal medications Gingko biloba, vitamin E, garlic, St. John's wort, Echinacea, fish oil	Inhibits platelet aggregation and function

Abbreviation: ADP, adenosine diphosphate.
Source: Calaitges, Silver (2005); Sharis, Cannon, Loscalzo (1998); Kaye, Clarke, Sabar (2000).

Patients should also be screened for implantable defibrillators and cardiac pacemakers. The use of electrosurgery in dermatologic procedures can cause potentially hazardous electrical interference with the function of pacemakers and implantable cardioverter defibrillators. Electrocautery, one form of electrosurgery, converts electrical energy into thermal energy by heating a metal tip, producing coagulation and tissue necrosis when held in contact with the tissue. It is considered the safest of the electrosurgical instruments used, as no current flows through the patient with this technique. For high frequency electrosurgery, the use of a bipolar instrument, such as coagulation forceps is recommended. In bipolar electrocoagulation, current is concentrated at the tips of the instrument, minimizing current leakage and potential interference with implantable devices. Electrosection or electrocutting poses the greatest risk to pacemakers and implantable defibrillators, as it delivers the highest current per unit time. CO_2 lasers could be also used as an alternative for hemostasis.

Patients should be screened on preoperative evaluation for hypertension. Those patients with severe hypertension may be at risk for excessive perioperative bleeding. Patients should be instructed to take their antihypertensive medications as prescribed prior to their surgery.

Hematologic Disease

Patients should be screened for history of any bleeding disorders and use of anticoagulant medications. Prospective patients should include a personal or family history of bleeding disorders, epistaxis, and excessive bleeding with prior surgical procedures. If there is any question of underlying bleeding problems, a clotting panel should be ordered, which includes platelets, bleeding time, prothrombin time (PT), partial thomboplastin time (PTT), and international normalization ratio (INR). If further workup of bleeding disorders is necessary, a formal hematology consultation should be obtained.

As an increasing number of patients are on anticoagulants, the surgeon must decide whether to stop these medications. Aspirin and nonsteroidal anti-inflammatory drugs (NSAIDs), both commonly prescribed over-the-counter medications, can interfere with the normal coagulation process, and cause significant perioperative bleeding. Other anticoagulants regularly used include warfarin, clopidogrel, dipyrimidamole, ticlopidine, low molecular weight heparin, or lovenox and heparin. Controversies persist whether to stop these medications before surgery. The common practice has been stopping aspirin and NSAIDs 7 to 10 days prior to surgery, which is largely based on the experience of major surgeries where the incidence of complications is higher in patients taking aspirin. However, many recent studies have shown that continuous treatment with blood thinners perioperatively in patients undergoing Mohs and cutaneous surgery is not associated with an increase in surgical complications. Studies have not shown increased bleeding complications of minor cutaneous surgery with aspirin use. Discontinuing these medications in the perioperative period may increase the risk of cerebral and cardiovascular complications in the patient. Otley et al. showed bleeding complications in patients taking blood thinners, such as increased intraoperative bleeding, hematoma, wound dehiscence, and necrosis of a flap or graft, were not significantly higher than the control patients.

In patients taking warfarin, monitoring the INR 24 hours prior to dermatologic surgery is recommended. An INR of 2.5 to 3.5 is considered safe for dermatologic surgery and recommended to prevent thromboembolic events such as stroke.

Multiple factors should be considered when deciding whether to continue or withhold the use of anticoagulants and antiplatelet agents, including the risk of hemorrhagic, thrombotic, neurological, cardiovascular, and other intraoperative complications versus the risk of perioperative bleeding.

Diabetes Mellitus

In a patient with diabetes, the goal of the preoperative evaluation is to assess the severity of diabetes, prior surgical complications, and the diabetic medications used. Diabetic patients can be at risk for hyperglycemia and hypoglycemia. Detailed instructions should be provided to the patient. They should be advised to take their diabetic medications per routine, to consume a light meal prior to surgery, and to carry snacks or necessary medications if the surgery is prolonged. Adjustments in medications should be made if patients are required to remain fasting or nothing per orum prior to surgery. The surgeon may also wish to store sweetened juices, food items, or glucose tablets in the office in the event of hypoglycemic episode.

Poorly controlled diabetics may have prolonged wound healing and increased propensities toward postoperative infections. The phagocytic and chemotactic functions of granulocytes are suppressed by hyperglycemia and collagen synthesis is reduced when glucose levels are higher than 200 mg/dL. Postoperative antibiotics and optimization of glucose control postoperatively may be useful to prevent wound infections and enhanced healing.

Renal Disease

During the preoperative evaluation, patients with renal disease should undergo a thorough interview, physical examination, and laboratory testing if necessary. Patients with end-stage renal disease can have serious comborbid conditions such as cardiovascular disease, coagulopathy and decreased ability to eliminate and excrete medications, including analgesics, antibiotics, and anesthetics. Uremic patients are also susceptible to increased bleeding tendency secondary to platelet dysfunction. These patients can be immunosuppressed and at increased risk for developing infections following surgery. The preoperative evaluation may entail coordination with patient's provider and laboratory tests, including a blood count, metabolic panel, serum magnesium, phosphorus, and coagulation profile. Depending on the severity of renal disease, careful adjustment of perioperative medications, and prevention of postoperative infections should be considered prior to surgery.

Pulmonary Disease

The preoperative assessment should review the patient's pulmonary status through medical history, medications, and presence of active respiratory symptoms. In patients with compromised function, key factors such as heavy cigarette smoking, frequent hospitalizations, intensive care unit admissions, steroid dependency, and recent upper respiratory infections should be elucidated. As most surgeries performed by dermatologists do not require sedation or general anesthesia, the perioperative and postoperative complications are fewer. However, factors such as stress, associated pain, positioning, and immobilization can potentially impact respiratory function. Patients with poor respiratory function should be encouraged to stop smoking eight weeks prior to surgery, and use bronchodilators, antibiotics, and supplemental oxygen when necessary. Additional coordination with the patient's pulmonologist or primary care physician may be necessary in patients with high risk factors.

In smokers undergoing major surgery, previous studies have shown that incidence of wound complications is higher when compared with nonsmokers. Specifically, the incidence of wound infections and wound dehiscence are increased in this population. Smoking is thought to affect tissue hypoxia, normal collagen regeneration, and the neutrophilic response towards pathogens. Patients should be encouraged to abstain from smoking four to eight weeks prior to surgery.

Psychiatric Disease

Psychiatric disease is composed of a broad and diverse group of illnesses, which includes disorders of mood and anxiety, psychotic disorders, disorders of cognition, substance abuse, and disorders of emotional function. The preoperative evaluation process requires that patients have normal cognitive and comprehension skills. In traditional psychiatric illness such as depression and schizophrenia, cognitive functioning is usually intact. These patients are typically able to answer questions regarding medical history and provide consent for surgery. Cognitive functions of orientation, memory, and concentration remain unaltered. However, in conditions such as delirium, dementia, and autism, cognitive functioning is impaired. If a patient does not have the capacity to make a medical decision, an alternative mode of decision making must be employed. Patients with underlying psychiatric disorders may have difficulty coping with the stress and strain of surgery and should be addressed with respect and consideration. Additional reassurance and handholding is necessary especially for the depressed and anxious patient. For those with cognitive impairment, repeated explanation of the surgical procedure and an alternative decision maker may be necessary.

The preoperative evaluation should also screen for patients with body dysmorphic disorder. Most often, patients seek out a dermatologist or plastic surgeon rather than a psychiatrist for treatment of their "defect". Patients who present with an intense preoccupation with minor or nonexistent defects in appearance should prompt further evaluation and referral to a psychiatrist. Characteristic features of these patients include camouflaging, difficulty in functioning, dissatisfaction with previous dermatological or surgical procedures, and unusual or excessive requests for cosmetic procedures. Procedures in these patients should be avoided and patients should be counseled to see a psychiatrist.

Pregnancy

Women of childbearing age should be asked about pregnancy. Any doubts should prompt pregnancy testing. Surgery in the pregnant patient should be approached with caution and the risks and benefits of the surgery should be weighed. If the surgery is purely elective, and can be delayed without added harm to the patient, the surgery should be performed after delivery. The surgeon should realize that the effect of surgery, anesthesia, and other perioperative medications could have potential effects on the developing fetus and the potential to trigger preterm labor. The ability of local anesthetics to cross the placenta is estimated to lead to exposure in the fetus in 11% to 23% of pregnancies. Most elective surgeries should be postponed until after the first trimester after fetal organogenesis is complete. Etidocaine, lidocaine, and prilocaine are classified as pregnancy category B, whereas bupivicaine and mepivicaine are pregnancy class C, secondary to its association with fetal bradycardia. A large study by Heinonen et al. showed that exposure to lidocaine, benzocaine, propoxycaine, or tetracaine in the first four months of pregnancy was not related to the development of any particular congenital malformation. Women should be asked if they are breastfeeding, as local anesthetics and other medications may be excreted in breast milk. Ester-based anesthetic or "noncaine" anesthetics such as saline with benzyl alcohol should be used as alternatives in these patients.

Liver Disease

Risk factors for liver disease should be assessed in all patients during the medical interview. Risk factors for liver disease include previous blood transfusions, tattoos, illicit drug use, sexual promiscuity, family history of jaundice, alcohol use, and a complete review of medications. The physical examination should evaluate patients with hepatic disease for signs of jaundice, palmar erythema, hepatosplenomegaly, spider telengiectases, increased abdominal girth and gynecomastia and testicular atrophy in males. Liver function tests, coagulation times (PT, PTT, and bleeding time), and platelets should be checked. The synthesis of most serum proteins, metabolism of nutrients and drugs, and excretion and detoxification of toxins can be impaired in patients with liver disease. As a result, anesthetics and analgesics can be affected by changes in binding to plasma proteins, detoxification, and excretion. Elective surgery is contraindicated in patients with acute viral and alcoholic hepatitis, fulminant hepatic failure, severe chronic hepatitis, and severe coagulopathy (prolongation of PT for 3 seconds despite vitamin K repletion, platelet count < 50,000). In patients with chronic liver disease such as hepatitis C, fatty liver, in which liver function is preserved, operative risk for elective surgeries is not significantly increased.

Immunocompromised/Immunosupressed Patients

In patients with HIV infection or AIDS postoperative complications such as poor wound healing and postoperative wound infections can occur in patients with decreased total white blood cell counts, and low CD4 lymphocyte counts. Recent studies in patients with HIV/AIDS suggest the viral load followed by CD4 counts, neopterin levels, B2 microglobulin, and fever or thrush are the best prognostic indicators for surgical outcome. Patients on chronic steroids or chemotherapeutics are at also significantly increased risk for postoperative wound infections. In chronic steroid use, the microbicidal capacity of immune system is decreased as the quantity of circulating monocytes, macrophages, and lymphocytes are reduced. Similarly, chemotherapeutic agents used in transplant recipients and cancer patients alter the immune system predisposing to opportunistic and other infections. Special considerations, such as preoperative antibiotics, and close monitoring should be performed in these patients.

SUMMARY

In summary a thorough and complete preoperative evaluation is important for successful surgical outcomes. Medical history and patient's functional status are two of the most important parameters that must be considered in the preoperative evaluation process. A complete preoperative assessment optimizes patient's satisfaction and comfort with his or her care and ensures a better outcome for both the surgeon and the patient.

BIBLIOGRAPHY

Alcalay J, Alcalay R. Controversies in perioperative management of blood thinners in dermatologic surgery: continue or discontinue? Derm and Surg 2004; 30:1091.

Alcalay J. Cutaneous surgery in patients receiving warfarin therapy. Dermatol Surg 2001; 27:256–258.

Bartlett GR. Does aspirin affect the outcome of minor cutaneous surgery? Br J Plast Surg 199; 52:214–216.

Bartley BG, Warndahl RA. Surgical bleeding associated with aspirin and nonsteroidal anti-inflammatory agents. Mayo Clin Proc 1992; 67:402–403.

Calaitges JG, Silver D. Antithrombotic therapy. In: Rutherford: Vascular Surgery. 5th ed. W.B. Saunders Company, 2005; Chapter 26:435–446.

Cassidy J, Marley RA. Preoperative assessment of the ambulatory patient. J Perianesth Nurs 1996; 11(5):334–343.

Collins S, Dufresne RG. Dietary supplements in the setting of Mohs surgery. Dermatol Surg 2002; 28(6):447–452.

Cook JL, Perone J. A prospective evaluation of the incidence of complications with Mohs micrographic surgery. Arch Dermatol 2003; 39(2):143–152.

Desan PH, Powsner. Assessment and management of patients with psychiatric disorders. Crit Care Med 2004; 32(4):S166–S171.

Eagle KA, Berger PB, Calkins H, et al. ACC/AHA Guideline update for perioperative cardiovascular evaluation for noncadiac surgery-executive summary. J Am Coll Cardiol 2002; 39:542–553.

Eagle KA, Rihal CS, Mickel MC, Holmes DR, Foster ED, Gersh BJ. Cardiac risk of noncardiac surgery: influence of coronary disease and type of surgery in 3368 operations. Circulation 1996; 96(6):118.

El-Gamal H, Dufresne RG, Saddler K. Electrosurgery, pacemakers, and ICDs: a survey of precautions, and complications experienced by cutaneous surgeons. Dermatol Surg 2001; 27:385–390.

Ferraris VA, Ferraris SP, Lough FC, Berry WR. Preoperative aspirin ingestion increases operative blood loss after coronary artery bypass grafting. Ann Thorac Surg 1988; 45:71–74.

Friedman LS. The risk of surgery in patients with liver disease. Hepatology 1999; 29(6):1617–1622.

Gholson CE, Provenza JM, Bacon BR. Hepatologic considerations in patients with parenchymal liver disease undergoing surgery. Am J Gastroenterol 1990; 85:487–496.

Greenberg SB. Infections in the immunocompromised rheumatological patient. Crit Care Clin 2002; 18(4):931–956.

Heinonen OP, Sloane D, Shapiro S. eds. Birth Defects and Drugs in Pregnancy. Littleton CO: Publishing Sciences Group, 1977:357–365.

Jensen JA, Goodson WH, Williams H, et al. Cigarette smoking decreases tissue oxygen. Arch Surg 1991; 126:1131–1134.

Jorgensen LN, Kallehave F, Christensen E, et al. Less collagen production in smokers. Surgery 1998; 123:450–455.

Joseph AJ, Cohn SL. Perioperative care of the patient with renal failure. Med Clin N Am 2003; 87:193–210.

Karnath BM. Preoperative cardiac risk assessment. Am Fam Physician 2002; 66:1889–1896.

Kaye AD, Clarke RC, Sabar R, et al. Herbal medicines: current trends in anesthesiology practice—a hospital survey. J Clin Anesth 2000; 12:468–441.

Keegan MT. The transplant recipient for nontransplant surgery. Anesth Clin N Am 2004; 22:821–861.

Kuczkowski KM. Nonobstetric surgery during pregnancy: what are the risks of anesthesia? Obstetr Gynec Survey 2003; 59(1):52–56.

Leshin B, Whitaker D, Swanson N. An approach to patient assessment and preparation in cutaneous onclology. J Am Acad Dermatol 1988; 19:1081–1088.

Levasseur JG, Kennard CD, Finley EM, Muse RK. Dermatologic electrosurgery in patients with implantable cardioverter-defibrillators and pacemakers. Dermatol Surg 1009; 24:233–240.

Martinelli PT, Schulze KE, Nelson BR. Mohs micrographic surgery in a patient with a deep brain stimulator: a review of the literature on implantable electrical devices.

McGillis ST, Stanton-Hicks U. The preoperative patient evaluation: preparing for surgery. 1998; 16:1–15.

Mellors JW, Rinaldo CR, Gupta P, et al. Prognosis in HIV-1 infection predicted by the quantity of virus in plasma. Science 1996; 272:1167–1170.

Moore PA. Selecting drugs for the pregnant dental patient. J Am Dental Assoc 1998; 129:1281–1286.

Otley CC, Fewkes JL, Frank W, Olbricht SM. Complications of cutaneous surgery in patients who are taking warfarin, aspirin, nonsteroidal anti-inflammatory drugs. Arch Dermatol 1996; 132:161–166.

Perkins SW, Sklarew EC. Prevention of facial herpetic infections after chemical peel and dermabrasion: new treatment strategies in the prophylaxis of patients undergoing procedures of the perioral area. Plas Reconst Surg 1996; 98: 427–435.

Phillips KA, Dufresne RG. Body dysmorphic disorder: a guide for dermatologists and cosmetic surgeons. Am J Clin Dermatol 2001; 1:235–243.

Richards KA, Stasko T. Dermatologic surgery and the pregnant patient. Dermatol Surg 2002; 28:248–256.

Riordan AT, Gamache C, Fosko SW. Electrosurgery and cardiac devices. J Am Acad Dermatol 1997; 37:250–255.

Schein OD, Katz J, Bass ER, et al. The value of routine perioperative medical testing before cataract surgery. New Eng J Med 2000; 342:169–175.

Schiff RL, Emanuelle MA. The surgical patient with diabetes mellitus. Guidelines for management. J Gen Intern Med 1995; 10:154–161.

Schiff RL, Welsh GA. Perioperative evaluation and management of the patient with endocrine dysfunction. Med Clin N Am 2003; 87:175–192.

Sebben JE. Electrosurgery and cardiac pacemakers. J Am Acad Dermatol 1983; 9:457–463.

Sharis PJ, Cannon CP, Loscalzo J. The antiplatelet effects of ticlopidine and clopidogrel. Ann Intern Med 1998; 129: 394–405.

Sheinfeld N, Yu T, Weinberg J, Norman, Alam M. Cutaneous oncologic and cosmetic surgery in geriatric patients. Dermatol Clin 2004; 22:97–113.

Skidmore RA, Patterson JD, Tomsick RS. Local anesthesia. Dermatol Surg 1996; 22:511–522.

Sorensen LT, Karlsmark T, Gottrup F. Abstinence from smoking reduces incisional wound infection: a randomized controlled trial. Ann Surgery 2003; 238(1):1–5.

Tamul PC, Peruzzi WT. Assessment and management of patients with pulmonary disease. Crit Care Med 2004; 32(4):S137–S145.

Thomas D, Ritchie CS. Preoperative assessment of older adults. J Am Geriatric Soc 1995; 43:811–821.

Tran HS, Moncure M, Tarnoff M, et al. Predictors of operative outcome in patients with human immunodeficiency virus or acquired immunodeficiency syndrome. Am J Surg 2000; 180:228–233.

Wilson JB, Arpey CJ. Body dysmorphic disorder: suggestions for detection and treatment in a surgical dermatology practice. Dermatol Surg 2004; 30(11):1391–1399.

5

Preoperative Psychological Evaluation

Hugh M. Gloster, Jr.
University of Cincinnati, Cincinnati, Ohio, U.S.A.

Randall K. Roenigk
Mayo Clinic, Rochester, Minnesota, U.S.A.

The preoperative evaluation of candidates for dermatologic surgery is often as important as the surgery itself. Fortunately, the risks and complications of minor skin surgery occur infrequently. Cosmetic surgery, however, requires a minimum risk of complications since patients' expectations are so high. Most dermatologic surgery can be performed under local anesthesia in an office or outpatient surgical suite without the need for general anesthesia or sedation. Therefore, even patients who have significant medical problems or are elderly can undergo these procedures safely. More time should be spent explaining a procedure and possible risks, because an anxious patient usually lacks understanding about what is going to happen. Patients are more cooperative and relaxed once they understand the procedure and its expected results.

The preoperative psychological management of patients undergoing skin surgery should be classified into three treatment groups: minor dermatologic surgery, oncologic dermatologic surgery, and cosmetic dermatologic surgery. Patients with skin cancer are highly motivated to undergo treatment as soon as possible. The final cosmetic result is usually secondary and not the main concern. Cosmetic dermatologic surgery patients may not have objective disease but are motivated to have surgery for a variety of reasons. Some patients want specific problems corrected, while others think they need "new skin." These patients may have unique personalities, and although all dermatologic surgeons may not find themselves qualified to evaluate them, time and experience are required to prepare patients for cosmetic surgery, lest one perform procedures on inappropriate patients.

The preoperative psychological evaluation of dermatologic surgery patients is difficult to teach and is learned through experience. Some surgeons never master this art of medicine and have difficulty communicating with patients. Patient satisfaction is determined not only by the technical quality of the surgery performed, but also by a good physician-patient relationship.

THE NONCOSMETIC CONSULTATION

Minor dermatologic surgery involves the removal of such benign neoplasms as nevi, cysts, and cherry angiomas. Removal of these lesions is done for both medical and cosmetic reasons but seldom involves stress on the part of the patient. Usually, patients understand the risks to be minimal and generally are not anxious about the results but do expect little or no resulting scar. Most malignant oncologic dermatologic surgery involves the treatment of basal cell carcinoma and squamous cell carcinoma. Simple outpatient therapy such as electrodesiccation and curettage seldom evokes emotional stress in patients, especially when a patient has been adequately instructed on the risk of these tumors. Finally, malignant melanoma is potentially life-threatening and requires more emotional support and discussion. Most dermatologists do not treat clinical stage II and III metastatic disease and therefore are not encumbered with handling the more emotional end stages and deaths in these patients. This is best left to the oncologist and others who deal with these problems routinely.

Once a diagnosis of basal cell carcinoma or squamous cell carcinoma has been made, it is important to explain the likely morbidity. The best approach is to be honest and give factual medical advice in a simplified fashion so that the patient understands completely. Of course, the patient may forget much of this information, and written material is always helpful. Apart from exceptional cases that require extensive surgery and reconstruction, reassurance about the out-come of basal cell carcinoma treatment is the best approach. The cosmetic result from reconstruction is secondary but important. The same can be said for most squamous cell carcinomas, since the risks for metastatic disease are minimal in most cases.

The treatment of nonmelanoma skin cancer can be thought of as a two-staged procedure. The first stage is treatment of the disease, and the second is reconstruction. Many patients are only concerned with the first stage and not with the cosmetic result when the diagnosis is first made. Most standard treatments for nonmelanoma skin cancer combine both stages. Electrodesiccation and curettage, fusiform excision, and cryosurgery often result in an excellent cosmetic scar that needs no further revision. Mohs micrographic surgery is generally reserved for more difficult tumors. The tumor-free margins obtained with Mohs micrographic surgery result in a defect that must be closed or allowed to heal by second intention. Reconstruction may involve the use of more advanced flaps or grafting procedures, and therefore a more complete discussion with the patient is required.

Patients with malignant melanoma have what might be a life-threatening tumor. The approach to these patients depends greatly on the clinical stage and histologic depth of the tumor. Most patients with thin melanomas (Breslow level less than 0.85 mm) classified as clinical stage I can be treated by simple excision with adequate margins and can expect very high cure rates. Despite the fact that we can reassure these patients, it is important to detail factual information about the long-term risks of this disease. Patients appreciate getting factual medical advice and simple, complete answers to their questions. In studies comparing patients with malignant melanoma and those with other dermatologic disorders, it has been shown that those with melanoma scored approximately equal to the general public and strikingly superior to other dermatologic patients in tests for emotional well-being. While patients with chronic dermatologic disease may have low self-esteem and self-image, patients with melanoma or other life-threatening cancer have the ability to "respond to the challenge" and emotionally "attack" the disease. Many cancer patients exhibit hopeful and goal-oriented thinking with a positive attitude.

In general, patients with skin cancer are anxious to be cured and require little discussion about whether surgery should be performed. Secondarily, they would like the final result to be cosmetically acceptable. When the cosmetic result takes precedence, there should be concern that the patient does not have a clear understanding about the tumor.

THE COSMETIC CONSULTATION

The preoperative consultation for patients undergoing cosmetic dermatologic surgery includes some basic determinations (Table 1). The first is the patient request, during which the patient describes the problem to be corrected. Second is the physical examination: the surgeon evaluates the patient based on his or her request and plans treatment. The third is a medical evaluation to determine if there are contraindications to the procedure. The final evaluation is the psychological assessment, which begins at the first meeting and continues through surgery and during all follow-up visits.

During the patient request, let the patient do all the talking. Give him or her a mirror and a pointer to show you the specific problems. The surgeon should listen to the patient's requests and not intercede with suggestions.

The physical examination is done to evaluate the patient and to determine if his or her request is reasonable. The surgeon can then point out additional problems that can be treated. The surgeon then plans his or her approach and tells the patient what can be done and what results can be expected. At this stage you must assess whether the patient has a reasonable understanding of what can be corrected based on the planned procedure. The patient must also demonstrate an understanding of the wound-healing process and the possible need for subsequent procedures. If a procedure can be performed, a determination of the patient's medical ability to undergo the operation is completed next (Chapter 5).

The preoperative psychological assessment includes an evaluation of the patient's expectations and motivations for surgery. At this time, the surgeon must develop insight into the patient's own body perception for a successful

Table 1 The Cosmetic Consultation

- Patient request
- Physical examination
- Medical evaluation
- Psychological assessment

Table 2 Important Aspects of the Preoperative Psychological Assessment of the Cosmetic Patient

- Motivation for surgery
- Expectations of surgery
- Understanding of the risks and implications of surgery
- Anxiety level
- Ego strength

surgical outcome. Important aspects of the preoperative psychological assessment of the cosmetic patient are listed in Table 2. It is necessary to determine the patient's motivations for surgery. A personal wish to change is essential to prevent later resentment. Patients who seek cosmetic surgery affecting body image for internal reasons are more likely to be pleased with their operation than those with externally directed motives. Internal motivations to undergo aesthetic surgery include a patient's desire to change his or her appearance in order to improve self-image or to meet a personal standard of physical attractiveness. Externally motivated patients, however, either respond to pressure from others (e.g., spouse, friend, or relative) to change their appearance or are driven to achieve some change external to themselves by undergoing surgery (e.g., to guarantee success in love and marriage). In other words, the disfigurement has become a focus for other psychological problems. The surgeon is usually unable to satisfy such patients. Preoperative assessment can provide the surgeon with information that allows the classification of patient motivations as internal or external. A direct way to evaluate patient motivations is to simply ask how and why they chose this time to undergo cosmetic surgery.

There is a developing consensus in the professional literature that the most important factor in the process of preoperative evaluation is the assessment of patient expectations regarding the outcome of aesthetic surgery. Expectations, which critically influence the patient's perception of surgical outcome, should be realistic, and the patient should not believe that surgery will improve occupational problems, solve financial difficulties, resolve personal conflicts, or render physical perfection. From a medical-legal standpoint, it is important that the patient understand what results can be expected, good or bad. The use of before and after photos and written material on a procedure may help to explain a cosmetic procedure. Adequate physician-patient communication cannot be stressed enough.

The patient must understand the risks and implications of surgery in order to be sufficiently well informed to make an intelligent decision about whether or not to proceed with the operation. It is often helpful to delay the patient's decision about whether to have surgery. After the consultation, the patient may not fully understand all of the risks, benefits, and alternatives and may think of other questions later. The patient needs to understand the procedure completely as well as the follow-up care expected. Patients should also understand that the surgeon cannot predict the final outcome precisely. It is therefore important to document the nature and purpose of the procedure and alternatives; the risks involved need to be discussed and documented in the chart. Well-written and specific informed consent is essential.

The patient's anxiety level should be assessed. No anxiety indicates denial and a possible failure of the patient to fully comprehend the risks of surgery. Unwarranted, excessive anxiety may result in a decision to cancel surgery unnecessarily.

Finally, the surgeon must determine the patient's ego strength. An individual with normal ego strength is stable, capable of tolerating the stress of surgery, and will not be governed by irrational fears or fantasies.

To do an adequate consultation, it is not reasonable to see patients briefly. Cosmetic surgery consultations should be scheduled and uninterrupted (30–45 min). The consultation should not be hurried. If there is not enough time, the cosmetic surgery consultation should be rescheduled. During an extended discussion, the patient reveals more to the physician. If there are psychosocial motivations for surgery, these can be discussed. If the patient does not understand what can be expected, the procedure can be delayed. In addition, if complications occur later, the patient knows the surgeon better and recognizes that the surgeon wants to help him or her through the problem.

Dermatologic surgeons are not trained in psychology but deal with these issues routinely. A psychiatrist or psychologist can evaluate the patient in special situations, but generally this is not necessary if the surgeon pays particular attention to this part of the evaluation. If the patient is already under the care of a psychologist or psychiatrist, he or she should be contacted before the surgeon agrees to proceed with cosmetic surgery.

GOOD CANDIDATES FOR COSMETIC SURGERY

Good candidates for cosmetic surgery can be grouped as having either major or minor disfigurements (Table 3). Examples of patients with major disfigurements include those with severe acne scarring, neurofibromatosis, multiple cylindromas, and scarring alopecia. These patients have a physical deformity, and surgery may be considered reconstructive in most cases. They have the greatest need for help and have the best chance for physical improvement. Psychiatric issues regarding the surgery are minimal since the disfigurement has already created a problem that may be improved by the operation.

Patients with minor disfigurements can also be good candidates for cosmetic surgery. Examples are patients with small nevi, Norwood's type I-III male pattern alopecia, or superficial rhytids that require soft tissue augmentation. Correction of a specific problem can be very satisfying. Inquire why the patient wants surgery performed. Patients who work in public contact occupations are good candidates, because they have strong motivation. Older patients who simply do not like their aging appearance are appropriately motivated: they see specific changes over the years that can be corrected. Another good candidate is the information seeker. These patients consider surgery for many years, read all they can, and seek the consultation of several surgeons. Once the information seeker decides to undergo surgery, he or she already has a good understanding of what can be expected.

It is difficult to be certain who will be the best candidate for cosmetic surgery. The close relationship between cosmetic surgery and psychological factors has long been recognized. Early investigators felt that the desire to change the appearance of the body may reflect failure to resolve underlying psychological conflicts. Requests for cosmetic surgery were thus interpreted as a symptom of neurosis. Several studies performed 25 to 30 years ago investigated the mental status of patients seeking aesthetic surgery. Forty to seventy two percent of patients were classified as either psychotic, neurotic, or having a personality trait disorder. Nevertheless, it has been determined that despite the high incidence of psychopathology preoperatively, most cosmetic patients are satisfied with their operation. As a result, cosmetic surgery often promotes positive changes in many aspects of psychosocial functioning, such as self-confidence and self-esteem. Patients usually become more socially outgoing and have an increased sense of well-being after aesthetic surgery. Thus, a history of psychiatric disease should not be an absolute contraindication to cosmetic surgery since well-chosen cases may have positive benefits on the overall adjustment of the individual.

A more recent evaluation of patients seeking cosmetic surgery showed that approximately 25% had psychological abnormalities as measured by the Minnesota Multiphasic Personality Inventory. This decline in the number of patients with an "abnormal" psychological profile seeking cosmetic surgery reflects current social changes such as the high value placed on physical attributes, the emphasis on youthfulness as being synonymous with capability at the workplace, the greater exposure of the body in modern clothing and sport trends, and increasing public awareness that cosmetic surgery procedures are readily available. In fact, there has been an astounding increase in the demand for such surgery over the past 20 years.

On the basis of a questionnaire and interview study of more than 60 consecutive cosmetic surgery patients, one author (RKR) found that the average patient who had cosmetic surgery performed would be approximately 40 years old, female, and having attained only a high school education. These patients are likely to be in public contact occupations. They feel average or normally attractive and are slightly concerned about their appearance. These patients have considered surgery for three to four years before one or two consultations are obtained. The patient expects some improvement in physical appearance but still expects to be basically the same person after surgery. An improved sense of self-esteem is expected by the patient, but this is subjective. These patients do not expect that cosmetic surgery will improve their occupation but often consider this possibility. The primary reason for undergoing the surgery is that the patient alone will notice the improved appearance and feel better about himself or herself, thus enhancing the quality of life.

POOR CANDIDATES FOR COSMETIC SURGERY

Though most patients do benefit from cosmetic surgery, a small number of individuals will not be satisfied with the outcome of well-executed surgical procedures. An even smaller minority may be psychologically harmed by aesthetic surgery. The profiles of poor candidates for cosmetic surgery are listed in Table 4. Patients with recurrent psychiatric illness, especially those requiring hospitalization, should be carefully evaluated. Psychiatric disease is not an absolute contraindication to cosmetic surgery, and a

Table 3 Good Candidates for Cosmetic Surgery

Major disfigurement	Minor disfigurement
Most accepting	Public appearance occupation (solid motive)
Greatest need	Do not like aging appearance
Best chance for improvement	The information seeker
Psychiatric issues relate to the disease, not surgery	

Table 4 Poor Candidates for Cosmetic Surgery

Recurrent psychiatric illness/hospitalization
The minimal defect patient
Surgeon shopping: seeing more than three surgeons reflects patient
  indecision
The sudden whim
Unreasonable motive: "My husband will stop cheating on me ..."
The solution to all problems

pleasing outcome can result. Neurotic patients may be anxious and worry. Somatic complaints are a defense against this stress. With adequate counseling, treatment with surgical intervention of a monosymptomatic neurosis directed at a cosmetic problem may result in improvement.

Psychotic patients have escaped into their own psychological island without stress, conflict, or reality checks. Psychiatric consultation for these patients is important. Some people feel that the danger of operating on psychotics is exaggerated, and sometimes psychological improvement is realized postoperatively. However, schizophrenics are characterized by disorganized thought, and paranoid schizophrenics can be dangerous. Surgery is best avoided in these patients. In general, surgery for psychotic patients should be limited to severe deformities that are not involved in the patient's delusions or hallucinations. Close liaison between the surgeon and the psychiatrist is necessary to manage such patients.

Patients with personality disorders, including those with maladaptive behavior or who are sociopathic, can easily disguise their problem and persuade a surgeon to operate. The surgery will not affect their behavior, and these patients are prone to sue for medical malpractice. Under no circumstances should the surgeon operate with the intent to treat a patient's personality problem. Other patients with personality disorders to be aware of include the obsessive-compulsive or hysterical patient. These patients may be flighty, reactive, and compulsive with excessive anxiety. They may have a positive response to surgery, but the course can be rocky and emotional. It is also important to be familiar with the poly surgical syndrome (Munchausen's syndrome) or the surgical addict. These patients give a history of surgical failures and a futile outlook. Surgery is fantasy for them, and it is important to resist their pleas for further procedures.

Certain patients seeking cosmetic surgery present to the surgeon with a conviction of having a physical defect, although their appearance is normal or very close to normal. These patients focus on one aspect of their body, which they find distasteful. This delusional preoccupation with some imagined defect in a normal-appearing person is called "dysmorphophobia," and most of these patients have a severe personality disorder or frank schizophrenia. Invariably, such patients are not pleased with surgery.

Besides the patient with specific psychopathology, another poor candidate for cosmetic surgery is the patient who gives a history of repeated surgery resulting in dissatisfaction and makes comments such as "the last doctor did it wrong" or "just a little change is needed here." The patient may be correct in believing that the last doctor did it wrong or that some modification may be required, but this should arouse suspicion that you, too, may not be able to meet the patient's expectations. In general, these patients have a severe disturbance in their object relations and carry a diagnosis of personality disorder with sadomasochistic, borderline, narcissistic, or antisocial traits.

The surgeon shopper is another patient to avoid. This is the patient who cannot make up his or her mind to have the procedure performed but seeks a number of consultations. After seeing two or three surgeons, most patients should be able to come to a decision. Indecision on the part of the patient may result in regret after the surgery has been performed. This decision is important, and if the patient is uncertain, a delay is warranted. Conversely, patients with the sudden whim to have cosmetic surgery should be considered poor candidates. An advertisement the patient saw in last week's Sunday sports section is unlikely to provoke serious thought about the consequences of his or her decision.

Some patients have unreasonable motives for having cosmetic surgery performed: "My husband will stop cheating on me if only I get this fixed." No cosmetic surgical procedure can be the solution to psychosocial or economic problems. It is unlikely that the surgeon will be able to meet such expectations.

Males requesting aesthetic surgery have traditionally been viewed suspiciously. Malignantly dissatisfied patients who tend to have aberrant reactions to cosmetic surgery are more likely to be men. Also, male cosmetic surgery patients appear to be more emotionally unstable than female patients. Changing sociocultural trends have lessened these concerns about the male psyche since it is currently more acceptable for men to want to alter their physical appearance. Hair replacement surgery is among the most commonly performed procedures today.

If, after the preoperative assessment, the surgeon is concerned about the presence of psycho-pathology in a patient, it is worthwhile to seek psychiatric consultation. A thorough preoperative evaluation by a psychiatrist is better patient care, and high-risk patients can be screened. The psychiatrist is better qualified to clarify the patient's mental health, motivations, expectations, personality make-up, anxiety level, ego strength, and ability to understand the risks and implications of surgery. After the preoperative assessment, the surgeon and/or the psychiatrist may feel that the patient is not an ideal candidate for cosmetic surgery. In such cases, the following courses of action may be taken, each requiring the participation of the surgeon and psychiatrist:

1. A decision against surgery based on the patient's impaired psychological functioning along with a recommendation that the patient seek further psychiatric treatment. This course is most commonly chosen when the patient is externally motivated, unable to understand the procedure, or when the body image goal is surgically unfeasible and linked with other psychopathology.
2. Deferring surgery for several months and, in the meantime, offering psychotherapy to clarify expectations and motivations for surgery.
3. Deciding not to perform surgery unless the patient agrees to psychiatric follow-up postoperatively.
4. Deciding not to perform surgery on the basis of the surgeon's belief that the operation would be of no benefit (e.g., the "minimal defect" patient).
5. Recommending preoperative supportive treatment.
6. Referral to another surgeon. This is done when the patient is a good candidate but has a poor personality fit with the first surgeon. The patient's willingness to accept consultation has been positively correlated with the ability to accept surgical results.

THE DAY OF SURGERY

Although the psychological evaluation should be complete by the time surgery is performed, a relationship between the surgeon and patient continues. The patient has placed his or her confidence in the surgeon and expects technical perfection. Patients have few ways of evaluating surgical expertise and rely heavily on how the surgeon appears or whether they like the surgeon. On the day of surgery, the surgeon should appear happy, efficient, and organized. The surgeon should greet the patient and establish that the surgery is a happy event. The surgeon's perspective about the operative outcome can strongly influence the patient's reactions to the operative results. Patient anxiety is normal and should be expected. Most patients want to know that everything is going as it should on a routine basis. As most dermatologic surgery is performed with local anesthesia, the patient is acutely aware of all that is said during the procedure. It is important that intraoperative problems be dealt with quietly and efficiently. Patients are unsettled by complications and would rather be assured that everything is proceeding routinely (never say "oops" during the procedure).

FOLLOW-UP

Follow-up care is just as important as the preoperative consultation. Wound care is dealt with elsewhere in this book, but in addition to medical treatment, the patient must also be given psychological support. If there is a problem and the patient is dissatisfied, listen to the patient's complaint and do not try to argue. Although the patient may be disappointed, he or she still wants your help through the follow-up care. Most dissatisfied patients are not litigious and simply want the doctor to stand by and be attentive to their feelings of disappointment. Recent research has shown that the majority of patients are in the physician's corner and not "out to get them." If the patient becomes troublesome, resist the temptation not to schedule follow-up appointments. It would be more prudent to schedule more frequent visits and give the patient more time. If the surgeon is dissatisfied with the results, his or her feelings should be dealt with away from the patient. Once the surgeon is relaxed, he or she can then better deal with the patient's problem. Never completely dismiss a post-cosmetic surgery patient. Always leave the door open for later consultation and re-evaluation.

The three main causes of patient dissatisfaction with the outcome of cosmetic surgery are listed in Table 5. Physical complications must be discussed in a straightforward manner with the patient. The surgeon should not deny the existence of a complication, as this implies guilt and projects blame to the patient. The surgeon must re-establish the patient's confidence so the patient will be receptive to a secondary, corrective procedure.

Postoperatively, it is difficult to deal with the patient who is dissatisfied as a result of unrealistic expectations. It is easier to screen such patients during the preoperative assessment. After carefully listening to the patient's complaints, the surgeon should simply state what he or she is capable of doing without dwelling on the patient's unreasonable arguments.

Table 5 Reasons for Patient Dissatisfaction with Surgery

Physical complication or disappointment in anatomic change
Unrealistic psychological expectations
Lack of rapport between the physician and the patient

Because lack of rapport between the patient and physician has been documented as the major cause of medical malpractice suits, it is critical that the surgeon establish a good relationship with the patient. This can be done by listening to the patient and responding to complaints and concerns in an understanding rather than defensive manner.

The occasional patient may become malignantly dissatisfied with cosmetic surgery. Such patients tend to be male and may react psychopathologically to surgery with suicide attempts, delusional fixation upon the "damaged" organ, pursuit of further operations, or paranoid attitudes toward successive physicians. The occasional murder of physicians by such patients should provide ample incentive for surgeons performing cosmetic procedures to be adept at recognizing this potentially dangerous personality trait.

Cosmetic surgery may result in a significant change in body image, which requires psychological readjustment and adaptation to a new appearance. Therefore, most patients experience a transient, brief psychiatric disturbance in the immediate postoperative period, which may be manifested by irritability, emotional liability, and interpersonal conflict. Patients who are forewarned about these kinds of emotional fluctuations are more likely to have an easier time adjusting to them if they occur. These preoperative presence of psychosis or neurosis may intensify emotional disturbances during the postoperative period. Alternatively, hidden psychiatric disease may be unmasked following an operation.

Postoperative depression is a common phenomenon. In one study, varying degrees of depression occurred at a rate of 57%. In that study, 19% of patients required hospitalization for psychiatric observation. Transient postoperative depression usually occurs at rates of 12% to 16% 5 to 14 days (rarely longer) after surgery. Surgeons should be aware that when a patient is depressed preoperatively, the depression will likely intensify postoperatively. Some dermatologic surgical procedures such as dermabrasion and deep chemical peel result in erythema that persists for two to three months. Although many patients understand this preoperatively, it is reasonable to expect them to feel disappointed at some point that the wound healing is not more expeditious.

Patient satisfaction with cosmetic surgery sometimes fails to correlate with the technical quality of the surgery performed. This paradox is perplexing. The use of good preoperative and postoperative photos is valuable as documentation of what has been achieved, good or bad. Generally, when a patient is well informed and the procedure is performed satisfactorily, the surgeon and patient are happy with the results. Predictably, when problems arise, the patient may be disappointed, but when treated appropriately he or she may still be pleased with the outcome. It is surprising that surgery performed poorly with substandard results may be acceptable to some patients. The problem occurs when patients are never pleased despite flawless technique and excellent results. It is therefore imperative that some assessment of patients' expectations and psyche be made during the preoperative consultation to determine whether or not the surgeon is capable of improving the perceived problem. Judging patients' psyches is an inexact science at best. This problem is more profound for the cosmetic surgery patient than the oncologic patient. However, understanding patients' expectations helps surgeons to prevent dissatisfaction postoperatively.

BIBLIOGRAPHY

Adams GR. The effects of physical attractiveness on socialization process. In: Lucker GW, Ribbens KA, McNamara JA

Jr., eds. Psychological Aspects of Facial Form. Ann Arbor, MI: Center for Human Growth and Development, 1981.

Arndt EM, Travis F, Lefebvre A, et al. Beauty and the eye of the beholder: social consequences and personal adjustments for facial patients. Br J Plast Surg 1984; 37:313–318.

Baker JT. Patient selection and psychological evaluation. In: Webster R, ed. Clinics in Plastic Surgery: The Aging Face. Philadelphia; Saunders, 1978, 3–15.

Belfer ML, Mulliken JB, Cochran TC. Cosmetic surgery as an antecedent of life change. Am J Psychiatry 1979; 136:199–201.

Berscheid E, Gangestad S. The social psychological implications of facial physical attractiveness. clin Plast Surg 1982; 9(3):289–296.

Cassileth BR, Zupkis RV, Sutton-Smith K, et al. Information and participation preferences among cancer patients. Ann Intern Med 1980; 92:832–836.

Cassileth BR, Lusk EJ, Tenaglia AN. A psychological comparison of patients with malignant melanoma and other dermatologic disorders. J Am Acad Dermatol 1982; 7:742–746.

Cone JCP, Hueson JT. Psychological aspects of hand surgery. Med J Aust 1974; 1:104–108.

Connolly FH, Gipson M. Dysmorphophobia-a long-term study. Br J Psych 1978; 132:568–570.

Deaton AV, Langman MI. The contribution of psychologists to the treatment of plastic surgery patients. Prof Psychol: Res Pract 1986; 17(3):179–184.

Edgerton MT, Jacobson WE, Meyer E. Surgical-psychiatric sutdy of patients seeking plastic (cosmetic) surgery: ninety-eight consecutive patients with minimal deformity. Br J Plast Surg 1961; 13:136–145.

Edgerton MT, Knorr NJ. Motivational patterns of patients seeking cosmetic (aesthetic) surgery. Plast Reconstr Surg 1971; 48:551–557.

Gifford S. Cosmetic surgery and personality change: a review and some clinical observations. In:Goldwyn RM, ed. The Unfavourable Result in Plastic Surgery. Boston:Little, Brown and Company, 1972:11–35.

Goin JM, Goin MK. Changing the Body. In: Psychological Aspects of Plastic Surgery. Baltimore: Williams and Wilkins, 1981.

Goin MK, Burgoyne RK, Goin JM. Face-lift operations: The patient's secret motivations and reactions to informed consent. Plast Reconstr Surg 1976; 58:273–279.

Goin MK, Burgoyne RW, Goin JM, Staples FR. A prospective psychological study of 50 female facelift patients. Plast Reconstr Surg 1980; 65:436–442.

Goldwyn RM. The consultant and the unfavorable result. In: Goldwyn RM, ed. The Unfavorable Result in Plastic Surgery. Boston: Little Brown and Company, 1972:1–4.

Hay GG, Heather BB. Changes in psychometric test results following cosmetic nasal operations. Br J Psychiatr 1973; 122:89–90.

Hay GG. Psychiatric aspects of cosmetic nasal operations. Br J Psychiat 1970; 116:85–97.

Hazards of cosmetic surgery. Editorial. Br Med J 1967; 1:381.

Hill G, Silver AG. Psychodynamic and esthetic motivations for plastic surgery. Psychosom Med 1950; 12:345–355.

Hueston J, Dennerstein L, Gotts G. Psychological aspects of cosmetic surgery. J Psych ObGyn 1985; 4:335–346.

Jacobson WE, Edgerton MT, Meyer E, et al. Psychiatric evaluation of male patients seeking cosmetic surgery. Plast Reconstr Surg 1960;26:356–372.

Knorr NJ, Edgerton MT, Hoopes JE. The "insatiable" cosmetic surgery patient. Plast Reconstr Surg 1967; 40:285–289.

Marcus P. Psychological aspects of cosmetic rhinoplasty. Br J Plast Surg 1984; 37:313–318.

Merloo JAM. The fate of one's face with some remarks on the implications of plastic surgery. Psychiatr Q 1956; 30:31–43.

Mohl PC. Psychiatric consultation in plastic surgery: The psychiatrist's perspective. Psychosomatics 1984; 25(6):471–476.

Pruzinsky T, Persing JR. Psychological perspectives on aesthetic applications of reconstructive surgery techniques. In: Ousterhout DK, ed. Aesthetic Applications of Craniofacial Techniques. Boston: Little, Brown and Company, 1991:43–56.

Pruzinsky T. Psychological factors in cosmetic plastic surgery: recent developments in patient care. Plast Surg Nurs 1993; 13(2):64–72.

Reich J. Aesthetic plastic surgery development and place in medical practice. Med J Aust 1972; 1:1152–1156.

Reich J. The surgery of appearance: psychological and related aspects. Med J Aust 1969; 2:5–13.

Rosenthal GK. Preventing malpractice claims. Washington University Magazine 1977; 47:7–13.

Schneitzer I, Hirschfeld JJ. Post-rhytidectomy psychosis: a rare complication. Plast Reconstr Surg 1984; 74:419–422.

Schneitzer I. The psychiatric assessment of the patient requesting facial surgery. Aust NZ J Psychiatry 1989; 23:249–254.

Shulman BH. Psychiatric assessment of the candidate for cosmetic surgery. Otolaryngol Clin North Am 1980; 12(2):383–389.

Sihm F, Jagd M, Pers M. Psychological assessment before and after augmentation mammoplasty. Scand J Plast Reconstr Surg 1978; 12:295–298.

Wright MR, Wright WK. A psychological study of patients undergoing cosmetic surgery. Arch Otolaryngol 1975; 101:145–151.

Wright MR. How to recognize and control the problem patient. J Dermatol Surg Oncol 1984; 10(5):389–395.

Wright MR. Management of patient dissatisfaction with results of cosmetic procedures. Arch Otolaryngol 1980; 106:446–471.

Young JK. Lay-professional conflict in a Canadian community health center. Med Care 1975; 13:897–904.

6

Informed Consent

Abel Torres
Loma Linda University School of Medicine, Loma Linda, California, U.S.A.

Richard F. Wagner, Jr.
University of Texas Medical Branch, Galveston, Texas, U.S.A.

Steven Proper
University of Florida School of Medicine, Tampa, Florida, U.S.A.

INTRODUCTION

Physicians practicing medicine in the United States today are not usually free to render treatment until the patient's consent is obtained. Simple consent, i.e., only obtaining the patient's agreement to contemplated treatment without discussion of risks, benefits, or alternatives is no longer adequate to shield a healthcare practitioner from liability or medical malpractice. In general, in addition to a patient giving consent for a contemplated procedure, consent must also be "informed." This informed consent, which is an ever evolving legal doctrine, that was formulated and realized over the later half of the 20th century includes not only the type of procedure that is planned for the patient but also enumerates the risks and alternatives associated with the treatment. This issue has been formulated into a legal concept called the Doctrine of Informed Consent. The Doctrine is predicated on an individual's right to determine what happens to his or her body.

Full informed consent consists of three material elements: (i) informed exercise of choice after receiving the diagnosis or nature of the specific condition requiring treatment as well as the purpose and distinct nature of the treatment; (ii) opportunity to knowledgeably evaluate the available options or alternative treatments, the probability of success of the proposed procedure and the option of refusing all treatment; and (iii) understand the attendant relative risks and benefits. The information must be sufficient to make the agreement meaningful. The right to agree (consent) to treatment is based on the right to self-determination (autonomy), the law of negligence, and the law of battery.

The American Hospital Association published "A patient's Bill of Rights," which clearly summarizes the information that a patient has a right to expect before undergoing medical treatment or a surgical procedure: "The patient has the right to receive from his physician, information necessary to give informed consent prior to the start of any procedure and/or treatment. Except in emergencies, such information for informed consent should include but not necessarily be limited to the specific procedure and/or treatment, the medically significant risks involved, and the probable duration of incapacitation. Where medically significant alternatives for care or treatment exist, or when the patient requests information concerning medical alternatives, the patient has the right to such information. The patient also has the right to know the name of the person responsible for the procedures and/or treatment."

The detailed discussion below will focus on the application of the informed consent concept as related to medical dermatology and dermatological and cosmetic surgical practice with detailed description of the consent topic, including its relationship to the tort of battery and professional negligence (medical malpractice).

SIMPLE CONSENT

The right to consent is best exemplified by the 1914 case of *Schoendorff versus Society of New York Hospital*. In that case, Justice Cardozo declared that "every human being of adult years and sound mind has a right to determine what shall be done with his own body: and a surgeon who performs an operation without his patient's consent commits an assault, for which he is liable in damages". This "unauthorized touching" (surgery or procedure) gives rise to a legal action for "battery" because the latter is defined as the use of force upon or intentional touching of another person without the person's consent. Exemplifying this concept is the case of *Mohr versus Williams* where, a physician was found liable for operating on a left ear when permission was given for surgery on the right ear only.

A battery may also occur when a physician exceeds the scope of the patient's consent such as when the wrong procedure is performed or a procedure is performed by a different physician without giving prior notice to the patient. In the legal case of *Perna versus Pirozzi*, defendant urologists were part of a self-described team that included decisions to designate a specific member of the group to perform surgery but failed to inform the patient of this policy. Thus, when the patient signed a consent designating one physician as surgeon but having the operation performed by two other physicians, the court found that this "ghost surgery" was a violation of consent. Thus, physicians should be cautious in a setting where they allow other physicians, e.g., their residents or fellows, to perform procedures or treatments on their patients without adequately informing the patient.

If a battery is alleged by a patient, he or she can seek ordinary and or punitive damages whether or not the procedure was properly performed. Such damages, if awarded by a court may not be covered by malpractice insurance. The absolute nature of a battery together with its narrow remedies and defenses could result in a doctor being found liable for significant damages even if the medical care was faultless. Recognizing that doctors ordinarily lack the "intent" to harm as defined by the tort of battery, and that physicians have a professional duty to treat a patient with due care, and the failure to give adequate informed consent is a breach of that duty, it rationally follows that the courts have come to see an action in negligence as a better fit than an action in battery, particularly when it comes to the nuances of the physician–patient relationship.

The physician in control of the recommended procedure/treatment has the duty of obtaining informed consent (see below). For example, a consulting physician who only advises the referring physician is not under an affirmative duty to obtain informed consent from the patient consulted. On the other hand, if the referring physician does not participate in controlling the treatment recommended and prescribed by the consulting physician specialist, then the consulting physician is obligated to secure informed consent. Furthermore, a hospital has no independent obligation to procure a patient's informed consent in lieu of the treating physician.

Consent can be implied or express. Implied consent occurs when the conduct of the patient indicates awareness of the planned treatment by the patient's willingness to submit to a particular treatment or by the patient's failure to object to the recommended procedure. Implied consent has also been found when the patient signs a general authorization to act or consent permitting additional related unnamed procedures as extending an incision or surgical procedure. For example, while performing an appendectomy, a physician may have the privilege of treating an incidental finding of a ruptured ovarian cyst. In Florida, implied consent may be valid if it was impracticable to have obtained actual consent. Unless consent is implied by statute, the burden will generally rest on the physician to prove that the patient's conduct implied consent. To buttress the implied consent, it would benefit the physician to show that there was no feasible way to obtain substituted consent by an appropriate party, such as a parent, in the case of a minor, before performing an elective procedure. Thus, a physician should realize that relying on implied consent is very risky and could result in unexpected professional liability and malpractice based on the Doctrine of Informed Consent. When a particular medical technique is performed, it is held that a physician may be authorized to do what is reasonably necessary and appropriate to achieve the expected result.

Express consent requires oral or written authorization by the patient. *Oral consent* is valid if the necessary information is related to the patient and the patient is given an opportunity to ask questions coupled with adequate answers by the practitioner. Oral consent poses the problem that the patient could later deny that he or she was properly informed and that the witnesses to the incident may no longer be available if subsequently needed to attest to the consent.

Written consent provides physical evidence of consent but, as will be discussed below, may not necessarily establish "informed consent." If a physician obtains consent for treatment of a condition rather than a specific procedure, this may help avoid a scope of consent issue. Nevertheless, if the condition is treated in multiple steps that cannot be

terminated once begun, the patient must be informed of all the steps and risks associated therein. Often a vague and broad general consent form or a form not written in ordinary lay language may not represent adequate informed consent exposing the physician to liability.

The scope of the consent does not require that the patient be informed of every possible side effect or of comparative risk statistics. The physician is not expected to give a minicourse on medicine, pharmacology, or surgery in obtaining informed consent (see below).

Specifically, the patient should receive information concerning the character and seriousness of the ailment, general facts, and risks of the anticipated procedure, the chances of success, the hazards of refusing or not undergoing the procedure, the alternative treatments, and the experimental nature of the proposed treatment, if applicable. Exposing all the risks to the patient prior to treatment is not practical or sensible, but the "material" risks must be communicated to effectuate adequate informed consent, including the risk of contracting HIV from a HIV-positive surgeon. Even if no transmission of the disease occurs, a patient has a cause of action in negligence because of infliction of emotional distress.

Although the physician does not have an affirmative duty to disclose his or her qualifications (or lack thereof), a patient may claim that he or she would not have undertaken the procedure if he or she knew of the lack of experience or qualification of the operating surgeon (see below).

VALIDITY OF CONSENT
Fraud, Duress, Mistake, Competency, Nondisclosure of Conflicts of Interest

When a consent is obtained by fraud, duress, mistaken belief of which the defendant was aware, or where the patient is a minor, incompetent, or in an incoherent state, the consent is invalid. Consent must be obtained from a competent adult or, in the case of minors or incompetent adults, from authorized decision makers. However, this may be circumvented by proving an emergency existed (see below) and that there was no practicable way to procure consent from either the patient or the guardian. Additionally, where a minor is legally emancipated, where the minor is married with/without children, or enlisted in the military, valid consent may be obtained. For example, some states have enacted special legislation rendering a minor's consent valid for examination and treatment of venereal disease, treatment of the minor's children, pregnancy care, abortion, drug and alcoholic dependency treatment, donations of blood, rape kit examination, and birth control pill prescriptions. It is incumbent upon practicing physicians to be familiar with the laws of their state, which define competent adult and authorized decision makers for minors or incompetent adults. If there is a question of incompetency, the judicious physician should seek appropriate authorized consent.

DISCLOSURE OF ALTERNATIVE TREATMENTS

A patient can allege that failure by a physician to disclose alternative treatment options is a defect that invalidated his or her consent to treatment and deprived the patient of the right to select another treatment. Although some states uphold a subjective or good faith standard of proof as to the patient's informed consent validity, most courts require an objective standard or the reasonable prudent person standard to determine the ruling as to those complaints by patients that claim: "I would have never have agreed to the procedure had I'd known of all the risks and the availability of less risky alternatives" (see below).

In general, courts recognize no liability where there is more than one recognized and acceptable method of diagnosis or therapy, and the physician was not considered to have been negligent if, while exercising best judgment, he or she selected a method that later turned out to have been unsuccessful or mistaken. However, the other question that can still be raised is whether a physician is expected to inform the patient of procedures (alternatives) that are not recommended. Generally, appellate courts have rejected a general duty of disclosure concerning a treatment or procedure that a physician does not recommend because the landmark court case of *Cobbs versus Grant* (Cal. 1972) stated that informed disclosure and consent laws "do not require a minicourse in medical science" (see above). This type of reasoning has been recently validated in a California appeals court case from *Purris versus Sands*, which held that the doctor was not obligated to inform the patient of a treatment he did not recommend. Thus, failure by the physician to discuss all possible medical treatment options may not constitute a lack of informed consent. However, as articulated in the Connecticut Supreme Court case of *Logan versus Greenwich Hospital Association*, a patient might be found to reasonably rely upon a specialist to provide such information. This is somewhat supported by the California *Parris versus Sands* court case cited above, which implied that a case involving surgery, cancer diagnosis, cancer treatment, or other life-threatening procedures might bring a different conclusion to the scope of discussion of alternative treatments. With this in mind, specialists, such as dermatologic or Mohs micrographic surgeons, should be careful when choosing not to discuss alternative treatments they do not recommend, e.g., radiation therapy, cryosurgery, or topical chemotherapy. In addition, if the physician is unaware of possible medical treatment options because he or she has not kept reasonably abreast of medical advances, then there may arise a standard of care issue exposing the physician to liability.

INFORMED REFUSAL

The premise underlying the informed consent/informed refusal doctrine in many states is that patients should receive enough information about their condition to permit them to choose among potential interventions, including the option of no further treatment. It calls for a balancing of the doctor's perception of what is an appropriate amount of information versus the patient's need for enough information to make an informed decision. In the extreme, a competent patient's autonomy permits him or her to refuse treatment for a potentially deadly but curable disease, even if the cure is minimally intrusive and well accepted by the medical community.

Informed consent constitutes an affirmative decision by a competent adult, which permits the physician to treat the patient in an agreed manner. Selecting one treatment after informed consent results in the "refusal" of another intervention. Thus, the concept of informed refusal is logically linked to that of informed consent.

In contrast, an informed refusal situation is usually encountered when a competent adult decides to forego (refuse) a recommended test or treatment. Conflict around informed consent and informed refusal can arise when well-meaning physician interventions deprive a patient of his or her autonomy, especially when damage (injury, harm) ensues.

In the context of posttreatment injury, the patient is likely to learn about previously undisclosed alternative treatment options or risks. Under such circumstances, the patient may conclude that had these relevant facts been explained, he or she would have selected a different treatment and the complication might have been avoided (see above).

To educate patients and protect patient autonomy in medical decision-making, some states require physicians to distribute a written list of treatment options to patients who have or are suspected of having certain diseases.

The best way for physicians to avoid problems with informed consent and informed refusal issues is to fully communicate to patients the diagnosis or potential diagnosis, its natural course if untreated, the recommended treatment along with its potential benefits and risks, and the alternative treatments including their potential benefits and risks. Specialists often are held to a special responsibility for detailing available treatment options before undertaking treatment. Physicians' failure to obtain informed consent or informed refusal could potentially result in legal allegations of an intentional tort (assault, battery), breach of contract (particularly, if the physician proposes any guarantees), or negligence.

Negligence appears to be the most frequently employed allegation in instances where informed consent or informed refusal was not obtained, or was defective.

Two key legal components required to prove that a physician was negligent in rendering medical care are: first, to establish that the physician owed a particular duty to the patient, and second, to show that the physician breached that duty through an act of commission or an omission. When a physician is accused of failing to obtain informed consent or informed refusal, it amounts to a claim that the physician had a duty to disclose more information to the patient but failed to do so. The patient must then prove that the doctor withheld pertinent medical information concerning the risks and alternatives of the treatment or procedure, or potential results if the treatment or procedure was not performed.

The legal literature is full of reports where rare but serious potential complications were not disclosed to patients during the informed consent process. Although physicians are not held to the standard of disclosing every possible complication of a treatment, dermatology practitioners should remember that the risk of life-threatening or potentially disabling or disfiguring outcomes are well recognized, and as such, they should be disclosed to, and understood by, the patient prior to treatment. Likewise, treatments involving medicines as well as medical and surgical procedures are subject to informed consent requirements. Yet, the courts have ruled that when it comes to distinctly uncommon side effects, physicians are not required under accepted medical practice to warn patients.

Exceptions to informed consent and informed refusal doctrine exist. Medical and surgical emergencies, especially when the patient is unconscious or incompetent to make medical decisions and no authorized person with decisional capacity is available, tend to diminish or negate the need to meet the simple consent or informed consent requirements (see above). However, such "emergency" situations are rare in dermatology practice. Medical information that is generally known by the lay public is also often exempted from informed consent requirements. However, physician reliance on this exception will be retroactively scrutinized in the event of a lawsuit. Thus, it is usually better for the physician to assume the outlook of some courts and presume that the patient has no knowledge about his or her condition or what risks the treatment will entail. This cautious approach places responsibility on the physician to explain more information to the patient so that the patient can make an informed choice about his or her healthcare.

Many in the field of healthcare risk management prefer some form of written informed consent or informed refusal that is signed by the patient before treatment is given or withheld. A writing of this nature in the medical record documents that informed consent or informed refusal was obtained from the patient. Also signing a standardized informed consent or informed refusal form may diminish a patient's perception of his or her chance for successful litigation. In some states, such as California, written documentation of informed consent is required for procedures, such as blood transfusions, sterilizations, and breast biopsies. However, because informed consent and informed refusal is really a process, defects in the process can serve to invalidate signed documents. A defect in the process that can serve to invalidate informed consent centers on the issue of who is responsible for obtaining informed consent. Although nurses and other nonphysicians can help inform the patient, the courts have generally placed the responsibility for obtaining informed consent on the treating physician.

Some institutions prefer to use a note in the patient's medical record, by the physician, detailing the informed consent or refusal in place of having the patient sign a document. Others advocate that the patient sign or initial that note to acknowledge the informed consent process. Still, others advocate the note and a signed consent document. In any case, all of these approaches have the merit of asking the physician to actively participate and document his or her role in the informed consent process.

Various approaches to the doctor–patient relationship may affect the informed consent and informed refusal processes. In an effort to determine the ideal relationship between patients and physicians, Emanuel and Emanuel (1992) delineated four theoretical models of interaction between the physician and patient: (i) paternalism, (ii) informative, (iii) interpretive, and (iv) deliberative.

The *paternalistic* model is problematic for both informed consent and informed refusal processes because paternalism or beneficence is based upon the physician's perceptions about what is best for the patient. Early on, as the doctrine of informed consent evolved, courts held that a doctor's disclosure was "limited to those disclosures which a reasonable medical practitioner would make under the same or similar circumstances". This is the "professional standard" which is followed by very few jurisdictions today as the doctrine has evolved into the "materiality of risk" or "prudent patient" standard.

The currently dominant *informative* model views the physician as a competent technician who provides essential information to the patient and then implements the patient's decision. This standard requires a physician to disclose material information to the patient even if the patient does not ask questions. Material information is defined as when a reasonable patient, would be likely to attach significance to the risk in deciding whether to submit to or forego a proposed therapy in what the physician knows or should know to be the patient's position. In the *interpretive* model, the physician serves as a counselor to the patient, helping to clarify values and desires and then aiding the patient in the selection of treatment that is consistent with his or her outlook. Some authors conclude that the *deliberative*

model, where the physician acts as a friend or teacher is preferable because conversation between the patient and physician may help the patient to select the best treatment. Adoption of the deliberative model could potentially improve the informed consent process but care must be taken by the physician to avoid imposing an undesired intervention upon the patient.

The dermatological surgeon routinely assesses his patient's personality, knowledge, intelligence, and needs. The dermatologist's familiarity with the patient's expectations as well as the patient's functional and aesthetic needs are helpful in determining which interactive model would best be suited for his or her patient. Often, the patient expects the physician to make a good faith decision based on the doctor's experience. Thus, the paternalistic model or a hybrid of this and other models is commonly invoked and is especially appropriate in those jurisdictions where the professional standard is held.

Therefore, identifying potential conflicts of interest between a physician and patient may permit greater appreciation of why problems with informed consent may arise. Trust is required for a successful physician–patient relationship, and undisclosed conflicts of interest tend to undermine trust. Identifying and disclosing any potential conflicts of interest with the patient during the informed consent process, the physician is likely to gain the patient's respect and trust appropriately and, at the same time, improve the chances that a valid informed consent will be obtained.

TRANSLATION AND INFORMED CONSENT

The United States continues to become more multicultural. Encountering patients who do not speak or understand English is increasingly common. When it is necessary to employ a translator in order to communicate with a patient, it is usually a better medical practice to use a bilingual employee or translation service rather than to use a patient's friend, employee, or family member.

In a recent lawsuit, a plastic surgeon amputated the toe of a non–English-speaking patient for the purpose of replacing a thumb lost to traumatic amputation. The patient did not speak English, so the patient's friend translated and the surgeon was satisfied that he had obtained adequate consent. However, the patient later claimed that he had agreed to skin grafting and not to amputation of his toe. A jury awarded this patient $413,000 in damages in addition to interest. In another case, a plaintiff whose native language was French and possessed a sixth grade education signed a consent form just after being awakened following sedation, the court held that proper informed consent was not obtained.

MISREPRESENTATION OF CREDENTIALS

At least one jurisdiction has allowed a claim of lack of informed consent when a physician misrepresents his credentials or experience. In the case of *Jóhnson versus Kokemoor* in Wisconsin, the court found that a reasonable person would have considered information regarding a doctor's relative lack of experience in performing surgery to be material in making an intelligent and informed decision. However, the courts have not allowed actions for "fraud" on issues such as whether the physician failed to disclose whether he had board certification as a plastic surgeon versus another board certification, or concealment of malpractice. Similarly, other courts have not held that "a doctor has a duty to detail his background and experience as part of the required informed consent," and courts have generally held that claims of lack of informed consent based on failure to disclose professional background information are without merit. Yet in *Johnson versus Kokemoor* (see above) the situation was different in that the physician had misrepresented his experience in response to a direct question and the courts have held that in certain circumstances misrepresentation concerning the quality or extent of a physician's professional experience can be "material." However, at least one court has ruled that misrepresented or exaggerated physician experience would have to undergo a two-step proximate cause analysis looking at: (i) whether the more limited experience or credentials could have substantially increased the plaintiff's risk, and (ii) whether that substantially increased risk would cause a reasonably prudent person not to consent to undergo the procedure. Similarly, the courts have found liability where the doctor misrepresents information to induce the patient to proceed with unnecessary surgery for personal gain.

ESTABLISHING MEDICAL NEGLIGENCE

To establish medical negligence based on a theory of lack of informed consent, the plaintiff must show, that the physician breached his or her duty to the patient and "(i) failed to comply with the reasonably prudent patient standard for disclosure; (ii) the undisclosed risk was material and reasonably foreseeable, occurred, and harmed the plaintiff; (iii) a reasonable person under the circumstances would not have consented and submitted to the operation or surgical procedure had he or she been so informed; and (iv) the operation or surgical procedure was a proximate cause of the plaintiffs' injuries."

Under the prudent patient standard, the sufficiency of disclosure requires that the disclosure be viewed through the eyes of the patient and not the doctor. Thus, expert testimony is not usually required to establish a medical community's standard for disclosure. However, many states' apply the objective professional standard of disclosure whereby the patient must produce an expert to show what procedures, alternatives, and risks a reasonable practitioner under similar circumstances would disclose to the patient. The plaintiff must prove the lack of informed consent "by competent expert testimony" demonstrating the defendant physician failed to give adequate informed consent about the medical treatment given and its "recognized and defined risks of adverse consequences."

The last part of this analysis emphasizes that there must be a causal connection between the injury sustained and the undisclosed risk. This is a two-pronged test of proximate causation where the plaintiff must prove that the undisclosed risk, (i) actually materialized, and (ii) it was medically caused by the treatment. However, the plaintiff does not have to prove that the physician deviated from the standard of care in performing the treatment but rather that the damages derive from the harm to the patient caused by the inadequate disclosure and in some states, causation is determined by what a prudent person in the patient's position would have decided if adequately informed of all significant risks.

BIBLIOGRAPHY

Arato vs. Avedon. 5 Cal. 4th 1172. 23 Cal Rptr 2d 131, 858 P.2d 598 (1993).

Auler vs. Van Natta, 686 N.E.2d 172, 175–176 (Ind. App. 1997).

Boumil MM, Elias CE, Moes DB. Medical Liability in a Nutshell. In: St. Paul: West Thomson Business Publications, 2003:96.

Canterbury vs. Spence, 464 F. 2d 772 (D.C. Cir.), cert. denied 409 U.S. 1064 (1972). Fourth Circuit: Canterbury vs. Spence, 464 F. 2d 722, 728, cert.

Cobbs vs. Grant 8 Cal.3d 229, 104 Cal Rptr 505, P.2d 1 (1972).

Cooper vs. United States. 903 F. Supp. 953, 956–957 (D. S.C. 1995).

Demers vs. Gerety, 85 N.M. 641, 515 P.2d 645 (Ct. App. 1973), rev'd on other grounds, 86 N.M. 141, 520 P.2d 869 (1974).

Ditto vs. McCurdy, 86 Hawaii 84, 947 P. 2d 952, 958–959 (1997) (cosmetic surgeon did not inform patient that he was not a plastic surgeon nor had hospital privileges).

Emanuel EJ, Emmanuel LL. Four Models of the physician-patient relationship. JAMA 1992; 267(10):2221–2226.

Faya vs. Almaraz. 329 Md. 435, 448.455–456 620 A. 2d 327, 333, 336–337 (1993).

Faya vs. Almaraz, 329 Md. 435, 620 A.2d 327 (Md. 1993) 87, 117.

Febus vs. Barot 260 N.J.Super.322, 616 A.2d 933 (1992) (quoting Calabrese vs. Trenton State College, 162 N.J. Super. 145, 156, 392, A.2d 600 (App. Div. 1978), aff'd 82 N.J. 321, 413 A.2d 315 (1980).

Feeley vs. Baer, 424 Mass. 875. 877, 679 N.E.2d 180, 182 n.3 (1997).

French vs. Fischer, 50 Teen.App. 587, 362 S.W.2d 414, 417 (1991), Wotten vs. Curry, 50 Tenn.App. 549, 362 S.W.2d 820, 822 (1961), McPeak vs. Vanderbilt University Hospital, 33 Tenn.App. 549, 362 S.W.2d 150 (1950).

Howard vs. University of Med. & Dentistry of New Jersey, 172 N.J. 537, 800 A.2d 73 (N.J.2002), 105 (lack of informed consent claim where defendant was not board certified and had performed type of surgery only a couple dozen times rather than the sixty he claimed); (quoting Perna vs. Pirozzi, 92 N.J. 460, 457 A.2d 431 (1983).

Id. Natanson vs. Kline, 186 Kan. 393, 350 P.2d 1093, 1106 modified on other grounds, 187 Kan. 186, 354 P. 2d 671–672 (1960).

Johnson vs. Kokemoor, 199 Wis.2d 615, 545 N.W.2d 495, 498 (Wis. 1996).

K.A.C. vs. Benson. 527 N.W.2d 553. 561 (Minn. 1995).

Keane vs. Sloan-Kettering Institute for Cancer Research, 96 A.D.2d 505, 464 N.Y.S. 2d 548 (1983).

Kennedy vs. Parrott, 243 N.C. 355, 90 S.E.2d 754 (1956).

Ketchup vs. Howard 543 S.E.2d 371 (Ga. App. 2000) (Georgia courts analysis of the informed consent doctrine in each state).

King JH Jr. The Law of Medical Malpractice in a Nutshell. St. Paul: West Publishing Co., 1977:139.

Largey vs. Rothman, 110 N.J. 211–212, 540 A.2d 504 (1988).

Lasley vs. Georgetown University, 842 F. Supp. 593 (D.D.C. 1994).

Logan vs. Greenwich Hospital Association, 191 Conn 282 (1983).

Lowney vs. Arciom 232 III App.3d 715, 173 Ill. Dec. 843, 597 N.E.2d 817, 819 (1992)

Marjorie Maguire Schultz. In: Informed Consent to Patient Choice: A New Protected Interest, Yale L.J. 1985; 95: 219, 225.

Martin by Scoptur vs. Richards. 531 N.W.2d 70. 77 (Wis. 1995).

McGuire vs. Rix, 118 Neb. 434, 225 N.W.120 (1929).

Mohr vs. Williams, 95 Minn. 261. 104 N.W.12, 14–15 (1905).

Mole vs. Jutton. 846 A.2d 1035 (Md. 2004).

Moss vs. Rishworth, 222 S.W.225 (Tex. Civ. App. 1920).

Natanson vs. Kline, 186 Kan. 393, 350 P.2d 1093, 1106 modified on other grounds, 187 Kan. 186, 354 P.2d 671–672 (1960).

Nogowski vs. Alemo-Hammad, 691 A.2d 950,957 (Pa Super 1997).

O'Neal vs. Hammer, 87 Hawaii 183,953 P.2d 561, 568 (1998).

Parris vs. Sands 93 Daily J DAR 16233.

Perna vs. Pirozzi, 92 N.J.446, 457 A. 2d 431 (N.J. 1983), 68.

Rodriguez vs. Pino. 634 So.2d 681, 687 (Fla. App. 1994).

Salgo vs. Leland Standford, Jr. University Board of Trustees, 317 P.2d 170, 181 (Cal. App. Ct. 1957).

Salgo vs. Leland Stanford Jr. Univ Bd of Trustees, 154 Cal.App.2d 560, 317 P.2d 170. 181 (Cal.App.1957).

Schoendorff vs. Society of New York Hospital case (211 N.Y. 125, 105 N.E. 92, 93 (N.Y. 1914).

Shandell RE, Smith P, Schulman FA. The Preparation and Trial of Medical Malpractice Cases. New York: Law J Press, 2005.

Shinn vs. St. James Mercy Hospital, 675 F. Supp 94 (W.D.N.Y.), aff'd 847 F.2d 836 (2d Cir. 1988).

Shkolnik vs. Hospital for Joint Diseases Orthopedic Institute 627 N.Y.S.2d 353. 355 (App. Div. 1st Dept. 1995).

Tonelli vs. Khanna, 238 N.J. Super. At 128, 569 A.2d 282 (App.-Div.) cert. denied, 121 N.J. 657, 583 A.2d 344 (1990).

Watkins vs. United States, 482 F. Supp 1006.

Wilkerson vs. Mid-America Cardiology, 908 S.W.Zd 691. 700 (Mo. App. 1995).

Wuerz vs. Huffaker, 42 S.W.3d 652 (Mo. App. 2001).

Zoski vs. Gaines, 271 Mich. 1, 260 N.W. 99 (Mich. 1935), 96.

7

Standard Precautions

Clifford S. Perlis
Fox Chase Cancer Center, Philadelphia, Pennsylvania, U.S.A.

Raymond G. Dufresne, Jr.
*Department of Dermatology, Brown Medical School, Brown University,
Providence, Rhode Island, U.S.A.*

INTRODUCTION

Isolation techniques, as codified in Standard Precautions, protect patients and health-care workers from blood- and body fluid-borne pathogen transmission. Standard Precautions should be adhered to in the care of every patient, because it is frequently impossible to recognize a patient's infectious status without serological testing. Careful use of sharps (including needles and scalpels), wearing personal protective equipment (i.e., gloves, masks, gowns, and eye protection as indicated), and frequent hand washing form the core of Standard Precautions. Dermatologists may take several steps to ensure compliance and create a safer work environment with Standard Precautions.

HISTORY

Standard Precautions represent the most recent step in the evolution of measures to isolate infectious diseases in patients. Early and current measures focus on hospitalized patients. The first published infection control isolation guidelines in the United States appeared in 1877. This hospital handbook suggested separating patients with infectious diseases in different facilities . This basic approach of isolating infectious patients from other susceptible patients evolved through the "cubicle system" of multibed wards in the early 1900s to the first published, detailed manual by the Centers for Disease Control (CDC) in 1970. This manual, *Isolation Techniques for Use in Hospitals*, provided detailed isolation precaution guidelines for general hospitals. Accumulating epidemiologic data led to several subsequent revisions of the CDC guidelines.

The emergence of human immunodeficiency virus (HIV) in the 1980s precipitated a fundamental shift in the aim of isolation precautions. Anecdotes of health-care providers contracting HIV through needle-stick injuries and blood exposure generated renewed interest in isolation procedures. Whereas previous measures emphasized limiting patient-to-patient transmission of disease, new revisions focused on protecting hospital personnel from infected patients. The CDC introduced a new approach to isolation practices in 1985 called Universal Precautions. The title "Universal" came from the realization that individuals infected with blood-borne pathogens are not always recognized as such. Consequently, all patients should be treated according to the prescribed Universal Precautions. These precautions described methods to limit the exposure to blood and body fluids through the use of gloves, gowns, masks, and eye protection, as well as steps to reduce injuries from sharps. The introduction of another isolation system, Body Substance Isolation, in 1987 eventually led to confusion, disagreement, and inconsistent application of isolation precautions.

Combining key features of both Body Substance Isolation and Universal Precautions, the current CDC recommendations are called "Standard Precautions". These precautions provide general directions for the care of all hospitalized patients as well as simplified guidelines for specific diseases and syndromes. Even though the Standard Precautions were designed for limiting disease transmission in hospitalized patients, they serve an important role in cutaneous surgery. Adherence to the guidelines decreases the risk of health-care personnel and patients contracting blood- or body fluid-borne pathogens from other patients.

PURPOSE

Dermatologic surgery is almost always carried out on an elective basis. Accordingly, patients have been evaluated prior to surgery and were found healthy enough to withstand the stresses of cutaneous surgery. Although most dermatologic surgery patients have been evaluated prior to surgery, many patients may not have overt signs of infection. However, several blood-borne infections lack overt clinical signs during early stages of disease. For these situations, Standard Precautions apply particularly well. The three major blood-borne pathogens transmissible through a sharps injury are Hepatitis B virus (HBV), Hepatitis C virus (HCV), and HIV. These viruses pose substantial threats because they are prevalent in the population, and infection may lead to serious disability and death. A male prison population sample revealed prevalences of HIV of 1.8%, HBV 20.2%, and HCV 23.1%. Even among other populations preselected to have a low risk of blood-borne pathogens, a significant risk persists. In an American Red Cross sample of first-time whole blood donors in 2002, the prevalence of antibodies toward HIV was 0.0120%, toward HBV 0.0703%, and toward HCV 0.2556%.

While much of the public discussion has focused on HIV transmission, the rates for occupational transmission from percutaneous exposure to viral pathogens is higher for HBV and HCV than it is for HIV. The rate of occupational transmission from a HBV-positive source to a nonimmunized recipient is 6% to 24%. Hepatitis B immunization substantially decreases transmission rates. Routine immunization

Table 1 Standard Precautions

A. Hand washing
   1. Wash hands after touching blood, body fluids, secretions, excretions, and contaminated items, whether or not gloves are worn.
   2. Wash hands immediately after gloves are removed, between patient contacts, and when otherwise indicated to avoid transfer of microorganisms to other patients or environments.
   3. It may be necessary to wash hands between tasks and procedures on the same patient to prevent cross-contamination of different body sites.
   4. Use a plain (nonantimicrobial) soap for routine hand washing.
   5. Use an antimicrobial agent or a waterless antiseptic agent for special circumstances (e.g., control of outbreaks or hyperendemic infections), as defined by the infection control program.

B. Gloves
   1. Wear gloves (clean, nonsterile gloves are adequate) when touching blood, body fluids, secretions, excretions, and contaminated items.
   2. Put on clean gloves just before touching mucous membranes and nonintact skin.
   3. Change gloves between tasks and procedures on the same patient after contact with material that may contain a high concentration of microorganisms.
   4. Remove gloves promptly after use, before touching noncontaminated items and environmental surfaces, and before going to another patient, and wash hands immediately to avoid transfer of microorganisms to other patients or environments.

C. Mask, eye protection, face shield
   1. Wear a mask and eye protection or a face shield to protect mucous membranes of the eyes, nose, and mouth during procedures and patient-care activities, which are likely to generate splashes or sprays of blood, body fluids, secretions, and excretions.

D. Gown
   1. Wear a gown (a clean, nonsterile gown is adequate) to protect skin and to prevent soiling of clothing during procedures and patient-care activities, which are likely to generate splashes or sprays of blood, body fluids, secretions, or excretions.
   2. Select a gown that is appropriate for the activity and amount of fluid likely to be encountered.
   3. Remove a soiled gown as promptly as possible, and wash hands to avoid transfer of microorganisms to other patients or environments.

E. Patient-care equipment
   1. Handle used patient-care equipment soiled with blood, body fluids, secretions, and excretions in a manner that prevents skin and mucous membrane exposures, contamination of clothing, and transfer, of microorganisms to other patients and environments.
   2. Ensure that reusable equipment is not used for the care of another patient until it has been cleaned and reprocessed appropriately.
   3. Ensure that single-use items are discarded properly.

F. Environmental control
   1. Ensure that the hospital has adequate procedures for the routine care, cleaning, and disinfection of environmental surfaces, beds, bed rails, bedside equipment, and other frequently touched surfaces, and ensure that these procedures are being followed.

G. Linen
   1. Handle, transport, and process used linen soiled with blood, body fluids, secretions, and excretions in a manner that prevents skin and mucous membrane exposures and contamination of clothing, and
      that avoids transfer of microorganisms to other patients and environments.

H. Occupational health and blood-borne pathogens
   1. Take care to prevent injuries when using needles, scalpels, and other sharp instruments or devices; when handling sharp instruments after procedures; when cleaning used instruments; and when disposing used needles.
   2. Never recap used needles, or otherwise manipulate them using both hands, or use any other technique that involves directing the point of a needle toward any part of the body; rather, use either a one-handed "scoop" technique or a mechanical device designed for holding the needle sheath.
   3. Do not remove used needles from disposable syringes by hand, and do not bend, break, or otherwise manipulate used needles by hand.
   4. Place used disposable syringes and needles, scalpel blades, and other sharp items in appropriate puncture-resistant containers, which are located as close as practical to the area in which the items were used, and place reusable syringes and needles in a puncture-resistant container for transport to the reprocessing area.
   5. Use mouthpieces, resuscitation bags, or other ventilation devices as an alternative to mouth-to-mouth resuscitation methods in areas where the need for resuscitation is predictable.

I. Patient placement
   1. Place a patient who contaminates the environment or who does not (or cannot be expected to) assist in maintaining appropriate hygiene or environmental control in a private room.
   2. If a private room is not available, consult with infection control professionals regarding patient placement or other alternatives.

Source: From Garner, Hierholzer, McCormick, et al. (1996).

of Taiwanese children reduced the prevalence of HBV infection by 93%. Furthermore, passive administration of hepatitis B surface antigen antibody following HBV exposure can also help prevent disease transmission. The rate of occupational transmission following exposure to HCV is 1% to 10%. By contrast, the rate following percutaneous exposure to HIV is 0.3% and 0.09% for mucus membrane exposure. These transmission rates vary somewhat according to the viral titer of the source and type of sharps injury. Sources with elevated viral titers confer higher risks of

transmission. Larger volumes of blood, such as those contained in hollow- versus solid-bore needles, also confer a higher risk of transmission. In addition to helping to protect health-care workers, Standard Precautions also protect patients from accidental infection by health-care workers.

STANDARD PRECAUTIONS

Standard precautions are intended to be applied in the care of all patients. Table 1 lists the precautions as described by the CDC.

Table 2 Recommendations for Adherence to Standard Precautions

1. Promote a culture of compliance by ensuring employee knowledge of Standard Precautions through regular educational and reinforcement activities.
2. Post a list of the key provisions of Standard Precautions in a highly visible location.
3. For each patient-care room, provide easily accessible sinks, hand washing soap, gloves (in several sizes), eye protection, masks, gowns, puncture-resistant sharps containers, and biohazardous waste containers.
4. Encourage the use of safety needles and other innovative safety devices as appropriate.
5. Clearly and comprehensively record breaches in compliance with Standard Precautions so problematic factors may be identified and remedied.

COMPLIANCE WITH STANDARD PRECAUTIONS

Standard precautions are recommended for the care of all patients, but health-care personnel's compliance with the recommendations is inconsistent. Several studies document poor compliance with Standard Precautions, and its predecessor Universal Precautions, among health-care workers. One survey of hospital-based health-care workers revealed especially low rates of compliance for wearing protective gowns (62.0%), eye shields (63.1%), and face masks (55.5%). Furthermore, self-reported rates of compliance exceed those recorded by direct observation. Direct observation of employees in a hospital emergency department revealed rates of compliance for the use of personal protective equipment to be 12% for protective gowns, 13% for eye shields, and 1% for face masks.

There are several factors associated with poor compliance with Standard Precautions. These factors may relate to the equipment itself, personality traits of the health-care employee, and work environment itself. One factor is the belief that adherence to Universal Precautions interferes with performing patient-care procedures. Another factor reportedly associated with poor compliance is a health-care worker's high score on a risk-taking personality profile.

Dermatologists can take several steps to improve compliance with Standard Precautions and safety in dermatologic surgery. One study found that the perception that senior management supports the practice of Standard Precautions is the most effective way to promote compliance with them. Table 2 provides several recommendations for promoting adherence to Standard Precautions.

SUMMARY

Standard Precautions represent the most recent evolution of isolation techniques designed to protect patients and health-care workers from the transmission of diseases through blood- and body fluid-borne pathogens. Because it cannot always be reliably known the infection status of a patient or health-care provider, Standard Precautions should be applied to the care of every patient. Key provisions include the use of gloves and other personal protective equipment (i.e., masks, gowns, and eye protection as appropriate), frequent hand washing, and measures to decrease the risk of injuries from sharps. While studies have documented poor compliance with Standard Precautions, dermatologists may take several steps to boost compliance and safety.

BIBLIOGRAPHY

Alter MJ. Epidemiology and prevention of hepatitis B. Semin Liver Disease 2003; 23(1):35–46.
Angtuaco TL, Oprescu FG, Lal SK, et al. Universal precautions guideline: self-reported compliance by gastroenterologists and gastrointestinal endoscopy nurses—a decade's lack of progress. Am J Gastroenterol 2003; 98:2420–2423.
Barraf J, Talan D. Compliance with universal precautions in a university hospital emergency department. Ann Emerg Med 1989; 18:654–657.
Cardo DM, Culver DH, Ciesielski CA, et al. A case-control study of HIV seroconversion in health care workers after percutaneous exposure. N Engl J Med 1997; 337:1485–1490.
Centers for Disease Control. Recommendations for preventing transmission of infection with human T-lymphotropic virus type II/ lymphadenopathy-associated virus in the workplace. MMWR 1985; 34:681–686, 691–695.
Garner J, Hierholzer W, McCormick R, et al. Guideline for isolation precaution in hospitals. Am J Infect Control 1996; 24:24–52.
Gershon R, Karkashian CD, Grosch JW, et al. Hospital safety climate and its relationships with safe work practices and workplace exposure incidents. Am J Infect Control 2000; 28:211–221.
Gershon R, Vlahov D, Felknor S, et al. Compliance with universal precautions among health care workers at three regional hospitals. Am J Infect Control 1995; 23:225–236.
Godin G, Nacach H, Morel S, Ebacher MF. Determinants of nurses' adherence to universal precautions for venipunctures. Am J Infect Control 2000; 28:359–364.
Gorse G, Messner R. Infection control practices in gastrointestinal endoscopy in the United States: a national survey. Infect Control Hosp Epidemiol 1991; 12:289–296.
Henry K, Campbell S, Maki M. A comparison of observed and self-reported compliance with universal precautions among emergency department personnel at a Minnesota public teaching hospital: implications for assessing infection control programs. Ann Emerg Med 1992; 21:940–946.
http://www.emedicine.com/emerg/topic333.htm
Jackson MM, Lynch P. An attempt to make an issue less murky: a comparison of four systems for infection precautions. Infect Control Hosp Epidemiol 1991; 12:448–450.
Lynch T. Communicable Disease Nursing. St. Louis, MO: Mosby, 1949.
Macalino GE, Viahov D, Sanford-Colby S, et al. Prevalence and incidence of HIV, hepatitis B virus, and hepatitis C virus infections among males in Rhode Island prisons. Am J Public Health 2004; 94:1218–1223.
Ni YH, Chang MH, Huang LM, et al. Hepatitis B virus infection in children and adolescents in a hyperendemic area: 15 years after mass hepatitis B vaccination. Ann Intern Med 2001; 135:796–800.
Ros S, Carrera-Ros B. Poor compliance with universal precautions: a universal phenomenon? Pediatr Emerg Care 1990; 6:183–185.
Zou S, Notari E, Stramer S, et al. Patterns of age- and sex-specific prevalence of major blood-borne infections in United States blood donors, 1995–2002: American Red Cross blood donor study. Transfusion 2004; 44:1640–1647.

8

Cutaneous Anesthesia

Andrea Willey and Peter K. Lee

Department of Dermatology, University of Minnesota, Minneapolis, Minnesota, U.S.A.

INTRODUCTION

Effective cutaneous anesthesia is a central component of dermatologic surgery. Current use of local anesthetics provides anesthesia necessary for a variety of diagnostic and therapeutic procedures in dermatology while avoiding the potential risks associated with general anesthesia. In recent years new anesthetic formulations and techniques of administration have accompanied advances in procedural dermatology. Several anesthetic agents are available with varying pharmacologic properties suited for different applications and techniques of administration. Proper selection and administration of anesthesia is essential to ensure efficacy, safety, and patient comfort.

HISTORY

A rich history of the development of local anesthetics exists and has been recently chronicled. Briefly reviewing this history reveals the following highlights. Albert Neiman first isolated the alkaloid cocaine from the *Erythroxylon coca* plant in 1860. However, it was not until 1884 that Carl Koller performed the first operation for glaucoma using cocaine. News of Koller's work sparked further development of local anesthetics. As the toxic and addictive affects of cocaine became apparent, the development of synthetic ester anesthetics, procaine, and tetracaine, soon followed. The emerging toxicities and allergic potential of ester anesthetics then led to the exploration of alternative anesthetics. In 1946, Nils Löfgren and Bengt Lundquist developed the xylidine derivative, lidocaine, with greater efficacy and scant allergic potential. The superior safety and efficacy of lidocaine led to its widespread use, as well as the development of additional amide anesthetics with varying properties aimed at optimizing efficacy and Systemic Toxicity. Mepivicaine, bupivacaine, prilocaine, and etidocaine followed; articaine, the most recent anesthetic emerged in 1972.

MECHANISM OF ACTION

Local anesthetics exhibit their clinical effects on peripheral nerves by temporarily inhibiting the influx of sodium ions required for the generation and propagation of action potentials across the nerve cell membrane, thus preventing the conduction of nerve impulses. Anesthetic actions result from both complex interactions with specific sites on the voltage-gated sodium ion channels as well as intrinsic impulse inhibition of some anesthetics. Sensations of pain and temperature are conducted by small unmyelinated type-C fibers, as well as myelinated type-A delta fibers. It is generally accepted that these smaller fibers are most susceptible to the effects of anesthetics, leading to the relative preservation of pressure sensation during procedures.

The clinical effects of local anesthetics depend on their ability to diffuse across nerve cell membranes and to bind sodium ion channels, blocking sodium influx and nerve depolarization. The molecular structure of local anesthetics allows for these amphipathic characteristics, and determines the pharmacologic properties of individual agents (Table 1). The pharmacologic properties of local anesthetics are determined by their solubility in lipid and aqueous environments and their avidity for proteins on sodium ion channels. The structure of local anesthetics can be divided into three parts: an aromatic ring separated from a tertiary amine by an intermediate ester or amide linkage (Fig. 1). The lipophilic nature of anesthetics is determined by the size the alkyl substituents on both the tertiary amine and aromatic moieties. Lipid solubility and the tendency to associate with lipophilic nerve membranes determines the potency of local anesthetics. The avidity for binding proteins on sodium ion channel determines the duration of anesthetic effect. Both the aromatic and amine moieties participate in protein binding.

The pK_a of local anesthetics determines the proportion of the agent in the uncharged base and protonated cation forms in aqueous solution. Agents with a lower pK_a have a greater proportion in the uncharged base form, which diffuses more readily across lipid membranes, yielding a faster onset of action. However, once anesthetics cross the nerve membrane, the cationic form actively binds membrane receptors, thus moderate hydrophobicity is optimal for local anesthetic efficacy. Low-tissue pH associated with local infection leads to a greater proportion of cationic forms, which may reduce the efficacy of local anesthetics.

The intermediate ester or amide linkage determines anesthetic metabolism and propensity for hypersensitivity. Esters are readily metabolized by plasma pseudocholinesterases and the metabolites are renally excreted. Paraaminobenzoic acid is the major metabolite responsible for high incidence of allergic reactions associated with ester anesthetics. In contrast, amides anesthetics are dealkylinated and hydrolyzed by liver microsomal enzymes prior to renal excretion. Compromised liver function may increase susceptibility to toxic effects of amide anesthetics. Lidocaine is the most commonly used amide anesthetic with intermediate duration of action and low antigenicity.

ADDITIVES TO LOCAL ANESTHETICS

Most local anesthetics, except for cocaine, produce smooth muscle relaxation and vasodilation, which leads to increased bleeding and enhanced absorption of the

Table 1 Anesthetics and Properties

Amides

Anesthetic	pk$_a$	Onset (min)	Duration (hr)	Duration with epinephrine (hr)	Maximum dose (mg/kg)	Maximum dose with epinephrine (mg/kg)
Lidocaine	7.86	<1	2	4	4.5	7
Mepivicaine	7.6	3–20	2–2.5		7	7
Prilocaine	7.89	5–6	1–1.5	2	8	8
Bupivacaine	8.1	4–10	1–3	2–4	2	2
Etidocaine	7.74	3–5	2–4	4	6	8
Ropivacaine	8.07	1–15	2–6	–	3.5	–
Levobupivacaine	8.1	4–10	2–4	–	2	–
Articaine	7.8	1–6	–	1	7	–
Esters						
Procaine	8.9	2–5	0.5–1.5	0.25–0.5	10	14
Chloroprocaine	9.1	6–12	–	Up to 1	11	14
Tetracaine	8.4	7	–	2–3	2	2

anesthetic. Vasoconstrictors are commonly added to local anesthetics to minimize hemorrhage, increase the duration of action, and decrease the amount of anesthetic needed, and thus the potential for toxic side effects. Epinephrine is the most frequently used vasoconstrictor used with local anesthesia. Other vasoconstrictors include norepinephrine, phenylephrine, and levonordefrin. Most local anesthetics are available premixed with epinephrine at a concentration of 1:100,000 (1 mg/100 mL) or 1:200,000. The lower pH of premixed lidocaine epinephrine solutions, which contain antioxidants to stabilize epinephrine, increases the pain of injection. To minimize pain associated with low pH, lidocaine epinephrine solutions can be freshly prepared prior to surgical procedures. Alternatively, premixed solutions can be buffered with a 1:10 dilution of sodium bicarbonate: lidocaine with epinephrine.

TOXICITY

Local anesthetics are generally safe; however, local reactions and systemic toxicity can be associated with anesthetics and additives. Clinicians should be familiar with the toxicity of local anesthetics and be able to recognize and skillfully manage symptoms of toxicity should they occur. The smallest amount of anesthetic agent should be used to achieve anesthesia and minimize potential side effects. When large areas are anesthetized, large volumes of dilute solutions can be used, and regional blocks and ring blocks can be performed to minimize the amount of anesthetic administered. A 1:200,000 dilution of lidocaine epinephrine is effective for most cutaneous surgeries. Stronger solutions may be associated with

tissue necrosis. Localized tumescent techniques using 0.5% lidocaine epinephrine have more recently been advocated for use with Mohs surgery and other facial procedures.

LOCAL REACTIONS

Local reactions to anesthetics include pain upon infiltration, ecchymosis, hematoma, and nerve injury. Inadvertent injection of vessels in highly vascularized areas such as the face can lead to ecchymosis or hematoma. Local nerve injury can result from inadvertent nerve transection or local ischemia. Acute pain during injection may indicate intraneural injection. Direct injection into nerve foramina should be avoided.

ALLERGIC REACTIONS

Immediate allergic reactions are most common with ester anesthetics, which are metabolized to para-aminobenzoic acid. True allergic reactions to amide anesthetics are rare; however, may be associated with hypersensitivity to preservatives of multidose vials, including methylparabens and sodium metabisulfite . Cross-reactions with ester anesthetics have occurred with sulfonamide medications and paraphenylenediamines. If allergy to lidocaine is suspected, patch testing can be performed with intradermal challenge using preservative-free lidocaine to confirm positive patch results. Single-dose vials of preservative-free lidocaine are available for use in allergic patients. In addition, bacteriostatic saline that contains benzyl alcohol can be used for minor procedures. Symptoms of immediate type-I hypersensitivity reactions include urticaria, angioedema, nausea, dyspnea, and anaphylaxis with associated hypotension and tachycardia. Side effects of epinephrine can be confused with symptoms of anesthetic allergy; however, the presence of hypertension is distinguishing. Antihistamines and corticosteroids can be given for mild type-I hypersensitivity reactions. More serious reactions require administration of epinephrine and basic life support. Delayed type-II hypersensitivity reactions that presents as allergic contact dermatitis can occur with both ester and amide anesthetics.

SYSTEMIC TOXICITY

Systemic toxicity to local anesthetics associated with increased blood levels affects the central nervous and cardiac systems. Increased blood levels can occur with administration of excessive volumes, in advertent intravenous injection, rapid absorption of topical anesthetics

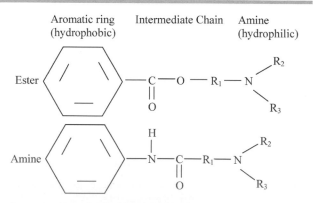

Figure 1 Basic structure of ester and amide anesthetic molecules.

Table 2 Central Nervous System (CNS) Toxicity Associated with Increased Blood Levels of Lidocaine

1–5 µg/mL	5–8 µg/mL	8–12 µg/mL	20–25 µg/mL
Ringing in ears	Nystagmus	Seizures	Respiratory depression
Circumoral tingling	Slurred speech		Coma
Metallic taste	Hallucinations		
Light-headedness	Muscle twitching		
Talkativeness	Tremor		
Nausea/emesis			
Double vision			

from mucosal surfaces, pseudocholinesterase deficiency, or impaired metabolism associated with liver disease or decreased blood flow to the liver associated with congestive heart failure or beta-blocker medications. The central nervous system (CNS) toxicity of lidocaine is dose dependent (Table 2). Importantly, anesthetics with greater potency, such as etidocaine and bupivacaine, induce CNS toxicity at lower levels than lidocaine and may have a greater risk of cardiac toxicity through direct interaction with cardiac muscle. Using the smallest amount of local anesthetic necessary for a given procedure and monitoring for signs of toxicity is important to minimize the risk of anesthetic toxicity.

PREGNANCY AND LACTATION

Local anesthetics can cross the placenta by passive diffusion; however, their judicious use during pregnancy is generally considered to be safe. Lidocaine, etidocaine, levobupivacaine, prilocaine, and procaine are labeled pregnancy category B. Bupivacaine, mepivacaine, articaine, tetracaine, and chloroprocaine are labeled category C. Local anesthetics are excreted in breast milk and caution must be used when administering during lactation. The use of ester anesthetics with rapid metabolism or the use of alternate agents such as 9% saline with benzyl alcohol has been recommended to minimize fetal exposure during lactation. Epinephrine is labeled category C and is excreted in breast milk, and, thus, must be used cautiously. Large doses of epinephrine may lead to decreased placental perfusion.

EPINEPHRINE TOXICITY

Systemic toxicity of epinephrine also affects the cardiovascular and central nervous systems. The maximal dose of epinephrine in normal patients is 1 mg (100 mL of 1:100,000 solution). Dilutions of 1:300,000 with a maximal dose of 0.2 mg has been recommended for patients with unstable angina or a history of cardiac arrhythmia. Absolute contraindications include severe cardiovascular disease, hypertension, and peripheral vascular disease, hyperthyroidism, and pheochromocytoma. Relative contraindications include use during pregnancy, in areas of compromised vasculature, and in patients taking beta-blocker medications. Marked paradoxical hypertension followed by reflex bradycardia due to unopposed α-1 blockade may occur in patients taking beta-blockers, which may lead to cardiac arrest or hypertensive stroke. In patients taking beta-blockers, blood pressure monitoring and use of dilute solutions of epinephrine is prudent. Gradual discontinuation of beta-blocker medications may be indicated in some patients.

The use of epinephrine containing anesthetics for digital blocks has been limited due to concerns of vasoconstrictor-induced ischemia; however, this concept has been debated. Recent studies demonstrate vasoconstrictor effects are reversible and appear safe in healthy subjects. Some caution may be advised in the setting of peripheral and microvascular disease.

ADMINISTRATION

Topical Anesthetics

The increased frequency of laser surgery and aesthetic procedures has expanded the use of topical anesthesia in procedural dermatology and led to the development of novel formulations that increase the penetration and improve the application of topical anesthetics. Various formulations have been developed to improve penetration through the stratum corneum and improve the efficacy of topical anesthetics on keratinizing skin surfaces (Table 3). Caution must be used on large surface areas and on mucosal surfaces in which rapid absorption may lead to high serum levels of anesthetic.

EMLA (AstraZeneca) is as a eutectic mixture of 2.5% lidocaine and 2.5% prilocaine and emulsifiers that enhances penetration and concentrate anesthetic agent within the oil component of the emulsion to improve penetration and reduce toxicity. Application for one to two hours under occlusion leads to peak anesthesia that persists for one to two hours. The depth of penetration is proportional to time of contact. Vasoconstrictive effects may be seen that peak at 1.5 hours. Onset of anesthesia is 5 to 15 minutes on mucous membranes. Maximum dose recommendation is based on age and weight. There is a risk of methemoglobinemia with the use of EMLA cream and, thus it should not be used in those with G6PD deficiency or persons taking methemoglobin-inducing agents. The maximum dose in infants less than three months age is 1 g applied for one hour. Application near the eyes is avoided due to potential for chemical injury to the cornea and conjunctiva.

LMX™ (Ferndale) is a 4% or 5% lidocaine cream formulated in a liposomal delivery system that facilitates cutaneous penetration and increased duration of action. Application for 30 minutes without occlusion leads to anesthesia comparable to EMLA. Use on mucous membranes is not recommended due to increased absorption. There is no risk of methemoglobinemia; however, application is limited to an area 100 cm² in children less than 20 kg.

The S-Caine peel (TetraPeel™ ZARS) is a eutectic mixture of 7% lidocaine and 7% tetracaine cream that dries into a film that is easily peeled off. A 20- to 30-minute application has been found to be effective for use with several laser procedures. Lidocaine 30% hydrophilic mixtures such as Acid Mantle™ (Doak Dermatologics) or Velvachol™ (Novartis) that hydrate the stratum corneum for improved penetration have also been useful for various laser procedures.

Topical ophthalmic anesthetic preparations are useful for periocular surgical and laser procedures and for placement of corneal shields. Proparacaine 0.5% and tetracaine 0.5% solutions are commonly used preparations that provide rapid anesthesia lasting 15 to 45 minutes. Stinging upon application is common.

LOCAL INFILTRATION

Local infiltration is the most commonly used technique to achieve cutaneous anesthesia in dermatologic surgery. Anesthetic agents may be injected intradermally or subcutaneously. Intradermal injection leads to immediate onset of action; however, can be painful if injection is rapid and usually involves some degree of tissue distortion. Subcutaneous

Table 3 Topical Anesthetics

Proprietary name	Anesthetic	Formulation	Application (min)	Duration (min.)	Max. dose
EMLA (AstraZeneca)	Lidocaine 2.5% Prilocaine 2.5%	Eutectic emulsion	60–120 (occlusion) (5–10 mucosa)	60–120 hrs (15–20 mucosa)	Children: dose limitations
LMX™ 4/5[a] (Ferndale Labs)	Lidocaine 4%/5%	Liposomal	30	–	No mucosa Child <20 kg <100 cm^2
Topicaine[a] (Esba Labs)	Lidocaine 4%, 5%	Microemulsion	30–60 (occlusion)	30	Adult 600 cm^2 Child 100 cm^2
Betacaine Enhanced Gel[a] (Thermaderm)	Lidocaine 5%	Alcohol gel petrolatum emulsion	30	–	–
Betacaine LA[c]	Lidocaine Prilocaine Dibucaine	Petrolatum	30–45	–	300 cm^2 Child not studied
Lidocaine Ointment[b]	Lidocaine 30%	Petrolatum	–	–	–
Photocaine[b]	Lidocaine 6% Tetracaine 6%	Proprietary	–	–	–
Tetracaine Gel	Tetracaine 4%	Lecithin gel	60 (occlusion)	–	–
S-Caine peel[c] (ZARS Inc.)	Lidocaine 7% Tetracaine 7%	Cream-Film	60	–	–

[a]Over-the-counter.
[b]Compounded.
[c]Not FDA approved.

injections are less painful; however, onset of action is delayed and the duration is shorter due to increased absorption. Using a small needle (1 in. 30-gauge needle is most often used) and injecting slowly into a previously numbed area can minimize pain associated with infiltration anesthesia. Using a smaller syringe may also be helpful by decreasing the rate of injection. Although intradermal infiltration results in immediate anesthesia, the vasoconstrictive properties of epinephrine may require up to 15 minutes for full effect. Pretreatment with topical anesthetics or ice packs and the use of counter stimulus techniques such as pinching the skin can also be helpful in reducing patient discomfort. Circumferential infiltration of anesthesia, or a ring block, may be used to reduce the amount of anesthesia required for large areas or when direct injection into a lesion is avoided. Injection into both superficial and deep planes is required for an effective ring block. Use of tumescent anesthesia using large volumes of dilute anesthetic agents, initially developed for use in liposuction, is now used for many dermatologic procedures and is discussed elsewhere in this book.

REGIONAL BLOCKS

Regional anesthesia of the face is useful for anesthetizing large areas and can minimize pain of local infiltration. Smaller amounts of anesthetic agents in higher concentration may be used to achieve regional anesthesia; however, local infiltration of anesthetic containing epinephrine is required for vasoconstrictive effects. Local infiltration with minimal pain can be performed following the onset of regional blockade, which is approximately 5 to 10 minutes following injection. Withdrawal prior to injection near regional nerve trunks is essential to avoid inadvertent intravenous injection. Use of a 25-gauge needle has also been advocated to ensure sanguinous withdrawal is visualized. Knowledge of the neuroanatomy of the face and neck is necessary to achieve effective regional anesthesia and minimize risks of nerve injury.

Sensory innervation of the face and neck is supplied by the three divisions of the trigeminal nerve, the ophthalmic, maxillary, and mandibular nerves, and superior branches of the cervical plexus (Figure 2). Motor branches of the

trigeminal nerve supply the muscles of mastication. Regional blocks of the three major branches of the trigeminal nerve are frequently performed where each of the three branches exits their respective bony foramina. Minor blocks of smaller branches of the trigeminal and cervical nerves are also useful and are described here.

THE OPHTHALMIC NERVE

The ophthalmic division of the trigeminal nerve further divides into the supraorbital, supratrochlear, infratrochlear, lacrimal, and external nasal branches. The supraorbital, supratrochlear, and infratrochlear branches of the ophthalmic division innervate the forehead, anterior scalp to the vertex, upper eyelid, and medial canthus and can be anesthetized with a single injection. The supraorbital nerve

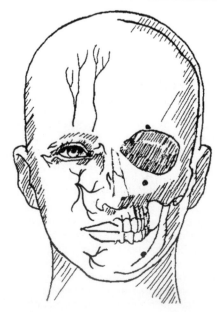

Figure 2 Cutaneous sensory nerves. *Source*: Illustration by Sheila Belkin.

exits the supraorbital foramen, or notch, 2.5 cm from the midline along the supraorbital rim; the supratrochlear nerve lies 1.5-cm medially. The infratrochlear nerve exits the orbit above the medial canthus. Regional blockade of both of these branches can be achieved by entering lateral to the supraorbital notch, advancing medially approximately 2 cm in the submuscular plane and injecting 1 to 2 mL anesthetic. The palpebral branch of the lacrimal nerve innervates the lateral upper eyelid and brow. Anesthesia of this nerve can be achieved by injecting approximately 1 mL anesthetic just above the lateral canthus. The external nasal nerve innervates the nasal tip and dorsum. Anesthesia can be achieved by injecting 1 mL anesthetic inferolaterally from the junction of the nasal bone and cartilage.

THE MAXILLARY NERVE

The infraorbital branch of the maxillary division innervates the lower eyelid, nasal sidewall and ala, columella, medial cheek, and upper lip. The infraorbital nerve exits the skull through the infraorbital foramen 1 cm below the orbital rim just medial to the mid-pupillary line. Regional block of this nerve can be achieved by injecting approximately 2 to 3 mL anesthetic transcutaneously or intraorally. Intra-oral injections are placed in the gingival sulcus superior to the canine tooth and advancing approximately 1 cm. Injecting a small amount of anesthetic into the mucosal sulcus prior to advancing the needle can minimize patient discomfort.

THE MANDIBULAR NERVE

The mental branch of the mandibular division innervates the lower lip and chin. This branch exits the mental foramen in the mid-mandible just medial to the mid-pupillary line. The nerve can be approached intraorally by entering the lower gingival sulcus at the apex of the second premolar and advancing approximately 0.5 cm and injecting approximately 2 mL anesthetic. The auriculotemporal nerve courses superiorly from just anterior to the tragus to innervate the temporal scalp, temple, and preauricular cheek. Anesthesia can be achieved by injecting over the zygomatic arch superior to the temporomandibular joint. The buccal nerve innervates the lateral cheek from the oral commissure to the ramus of the mandible. Anesthesia can be achieved by injecting 2 to 4 cc anesthetic half way along a line from the tragus to the oral commissure just beyond the border of the masseter muscle.

THE CERVICAL PLEXUS

The greater auricular and transverse cervical nerves emerge from midway along the posterior border of the sternocleidomastoid muscle (Erb's point) traveling superior and inferomedial, respectively, to innervate the skin overlying the posterior ear, submandibular lateral and central neck. Anesthesia can be achieved by injecting anteriorly from the lateral border of the muscle.

DIGITAL BLOCK

Digits are innervated by dorsal and ventral nerves that run laterally along each digit. Anesthesia is achieved by injecting a small volume of anesthesia at the dorsolateral aspect of the base of the digit then advancing ventrally to inject the ventrolateral aspect at the base.

BIBLIOGRAPHY

Altinyazar HC, Ozdemir H, Koca R, Hosnuter M, Demirel CB, Gundogdu S. Epinephrine in digital block: color Doppler flow imaging. Dermatol Surg 2004; 30(4 Pt 1):508–511.

Amin SP, Goldberg DJ. Topical anesthetics for cosmetic and laser dermatology. J Drugs Dermatol 2005; 4(4):455–461.

Auletta MJ, Grekin RC. Local Anesthesia for Dermatologic Surgery. New York, NY: Churchill Livingstone, 1991.

Behroozan DS, Goldberg LH. Dermal tumescent local anesthesia in cutaneous surgery. J Am Acad Dermatol 2005; 53(5):828–830.

Bjerring P, Arendt-Nielsen L. Depth and duration of skin analgesia to needle insertion after topical application of EMLA cream. Br J Anaesth 1990; 64(2):173–177.

Calatayud J, Gonzalez A. History of the development and evolution of local anesthesia since the coca leaf. Anesthesiology 2003; 98:1503–1508.

Covino BG. Local anesthesia (First of two parts). N Engl J Med 1972; 286(18):975–983.

Covino BG. Local anesthesia 2. N Engl J Med 1972; 286(19):1035–1042.

Covino BG. Pharmacology of local anaesthetic agents. Br J Anaesth 1986; 58(7):701–716.

EMLA package insert. Wilmington, DE: AstraZeneca LP, 2005.

Eaglstein NF. Chemical injury to the eye from EMLA cream during erbium laser resurfacing. Dermatol Surg 1999; 25(7):590–591.

Eaton JS, Grekin RC. Regional anesthesia of the face. Dermatol Surg 2001; 27(12):1006–1009.

Friedman PM, Mafong EA, Friedman ES, Geronemus RG. Topical anesthetics update: EMLA and beyond. Dermatol Surg 2001; 27(12):1019–1026.

Grekin RC, Auletta MJ. Local anesthesia in dermatologic surgery. J Am Acad Dermatol 1988; 19(4):599–614.

Hanke CW. The tumescent facial block: tumescent local anesthesia and nerve block anesthesia for full-face laser resurfacing. Dermatol Surg 2001; 27(12):1003–1005.

Huang W, Vidimos A. Topical anesthetics in dermatology. J Am Acad Dermatol 2000; 43(2 Pt 1):286–298.

LMX-4 package insert. Ferndale, MI: Ferndale labs. 2005.

Mackley CL, Marks JG Jr., Anderson BE. Delayed-type hypersensitivity to lidocaine. Arch Dermatol 2003; 139(3):343–346.

Naguib M, Magboul MM, Samarkandi AH, Attia M. Adverse effects and drug interactions associated with local and regional anaesthesia. Drug Saf 1998; 4:221–250.

Nau C, Wang GK. Interactions of local anesthetics with voltage-gated Na channels. J Membr Biol 2004; 201(1):1–8.

Randle HW, Salassa JR, Roenigk RK. Know your anatomy. Local anesthesia for cutaneous lesions of the head and neck–practical applications of peripheral nerve blocks. J Dermatol Surg Oncol 1992; 18(3):231–235.

Richards KA, Stasko T. Dermatologic surgery and the pregnant patient. Dermatol Surg 2002; 28(3):248–256.

Skidmore RA, Patterson JD, Tomsick RS. Local anesthetics. Dermatol Surg 1996; 22(6):511–522; quiz 523–524.

Strichartz GR, Berde C. Local anesthetics. In: Miller RD, ed. Miller's Anesthesia. 6th ed. Philadelphia, PA: Churchill Livingstone, 2005:573–603.

Wilhelmi BJ, Blackwell SJ, Miller JH, et al. Do not use epinephrine in digital blocks: myth or truth? Plast Reconstr Surg 2001; 107(2):393–397.

9

Tumescent Anesthesia

P. Lillis
University of Colorado Health Sciences Center, Denver, Colorado, U.S.A.

INTRODUCTION

The intelligent and efficient use of local anesthesia for soft-tissue surgery has been greatly influenced by dermatologists since dermatologic surgery became an integral part of our specialty. Dermatologic surgeons have been at the forefront in pioneering office-based local anesthesia for procedures previously performed in hospital operating rooms under general anesthesia.

During the 1970s and early 1980s, there was little incentive for hospital-based surgeons to perform office surgery. Cost containment was not an important issue, and physicians predictably practiced in the manner in which they were trained.

In the early 1970s, dermatologic surgery began to play a more prominent role in the specialty of dermatology. Sophisticated surgical training became available in many dermatology residencies and at various dermatology meetings. The dermatologist's anatomical, clinical, and histologic knowledge of the skin placed him or her in a uniquely advantageous position to render appropriate surgical treatment of skin problems.

Dermatologists treat the vast majority of skin cancers in an in-office outpatient setting. Even dermatologists who have acquired hospital surgical privileges rarely treat cases in the hospital. Efficiency, convenience for both doctor and patient, a lower infection rate, and cost savings are noted as primary reasons to provide office-based surgery. Dermatologic surgeons have now been routinely performing in-office, sophisticated surgical procedures under local anesthesia for more than three decades.

Full-face dermabrasion and ablative laser resurfacing, for example, have traditionally been considered a general anesthesia procedure when performed by nondermatologists. Dermatologic surgeons, however, have traditionally used a combination of methods (ice-packs, refrigerant sprays, nerve blocks, EMLA, and tumescent anesthesia) to make this an office-based local anesthetic procedure.

In the mid-1980s, Dr. Jeffrey Klein, the founder of tumescent liposuction, suspected that the 5 to 7 mg/kg limit for lidocaine that had been accepted as gospel was not valid. In researching his suspicions, he discovered that in their 1948 application for Food and Drug Administration approval, Astra Pharmaceuticals had merely indicated that the safe dose of lidocaine was probably equivalent to the safe dose of procaine.

No specific studies had been performed. No consideration was given to the vascularity of the area to be anesthetized, the concentration of lidocaine, the inclusion of epinephrine, or the rate of injection. Dr. Klein initiated a study of 26 patients in which a relatively large volume of very dilute lidocaine or epinephrine solution was used to anesthetize sites prior to liposuction.

Dr. Klein instilled an average of 2 Vol% times the recommended upper limit of lidocaine and measured blood levels of lidocaine up to one-hour postinjection. Surprisingly, the average lidocaine levels obtained did not approach even one-tenth of the low toxicity range of 5 ng/mL.

The implications of these findings were profound but not generally appreciated by dermatologists, let alone the medical community at large. At the time, most dermatologists had little training in sophisticated surgical techniques and even fewer had exposure or interest in liposuction. Nearly all liposuction at that time was performed under general anesthesia, and the specialists performing liposuction had no interest in and for years were unaware of Klein's discoveries.

During the 1970s and early 1980s, there was little incentive for hospital-based surgeons to perform office surgery. Cost containment was not an important issue, and physicians predictably practiced in the manner in which they were trained.

Dermatologists in general performed very little surgery through the 1960s and early 1970s. In the mid-1970s, the American Society of Dermatologic Surgery was formed by a small group of surgically oriented dermatologists. Even at that time, dermatologists who were considered "Dermatologic surgeons" performed primarily excisions, nail surgery, perhaps, dermabrasion, and hair transplantation.

The advent of fresh tissue Mohs surgery pioneered by the studies of Tromovitch and Stegman was more responsible than any other factor in accelerating the advances in Dermatologic surgery. Dermatologic surgeons were now inspired to learn and develop new reconstructive techniques for closure of skin cancer defects. This naturally led to the extension of these skills into the cosmetic arena.

The expansion of dermatologic surgery over the past decade has been astounding, especially in the field of lasers. Enthusiasm for training in liposuction by dermatologists is less than what it was 10 years ago. Reasons for this may include the perception of liposuction as being a risky procedure. Turf pressure from other specialists may to some degree intimidate a dermatologist from starting or pursuing liposuction in one's practice. Many malpractice insurance companies either do not appreciate the safety of tumescent liposuction with local anesthesia compared to the not uncommon significant complications of liposuction under general anesthesia or IV sedation or are influenced by physicians in positions of power who are motivated by turf protection issues.

In my opinion, the most significant factor in the decreased popularity of liposuction among dermatologic surgeons is the development of "minimally invasive techniques," which have a hi-tech appeal and appear to have little downside. Intense pulse light sources, vascular lasers, various fillers, radiofrequency skin tightening, suture suspension lifts, etc., appear to be safer and have a shorter learning curve than liposuction.

Although these techniques, most of which have either been developed or significantly advanced by dermatologists, are significant advancements in dermatologic surgery, many times the degree of improvement obtained with these techniques is subtle or occasionally nonexistent.

In my experience (over 8000 cases in approximately 25,000 body sites), liposuction results in a "home run" in the vast majority of cases. Rarely is the improvement subtle unless the patient is "nearly perfect" to begin with.

Liposuction by the tumescent technique with only oral and/or intramuscular sedation is perfectly suited to the Dermatologic surgery office-based practice. In addition to the consistently significant improvement obtained, the safety record of liposuction performed in this manner is very impressive. Equipment needed to perform liposuction is modestly priced, and the cost of disposables needed for liposuction is comparatively low. Compare this to the fixed costs of lasers, LPL, radiofrequency skin tightening, etc.

Those of us in Dermatologic surgery who perform liposuction generally get consistently excellent results with an unparalleled safety record. Our patients experience less postoperative morbidity, and this approach is more cost efficient. In my opinion, tumescent liposuction is second only to Mohs surgery as the ideal Dermatologic surgery procedure. The principles of tumescent anesthesia developed for liposuction have been proven to enhance hemostasis and prolong anesthesia. These principles can be applied to many other types of soft-tissue surgery.

DEVELOPMENT OF THE TUMESCENT TECHNIQUE

The development of the tumescent technique has been the most significant contribution to liposuction surgery since the development of liposuction in Europe in the late 1970s. Dr. Jeffrey Klein is the originator of the tumescent technique. I was influenced by Dr. Klein in the "early days" of the development of the tumescent technique and have been in a position to contribute to the profound implications of Dr. Klein's work. I will convey from my perspective the history of the tumescent technique.

The Second World Congress of Liposuction was held in June 1986 in Philadelphia, Pennsylvania. At this meeting, Dr. Klein presented the tumescent technique for liposuction surgery. Dr. Klein described a modification of the "wet technique" in which a very large volume of extremely dilute lidocaine or epinephrine solution was injected into subcutaneous tissue to the extent that swelling and firmness occurred. At this meeting, Dr. Klein also unveiled a specially designed device to efficiently infiltrate large quantities of the tumescent solution into the subcutaneous tissue. The "Klein needle," a blunt-tipped 30 cm long, 4.7 mm diameter cannula contains a port into which a 60 cc syringe is inserted. One liter of dilute lidocaine or epinephrine solution is connected to the syringe by an intravenous line. The "needle" is inserted into the same incision site used for introduction of the suction cannula. The lidocaine or epinephrine solution is injected along a pathway in which the suction cannula will follow.

Klein reported that, by injecting a solution of 0.1% lidocaine with 1:1,000,000 epinephrine into 26 patients, he was able to infiltrate a mean lidocaine dose of 1250 mg (18.4 mg/kg), which was more than twice the recommended maximal dose of lidocaine (5–7 mg/kg). Blood lidocaine measurements at one-hour postinfiltration yielded a mean serum lidocaine level of 0.36 μg/mL (toxicity range begins at approximately 5.0 μg/mL). The highest serum lidocaine level recorded in his patients was 0.614 μg/mL. In Klein's study, the mean volume of fat extracted was 915 mL. There was no apparent change in hematocrits measured 48 to 72 hours postsurgery, indicating a significant decrease in expected blood loss.

Surprisingly, Klein's presentation generated little interest or discussion at this meeting. In retrospect, the lack of interest is understandable. The majority of those attending this conference were hospital-based surgeons trained in performing most procedures under general anesthesia.

Prior to the conference, I performed most of my liposuction surgery under general anesthesia in a hospital setting. Smaller cases were performed in my office with local anesthesia. These cases required a considerable amount of time to obtain adequate local anesthesia with a standard syringe and 25 gauge needle. I immediately realized the potential of the Klein needle for efficient delivery of local anesthetic. Klein's data on low serum lidocaine levels after subcutaneous injection of high doses of lidocaine were both promising and intriguing.

Over the ensuing 14 months, I began performing larger-volume liposuction cases in my office using progressively larger doses of lidocaine and periodically checking 30- and 60-minute postinfiltration serum lidocaine levels. Results were consistently found to be less than 1 μg/mL, even after greatly exceeding the recommended upper limit of 5 to 7 mg/kg.

High-volume liposuction cases were still performed under general anesthesia in a hospital operating room, but I now treated moderate-sized cases in my office with a combination of epidural anesthesia, supplemented by tumescent anesthesia (for areas superior to those anesthetized by the epidural block). Smaller-volume cases were performed totally by the tumescent technique.

In cases using both epidural block and tumescent anesthesia, there was a striking difference between areas suctioned. The epidural block areas yielded grossly bloody aspirate, whereas the tumescent areas yielded bright yellow bloodless fat. Realizing the potential for decreased blood loss, I began injecting tumescent solution into areas suctioned in cases performed under general anesthesia. During my first case using tumescent anesthesia with general anesthesia, the anesthesiologist immediately commented on the noticeable absence of blood in the aspirate.

In March 1988, 1 initiated a study of 20 consecutive patients in which a minimum of 1500 cc of fat was removed to determine serum lidocaine levels and blood loss with the tumescent technique. The results of the study not only confirmed Dr. Klein's work, but also showed that much larger doses of lidocaine could be safely administered, allowing a larger volume of fat removal.

The average volume of fat removed in this study was approximately 2000 cc. The average preoperative hematocrit was 40.3 followed by an average one-week postoperative hematocrit of 40.0. Prior to this study, the most complete work on blood loss in liposuction surgery indicated that the average total blood loss (blood in the aspirate plus third space blood loss) in females would decrease the one-week postoperative hematocrit by 0.5 for every 100 cc of aspirate. The predicted decrease in hematocrit in my study, with an average aspirate of 2800 cc, therefore would have been 14. Subsequent clinical experience has confirmed this virtual absence of significant blood loss with liposuction by the tumescent technique.

My study and Klein's "Anesthesia for Liposuction and Dermatologic Surgery" were published in October 1988. At the time of publication we believed that the reason we were able to use such large doses of lidocaine was a combination of decreased concentration of lidocaine, vasoconstriction induced by epinephrine, and the relative avascularity of the adipose tissue preventing lidocaine from rapidly entering the bloodstream. We then assumed that we were removing most of the lidocaine during the liposuction process.

At the 1988 International Society of Dermatologic Surgery meeting, a presentation was given by Dr. John Skouge of Johns Hopkins University, who had measured the amount of lidocaine in liposuction aspirate. Skouge noted that only 5% of injected lidocaine was removed with the aspirate. These findings were subsequently confirmed by Bridenstine.

Klein subsequently performed a study in which a small number of patients were infiltrated with tumescent solution, and liposuction was not performed. The same patients were later infiltrated with an identical amount of the same solution and liposuction was performed. Blood lidocaine levels were obtained at regular intervals for 24 hours in both situations. Klein felt that the rate of absorption and peak lidocaine levels were a function of concentration of lidocaine and the rate of injection. Lower lidocaine concentration and slower injection would produce delayed and lower peak concentration. His study indicated that blood lidocaine levels peaked at approximately 12 hours, returning to zero by 24 hours. Peak levels did not vary greatly whether or not liposuction was performed.

It also became apparent that when large volumes of fluid were injected into the fat, third spacing of vascular fluid into the treated areas was prevented. The injected fluid not only prevented third spacing but also was absorbed into the vascular space if needed for fluid replacement. The need for estimating and providing intravenous fluid replacement was therefore eliminated.

An additional unexpected finding was the prolonged anesthesia that resulted with the tumescent technique. Prior to the tumescent technique, liposuction performed under general anesthesia would routinely cause patients to awaken in the recovery room in severe pain, usually with shaking chills. When I initially used the tumescent technique, I did not appreciate the prolonged anesthesia that resulted and would routinely place patients on postoperative narcotic analgesics. Postoperative nausea and vomiting was not uncommon. It was not clear to me whether this was due to rising blood levels of lidocaine or to the postoperative narcotic analgesics. Once the 12 to 18 hours duration of local anesthesia was appreciated and postoperative narcotics were no longer given, problems with postoperative nausea were virtually eliminated.

Prior to the development of the tumescent technique, Fournier and others advocated chilling the local anesthetic before injection to induce vasoconstriction, thereby decreasing blood loss. This practice would significantly lower body core temperature, producing shaking chills. The development of the tumescent technique solved the problem of blood loss. It was noted, however, that even injecting large volumes of fluid at room temperature would frequently produce shaking chills. Heating the tumescent solution to body temperature greatly improved patient comfort.

The discovery that the addition of bicarbonate to local anesthetic significantly decreased the pain of injection by neutralizing the pH of lidocaine found immediate application in liposuction surgery. The decrease in discomfort when injecting buffered versus nonbuffered lidocaine was dramatic. Although the rate of infection with liposuction surgery was always quite low, the discovery that buffering lidocaine greatly enhanced its antibacterial properties is possibly responsible for the very low infection rate with the tumescent technique.

A final serendipitous finding with the tumescent technique was the discovery that by magnifying the subcutaneous compartment by installation of copious amounts of fluid, fat extraction was not only physically easier to perform, but was also more accurate and uniform. Ridges and irregularities, which were commonly seen prior to the tumescent technique due to locally excessive fat extraction, were uncommon with the tumescent technique. The ease of fat extraction led to the development of significantly smaller cannulas, further reducing the incidence of these irregularities. During 1989 and 1990, many dermatologists attempted liposuction by the tumescent technique. My colleagues related in many instances the inability to obtain adequate anesthesia. The magnitude of tumescent solution required for this technique was difficult to comprehend. Once the concept was fully understood and mastered, this method proved a vast improvement over any previous attempts at local anesthesia.

Tumescent technique liposuction became "state of the art" for dermatologic surgeons by 1990. In spite of this, other specialties were basically unaware of the existence or advantages of this approach.

At a 1990 workshop in Houston, Texas, conducted by Dr. Gary Fenno, I performed liposuction by tumescent technique under local anesthesia. Dr. Howard Tobin and Dr. Richard Dolsky, two prominent leaders in cosmetic surgery, were present. After observing this case, Drs. Tobin, Dolsky, and Fenno adopted the tumescent technique in conjunction with general anesthesia. They were instrumental in spreading the word to other cosmetic surgeons about the advantages of using tumescent anesthesia whether liposuction was performed by local, epidural, or general anesthesia.

The speciality of plastic surgery remained basically unaware of the tumescent technique until the publication of Pitman's textbook and Repiogle's paper. As late as June 1992, Courtiss published "Large Volume Lipectomy-A Retrospective Analysis of 108 Patients." This article was a review of Courtiss's "high-volume" liposuction. "High volume" consisted of more than 1500 mL of aspirate, Courtiss's average volume removed was approximately 2700 cc. My paper, published four years earlier, also included patients with extracted fat volume greater than 1500 cc. My average extracted volume was coincidentally also approximately 2700 cc.

All of Courtiss's cases were performed in a hospital setting. About 44% of his patients were admitted for at least one night postoperatively. About 227 units of autologous and two units of homologous blood were transfused. His average patient lost 2 L of blood, which accounted for an average of 40% of the total patient blood volume.

The percentages of blood aspirate by body area consisted of thighs- 30%, hips- 35%, abdomen- 45%, and flanks- 46%. In spite of this significant blood loss, Courtiss concluded that high-volume liposuction was a "safe procedure." Our studies demonstrated total blood loss by tumescent technique to be less than 1%.

LIDOCAINE

The two major types of local anesthetic are amides and esters. Esters (e.g., procaine) have a lower toxicity potential than amides (e.g., lidocaine). Esters have a much higher allergenic potential. The esters are hydrolyzed in the plasma by pseudocholinesterase and the amides are metabolized hepatically. Most studies to date with tumescent anesthesia involve lidocaine and to a lesser degree prilocaine. Properties of local anesthetics other than lidocaine will not be discussed. Anesthesia for cutaneous surgery may be local, regional, or general. Ideally, the safest method of anesthesia should be selected. General anesthesia carries a greater risk of morbidity and mortality than local anesthesia. Many procedures that were previously carried out under general anesthesia are now performed with regional or local anesthesia.

Use of local anesthesia on high-risk cardiac patients substantially reduces the risk of infarction when compared to general anesthesia. When using local anesthesia, the cardiovascular and respiratory systems are not compromised. The development of tumescent anesthesia has eliminated the need for general anesthesia and regional anesthesia in many procedures in which excessive amounts of local anesthesia would previously have been necessary.

The unquestioned advantages of tumescent anesthesia are decreased blood loss and bruising in all types of soft-tissue surgery involving larger areas. Potential disadvantages of Tumescent anesthesia may include fluid volume overload, increased time required to administer adequate local anesthesia, prolonged drainage, and elevated plasma levels of lidocaine, which could occur hours after discharge. The latter has been the subject of much discussion. Predicting at what mg/kg dose lidocaine toxicity will occur in a particular individual is complex and imprecise. Many factors must be taken into account.

Plasma concentrations of lidocaine are affected not only by the mg/kg dose given but also by the vascularity of the site of injection, the presence of vasoconstriction, the body fat percentage of the patient, and hepatic function. Injection into more vascular areas of subcutaneous tissue (e.g., face) probably results in higher and earlier peaks of plasma lidocaine values, although to my knowledge this has not been studied in regard to tumescent anesthesia.

Although total plasma lidocaine is what has been measured in studies, it is the unbound free lidocaine that is active. The bound portion of lidocaine is associated with the acute-phase protein alpha-1 acid glycoprotein (AAG). Albumin also binds a small portion of plasma lidocaine. A decrease in AAG or albumin may therefore cause an increased percentage of free unbound lidocaine for an equivalent total plasma lidocaine value.

Lidocaine clearance may also be influenced by decreased hepatic perfusion and drug interactions. Decreased hepatic perfusion may be due to liver disease, beta blockers, or decreased cardiac output with congestive heart failure or shock.

Drug interactions influencing decreased lidocaine clearance rates primarily involve the cytochrome P450 oxidase system. Lidocaine is metabolized to Monoethylglycinexylidide (MEGX). MEGX is further metabolized to glycinexylidide, xylidide, 4-hydroxylidide, and 3-hydroxylidocaine. 4-hydroxylidide is the primary urinary metabolite.

Klein, among others, has written on the potential for drugs, which inhibit the P450 3A4 isoenzymes to decrease hepatic clearance of lidocaine. These drugs include antibiotics such as erythromycin, clarithromycin, and ciprofloxacin. Antifungals fluconazole, ketoconazole, and itraconazole as well as all of the SSRI antidepressants and nefazodone may also inhibit P450 3A4. Calcium channel blocker bromocriptine, cimetidine, cyclosporin, grapefruit juice, methadone, methylprednisolone, tamoxifen, valproic acid, and zafirlukast are also P450 3A4 inhibitors.

Recent studies have shown that P450 1A2 may be more responsible for the metabolism of lidocaine to MEGX. Studies have demonstrated that potent P450 3A4 inhibitors erythromycin and itraconazole had little effect on plasma lidocaine concentrations. Fluvoxamine, a P450 1A2 inhibitor did, however, significantly reduce lidocaine clearance resulting in elevated plasma lidocaine measurements. Other P450 1A2 inhibitors are drugs, which also inhibit P450 3A4 enzymes. Hopefully future studies will more clearly elucidate the role of the P450 3A4 and 1A2 systems.

Plasma lidocaine levels of 3 to 5 ng/mL may produce annoying subjective symptoms such as a metallic taste, circumoral numbness, tinnitus, agitation, and nausea. Levels of about 5 to 6 ng/mL may produce tremors and shaking. Above 9 ng/mL seizures, cardiotoxicity, coma, and cardiac or respiratory arrest may occur.

Klein's article "Tumescent technique for regional anesthesia permits lidocaine doses of 35 mg/kg for liposuction" published in 1990 established this level as generally safe. Ostad et al. in 1996 demonstrated that a level of 55 mg/kg of lidocaine can be safely administered under ideal conditions. This is the upper limit now generally accepted in state and society guidelines. Although much higher doses of lidocaine have been used on numerous occasions since 1988 without significant sequelae, because of unique individual variations it is prudent to adhere to these established guidelines.

TUMESCENT ANESTHESIA

One of the most important aspects of tumescent anesthesia is formulating the ingredients correctly. Improper mixing of the tumescent solution is probably the riskiest part of liposuction with tumescent anesthesia.

I have had at least three personal experiences in which colleagues have sought my opinion during or shortly after a procedure. In one instance, a patient displayed signs of mild lidocaine toxicity even though slightly less than 40 mg/kg had been given. The physician obtained a plasma lidocaine level, which was greater than 6 ng/mL. Fortunately, he had not discarded the remainder of the tumescent solution. When this was analyzed, no epinephrine was present in the solution. This had allowed the lidocaine to be absorbed much more rapidly yielding an earlier and higher peak concentration.

On another occasion, a colleague called and stated that one of his young male patients had experienced a severe tachycardia requiring resuscitation after rapid infiltration of tumescent solution under general anesthesia. At this particular institution, it was required that the pharmacy mix up the solution. Apparently 10 amps of 1:1,000 epinephrine had been placed in 1 L of saline rather than the customary 1 amp.

On another occasion, a plastic surgeon's nurse mixed up a 1% concentration of lidocaine rather than the requested 0.2% concentration. Under IV sedation, the patient was rapidly given slightly greater than 100 mg/kg resulting in a fatal outcome.

Klein's original tumescent formula consisted of adding 1000 mg of lidocaine (100 cc of 1% lidocaine or 50 cc of 2% lidocaine) and 1 amp of 1:1,000 epinephrine to a liter of normal saline. This produced a 0.1% lidocaine with 1:1,000,000 epinephrine concentration. Eventually the use of 500 mg lidocaine/L of saline became a more commonly used concentration. For the past 7 to 10 years, I have used exclusively a 0.05% concentration with 1:1,000 epinephrine and have found this adequate in all situations.

In 1988 after a publication by McKay W. et al., in anesthesia and analgesia, I started adding about 12 mg/L of sodium bicarbonate to the tumescent solution. The decreased pain on injection was immediately apparent. Later studies demonstrated that lidocaine buffered in this manner is bacteriostatic against a wide range of organisms. A 0.5% concentration of lidocaine provides a dose-dependent inhibition of bacterial growth with gram-negative inhibition being greater than gram-positive inhibition. About 0.05% lidocaine is bacteriostatic for *Staphylococcus aurous*.

During the 1990s, Dr. Klein suggested adding 10 mg/cc of triamcinolone to the tumescent solution. A small percentage of his patients had experienced sterile subcutaneous inflammatory nodules unresponsive to antibiotics. With Dr. Klein's suggestion, many of us started adding triamcinolone to our formulations. Sometime thereafter, Dr. Klein stopped adding triamcinolone. He felt that the "post liposuction panniculitis" that seemed to be prevented by triamcinolone was actually related to the use of "open drainage and bimodal compression" which he coincidentally had initiated at about the same time he started adding triamcinolone.

In my experience, I felt that when I initiated the use of triamcinolone, my patients seemed to have less post-op morbidity. When I stopped using it, both I and my staff felt that our patients in general were more uncomfortable during their early post op course. When I reinstituted the use of triamcinolone, it was again my impression that it was of worthwhile benefit. I have continued to use triamcinolone 10 mg/L as part of my tumescent solution except in areas that will be used for fat transfer.

Warming of the tumescent solution to body temperature is helpful in both decreasing the discomfort of infiltration and decreasing loss of body heat. Uncomfortable chilling is still intermittently a problem but much less so than when tumescent solution is instilled at room temperature. Whenever I have tried to infiltrate tumescent solution warmed up to 105°F (to help decrease loss of body heat), the solution seemed to have a decreased analgesic effect. I have heard this opinion expressed by a few other physicians.

The role of epinephrine in tumescent solution is critical. Without epinephrine, blood loss would be significant (although not to the degree encountered in the "dry technique") and lidocaine would be absorbed too readily into the systemic circulation. The most commonly used concentration of epinephrine is 1:1,000,000. Studies have shown that even a concentration of 1:2,000,000 is effective. It is not known how quickly epinephrine is metabolized, but epinephrine toxicity has not, to my knowledge, occurred at this concentration. Typically an Iccamp of 1:1,000 epinephrine is added to the tumescent solution rather than epinephrine already previously mixed with lidocaine.

TECHNIQUE

The patient is marked preoperatively in the standing position with a "Sharpie" marker. Most experienced liposuction surgeons have developed their own marking systems, which have evolved over time. Accurate marking is essential. Once the area treated is tumesced, all physical landmarks will be erased.

My particular marking system is quite simple. The areas to be suctioned are outlined. X's are placed over the areas of greatest lipodystrophy, the larger the X's, the thicker the fat pad. If there is a sharp demarcation of the area to be treated with the surrounding area, a solid line is used. Dotted lines or dotted lines beyond the solid lines indicate areas where blending is optimal. Areas not to be entered (e.g., depressions) will have the word "NO" written on them (Figs. 1 and 2).

Prepping is done with standard solutions such as Hibiclens or Betadine followed by the use of sterile drapes over the surrounding areas not to be treated. Areas distant from treated areas may be covered with blankets, caps, booties, etc. Many devices are available to help with warming. Typically we use the "Bair Hugger Warmer" and place a hot water bottle on the patient's chest (Fig. 3). A blanket warming cabinet is also very helpful in this regard (Fig. 4).

As mentioned previously, the "Klein needle" was a significant advancement over syringe/needle delivery of anesthesia. The use of peristaltic pumps has greatly decreased the discomfort of the administration of tumescent anesthesia and significantly shortened the time to obtain adequate anesthesia (Fig. 5). It has also greatly decreased the workload for those administering anesthesia.

Peristaltic pumps have a dial in feature, which controls the rate of infusion. The rate of infusion will vary depending on the degree of sedation, the patient's tolerance, and the areas being infiltrated. Areas that are more fibrous

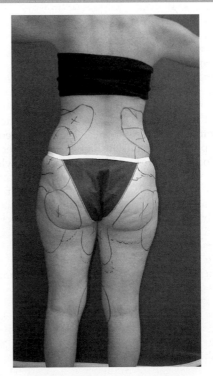

Figure 1 Preoperative marking.

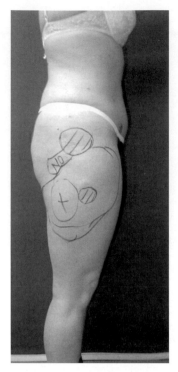

Figure 2   Preoperative marking.

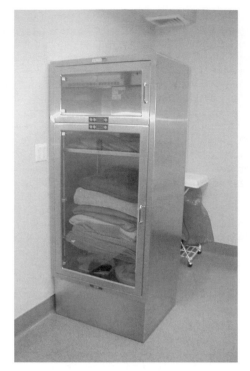

Figure 4   Blanket warming cabinet.

usually are more uncomfortable to anesthetize. Touch-up areas are frequently more uncomfortable to anesthetize due to the presence of scar tissue from previous procedures. Younger patients, especially if lean, have tighter, tauter tissues, which create more resistance to the diffusion and expansion of the tumescent solution.

Having two assistants delivering tumescent anesthesia simultaneously does not increase the discomfort (Fig. 6). The duration of delivery of tumescent anesthesia is nearly halved. The end point is the absence of burning, stinging, or sharpness. Occasionally, total tumescence will be achieved without adequate anesthesia. In this instance, a disposable McGhan's spring-loaded tissue expander is used to precisely anesthetize any remaining "hot spots" without administering

excessive solution (Fig. 7). The patient must be aware that sensations of pulling, tugging, pressure, and vibration will not be eliminated. The McGhan syringe is also useful for anesthetizing small areas such as neck/jowls or inner knees (Fig. 8).

Infusion cannulas for delivery of tumescent anesthesia are usually of the "garden spray" variety (Fig. 9). These are blunt tipped 12 to 14 gauge, 6- to 12-inch long cannulas, with small holes a variable length of the way down the shaft. About 18 to 20 gauge spinal needles have also been commonly used. There is obviously an inherent risk in their use. In our office, spinal needles are used commonly to start the procedure and infiltrate into the superficial and upper mid-fat. Only assistants with vast experience in

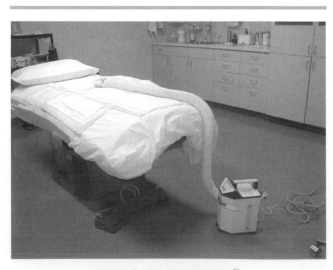

Figure 3   Bair Hugger warmer®

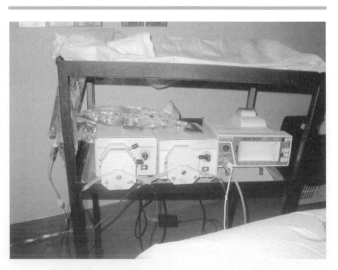

Figure 5   Peristaltic pump for delivery of anesthesia.

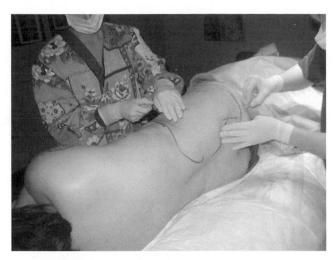

Figure 6 Two assistants delivering tumescent anethesia.

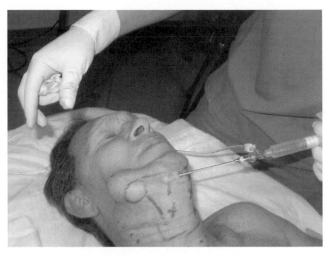

Figure 8 McGhar Sylinge.

administering tumescent anesthesia are allowed to use spinal needles.

Incision sites for administering tumescent anesthesia are made with a #11 blade on "nondrainage sites" and with a 1.5 to 2.0 mm punch on dependent "drainage sites" to facilitate thorough evacuation of tumescent fluid. Thorough evacuation of tumescent fluid postoperatively is important in obtaining optimum cosmetic results and decreasing morbidity. It is my practice to insert the largest cannula I will use in a particular case into the most camouflaged sites (usually suprapubic) to open them to a greater degree thereby maximizing and prolonging drainage.

It is important to stress repeatedly to the patient and the patient's companion that during the first evening, drainage may seem overwhelming. This is especially true after abdominal liposuction and even more so for large volume abdominal liposuction. The patient should be told that the drainage will look like blood but is actually 99% water. It is important to stress to the patient (and companion) that the more drainage there is, the better it will be for both rapid recovery and potential cosmetic outcome. Hopefully this will put a "positive spin" on a potentially disconcerting occurrence.

Skilled administration of tumescent anesthesia is more difficult than it appears. The beginner will typically leave numerous "hot spots." With experience, most will

acquire a sense for administering tumescent anesthesia effectively and efficiently. In my experience the "hot spots" I encounter most commonly are the periumbilical region, the posterior upper inner thigh area, and the deep flank or waist fat. I routinely test these areas gently before proceeding.

With experience, one will usually be able to estimate how much tumescent anesthesia will be necessary to anesthetize a particular area or areas. The situation in which I most commonly underestimate the amount of fat present is in patients with very good skin tone. The thickness of the dermis and lack of "sag" can effectively hide the amount of subcutaneous adipose tissue present.

In my experience, "hot spots" are found on large abdomens more commonly than on any other areas. It is not uncommon to add a significant amount of tumescent anesthesia to the sensitive areas encountered during the liposuction procedure. For this reason, I reduce the amount of tumescent anesthesia my assistants are allowed to deliver if a large abdomen and other areas are treated during the same session. More tumescent solution will then be in reserve, if necessary, to adequately anesthetize any remaining sensitive areas and at the same time avoid exceeding the recommended guidelines of lidocaine administration.

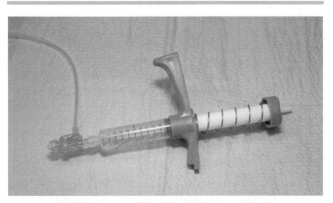

Figure 7 McGhan spring-loaded tissue expander.

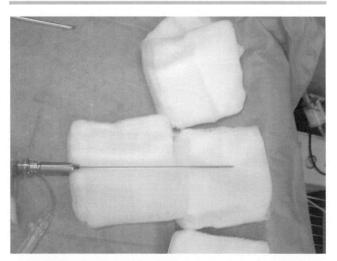

Figure 9 Infusion cannula for delivery of tumescent anesthesia.

Although tumescent anesthesia may effectively numb subcutaneous tissue within 15 to 20 minutes, and epinephrine may produce adequate hemostasis in 20 to 30 minutes, it is often helpful to wait 40 to 60 minutes after infusion to begin liposuction. Skin overlying tumesced areas, especially at the periphery, may take up to an hour to become numb. It is not uncommon for the patient to feel the puncture on the skin surface even though the subcutaneous tissue is adequately anesthetized. This is not often a problem when multiple areas are treated during the same session if the sequence of liposuction is done in the same order that the individual areas are anesthetized.

Tumescent solution accumulates around the interstitial spaces surrounding the adipocytes. When one does excisional surgery after tumescent anesthesia, the absolute lack of capillary and venous oozing is striking. The appearance of the fat is swollen and gelatinous.

OTHER USES

The beneficial features of tumescent anesthesia for other soft-tissue surgery are apparent. Large doses of local anesthesia can be safely administered, achieving profound hemostasis and prolonged postoperative analgesia.

Tumescent anesthesia changed liposuction from a general anesthetic procedure with significant blood loss to a walk in/walk out local anesthetic procedure where significant blood loss is absent. The use of tumescent anesthesia to perform other soft tissue surgical procedures can include facial flap surgery, scalp surgery, facelifts, rhinophyma, hair transplantation, dermabrasion, treatment of axillary hyperhidrosis, treatment of varicose veins, excision of lipomas and other soft tissue masses, outpatient proctologic procedures, anesthesia for axillary hair removal, anesthesia for burn debridement, and skin graft harvesting as well as other uses.

In applying the principles of tumescent anesthesia to scalp surgery (scalp flap, scalp reduction, and hair transplantation) profound hemostasis achieved is a significant benefit. Hydrodissection of the galea from the periosteum facilitates subgaleal undermining in scalp reduction and scalp flaps. In hair transplantation, the tumescence of donor tissue mimics a common practice of instilling saline in the donor areas prior to harvesting. Total anesthesia lasts hours longer than traditional local anesthesia. Coleman elicited feedback from 10 consecutive hair transplant patients all who had previously undergone hair transplantation with traditional local anesthesia. All preferred tumescent anesthesia.

Tumescent anesthesia provides many advantages when used in facial dermabrasion. The firmness provided by "tumescing" the tissues eliminates the need for cryogens. Cryosurgical preparation of the skin prior to dermabrasion may increase the risk of scarring (especially over the bony prominences), pigmentary disturbances, and postoperative swelling and edema.

When tumescent anesthesia is used in rhinophyma or postsurgical dermabrasion of nasal scars and sebaceous skin, dermabrasion is facilitated. Significant hemostasis allows one to effectively dermabrade thick sebaceous skin eliminating the considerable risk of scarring encountered in electrosurgery. Dermabrasion for acne scarring, wrinkles, actinic damage, and appendageal tumors such as neurofibromas and angiofibromas may also be performed with tumescent anesthesia.

The amount of local anesthetic needed for a facelift and other facial reconstructive procedures is reduced by the use of tumescent anesthesia. Profound hemostasis and profound anesthesia allow for a more uneventful and comfortable postoperative course. Risk of hematoma formation is decreased, and there is a definite reduction in bruising.

Tumescent anesthesia has improved the treatment of severe axillary hyperhidrosis. Prior to the development of tumescent anesthesia, severe, recalcitrant axillary hyperhidrosis was routinely treated by axillary excision. Postoperative infections were frequent. Hematomas and wound dehiscence were not uncommon. Scar contractures would often limit range of motion at least to a minor degree. Unattractive scars were often a cosmetic problem, especially in female patients.

Liposuction of the axilla after tumescent anesthesia is an efficient simple procedure, with nearly 100% success rate when executed properly. Scars are two to three in number, one-eighth to one-quarter of an inch in diameter, and are well hidden. Infections are almost never encountered. Recovery is rapid, and scar contracture does not occur. Profound hemostasis virtually eliminates the risk of hematoma formation. Prolonged anesthesia provides for a comfortable postoperative recovery.

Proebstle reported the use for tumescent anesthesia for subdermal curettage for axillary hyperhidrosis. In August 2004 J Am Acad of Derm, Krejci-Manwaring et al. reported on the use of tumescent anesthesia to eliminate the pain of axillary hair removal. I have used tumescent anesthesia prior to axillary Botox injections for hyperhidrosis with positive patient feedback. The axillary vault is easily distensible. The delivery of tumescent anesthesia to the axilla is rapid and relatively painless.

Tumescent anesthesia may also be used during Mohs' surgery especially in large lesions when the amount of local anesthetic to be repeatedly injected surpasses the recommended maximum of 5 to 7 mg/kg. Tumescent anesthesia is also useful for raising perichondrium off of cartilage. Anesthesia is prolonged, and capillary oozing is virtually eliminated.

Use of tumescent anesthesia for ambulatory phlebectomy has been described by Seiger et al. Regional or general anesthesia is unnecessary when performing this procedure in this manner. Proebstle reported in Dermal Surgery on using exclusively tumescent anesthesia for subfascial endoscopic perforator surgery in nearly all of 40 patients. Five patients required additional intravenous analgesics. Four of the five had marked dermatosclerosis.

Balducci reported on 80 cases in which ambulatory saphenectomy (saphenous stripping) was performed with tumescent anesthesia. Brief propofol sedation was required in some patients. They concluded that tumescent anesthesia resulted in less bleeding during and after surgery in all patients by visual observation of ecchymoses at 3 and 7 days. All patients experienced good postsurgical analgesia without functional impairment.

Eichhorn reported on the use of tumescent anesthesia in 195 patients undergoing sentinel lymph node biopsy of the axilla or groin. About 75% of the patients required only tumescent anesthesia. Bassen et al. performed 50 proctologic procedures with tumescent anesthesia. Procedures included perianal vein thrombectomy, subanodermal fistula resection, anal polyp resection, fissurectomy, perianal abscess revision, excision of anal skin, hemorrhoidectomy, intersphincteric fistula extirpation and pilonidal sinus, and perianal tumor excisions.

In December 2003, Bussolin et al. reported in the Journal of Anesthesiology on the use of tumescent anesthesia in pediatric burn patients. In 30 consecutive Class 1 or II burn patients 1 month to 10 years old, induction of anesthesia with nitrous oxide–oxygen–seroflurane was followed by infiltration of tumescent anesthesia. The maximum dose given was 7 mg/kg. After the initial incision for debridement or autologous graft harvesting, no response to painful stimuli was observed and there were no complications. Only five patients required analgesia postoperatively and this was limited to oral acetominophen.

There are undoubtedly numerous other potential applications for the use of tumescent anesthesia. As other specialties become more aware of the unique characteristics of tumescent anesthesia, other applications will be discovered. Dr. Jeffrey Klein's contribution has undoubtedly not only decreased the morbidity of liposuction (and other procedures) but has also significantly decreased mortality. For a detailed scholarly discussion of liposuction and tumescent anesthesia, I would highly recommend Dr. Klein's textbook *Tumescent Technique* (by C.V. Mosby, Inc.).

BIBLIOGRAPHY

Albright GA. Cardiac arrest following regional anesthesia with etidocaine or bupivacaine. Anesthesiology 1979; 51:285.

Allen GD. Nitrous oxide-oxygen sedation machines and devices.
J Am Dent Assoc 1974; 88:611.

Balducci D. Ambulatory saphenectomy: 80 operated cases using tumescent anesthesia. Chir Ital 2002; 54(1):77–82.

Bargetzi MJ, Aoyama T, Gonzalez FJ, et al. Lidocaine metabolism in human liver microsomes by cytochrome P450II1A4. Clin Pharmacol Ther 1989; 46:521–527.

Bieter RN. Applied pharmacology of local anesthetics. Am J Surg 1936; 34:500.

Bill TJ, Clayman MA, Morgan RF, Gampper TJ. Lidocaine metabolism: patho-physiology, drug interactions and surgical implications. Aesth Surg J 2004:307–311.

Bridenstine J. Letter to the editor. J Dermatol Surg Oncol 1989; 15(7):775–776.

Bussen D. Tumescent local anesthesia in proctologic surgery. Chirurg 2003; 74(9):839–843.

Bussolin L, Busoni P, Giorgi L, Crescioli M, Messeri A. Pain and regional anesthesia: tumescent local anesthesia for the surgical treatment of burns and postburn sequelae in pediatric patients. Anesthesiology 2003; 99(6):1371–1375.

Coleman WP III, Klein JA. Use of tumescent technique for scalp surgery, dermabrasion and soft tissue reconstruction. J Dermatol Surg Oncol 1992; 18:130–135.

Courtiss EH, Choucair RF, Donelan MB. Large volume suction lipectomy: an analysis of 108 patients. Plast Reconstr Surg 1992; 89:1080–1082.

Cozza KL, Armstrong SC. The Cytochrome p450 System: Drug Interaction Principles for Medical Practice. Washington, D.C.: American Psychiatric Publishing, 2001:47–68.

Dolsky R, Fetzek J, Anderson R. Evaluation of blood loss during liposuction surgery. Am J Cosm Surgery 1987; 4:257–261.

Eichhorn K. Sentinel node biopsy in melanoma of the trunk and the extremities in tumescent local anesthesia. Dermatol Surg 2004; 30(2 Pt 2):253–256.

Gajraj RJ, Hodson MJ, Gillespie JA, et al. Antibacterial activity of lidocaine in mixtures with Diprivan. Br J Anaesth 1998; 81:444.

Grazer FM, de Jong RH. Fatal outcomes from liposuction: census survey of cosmetic surgeons. Plast Reconstr Surg 2000; 105:436–448.

Imaoka S, Enomoto K, Oda Y, et al. Lidocaine metabolism by human cytochrome P-450s purified from hepatic microsomes: comparison of those with rat hepatic cytochrome P-450S. J Pharmacol Exp Ther 1990; 255:1385–1391.

Isohanni MH, Neuvonen PJ, Palkama VJ, et al. Effect of erythromycin and itraconazole on the pharmacokinetics of intravenous lignocaine. Eur J Clin Pharmacol 1998; 54:561–565.

Kaplan B, Moy RL. Comparison of room temperature and warmed local anesthetic solution for tumescent liposuction. Dermatol Surg 1996; 22:707–709.

Karlsson E, Collste R, Rawlins MD. Plasma levels of lidocaine during combined treatment with phenytoin and procainamide. Eur J Clin Pharmacol 1974; 7:455.

Kharasch ED, Mulroy M, Apfelbaum J. Commentary: lidocaine metabolism: patho-physiology, drug interactions and surgical implications. Aesth Surg J 2004:311–313.

Kiak GA, Koontz FF, Chavez AJ. Lidocaine inhibits growth of *Staphylococcus aureus* in propofol. Anesthesiology 1992; 77:A407.

Klein J. Tumescent technique. Am J Cosm Surg 1987; 4:263–267.

Klein JA. Anesthesia for liposuction and dermatologic surgery. J Dermatol Surg Oncol 1988; 14:1124–1132.

Klein JA. Antibacterial effects of tumescent lidocaine. Plast Reconstr Surg 1996; 104(6):1934–1936.

Klein JA. Tumescent technique for local anesthesia: improved safety in large volume liposuction. J Plast Reconstr Surg 1993; 92:1085–1098.

Klein JA. Tumescent technique for regional anesthesia permits lidocaine doses of 35 mg/kg for liposuction. J Dermatol Surg Oncol 1990; 16:248–263.

Klingenstrom P, Westermark L. Local effects of adrenalin and phenylalanyl-lysyl-vasopressin in local anesthesia. Acta Anaesthesiol Scand 1963; 7:131.

Krejci-Manwaring J, Markus J, Goldberg L, Friedman P, Markus R. Surgical pearl: tumescent anesthesia reduces pain of axillary laser hair removal. J Am Acad of Dermatol 2004; 51(2).

Lillis PJ, Coleman WP III. Liposuction for treatment of axillary hyperhidrosis. In: Lillis PJ, Coieman WP III, eds. Dermatologic Clinics: Liposuction. Philadelphia: Saunders, 1990; 8(3):479–482.

Lillis PJ. The tumescent technique for liposuction surgery. Dermatologic Clinics: Liposuction. Philadelphia: Saunders 1990; 8(3):439–450.

Lillis PJ. Liposuction surgery under local anesthesia: limited blood loss and minimal lidocaine absorption. J Dermatol Surg Oncol 1988; 14:1145–1148.

Lunn JN, Mushin WW. Mortality associated with anesthesia. Anesthesiology 1982; 37:856.

Matarasso A. Superwet anesthesia redefines large-volume liposuction. Aesth Surg J 1997; 17:358–364.

McKay W, Morris R, Mushlin P. Sodium bicarbonate attenuates pain on skin infiltration with lidocaine with or without epinephrine. Anesth Analg 1987; 65:572.

Metz H III, Gilliland M, Patronella C. Abdominal etching: differential liposuction to detail abdominal musculature. Aesthetic Plast Surg 1993; 17:287–290.

Miller MA, Shell WB. Antimicrobial properties of lidocaine on bacteria isolated from dermal lesions. Arch Dermatol 1985; 121:1157.

Nattel S, Rinkenberger RL, Lehrman LL, Zipes DP. Therapeutic blood lidocaine concentrations after local anesthesia for cardiac electrophysiologic studies. N Engl J Med 1979; 301:418.

Orlando R, Piccoli P, De Martin S, et al. Effect of the CYP3A4 inhibitor erythromycin on the pharmacokinetics of lignocaine and its pharmacologically active metabolites in subjects with normal and impaired liver function. Br J Clin Pharmacol 2003; 55:86–93.

Ostad A, Kageyama N, Moy RL. Tumescent anesthesia with a lidocaine dose of 55 mg/kg is safe for liposuction. Dermatol Surg 1996; 22:921–927.

Park BK, Pirmohamed M, Kitteringham NR. The role of cytochrome P450 enzymes in hepatic and extrahepatic human drug toxicity. Pharmacol Ther 1995; 68:385–424.

Parr AM, Zoutman DE, Davidson JSD. Antimicrobial activity of lidocaine against bacteria associated with nosocomial wound infection. Ann Plast Surg 1999; 43:239–245.

Physician's Desk Reference. Oradell, NJ: Medical Economics Co, Inc., 1989:640.

Proebstle TM. Gravimetrically controlled efficacy of subcorial curettage: a prospective study for treatment of axillary hyperhidrosis. Dermatol Surg 2002; 28(11):1022–1026.

Proebstle TM. Subfascial endoscopic perforator surgery with tumescent local anesthesia. Dermatol Surg 2002; 28(8): 689–693.

Rao RB, Ely SF, Hoffman RS. Deaths related to liposuction. N Engl J Med 1999; 340:1471–1475.

Replogle S. Experience with tumescent technique in lipoplasty. Aesthetic Plast Surg 1993; 17:205–209.

Scott DB, Jebson P Jr., Braid DP, Ortengren B. Factors affecting plasma lidocaine levels of lignocaine and prilocaine. Br J Anesth 1972; 44:1040.

Seiger E, Goldman S, Cohn M. Ambulatory phlebectomy using the tumescent technique for local anesthesia. J Dermatol Surg 1995.

Singer Ml, Shapiro LE, Shear NH. Cytochrome P450 3A: interactions with dermatologic therapies. J Am Acad Dermatol 1997; 37:765–771.

Steen PA, Tinker JH, Tarhan S. Myocardial reinfarction after anesthesia and surgery. JAMA 1978; 239:25–66.

Stenson RE, Constantino RT, Harrison DC. Interrelationships of hepatic blood flow, cardiac output, and blood levels of lidocaine in man. Circulation 1971; 43:205–211.

Sung CY, Truant AP. The physiological disposition of lidocaine and its comparison in some respects with procaine. J Pharmacol Exp Ther 1954; 112:432.

Swart EL, van der Hoven B, Groeneveld AB, et al. Correlation between midazolam and lignocaine pharmacokinetics and MEGX formation in healthy volunteers. Br J Clin Pharmacol 2002; 53:133–139.

Thompson K, Welykyj S, Massa M. Antibacterial activity of lidocaine in combination with a bicarbonate buffer. J Dermatol Surg Oncol 1993; 19:216–220.

Tucker GT, Mather LE. Pharmacokinetics of local anaesthetic agents. Br J Anaesth 1975; 47:213–224.

Wang JS, Backman JT, Taavitsainen P, et al. Involvement of CYP1A2 and CYP3A4 in lidocaine N-deethylation and 3-hydroxylation in humans. Drug Metab Dispos 2000; 28:959–965.

10

Wound Healing

Hann Lee, Yong Li, Tania Phillips, and David T. Woodley
The Division of Dermatology and the Section of Plastic Surgery, The Keck School of Medicine
University of Southern California, Los Angeles, California, U.S.A.

INTRODUCTION

Skin wounds are a major clinical problem in medicine. The wounds can be pathogenic such as the estimated annual 1.25 million burn victims or the 6.5 million patients with chronic skin ulcers, or they can be iatrogenic from surgical procedures. The average dermatologist performs 700 to 1000 skin biopsies or excisions per year and all surgical specialties must create skin wounds in the course of their routine surgical procedures. Wound healing in the skin is a complex orchestration of cellular processes that have been efficiently perfected throughout the eons of phylogeny. So many coordinated biological processes are invoked both simultaneously and in a regulated orderly fashion, that it has been likened to a recapitulation of gestation. Part of the problem with studying wound healing is dissecting out the processes independently and then seeing how they fit together and influence each other. In this chapter, we will review selected aspects of the known biology of skin wound healing, present some contemporary clinical therapies for skin wounds, and then end with newer scientific observations that provide insight into the biology of human skin wound healing.

PHASES OF WOUND HEALING

According to Singer and Clark, the healing of skin wounds can be subdivided into three stages that overlap in time. Stage I is clotting and Inflammation. This occurs immediately after the wound is made and the clotting cascade is invoked by the disruption of blood vessels. During this time, the skin tissues, which are usually bathed in plasma, are now suddenly bathed in serum. In serum, the clotting proteins have been consumed and the contents of platelets are extruded releasing platelet-derived growth factors (PDGF) into the serum. Note that epidermal growth factor (EGF), PDGF, and transforming growth factor α (TGF-α) are significantly higher in serum than plasma. These soluble growth factors may play important roles in the ultimate healing of the skin wound. For example, macrophages and fibroblasts are activated and attracted by soluble cytokines and growth factors, which are generated from the coagulation and platelet clotting processes. These factors also are proinflammatory, activate complement, and recruit leukocytes to the site of injury. The plasma-to-serum transition also creates a clot within the wound space that serves as a primordial nidus of solid material that will provide a provisional matrix, which becomes granulation tissue, a neodermis, and ultimately a healed reconstituted dermis.

The clot forms the provisional matrix that keratinocytes migrate over to reepithelialize the wound, and during this process migrating keratinocytes are in contact with fibrin, fibrinogen, fibronectin, and fragments of collagen.

Stage II has been called the stage of tissue formation or granulation tissue formation. In this stage, much is happening at the same time. Endothelial cells are coming into the clot/provisional matrix to form new vascular tubes, a process called "neovascularization." At the same time, fibroblast that are resident around the clot and wound also migrate into the clot to begin to lay down new collagen, fibronectin, hyaluronic acid, and other dermal matrix molecules; this process is called "fibroplasia." Although keratinocytes at the margins of the wound and at the cut edges of skin appendages begin to move within the first 24 to 72 hours of wounding, reepithelialization, which started as in Stage I, reaches its full capacity during Stage II. Also, during this stage, keratinocytes in the stationary epidermis just behind the advancing epidermal tongue begin to proliferate and contribute additional keratinocytes to the migrating epithelial advancing tongue.

During this stage, PDGF is responsible for the fibroblast ingress into the clot/granulation tissue and the presence of transforming growth factor β (TGF-β) stimulates the fibroblasts to synthesize and deposit matrix macromolecules such as collagen and fibronectin.

Stage III of wound healing has been called the stage of wound contraction and tissue remodeling. This is the longest of the three phases and may continue for up to a year. Interestingly, the tensile strength of the healed wound skin never gets made to that of a unwounded skin. During the beginning of the phase, at roughly days 7 to 10 after the wound, some fibroblasts change their phenotype to become myofibroblasts, which can be recognized by containing large bundles of actin-containing microfilaments.

CLINICAL ADVANCES IN WOUND HEALING

Likely because of natural selection, living creatures are very adept at healing cutaneous wounds. Although many components of the wound-healing cascade have been characterized, the use of these mediators to improve the wound healing has not been universally successful. Recombinant EGF has been shown to spend the healing of skin graft donor sites and human recombinant-PDGF (rh-PDGF) increases the efficiency of healing when healing is impaired, such as in diabetic foot ulcers or pressure ulcers. However, many other proteins have been tested and not been found to significantly alter the wound healing. Further, when the mediators affect healing in clinical studies or experimental models, the gain in wound-healing time is minimal. Because they are quite expensive, the cost benefit ratio is not favorable. It has been difficult for biotechnology advances to improve on the designs of Mother Nature. As pointed out by Singer and Clark, "The overall clinical experience with growth factors and other mediators to accelerate wound healing has been discouraging."

Another confounding factor that makes the true data-driven conclusions about the healing of human skin wounds is the paucity of controlled studies. Using historical controls is fraught with errors. This is because when a patient with a chronic skin wound is entered into a study, they tend to do much better than historical controls in the general population even if they are getting the placebo agent, because they and the study team are paying great attention to the wound and compliance for general wound care, which goes way up compared with similar patients not in the study. Another confounding variable is the fact that it is almost impossible to test identical wounds in a study, in the same patient or paired patients. The history of a wound and its size and shape and bacterial colonization, anatomical location, and vessel and nerve innervation are relatively singular. Wound-healing comparison studies in humans are difficult to control adequately. This makes evidence-based medicine for human skin wounds problematic. This also means in terms of therapy for acute and chronic wounds. There is more tradition and art than much evidence-based support for a given therapy. Perhaps, one of the most notable examples of this is the use of hydrogen peroxide as a recommended part of a patient's wound care regime. Hydrogen peroxide is not a particularly good antiseptic or debridement reagent. It likely gives the patient something to do and usually is harmless when used on the head and neck. Nevertheless, it has been shown that hydrogen peroxide in concentrations used clinically likely inhibits the migration of human keratinocytes. Table 1 summorizes current techniques and products for wound healing.

Autologous Cultured Keratinocytes for Burn Wounds

Since the development of techniques to culture epidermal keratinocytes, autologous cultured keratinocyte sheets have been used to heal burn wounds in children and adults. These have a theoretical advantage, as a small skin biopsy could be used to introduce the keratinocytes into tissue culture and expanded over two to four weeks into large sheets of epidermis that could be transplanted back onto prepared wound sites on the patient. These are currently commercially available (Genzyme). Despite clinical success and the survival of patients with greater than 90% body surface area burns, the technique has not been generally accepted. The technical demands of a meticulously prepared burn wound site, the delay of two to four weeks for the cultures to expand, and the lack of improved outcome has limited the impact of this technique.

Cultured Allogeneic Keratinocyte Sheets for Wounds

Allogeneic cultured keratinocyte grafts have been used to heal a variety of chronic cutaneous wounds including venous stasis ulcers, allogeneic, and even pyoderma gangrenosum. Because the grafts come from the same species but not the same person, the grafts take, but do not persist. Nevertheless, their presence on the wound even for a short period of time has beneficial effects. The grafts provide protection to the wound from desiccation, reduce pain, condition the wound bed, and provide keratinocyte-derived

growth factors such as PDGF and EGF that may help accelerate the wound-healing process.

Allogeneic and Xenogeneic Dermis to Cover Wounds

In a somewhat analogous manner, wound beds can be "conditioned" to promote wound healing or to accept autologous split-thickness skin grafts by the temporary grafting of allogeneic human cadaver dermis or even xenogeneic pig dermis. This temporary cover appears to have the effect of down regulating the wound inflammatory process and firms the wound bed. It also provides a temporary cover to protect the wound victim and diminishes the pain at the wound site. Although most dermal graft covers are treated by freezing and thawing and/or gamma irradiation to get rid of the cellular components of the dermis, there may be some residual cells that survive these measures and are able to contribute growth factors to the wound bed as well.

The Role of Antibiotics in Wounds

When wound healing is delayed or fails, local wound infection is usually a contributor. Many practitioners find that many chronic wounds heal simply by daily treatment with broad-spectrum topical antibiotics, such as Silvadene. These daily dressings have the disadvantage of requiring repeated, painful, and messy dressings. A recently developed alternative is the use of silver-releasing dressings. The best known and studied of these, Acticoat, has a broad-spectrum of activity against resistant gram-positive and gram-negative pathogens and releases antibacterial levels of silver for three to seven days, depending on the particular product. This allows antibacterial treatment without the need for frequent dressings. Further, the silver appears to displace the zinc ions in matrix metalloproteinases linked to wound chronicity (Greg Schultz PhD, University of Florida, personal communication).

Although appropriate antibacterial treatment can be essential for wound treatment, certain antibiotics applied topically to wounds can inhibit wound healing. Povidone iodine, for example, is known to inhibit the wound from healing. Nevertheless, a newer formulation of iodine, cadexomer iodine, is a slow release agent in which the iodine is released into the wound in small amounts from dextrin beads. In a recent study, Zhoe and coworkers showed that this type of slow release iodine preparation is not toxic to skin cells at the concentrations used clinically, does not inhibit keratinocyte migration, and does not depress the proliferative capacity of fibroblasts. This finding is consistent with clinical studies that indicate that cadexomer iodine is useful in venous stasis ulcers and other types of skin ulcers.

Venous Ulcers

The cornerstone of therapy for venous ulcers remains compression. It is generally agreed that venous ulcers heal more rapidly with compression than without, and that high compression is better than low compression.

In the United States, inelastic compression with the Una boot or Duke boot tends to be favored. In the United Kingdom, multilayered elastic compression bandaging is the treatment of choice, while in Europe and Australia, short stretch bandages are used. There are no clear data as to which is the optimal type of compression system.

For immobile patients, elastic bandages are recommended because inelastic bandages will fail to generate adequate compression if the calf muscle pump is weak or ineffective. For patients with a degree of arterial insufficiency, inelastic bandages, which exert low pressure at rest,

Table 1 Current Products to Aid Wound Healing

Name	Description	Advantage	Disadvantage	Clinical experience
		Epidermal		
EpiDex (IsoTis SA, Lausanne, Switzerland)	Tissue engineered, fully differentiated, autologous epidermal equivalent derived from QRS[a] keratinocytes of plucked anagen hair follicles	Easy application; Outpatient procedure; Rapidly growing stem cell; Relieves pain; As effective as skin graft	Limited controlled studies	Recurrent venous or arterial ulcer; Failed MSTSG[a]
Allogeneic keratinocyte sheets CEC[a]	Allogeneic keratinocyte culture derived from neonatal foreskin screened for HIV (PCR), and other virus and bacteria	Rapid in vitro growth; Immediate availability; No need for biopsy; Longer storage time (indefinite at −120°C and 6 mo at −20°C); Low cost and effective on ulcers of different etiology	Lack of dermal component; Not commercially available; Limited controlled trials	Burn, venous and diabetic ulcer, STSC donor site, epidermolysis bullosa, post-Mohs, decubitus ulcer, laser, and dermabrasion wounds
Autologous (keratinocyte culture) Epicel	Autologous skin keratinocyte cultures derived from biopsy	Effective on ulcers of different etiologies	Biopsy needed; Not immediately available	Burns, venous ulcer, vibligo, mastoid cavity for chronic otorrhea, epidermolysis bullosa, pyoderma gangrenosum
		Dermal		
Biodegradable mesh with allogenic fibroblast culture Dermagraft	Biodegradable mesh of PGA[b] or PGL190[c] containing allogenic fibroblasts	Immediate availability; No need for biopsy; Full-thickness wounds; Excellent cosmetic and functional result	Needs multiple applications; Contraindicated in allergy to bovine protein	Burns; Diabetic ulcer; Full-thickness wounds
Allogeneic dermis Alloderm	Human allograft skin treated with decellularization, matrix stabilization and freeze drying	Immediate availability; Allows ultrathin STSG with less scarring; immunologically inert	Allograft procurement, virus screening	Surgical wounds
Integra	Bovine collagen and chondroitin sulfate over Silastic	Bovine collagen and chondroitin sulfate over silastic	Integral susceptibility to infection, complete wound excision before application, expensive, contraindicated in allergy to bovine proteins	Excised burn wounds
		Composite (epidermal and dermal)		
Living skin equivalent (LSE) Apligraf	Bilayered construct of human keratinocytes and dermal fibroblast with bovine Type I collagen. Matrix proteins and cytokines, lacks langerhans cells and melanocyte	Immediate availability; Easy handling; Does not require subsequent skin graft	Contraindicated in hypersensitivity to bovine product; Limited viability	Venous ulcers; Full-thickness diabetic ulcer
Skin equivalent OrCell	Bilayered cellular matrix with human keratinocyte and fibroblast in separate layers on a bioabsorbable matrix made of bovine Type I collagen	Immediate availability	Contraindicated in hypersensitivity to bovine proteins	Split-thickness donor sites in burn patients

[a]Cryopreserved epithelial culture; [b]Polyglycolic acid; [c]Polyglactin-910.

are preferable (EWMA position document: Medical Education Partnership, Ltd., London, U.K., 2003). Recurrence rates of venous ulcers are high (26%–28% in 12 months). Surgery can be helpful in reducing recurrence rates, especially in patients who have superficial venous incompetence. A recent study of 500 venous ulcer patients, which compared surgery and compression with compression alone, showed that surgical correction of superficial venous reflux could reduce 12-month ulcer recurrence. Overall 24-week healing rates were similar in the two treatment groups (65%) but 12-month recurrence rates were significantly reduced in the compression and surgery group compared to compression alone (12% vs. 28%). Thus most patients with chronic venous ulceration will benefit from the addition of simple venous surgery.

New technologies such as skin substitutes are Food and Drug Administration (FDA) approved for venous ulcers but is expensive and should be reserved for hard to heal wounds. Poor prognostic indicators for venous ulcers include large size, long duration, deep vein involvement, poor mobility, fibrin on the wound surface, ankle-brachial index (ABI) of less than 0.8, and a history of hip or knee replacement.

The rate of ulcer healing after initiation of compression therapy is also a predictor of healing; ulcers which heal slowly (less than 40% size reduction by three weeks of compression therapy or less than 0.05 cm/wk) are unlikely to heal and would likely benefit from intervention of advanced technologies.

Arterial Ulcers

In patients with arterial ulcers, surgical reestablishment of an adequate vascular supply should be performed whenever possible. Medical management includes control of diabetes mellitus or hypertension, smoking cessation, and moderate exercise. Cilostazol is a phosphodiesterase inhibitor, which has antiaggregation effects on platelets, beneficial effects on serum lipids, and vasodilator effects. This drug has been approved by the FDA for the treatment of intermittent claudication.

In a double blind randomized placebo controlled trial to evaluate the relative efficacy and safety of cilostazol versus pentoxifylline, 698 patients with moderate to severe claudication were randomly assigned to blinded treatment with either cilostazol 100 mg b.i.d., pentoxifylline 400 mg t.i.d., or placebo. Cilostazol was significantly better than pentoxifylline or placebo for increased walking distance in patients with intermittent claudication. It was, however, associated with a greater frequency of minor side effects, including headache, palpitations, and diarrhea. Pentoxifylline and placebo had similar effects. Cilostazol is currently being evaluated in a multicenter trial for arterial ulcers.

Diabetic Foot Ulcer

Neuropathic diabetic foot ulcers are a leading cause of morbidity in patients with diabetes. They develop in approximately 15% of patients with diabetes and 85% of lower limb amputations in patients with diabetes are preceded by foot ulceration. Ulceration is principally caused by neuropathy, but other causes include peripheral vascular disease, callus, edema, and deformity.

Management of diabetic neuropathic ulcers includes treatment of infection, debridement of the wound, correction of any arterial disease, and removal of pressure from the ulcer. Glycemic control should be optimized, and patients should be advised to stop smoking. Regular sharp

debridement of ulcers has been shown to promote healing. Treatment of local edema with a pneumatic compression pump in addition to debridement has been shown to improve healing compared to debridement alone. Pressure can be offloaded from the diabetic foot ulcer using a variety of modalities such as contact casting, boots, half shoes, sandals, or foam dressings. A variety of dressings are available to provide a moist wound environment, but there are few randomized controlled trials to assess their efficacy. Dressings containing antibacterial agents such as silver or iodine in slow release formulation may be helpful for superficially infected wounds.

Pexiganan is a 22 aminoacid antimicrobial peptide derived from magainin peptides isolated from the skin of the African clawed frog. It demonstrates antimicrobial activity against a broad range of organisms including gram-positive aerobes and anaerobes, including *Staphylococcus, Streptococcus, Enterococcus, Corynebacterium, Pseudomonas, Acinetobacter, Stenotrophomonas, Bacteroides,* and other species.

A randomized controlled trial of topical pexiganan compared to treatment with oral ofloxacin in mildly infected diabetic foot ulcers showed clinically equivalent response with equivalent healing rates.

For clinically infected wounds, culture guided therapy with systemic antibiotics is required. Linezolid (Zyvox) is the only oral antibiotic approved for the treatment of methocillin resistance *Staphylococcus aureus* infections, and has been recently approved by the FDA to treat diabetic foot infections. In a randomized controlled trial, 371 patients with diabetic foot infections were randomly assigned to receive linezolid versus standard amino penicillin therapy of aminopenicillin/beta lactamase inhibitor ± vancomycin. There was 83% efficiency in the linezolid arm versus 73% in the control group.

Additional therapies may be helpful in the treatment of diabetic foot ulcers, which are slow to respond to traditional care. rh-PDGF has been approved by the FDA for the treatment of neuropathic foot ulcers in diabetic patients.

Two-tissue engineered skin products have been approved by the FDA for adjunctive treatment of diabetic foot ulcers. In a randomized trial of a bilayered skin construct, (Apligraf, Organogenesis, Inc.) higher healing rates, lower incidence of osteomyelitis, and less lower limb amputation were found in the active treatment group compared to the control group.

A dermal equivalent (Dermagraft, Smith and Nephew) has also been FDA approved for the treatment of diabetic foot ulcers.

Antimicrobial Dressings

When chronic wounds fail to heal yet do not show clinical signs of systemic infection, there may be heavy bacterial contamination, principally located in the superficial zone of the wound. Topical antimicrobial agents can be used in this situation to reduce the wound bioburden and facilitate healing.

There has been a resurgence of interest in the use of topical antiseptics such as iodine and silver to control wound bioburden. These agents have a broad-spectrum of antibacterial activity and are less likely to induce bacterial resistance than antibiotics.

New dressing formulations have been developed, which allow slow release of antibacterial agents such as silver and iodine in concentrations that are non toxic to cells within the wound yet have antibacterial activity. Silver has been used for centuries to prevent and treat a variety of diseases. Silver was used in ancient Greece and Rome when silver coins were placed in jars of water to maintain sterility,

Silver ions can kill microorganisms by blocking respiratory enzyme systems and appear to have no negative effects on human cells. Silver has been demonstrated to be effective in killing antibiotic resistant bacteria such as methicillin resistant staphylococcus aureus and vancomycin resistant enterococcus.

In a study of patients with symmetric burn wounds randomized to treatment with 0.5% silver nitrate solution versus nanocrystaline silver dressing, burn wound sepsis and secondary bacteremias were reduced in the silver dressing group. In addition, dressing removal was less painful than with the silver nitrate solution. Silver dressings may also alter the inflammatory environment of the chronic wound. It has been shown that wounds treated with nanocrystalline silver dressings have decreased levels of matrix metalloproteinases, which are usually upregulated in chronic wounds.

Cadexomer iodine is a three-dimensional starch lattice formed into spherical micro beads. Iodine is trapped within this lattice at 0.9% weight per volume. This has a high absorptive capacity. It absorbs exudate from the wound and gradually releases iodine from the resulting gel. In a randomized controlled trial in 38 venous ulcer patients, topical Cadexomer iodine reduced colonization with *S. aureus*, beta hemolytic *Streptococcus*, *Proteus*, and *Klebsiella* ($p > 0.001$). There was a correlation between *S. aureus* removal and the healing rate of the wounds.

These dressings are clinically very promising, but larger randomized trials in different patient groups are required.

SELECTED SCIENTIFIC OBSERVATIONS
What Ate the Pro-Healing Intrinsic Elements in Skin?

The first phase of wound healing includes clotting of the blood, aggregation of platelets, release of platelet contents, the transformation of plasma into serum, and inflammation. Wound healing of skin is often thought of as the recapitulation of gestation, which involves so many processes that it is difficult to determine the origins of biological elements within a complex wound. To get around this problem, investigators have attempted to isolate processes in vitro and dissect what a given cell or tissue can contribute. Falanga and coworkers have been working with a commercially available, three-dimensional skin substitute, Apligraf (Organogenesis, Canton, Massachusetts). This construct consists of a collagen lattice gel containing human dermal fibroblasts overlaid with human keratinocytes. After appropriate culture including time for keratinocyte expansion and a period of air-fluid culture to stratify and mature the differentiation of the keratinocytes, the construct consists of a bilayer of a neodermis covered with a stratified epithelium of human keratinocytes. This skin equivalent construct can then be used for grafting onto human skin wounds. Although the construct does not engraft permanently on the human recipient because it is made of allogeneic cells, its presence in human wounds for a period of time is thought to promote wound healing by the provision of growth factors, cytokine release, structural support, and a moist wound environment. The skin equivalent in culture obviously does not have all of the inflammatory or clotting elements involved in an acute human skin wound such as platelets or inflammatory cells. Therefore, the skin equivalent provides an opportunity to see what the intrinsic cells of the construct can contribute to the wound by wounding the construct in vitro. The skin equivalent can be wounded in vitro by

meshing the construct as a surgeon would do for the preparation of split-thickness skin for mesh grafts on burn wounds or by creating a scalpel incision wound into the construct. It was found that the skin equivalent stimulated by wounding produced an ordered and reproducible cytokine profile reminiscent to that seen in human skin wounds. Interleukin-1 beta was expressed 12 hours after wounding while interleukin-1 alpha and transforming growth factor-alpha expression peaked at 24 hours. Other cytokines were expressed as well, but later in the sequence, including transforming growth factor-beta and insulin-like growth factor-2 at 48 hours, and platelet derived growth factor-B at 72 hours. The specificity of this cytokine staged progression was suggested not only by the reproducibility of the timing, but because certain cytokines did not change at all during the post-wound period of observation. This model makes it clear that two predominant cells intrinsic to the skin, namely keratinocytes and dermal fibroblasts, are capable of contributing growth factors and cytokines thought to be essential to wound healing. Interestingly, the expression of the keratinocyte and fibroblast-derived cytokines were associated with a functional component within the skin equivalent: the transformation of the keratinocytes from a differentiation or proliferative mode into a mode of cell migration. Associated with the order cytokine progression, there was decreased keratinocyte proliferation and a coordinate increase in keratinocyte motility and reepithelialization. Sarret and coworkers showed that the proliferative potential of human keratinocytes could be driven essentially to zero by the presence of TGF-β and yet the keratinocytes were readily capable of cell migration on promigratory extracellular matrices such as Type I collagen and fibronectin. This suggests that keratinocytes can either be in a proliferative mode or a migratory mode but cannot do both biological functions at the same time. The TGF-β expression within the skin equivalent like contributes to the keratinocyte hypo-proliferative and promigratory mode associated with re-epithelialization of the incision or mesh wound. It has been demonstrated that EGF, transforming growth factor-alpha, and interleukin-1 alpha all promote human keratinocyte migration if the cells are apposed to a promotility matrix. These selected cytokines and growth factors are expressed strongly in the postwound period of the skin equivalent at a time when the keratinocytes in the construct are involved in reepithelialization. This model does increase our understanding of the healing of skin wounds because it dissects the wound-healing process in a clear fashion. Clinically, we know that when patients have had chemotherapy and bone marrow ablation for stem cell or bone marrow transplantation, these procedures are not associated with delayed healing of skin wounds in any significant or consistent manner.

Serum vs. Plasma

A simplistic or even childish view of the influences upon cells in a wound could be that there are essentially two elements: small soluble factors such as cytokines and growth factors or large connective tissue macromolecules such as extracellular matrix components. The nutrients supplied to keratinocytes, fibroblasts, melanocytes, Merkel cells, Langerhans cells, and endothelial cells in unwounded normal skin come from a filtrate of plasma. The proteins within the plasma of the circulation must pass through a basement membrane zone (BMZ) that surrounds each dermal blood vessel. These proteins are then available to bathe and influence the biology of dermal fibroblasts. The same proteins may diffuse from the dermis, cross the dermal epidermal junction where lies another basement membrane zone and enter the epidermis where they may influence the biology of epidermal cells. Interestingly, little is known about what plasma proteins selectively diffuse through the vascular basement membranes and influence the dermal cells versus the plasma proteins that selectively diffuse through the basement membrane zone at the dermal epidermal junction and influence the epidermal cells. This question is interesting because the vascular BMZ and the BMZ of the dermal epidermal junction have both common and different elements. In common are Type IV collagen, laminin-1 and heparan sulfate proteoglycans. The BMZ at the dermal epidermal junction, however, also contains Type VII collagen, Type XVII collagen, and anchoring filament proteins such as laminin-5. During wounding, the blood vessels are cut, clotting mechanisms are invoked, platelets aggregate releasing their contents, and the plasma is converted into serum. The skin cells in a wound, therefore, for the first time are confronted with serum rather than plasma. In most in vitro keratinocyte motility assays, bovine pituitary extract (BPE) is present as a source of growth factors. This is because of a long tradition of culturing human keratinocytes in low calcium, serum-free conditions as established by Boyce and Ham. In this keratinocyte culture medium, the medium is supplemented with BPE, transferrin, hydrocortisone, and EGF. Nevertheless, surprising little is known about the contents of BPE except that it contains keratinocyte growth factor-2 (aka fibroblast growth factor 10) and basic fibroblast growth factor (bFGF). Henry and coworkers studied standard keratinocyte migration assays but used human serum, human plasma or BPE as a source of growth factors for keratinocytes migrating on promigratory matrices such as collagen J, collagen IV, and fibronectin. The investigators found that human serum augmented human keratinocyte migration on these matrices whereas plasma was incapable of promoting cellular motility. It found that serum did this by at least two mechanisms: promoting the keratinocyte derived expression of metalloproteinases and promoting the p38 MAP kinase signaling pathway, both thought to be important for human keratinocyte motility. These laboratory findings are interesting because they make sense with what we know about real human skin wounds. It also raises the next important question: what is in human serum that augments ECM-driven human keratinocyte migration in the wound?

Human keratinocytes must migrate from the cut edges of the wound and from the cut epidermal appendages to reepithelialize, resurface, and close human skin wounds. Therefore, these cells are transformed from cells destined to a tightly regulated program of terminal differentiation into dead *Stratum corneum* cells, the most external layer of skin that provides humans with a critical permeability barrier. In addition to keratinocytes being transformed into a migratory cell type, within the dermis and wound bed, fibroblasts too must be stimulated to migrate. Fibroblasts in the unwounded dermis juxtaposed to the clot and wound bed, must migrate into the wound bed and begin to contribute cytokines and growth factors, release metalloproteinases to help clear the wound debris and begin to lay down essential extracellular matrix macromolecules to form the neodermis which will then undergo a long process of remodeling. As mentioned above, the wound bed is swamped by serum and dermal fibroblasts experience serum rather than plasma in the wound setting. Fibroblasts, like keratinocytes, become migratory in the setting of a cutaneous wound. Recently, Li and coworkers

demonstrated that the element within human serum that enhances dermal fibroblast motility is PDGF-BB. PDGF-BB can completely replace serum in terms of promoting human dermal fibroblast migration on a Type I collagen matrix. Likewise, the promotility activity in human serum for dermal fibroblasts is completely blocked by the presence of functional antibodies to PDGF-BB in the migration assays. Therefore, the element within human serum responsible for human dermal fibroblast migration has been identified.

The Role of Soluble Growth Factors and Extracellular Matrix in Skin Motility

The scientific literature on human keratinocyte and human fibroblast migration could make one believe that small soluble growth factors or cytokines can alone induce cell migration. This is a false impression. We do not believe that any soluble cytokine or growth factor can alone make fibroblasts or keratinocytes migrate on the bottom of a Petri dish (tissue culture polystyrene plastic), or a Petri dish coated with albumin, laminin-1, processed laminin-5, or any substratum that allows cell attachment but is not intrinsically promotility. For example, keratinocytes can be initiated to migrate significantly by apposition to promotile matrices such as collagen I and fibronectin even in the total absence of added growth factors. The addition of promotility soluble factors such as serum, EGF, or IL-1 alpha enhances the matrix initiated cell motility and gives the cells polarity and direction. If the cells themselves contribute small soluble factors as autocrines, these factors are unable to optimize the matrix-initiated motility or give the cells directionality. In a real skin wound, the cells are obviously influenced by both contacts with extracellular matrices in the wound bed and by soluble growth factors within the microenvironment of the wound including those in serum. Nevertheless, it is interesting that extracellular matrix provides the stimulus and activates the necessary signaling pathways via integrin receptors to initiate the cell motility of skin cells. It is likely that the presence of growth factors and cytokines then initiate other signaling pathways via activation of their tyrosine kinase receptors and in a still to be defined mechanism, the matrix initiating and the growth factor enhancing signals like cross-talk in an orchestrated manner to optimize cell migration. Li et al. have shown that the signals from matrix that initiate keratinocyte and fibroblast motility and the signals from growth factors that enhance and optimize matrix-initiated motility use common and disparate signaling pathways within the cytosol of the cell.

Oxygen Tension and Wound Healing

It is believed that low oxygen tension in the long run inhibits wound closure. Although there are precious few controlled blinded studies, hyperbaric oxygen chambers have been employed to help heal chronic wounds, particularly when it is believed that arterial disease hampers the delivery of oxygen to the wound tissue. Nevertheless, during an acute wound, the periwound tissues experience sudden and extreme hypoxia. Many signaling pathways in cells are activated by nonspecific stress signals that in turn activate survival genes. Keratinocytes next to the wound and fibroblasts around the dermal defect likely experience acute hypoxia because all of the blood vessels are rapidly clotted to prevent the organisms from exsanguination. Therefore, red blood cells and hemoglobin are not getting to these tissues. It is conceivable that this situation creates stress signals that, at least in the short-run, promote the transformation of keratinocytes and fibroblasts into migratory cells and cells that help initiate the healing of the wound. For example, it is known that TGF-β produced by dermal fibroblasts increases the extracellular matrix by causing the same cells to synthesize more matrix macromolecules such as collagens and synthesize and secrete less matrix degrading enzymes such as collagenases (matrix metalloproteinases). Falanga et al. have shown that hypoxia upregulates the synthesis of TGF-β 1 by human dermal fibroblasts. Therefore, this important wound-healing growth factor would be available within the wound to stimulate cells to make more extracellular matrix and fill in the rent in the skin. In addition, a hypoxic environment promotes the growth potential of fibroblasts and helps them avoid senescence.

In the case of keratinocytes, it has been shown that human keratinocytes migrate better on collagen I, collagen IV, and fibronectin under hypoxic conditions compared with normoxia. This superior migration under hypoxia is associated with an upregulation in proteins that build cell lamillipodia and with increased keratinocyte expression of collagenases—both elements that promote cellular locomotion.

Our view of these data is that hypoxia in acute wounds may serve as a stress signal to the wound cells and invokes a series of signaling pathways that transform the cells from maintenance skin cells into cells that are activated and migratory to begin healing the wound.

The Origin of Stem Cells in Healing Skin Wounds

Stem cells are slow cycling cells that are considered the "mother cells" that give rise to a progeny of cells. Keratinocyte stem cells are located within the basal keratinocyte layer and within the bulge region of the pilosebaceous unit. The general view of healing skin wounds has been that the healing is generated by local cells at the site of the wound. Nevertheless, this view may need to be modified. Investigators have taken bone marrow cells from one animal and by transfection methods induced the cells in culture to express green fluorescent protein (GFP). They took these GFP positive bone marrow cells and injected them into the circulation of a mouse of identical species. They wounded this mouse and noted that a large number of the GFP positive cells homed to the wound and were involved in the wound-healing process. Along similar lines, patients with nonhealing wounds have had their wounds treated with autologous bone marrow cells—either by direct inoculation of the wound with bone marrow aspirates or with bone marrow cells after culturing. Although the number of patients was very small and the results uncontrolled, wounds that had not healed for over one year healed by these maneuvers. These observations, while preliminary, are very encouraging and potentially open a whole new way of looking at the wound-healing process and strategies for healing large nonhealing wounds.

BIBLIOGRAPHY

AK Touche, M Skaria, L Bohlen, et al. An autologous epidermal equivalent tissue-engineered from follicular outer loot sheath keratinocytes is as effective as split-thickness skin autograft in recalcitrant vascular leg ulcer. Wound Repair Regen 2003; (11):248–252.

Armstrong DG, Nguyen HC. Improvement in healing with aggressive edema reduction after debridement of foot infection in persons with diabetes. Arch Surg 2000; 135(12): 1405–1409.

Badiavas EV, Abedi M, Butmarc J, Falanga V, Quesenberry P. Participation of bone marrow derived cells in cutaneous wound healing. J Cell Physiol 2003; 196:245–250.

Badiavas EV, Falanga V. Treatment of chronic wounds with bone marrow-derived cells. Arch Dermato 2003; 139:510–516.

Barwell JR, Davies CE, Deacon J, et al. Comparison of surgery and compression with compression alone in chronic venous ulceration (ESCHAR Study): randomized controlled trial. Lancet 2004; 363:1854–1859.

Bello YM, Phillips TJ. Recent Advances in Wound Healing. JAMA 2000; 283:716–718.

Boulton AJN, Kirsner RS, Vileikyte L. Neuropathic diabetic foot ulcers. NEJM 2004; 351:48–55.

Bowler PG, Duerden BI, Armstrong DG. Wound microbiology and associated approaches to wound management. Clin Microbiol Review 2001; 14:244–269.

Boyce ST, Ham RG. Calcium-regulated differentiation normal human epidermal keratinocytes in chemically defined clonal culture and serum-free serial culture. J Invest Dermatol 1983; 81(suppl):33–40.

Brown GL, Nanny LF, Griffen J, et al. Enhancement of wound healing by topical treatment with epidermal growth factor. N Engl J Med 1989; 321.76–79.

Cha D, O'Brian P, O'Toole EA, Woodley DT, Hudson LG. Enhanced modulation of keratinocyte motility by transforming growth factor-alpha (TGF-alpha) relative to epidermal growth factor (EGF). J Invest Dermatol 1996; 106:590–597.

Chen JD, Kim JP, Zhang K, et al. Epidermal growth factor (EGF) promotes human keratinocyte locomotion on collagen by increasing the alpha 2 integrin subunit. Exp Cell Res 1993; 209:216–223.

Chen TO, Lapiere JC, Sauder DN, Peavey C, Woodley DT. Interleukin 1 alpha stimulates keratinocyte migration through and epidermal growth factor/transforming growth factor alpha-independent pathway. J Invest Dermatol 1995; 104:729–733.

Cotsarelis G, Sun TT, Lavaker RM. Label-retaining cells reside in the bulge area of the pilosebaceous unit: implications for follicular stem cells, hair cycle and skin carcinogenesis. Cell 1990; 61:1329–1337.

Cullum N, Nelson EA, Fletcher AW, Sheldon TA, Cocbrane database of systematic reviews, 2004.

Dawson DL, Cutler BS, Hiatt WR, et al: A comparison of Cilostazol and pentoxyfilline for treating intermittent claudication. Am J Med 2000; 109:523–530.

Demling RH, Desan TL. The role of silver in wound healing. Wounds 2001; 13:5–15.

Falanga V, Margolis D, Alvarez D, et al. Rapid healing of venous leg ulcers and lack of clinical rejection with an allogeneic cultured human skin equivalent. Arch Dermatol 1997; 134:293–300.

Falanga V, Qian SW, Danielpour D, et al. Hypoxia upregulates the synthesis of TGF-beta 1 by human dermal fibroblasts. J Invest Dermatol 1991; 97:634–637.

Falanga V, Kirsner RS. Low oxygen stimulates proliferation of fibroblasts seeded as single cells. J Cell Physiol 1993; 54:506–510.

Gallico GG, O'Connor NE. Cultured epithelium as a skin substitute. Clin Plast Surg 1985; 12:149–157.

Ge Y, MacDonald D, Henry MM, et al. In vitro susceptibility to pexiganan of bacteria isolated from infected diabetic foot ulcers. Diagn Microbiol Infect Dis 1999; 35(l):45–53.

Ge Y, MacDonald DL, Holroyd KJ, Thomsberry C, Wexler H, Zasloff M. In vitro properties of pexiganan, an analog of magainin. Antimicrob Agents Chemother 1999; 43:782–788.

Hansborough J, Cooper M, Gohen R, et al. Evaluation of biodegradable matrix containing cultured human fibroblast as a dermal replacement beneath meshed skin graft on athymic mice. Surgery 1992; 111:439–446.

Henry G, Li W, Garner W, Woodley DT. Migration of human keratinocytes in plasma and serum and wound re-epithelialization. Lancet 2003; 361:574–576.

Holder IA, Durkee P, Supp AP, Boyce ST. Assessment of a silver-coated barrier dressing for potential use with skin grafts on excised burns. Burns 2003; 29:445–448.

Holloway GA, Johansen KH, Barnes RW, et al. Multicenter trial of cadexomer iodine to treat venous stasis ulcers. West J Med 1989; 151:35–38.

Jones SA, Bowler PG, Walker M, Parsons D. Controlling wound bioburden with a novel silver containing hydrofiber dressing. Wound Repair Regen 2004; 12:288–294.

Khachemount A, Bello Y, Phillips T. Factors that influence healing in chronic venous ulcers treated with cryopreserved human epidermal culture. Dermatol Surg 2002; 28:274–276.

Kirsner RS, Orsted H, Wright JB. Matrix metalloproteinases in normal and impaired wound healing: a potential of nanocrystalline silver. Wounds 2001; 13:5–12.

Kolenic SA Leffell DJ. The use of cryopreserved human skin allografts in wound healing following mohs surgery. Dermatol Surg 1995; 21:615–620.

Li W, Fan J, Chen M, et al. Mechanism of human dermal fibroblast migration driven by Type I collagen and platelet-derived growth factor-BB, Molecular Biology of the Cell 2004; 15:294–309.

Li W, Henry G, Fan J, et al. Signals that initiate, augment and provide directionality for human keratinocyte motility. J Invest Dermatol. In press.

Limat A, French L, Blat L, Saurat J, Hunziker T, Soloman D. Organotypic cultures of autologous hair follicle keratinocytes for the treatment of recurrent leg ulcers. JAAD 2003; 48:207–214.

Lipkin, E Chaikof, Z Isseroff, P Silverstain. Effectiveness of bilayered cellular matrix in healing of neuropathic diabetic foot ulcers: results of multicenter pilot trial. Wounds 2003; 15:230–236.

Lipsky BA, Itani K, Norden C. Treating foot infections in diabetic patients. A randomized, multicenter, open label trial of Linezolid versus ampicillin sulbactam/amoxicillin clavulanate. Clin Infect Dis 2004; 38:17–24.

Lipsky BA, McDonald D, Litka PA. Treatment of infected diabetic foot ulcers, topical MSI-78 vs. oral ofloxacin. Diabetologica 1997; 40:482.

Margolis DM, Berlin JA, Strom BL. Risk factors associated with the failure of venous leg ulcer to heal. Arch Dermatol 1999; 135(8):920–926.

Marston WA, Hanst J, Norwood P, Pollack R. The efficacy and safety of Dermagraft in improving the healing of chronic diabetic foot ulcers: results of a prospective randomized trial. Diabetes Care 2003; 26:1701–705.

Mober S, Hoffman L, Grennert ML, et al. A randomized trial of cadexomer iodine in decubitus ulcers. J Am Qeriatr Soc 1983; 31:462–465.

O'Toole EA, Marinkovich MP, Peavy CL, et al. Hypoxia increases human keratinocyte motility on connective tissue. J Clin Invest 1997; 100:2881–2891.

O'Toole EA, Goel M, Woodley DT. Hydrogen peroxide inhibits human keratinocyte migration. Dermatol Surg 1996; 22:525–529.

Ormiston MC, Seymour MT, Venn GE, et al. Controlled trial of Iodosorb in chronic venous ulcers. Sri Med J 1985; 291: 308–310.

Paddle-Ledinek JE, Cruickshank DG, Masterton JP. Skin replacement by cultured keratinocyte grafts: an Australian experience. Burns 1997; 23(3):204–211.

Palumbo PJ, Nelzen LJ III. Peripheral vascular disease and diabetes. In: Diabetes and America. Diabetes data compiled

1984: Washington, DC. Government Printing Office, August 1985. 15–1-15–21. NIH publication #85–1468.

Phillips TJ, Machado F, Trout R, et al. Prognostic indicators for venous ulcers: analysis of a randomized, double blind, placebo controlled study. J Amer Acad Dermatol 2000; 43:627–630.

Phillips TJ, Manzoor J, Rojas A, et al. The longevity of a bilayered skin substitute after application to venous ulcers. Arch Derm 2002; 138:1079–1081.

Phillips T, Provan A, Colbert D, Easley KW. A randomized single-blind controlled study of cultured epidermal allografts in the treatment of split-thickness skin graft donor sites. Arch Dermatol 1993; 129:879–882.

Pollak R, Edingtin H, Jenson J, Kroeker R, Gentzkow G. A human dermal replacement for the treatment of diabetic foot ulcer. Wound 1997; 9:175–182.

Robson MC, Phillips LG, Thompson A, et al. Platelet-derived growth factor BB for the treatment of chronic pressure ulcers. Lancet 1992; 339:23–25.

Robson MC. Wound infection: a failure of wound healing caused by an imbalance of bacteria. Surg Clin North Am 1997; 77:637–650.

Sarret Y, Woodley DT, Grigsby K, Wynn K, O'Keefe EJ. Human keratinocyte locomotion: The effect of selected cytokines. J Invest Dermatol 1992; 98:12–16.

Singer AJ, Clark RAF. Cutaneous wound healing. N Engl J Med 1999; 341:738–746.

Skog E, Arnesjo B, Troeng T, et al. A randomized trial comparing Cadexomer iodine and standard treatment in the outpatient management of chronic venous ulcers. Br J Derm 1983; 109:77–83.

Steed DL, Donohoe D, Webster MW, Lindsley L. Effect of extensive debridement and treatment on the healing of diabetic foot ulcers. J Am Coll Surg 1996; 183:61–64.

Taylor G, Lehrer MS, Jensen PJ, Sun TT, Lavker RM. Involvement of follicular stem cells in forming not only the follicle but also we epidermis. Cell 2000; 102:451–461.

Tredget E, Shankowsky HA, Groeneveld A, Burrell R. A matched pair randomized study evaluating the efficacy and safety of Acticoat silver-coated dressing for the treatment of burn wounds. J Burn Care Rehab 1998; 19:532–537.

Veves A, Falanga V, Armstrong DG, Sabolinski ML. Apligraf Diabetic Foot Ulcer Study. Graftskin, a human skin equivalent, is effective in the management of noninfected neuropathic diabetic foot ulcers: a prospective randomized multicenter clinical trial. Diabetes Care 2001; 24(2):290–295.

Veves A, Falanga A, Armstrong DG, Sabolinsky ML. Graftskin, a human skin equivalent is effective in the management of noninfected neuropathic diabetic foot ulcers, a prospective, randomized, multicenter clinical trial. Diabetes Care 2001; 24:290–295.

White R, Cooper R, Kingsly A. Wound colonization and infection: The role of topical antimicrobials and guidelines in management. Br J Nursing 2001; 10:563–578.

Wieman TJ, Smiell JN et al. Efficacy and safety of a topical gel formulation of recombinant human platelet derived growth factor BB (Bercaplamin) in patients with chronic neuropathic diabetic ulcers. A phase III randomized, placebo controlled, double blind study. Diabetes Care 1998; 21:822–827.

Woodley DT, Peterson HD, Herzog SR, et al. Burn wounds resurfaced by cultured epidermal autografts show abnormal reconstitution of anchoring fibrils, JAMA 1988; 259:2566–2571.

Wright JB, Lam K, Burrell RE. Wound management in an era of increasing bacterial antibiotic resistance: a role for topical silver treatment. Am J Infection Control 1998; 26:572–577.

Zhou LH, Nahm WK, Badiavas E, Yufit T, Falanga V. Slow release iodine preparation and wound healing: in vitro effects consistent with lack of in vivo toxicity in human chronic wounds. Br J Dermatol 2002; 146(3):365–374.

11

Complications in Cutaneous Procedures

Thomas Stasko
Vanderbilt University Medical Center, Nashville, Tennessee, U.S.A.

William B. Henghold
The Skin Cancer Center of Northwest Florida, Pensacola, Florida, U.S.A.

The word *complicate* comes from the Latin *complicare*, meaning to fold up, or in other words to make or become complex or intricate. In medicine a complication is a secondary disease or condition aggravating a previous one. A surgical complication is a deviation from the original planned outcome. It may be one small event that leads directly to a single change in outcome, or more commonly from a combination of seemingly unrelated factors that cascades to the undesired result. The field of dermatologic surgery encompasses multiple distinct procedures, each with its own unique complications. The four major acute complications encountered in dermatologic surgery (hemorrhage, infection, necrosis, and dehiscence) are referred to as the "terrible tetrad." Each can singly or in combination lead to failure of the desired outcome, optimal wound healing (Fig. 1). Not surprisingly, the occurrence of one complication lowers the threshold for the development of others.

An old surgical adage is that if a surgeon has not experienced a complication with a particular procedure, then he or she has not performed enough of them. Some complications are the unavoidable result of factors beyond the control of the surgeon or the patient. An integral part of the informed consent process prior to performing any procedure is the discussion of the inherent risks and potential complications, and each patient and each procedure present unique considerations. The chance of a complication occurring with any given procedure is dependent on the interplay of three primary factors, each of which has a number of cofactors: (i) patient related (e.g., age, general health, medical comorbidities, medications, ability to follow instructions); (ii) surgeon and medical staff related (e.g., training, skill, attention to detail); and (iii) procedure related (e.g., type of procedure, office or hospital setting, level of anesthesia, anatomic location, duration).

In spite of optimal planning and care, the diversity of human response to injury and disease yields an outcome different from that intended and results in additional problems requiring attention. But it must be stated from the outset that the best treatment for any complication is prevention. Avoidance of even one or two of the small events that contribute to an adverse result can abort the complication cascade. Strict attention to each individual, routine detail is probably the best means of preventing complications. Bending the rules to accommodate a particular patient's needs or desires or changing the routine to fit unusual circumstances is a particularly insidious genesis for a complication. The surgeon can be flexible but must be aware of the consequences of any alterations to the routine.

Ultimately, complications are events that threaten the patient's life, efficient wound healing, cosmesis, and/or litigation. Fortunately, emergencies in cutaneous surgery are extremely rare, but the surgeon must be prepared to deal with acute cardiac problems, seizures, reactions to anesthesia, and the like. The details of developing a plan to prevent such emergencies and deal with those that do arise are covered in Chapter 7. Also of serious concern is the possible development of bacterial endocarditis or infection of prosthetic devices as a result of bacteremia from skin surgery. The prophylactic use of antibiotics in such situations is discussed in Chapter 5.

THE SAFETY OF OFFICE-BASED SURGERY

The number of cutaneous procedures performed and the number of practitioners performing them has increased dramatically over the past several decades. A survey conducted by the American Society for Dermatologic Surgery in 2003 found that its members performed 4.1 million skin surgery procedures, an 11% increase from 2001. Over 1.6 million were for treatment of skin cancer. Recently there has been a trend toward a critical evaluation of the safety of office-based surgical practice, driven in part by legislative threats to limit office-based surgery. Since March 2000 the state of Florida has required mandatory, prospective reporting of all adverse office-based surgical incidents resulting in patient injury or death. Coldiron et al. reported on three years of Florida adverse event data, confirming the safety of office-based surgery as currently practiced by dermatologic surgeons. Over that time period there were 13 procedure-related deaths and 43 procedure-related complications necessitating hospital transfer. Seven of the 13 deaths occurred in the office setting. No dermatologists were involved in any of the deaths and only two of the complications involved dermatologists.

The first comprehensive prospective assessment of the incidence of a variety of complications was reported by Cook and Perone in 2003. This noncomparative study was performed over a one-year period and detailed the incidence and nature of complications in a Mohs micrographic surgery (MMS) practice. The overall incidence of complications was 1.64% (22 occurences in 1343 cases). No

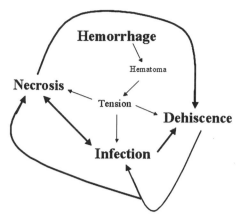

Figure 1   The "terrible tetrad" of acute surgical complications.

complication was significant enough to require hospitalization or transfer of care to another specialist. The complications encountered consisted of postoperative hemorrhage ($N=2$), hematoma formation ($N=7$), wound dehiscence ($N=1$), wound infection ($N=1$), necrosis of flap ($N=5$), and necrosis of skin graft ($N=6$). Dermatologic surgeons have always had the general impression that cutaneous procedures performed in the office setting are safe for patients. This impression is now increasingly being supported by solid evidence-based data.

COMPLICATIONS THAT THREATEN EFFICIENT WOUND HEALING
Wound Healing Basics
Wounding of the skin initiates a remarkable series of events at a molecular and cellular level that ultimately lead to repair of the injury. The inflammatory phase follows closely the formation of a hemostatic clot that occurs initially after wounding. This phase then leads to the formation of granulation tissue, re-epithelization, neovascularization, and fibroplasia. Finally, the extracellular matrix is rebuilt and remodeled. The details of our current understanding of wound healing are covered in Chapter 9, but on a more macroscopic level it is intuitive that events which disrupt this orderly progression will inhibit wound healing and lead to complications.

Mechanisms of Hemostasis
The human hemostatic mechanism is a highly complex process of interrelated events involving procoagulant factors and coagulation inhibitors. When the system functions as designed, blood is maintained in a fluid state intravascularly, yet rapidly coagulates to prevent extravascular loss in the event of an injury. Early theories on coagulation envisioned an orderly cascade of events involving somewhat distinct intrinsic, extrinsic, common, and platelet pathways. It is now evident that the entire process is an interrelated, tightly interwoven sequence of events to halt the blood loss and begin repair of the wounded site.

The initial response to the transection of a vessel is vasoconstriction. This reduces the area of transected vessel that must be filled with aggregated platelets and reduces blood loss prior to formation of the platelet plug. Vasoconstriction also slows blood flow and prolongs the exposure to subendothelial collagen and coagulation factors, resulting

in enhanced platelet adherence to the injury site. Most local anesthetics, with the exception of cocaine, produce vasodilatation as a result of the relaxation of the smooth muscle of the vessel wall. It is essential for the surgeon to remember this action when using local anesthesia without epinephrine. Epinephrine is routinely added to local anesthetic solution to counteract this action and provide additional vasoconstriction. The use of epinephrine in a concentration as low as 1:500,000 can provide potent vasoconstriction and a much drier surgical field. The surgeon must be aware that this effect is time-limited and fresh bleeding may occur when the vessel returns to its normal diameter. Such bleeding may occur during the final stages of a prolonged procedure or in the immediate postoperative period.

The goal of hemostasis is to produce a solid fibrin/platelet clot at the site of vessel injury. The major initiating event in hemostasis is the formation of a factor VIIa-tissue factor (TF) complex at the site of injury. This catalyzes several important reactions, the result of which is to generate thrombin and activate platelets. The generation of thrombin catalyzes the conversion of fibrinogen to fibrin monomers, which then spontaneously polymerize to form a fibrin plug. Binding of fibrinogen to platelet glycoprotein (Gp) IIb/IIIa leads to platelet aggregation by cross-linking of GpIIb/IIIa molecules on individual platelets. Platelets aggregate at the same sites where TF is exposed. TF is expressed in the adventitia of blood vessels (subendothelial collagen) as well as by epidermal cells and extravacular connective tissue. Endothelial cells make and secrete von Willebrand's factor (vWf), which also enhances platelet adherence by forming a cross-link between TF and vWf receptors on the surface of activated platelets (Fig. 2).

Drugs and Other Agents that Interfere with Hemostasis
It is not uncommon to find patients on more than one blood thinner at a time, to include over-the-counter medications or dietary supplements with anticoagulant properties. In a survey of 100 consecutive patients undergoing Mohs surgery, 48% were taking medications such as aspirin, nonsteroidal anti-inflammatory drugs (NSAIDs), clopidogrel bisulfate, or warfarin, 49% were taking dietary supplements, and 21% were taking both prescription and over-the-counter medications with anticoagulant properties. Two-thirds of patients did not self-report their use of dietary supplements, emphasizing the importance of directed questioning on the part of the health care provider. The list of drugs that interferes with the normal hemostatic machinery is lengthy, but only a limited number of common medications are usually of concern in cutaneous surgery.

Antiplatelet Drugs
Aspirin
Aspirin is by far the most commonly prescribed antiplatelet agent. By irreversibly inactivating platelet cyclooxygenase, aspirin prevents the synthesis of thromboxane A2, a powerful platelet agonist. As the platelet cannot replace the defective enzyme, the effect persists as long as the platelet survives. A single dose of aspirin will impair platelet function for the entire 9.5-day platelet lifespan. The increased bleeding from aspirin can be difficult to control in the form of diffuse oozing at the time of surgery and can lead to postoperative bleeding and more extensive ecchymoses than are usual. Aspirin ingestion postoperatively will not affect a well established fibrin-platelet clot.

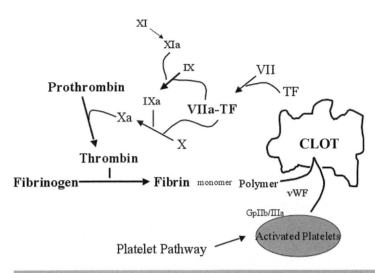

Figure 2 Simplified schematic for the formation of a platelet–fibrin clot.

NSAIDs

Most NSAIDs act on platelets in a manner similar to that of aspirin (inhibition of cyclooxygenase), but the effect is usually less potent and is reversible. The duration of the effect is related to the half-life of the drug and only continues if adequate blood levels are maintained.

Thienopyridines (Ticlopidine Hydrochloride and Clopidogrel Bisulfate)

This novel class of antiplatelet agents interferes with ADP-mediated platelet activation and leads to irreversible inhibition of platelet aggregation. Thienopyridines are commonly prescribed in combination with aspirin as clinical trials have demonstrated an impressive benefit with dual therapy. The data shows the benefit of early antiplatelet therapy and the incremental benefit of continuing this therapy for many months after a myocardial infarction or therapeutic cardiovascular procedure. Ongoing trials investigating this strategy in other patient populations are likely to expand their clinical use. Clopidogrel (Plavix®) is emerging as the preferred drug in this class Importantly, there is evidence that clopidogrel may be associated with a higher risk of bleeding complications in the perioperative setting. Although coronary artery bypass patients as a whole benefited from the addition of clopidogrel, treatment within five days of bypass surgery created a trend toward higher rates of major bleeding. In addition, retrospective studies have suggested higher rates of surgical re-exploration for bleeding when clopidogrel is administered within seven days of surgery. To date, almost all of the dermatologic surgery literature regarding perioperative complications with blood thinners deals with aspirin, NSAIDs, and warfarin. There may be an increase in the reports of bleeding complications with clopidogrel as its use becomes more widespread.

Dipyridamole

Dipyridamole interferes with ADP-induced platelet aggregation. Dipyridamole usually does not alter platelet function to such an extent that the effect is noticeable at the time of surgery, but may lead to postoperative bleeding.

Antibiotics

Many antibiotics can interfere with platelet aggregation and platelet granule release. Any resulting dysfunction is usually minor. However, at therapeutic dosages carbenicillin and other beta-lactam antibiotics may have sufficient effect to prolong bleeding times and produce an increased risk of bleeding.

Anticoagulants

Warfarin

Warfarin, a structural analog of vitamin K, disrupts the vitamin K-dependent components of the coagulation cascade: factors II (prothrombin), VII, IX, and X. Warfarin competitively inhibits the hepatic enzyme vitamin K-2,3-epoxide reductase, which converts vitamin K to its active form. The most common indications for warfarin therapy are atrial fibrillation, the presence of a mechanical heart valve, and treatment of or prophylaxis for venous thromboembolism (VTE). Table 1 lists the most common indications for warfarin therapy.

Heparin is a parenteral antithrombin agent that exerts its anticoagulant effect by enhancing the inactivation by antithrombin III of thrombin, factor Xa, and factor IXa. Unfractionated heparin (UFH) is rapidly being replaced by low molecular weight heparins (LMWH) for clinical use. The unique pharmacokinetic properties of LMWH including a very high bioavailability (greater than 90%) after subcutaneous injection, a longer half-life than UFH, and much less variation in the anticoagulant effect to a given

Table 1 The Most Common Indications for Warfarin Anticoagulation

Indication	Target INR	Perioperative annual risk without therapy
Acute venous thromboembolism	2.0–3.0	Month 1: High (40%)
		Month 3: Intermediate
Recurrent venous thromboembolism	2.0–3.0	High (15%)
Nonvalvular atrial fibrillation	2.0–3.0	Intermediate (4.5%)
Nonvalvular atrial fibrillation with previous embolism	2.0–3.0	High (12%)
Cardiomyopathy without atrial fibrillation	2.0–3.0	Low (<4%)
Valvular heart disease	2.0–3.0	Low (<4%)
Tissue prosthetic valve	2.0–3.0	Low (<4% annual risk)
Mechanical prosthetic valve	2.5–3.5	Aortic: Intermediate (4–7%)
		Mitral: High (8%)

Abbreviation: INR = International normalized ratio.
Source: From Hirsh, Dalen, Deykin, Poller, Bussey (1995); Chong, Mohr (2005); Kearon, Hirsh (1997); Dunn, Turpie (2003).

dose make it superior to its parent. The anticoagulant response to a fixed dose of LMWH is highly correlated with body weight. LMWH is cleared mainly by the kidneys; therefore, dosage adjustments are necessary in patients with renal failure. The anticoagulant effect of LMWH is not completely neutralized by protamine sulfate, but administration may still decrease the hemorrhagic effect. Because LMWH is given by subcutaneous injection once or twice daily and usually does not require laboratory monitoring of the anticoagulant effect it enables many patients who require heparin anticoagulation to be treated in an outpatient setting. LMWH also has a much lower risk of thrombocytopenia than UFH. Traditionally UFH has been utilized for patients who require a procedure, but can only be without anticoagulation for very limited periods of time. The patient is hospitalized and heparin substituted for warfarin. The heparin may then be discontinued just hours before surgery (or reversed with protamine sulfate) and the procedure performed. With LMWH this substitution can be performed in the outpatient setting. The activated partial thromboplastin time (aPTT) is the test most commonly used to monitor heparin treatment.

Dietary Supplements and Herbal Medications

The use of dietary supplements and alternative medications is on the rise. The most extensive survey on the use of alternative medicine showed an increase of 380% in herbal remedies and 130% in high-dose vitamin use between 1990 and 1997. A review by Ang-Lee et al. identified eight herbal medications (not including nonherbal dietary supplements such as vitamins) that pose the greatest risk to patients in the perioperative setting. These eight herbs account for more than 50% of the over 1500 herbal medications sold in the United States. Of the eight, garlic, ginkgo, and ginseng have been recognized as having antiplatelet activity, and there are a number of reports in the literature implicating these agents in bleeding complications. Although not associated with bleeding complications, ephedra (ma huang) is another herbal remedy clinically relevant to the dermatologic surgeon due to its potential interaction with epinephrine. Ephedra exhibits sympathomimetic effects in a dose-dependent fashion and has been associated with numerous complications including fatal heart attacks and strokes. As patients uniformly take these agents for

noncritical indications, they should be discontinued at least 7 days (for garlic and ginseng) and 36 hours (for ginkgo) prior to any surgery.

Chang and Whitaker reviewed the literature and identified ginger, feverfew, and vitamin E (in addition to garlic, ginkgo, and ginseng) as nonprescription, noncritical medications that should be discontinued prior to surgery to minimize the potential for bleeding problems. All of the identified agents possess antiplatelet activity via a variety of mechanisms. Vitamin E (alpha-tocopherol) has been advocated for the prevention of cancer and cardiovascular adverse events (heart attacks and strokes), but recent evidence has shown that it does not reduce the risk of either, at least in terms of mortality. In fact, it has been associated with an increased risk of death from hemorrhagic stroke in male smokers. Ingestion of large amounts of certain fish oils (omega-3 fatty acids) may increase BT by interfering with platelet function. This effect may also be additive with aspirin. Table 2 lists the most commonly used herbal medications and dietary supplements that may present problems in the perioperative setting.

Ethanol

Ethanol inhibits ADP-induced platelet aggregation and platelet granule release. By itself this effect is minor, but ethanol does appear to accentuate the increase in BT caused by aspirin. Alcohol is also a potent vasodilator. The ingestion of alcohol in the postoperative period may result in fresh bleeding from dilated vessels. This effect plus the possible loss of protective inhibitions with alcohol consumption make it important to prohibit drinking in the postoperative period.

The Preoperative Evaluation

The evaluation of a patient prior to surgery with regard to the risk for excessive bleeding should begin with a brief but thorough history. The use of prescription drugs is usually easy to elicit, but covering all of the over-the-counter medications can take some time and patience. A large number of inherited and acquired medical problems may also result in coagulation defects. Obviously, the patient should be asked whether he has any known defect of coagulation. The patient should also be questioned about bleeding with previous surgical or dental procedures, trauma and the like. Does the patient have prolonged bleeding with minor cuts and scratches? Does the patient develop large ecchymoses

Table 2   Dietary Supplements and Herbal Medicines Relevant to the Dermatologic Surgeon

Name	Pharmacologic effect	Perioperative effect	Discontinue
Echinacea	Immunosuppression with long-term use	Poor wound healing	No data
Ephedra	Sympathomimetic	Potentiates epinephrine effect	24 hrs prior to surgery
Feverfew	Inhibits platelet aggregation	Bleeding risk	No data
Fish oil	Inhibits platelet aggregation	Bleeding risk	No data
Garlic	Inhibits platelet aggregation	Bleeding risk	7 days prior to surgery
Ginger	Inhibits platelet aggregation	Bleeding risk	Avoid doses over 2 g several days prior to surgery
Ginkgo	Inhibits platelet aggregation	Bleeding risk	36 hrs prior to surgery
Ginseng	Inhibits platelet aggregation	Bleeding risk	7 days prior to surgery
Green tea	Inhibits platelet aggregation	Bleeding risk	No data
Kava	Sedation	Increases sedative effect of anesthetics	24 hrs prior to surgery
St. John's wort	Cytochrome P450 inducer	May affect lidocaine metabolism	5 days prior to surgery
Valerian	Sedation	Increases sedative effect of anesthetics	No data
Vitamin E	Inhibits platelet aggregation	Bleeding risk	7 days prior to surgery

Source: From Collins, Dufresne (2002); Eisenberg, Davis, Ettner (1998); Hopkins, Androff, Benninghoff (1988).

(greater than the size of a half-dollar) without known trauma? If the patient answers in the negative to all of these questions and has had a history of sufficient hemostatic challenge, then no further preoperative workup is required. If the patient has a known defect of coagulation abilities, consultation with the patient's appropriate specialist is in order. If the history reveals only a general sense of "easy bleeding," without a contributing drug or medical history, some formal preoperative evaluation may be warranted. Screening the patient with a complete blood count including a platelet count can exclude chronic blood loss sufficient to cause anemia and provide a quantitative evaluation of platelets. INR and PFA-100 determinations may be indicated.

International Normalized Ratio

The prothrombin time (PT) is the test most commonly used to monitor warfarin therapy. It is performed by adding tissue thromboplastin (tissue factor) and other reagents to the patient's serum. Different thromboplastins vary markedly in their responsiveness to the effect of anticoagulants. The international sensitivity index (ISI) is a measure of the responsiveness of a given thromboplastin to the effect of warfarin. Owing to the variability of the ISI, the PT results from one laboratory are not comparable with that of another. The INR was developed as a means to promote the worldwide standardization of oral anticoagulant control. The World Health Organization developed a reference tissue factor, prepared from human brain. The INR is now the preferred method of reporting the PT. The majority of both minor and major bleeding problems reported in patients on anticoagulation occur when the INR is greater than 3.5, and for this reason some authors advocate preoperative INR measurement for every patient undergoing even minor surgery. A study by Syed et al. showed significantly more episodes of minor bleeding in the patients on warfarin compared with controls. There were no major bleeding episodes reported. The majority of the warfarin patients who experienced bleeding (9 of 12) had INRs >3.5. A simple and quick, in-office method for measuring a patient's INR preoperatively has been described.

Platelet Function Analyzer (PFA-100)

The BT assay has been supplanted by other technology, such as PFA-100 analysis. The PFA-100 is an in vitro device that simulates in vivo primary hemostasis. The test result is measured in seconds and reported as the closure time (CT). PFA-100 offers a number of advantages over BT assays. It does not require the patient to be present, and it can be performed on those who are difficult to study with BT assays (e.g., pediatric patients). As a screening test for the most common inherited abnormality of coagulation, von Willebrand disease, the PFA-100 is significantly more sensitive than the BT. It is also an excellent screen for intrinsic platelet aggregation disorders.

The Perioperative Management of Blood Thinners

The question of whether to withhold anticoagulant or antiplatelet medications prior to cutaneous surgery has been debated for over a decade in the dermatologic surgery literature. A recent report by Kovich and Otley shows that the majority of dermatologic surgeons discontinue blood thinners prior to surgery at least some of the time. Importantly, the weight of the literature now appears to be firmly in favor of maintaining patients on their prescribed medication. The rationale for this is twofold. First, a number of studies, both

prospective and retrospective, have demonstrated no increase in bleeding complications in patients on blood thinners undergoing cutaneous surgery. Secondly, there are now multiple reports detailing perioperative thromboembolic events in patients whose blood thinners were withheld prior to surgery. Alcalay and Alkalay performed a prospective study and found no bleeding complications in 68 consecutive patients on blood thinners undergoing MMS or other dermatologic surgery. All patients who were on warfarin had INRs less than 3.5. A prospective study by Billingsley and Maloney of 109 patients on aspirin, NSAIDs, or warfarin compared with 213 control patients found no statistically significant difference in postoperative bleeding complications after MMS with flap and graft repair. Otley et al. performed a retrospective study analyzing complications in patients taking platelet inhibitors or warfarin who underwent cutaneous surgery and found no statistical difference in the complication rate between patients on or off blood thinners. A study by Bartlett found no significant difference in bleeding complications between patients on aspirin and control patients undergoing minor cutaneous plastic surgery. A number of other procedural subspecialties, including oral maxillofacial surgery, ophthalmology, gastroenterology, urology, cardiothoracic surgery, and vascular surgery have reported no significant postoperative bleeding complications in patients on warfarin. In a retrospective literature review concerning dental procedures and warfarin, there were no reports of serious bleeding complications in patients receiving anticoagulation, but there were several documented cases of serious embolic events in patients whose warfarin was withheld prior to surgery. In the report, 12 of 774 patients (1.5%) had a postoperative bleeding complication requiring control by other than local measures (usually requiring administration of vitamin K). Five of the 12 had INRs above 3.5. In patients whose warfarin was withdrawn prior to surgery, 5 of 493 (1%) had a serious embolic complication, with 4 deaths.

Schanbacher and Bennett reported two patients, one with a mechanical heart valve and the other with atrial fibrillation, who underwent MMS and had their warfarin discontinued one week prior to surgery and resumed one day after surgery. Both suffered strokes within several days after surgery. Alam and Goldberg also reported two patients who underwent MMS and suffered thromboembolic events after discontinuation of their blood thinners. Kovich and Otley queried members of the American College of Mohs Micrographic Surgery and Cutaneous Oncology regarding thromboembolic complications in their patients whose blood thinners were withheld perioperatively. A total of 46 events were reported, 25 from discontinuation of warfarin and 18 when aspirin was stopped. Of the total, there were 24 strokes, 3 cerebral emboli, 5 heart attacks, 8 transient ischemic attacks, 3 deep nervous thrombosis, 2 pulmonary embolism, and 1 retinal artery occlusion resulting in blindness. Three of the events resulted in death. The estimated risk of a thromboembolic complication was 1 in 12,816 operations (1 event per 6219 for warfarin and 1 per 21,448 for aspirin discontinuation).

The weight of the evidence in the medical literature favors maintaining a patient on blood thinners prior to surgery. Independent of the intensity of anticoagulation, an increased risk for thromboembolism appears to exist in the perioperative setting, either due to rebound hypercoagulation from abrupt medication withdrawl, unmasking of the patient's primary thromboembolic risk, a prothrombotic state induced by the surgical setting, or a combination of the three. While thromboembolic events after discontinuation of anticoagulation are rare, major bleeding complications associated with continuation of blood thinners are rarer still.

Available evidence suggests that the vast majority of cutaneous surgery cases can be performed with the patient on blood thinners without significant bleeding complications. This counterintuitive finding may result from the fact that bleeding from cutaneous surgery can usually be readily identified and managed. However, for patients who take herbal preparations or routine aspirin prophylaxis in the absence of known preexisting disease, it is reasonable to stop the medications prior to surgery. In addition, some alterations in therapy might be considered in patients on multiple anticoagulants. In cases with a higher bleeding complication risk, such as extirpation of a large tumor in a vascular area or when a complex reconstruction is the best repair option, more detailed consideration should be given. Dunn and Turpie performed a detailed review of the available medical literature on the perioperative management of patients on OACs and, while acknowledging the overall poor quality of the studies available, determined that OAC can be continued without increasing the risk of serious bleeding complications for dental procedures, joint and soft tissue injections and arthrocentesis, cataract surgery, and gastrointestinal endoscopy with or without biopsy, as long as the INR was within therapeutic range. For all other procedures (including dermatologic surgery), they recommend an individualized strategy based on the estimation of the patient's risk of thromboembolism off anticoagulation. For those with a low annual risk ($<4\%$; e.g., atrial fibrillation without a prior thromboembolic event) OAC can be withheld without administration of heparin. For those with a high annual risk ($>7\%$; e.g., mechanical mitral valve and atrial fibrillation with prior thromboembolism), intravenous heparin or subcutaneous LMWH should be administered for the entire period that the INR is subtherapeutic. For those with a moderate thromboembolic risk ($4–7\%$; e.g., mechanical aortic valve), administration of heparin was deemed optional. Despite these recommendations, the authors did point out that the perioperative thromboembolic rate appears to be substantially higher for patients whose OAC is withheld, with or without the administration of heparin, than would be predicted for nonanticoagulated patients with atrial fibrillation or mechanical heart valves in nonsurgical settings. The reasons for this are unclear, but again rebound hypercoagulability from warfarin discontinuation and the particularities of the surgical setting are implicated. Table 1 lists the most common indications for anticoagulant therapy along with the perioperative thromboembolic risk if therapy is discontinued.

The decision to withhold blood thinners prior to surgery should always be made in consultation with the patient's prescribing physician. Several patient management strategies exist: (i) continue blood thinners at the same or reduced dose, (ii) discontinue blood thinners and add nothing, (iii) discontinue and add intravenous or subcutaneous UFH, or (iv) discontinue and add subcutaneous low-molecular-weight heparin (LMWH). Unfortunately, no randomized controlled trials have been performed to help guide the selection of a management plan. In the prospective but nonblinded, nonrandomized study by Cook and Perone, the authors chose to limit the use of anticoagulant and antiplatelet medications preoperatively, in consultation with the prescribing physician, and did not use heparin perioperatively. No thromboembolic complications were reported. Marietta et al. studied the safety and effectiveness of a protocol for reducing but not eliminating anticoagulation

prior to minor surgery. Eighty consecutive anticoagulated patients had their warfarin doses reduced by 50% on days 4, 3, and 2 before surgery, restoring the original dose the day before surgery. Patients then took a double dose the evening after surgery, and thereafter the usual dose was continued. There were no minor or major bleeding complications, and no thromboembolic events reported. There was also no evidence of induction of a hypercoagulable state as measured by prothrombin fragment assay. The mean INR values one week before surgery, the day of surgery, and one week after surgery were 2.63, 1.68, and 2.43, respectively.

Managing Bleeding Complications
Exsanguination
Although it is possible for bleeding from cutaneous surgery to reach levels at which it presents with hemodynamic significance, this situation is extremely rare. The unusual cases in which such a situation might occur include some Mohs' procedures in which tumors might be traced to depths at which large major vessels could be encountered (e.g., the carotid artery, femoral artery, etc.), scalp procedures without suturing (e.g., hair transplants), and surgery in which bleeding into a large dead-space is possible. This situation can always be aggravated by pre-existing hematalogic abnormalities and drug-induced coagulopathies.

Intraoperative Bleeding
Intraoperative bleeding can distress the surgeon and the patient. Even for experienced surgeons bleeding raises the general anxiety level in the operating room and flowing blood can be very distressing to the patient. Blood obscuring the operative site can interfere with the careful dissection desirable. By minimizing the potential causes of increased bleeding and using epinephrine, the surgeon can decrease the effects of this blood loss. The use of suction can help maintain good visualization in a bloody field. Immediate drying of the surgical field can sometimes be obtained by applying pressure to the periphery of the operative site. An assistant can provide traction across the wound surface with gloved hands or a ringed instrument, such as a scissors handle (Fig. 3). This can allow the completion of the immediate portion of the procedure. Intraoperative bleeding can then be controlled as soon as practical. Individual small vessels should be isolated and cauterized with electrocoagulation or hot-tipped cautery. Various devices are available for this purpose, each with advantages and disadvantages as discussed in Chapter 15. Such hemostasis should be as precise as possible to avoid unnecessary tissue destruction that leaves excessive char in the operative site, causing increased inflammation and a possible nidus for infection.

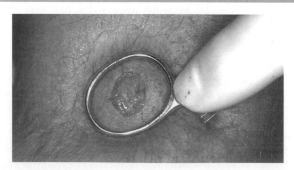

Figure 3 The use of a ringed instrument handle to help dry the operative field.

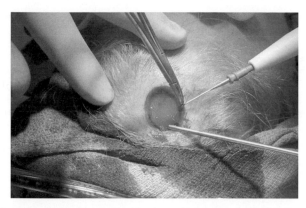

Figure 4 Electrocoagulation of a larger caliber vessel with the aid of a hemostat.

Slightly larger vessels should be grasped with an appropriately sized hemostat and then cauterized (Fig. 4). This maneuver tends to limit the extent of the destruction. Larger, muscular vessels should be ligated with ties of absorbable sutures. Coagulation of such vessels may provide immediate hemostasis, but can lead to delayed bleeding if the clot retracts into the large vessel lumen. The surgical field should be as dry as possible prior to closure. Particular attention should be paid to the apices of ellipses and flaps. In addition, cut muscle may have multiple small bleeding points.

If bleeding has been particularly difficult to control during the initial portion of a procedure, the surgeon may wish to consider modifying the extent of the ultimate operation. Limiting undermining or choosing a linear closure rather than a flap or graft will limit the potential "dead space" in which blood may accumulate postoperatively. If bleeding has been difficult to control during the performance of a flap or a large multilayered closure, the placement of a drain may prevent hematoma formation. A simple drain may be created from a sterilized rubber band, a fenistrated penrose drain may be placed, or a more elaborate drain such as a Jackson-Pratt drain may be utilized. Such a drain can usually be removed 24 to 48 hours after the procedure. Although placement of a drain may cause a small delay in healing and slightly increase the risk of infection, some surgeons choose to place drains after any extensive procedure to allow for small amounts of postoperative bleeding.

Postoperative Care

A layered pressure dressing can aid in hemostasis. This firmly applied series of bandages can also wick away small amounts of bleeding from the wound site. However, if the dressing becomes saturated with blood, it rapidly loses any compressive qualities and will not impede bleeding. Dressings and/or splints may also be utilized to decrease wound site motion after a procedure. Movement of the site may dislodge clots or electrocoagulation char and precipitate new bleeding. The proper application of a dressing can protect the wound site from external trauma with its resulting risk of bleeding. The patient should be given strict, explicit instructions regarding activity after each procedure. These instructions may range from essentially only restrictions on wetting the area for simple shave procedures to modified bedrest for large, extensive flaps. The patient should be instructed in such circumstances to avoid putting

the wound in dependent positions. Perioral wounds may require a soft diet and restriction on talking. Lower extremity wounds may require limitations on standing and walking. The patient needs to be told when and at what level normal activities can be resumed. Especially now that regular exercise is an important part of many patients' routines, a simple "take it easy" may be insufficient in many circumstances.

Postoperative Bleeding

In spite of careful preoperative evaluation, precise intraoperative hemostasis, and limitation of a patient's activities, postoperative bleeding will occur in a small number of cases. The bleeding may be a continuation of a slow ooze which was present at the end of the procedure, or it may have begun fresh. The first few hours after surgery present the greatest risk. As the patient returns home after surgery the clots are still fragile, and sudden movements or elevations in blood pressure may precipitate new bleeding. In addition, the loss of the epinephrine effect may yield small vessel bleeding. The patient should be instructed that a small amount of blood on the wound dressing is normal. If the bloodied area is increasing or blood is dripping from the dressing, the patient should be instructed to apply firm pressure directly to the wound site for 20 minutes. The patient must be instructed not to remove pressure to look at the site during this period. If not measured by a clock, the time will likely be underestimated. If the dressing was saturated with blood, the dressing should be removed prior to applying pressure and replaced with sterile dry dressing material. If the pressure is successful in stopping the bleeding, this dressing or the original one can be reinforced with additional gauze and tape.

If the bleeding persists, the surgeon should evaluate the patient. A trial of direct pressure can again be initiated. If this fails, the wound must be opened and explored for the source of the bleeding. The infiltration of local anesthesia is usually necessary prior to such exploration. The use of epinephrine in the anesthesia mix will provide a drier field, but may obscure the bleeding sites. Rarely, the bleeding may be from a single large vessel. In this event, the vessel should be isolated and cauterized or ligated as appropriate. The wound can then be resutured. In most cases, the bleeding is from multiple small vessels. These bleeding points should be isolated and cauterized. If a very dry surgical field is not obtainable, consideration should be given to the placement of a surgical drain.

Postoperative Bleeding in the Anticoagulated Patient

In the event of a severe bleeding complication due to warfarin hyperanticoagulation, immediate warfarin reversal is achieved with prothrombin complex concentrate (PCC) and fresh frozen plasma (FFP). PCC contains factors II, IX and X, and low levels of factor VII. FFP is added as an additional source of factor VII. Vitamin K is essential for sustaining the reversal achieved by PCC and FFP. An intravenous dose of 0.5 mg vitamin K seems sufficient to achieve an INR in the therapeutic range in most patients within 24 hours; however, this route of administration should be avoided if possible, since anaphylactic reactions have been described. Vitamin K may be delivered subcutaneously, but oral vitamin K has been shown to lower INR more rapidly. For ease of administration, the injectable formulation of the drug can be delivered orally. To temporarily reverse the effect of anticoagulation, vitamin K should be given in a dose that will quickly lower the INR to a safe, but not subtherapeutic, range and will not cause resistance once warfarin is reinstated. Weibert et al. have demonstrated successful correction of excessive anticoagulant effect using a single fixed dose of 2.5 mg of oral vitamin K after eliminating one or two doses of the daily warfarin regimen. Higher vitamin K doses are required during the correction of an excessive INR when warfarin therapy is not interrupted.

Hematoma

Bleeding through a sutured wound is troublesome, but blood collecting as a large clot in the dead space of a wound can cause even greater problems. The development of a hematoma may be accompanied by external bleeding but most often it is not. The most frequent symptom of a large, expanding hematoma is the onset of new, often throbbing, pain, but if the hematoma is small the patient may sense only increased pressure. Removal of the dressing will reveal an ecchymotic, sometimes oozing, firm, yet fluctuant mass under all or part of the wound (Fig. 5). Early hematomas should be evacuated. The thick clot provides a barrier to immune surveillance and therefore an excellent medium for the growth of bacteria. In addition, adequate wound healing is impaired and can lead to dehiscence after suture removal. Also, a large or expanding hematoma increases tension across the wound edge or the flap pedicle, impairing blood flow and leading to necrosis and wound dehiscence.

Applying pressure to the wound may express small amounts of blood, but the hematoma itself cannot usually be evacuated in this manner. The early hematoma has the consistency of gelatin. By removing several sutures and opening a tract to the dead-space of the wound with scissors or a hemostat, large portions of the hematoma may be evacuated (Fig. 6). The bulk of it is often fragmented into numerous smaller clots, and the wound may need to be widely opened to remove the entire contents of the hematoma pocket. The site should then be irrigated and inspected for bleeding sites. Local anesthesia is generally always required. The surgeon should be aware that the walls of the wound abutting the hematoma now have a dusky, ecchymotic appearance rather than pink and fresh as at the initial surgery. Again, a single bleeding vessel may be found, but most often there are multiple small bleeding points requiring attention. After diligent hemostasis, the

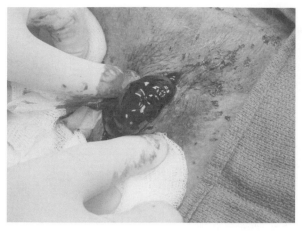

Figure 6 Gelatin-like clots of a hematoma being expressed after removal of several staples. (*See color insert.*)

wound may be resutured. Strict attention should be paid to repair of any dead-space. If there is any difficulty obtaining a dry field, a drain should be placed (Fig. 7). Because of the increased risk of wound infection antibiotic prophylaxis is indicated.

If the hematoma is not recognized or treated early, within several days the clot becomes organized. It develops a thick fibrous texture and adheres to the surrounding tissue. Large or expanding hematomas are probably best still evacuated at this stage to decrease the risk of infection and limit necrosis from increased wound tension. After the infiltration of local anesthesia, the area over the hematoma is opened and as much of the organized clot is removed as is possible. The original source of the bleeding has most often stopped, but fresh bleeding may be caused by the removal of the adherent material. Most often the wound is not resutured but is allowed to heal by second intention. Because dead-space is created by the evacuation of the hematoma, such a wound often requires packing with daily changes of the packing material.

A small, stable hematoma may be observed rather than operatively evacuated. This hematoma will be quite firm with an ecchymotic appearance (Fig. 8). Gentle heat applied at 30 to 60 minute intervals several times each day may speed resolution. With time the hematoma is liquefied by the action of the fibrinolytic system. Small hematomas may be completely reabsorbed by the body in this manner. Larger

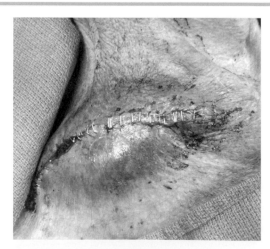

Figure 5 Acute hematoma presenting 24 hours postoperatively at supraclavicular full thickness skin graft donor site. (*See color insert.*)

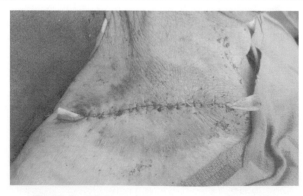

Figure 7 A Penrose drain in place. (*See color insert.*)

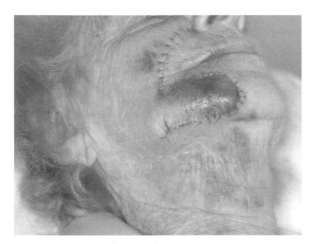

Figure 8 Organized hematoma at postoperative day 7. (*See color insert.*)

hematomas may develop a fluctuant mass that requires aspiration approximately one to two weeks after surgery. Aspiration can usually be accomplished with a large bore needle (16 to 18 gauge) without opening the wound, but may have to be repeated over several days.

Ecchymosis

Ecchymosis, or bruising, is caused by the leakage of small amounts of blood into the interstitial space. Ecchymoses often develop after surgical procedures, especially in areas of loose, distensible tissue (e.g., periorbital region or on the chest or forearms in elderly individuals), and may appear in these areas even with surgery performed at relatively distant sites (Fig. 9). The trauma of skin surgery, beginning with the distention of the tissue with the injection of local anesthesia, can immediately lead to ecchymoses in the surgical area. The area of bruising initially is black and blue from the reduced hemoglobin in extravasated blood. Over the ensuing days as the hemoglobin is degraded to bilirubin, the colors change to green and yellow and finally dissipate by two weeks, if not sooner. Ecchymoses may be quite alarming to the patient, especially in the periorbital area, but will resolve quickly and usually with no sequelae.

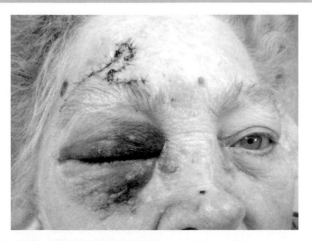

Figure 9 Periorbital edema and ecchymoses the day after a procedure on the forehead. (*See color insert.*)

INFECTION

The risk of infection in cutaneous surgery is generally very low, but when it develops, it can lead to severe problems in wound healing. Disruption of all or part of the repair may occur, leading to an unacceptable scar. In rare circumstances, systemic dissemination may take place leading to even more serious consequences. Infectious risk is directly proportional to the degree of wound contamination (the "dose" and virulence of the infecting organism) and inversely proportional to the body's level of tissue defense.

A few detailed studies are available in the dermatologic surgical literature to help predict surgical site infection (SSI) rates for outpatient cutaneous surgery. It is generally felt that the rate of significant infections is less than 5% and most often 1% to 2%. In a prospective study by Whitaker et al. performed over a 30-month period, an infection rate of 0.7% (27/3961) was seen for class I (excsional surgical wounds with immediate or same day closure) and class II (excisional or other procedures with delayed closure or second intention healing) wounds. No infections were reported in over 6000 class III procedures (no full-thickness penetration of dermis). No patients included in the study received antibiotic prophylaxis. In a retrospective review, Futoryan and Grande reported a wound infection rate of 2.3% (24/1047) in cases involving MMS and other excisional surgery. Patients on antibiotic prophylaxis for pre-existing medical conditions were excluded from the study, but patients given perioperative antibiotics for large defects or prolonged operative time were not. In the study by Cook and Perone, postoperative wound infection occurred in just one case (out of 1343), yielding an unexpectedly low infectious complication rate of 0.07%; however, the investigators chose to administer postoperative antibiotics to all patients who underwent flap or graft repair ($N = 578$).

The SSI rates reported in these studies compare favorably with those of in-hospital procedures. Unfortunately, these perceived rates do not adequately distinguish between patients who receive prophylactic antibiotics and those who do not. This low apparent rate of infection makes studies on the effectiveness of prophylactic antibiotics and other preventive measures difficult due to the large numbers of patients required to detect a statistical difference between randomized groups. In addition, this brings into question the dermatologic surgeon's sense of having prevented infections by employing antibiotics prophylactically.

Etiology and Risk Factors for SSI

When the patient's natural barrier to infection is disrupted by a surgical incision, the underlying tissues are exposed to contamination by both endogenous and exogenous flora. Most SSIs are derived from the microbial flora of the patient's own skin or mucous membranes. Coagulase negative staphylococci (e.g., *Staphylococcus epidermidis*) constitutes more than 50% of the resident skin flora, but result in far fewer SSIs. *Staphylococcus aureus* is not part of the endogenous flora of glabrous skin but is found in the nasal passages and perineal areas of 20% to 40% of normal adults, and it is also present in high concentrations on diseased skin. Carriers of *S. aureus* have an up to ninefold increase in the risk of SSI. *S. aureus* is consistently the most commonly isolated pathogen in SSI, and is typically more virulent than other frequent causes, such as coagulase-negative staphylococci and enterococci. When incisions are made near the perineum or groin, anaerobic and gram-negative aerobic bacteria are encountered. *Pseudomonas aeruginosa* infection

Table 3 Percentage of Isolates From Surgical Site Infections, 1986–1996

Pathogen	% (N = 17,671)
Staphylococcus aureus	20
Coagulase-negative staphylococci	14
Enterococcus spp.	12
Escherichia coli	8
Pseudomonas aeruginosa	8
Enterobacter spp.	7
Proteus mirabilis	3
Klebsiella pneumoniae	3
Other *Streptococcus* spp.	3
Candida albicans	3
Group D *Streptococcus*	2
Other gram-positive aerobes	2
Bacteroides fragilis	2
Gram-positive anaerobes	1
Other *Candida* spp.	1
Acinetobacter spp.	1
Serratia marcescens	1
Citrobacter spp.	1
Other enterobacteriaceae aerobes	1
Other nonenterobacteriaceae aerobes	1
Group B *Streptococcus*	1
Other *Klebsiella* spp.	1

Source: From Centers for Disease and Control Prevention (1996); Mangram, Horan, Pearson, Silver, Jarvis (1999).

complicates surgical procedures performed on the ear with increased frequency and is possibly related to the bacteria's tropism for the epithelium of the external auditory canal. Table 3 lists the frequency of isolates from documented SSIs as tabulated by the National Nosocomial Infections Surveillance System from 1986 to 1996.

A number of other endogenous (patient) and exogenous (surgeon/staff and procedure-related) factors have been shown to play an important role in the risk of SSI development (Table 4). With the interplay of so many variables, it is often difficult to directly implicate any single factor when a wound infection does develop. An adequate knowledge of the inherent risks is critical to proper pre- and postoperative planning. It also underscores the importance of tracking SSIs as part of a regular invasive procedure review. If a trend is identified, a detailed examination of all possibly implicated factors is warranted.

Pre-existing bacterial infection at the operative site such as an infected epidermoid cyst or a necrotic tumor or

Table 4 Factors Relevant to the Development of Surgical Site Infection

Patient related	Surgeon/staff related	Operation
Concurrent remote infection	Aseptic technique	Operative facility
Bacterial colonization	Surgical attire	Anatomic location
Diabetes mellitus	Surgical scrub	Duration of operation
Cigarette smoking	Surgical drapes	Complexity of operation
Systemic steroid use	Patient skin prep	Antibiotic prophylaxis
Obesity	Instrument sterilization	Use of
Renal failure	Surgical technique	Timing of
Extremes of age	Tissue handling	
Poor nutritional status	Hemostasis	
Immunosuppression	Minimizing dead space	
Preoperative hospitalization	Choice of materials	
Postoperative wound care		

even an infection at a separate, remote site can greatly increase the risk of wound infection. If possible, such infections should be completely treated prior to elective procedures. As mentioned, bacterial colonization (especially by *S. aureus*) is one of the most important risk factors for SSI. In the same manner, prolonged preoperative hospitalization is associated with an increased risk of SSI, possibly secondary to colonization of the patient with pathogenic microorganisms, although such patients would be expected to be more seriously ill and therefore more susceptible to infection.

The postoperative period is not commonly associated with the initiation of wound infections; however, early contamination of wounds is possible if poor wound care practices are followed. Failure to remove blood-soaked dressings increases the risk of bacterial infection. The site may also be contaminated due to a patient's poor handwashing with dressing changes or by excessive manipulation or exposure of the wound during the first 24 to 48 hours after the procedure. After this time the wound is more resistant to contamination. Specific wound care instructions should be provided to every patient verbally and in writing.

It has been shown that a host of independent systemic factors can lower a patient's resistance to the development of infection. Poor control of blood glucose in the immediate postoperative period has been associated with an increased risk for SSI. Cigarette smoking, obesity, renal failure, and malnutrition may all contribute to an increased risk of infection. Any abnormality that alters the immune system by reducing the number or effectiveness of granulocytes or lymphocytes may lead to infection with common and unusual pathogens in both the surgical and nonsurgical settings. Patients with AIDS certainly have an increased risk of many infections; however, the risk of developing infections after cutaneous procedures has not been quantitated. Processes that alter the body's ability to produce effective immunoglobulins, may also predispose an individual to infection. Immune defenses may also be compromised by systemic medications. Corticosteroids, immunosuppressants, and cytotoxic agents may all increase the risk of infection. Increasing numbers of patients are now receiving long-term immunosuppression for organ transplantation, onconologic, rheumatologic and dermatologic conditions.

Proper aseptic and surgical technique is paramount to minimizing the risk of infectious problems. Proper handwashing before the first case and between cases should be a ritual for the entire surgical team. The surgeon's first surgical scrub of the day should last for at least two minutes and consist of a thorough cleaning underneath the fingernails. For subsequent handwashing, the use of an alcohol-based hand rinse has been shown to be a more effective microbicide with less potential for emergence of resistant strains and to cause less skin damage than traditional detergent-based scrubs. The proper surgical attire (caps, masks, sterile gloves, protective clothing) should be worn in an effort to prevent contamination of the operative site and for protection of surgical personnel. Preparation of the surgical site is most commonly performed with chlorhexidine gluconate or povidone-iodine. Chlorhexidine may be the superior agent as it has been shown to produce a greater reduction in skin flora than povidone-iodine, and also since povidone-iodine is inactivated by blood. Preoperative shaving of the operative site with a razor, especially if performed the prior evening, is associated with a significantly increased risk of SSI. Hair should only be removed if it will grossly interfere with the surgical procedure. In that event, it is preferably clipped with scissors or a depilatory employed just prior to the procedure.

Improperly sterilized surgical instruments and other materials used intraoperatively has been associated with a host of common and unusual infectious problems. Sterilization of instruments by steam autoclaving at 121°C at a pressure of 15 pounds per square inch for 15 minutes has been shown to be effective in killing all microorganisms; however, microbial monitoring of steam autoclave performance is necessary and can be accomplished with the use of commercially available biologic indicators.

Local wound factors created or exacerbated by poor surgical technique can increase the risk for SSI. As discussed previously, a hematoma is resistant to penetration by the body's immune response and can thus serve as a favorable media for bacterial growth. Excessive tension on the skin from a poorly executed closure or an expanding hematoma may decrease the blood supply to a wound, providing devitalized tissue as a nidus for infection. Improper wound closure resulting in a potential space promotes seroma or hematoma formation. Foreign bodies such as suture and excessive char from electrocoagulation may incite an inflammatory response and also serve as a focus for infection. Inappropriate tissue handling by crushing the edges of a wound with forceps may result in ischemia and subsequent necrosis.

Anatomic location is another important consideration when assessing the risk of SSI. In the study by Futoryan and Grande, MMS performed on the ear was noted to produce a high percentage of wound infections compared with all other body sites (6/13 or 46%). For all Mohs cases performed on the ear, there was an infection rate of 12.5% (6/48). If the plane of excision was taken to the level of the cartilage, 28.6% of the ear cases became infected. Other sites such as the mouth, axilla, and groin carry an increased risk of SSI likely due to the resident flora there. Operative time longer than three hours also increases the risk of SSI.

The procedure room environment is also important to consider when minimizing the risk of SSI. Bacteria and other microbes are present at variable levels in dust, respiratory droplets, and airborne exfoliated skin cells. The concentration of microorganisms in the air is directly proportional to the number of people moving about in the room; therefore, flow of personnel in and out of the room should be kept to a

minimum during any operation. Specific techniques for preparation for surgery and maintenance of a clean operative field are discussed in detail in an earlier chapter and should be followed closely.

Evaluation and Management of SSI

A wound infection is heralded by the four cardinal signs of inflammation as enunciated by Celcius: *calor* (heat), *dolor* (pain), *rubor* (redness), and *tumor* (swelling) (Fig. 10). The signs and symptoms of an early wound infection are exaggerations of the inflammatory phase of normal wound healing. In the majority of cases an infection begins at some point during the operation, but most wound infections do not become evident until at least four days postoperatively. Rarely there may be delayed presentation, such as several days after suture removal. In most cases, pain and tenderness increase quickly, reversing the normal postoperative course. Erythema may extend rapidly with red streaks of lymphangitis becoming evident and lymphadenopathy developing as well. Firm swelling at the wound site may give way to fluctuance and purulent material may be discharged or expressed from the wound margins. Systemic symptoms including fever and chills herald spreading infection. If the patient reports at any time in the perioperative course the sudden or gradual onset of erythema, pain, swelling, or discharge, the wound should be examined promptly by the surgeon.

The treatment of an established wound infection should follow the principles established in general surgery of drainage, heat, elevation, and rest. For a red, warm wound with prulent drainage, the precept of draining the infection should be followed. Any remaining sutures should be removed and if an abscess is present, it should be opened and drained. In this situation deep absorbable sutures may also require removal, as they can be a further nidus for infection. The wound should be left open to allow additional drainage and if deep cavities are present the wound should be packed lightly with iodoform gauze to maintain drainage. Packing should be changed daily and the wound cleaned until the discharge ceases. Gentle heat to the area may hasten resolution of the infection by increasing local blood flow. Appropriate antibiotic measures should be initiated promptly. If a discharge or other exudative material is present, a specimen for culture and sensitivity should be submitted. A Gram's stain should be performed to aid with antibiotic selection. In the face of spreading erythema, exudate, or induration, remaining sutures should be removed, and if the wound dehisces it should be treated as mentioned. If only mild erythema is present, sutures that can be safely removed without causing dehiscence should be so. Antibiotic treatment should be initiated and the wound closely observed. If the infection is controlled by such measures, the remaining sutures can be removed at the usual time.

In the absence of a Gram's stain and while waiting for culture results, initial antibiotic selection is based on the anatomic site, the patient's overall medical condition, and the surgeon's local experience with wound infection. If *S. aureus* is suspected, a penicillinase-resistant penicillin or a first-generation cephalosporin (e.g., cephalexin) should be prescribed. Cephalosporins are among the most widely used and thoroughly studied antibiotics. Their demonstrated safety and cost-effectiveness make them, with few exceptions, the preferred choice for the initiation of antibiotic therapy for suspected SSI caused by gram-positive or gram-negative infections. The first-generation agents are most

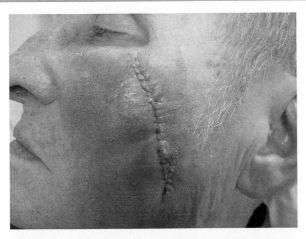

Figure 10 Acute wound infection presenting several days postoperatively. The area is red, warm, swollen, and tender. (*See color insert.*)

active against *S. aureus* and other gram-positive organisms. With each succeeding generation, gram-negative activity tends to improve but at the expense of gram-positive activity. The cephalosporins lack activity against methicillin-resistant *S. aureus* (MRSA) and *Enterococcus* spp.

If *Pseudomanas* infection is suspected, a fluoroquinolone or third-generation cephalosporin antibiotic is the preferred initial agent. Of the fluoroquinolones, ciprofloxacin is the most active against *P. aeruginosa*. However, resistance is an increasing problem indicating that ciprofloxacin may no longer provide assured empiric monotherapy. The newer fluoroquinolones (e.g., levofloxacin, moxifloxacin, gatifloxacin) have enhanced activity against gram-positive bacteria in addition to satisfactory aerobic gram-negative activity, and are FDA approved for use in uncomplicated skin and soft-tissue infections.

In certain geographic locations and patient populations the prevalence of MRSA and other antibiotic resistant organisms presents a special challenge. Rather than a first-generation cephalosporin, the first choice for empiric therapy may be clindamycin or trimethoprim-sulfamethoxazole if the frequency of MRSA isolates is especially high in the practice area. The surgeon should always be aware of any trends in terms of organism type and frequency of isolation for the more problematic pathogens. Keeping regular contact with the local microbiology lab or an infectious disease expert in the community is an excellent habit to develop.

Vancomycin is still considered the drug of last defense for multidrug-resistant gram-positive bacteria, but resistance to even this drug is on the rise, and therefore its use should be strictly limited to complicated wound infections posing significant morbidity or threat to life. Several novel antibacterial agents with activity against vancomycin-resistant strains of *S. aureus* and enterococcus, in addition to MRSA, are now available for the treatment of complicated skin infections. These include linezolid, quinupristin-dalfopristin, and daptomycin.

In all cases of suspected infection, further antimicrobial therapy should be guided by the culture and sensitivity and the clinical response to treatment. Early or mild infection should be treated aggressively. If available in the clinic, a loading dose with a parenteral antibiotic preparation is helpful. In a patient with a rapidly spreading infection, extensive lymphangitis, or systemic symptoms hospital admission for parenteral antibiotics and aggressive wound care should be strongly considered. Immunosuppression and poor general health are factors predisposing a patient to a severe infection and possible inadequate response to oral antibiotic therapy.

It is important to consider that conditions other than bacterial infections may also present with similar signs and symptoms. If the skin surrounding the wound has vesicles, pustules or scale in addition to erythema, one must consider a fungal etiology, especially *Candida*. An increasing proportion of SSIs due to *Candida albicans* is being seen, possibly as a result of the overuse of broad-spectrum antibiotics. A KOH examination and culture will aid in the evaluation in such circumstances. The occlusive dressings often used after surgery may provide the proper conditions for the growth of these organisms.

If the erythema closely corresponds to the area to which the antibiotic cream or ointment has been applied, contact dermatitis must be considered (Fig. 11). Occlusive dressings may provide a "patch test" environment. In a similar manner, if the erythema follows the contact areas of the dressing adhesive, an irritant or allergic contact

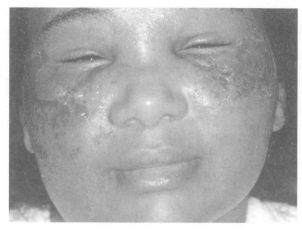

Figure 11 Allergic contact dermatitis to topical antibiotic applied to periocular wounds. (*See color insert.*)

sensitivity reaction is likely. Scale and vesiculation may also be present if the reaction is vigorous. Pruritus often accompanies irritant and allergic reactions rather than increased pain. Allergic and irritant reactions can be minimized by avoiding commonly sensitizing agents whenever possible. Neomycin, present in Neosporin® and other "triple antibiotic" ointments, is the third most common allergen in North America. Bacitracin, a component of Polysporin®, is also a potent allergen although its use as a topical antibiotic after skin surgery is still widespread. In fact, many patients sensitive to neomycin are also sensitive to bacitracin. If contact sensitivity is suspected, the antibiotic ointment should be discontinued. If possible the wound should be left open and a mild to medium potency topical steroid may be applied to the area surrounding the wound.

An inflammatory reaction to suture material may also be mistaken for a wound infection. Erythema or an erythematous papule may develop at each suture site. At its extreme, small pustules may be observed. Such reaction may be recognized by its localization to the site of the individual sutures (Fig. 12) The reaction is aborted by the removal of the sutures.

Indications for Antibiotic Prophylaxis

In dermatologic surgery, antimicrobial prophylaxis (AMP) is routinely employed for the prevention of SSI, endocarditis,

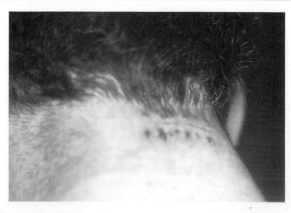

Figure 12 Brightly erythematous suture reaction. (*See color insert.*)

and prosthesis infection. There is no universally accepted standard of care for AMP in dermatologic surgery. Rather, a handful of nonevidence based guidelines, which lack specialty-specific data, serve as direction. The surgeon must balance the risk of adverse drug reactions and the ever-increasing problem of multiple drug resistant organisms due to widespread antibiotic usage with the benefit of infection prevention. As previously mentioned, the use of antibiotic prophylaxis for the prevention of endocarditis and prosthesis infection is discussed in Chapter 5. To help predict infection risk, surgical wounds were first classified in the general surgical literature as outlined in Table 5. This convention has found widespread use across surgical subspecialties. The vast majority of wounds in dermatologic surgery are either class I or class II wounds. MMS is an example of a class II wound given that strict sterile technique is generally not maintained; however, the observed infection rate in MMS, even in the absence of AMP, is generally much lower than what would be predicted by the classification. In this situation, AMP is probably not indicated in the absence of other compounding factors such as those listed in Table 5. Of important note, the use of antibiotics in class III and class IV wounds is considered therapeutic rather than prophylactic.

Prophylactic antibiotics are most effective if administered within two hours prior to surgical wounding. Typically, parenteral antibiotics are given within 30 minutes of the start of a procedure, and oral antibiotics should be administered approximately one hour before surgery given the delay in systemic absorption. Two randomized, prospective, blinded studies by Zitelli and coworkers show that a single, intraincisional injection of antibiotic (either nafcillin or clindamycin) mixed with local anesthetic and administered approximately 15 minutes prior to reconstruction of MMS defects is effective in reducing the risk of SSI. The duration of AMP is less well documented, but should probably be much shorter than is generally employed in current dermatologic practice. Some studies have suggested that the single preoperative dose is optimal, while other reports suggest that a second dose is helpful in prolonged procedures. There is no evidence to suggest that the extension of prophylactic antibiotic coverage beyond 24 hours is required. While it has long been recognized that having antibiotics in the surgical site prior to wounding is optimal, postoperative administration of AMP, common in dermatologic surgery, still reduces wound infection rates in a significant manner.

The choice of antibiotic for AMP should naturally be made on the basis of the most likely causal organism. Attention should also be paid to less frequently encountered but more potentially morbid situations. For example, AMP prior to surgery on the ear may be considered for prevention of liquefying chondritis caused by *P. aeruginosa*.

Topical antibiotic ointments and creams are commonly utilized to prevent wound infection and promote wound healing. Topical antibiotics can reduce bacterial counts in open wounds and around catheter sites, but there is not substantial evidence that wound infections are prevented with routine topical use. Given their propensity for contact allergy, the use of topical antibiotics for the prevention of wound infection is somewhat controversial, especially when used for wound care after clean procedures. There is evidence-based data to promote the discontinuation of topical antibiotics for aftercare of clean surgical procedures. In a large randomized, double-blind, prospective trial of 922 patients with 1249 surgical wounds, white petrolatum was demonstrated to be safe and effective with no case of contact dermatitis or anaphylaxis and no statistically significant increase in wound infection or impairment in wound healing when compared with bacitracin.

Preoperative antiseptic showering with chlorhexidine several nights prior to surgery greatly reduces skin bacterial counts but does not significantly reduce SSI rates in patients undergoing major surgery. In contrast, the topical application of benzoyl peroxide for seven days prior to surgery has been shown to reduce the rate of wound infection in surgical procedures to the centrofacial area.

In several studies, suppression or eradication of *S. aureus* nasal carriage has been associated with reduced rates of SSI compared with historical controls. However, in a recent randomized, double-blind, placebo-controlled trial evaluating the effectiveness of mupirocin ointment in preventing SSI, prophylactic intranasal application of mupirocin did not significantly reduce the rate of *S. aureus* SSI overall, but it did significantly decrease the rate of all nosocomial *S. aureus* infections among the patients who were *S. aureus* carriers.

Determining when antibiotic prophylaxis for SSI prevention in dermatologic surgery is necessary is difficult without a clear guideline developed from evidence-based studies. Given the overall very low risk of wound infection, it is clear that the routine, indiscriminate use of antibiotics is not indicated. The decision to use AMP should be individualized to the patient and procedure.

Necrosis

Necrosis is the death of previously viable tissue and results from circulatory failure at the operative site. Any event that compromises blood flow, whether initiated at the time of surgery or arising postoperatively as a consequence of other complications, can result in wound necrosis. The best treatment is prevention and many potential problems can be averted with proper surgical planning and technique.

The cutaneous blood supply comes primarily from a subdermal arterial plexus that in turn is supplied by small segmental arteries. These arteries are termed musculocutaneous, which pass through muscle to supply the overlying skin, and septocutaneous (also called direct cutaneous arteries), perforating vessels traveling through fascia dividing muscular segments. The subdermal plexus gives rise to a horizontal dermal plexus and plexuses around the hair follicles and other adnexal structures. Interruption of the segmental arteries may lead to areas of necrosis of several

Table 5 Operative Wound Classification

Classification	Characteristics	Risk of infection
1. Clean	No break in technique No inflammation Respiratory, GI, GU tracts not entered	1–4 %
2. Clean-contaminated	Minor break in technique Non-infected respiratory, GI or GU tract entered without gross spillage	5–15%
3. Contaminated	Major break in technique Gross spillage from respiratory, GI or GU tract	6–25%
4. Dirty and infected	Surgical wound includes acute bacterial infection with or without pus	> 25%(?100%)

Abbreviations: GI, gastrointestinal; GU, genitourinary.

Table 6 Factors that Increase the Risk of Necrosis

Systemic factors
    Arteriosclerotic vascular disease
    Diabetes
    Collagen-vascular disease
    Systemic vasculitis
    Smoking
Local factors
    Location: lower extremities, acral locations (fingers, toes, ears)
    Radiation dermatitis
    Lymphedema
    Stasis dermatitis
Wound complications
    Hematoma
    Infection
    Edema
    Venous congestion
    Excessive wound tension
    Tight sutures
    Excessive undermining
    Inadequate random flap pedicle width
    Compromise of blood flow in arterial-based flap

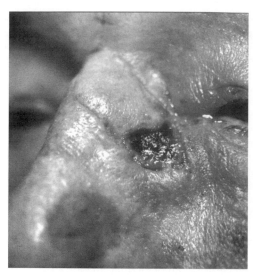

Figure 13 Necrosis of the distal portion of a transposition flap. Note also the hyperpigmentation from a full-thickness graft on the distal nose. (*See color insert.*)

centimeters. However, the blood supply to most skin areas in the absence of other disease processes is quite rich with multiple anastamoses. As a result the subdermal plexus continues to be supplied, albeit from a distance. A number of factors may decrease blood supply to the skin, thereby increasing the risk of necrosis (Table 6). With regard to tobacco use, patients should always be strongly advised to quit smoking several days prior to surgery and extending through the postoperative period. If the patient is unable to do so, decreasing smoking to less than one pack of cigarettes a day may be helpful in decreasing the risk of necrosis. Goldminz and Bennett retrospectively noted that heavy smokers (one or more packs per day) have a wound necrosis rate three-times higher than non-, former, or lighter smokers.

Extensive undermining of wounds decreases the circulation to the distal wound margins. Too superficial a level of undermining may damage the subdermal plexus as well as the segmental arteries. Any situation that will further decrease blood flow may cause a sufficient loss of perfusion and result in necrosis. Wound swelling from edema or venous congestion may tamponade the arterioles and capillaries and diminish the blood flow. A hematoma may take this pressure to the extreme. Even the tension on the wound edge created as the wound is closed will stretch the vessels and decrease flow. Small areas of blood flow may be completely obstructed by tight or improperly placed sutures. The orientation of the blood vessels in the dermis and the subdermis should be kept in mind and looping horizontally oriented sutures that have the potential to occlude portions of the plexuses should be avoided. As much tension as possible should be relieved from the skin edges by the placement of subcutaneous and deep dermal sutures. In addition, allowance should be made for the increased suture tension that results from postoperative wound edema. The use of suture material that stretches slightly, such as monofilament polypropylene or nylon, can relieve some of this tension. Employing a "loop stitch" compensates for excess tension from postoperative edema. A small 1 to 2 mm "loop" between the first and second throws of the knot allows room for tissue expansion.

Flaps may also suffer from an inherent inadequate blood supply. Many flaps in dermatologic surgery are based not on the preservation and supply of a named blood vessel but on a random blood supply to the subdermal plexus. In general, with a good blood supply the width of the pedicle of a random pattern flap should be at least one-third the length of the flap. If the width is not sufficient, distal necrosis may result (Fig. 13). In addition, rotation and transposition flap movement may create a standing cutaneous cone (dog-ear) at the base of the flap. Removal of this excess tissue must be taken in a manner such that the pedicle is not decreased in width or the flap elongated to the point that the 1:3 ratio is exceeded. In many cases removal of this redundancy should be delayed until the distal flap has developed new collateral circulation. Axial pattern flaps, such as the paramedian forehead flap, designed to preserve and transfer a specific blood supply with the tissue have become much more common in dermatologic surgery. When flaps are based on an isolated blood vessel pair, extreme care must be exercised in the handling of the pedicle that contains the vessel. Stretching or twisting the pedicle to mobilize the flap may compromise blood flow.

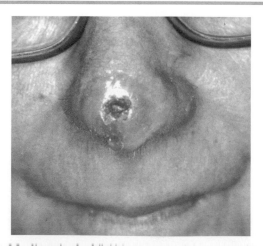

Figure 14 Necrosis of a full-thickness skin graft in an area placed over exposed cartilage. (*See color insert.*)

A full-thickness or split-thickness skin graft will necrosis if it fails to establish a blood supply from the underlying wound bed. If a properly harvested and prepared graft fails, one of two events may have occurred. First, the underlying bed may have insufficient vasculature to support the graft. Grafts placed over areas with greater than one square centimeter of bare cartilage or bone will often show areas of necrosis (Fig. 14). Grafts placed on sites that have previously been exposed to therapeutic radiation will frequently fail. Second, accumulated blood or serous fluid may have prevented the graft from adhering to the wound bed. Assuring a dry operative field prior to the placement of the graft and the use of basting sutures and tie-down bolsters can decrease the risk of necrosis due to this cause. Excessive physical activity by the patient can also interfere with adherence of the graft to the recipient site. Reported necrosis of flaps and graphs in dermatologic surgery has ranged from 1.9% to 10.4%.

The earliest sign of vascular insufficiency may be pallor that fails to resolve after the epinephrine effect of the local anesthesia has dissipated. More commonly, there is also venous insufficiency that presents as cyanotic swelling of the wound edge or flap. At this early stage, intervention may aid in aborting necrosis. A hematoma, if present, should be evacuated. Wound tension or pressure that can be relieved by judicious suture removal or replacement should be done. Gentle heat to the area may increase blood flow. Hyperbaric oxygen, if available, may also increase tissue survival. The use of 2% nitroglycerin ointment was not shown to be effective in reducing the incidence of necrosis in flap and graft repair after MMS in a prospective, blinded study.

After necrosis has begun, observation is usually the best course of action. The tissue loss may vary in depth from a superficial epidermal slough to full-thickness loss of the skin and subcutaneous tissue. If infection does not further complicate the wound, an eschar will form. The area of necrosis should be allowed to demarcate with only minimal cleaning and debridement. The extent of necrosis may be less than initially predicted and vigorous debridement may only further impair blood flow and extend the process.

The eschar will ultimately separate from the wound bed as the base heals by second intention.

DEHISCENCE

Dehiscence is the separation of the surgical wound. Any factor that impairs healing or imparts undue wound tension can lead to dehiscence, and as such it is seldom an isolated event. Patients will often present with a gapping of the surgical wound at an area of necrosis (Fig. 15). An infection or hematoma may lead to secondary wound separation even before sutures are removed to treat the primary problem. Again it is evident that prevention of one problem may help avoid another.

Even in the absence of a confounding problem, a wound may dehisce in the immediate period or shortly after regularly scheduled suture removal. The most common cause of wound dehiscence is excessive wound tension. Unlike other types of surgery that require a skin incision but no loss of cutaneous tissue, dermatologic surgery almost always involves the removal of a significant amount of skin tissue. Repair of the resultant defect is accomplished by recruitment of surrounding tissue in the form of a primary closure or local flap, which places tension on the wound edges. If the tension is significant, the wound may not be strong enough at the time of suture removal to keep the edges apposed. There is a lag between wounding and the development of wound tensile strength (Table 7). As most skin sutures are removed between 5 and 14 days, it is not surprising that some wounds reopen. At this point, little fibroplasia has occurred and the wound surface is held only by the newly bridged epithelium, wound coagulum, and early neovascularization. Judicious undermining and the proper placement of buried, absorbable sutures are essential to reduce tension and provide the necessary support to keep the wound edges approximated. Superficial stitches left in place for prolonged periods may decrease the risk of dehiscence but runs the risk of permanent suture tracks. The practice of removing sutures in stages at intervals of several days can help minimize this problem while providing prolonged support. Adhesive strips provide some support after suture removal, but they will not prolong protection in the face of significant wound tension.

Trauma, excessive wound movement, excessive use of electrocoagulation, or use of the CO_2 laser may delay the development of tensile strength and lead to dehiscence. Cigarette smoking is a potentially controllable factor that leads to impaired wound healing. Other patient factors such as advanced age, chronic disease, poor nutrition, infection, and steroid use all impair normal wound healing and increase the risk of dehiscence.

The treatment of wound dehiscence varies with the cause. If secondary to infection or significant necrosis, the wound should be left open for drainage and allowed to heal by second intention. A delayed closure or scar revision can be considered after resolution of the primary problem. If dehiscence occurs due to wound trauma or excessive

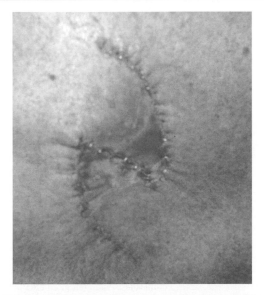

Figure 15 Dehiscence at the site of necrosis. (*See color insert.*)

Table 7 Wound Tensile Strength as a Percentage of Unwounded Skin

Time after wounding	Tensile strength (%)
2 wks	3–5
3 wks	15
4 wks	35
Final (1 yr)	80

closure tension in the first 48 hours after surgery, immediate reapproximation of the wound edges can be performed if there is no evidence of infection. Freshening of the wound edges should be kept to a minimum, removing only nonviable tissue. Otherwise, the lag period to fibroplasia is reset, delaying the development of tensile strength. Reclosure of dehisced wounds may greatly reduce healing times as opposed to allowing the area to heal by second intention.

NERVE DEFICITS

Sensory and motor nerves may be transected or injured during cutaneous surgery. Most areas of the skin and the underlying muscles have diverse nerve innervation and unless a major nerve is injured, there is little permanent effect. The transection of cutaneous sensory nerves happens with any skin incision. Patients may have relative anesthesia in the skin at primary closure sites and in the area of flaps. There will be hypoesthesia in any grafts. Sensory nerves readily regenerate and reinnervate in areas of wounding. This action may take many months to complete, and the healing process may be accompanied by troublesome paresthesias. In the case of grafts, sensation may never return completely to the preoperative state. In some locations larger sensory nerves may be injured leading to sensory deficits distal to the injury site. The most common sites for such injuries are on the forehead and anterior scalp, the posterior scalp, and the digits. The patient should be warned of the possibility of such nerve injuries prior to the procedure. With time, most of theses deficits at least partially resolve.

Injury or transection of motor nerves can be functionally and cosmetically devastating complications. A detailed understanding of the relevant anatomy is critical to the success of any surgical procedure, especially those performed on the head and neck. In general, the more proximal the nerve injury, the more severe the deficit. For example, injury to branches of the facial nerve medial to a line drawn from the lateral canthus to the angle of the mouth are unlikely to lead to severe consequences, while transection lateral to this area may lead to significant paralysis. Fortunately, most of the larger, more proximal nerve branches are relatively deep and well protected. The most common injury to a major branch of the facial nerve is to the temporal branch as it crosses the zygomatic arch. Here the nerve is superficial and covered only by the superficial temporalis fascia. Transection leads to paralysis of the frontalis muscle and loss of the ability to elevate the forehead on the affected side. Unless there is pre-existing brow ptosis, this loss is usually only of cosmetic consequence, but it can be surgically corrected if necessary with a brow lift procedure. The marginal mandibular branch of the facial nerve may be encountered as it crosses the mandible, near the facial artery and vein. It is superficial at this point, covered only by skin and the platysma. Loss of this nerve paralyzes the lip depressors and can give the face a distorted appearance with smiling and other facial movements. There may be some interference with mouth function as well. Injuries to the zygomatic and buccal branches or the main trunk of the facial nerve are rare but can have significant sequelae. Loss of function of the muscles around the eye and the mouth with resulting inability to close the eye, drooling from loss of oral spincter control, and a distorted facial appearance can occur (Fig. 16). The spinal accessory nerve may be injured in the posterior triangle of the neck at Erb's

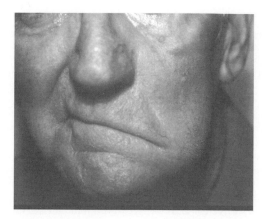

Figure 16 Paralysis of the main trunk of the facial nerve due to local anesthesia.

point where it exits from behind the sternocleidomastoid muscle. Damage to this nerve can lead to a paralysis of the trapezius muscle with resultant winging of the scapula, difficulty abducting the arm, and chronic shoulder pain. A dilemma results when tumor involves the area of a major nerve. If isolation of the nerve from the tumor is possible, nerve preservation should be attempted. If this is not possible, either the nerve must be removed or alternative therapy for the residual tumor (such as radiation therapy) must be planned. There may be some regrowth and return of function when major branches are injured; however, when major branches are transected, consideration must be given to repair with reapproximation and/or nerve grafts. In addition, muscle stimulation may be necessary to forestall muscle atrophy while awaiting return of function.

By design, local anesthesia will cause the temporary loss of function of sensory and motor nerves. If a major nerve is affected by the infiltration of local anesthesia or the nerve is only injured, but not severed by the procedure, it may not be possible at the conclusion of a procedure to fully assess the residual nerve function. The loss of function may be of varying duration (Table 8). While waiting to delineate the extent of any deficit, care must be taken to provide for the necessary functions provided by the nerve. The eye may need to be patched if the ability to close the eye is lost, and artificial tears may be required to keep the cornea moist. The patient must be warned to avoid hot liquids and chewing if perioral sensation is compromised. In most circumstances function will rapidly return, but the patient must be followed closely to assure that this is the case.

PROBLEMS OF WOUND APPEARANCE
Suture Problems
Buried sutures can cause a variety of problems prior to their total absorption. Plain gut or chromic gut sutures are

Table 8 Duration of Nerve Deficits

Injury	Duration
Local anesthesia	~6 hr
Nerve block	~12 hr
Neuropraxia	Up to 6 months
Transection	May be permanent

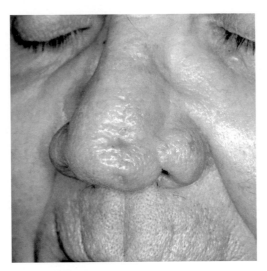

Figure 17 "Spitting" of Vicryl suture.

digested by neutrophils. As this digestion takes place a sterile abscess may form. Pustules may be opened and the remaining suture gently removed. Newer synthetic, absorbable sutures are absorbed without enzymatic action by hydrolysis. These sutures rarely result in pustules but may form firm papules in the suture line, and are most commonly evident six weeks after surgery. If the papule is deep, the skin cancer patient may be concerned that this thickening represents a return of the tumor. The papule usually resolves with time, but self-administered gentle massage may speed resolution. If the papule is near the skin surface, the suture may be extruded through the wound. Such a papule usually appears with little inflammation, and a small tuft of suture may protrude. It has been proposed that the spitting of absorbable sutures is the result of them placed too close to the surface or the knots tied towards the surface rather than buried. Although these factors may account for some instances of suture extrusion, at times properly placed deep sutures will "spit" (Fig. 17). If the suture is loose, it should be removed. If the loop is intact, the suture should be elevated with forceps and as much as possible should be clipped with scissors, allowing the remaining suture to retract into the wound to be absorbed. The ultimate wound appearance is usually unaffected by this event.

The placement of skin sutures through the epithelium creates a tract for epithelial cell migration. Epithelization around the suture occurs between the third and eight day. If the sutures are removed prior to complete epithelization, the track regresses. If the track completely epithelizes, several problems can develop. The keratinizing cells can incite

an inflammatory response that may persist after suture removal. This erythema may be confused with infection (Fig. 14). The inflammation may lead to scarring around the suture tracks with the development of pitted scars at the site. If the suture has also pressed tightly on the skin, it may create a linear scar linking the suture track scars and yielding a "railroad track" appearance (Fig. 18). The longer sutures are in place, the more likely such marks are to develop. In addition, some anatomic sites are more prone to the development of suture reactions than others. The risk is higher on sebaceous areas of the face, the chest, back, and extremities and lower on the eyelids, palms, and soles. The best way to avoid cutaneous suture reactions is through early suture removal, which is facilitated by minimizing wound edge tension through good surgical planning and the proper placement of buried sutures.

Hypertrophic Scars and Keloids

Any injury that extends into the dermis will heal with a scar. Hypertrophic scars and keloids result from an excessive accumulation of collagen at the site of wounding. Although their exact pathogenesis is unknown, they are very common, with an estimated incidence ranging from 4.5% to 16% depending on the population studied. Both types of scars are initially erythematous to purple, raised, and indurated, but by definition hypertrophic scars remain within the boundaries of the original wound while keloids extend beyond it. Relating to its clinical appearance, the word *keloid* comes from the Greek *chele*, meaning crab claw. Although keloids are most prevalent in dark-skinned races, they occur in all racial and ethnic groups. A patient with a personal or family history of keloids is at risk of developing one with any wounding injury. Hypertrophic scars and keloids may appear anywhere on the body, but they are especially prone to develop in areas under tension or subject to increased movement, such as the chest (including the breasts), back, and shoulders. They are very unusual on the central face, eyelids, palms and soles, and genetalia. Both are disfiguring and frequently pruritic and painful, and so patients often seek treatment. In predisposed individuals and on predisposed body sites, even small procedures such as shave or punch biopsies can lead to unsightly hypertrophic scars or keloids, and patients must be informed of this possibility (Fig. 19).

The treatment strategies for hypertrophic and keloid scars are the same. A variety of treatments have been employed with varying degrees of success (Table 9). An important difference to keep in mind is that hypertrophic scars usually resolve without treatment given sufficient time

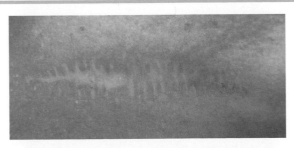

Figure 18 "Railroad tracking" at suture sites and early scar spreading. (*See color insert.*)

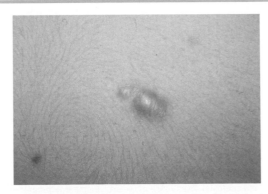

Figure 19 Keloid formation at punch biopsy site. (*See color insert.*)

Table 9   Treatment Modalities for Keloids

Surgical
  Cryosurgery
  Laser surgery
    CO_2
    Neodynium:YAG
    Pulsed-dye laser
  Surgical excision
  Replacement with flaps and/or grafts
Nonsurgical
  Radiation therapy
  Pressure garments
  Silicone gel sheeting
  Hydration and occlusion
  Steroids—Topical or intralesional
  Intralesional steroids plus hyaluronidase
  Topical retinoic acid
  Intralesional 5-fluorouracil
  Intralesional Interferon-gamma and alpha 2-b
  Imiquimod
Systemic medications
  Colchicine
  Methotrexate
  Penicillamine

(although the larger and firmer they become the more likely they are to result in a scar that is wide, with an irregular surface texture from loss of adnexal structures) (Fig. 20) and keloids are ultimately treatment resistant, with a high recurrence rate. Often combining various treatment modalities yields the best results. Intervention at the early stages of hypertrophic scar formation may yield a more acceptable scar. High potency topical steroids or intralesional steroid injections may decrease the thickness of the scar and bring symptomatic relief; however, the use of steroids may lead to unsightly telangectasias and an atrophic, widened scar. Smaller, less significant hypertrophic scars may respond to gentle massage. The etiology, pathogenesis, and treatment of keloids is covered in detail in Chapter 36.

Spread Scars

Even the most finely approximated incison line, with perfect wound edge eversion, can result in a spread scar if significant tension across the wound exists. Cosmetically objectionable scar spread can occur in any wound, but it is most common on locations subject to excess tension and frequent movement such as the neck, shoulders, back, and chest. Scar spread is also more common in skin with less elasticity (a thicker dermis) and fewer adnexal structures. Vigorous activity involving the area of wounding may also increase the degree of wound spread. It is important to recognize the risk of widened scars in such locations and situations and counsel the patient appropriately prior to the procedure. With this knowledge, some cosmetic procedures in these locations may be deferred.

Most scar widening takes place in the first six months postoperatively, after which time sufficient tensile strength has developed to prevent further spread. Certain operative maneuvers designed to reduce wound tension, such as wide undermining, can reduce the degree of spread. Also, subcutaneous placement of longer-lasting absorbable sutures, such as polydioxanone (PDS®) or glycolic acid (Maxon®) may retard spread. Use of nonabsorbable material such as clear nylon (Ethilon®), polypropylene (Prolene®), or polyester (Mersilene®) for deep, buried sutures also provides prolonged support to prevent wound spreading (but with the trade-off of an increased risk of suture reactions). A prolonged, six-month, placement of a running intradermal polypropylene suture may also reduce scar spread. Careful consideration must be given to revising a spread scar by re-excision, especially in a location prone to its development, as it will usually provide only minimal, if any, improvement. Success is possible with a Z-plasty type repair, which changes the direction of closure and can remove significant wound tension.

Prominent Scar Lines

The ideal scar is perfectly flat with no separation. However, some scar lines may be raised (but not classically hypertrophic) or depressed, and therefore prominent primarily due to the shadows they cast. At times the two sides of the scar appear uneven. Such a situation may follow planned primary closures, flaps, grafts, or the repair of traumatic injuries. This type of scar also seems to be more common in younger individuals who exhibit more exuberant healing. Resurfacing of the scar line between four and eight weeks after the original wounding appears to have a positive effect on the appearance of prominent scars. The beneficial effect may be diminished if dermabrasion is delayed beyond six to eight weeks. Immediate postoperative resurfacing of wounds, especially those which will undergo second intention healing, has been demonstrated to improve the overall scar appearance. Scar revision techniques are discussed in detail in Chapters 51 and 52.

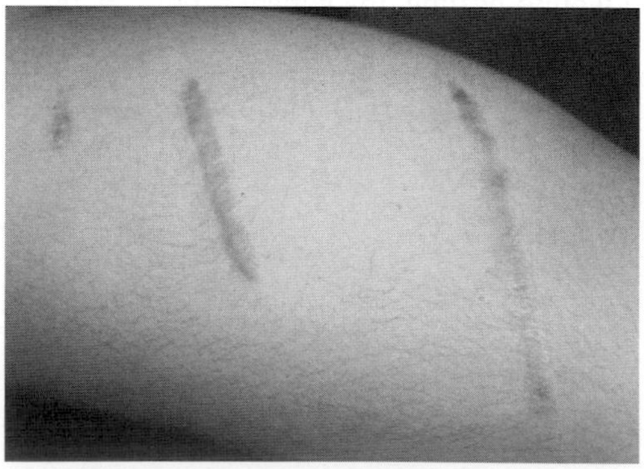

Figure 20   Hypertrophic scars from traumatic lacerations. Note the widened and stretched appearance of the scar as the hypertrophic elements regress (the longer scar).

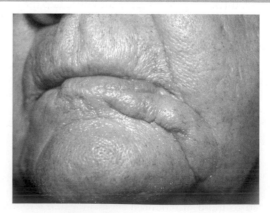

Figure 21   Trapdoor deformity.

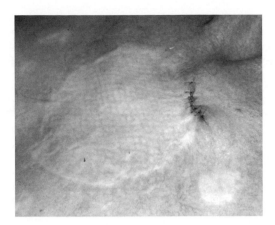

Figure 22 Hypopigmentation of a skin graft on the chest.

Trapdoor Deformity

During the first few weeks after surgery, repaired wounds may take on a bulky appearance known as a trapdoor or pincushion deformity. Transposition flap repairs are especially prone to this complication. The central portion of the flap may develop an elevated, somewhat dome shape which recedes towards the inverted-appearing wound margins (Fig. 21). Although the etiology of the trapdoor deformity has not been convincingly demonstrated, it probably results at least in part from contraction of the wound bed upon which the flap has been transposed. Careful surgical planning and execution are critical to reducing the risk of this esthetically displeasing problem.

Wide undermining of the skin edges of the defect to be filled by the flap or graft better distributes wound contracture and may minimize trapdooring. Sharply angulated incisions, as opposed to rounded ones, help limit the distortion as well. For instance, after Mohs surgery the resultant wound defect is typically round. If a rhombic flap is planned, maintaining the sharp angles of the flap by further trimming the defect as opposed to the flap results in angles of contraction in various directions as opposed to directed in a radial fashion. In order to reduce redundant tissue, flaps should be designed and cut such that they have to be stretched slightly to fit the defect. Trimming the underside of the flap of excess subcutaneous tissue also seems to inhibit trapdoor formation.

Postoperative revision techniques may be helpful should trapdooring occur. Steroid injections of the wound margins and the central flap may reduce wound contraction and tissue thickening. Massage to the entire flap may also be useful. After the flap and the deformity have matured (six months to one year), a procedure to undermine, defat, and trim the flap may provide further improvement.

Pigmentary Alterations

Epidermal wounding may result in changes in pigment. As skin pigmentation is produced by epidermal melanocytes, the broader the epidermal wound site, the more likely the pigmentary alteration. Wounds closed primarily may produce a hypopigmented or hyperpigmented scar line, but rarely a more extensive deformity. Broader based epidermal or full-thickness injuries such as those produced by electrosurgery, cryosurgery, CO_2 laser ablation or dermabrasion may lead to more pronounced pigmentary alterations. The degree of melanocytic injury seems to play a role as to whether hyperpigmentation or hypopigmentation results. Injury that destroys melanocytes such as deep cryosurgery leads to hypopigmentation. Partial injury, such as a superficial abrasion, often results in accelerated melanocytic activity in the recovery period and hyperpigmentation. Because wounds may often involve both melanocytic destruction and partial injury, many wounds develop mottled pigmentation. Hpyopigmentation is obviously most noticeable in dark-skinned individuals. Because of the ability of the melanocytes in dark-skinned people to react so vigorously to stimulation, hyperpigmentation can also be very prominent.

Patients undergoing procedures likely to result in pigmentary changes should be advised to practice strict sun protection. UV exposure will accentuate pigmentary changes by augmenting hyperpigmentation and providing additional contrast to areas of hypopigmentation. Patients should be advised to avoid intentional tanning and wear high-grade sun blocks for at least a year after the procedure. Consideration should be given to not performing elective procedures with a high risk of pigmentary alteration (such as dermabrasion) during the summer months. Full-thickness and split-thickness grafts are also prone to irregular pigmentation and should have strict photo protection (Fig. 22). Early or established hyperpigmentation may be treated with topical hydroquinones. Camouflage make-up may also be helpful.Tattooing may also occur in surgical scars from chemical cauterants such as ferrous subsulfate (Monsel's solution) or silver nitrate. Such tattooing is usually permanent, unless treated by excision or laser.

Surgeon–Patient Complications

A surgical scar is ultimately the result of an interplay of the action of the surgeon, the patient, and nature. The patient's role must begin at the decision to proceed with surgery and continue through the postoperative period. Although informed consent has legal meanings and implications, it truly should mean that the surgeon shares with the patient what he knows, expects, and is concerned about so that the patient can participate in his own care. The patient must be informed what results are reasonably expected and what might occur if complications arise. The patient may worry about how the procedure might affect his general health, appearance, or well-being. The surgeon must anticipate and address those concerns. The patient must also accept responsibility for his portion of preoperative preparation, cooperation with the surgical procedure, wound care and having realistic long-term expectations. If lifestyle habits such as smoking or drinking alcohol may be expected to affect wound healing, the patient should be instructed as to how altering behaviors might improve the outcome. The surgeon must provide detailed information, both oral and written to help the patient with these responsibilities. If complications arise, the complication, its treatment and the expected long-term result should be fully shared with the patient. Every surgeon has complications and every patient can potentially have a complication. Through truly informed consent, good doctor–patient communication, and involving the patient in his or her own care, the additional complication of litigation can be avoided in most circumstances.

BIBLIOGRAPHY

Ayliffe GA. Role of the environment of the operating suite in surgical wound infection. Rev Infect Dis 1991; 13(Suppl 10): S800–S804.

Ammirati CT, Cottingham TJ, Hruza GJ. Immediate postoperative laser resurfacing improves second intention healing on the nose: 5-year experience. Dermatol Surg 2001; 27:147–152.

Ang-Lee MK, Moss J, Yuan CS. Herbal medicines and perioperative care. JAMA 2001; 286:208–216.

Apitz-Castro R, Escalante J, Vargas R, Jain MK. Ajoene, the antiplatelet principle of garlic, synergistically potentiates the antiaggregatory action of prostacyclin, forskolin, indomethacin, and dypiridamole on human platelets. Thromb Res 1986; 42:303–311.

Alcalay J, Alkalay R. Controversies in perioperative management of blood thinners in dermatologic surgery: continue or discontinue? Dermatol Surg 2004; 30:1091–1094.

Aly R, Maibach HI. Comparative antibacterial efficacy of a 2-minute surgical scrub with chlorhexidine gluconate, povidone-iodine, and chloroxylenol sponge-brushes. Am J Infect Control 1988; 16:173–177.

Ah-Weng A, Natarajan S, Velangi S, Langtry JAA. Preoperative monitoring of warfarin in cutaneous surgery. Br J Dermatol 2003; 48:386–389.

Altemeier WA, Culbertson WR, Hummel RP. Surgical considerations of endogenous infections—sources, types, and methods of control. Surg Clin North Am 1968; 48:227–240.

Alam M, Goldberg LH. Serious adverse vascular events associated with perioperative interruption of antiplatelet and anticoagulant therapy. Dermatol Surg 2002; 28:992–998.

Bernstein G. The loop stitch. J Dermatol Surg Oncol 1984;10:587.

Bhatt DL, Bertrand ME, Berger PB. Meta-analysis of randomized and registry comparisons of ticlopidine with clopidogrel after stenting. J Am Coll Cardiol 2002; 39:9–14.

Burke JF. Infection. In: Hunt TK, Dunphy JE, eds. Fundamentals of Wound Management. New York: Appleton-Century-Crofts, 1979:170–240.

Bassetti M, Dembry LM, Farrel PA, Callan DA, Andriole VT. Comparative antimicrobial activity of gatifloxacin with ciprofloxacin and beta-lactams against gram-positive bacteria. Diagn Microbiol Infect Dis 2001; 41:143–148.

Bencini PL, Galimberti M, Signorini M, Crosti C. Antibiotic prophylaxis of wound infections in skin surgery. Arch Dermatol 1991; 127:1357–1360.

Bartlett GR. Does aspirin affect the outcome of minor cutaneous surgery? Br J Plast Surg 1999; 52:214–216.

Bencini PL, Galimberti M, Signorini M. Utility of topical benzoyl peroxide for prevention of surgical skin wound infection. J Dermatol Surg Oncol 1994; 20:538–540.

Burke JF. The effective period of preventive antibiotic action in experimental incisions and dermal lesions. Surgery 1961; 50:161–163.

Baker RI, Coughlin PB, Gallus AS, Harper PL, Salem HH, Wood EM. Warfarin Reversal Consensus Group. Warfarin reversal: consensus guidelines, on behalf of the Australasian Society of Thrombosis and Haemostasis. Med J Aust 2004; 181:492–497.

Bithell TC. Qualitative disorders of platelet dysfunction. In: Lee RG, et al., eds. Wintrobe's Clinical Hematology. Philadelphia: Lea & Febiger, 1993:1397–1421.

Billingsley EM, Maloney ME. Intraoperative and postoperative bleeding problems in patients taking warfarin, aspirin, and nonsteroidal anti-inflammatory agents. Dermatol Surg 1997; 23:381–385.

Crowther MA, Wilson S. Vitamin K for the treatment of asymptomatic coagulopathy associated with oral anticoagulant therapy. J Thromb Thrombolysis 2003; 16:69–72.

Catella-Lawson F, Reilly MP, Kapoor SC. Cycloxygenase inhibitors and the antiplatelet effects of aspirin. N Engl J Med 2001; 345:1809–1817.

Cimochowski GE, Harostock MD, Brown R, Bernardi M, Alonzo N, Coyle K. Intranasal mupirocin reduces sternal wound infection after open heart surgery in diabetics and nondiabetics. Ann Thorac Surg 2001; 71:1572–1579.

Chong JY, Mohr JP. Anticoagulation and platelet antiaggregation therapy in stroke prevention. Curr Opin Neurol 2005; 18: 53–57.

Classen DC, Evans RS, Pestotnik SL, Horn SD, Menlove RL, Burke JP. The timing of prophylactic administration of antibiotics and the risk of surgical wound infection. N Engl J Med 1992; 236:337–339.

Cupp MJ. Herbal remedies: adverse effects and drug interactions. Am Fam Physician 1999; 59:1239–1245.

Collins SC, Dufresne RG Jr. Dietary supplements in the setting of Mohs surgery. Dermatol Surg 2002; 28:447–452.

Crowe HM, Quintilliani R. Antibiotic formulary selection. Med Clin North Am 1995; 79:463–476.

Cook JL, Perone JB. A prospective evaluation of the incidence of complications associated with Mohs micrographic surgery. Arch Dermatol 2003; 139:143–152.

Chang LK, Whitaker DC. The impact of herbal medicines on dermatologic surgery. Dermatol Surg 2001; 27:759–763.

Coldiron B, Shreve E, Balkrishnan R. Patient injuries from surgical procedures performed in medical offices: three years of Florida data. Dermatol Surg 2004; 30:1435–1443.

Cheung AH, Wong LM. Surgical infections in patients with chronic renal failure. Infect Dis Clin North Am 2001; 15:775–776.

Crowther MA, Douketis JD, Schnurr T, et al. Oral vitamin K lowers the international normalized ratio more rapidly than subcutaneous vitamin K in the treatment of warfarin-associated coagulopathy. A randomized, controlled trial. Ann Intern Med 2002; 137:251–254.

Centers for Disease and Control Prevention. National Nosocomial Infections Surveillance (NNIS) report, data summary from October 1986-April 1996, issued May 1996. A report from the National Nosocomial Infections Surveillance (NNIS) System. Am J Infect Control 1996; 24:380–388.

Caliendo FJ, Halpern VJ, Marini CP, et al. Warfarin anticoagulation in the perioperative period: Is it safe? Ann Vasc Surg 1999; 13:11–16.

Clark RAF. Basics of cutaneous wound repair. J Dermatol Surg Oncol 1993; 19:693–706.

Chung KF, Dent G, McCusker M, Guinot P, Page CP, Barnes PJ. Effect of a ginkgolide mixture (BN 52063) in antagonizing skin and platelet responses to platelet activating factor in man. Lancet 1987; 1:248–251.

Dietrich W, Dilthey G, Spannagl M, et al. Warfarin pretreatment does not lead to increased bleeding tendency during cardiac surgery. J Cardiothor Vasc Anesth 1995; 9:250–254.

Dunn CL, Brodland DG, Griego RD, Huether MJ, Fazio MJ, Zitelli JA. A single postoperative application of nitroglycerin ointment does not increase survival of cutaneous flaps and grafts. Dermatol Surg 2000; 26:425–427.

Dellinger EP. Antibiotic prophylaxis of wound infections in skin surgery: is 4 days too much? Arch Dermatol 1991; 127: 1394–1395.

Dzubow LM. Facial Flaps: Biomechanics and Regional Application. Norwalk, Connecticut: Appleton & Lange, 1990.

Deykin D, Janson P, McMahon L. Ethanol potentiation of asprin-induced prolongation of the bleeding time. N Eng. J Med 1982;306:852.

Dodson MK, Magann EF, Meeks GR. A randomized comparison of secondary closure and secondary intention in patients with superficial wound dehiscence. Obstet Gynecol 1992; 80:321–324.

Dunn AS, Turpie AGG. Perioperative management of patients receiving oral anticoagulants: a systematic review. Arch Intern Med 2003; 163:901–908.

Eisenberg DM, Davis RB, Ettner SL, et al. Trends in alternative medicine use in the United States, 1990–1997: Results of a follow-up national survey. JAMA 1998; 280:1569–1575.

Elliot D, Mahaffey PJ. The stretched scar: the benefit of prolonged dermal support. Br J Plast Surg 1989; 42:74–78.

Epstein ME, Amodio-Groton M, Sadick NS. Antimicrobial agents for the dermatologist. II. Macrolides, fluoroquinolones, rifamycins, tetracyclins, trimethoprim-sulfamethoxazole, and clindamycin. J Am Acad Dermatol 1997; 37:365–381.

Epstein ME, Amodio-Groton M, Sadick NS. Antimicrobial agents for the dermatologist. I. β-Lactam antibiotics and related compounds. J Am Acad Dermatol 1997; 37:149–165.

Futoryan T, Grande D. Postoperative wound infection rates in dermatologic surgery. Dermatol Surg 1995; 21:509–514.

Fitzgerald GA. Dipyridamole. N Engl J Med 1987; 316:1247–1257.

Griego RD, Zitelli JA. Intra-incisional prophylactic antibiotics for dermatologic surgery. Arch Dermatol 1998; 134:688–692.

Grabb WC. A concentration of 1:500,000 epinephrine in a local anesthetic solution is sufficient to provide excellent hemostasis. Plast Recconstr Surg 1979; 63:834.

Genkinger JM, Platz EA, Hoffman SC, et al. Fruit, vegetable, and antioxidant intake and all-cause, cancer, and cardiovascular disease mortality in a community-dwelling population in Washington County, Maryland. Am J Epidemiol 2004; 160:1223–1233.

Goldsmith SM, Leshin B, Owen J. Management of patients taking anticoagulants and platelet inhibitors prior to dermatologic surgery. J Dermatol Surg Oncol 1993; 19:578–581.

Gainey SP, Robertson DM, Fay W, et al. Ocular surgery on patients receiving long-term warfarin therapy. Am J Ophthalmol 1989; 108:142–146.

Gerson LB, Gage BF, Owens DK, Triadafilopoulos G. Effect and outcomes of the periendoscopic management of patients who take anticoagulants. Am J Gastroenterol 2000; 95:1717–1724.

Genewein U, Haeberli A, Straub PW, Beer JH. Rebound after cessation of oral anticoagulant therapy: the biochemical evidence. Br J Haematol 1996; 92:479–485.

Grip L, Blomback M, Schulman S. Hypercoagulable state and thromboembolism following warfarin withdrawl in post-myocardial infarction patients. Eur Heart J 1991; 12:1225–1233.

Gil-Egea MJ, Pi-Sunyer MT, Verdaguer A, Sanz F, Sitges-Serra A, Eleizegui LT. Surgical wound infections: prospective study of 4,486 clean wounds. Infect Control 1987; 8:277–280.

Garman ME, Orengo I. Unusual infectious complications of dermatologic procedures. Dermatol Clin 2003; 21:321–335.

Giandoni MB, Grabski WJ. Cutaneous candidiasis as a cause of delayed surgical wound healing. J Am Acad Dermatol 1994; 30:981–984.

Gette MT, Marks JG, Maloney ME. The frequency of postoperative allergic contact dermatitis to topical antibiotics. Arch Dermatol 1992; 128:365–367.

Gloster HM, Twersky J. Surgical pearl: the use of the Coagu-Chek S system for the preoperative evaluation of patients taking warfarin. J Am Acad Dermatol 2004; 50:439–441.

Goding GS Jr., Hom DB. Skin flap physiology. In: Baker SR, Swanson NA, eds. Local flaps in facial reconstruction. St. Louis: Mosby, 1995:16.

Goldminz D, Bennett RG. Cigarette smoking and flap and full-thickness graft necrosis. Arch Dermatol 1991;127:1012–101.

Hirsh J, Warkentin TE, Raschke R. Heparin and low-molecular-weight heparin: mechanisms of action, pharmacokinetics, dosing considerations, monitoring, efficacy, and safety. Chest 1998; 114(suppl.):S489–S510.

Hopkins MP, Androff L, Benninghoff AS. Ginseng face cream and unexplained vaginal bleeding. Am J Obstet Gynecol 1988; 159:1121–1122.

Hollopeter G, Jantzen HM, Vincent D. Identification of the platelet ADP receptor targeted by antithrombotic drugs. Nature 2001; 409:202–207.

Huether MJ, Griego RD, Brodland DG, Zitelli JA. Clindamycin for intraincisional antibiotic prophylaxis in dermatologic surgery. Arch Dermatol 2002; 138:1145–1148.

Harris DR. Healing of the surgical wound. I. Basic considerations. J Am Acad Dermatol 1979; 1:197–207.

Hirschmann JV. Topical antibiotics in Dermatology. Arch Dermatol 1988; 124:1691–1700.

Hongo RH, Ley J, Dick SE, Yee RR. The effect of clopidogrel in combination with aspirin when given before coronary artery bypass grafting. J Am Coll Cardiol 2002; 40:231–237.

Haas AF, Grekin RC. Antibiotic prophylaxis in dermatologic surgery. J Am Acad Dermatol 1995; 32:155–176.

Hirsh J, Dalen JE, Deykin D, Poller L, Bussey H. Oral anticoagulants: mechanism of action, clinical effectiveness, and optimal therapeutic range. Chest 1995; 108(suppl.):231S–246S.

Jarvis WR. Epidemiology of nosocomial fungal infections, with emphasis on *Candida* species. Clin Infect Dis 1995; 20:1526–1530.

Jacob SE, James WD. Bacitracin after clean surgical procedures may be risky. J Am Acad Dermatol 2004;51:1036.

Jones RN, Pfaller MA. Ciprofloxacin as broad-spectrum empiric therapy—are fluoroquinolones still viable monotherapeutic agents compared with beta-lactams: data from the MYSTIC Program (US)? Diagn Microbiol Infect Dis 2002; 42:213–215.

Katz BE, Oca AG. A controlled study of the effectiveness of spot dermabrasion ('scarabrasion') on the appearance of surgical scars. J Am Acad Dermatol 1991; 24:462–466.

Kearon C, Hirsh J. Management of anticoagulation before and after elective surgery. N Engl J Med 1997; 336:1506–1511.

Kovich O, Otley CC. Thrombotic complications related to discontinuation of warfarin and aspirin therapy perioperatively for cutaneous operation. J Am Acad Dermatol 2003; 48:233–237.

Ketchum LD, Cohen IK, Masters FW. Hypertrophic scars and keloids. Plast Reconstr Surg 1974; 53:140–154.

Kluytmans J, van Belkum A, Verbrugh H. Nasal carriage of *Staphylococcus aureus*: epidemiology, underlying mechanisms, and associated risks. Clin Microbiol Rev 1997; 10:505–520.

Kluytmans JAJW, Mouton JW, VandenBergh MFQ, et al. Reduction of surgical-site infections in cardiothoracic surgery by elimination of nasal carriage of Staphylococcus aureus. Infect Control Hosp Epidemiol 1996; 17:780–785.

Kovich O, Otley CC. Perioperative management of anticoagulants and platelet inhibitors for cutaneous surgery: a survey of current practice. Dermatol Surg 2002; 28:513–517.

Koval KJ, Maurer SG, Su ET, et al. The effect of nutritional status on outcome after hip fracture. J Orthop Trauma 1999; 13:164–169.

Karchmer AW. Fluoroquinolone treatment of skin and skin structure infections. Drugs 1999;58:S82-S84.

Kimyai-Asadi A, Jih MH, Goldberg LH. Perioperative primary stroke: is aspirin cessation to blame? Dermatol Surg 2004; 30:1526–1529.

Larson EL, Aiello AE, Heilman JM, et al. Comparison of different regimens for surgical hand preparation. AORN J 2001;73:412–4, 417–8, 420.

Leigh DA, Stronge JL, Marriner J, Sedgwick J. Total body bathing with 'Hibiscrub' (chlorhexidine) in surgical patients: a controlled trial. J Hosp Infect 1983; 4:229–235.

Manuskiatti W, Fitzpatrick RE. Treatment response of keloidal and hypertrophic sternotomy scars: comparison among intralesional corticosteroid, 5-fluorouracil, and 585-nm flashlamp-pumped pulsed-dye laser treatments. Arch Dermatol 2002; 138:1149–1155.

Marietta M, Bertesi M, Simoni L, et al. A simple and safe nomogram for the management of oral anticoagulation prior to minor surgery. Clin Lab Haem 2003; 25:127–130.

Maragh SL, Otley CC, Roenigk RK, Phillips PK. Antibiotic prophylaxis in dermatologic surgery: updated guidelines. Dermatol Surg 2005; 31:83–93.

Mangram AJ, Horan TC, Pearson ML, Silver LC, Jarvis WR. The Hospital Infection Control Practices Advisory Committee. Guideline for prevention of surgical site infection, 1999. Infect Control Hosp Epidemiol 1999; 20:247–278.

Mishriki SF, Law DJ, Jeffery PJ. Factors affecting the incidence of postoperative wound infection. J Hosp Infect 1990; 16:223–230.

Marks JG Jr, Besito DV, DeReo VA, et al. North American Contact Dermatitis Group patch-test results 1998–2000. Am J Contact Dermatitis 2003; 14:59–62.

Mohr JF, Jones A, Ostrosky-Zeichner L, Wanger A, Tillotson G. Associations between antibiotic use and changes in susceptibility patterns of *Pseudomonas aeruginosa* in a private, university-affiliated teaching hospital: an 8-year-experience: 1995–2002. Int J Antimicrob Agents 2004; 24:346–351.

Maloney ME. Management of surgical complications and suboptimal results. In: Wheeland RG, ed. Cutaneous Surgery. Philadelphia: W.B. Saunders Co., 1994:921–934.

Niessen FB, Spauwen PH, Schalkwijk J, Kon M. On the nature of hypertrophic scars and keloidal scars: a review. Plast Reconstr Surg 1999; 104:1435–1458.

Nanney LB. Biochemical and physiological aspects of wound healing. In: Wheeland RG, ed. Cutaneous Surgery Philadelphia: W.B. Saunders, 1994:113–121.

Nagachinta T, Stephens M, Reitz B, Polk BF. Risk factors for surgical wound infection following cardiac surgery. J Infect Dis 1987; 156:967–973.

Nichols RL. Surgical antibiotic prophylaxis. Med Clin North Am 1995; 79:509–522.

Otley CC, Fewkes JL, Frank W, et al. Complications of cutaneous surgery in patients who are taking warfarin, aspirin, or nonsteroidal anti-inflammatory drugs. Arch Dermatol 1996; 132:161–166.

Otley CC. Continuation of medically necessary aspirin and warfarin during cutaneous surgery. Mayo Clin Proc 2003; 78:1392–1396.

O'Reilly RA, Kearns P. Intravenous vitamin K: dangerous prophylaxis. Arch Intern Med 1995; 155:2127–2128.

O'Shaughnessy M, O'Malley VP, Corbett G, Given HF. Optimum duration of surgical scrub time. Br J Surg 1991; 78:685–686.

Poller L, Thomson J. Rebound hypercoagulability after stopping anticoagulants. Lancet 1964; 2:62–64.

Postlethwait RW, Johnson WD. Complications following surgery for duodenal ulcer in obese patients. Arch Surg 1972; 105:348–350.

Pellitteri PK, Kennedy TL, Youn BA. The influence of intensive hyperbaric oxygen therapy on skin flap survival in a swine model. Arch Otolaryngol 1992; 118:1050–1054.

Petry JJ. Garlic and postoperative bleeding. Plast Reconstr Surg 1995; 96:483–484.

Posan E, McBane RD II, Grill DE, et al. Comparison of PFA-100 testing and bleeding time for detecting platelet hypofunction and von Willebrand disease in clinical practice. Thromb Haemost 2003; 90:483–490.

Polk HC Jr., Simpson CJ, Simmons BP, Alexander JW. Guidelines for prevention of surgical wound infection. Arch Surg 1983; 118:1213–1217.

Palareti G, Legnani C, Guazzaloca G, et al. Activation of blood coagulation after abrupt or stepwise withdrawal of oral anticoagulants: a prospective study. Thrombosis and Haemostasis 1994; 72:222–226.

Perl TM, Cullen JJ, Wenzel RP, et al. Intranasal mupirocin to prevent postoperative Staphylococcus aureus infections. N Engl J Med 2002; 346:1871–1877.

Parr NJ, Loh CS, Desmond AD. Transurethral resection of the prostate and bladder tumour without withdrawl of warfarin therapy. Br J Urol 1989; 64:623–625.

Rabb DC, Lesher JL Jr. Antibiotic prophylaxis in cutaneous surgery. Dermatol Surg 1995; 21:550–554.

Roberts HR, Monroe DM III, Hoffman M. Molecular biology and biochemistry of the coagulation factors and pathways of hemostasis. In: Beutler E, Coller BS, Lichtman MA, Kipps TJ, Seligsohn U, eds. William's Hematology. 6th ed. New York: McGraw-Hill, 2001:1410–1430.

Ritter MA, French ML, Eitzen HE, Gioe TJ. The antimicrobial effectiveness of operative-site preparative agents: a microbiological and clinical study. J Bone Joint Surg Am 1980; 62:826–828.

Rosenblatt M, Mindel J. Spontaneous hyphema associated with ingestion of Ginkgo biloba extract. N Engl J Med 1997; 336:1108.

Rajagopal V, Bhatt DL. Controversies of oral antiplatelet therapy in acute coronary syndromes and percutaneous coronary intervention. Semin Thromb Hemost 2004; 30:649–655.

Roth RR, James WD. Microbiology of the skin: resident flora, ecology, infection. J Am Acad Dermatol 1989; 20:367–390.

Riou JP, Cohen JR, Johnson H. Factors influencing wound dehiscence. Am J Surg 1992; 163:324–330.

Salasche SJ. Acute surgical complications: cause, prevention, and treatment. J Am Acad Dermatol 1986; 15:1163–1185.

Sebben JE. Avoiding infection in office surgery. J Dermatol Surg Oncol 1982; 8:455–458.

Stedman's Medical Dictionary. 24th ed. Baltimore: Williams & Wilkins, 1982.

Souto JC, Oliver A, Zuazu-Jausoro I, et al. Oral surgery in anticoagulated patients without reducing the dose of oral anticoagulant: a prospective, randomized study. J Oral Maxillofac Surg 1996; 54:27–32.

Syed S, Adams BB, Liao W, et al. A prospective assessment of bleeding and international normalized ratio in warfarin anticoagulated patients having cutaneous surgery. J Am Acad Dermatol 2004; 51:955–957.

Sundstrom J, Agrup C, Kronvall G, Wretlind B. *Pseudomonas aeruginosa* adherence to external auditory canal epithelium. Arch Otolaryngol Head Neck Surg 1997; 123:1287–1292.

Sebben JE. Prophylactic antibiotics in cutaneous surgery. J Dermatol Surg Oncol 1985; 11:901–906.

Schweiger ES, Weinberg JM. Novel antibacterial agents for skin and skin structure infections. J Am Acad Dermatol 2004; 50:331–340.

Simmons BP. Guideline for prevention of surgical wound infections. Infect Control 1982; 3:185–196.

Sorensen LT, Horby J, Friis E, et al. Smoking as a risk factor for wound healing and infection in breast cancer surgery. Eur J Surg Oncol 2002;28:815–820.

Schanbacher CF, Bennett RG. Postoperative stroke after stopping warfarin for cutaneous surgery. Dermatol Surg 2000; 26:785–789.

Scherbenske JM, Winton GB, James WD. Acute pseudomomas infection of the external ear (malignant otitis externa). J Dermatol Surg Oncol 1988; 14:165–169.

Smack DP, Harrington AC, Dunn C, et al. Infection and allergy reaction in ambulatory surgery patients using white petrolatum vs. bacitracin ointment. JAMA 1996; 276:972–977.

Singer AJ, Clark RA. Cutaneous wound healing. N Engl J Med 1999; 341:738–746.

Salasche SJ, Bernstein G, Senkarik M. Surgical Anatomy of the Skin. Norwalk, Connecticut: Appleton and Lange, 1988.

Sommerlad BC, Creasey JM. The stretched scar: a clinical and histologic study. Br J Plast Surg 1978; 31:34–45.

Thorngren M, Shafi S, Born GV. Quantification of blood from skin bleeding time determinations: Effects of fish diet or acetylsalicylic acid. Haemostasis 1983;13:282.

Teng CM, Kuo SC, Ko FN, et al. Antiplatelet actions of panaxynol and ginsenosides isolated from ginseng. Biochim Biophys Acta 1989; 990:315–320.

Vale S. Subarachnoid haemorrhage associated with Ginkgo biloba. Lancet 1998;352:36.

Weibert RT, Dzung TL, Kayser SR, et al. Correction of excessive anticoagulation with low-dose oral vitamin K_1. Ann Intern Med 1997; 126:959–962.

Winton GB, Salasche SJ. Wound dressings for dermatologic surgery. J Am Acad Dermatol 1985; 13:1026–1044.

Wentzien TH, O'Reilly RA, Kearns PJ. Prospective evaluation of anticoagulant reversal with oral vitamin K while continuing warfarin therapy unchanged. Chest 1998; 114:1505–1508.

Wahl MJ. Dental surgery in anticoagulated patients. Arch Intern Med 1998; 158:1610–1616.

Whitaker DC, Grande DJ, Johnson SS. Wound infection rate in dermatologic surgery. J Dermatol Surg Oncol 1988; 14:525–528.

Wenzel RP, Perl TM. The significance of nasal carriage of *Staphylococcus aureus* and the incidence of postoperative wound infection. J Hosp Infect 1995; 31:13–24.

Warkentin TE, Levine MN, Hirsh J. Heparin-induced thrombocytopenia in patients treated with low-molecular-weight heparin or unfractionated heparin. N Engl J Med 1995; 332:1330–1335.

Winton GB. Anesthesia for dermatologic surgery. J Dermatol Surg Oncol 1988; 14:41–54.

www.aboutskinsurgery.com/MedicalArticles/ASDS2003Stats Report.pdf. Accessed January 2, 2005.

Yusuf S, Zhao F, Mehta SR. Effects of clopidogrel in addition to aspirin in patients with acute coronary syndromes without ST-segment elevation. N Engl J Med 2001; 345:494–502.

Yarbrorough JM. Ablation of facial scars by programmed dermabrasion. J Dermatol Surg Oncol 1988; 14:292–294.

Yende S, Wunderink RG. Effect of clopidogrel on bleeding after coronary artery bypass surgery. Crit Care Med 2001; 29:2271–2275.

Zerr KJ, Furnary AP, Grunkemeier GL, Bookin S, Kanhere V, Starr A. Glucose control lowers the risk of wound infection in diabetes after open heart operations. Ann Thorac Surg 1997; 63:356–361.

Zitelli JA. The nasolabial flap as a single stage procedure. Arch Dermatol 1990; 126:1445–1448.

12

Emergencies in the Dermatology Office

Christopher B. Kruse
Advanced Dermatology Surgery Center, Tinton Falls, New Jersey, U.S.A.

Joshua E. Lane
*Section of Dermatology, Department of Medicine, The Medical College of Georgia,
Augusta, Georgia, U.S.A.*

INTRODUCTION

It is inevitable that emergencies will occur over the course of one's practice and may include cardiac arrests, myocardial infarctions, strokes, syncope, seizures, allergic reactions, excessive bleeding, and drug toxicities. An organized response is critical to properly manage these events and obtain the best outcome for the patient.

Basic equipment and medicines are a necessity to successfully manage these events. All medical assistants and interested office staff should be trained in basic life support (BLS). Physicians, in addition to BLS should stay current with advanced cardiovascular life support procedures. These courses are offered by the American Heart Association. Certifications are valid for two years. Additionally, periodic review of emergency procedures with the office staff improves recall and increases confidence in times of need. Table 1 provides a list of items that every office should have.

In addition, the decision to have a crash cart or an automated external defibrillator (AED) is influenced by your proximity and availability to emergency medical services (EMS). An AED is simple to use and inexpensive to purchase and maintain. The curriculum of the American Heart Association now includes instruction on the use of AEDs as they have become more common. All items should be easily located by the entire staff in the event they are needed.

CARDIAC ARREST

In the event of a cardiac emergency, an office should have a predetermined plan to set into action. Everything begins with a call to action, whether it be a reserved signal activated by a button or a code announced over the office intercom. Following this, everyone should know his/her job and what to gather while responding to the distress call.

The goal is to maintain cerebral perfusion until cardiac function can be restored. The physician begins with assessing whether the patient is responsive and the circumstances leading to the event. If the patient is unresponsive, the evaluation begins with BLS protocols. Open the airway and check for breathing. If the patient is not breathing or is not breathing adequately, 911 should be called immediately to initiate an EMS response. While one is calling EMS, give two rescue breaths and check for a pulse. If there is a pulse, continue administering rescue breathing as needed while awaiting for the arrival of EMS. Check blood pressure and place in Trendelenburg's position if the patient is hypotensive. Also,

obtain intravenous access if a catheter is available. Review and organize any medical information that is available. If no pulse is identified, begin chest compressions in groups of 15 at a rate of 100/min. Provide two breaths between every group of fifteen compressions. If an AED is available, it should be used as soon as possible. The use of a crash cart and manual defibrillator requires training in advanced cardiac life support (ACLS).

Cardiac arrest is the most common cause of death in the United States. It most commonly affects those with pre-existing coronary artery disease; however, concurrent medical conditions and/or administered medications (including local anesthetics) may also be responsible in some patients. In fact, the most significant medical emergency in the United States is sudden death secondary to coronary artery disease. Over two-thirds of these sudden cardiac deaths occur outside of the hospital setting. The survival rate from cardiac arrest is directly related to immediate cardiopulmonary rescucitation efforts and care. This is exemplified by a study that demonstrates a survival rate of 18.2% if performed within two minutes of the arrest versus 12.8% if performed after two minutes.

Health professionals should be trained in both BLS and ACLS, both of which are offered by the American Heart Association. Certification in these courses is invaluable when needed. Eisenberg et al. demonstrated that the highest hospital discharge rates for patients who survived cardiac arrest were in those treated with basic life support.

Basic health care equipment such as a stethoscope, sphygmomanometer, face mask/Ambu bag, and oxygen with nasal canula/mask are mandatory in the event of a cardiac arrest. Additional equipment found in crash carts such as epinephrine, atropine, and manual defibrillator may be found in some offices. Importantly, the location of these supplies is critical as they are useless if not immediately accessible.

MYOCARDIAL INFARCTION

Patients with complaints of chest pain require immediate assessment. Common symptoms of myocardial infarction (MI) include sternal (crushing) pain to discomfort that may radiate to the arm, neck, back, and jaw. Treatment includes early recognition, initial assessment (vital signs, positioning in supine position), and sublingual nitroglycerin (unless contraindicated). Oxygen via nasal cannula as well as chewing baby aspirin (81 mg) may be useful. Activation of EMS

Table 1 Minimal Equipment Necessary for the Office

Stethoscope
Sphygmomanometer
Oxygen with nasal canula/mask
Face mask/Ambu bag
Epinephrine
Antihistamine (e.g., Benadryl)
Intravenous catheters

followed by subsequent evaluation by a cardiologist is critical. Morphine (1–3 mg) may be supplemented if the patient continues to experience pain. The ABCs of BLS and ACLS should always be utilized.

CEREBROVASCULAR ACCIDENT

Stroke is the third leading cause of death in the United States, with over 500,000 cases and 150,000 deaths annually. A cerebrovascular accident (CVA) is a sudden loss of blood flow to an area of the brain that results in a neurologic deficit. If these symptoms resolve spontaneously, the event is termed a transient ischemic attack (TIA). A CVA can be secondary to a number of pathophysiologic mechanisms, including thrombosis, embolism, and hemorrhage. It is categorized as hemorrhagic or ischemic. Ischemia from thrombosis or embolism accounts for the vast majority (~75%). Advancements in acute care have dramatically increased the likelihood of a favorable outcome of a CVA. This level of medical care necessitates prompt transfer to dedicated facilities. The use of tissue-type plasminogen activator (t-PA) has proven beneficial in selected patients. The role of the dermatologist is simple and limited—it involves prompt recognition of neurologic deficit followed by activation of the EMS system and BLS.

The clinical presentation of an acute CVA involves a sudden onset of a neurologic deficit and/or altered state of consciousness. Prompt recognition of this condition is paramount so that EMS can be activated immediately and the ABCs of emergency care addressed.

PRESYNCOPE AND SYNCOPE

Syncope is the transient loss of consciousness marked by an inability to maintain postural tone. This is followed by spontaneous recovery. Use of this term excludes other states that may cause a similar clinical picture, such as seizures, coma, shock, or altered consciousness from medication. There are multiple causes of syncope that may be divided into cardiac and noncardiac groups. Most syncope in the office is psychogenic (vasovagal). Presyncope is similar to syncope but does not result in loss of consciousness. Perhaps the most significant complication of syncope in the realm of dermatologic surgery is injury related to a fall. Thus, pre-emptive action is key to avoiding such injury. It should also be noted that age and sex are not good predictors of who will have a syncopal episode. It is prudent to treat all patients equally.

Clinical diagnosis of vasovagal syncope is usually straightforward. There is often a prodrome of nausea, lightheadedness, and general ill feeling that may be accompanied by pallor and diaphoresis. The patient experiences a momentary lapse in consciousness followed by spontaneous recovery. Placement of the patient in Trendelenberg's position and application of a damp towel to the forehead usually leads to a rapid recovery. Vital signs should be obtained to assure consistency with the diagnosis, verify adequate blood pressure and document the time to recovery. It is important to allow the patient to return to a seated position in a slow and monitored fashion in case of a second episode.

Injections and biopsies elicit most vasovagal syncope. Making it routine to have patients recumbent while performing procedures can help to avoid an episode and protect from secondary injury should there be a loss of consiousness. Subsequently, it is prudent to have patients return to a sitting position slowly to avoid such episodes.

History and physical examination of the syncopal patient allows distinction from other conditions including seizure. Unusual sensory prodromes, incontinence, or altered level of consciousness may suggest seizure activity.

SEIZURES

Seizures are an uncommon occurrence in the dermatology office. Proper recognition and management are important to best serve the patient through the episode and to assist in the investigation of an etiology if not already apparent.

A seizure is defined as a transient involuntary burst of cortical activity that results from a focal or generalized disturbance of brain function. They are classified as idiopathic or primary when the cause is unknown and symptomatic or secondary when the etiology is known. Those that are felt to be secondary but no cause has been identified are classified as cryptogenic. Seizures are further divided into two main categories, partial and generalized. Partial seizures initiate from a focus in one cerebral hemisphere and manifest as motor, sensory, or psychomotor phenomena. Generalized seizures result in loss of consciousness and motor function and begin from both hemispheres simultaneously with no evidence of focal onset. Partial seizures are categorized as simple if consciousness is preserved and complex if consciousness is lost.

Seizures can result from many causes including head trauma, metabolic disorders, CVAs, tumors, illicit drugs, medications, fevers, and infections. Different conditions can be confused with seizures. The most common within the context of a dermatology appointment is syncope. This is further confounded because one can lose continence during a syncopal episode and the decreased cerebral perfusion can elicit a seizure secondarily. The best indications of a true seizure are lateral tongue biting and postevent confusion.

Management of a seizure should begin with turning the patient onto one side to prevent aspiration, and assessing and supporting breathing and circulation as needed. Clothing around the neck should be loosened. Nothing should be inserted into the mouth to protect the tongue because this can cause more damage, especially to the teeth. Most seizures spontaneously abate. The only laboratory test that must be done immediately is a blood glucose level to determine and correct hypoglycemia if that is the cause. Serum electrolytes and levels of anticonvulant medications in those with a history of seizures should also be ordered. These additional tests should not delay treatment of a protracted seizure. Any seizure lasting more than five minutes is not likely to spontaneously break. Call EMS and treat the patient for status epilepticus if equipped. Benzodiazapines are the first line agents to stop a seizure . Lorazepam, 0.1 mg/kg (maximum 4 mg) intravenous push over two to five minutes stops 80% of episodes within three minutes. A second dose can be administered after 10 minutes if needed. Blood pressure should be monitored. If lorazepam is not available, diazepam can be used. In adults 5–10 mg of diazepam is given intravenously, at a rate that should not exceed 5 mg/min; this can be repeated in 10 to 20 minutes if needed. Pediatric dosing is 0.2–0.3 mg/kg given over two to three minutes and can be repeated in 15 to 30 minutes. If benzodiazepines fail to terminate the seizure, use of phenytoin is considered. Evaluation of the seizure and further management should be coordinated by the emergency department. The patient's medical history and a description of the surrounding events are useful for this purpose. An immediate postical exam may show a focal neurologic deficit that corresponds to a locus in the brain from where the seizure originated. A patient's first seizure should be evaluated and explained. Those with a history of seizures need follow-up to assess management and cause of the breakthrough.

ANAPHYLAXIS AND ANAPHYLACTOID REACTIONS

Anaphylaxis is a severe and life threatening IgE-mediated systemic allergic reaction. Anaphylactoid reactions present identically to anaphylaxis but are not mediated through an IgE antibody–antigen interaction.

Anaphylactoid reactions can occur from exercise, increased core body temperature, administration of immunoglobulins in treating patients with immunodeficiency, administration of contrast media, or from a direct activation of mast cells by certain drugs such as opiates in those who are susceptible. These effects are mediated directly through mast cell stimulation or activation of the complement pathway. An anaphylactoid reaction can also occur via anti-IgA antibodies after transfusion of blood products containing IgA into a patient who has an IgA deficiency.

Common triggers of anaphylaxis are certain foods, drugs, and insect venoms. The most common of which is penicillin, and this occurs in one in every 10,000 patients. Anaphylaxis has been estimated to cause 500 deaths per year in the United States.

Reactions are usually evident within seconds or minutes after exposure but can occur one to two days later. Usually the history and physical findings are sufficient for diagnosis. Signs and symptoms include pruritus, erythema, urticaria, angioedema, nasal congestion, rhinorrhea, wheezing, dyspnea, abdominal pain, nausea, vomiting, diarrhea, tachycardia, hypotension, and complete cardiovascular collapse.

Management depends on the severity of the reaction. The most important aspect of anaphylaxis is early detection. Treatment should commence immediately with attention to maintaining an airway and supporting circulation. EMS should be notified. Recline the patient into Trendelenburg's position and provide supplemental oxygen. If there is evidence of bronchial obstruction and/or hypotension, 0.2–0.5 mL of 1:1000 solution of epinephrine should be injected intramuscularly for adults and 0.01 mL/kg for children. Subcutaneous injection is less preferable because of variability in absorption. This dose can be repeated every 15 to 30 minutes as needed up to three doses. Intravenous access should be established for the administration of fluids and medications. The dose of epinephrine if given intravenously is 1–5 mL of 1:10000 solution for adults and 0.01–0.05 mL/kg for children and can be given every 5 to 10 minutes as needed. If the hypotension is severe and intravenous access is not established, the intramuscular dose of epinephrine can be administered into the posterior third of the sublingual area or the intravenous dose can be injected through an endotracheal tube. Ringer's lactate or normal saline should also be given to maintain pressure. Persistent hypotension may require the use of other vasopressors such as dopamine, 200 mg in 500 mL of dextrose in water at a rate of 3–20 µg/kg/min titrating to blood pressure. Hypotension may be refractory to the effects of sympathomimetics in patients taking beta-blockers. Use of glucagon in these patients may be of benefit. It is administered as a 50 µg/kg intravenous bolus over one minute or as a continuous infusion at 5–15 µg/min. Atropine may be given for bradycardia, 0.3–0.5 mg intramuscularly or subcutaneously.

Respiratory distress should be treated with nebulized albuterol, 10 mg/hr or 2.5 mg every 15 to 20 minutes. Intravenous aminophylline can be considered as a second line therapy. If the airway is threatened, intubation may be necessary. If unavailable or too difficult because of laryngeal edema, a cricothyroidotomy or tracheostomy must be done. A needle cricothyroidotomy using a 14 or 16 gauge needle can provide an emergency airway.

Diphenhydramine 25–50 mg intravenously, intramuscularly, or subcutaneously will help alleviate symptoms and possibly prevent additional histamine release. Use of an H_2 blocker such as ranitidine, 1 mg/kg intravenoulsly, or cimetidine, 4 mg/kg intravenously, may provide additional benefit.

If the reaction was from a sting or local injection, a tourniquet should be placed proximally at a pressure that obstructs venous but not arterial flow. The stinger can be removed with the edge of a blade or fingernail being careful to not release additional venom. Injection of 0.005 mL/kg of 1:1000 solution of epinephrine into the site (maximum of 0.25 mL) may help to slow absorption of the antigen.

Corticosteroids do not alleviate the acute symptoms of anaphylaxis and there is no good evidence supporting their use in preventing a recurrence for protracted anaphylaxis. However, they are often given. Hydrocortisone sodium succinate 250–500 mg IV every 4 to 6 hours (4–8 mg/kg for children) or methylprednisolone 60–125 mg IV (1–2 mg/kg for children) are two such regimens.

All patients who experience anaphylaxis should be monitored in the hospital for 24 hours after symptom resolution for the possibility of a recurrent episode. A shorter period may be acceptable for very mild reactions.

Once a person successfully recovers, it is important that he/she sees an allergist for further investigation and recommendations to prevent and/or treat a future episode.

LIDOCAINE TOXICITY

The majority of dermatologic procedures are performed under local anesthesia through direct infiltration, peripheral nerve blockade, or tumescence. Anesthetics are divided into two classes based upon their molecular structure, amides, and esters. The most popular agent used is lidocaine, an amide anesthetic. Others in this group include mepivocaine, prilocaine, bupivocaine, etidocaine, and ropivocaine. The ester group is composed of procaine, chlorprocaine, tetracaine, and cocaine. All the agents act by blocking impulse conduction through inhibition of sodium channels. The agents vary from one another in their potency, time to onset of action, duration of action, and side effect/toxicity profiles.

The two untoward reactions that are of concern to the dermatologist are allergy and systemic toxicity. True allergic reactions to lidocaine or bupivicaine are extremely rare. Allergy is more common with the ester agents because these are metabolized by plasma cholinesterase to the more common sensitizer, para-aminobenzoic acid (PABA). The amide anesthetics are metabolized by the liver into metabolites that are unrelated to PABA. Therefore, no cross-reactivity is observed between amide and ester anesthetics. Allergic reactions when using amides are most often to a methylparaben preservative rather than the anesthetic itself. This can be avoided by the use of a single dose, preservative-free formulation. Allergy to anesthetics is rare. True IgE allergy accounts for less than 1% of reported adverse reactions. Should you suspect an allergic reaction, stop the administration of anesthesia and treat accordingly (see Anaphylaxis and Anaphylactoid Reactions).

Toxicity results from using an excessive amount of an agent or through inadvertent intravascular injection of an agent. It is the latter that accounts for the majority of reported toxicities. Suggested maximum dosages of anesthetics depend on the agent and whether epinephrine is used. Epinephrine through its vasoconstriction, slows the systemic absorption of the anesthetic allowing for a longer duration of anesthesia and a lower peak serum concentration compared with the same dose administered without epinephrine. Tumescent anesthesia uses a very dilute preparation of lidocaine and epinephrine. Peak serum levels occur 12 to 14 hours after the start of infiltration but can occur up to 23 hours. This delay in absorption raises the limit on the amount of lidocaine that can be safely used to 35 mg/kg, and in some reports to 55 mg/kg.

Systemic reactions involve the central nervous system (CNS) and myocardium. CNS toxicity occurs at a lower serum concentration of anesthetic than does cardiac toxicity. The initial symptoms include tinnitus, lightheadedness, circumoral numbness, disorientation, confusion, visual disturbances, and lethargy. These usually manifest at serum lidocaine concentrations between 3 and 6 μg/mL. If toxicity progresses, one can see tremors, seizures, and respiratory arrest. Studies show that the serum concentration of lidocaine needed to elicit seizures is greater than 10 μg/mL. Other factors, though, can affect the concentration at which these events occur. The more rapid the rise in serum concentration, the lower the level needed to develop toxicity. Also, concurrent use of sedatives can raise the threshold for seizures while acidosis lowers the level needed for toxicity. If toxicity is suspected, no additional anesthetic should be given. Oxygen should be provided and vital signs monitored. ACLS procedures should be followed. Seizures are treated with barbiturates and benzodiazepines (see Seizures), and EMS should be notified.

The effects on the myocardium are more difficult to manage. These include decreased cardiac output, arrhythmias, and cardiac arrest. ECG changes are the earliest evidence of toxicity. Slowed conduction results in prolonged PR, QRS, and QT intervals. Cardiovascular toxicity is uncommon with the use of lidocaine because of the high concentration required to elicit this effect and the warning availed by the CNS symptoms at lower concentrations. The plasma level of lidocaine needs to be much greater than 10 μg/mL to observe cardiac toxicity but this threshold can be lowered by the additive effect from concurrent medications that depress cardiac conduction, e.g., calcium channel or beta-adrenergic blockers. Bupivocaine is more cardiotoxic than other local anesthetics, and toxicity occurs at a lower relative concentration compared with that needed to produce CNS symptoms as measured in animal models.

Treatment of cardiac toxicity should begin with correcting potentially exacerbating factors. Hypoxia and metabolic acidosis can worsen both CNS and cardiac toxicities. Supplemental oxygen should be provided along with standard cardiopulmonary support. Hypotension can be treated with alpha- and beta-adrenergic agonists, and bradycardia can be treated with atropine. Cardiopulmonary bypass for unresponsive cardiovascular collapse should be considered if available until sufficient redistribution and metabolism of the anesthetic has occurred.

HEMOSTASIS

Successful hemostasis requires knowledge of the patient's medical and pharmacologic history. Identification of the patient's medications and allergies allows the surgeon to decide which local anesthetic to use. Perhaps more importantly the surgeon decides what dilution of epinephrine is most appropriate for each patient. Patients with a history of atrial fibrillation may handle a procedure better without the routine addition of epinephrine as would an otherwise healthy patient.

Knowledge of implantable cardiac devices is an important component of the preoperative history. Electrosurgical units are commonly utilized in cutaneous surgery; however, these devices can stimulate defibrillators to activate and thus should not be used with these devices. Thermal cautery, however, does not pass a current through the patient and is safe. Pacemakers can also be affected by electrosurgery. The use of short bursts with electrodessication or bipolar forceps is considered safe for these patients.

The use of anticoagulant therapy has dramatically increased within the last decade. More recent data recommends continuation of anticoagulant therapy for patients taking such medications for cardiac and/or vascular reasons. Multiple studies have contended that the risk of postoperative bleeding complications from anticoagulant therapy is far outweighed by the potential risks of discontinuing these therapies. Thus, most dermatologic surgeons have focused on optimizing hemostatic techniques in the setting of continued anticoagulant therapy. This may impact reconstruction options.

EXPOSURES

Exposure to infectious agents can be life threatening. The Centers for Disease Control and Prevention (CDC) has proposed standard precautions to help safeguard from this risk. Standard precautions apply to all potentially infectious material including blood, tissue, all body fluids except sweat, nonintact skin, and mucous membranes. Precautionary measures include hand washing, use of gloves, masks, and gowns whenever there is an exposure to potentially infectious material.

Despite careful practice, however, accidental exposures occur. The infectious agents of greatest concern are hepatitis B (HBV), hepatitis C (HCV), and human immunodeficiency virus (HIV). It is important to have an established protocol to manage these incidents and to include this training for all who are at risk as the efficacy of postexposure prophylaxis (PEP) is dependent on prompt initiation. There are two main categories of exposures that place one at risk for disease transmission: percutaneous injuries, such as from a needle stick or sharp object, and contact of a mucous membrane or nonintact skin with potentially infectious material as blood, tissue, or body fluids. Vaccination against HBV has been recommended for healthcare personnel since the early 1980s. Currently there is no effective vaccine for HCV or HIV.

After any exposure, the wound should be cleaned with soap and water. If a mucous membrane contact occurred, copiously rinse the area with water. Assess the source person of exposure for a known history of HBV, HCV, or HIV. If not known, inform the source of the exposure and request consent for testing. Testing should be done immediately. Consult the proposed laboratory facility to determine the correct procedure and tests to order to assure the fastest response. If enzyme-linked immunosorbent assay for HIV status cannot be completed within 24 to 48 hours, consider using an FDA-approved rapid HIV antibody test kit. If testing cannot be done, gather all clinical, epidemiological, and laboratory information that is available

Table 2 Recommended Postexposure Prophylaxis for Exposure to Hepatitis B Virus

Vaccination and antibody response status of exposed workers[a]	Treatment		
	Source HBsAg[b] positive	Source HBsAg[b] negative	Source unknown or not available for testing
Unvaccinated	HBIG[c] × 1 and initiate HB vaccine series[d]	Initiate HB vaccine series	Initiate HE vaccine series
Previously vaccinated			
Known responder[e]	No treatment	No treatment	No treatment
Known nonresponder[f]	HBIG × 1 and initiate revaccination or HBIG × 2[g]	No treatment	If known high risk source, treat as if source were HBsAg positive
Antibody response unknown	Test exposed person for anti-HB[h] If adequate[e], no treatment is necessary If inadequate[f], administer HBIG × 1 and vaccine booster	No treatment	Test exposed person far anti-HBs If adequate[h], no treatment is necessary If inadequate[h], administer vaccine booster and recheck titer in 1–2 months

[a]Persons who have previously been infected with HBV are immune to reinfection and do not require postexposure prophylaxis.
[b]Hepatitis B surface antigen.
[c]Hepatitis B immune globulin; dose is 0.06 mL/kg intramuscularly.
[d]Hepatitis B vaccine.
[e]A responder is a person with adequate levels of serum antibody to HBsAg (i.e., anti-HBs $\geq$10 mIU/mL).
[f]A nonresponder is a person, with inadequate response to vaccination (i.e., serum anti-HBs <10 mIU/mL).
[g]The option of giving one dose of HBIG and reinitiating the vaccine series is preferred for nonresponders who have not completed a second 3-dose vaccine series. For persons who previously completed a second vaccine series but failed to respond, two doses of HBIG are preferred.
[h]Antibody to HBsAg.
Source: From CDC (1982).

to estimate the risk from exposure. The circumstances and management of the exposure should be documented in a medical record according to Occupational Safety and Health Administration (OSHA) and state requirements.

The risk of occupational transmission of HBV to an unvaccinated person depends on the type of exposure as well as the serology of the source person. Percutaneous injury with a needle contaminated with blood containing HBV leads to serologic evidence of HBV in the injured person in 23% to 37% of instances if the source blood is HBSAg-positive and HBeAg-negative and 37% to 62% if the source blood is positive for both HBSAg and HBeAg. The risk of clinical hepatitis is 1% to 6% and 22% to 31% respectively. Although percutaneous injury may pose the highest risk of HBV transmission as an individual event, it

is probable that the majority of transmissions occur through mucous membrane or nonintact skin because of the greater frequency of these exposures. The recommendations for PEP for HBV are summarized in Table 2.

The risk of HCV transmission is much less than that for HBV. No transmission has been documented from contact with nonintact skin, and it rarely occurs from mucous membrane exposure. Seroconversion occurs in 1.8% of percutaneous exposures. No study has evaluated use of antiviral agents as prophylaxis, and use of immunoglobulin in animal models has been unsuccessful. Currently, there is no recommended PEP. Baseline and follow-up testing for anti-HCV antibodies and liver function tests should be performed. Studies outside the United States suggest there may be benefit from interferon use early in the course of acute hepatitis C. An

Table 3 Recommended HIV Postexposure Prophylaxis for Percutaneous Injuries

Exposure type	Infection status of source				
	HIV-positive Class 1[a]	HIV-positive Class 2[a]	Source of unknown HIV status[b]	Unknown source[c]	HIV-negative
Less severe[d]	Recommend basic 2-drug PEP	Recommend expanded 3-drug PEP	Generally, no PEP warranted; however, consider basic 2-drug PEP[e] for source with HIV risk factors[f]	Generally, no PEP warranted; however, consider basic 2-drug PEP[e] in settings where exposure to HIV-infected persons is likely	No PEP warranted
More severe[g]	Recommend expanded 3-drug PEP	Recommend expanded 3-drug PEP	Generally, no PEP warranted; however, consider basic 2-drug PEP[e] for source with HIV risk factors[f]	Generally, no PEP warranted; however, consider basic 2-drug PEP[e] in settings where exposure to HIV-infected persons is likely	No PEP warranted

[a]HIV-Positive, Class 1—asymptomatic HIV infection or known low viral load (e.g., <1500 RNA copies/mL). HIV-Postive, Class 2—symptomatic HIV infection, AIDS, acute seroconversion, or known high viral load. If drug resistance is a concern, obtain expert consultation. Initiation of PEP should not be delayed pending expert consultation, and, because expert consultation alone cannot substitute for face-to-face counseling, resources should be available to provide immediate evaluation and follow-up care for all exposures.
[b]Source of unknown HIV status (e.g., deceased source person with no samples available for HIV testing).
[c]Unknown source (e.g., a needle from a sharps disposal containe).
[d]Less severe (e.g., solid needle and superficial injury).
[e]The designation "consider PEP" indicates that PEP is optional and should be based on an individualized decision between the exposed person and the treating clinician.
[f]If PEP is offered and taken and the source is later determined to be HIV-negative, PEP should be discontinued.
[g]More severe (e.g., large-bore hollow needle, deep puncture, visible blood on device, or needle used in patient's artery or vein).
Abbreviation: PEP, postexposure prophylaxis.
Source: From CDC (1982).

Table 4   Recommended HIV Postexposure Prophylaxis for Mucous Membrane Exposures and Nonintact Skin[a] Exposures

Exposure type	Infection status of source				
	HIV-positive Class 1[b]	HIV-positive Class 2[b]	Source of unknown HIV status[c]	Unknown source[d]	HIV-negative
Small volume[e]	Consider basic 2-drug PEP[f]	Recommend basic 2-drug PEP	Generally, no PEP warranted; however, consider basic 2-drug PEP[f] for source with HIV risk factors[g]	Generally, no PEP warranted; however, consider basic 2-drug PEP[f] in settings where exposure to HIV-infected persons is likely	No PEP warranted
Large volume[h]	Recommend basic 2-drug PEP	Recommend expanded 3-drug PEP	Generally, no PEP warranted; however, consider basic 2-drug PEP[f] for source with HIV risk factors[g]	Generally, no PEP warranted; however, consider basic 2-drug PEP[f] in settings where exposure to HIV-infected persons is likely	No PEP warranted

[a]For skin exposures, follow-up is indicated only if there is evidence of compromised skin integrity (e.g., dermatitis, abrasion, or open wound).
[b]HIV-positive, Class 1—asymptomatic HIV infection or known low viral load (e.g., <1500 RNA copies/mL). HIV-postive, Class 2—symptomatic HIV infection, AIDS, acute seroconversion, or known high viral load. If drug resistance is a concern, obtain expert consultation. Initiation of PEP should not be delayed pending expert consultation, and, because expert consultation alone cannot substitute for face-to-face counseling, resources should be available to provide immediate evaluation and follow-up care for all exposure.
[c]Source of unknown HIV status (e.g., deceased source person with no samples available for HIV testing).
[d]Unknown source (e.g., splash from inappropriatelty disposed blood).
[e]Small volume (i.e., a few drops).
[f]The designation "consider PEP" indicates that PEP is optional and should be based on an individualized decision between the exposed person and the treating clinician.
[g]If PEP is offered and taken and the source is later determined to be HIV-negative, PEP should be discontinued.
[h]Large volume (i.e., major blood splash).
Abbreviation: PEP, postexposure prophylaxis.
Source: From CDC (1982).

exposed person with any evidence of infection should be referred to a specialist for management.

Exposure to HIV in the hospital setting is a major concern for health care workers. As of June, 2001, 57 healthcare workers in the United States are documented to have acquired HIV through occupational exposure, and it is suspected that the actual number of transmitted infections is greater than 100. Risk of HIV transmission is 0.3% from a percutaneous injury and 0.09% from a mucous membrane contact. Although documented transmission has occurred from exposure on nonintact skin, it is estimated to be less common than for mucous membrane contact. The risk of transmission with a percutaneous injury is increased if inflicted by a large bore needle, blood visibly contaminates the sharp object, the needle was used in a vein or artery, or the source patient has a terminal illness. The latter may reflect a higher titer of HIV. PEP is recommended for HIV and routine protocols are established in most hospitals. Initiation of PEP is based on multiple factors including the exposure type (needle, non-needle sharp, splash), HIV status of the exposure source, time between exposure and medical evaluation, medical history of both the source patient and the exposed person, and side effects of medications. The use of PEP is best managed by a specialist. Two and three drug regimens are recommended based on the overall risk of exposure (Tables 3 and 4).

In all instances, proper counseling should be offered for exposed healthcare personnel and all source patients who have newly diagnosed conditions.

BIBLIOGRAPHY

Additional resources concerning postexposure management can be found online at www.needlestick.mednet.ucla.edu and from the National Clinican's Hotline (PEPline) at www.uscf.edu/hivcntr/resources/pep/index.html.

Aldrete IA, Johnson DA. Evaluation of intracutaneous testing for investigation of allergy to local anesthetic agents. Anesth Analg 1970; 49:173–181.

Alter MJ. The epidemiology of acute and chronic hepatitis C. Clin Liver Dis 1997; 1:559–568.

Albers GW, Amarenco P, Easton JD, Sacco RL, Teal P. Antithrombotic and thrombolytic therapy for ischemic stroke: the seventh ACCP conference on antithrombotic and thrombolytic therapy. Chest 2004; 126:483S–512S.

Alalay J, Alkalay R. Controversies in perioperative management of blood thinners in dermatologic surgery: continue or discontinue? Dermatol Surg 2004; 30:1091–1094.

Bosnjak Z, Stowe D, Kampine J. Comparison of lidocaine and bupivocaine depression of sinoatrial node activity during hypoxia and acidosis in adult and neonatal guinea pigs. Anesth Analg 1986; 65:911–917.

Bochner BS, Lichtenstein LM. Anaphylaxis. N Engl J Med 1991; 324:1785–1790.

Bell DM. Occupational risk of human immunodeficiency virus infection in healthcare workers: an overview. Am J Med 1997; 102(suppl. 5B):9–15.

Beers MH, Berkow R, et al. eds. The Merck Manual of Diagnosis and Therapy. 17th ed. West Point: Merck & Co, Inc, 1999.

Burk RW, Guzman-Stein G, Vasconez LO. Tumescent anesthesia with a lidocaine dose of 55 mg/kg is safe for liposuction. Dermatol Surg 1996; 22:921–927.

Bronner LL, Kanter DS, Manson JE. Primary prevention of stroke. N Engl J Med 1995; 333:1392–1400.

CDC. Recommendation of the Immunization Practices Advisory Committee (ACIP) inactivated hepatitis B virus vaccine. MMWR 1982; 31:317–328.

Centers for Disease Control and Prevention. Public health service guidelines for the management of health-care worker exposures to HIV and recommendations for postexposure prophylaxis. MMWR 1998; 47:1–33.

CDC. Update: human immunodeficiency virus infections in health-care workers exposed to blood of infected patients. MMWR 1987; 36:285–289.

Centers for Disease Control and Prevention. Preventing Occupational HIV Transmission to Healthcare Personnel, 2002 http://www.cdc.gov/hiv/pubs/facts/hcwprev.htm.

CDC. Updated U.S. Public Health Service Guidelines for the Management of Occupational Exposures to HBV, HCV, and HIV and Recommendations for Postexposure Prophylaxis. MMWR 2001; 50:1–42.

Cardo DM, Culver DH, Ciesielski CA, et al. A case–control study of HIV seroconversion in health care workers after percutaneous exposure. N Engl J Med 1997; 337:1485–1490.

Dambro MR, ed. Griffith's 5-Minute Clinical Consult. 13th ed. Lippincott Williams & Wilkins, 2005.

Emergency cardiac care committee and subcommittees. American Heart Association. JAMA 1992; 268:2171–2183.

Eisenberg MS, Bergner L, Hallstrom A. Cardiac resuscitation in the community. Importance of rapid provision and implications for program planning. JAMA 1979; 241:1905–1907.

Fisher JA, Baldor RA. Anaphylaxis and anaphylactoid reactions. In: David AK, Johnson TA Jr., Phillips DM, Scherger JE, eds. Family Medicine: Principles and Practice. 6th ed. New York: Springer-Verlag, 2003.

Fader DJ, Johnson TM. Medical issues and emergencies in the dermatology office. J Am Acad Dermatol 1997; 36:1–16.

Fried MW, Hoofnagle JH. Therapy of hepatitis C. Semin Liver Dis 1995; 15:82–91.

Guberman AH, Bruni J. Essentials of Clinical Epilepsy. 2nd ed. Boston: Butterworth Heinemann, 1999:1–199.

Hauser WA. Status epilepticus, epidemiologic considerations. Neurology 1990; 40(suppl. 2):9–13.

Ippolito G, Puro V, De Carli G, Italian Study Group on Occupational Risk of HIV Infection. The risk of occupational human immunodeficiency virus in health care workers. Arch Int Med 1993; 153:1451–1458.

Krawczynski K, Alter MJ, Tankersley DL, et al. Effect of immune globulin on the prevention of experimental hepatitis C virus infection. J Infect Dis 1996; 173:822–828.

Kaufman B, Wahlander S. Local anesthetics. In: Goldfrank LR, ed. Goldfrank's Toxicologic Emergencies. 7th ed. New York: The McGraw-Hill Companies, 2002:824–834.

Kemp SF, Lockey RF, Wolf BL, et al. Anaphylaxis: a review of 266 cases. Arch Intern Med 1995; 155:1749–1754.

Klein JA. The tumescent technique, anesthesia and modified liposuction technique. Dermatol Clin 1990; 8:425–437.

Lowenstein DH, Bleck T, Macdonald RL. It's time to revise the definition of status epilepticus. Epilepsia 1999; 40:120–122.

Lanphear BP, Linnemann CC Jr., Cannon CG, DeRonde MM, Pendy L, Kerley LM. Hepatitis C virus infection in healthcare workers: risk of exposure and infection. Infect Control Hosp Epidemiol 1994; 15:745–750.

Lane JE, Moore CC, Vogel RL, Stephens JL. Acceptance of HIV post-exposure prophylaxis according to occupation in the hospital setting. Int J Infect Dis 2004; 3.

Lieberman P. Anaphylaxis and anaphylactoid reactions. In: Middleton E, ed. Allergy: principles and practice. 5th ed. St. Louis: Mosby, 1998: 1079–1089.

Lempert T, Bauer M, Schmidt D. Syncope: a videometric analysis of 56 episodes of transient cerebral hypoxia. Ann Neurol 1994; 36:233–237.

Middleton DB. Seizure disorders. In: David AK, Johnson TA Jr., Phillips DM, Scherger JE, eds. Family Medicine: Principles and Practice. 6th ed. New York: Springer-Verlag, 2003.

Marcus R. The Centers for Disease Control and Prevention Cooperative Needlestick Surveillance Group. Surveillance of health care workers exposed to blood from patients infected with the human immunodeficiency virus. N Engl J Med 1988; 319:1118–1123.

Mitsui T, Iwano K, Masuko K, et al. Hepatitis C virus infection in medical personnel after needlestick accident. Hepatology 1992; 16:1109–1114.

Marick PE, Varon J. The management of status epilepticus. Chest 2004; 126:582–591.

Puro V, Petrosillo N, Ippolito G, Italian Study Group on Occupational Risk of HIV and Other Bloodborne Infections. Risk of hepatitis C seroconversion after occupational exposure in health care workers. Am J Infect Control 1995; 23:273–277.

Parkin JM, Murphy M, Anderson J, El-Gadi S, Forster G, Pinching AJ. Tolerability and side-effects of post-exposure prophylaxis for HIV infection. Lancet 2000; 355:722–723.

Quin JW. Interferon therapy for acute hepatitis C viral infection—a review by meta-analysis. Aust N Z J Med 1997; 27:611–617.

Rosen M, Thigpen J, Schnider S, et al. Bupivocaine-induced cardiotoxicity in hypoxic and acidotic sheep. Anesth Analg 1985; 64:1089–1096.

Rao RB, Ely SF, Hoffman RS. Deaths related to liposuction. N Engl J Med 1999; 340:1471–1475.

Sistrom MG, Coyner BJ, Gwaltney JM, Farr BM. Frequency of percutaneous injuries requiring postexposure prophylaxis for occupational exposure to human immunodeficiency virus. Infect Control Hosp Epidemiol 1998; 19:504–506.

Samdal F, Amland PF, Bugge JF. Plasma lidocaine levels during suction-assisted lipectomy using large doses of dilute lidocaine with epinephrine. Plastic Reconstr Surg 1994; 93:1217–1223.

Swanson JG. Assessment of allergy to local anesthetic. Ann Emerg Med 1983; 12:316–318.

Sabo-Grahm T, Seay AR. Management of status epilepticus in children. Pediatr Rev 1998; 19:306–309.

Smith PE, Cossburn MD. Seizures: assessment and management in the emergency unit. Clin Med 2004; 4:118–122.

Suraj A, Suriti K. Principles of office anesthesia: part I. infiltrative anesthesia. Am Fam Physician 2002; 66:91–94.

Tetzlaff JE. The pharmacology of local anesthetics. Anesth Clin North Am 2000; 18:217–233.

Tang AW. A practical guide to anaphylaxis. Am Fam Phys 2003; 68:1325–1332.

Terr AI. Anaphylaxis & urticaria. In: Parslow TG, Stites DP, Terr AI, Imboden JB, eds. Medical Immunology. 10th ed. New York: The McGraw-Hill Companies, Inc., 2001.

Vukmir RB. Sodium Bicarbonate Study Group. Witnessed arrest, but not delayed bystander cardiopulmonary resuscitation improves prehospital cardiac arrest survival. Emerg Med J 2004; 21:370–373.

Vogel W, Graziadei I, Umlauft F, et al. High-dose interferon-a_{2b} treatment prevents chronicity in acute hepatitis C: a pilot study. Dig Dis Sci 1996; 41(suppl. 12):81S–85S.

Werner BG, Grady GF. Accidental hepatitis-B-surface-antigen-positive inoculations: use of e antigen to estimate infectivity. Ann Intern Med 1982; 97:367–369.

Wheless JW. Acute management of seizures in the syndromes of idiopathic generalized epilepsies. Epilepsia 2003; 44(suppl. 2):2226.

White PF, Katzung BG. Local anesthetics. In: Katzung, BG, ed. Basic and Clinical Pharmacology. 9th. New York: The McGraw-Hill Companies, 2004.

www.cdc.gov.

13

Surgical Coding: Current Procedural Terminology

Brett Coldiron, Eric Adelman, and Vernell St. John
Health Policy and Practice, American Academy of Dermatology, Schaumburg, Illinois, U.S.A.

INTRODUCTION

Accurate surgical current procedural terminology (CPT) coding is essential for proper reimbursement and coupled with adequate documentation will fend off audits and refund claims. Readers should consult the current CPT book and ICD-9-CM (*International Classification of Diseases, Ninth Edition*) for reference. All providers/readers must have the current copy of each of these manuals for reference and become familiar with them to, report services provided. CPT and ICD-9-CM comprise the language which providers must use to communicate with insurers.

Keep in mind that the provider, not the billing clerk, is ultimately responsible for all claims errors. Billing errors can at best result in less payment, and at worst, audits, penalties, and claims of fraud.

In this chapter it is assumed that the reader knows and understands evaluation and management (E/M) coding, because this topic is complex and worthy of a chapter in itself. Medicare currently accepts the use of either the 1995 or 1997 documentation guidelines. Surgical dermatologists may find complying with the 1995 E/M guidelines most preferable. The 1997 documentation guidelines contain a single-organ system examination that requires a specific number of bullets per level of E/M service. However, use of either guideline is acceptable for selecting the level of evaluation and management services.

It must be noted, however, that it is reasonable and proper to report a new patient or consultation evaluation and management service the same day as a procedure is performed. A medically necessary and properly documented E/M service can be justified and should be reimbursed if the proper modifier(s) are appended to the E/M code.

RELATIVE VALUE UNITS

Relative value units (RVU) are a measurement of the work done related to a specific code. The payment amount reimbursed per code can be calculated by multiplying the RVU times the Medicare conversion factor for that year. For example, the biopsy code RVUs for a nonfacility totals 2.10. The Medicare conversion factor for 2005 is 37.8975. Thus, the reimbursement for a biopsy of one lesion in 2005 is $79.58 nationally. The geographic practice costs indices apply, which determine the local carrier reimbursement; and will cause minor differences in reimbursements. A list of codes and their corresponding RVUs are given in Table 1.

GLOBAL SURGICAL PACKAGE

The global surgical package is a payment policy of bundling payment for the various services associated with a procedure into a single payment. The RVUs of a global surgical package for a procedure include the preoperative, intraoperative, and postoperative work related to that procedure (e.g., preoperative work, follow-up visits relating to the procedure, suture removal, and wound care). The global period is the time allotted for the performance of the work related to the procedure. In order for a physician to report services provided unrelated to the original procedure during the global period, the services must be reported with the appropriate modifier(s). These modifiers notify the carrier that the work was unrelated to the global procedure or the usual work associated to the global procedure (see section on modifiers below). A few common procedures and their corresponding global periods are given in Table 2.

MODIFIERS

Modifiers provide the physician communication tools that are used to instruct the insurance carrier that a service or procedure has been performed under special circumstances. Private insurance carriers may have software designed that differs from Medicare. When billing for surgery on more than one site, for example, the carrier software will assume that the physician is double billing and deny the second site unless a modifier (-59 designating a separate surgery site in this case) is appended to the surgical CPT codes. It is imperative to know each carrier's guidelines on the use and acceptance of modifiers.

A brief overview of modifiers pertinent to surgical dermatology is given in the following sections.

Modifier -22: Unusual Procedural Services

Modifier -22 is used when a physician performs a service that is above and beyond the service described by the specific procedure code. The physician must attach a report to the claim explaining what was unusual about the service provided; that is, how the service provided was different from the norm. From our experience, this modifier describes more work but does not result in additional compensation. This modifier slows the adjudication of the claim and we suggest you not use it except under the most extraordinary circumstances.

Modifier -24: Unrelated Evaluation and Management Service by the Same Physician During a Postoperative Period

Modifier -24 is used when a patient presents with a different problem for an evaluation and management service during the postoperative period (global period) unrelated to the previously performed procedure. For example, one month ago a patient had a basal cell removed with the defect repaired

Table 1 Physician Work Relative Unit Values

CPT/HCPCS	Description	2006 physician work RVUs	2006 Non facility total RVUs	Global period
10040	Acne surgery	1.18	2.24	010
10060	Drainage of skin abscess	1.17	2.50	010
10061	Drainage of skin abscess	2.40	4.49	010
10080	Drainage of pilonidal cyst	1.17	4.39	010
10081	Drainage of pilonidal cyst	2.45	6.77	010
10120	Remove foreign body	1.22	3.52	010
10121	Remove foreign body	2.69	6.54	010
10140	Drainage of hematoma/fluid	1.53	3.50	010
10160	puncture dranage of lesion	1.20	2.94	010
10180	Complex drainage, wound	2.25	5.59	010
11000	Debride infected skin	0.60	1.25	000
11001	Debride infected skin add-on	0.30	0.57	ZZZ
11010	Debride skin, fx	4.19	11.74	010
11011	Debride skin/muscle, fx	4.94	13.86	000
11012	Debride skin/muscle/bone, fx	6.87	20.17	000
11040	Debride skin, partial	0.50	1.08	000
11041	Debride skin, full	0.82	1.58	000
11042	Debride skin/tissue	1.12	2.22	000
11100	Biopsy, skin lesion	0.81	2.09	000
11101	Biopsy, skin add-on	0.41	0.76	ZZZ
11200	Removal of skin tags	0.77	1.85	010
11201	Remove skin tags add-on	0.29	0.47	ZZZ
Shave codes:				
11300	Shave skin lesion	0.51	1.53	000
11301	Shave skin lesion	0.85	2.00	000
11302	Shave skin lesion	1.05	2.40	000
11303	Shave skin lesion	1.24	2.89	000
11305	Shave skin lesion	0.67	1.59	000
11306	Shave skin lesion	0.99	2.16	000
11307	Shave skin lesion	1.14	2.50	000
11308	Shave skin lesion	1.41	2.99	000
11310	Shave skin lesion	0.73	1.88	000
11311	Shave skin lesion	1.05	2.33	000
11312	Shave skin lesion	1.20	2.68	000
11313	Shave skin lesion	1.62	3.53	000
Benign excision codes:				
11400	Exctr-ext b9+marg 0.5 < cm	0.85	2.91	010
11401	Exctr-ext b9+marg 0.6–1 cm	1.23	3.39	010
11402	Exctr-ext b9+marg 1.1–2 cm	1.51	3.87	010
11403	Exctr-ext b9+marg 2.1–3 cm	1.79	4.36	010
11404	Exctr-ext b9+marg 3.1–4 cm	2.06	4.98	010
11406	Exctr-ext b9+marg > 4.0 cm	2.76	6.15	010
11420	Exch-f-nk-sp b9+marg 0.5 <	0.98	2.84	010
11421	Exc h-f-nk-sp b9+marg 0.6–1	1.42	3.62	010
11422	Exc h-f-nk-sp b9+marg 1.1–2	1.63	4.05	010
11423	Exch-f-nk-sp b9+marg 2.1–3	2.01	4.80	010
11424	Exch-f-nk-sp b9+marg 3.1–4	2.43	5.49	010
11426	Exc h-f-nk-sp b9+marg > 4 cm	3.77	7.70	010
11440	Exc face-mm b9+marg 0.5 < cm	1.06	3.35	010
11441	Exc face-mm b9+marg 0.6–1 cm	1.48	3.95	010
11442	Exc face-mm b9+marg 1.1–2 cm	1.72	4.43	010
11443	Exc face-mm b9+marg 2.1–3 cm	2.29	5.43	010
11444	Exc face-mm b9+marg 3.1–4 cm	3.14	6.92	010
11446	Exc face-mm b9+marg > 4 cm	4.48	8.96	010
Malignant excision codes:				
11600	Exc tr-ext mig+marg 0.5 < cm	1.31	4.05	010
11601	Exc tr-ext mig+marg 0.6–1 cm	1.60	4.63	010
11602	Exc tr-ext mig+marg 1.1–2 cm	1.95	4.90	010
11603	Exc tr-ext mig+marg 2.1–3 cm	2.19	5.43	010
11604	Exc tr-ext mig+marg 3.1–4 cm	2.40	6.98	010
11606	Exc tr-ext mig+marg > 4 cm	3.42	7.85	010

Table 1 Physician Work Relative Unit Values (*Continued*)

CPT/HCPCS	Description	2006 physician work RVUs	2006 Non facility total RVUs	Global period
11620	Exc h-f-nk-sp mlg+marg 0.5 <	1.19	3.88	010
11621	Exc h-f-nk-sp mlg+marg 0.6–1	1.76	4.59	010
11622	Exc h-f-nk-sp mig+marg 1.1–2	2.09	5.20	010
11623	Exc h-f-nk-sp mig+marg 2.1–3	2.61	6.15	010
11624	Exc h-f-nk-sp mig+marg 3.1–4	3.06	7.08	010
11626	Exc h-f-nksp mig+mar > 4 cm	4.29	9.38	010
11640	Exc face-mm malig+marg 0.5 <	1.35	4.12	010
11641	Exc face-mm malig+marg 0.6–1	2.16	5.35	010
11642	Exc face-mm malig+marg 1.1–2	2.59	6.19	010
11643	Exc face-mm malig+marg 2.1–3	3.10	7.17	010
11644	Exc face-mm malig+marg 2.1–3	4.02	9.08	010
11646	Exc face-mm mig+marg > 4 cm	5.94	12.32	010
Repair codes:				
12001	Repair superficial wound(s)	1.70	3.84	010
12002	Repair superficial wound(s)	1.86	4.08	010
12004	Repair superficial wound (s)	2.24	4.78	010
12005	Repair superficial wound (s)	2.86	5.96	010
12006	Repair superficial wound (s)	3.66	7.41	010
12007	Repair superficial wound (s)	4.11	8.39	010
12011	Repair superficial wound (s)	1.76	4.06	010
12013	Repair superficial wound (s)	1.99	4.45	010
12014	Repair superficial wound (s)	2.46	5.27	010
12015	Repair superficial wound (s)	3.19	6.62	010
12016	Repair superficial wound (s)	3.92	7.85	010
12017	Repair superficial wound (s)	4.70	NA	010
12018	Repair superficial wound (s)	5.52	NA	010
12020	Closure of spilt wound	2.62	6.75	010
12021	Closure of spilt wound	1.84	3.91	010
12031	Layer closure of wound(s)	2.15	4.61	010
12032	Layer closure of wound(s)	2.47	6.48	010
12034	Layer closure of wound(s)	2.92	6.37	010
12035	Layer closure of wound(s)	3.42	9.02	010
12036	Layer closure of wound(s)	4.04	10.16	010
12037	Layer closure of wound(s)	4.66	11.43	010
12041	Layer closure of wound(s)	2.37	5.11	010
12042	Layer closure of wound(s)	2.74	6.18	010
12044	Layer closure of wound(s)	3.14	6.63	010
12045	Layer closure of wound(s)	3.63	9.32	010
12046	Layer closure of wound(s)	4.24	11.30	010
12047	Layer closure of wound(s)	4.64	11.58	010
12051	Layer closure of wound(s)	2.47	5.95	010
12052	Layer closure of wound(s)	2.77	6.17	010
12053	Layer closure of wound(s)	3.12	6.60	010
12054	Layer closure of wound(s)	3.45	7.32	010
12055	Layer closure of wound(s)	4.42	9.36	010
12056	Layer closure of wound(s)	5.23	12.59	010
12057	Layer closure of wound(s)	5.95	12.66	010
13100	Repair of wound or lesion	3.12	7.44	010
13101	Repair of wound or lesion	3.91	8.84	010
13102	Repair of wound/lesion add-on	1.24	2.54	ZZZ
13120	Repair of wound or lesion	3.30	7.71	010
13121	Repair of wound or lesion	4.32	9.43	010
13122	Repair of wound/lesion add-on	1.44	3.10	ZZZ
13131	Repair of wound or lesion	3.78	8.41	010
13132	Repair of wound or lesion	5.94	12.18	010
13133	Repair of wound/lesion add-on	2.19	4.03	ZZZ
13150	Repair of wound or lesion	3.80	9.02	010
13151	Repair of wound or lesion	4.44	9.56	010
13152	Repair of wound or lesion	6.32	12.77	010
13153	Repair of wound/lesion add-on	2.38	4.56	ZZZ
13160	Late closure of wound	10.46	NA	090

(Continued)

(Continued)

Table 1 Physician Work Relative Unit Values (*Continued*)

CPT/HCPCS	Description	2006 physician work RVUs	2006 Non facility total RVUs	Global period
14000	Skin tissue rearrangement	5.88	14.34	090
14001	Skin tissue rearrangement	8.469	18.72	090
14020	Skin tissue rearrangement	6.58	15.85	090
14021	Skin tissue rearrangement	10.04	20.86	090
14040	Skin tissue rearrangement	7.86	17.31	090
14041	Skin tissue rearrangement	11.47	22.82	090
14060	Skin tissue rearrangement	8.49	17.98	090
14061	Skin tissue rearrangement	12.27	24.66	090
14300	Skin tissue rearrangement	11.74	24.06	090
14350	Skin tissue rearrangement	9.60	NA	090
15000	Wound prep, 1st 100 sq cm	3.99	8.33	000
15001	Wound prep, addl 100 sq cm	1.00	2.49	ZZZ
15040	Harvest cultured skin graft	2.00	6.81	000
10550	Skin pinch graft	4.29	11.79	090
15100	Skin splt grft, trnk/arm/leg	9.04	22.94	090
15101	Skin splt grft t/a/l add-on	1.72	5.70	ZZZ
15110	Epidrm autogrft trnk/arm/leg	9.50	21.51	090
15111	Epidrm autogrft t/a/l add-on	1.85	3.40	ZZZ
15115	Epidrm a-grft face/nck/hf/g	9.81	20.21	090
15116	Epidrm a-grft f/n/hf/g addl	2.50	4.41	ZZZ
15120	Skn splt a-grft fac/nck/hf/g	9.82	21.73	090
15121	Skn splt a-grft f/n/hf/g add	2.67	7.54	ZZZ
15130	Derm autograft, tmk/arm/leg	7.00	17.86	090
15131	Derm autograft t/a/l add-on	1.50	2.78	ZZZ
15135	Derm autograft face/nck/hf/g	10.50	21.63	090
15136	Derm autograft, f/n/hf/g add	1.50	2.59	ZZZ
15150	Cult epiderm grft t/arm/leg	8.26	17.87	090
15151	Cult epiderm grft t/a/l add	2.00	3.59	ZZZ
15152	Cult epiderm grft t/a/l+%	2.50	4.41	ZZZ
15155	Cult epiderm grft, f/n/hf/g	9.00	17.89	090
15156	Cult epiderm grft f/n/hf/g add	2.75	4.67	ZZZ
15157	Cult epiderm grft f/n/hfg+%	3.00	5.17	ZZZ
15170	Acell graft trunk/arms/legs	5.00	9.39	090
15171	Acell graft t/arm/leg add-on	1.55	2.42	ZZZ
15175	Acellular graft f/n/hf/g	7.00	13.26	090
15176	Acell graft, f/n/hf/g add-on	2.45	3.85	ZZZ
15200	Skin full graft, trunk	8.02	18.43	090
15201	Skin full graft, trunk add on	1.32	4.08	ZZZ
15220	Skin full graft sclp/arm/leg	7.86	17.91	090
15221	Skin full graft add-on	1.19	3.68	ZZZ
15240	Skin full graft face/genit/hf	9.03	20.18	090
15241	Skin full graft add-on	1.86	4.54	ZZZ
15260	Skin full graft een & lips	10.04	20.97	090
15261	Skin full graft add-on	2.23	5.14	ZZZ
15300	Apply skin allograft/arm/leg	3.99	7.69	090
15301	Apply skinallogrft/a/l addl	1.00	1.60	ZZZ
15320	Apply skin allogrft/n/hfg	4.70	8.91	090
15321	Aply sknallogrft f/n/hfg add	1.50	2.40	ZZZ
15330	Aply acell allogrft t/arm/leg	3.99	7.68	090
15331	Aply acell alogrft t/a/l add-on	1.00	1.60	ZZZ
15335	Apply-acell graft, f/n/hf/g	4.50	8.53	090
15336	Apply acell grft f/n/hf/g add	1.43	2.32	ZZZ
15340	Apply cult skin subsitute	3.72	8.14	010
15341	Apply cult skin sub add-on	0.50	1.17	ZZZ
15360	Apply cult derm sub, t/a/l	3.87	8.78	090
15361	Apply cult derm sub t/a/l add	1.15	1.87	ZZZ
15365	Apply cult derm sub f/n/hf/g	4.15	9.17	090
15366	Apply cult derm f/hf/g add	1.45	2.32	ZZZ
15400	Apply skin xenograft, t/a/l	3.99	8.48	090
15401	Apply skin xenograft t/a/l add	1.00	3.04	ZZZ
15420	Apply skin xgraft, f/n/hf/g	4.50	9.81	090

Table 1 Physician Work Relative Unit Values (*Continued*)

CPT/HCPCS	Description	2006 physician work RVUs	2006 Non facility total RVUs	Global period
15421	Apply skn xgraft t/n/hf/g add	1.50	3.03	ZZZ
15430	Apply acellular xenograft	5.75	13.33	090
15431	Apply acellular xgraft add	0.00	0.00	ZZZ
15570	From skin pedicle flap	9.20	21.87	090
15572	From skin pedicle flap	9.26	19.98	090
15574	From skin pedicle flap	9.87	21.78	090
15576	From skin pedicle flap	8.68	19.33	090
15600	Skin graft	1.91	9.80	090
15610	Skin graft	2.42	7.47	090
15620	Skin graft	2.94	11.09	090
15630	Skin graft	3.27	10.67	090
15650	Transfer skin pedicle flap	3.96	11.54	090
15732	Muscle-skin graft, head/neck	17.81	37.89	090
15734	Muscle-skin graft, trunk	17.76	38.53	090
15736	Muscle-skin graft, arm	16.26	36.98	090
15738	Muscle-skin graft, leg	17.89	38.56	090
15740	Island pedicle flap graft	10.23	21.02	090
15750	Neurovascular pedicle graft	11.39	NA	090
15756	Free myo/skin flap microvasc	35.18	NA	090
15757	Free skin flap, microvasc	35.18	NA	090
15758	Free fascial flap, microvasc	35.05	NA	090
15760	Composite skin graft	8.73	19.63	090
15770	Derma-fat-fascia graft	7.51	NA	090
15775	Hair transplant punch grafts	3.95	8.71	000
15776	Hair transplant punch grafts	5.53	11.62	000
15780	Abrasion treatment of skin	7.28	19.50	090
15781	Abrasion treatment of skin	4.84	12.11	090
15782	Abrasion treatment of skin	4.31	14.53	090
15783	Abrasion treatment of skin	4.28	11.45	090
15786	Abrasion, lesion, single	2.03	5.50	010
15787	Abrasions-lesions, add-on	0.33	1.46	ZZZ
15788	Chemical peel, face, epiderm	2.09	8.93	090
15789	Chemical peel, face, dermal	4.91	13.22	090
15792	Chemical peel, nonfacial	1.86	9.10	090
15793	Chemical peel, nonfacial	3.73	10.22	090
15819	Plastic surgery, neck	9.37	NA	090
15820	Revision of lower eyelid	5.14	12.53	090
15821	Revision of lower eyelid	5.71	13.53	090
15822	Revision of upper eyelid	4.44	10.66	090
15823	Revision of upper eyelid	7.04	15.41	090
15831	Excise excessive skin tissue	12.38	NA	090
15832	Excise excessive skin tissue	11.57	NA	090
15833	Excise excessive skin tissue	10.62	NA	090
15834	Excise excessive skin tissue	10.83	NA	090
15835	Excise excessive skin tissue	11.65	NA	090
15836	Excise excessive skin tissue	9.33	NA	090
15837	Excise excessive skin tissue	8.42	18.17	090
15838	Excise excessive skin tissue	7.12	NA	090
15839	Excise excessive skin tissue	9.37	19.44	090
15840	Graft for face nerve palsy	13.24	NA	090
15841	Graft for face nerve palsy	23.23	NA	090
15842	Flap for face nerve palsy	37.90	NA	090
15845	Skin and muscle repair, face	12.56	NA	090
15852	Dressing change not for burn	0.86	2.80	000
15860	Test for blood flow in graft	1.95	3.05	000
15920	Removal of tail bone ulcer	7.94	NA	090
15922	Removal of tail bone ulcer	9 89	NA	090
15931	Remove sacrum pressure sore	9.23	NA	090
15933	Remove sacrum pressure sore	10.83	NA	090
15934	Remove sacrum pressure sore	12.67	NA	090
15935	Remove sacrum pressure sore	14.55	NA	090

(Continued)

(Continued)

Table 1 Physician Work Relative Unit Values (*Continued*)

CPT/HCPCS	Description	2006 physician work RVUs	2006 Non facility total RVUs	Global period
15936	Remove sacrum pressure sore	12.36	NA	090
15937	Remove sacrum pressure sore	14.19	NA	090
15940	Remove hip pressure sore	9.33	NA	090
15941	Remove hip pressure sore	11.41	NA	090
15944	Remove hip pressure sore	11.44	NA	090
15945	Remove hip pressure sore	12.67	NA	090
15946	Remove hip pressure sore	21.54	NA	090
15950	Remove thigh pressure sore	7.53	NA	090
15961	Remove thigh pressure sore	10.70	NA	090
15952	Remove thigh pressure sore	11.37	NA	090
15953	Remove thigh pressure sore	12.61	NA	090
15956	Remove thigh pressure sore	15.50	NA	090
15958	Remove thigh pressure sore	15.46	NA	090
15999	Removal of pressure sore	0.00	0.00	YYY
Destruction codes:				
17000	Destroy benign/Premig lesion	060	1.60	010
17003	Destroy lesions, 2–14	0.15	0.27	ZZZ
17004	Destroy lesions, 15 or more	2.79	5.21	010
17106	Destruction of skin lesions	4.58	9.54	090
17107	Destruction of skin lesions	9.15	17.00	090
17108	Destruction of skin lesions	13.18	23.01	090
17110	Destruct lesion, 1–14	0.65	2.32	010
17111	Destruct lesion, 15 or more	0.92	2.64	010
17250	Chemical cautery, tissue	0.50	1.78	000
17260	Destruction of skin lesion*	0.91	2.23	010
17261	Destruction of skin lesions	1.17	2.83	010
17262	Destruction of skin lesions	1.55	3.53	010
17263	Destruction of skin lesions	1.79	3.92	010
17264	Destruction of skin lesions	1.94	4.25	010
17266	Destruction of skin lesions	2.34	4.94	010
17270	Destruction of skin lesions	1.32	3.07	010
17271	Destruction of skin lesions	1.49	3.33	010
17272	Destruction of skin lesions	1.77	3.84	010
17273	Destruction of skin lesions	2.05	4.34	010
17274	Destruction of skin lesions	2.59	5.26	010
17276	Destruction of skin lesions	3.20	6.31	010
17280	Destruction of skin lesions	1.17	2.83	010
17281	Destruction of skin lesions	1.72	3.70	010
17282	Destruction of skin lesions	2.04	4.28	010
17283	Destruction of skin lesions	2.64	5.30	010
17284	Destruction of skin lesions	3.21	6.27	010
17286	Destruction of skin lesions	4.43	8.34	010
Mohs codes:				
17304	1 stage Mohs, up to 5 spec	7.59	16.15	000
17305	2 stage Mohs, up to 5 spec	2.85	6.86	000
17306	3 stage Mohs, up to 5 spec	2.85	6.88	000
17307	Mohs addl stage up to 5 spec	2.65	6.53	000
17310	Mohs any stage > 5 spec	0.95	2.60	ZZZ
Misc. codes:				
17340	Cryotherapy of skin	0.76	1.18	010
17360	Skin peel therapy	1.43	2.93	010
40490	Biopsy of lip	1.22	2.90	000
40500	Partial excision of lip	4.27	11.56	090
40510	Partial excision of lip	4.69	11.81	090
40520	Partial excision of lip	4.66	12.74	090
40625	Reconstruct lip with flap	7.54	NA	090
40527	Reconstruct lip with flap	9.12	NA	090
40650	Repair lip	3.63	10.82	090
40652	Repair lip	4.25	12.53	090
40664	Repair lip	5.30	14.52	090
40808	Biopsy of mouth lesion	0.96	3.72	010

(*Continued*)

Table 1 Physician Work Relative Unit Values (*Continued*)

CPT/HCPCS	Description	2006 physician work RVUs	2006 Non facility total RVUs	Global period
40810	Excision of mouth lesion	1.31	4.33	010
40812	Excise/repair mouth lesion	2.31	6.32	010
40814	Excise/repair mouth lesion	3.41	8.77	090
40816	Excision of mouth lesion	3.66	9.24	090
64650	Botx Trtmt Hyperhidrosis axil	0.70	1.63	000
64653	Botx Trtmt Hyperhidrosis other	0.88	1.88	000
67961	Revision of eyelid	6.68	14.72	090
67966	Revision of eyelid	6.66	16.09	090
DermPath codes:				
88304 -26	Tissue exam by pathologist	0.22	0.32	XXX
88304 -TC	Tissue exam by pathologist	0.00	125	XXX
88304	Tissue exam by pathologist	0.22	1.57	XXX
88305 -26	Tissue exam by pathologist	0.75	1.11	XXX
68305 -TC	Tissue exam by pathologist	0.00	1.62	XXX
88305	Tissue exam by pathologist	0.75	2.73	XXX
88331 -26	Path consult intraop, 1 bloc	1.19	1.74	XXX
88331 -TC	Path consult intraop, 1 bloc	0.00	0.63	XXX
88331	Path consult intraop, 1 bloc	1.19	2.37	XXX
Light/laser codes:				
96567	Photodynamic tx, skin	0.00	2.00	XXX
96900	Ultraviolet light therapy	0.00	0.46	XXX
96902	Trichogram	0.41	0.60	XXX
96910	Photochemotherapy with UV-B	0.00	1.03	XXX
96912	Photochemotherapy with UV-A	0.00	1.31	XXX
96913	Photochemotherapy with UV-A or B	0.00	1.78	XXX
96920	Laser tx, skin < 250 sq cm	1.15	3.71	000
96921	Laser tx, skin 250–500 sq cm	1.17	3.81	000
96922	Laser tx, skin > 500 sq cm	2.10	5.63	000
Office visit codes:				
99201	Office/outpatient visit, new	0.45	0.97	XXX
99202	Office/outpatient visit, new	0.88	1.72	XXX
99203	Office/outpatient visit, new	1.34	2.56	XXX
99204	Office/outpatient visit, new	2.00	3.62	XXX
99205	Office/outpatient visit, new	2.67	4.60	XXX
99211	Office/outpatient visit, est	0.17	0.57	XXX
99212	Office/outpatient visit, est	0.45	1.02	XXX
99213	Office/outpatient visit, est	0.67	1.39	XXX
99214	Office/outpatient visit, est	1.10	2.18	XXX
99215	Office/outpatient visit, est	1.77	3.17	XXX
99241	Office consultation	0.64	1.33	XXX
99242	Office consultation	1.29	2.43	XXX
99243	Office consultation	1.72	3.24	XXX
99244	Office consultation	2.58	4.57	XXX
99245	Office consultation	3.42	5.91	XXX

Key: XXX, Global concept does not apply; YYY, The global period is to be set by the carrier; ZZZ, The code is related to another service that is always included.

with a flap, and today the patient presents with herpes zoster. The provider would report an E/M service at the appropriate level based on the documentation in the medical record. Modifier -24 would be appended to the E/M code because the encounter was for a new problem within the 90-day global period for the flap previously performed.

Modifier -25: Significant, Separate Evaluation and Management Service on the Same Day of the Procedure or Other Service

Modifier -25 is used when an E/M service is provided on the same day that a minor surgical procedure is performed. Medicare defines a minor procedure as one that has a 0- to

Table 2 Global Periods for Procedures

Shave skin lesion	113 XX	0 days
Mohs surgery	17304–17310	0 days
Biopsy skin lesion	11100	0 days
Acne surgery	10040	20 days
Excision benign/ malignant lesion	11400–11146/ 11600–11646	10 days
Freeze wart/AK	17000/172 XX	10 days
Simple/layered/ complex closure	12031–131 XX	10 days
Skin flap/graft	14 XXX–15845	90 days

10-day global period. For example, a patient presents for consultation for possible basal cell carcinoma. The appropriate E/M code should be appended with Modifier -25 if the basal cell is treated after the consultation. According to the descriptor of Modifier -25 in CPT, the E/M service provided may be the result of a condition or symptom of the procedure performed during the same encounter. Thus, a separate diagnosis is not a requirement for the use of modifier -25. The E/M service must be identified in the medical record as separately identifiable and medically necessary.

Modifier - 25 should not be abused. For example, a patient presents with multiple skin cancers. If it is in the patient's best interest to remove them a few at a time over several weeks, an E/M service would be unnecessary at the subsequent surgical visits. These were planned procedures and not new diagnoses, thus there is no medical necessity to justify the need for an E/M service each time.

Modifier -51: Multiple Procedures

Modifier -51 indicates that multiple procedures were performed by the same provider during the same operative session. "This code identifies a secondary service associated with less physician work and practice expense than if it were a primary service and, therefore, is usually reimbursed less than if it were a primary service". This code is rarely applied by the provider as most carriers' software systems append it automatically. Providers must know the individual carrier's rules regarding the application of modifier -51. This modifier should not be appended to codes listed in Appendix E of the CPT code book. Appendix E is a list of codes not subject to multiple-surgery reductions. In addition, Appendix D lists "add-on codes" that are not subject to multiple-surgery reductions. Add-on codes are identified in CPT with the + symbol preceding the code.

Medicare's multiple-surgery reduction rule is applied for reimbursement as follows: 100% for the first procedure and 50% for each subsequent procedure. If six or more procedures are performed during the same encounter, a report must be submitted with the Medicare claim. Private carriers may decrease the reimbursement to 25% on the third and subsequent procedures. Providers should be aware of multiple surgery rules that deviate from Medicare's multiple-surgery rule and work with those payers to adequately reimburse for services provided. Providers should also closely monitor explanation of benefit (EOB) forms and appeal those claims that aren't paid appropriately.

Some carriers may also inappropriately append the -51 to the most valuable service, in which case you may want to start appending the -51 yourself.

Modifier -52: Reduced Services

A provider may on occasion report a procedure that is less than the normal service. The Modifier -52 would be reported

in such an instance. An example would be when the procedure performed is less than usually included in the procedure. This modifier allows reporting the basic service even though the service was reduced.

Modifier -54: Surgical Care Only

This modifier is occasionally used by dermatologic surgeons who have patients from remote locations that are sent back to the referring physician following surgery for the necessary postoperative care. The use of this modifier affects the reimbursement of the operating physician. The reimbursement is based on a percentage amount that is linked to 10-day and 90-day global period codes. Medicare has assigned percentages as follows for integumentary codes:

	10-day global period	90-day global period
Preoperative	10%	10%
Intraoperative	80%	71%
Postoperative	10%	19%

The physician should report the date care was assumed and the date the care was relinquished according to the carrier's guidelines. Conversely, the physician providing the follow-up care must append modifier -55 to be reimbursed for the service provided.

Modifier -55: Postoperative Management Only

This modifier is used by the provider who did not perform the surgery but provides the necessary follow-up care.

The provider should report the date that care of the patient was assumed according to the carrier's guidelines. The provider reports the appropriate follow-up care codes with Modifier -55 and will be reimbursed the percentages of the total surgical procedure noted above instead of just an E/M visit.

Modifier -57: Decision for Surgery

Modifier -57 is a very useful code as it allows billing for the preoperative E/M or consultation on the same day as a major surgery. A major surgery is defined by Medicare as a surgical procedure with a 90-day global period. It is unreasonable to expect a patient to undergo a procedure without first discussing it with the treating physician. Therefore, reporting an appropriate level of service is justified.

An example of the use of Modifier -57 is when a new or established patient is evaluated for surgery on the same day as surgery. The provider discusses treatment options, alternatives, risks/benefits, and then the decision is made to do a procedure with a 90-day global period. In this instance, the appropriate level of a consultation or E/M visit is appended with Modifier -57. In the case of the patient being seen for Mohs (zero-day global period) or a minor procedure (10-day global period), the appropriate consultation or E/M service would be appended with Modifier -25 and if the defect was repaired with a graft or flap then an additional -57 would be appended.

Modifier -58: Staged/Related Procedure or Service by the Same Physician During the Postoperative Period

This modifier indicates that the procedure was either planned in stages, more extensive than the original procedure, or for therapy following a diagnostic surgical procedure.

For example, an excision of melanoma in-situ reveals positive margins. If the re-excision with wider margins is done during the 10-day global period, Modifier -58 must be appended to the excision code. Should the re-excision be performed after the 10-day global period, Modifier 58 is unnecessary, unless there is applicable global period for a previous procedure.

Another example of modifier -58 is when a partial closure is performed, with the plan for a delayed graft. Modifier -58 would be appended to the graft code at the time of the delayed procedure.

The modifier -58 should not adversely affect reimbursement; however, the lack of modifier -58 when necessary most likely will cause the claim to be denied.

Modifier -59: Distinct Procedural Service

Modifier -59 is perhaps the single most important surgical modifier for dermatologists. This modifier is used to indicate that the treatment of a specific procedure or service was independent of another procedure or service performed on the same day. The -59 modifier should be appended to the appropriate code according to the correct coding initiative (CCI) edits. The CCI edits may be downloaded from the CMS web site. Examples of the use of -59 Modifier are given in Table 3.

Modifier -79: Unrelated Procedure or Service in the Postoperative Period

"The physician may need to indicate that another procedure was performed during the postoperative period of the initial procedure". For example, a physician excised a basal cell carcinoma and repaired the wound with a graft, which has a 90-day global period. At the two-month follow-up visit, a new tumor is recognized. The biopsy and any subsequent treatment must be appended with a -79 to indicate to Medicare (and other carriers) that this service is unrelated to the previous procedure with the 90ay global period. It is important to append this modifier first when multiple modifiers are necessary during a global period. For example, if you are providing two new surgical services within a global procedure period from an <?show earlier procedure, you must append the -79 first then the -59, as appropriate. Global periods include routine follow-up care for the procedure performed.

Modifier -76: Repeat Procedure by Same Physician

Modifier -76 is used to report a procedure that was repeated subsequent to the original procedure. The modifier may also be used to report a second procedure after the first has failed. For example, if an initial flap fails and a second flap procedure is necessary to repair the defect, the second flap procedure would be appended with modifier -76. The proper ICD-9-CM code to use in this instance would be 996.52 or if within the 90-day global period the original diagnosis (skin malignancy) can be used.

Modifier -78: Return to Operating Room During the Postoperative Period

Modifier -78 is used only for procedures done in the operating room or ambulatory surgery center. This modifier is not appropriate to report for procedures performed in the physician's office.

Modifier -99: Multiple Modifiers

The CPT descriptor for Modifier -99 indicates this code should be used when two or more modifiers are necessary to describe the circumstances of a particular service. The

Table 3 Examples of Use of Modifier -59

An actinic keratosis on the face is destroyed and a separate suspicious growth on the face is biopsied during the same visit. Append -59 to the biopsy code so that the insurer does not assume the biopsy and destruction were on the same lesion. 17000, 11100 -59

A cyst on the back and a second cyst on the face are excised. In this case, a -59 is not necessary because the CPT codes for these two excisions, 11401 (back) and 11441 (face), differentiate the two procedures. However, if both cysts excised were within the same anatomical grouping, as noted in CPT, and the same size, modifier -59 would need to be appended to one of the excision codes to inform the payer that two distinct procedures were performed. *Note:* If the location modifiers can be used to describe the different locations, such modifiers should be used in lieu of Modifier -59. 11401, 11441

A basal cell carcinoma on the nose is excised and repaired with a flap, and a basal cell carcinoma on the leg is excised and closed with an intermediate layered closure. Append the -59 to the leg excision or it may be denied. The excision of the lesion on the face is not reported because lesion excision is included in the descriptor for the flap repair. Grafts and complex closures do not include the excision of the lesions, thus Modifier -59 would be appended as appropriate. 14060, 11601 -59, 12031

A basal cell carcinoma on the face is excised and closed with a layered closure and a basal cell carcinoma on the back is destroyed with electrodessication and curettage. Append the -59 to the destruction, to inform the carrier that the two tumors are separate sites. 1164x, 1726x -59

A keloid on the neck is injected and a shave removal of a lesion on the leg is performed. Append the -59 to the injection code. Injections reported with other procedures on the same day require Modifier -59 to notify the carrier that the injection was for another purpose other than the injection of local anesthesia for the surgical procedure performed.

Use Modifier -59 appropriately according to the correct coding initiative edits for all Medicare claims. Examples of fraud would be to report the excision and destruction of the same lesion or a biopsy and excision or destruction for the same lesion during the same encounter. Another example of fraud would be to report the injection code for the administration of local anesthesia. Do note that other insurance carriers may use modifier -59 differently than Medicare. Be knowledgeable of all payers' rules regarding modifiers.

Modifier -99 is appended to the service and the applicable modifiers would be either in the description area of the CMS-1500 claim form or in Box 19. Medicare carriers may vary on their guidelines regarding the use of the Modifier -99. Therefore, refer to the individual carrier's guidelines for directions for completing the claim form accurately.

Modifiers are essential for proper reimbursement. Modifiers indicate the specific circumstances to the payer for proper claim adjudication. The correct use of modifiers should not result in charges of fraud/abuse. Remember, payers may have rules for modifiers that differ from Medicare. Be astute and monitor EOBs for proper and accurate reimbursements.

It is important to note that some private carriers may not acknowledge certain modifiers such as -25 and -57; thus, the consultation or E/M service is bundled into the procedure. On appeal, these claims are usually paid. Or, carriers may acknowledge use of modifiers differently than Medicare. Knowing what each carrier requires will enable providers to submit accurate or "clean" claims.

CODING FOR MOHS MICROGRAPHIC SURGERY

Mohs surgery requires a single physician to act as both surgeon and pathologist. These codes are not appropriate if either responsibility is delegated to another physician. Even if the histologic examination includes enface or horizontal techniques and a map is made, it is not Mohs surgery unless the physician performs the surgery as well as the pathology. In those cases when the pathology services are performed by the pathologist in lieu of the surgeon, the surgeon reports only the appropriate excision code and repair codes if applicable.

Due to the recent five-year review of the Medicare Physician fee schedule, there have been some changes to the Mohs surgery codes. The new codes have been changed to reflect the specific site on which Mohs surgery is being performed, and to differentiate between tumors located on the head, neck, hands, feet, genitalia or any location directly involving muscle, cartilage, bone, tendon, major nerves or vessels (codes 17311–17312) from surgery performed on the trunk, arms, and legs (codes 17313–17314). Additionally, CPT 17310 was replaced by 17315.

17311 and 17313: These codes are used for the first layer of Mohs micrographic surgery and include the preservice, intraservice, and postservice work. Again, CPT 17311 corresponds to tumors removed from the head, neck, hands, feet, genitalia, or any location directly involving muscle, cartilage, bone, tendon, major nerves, or vessels; CPT 17313 corresponds to tumors located on the trunk, arms, and legs.

The preservice work includes explanation of the procedure, obtaining informed consent, and preparation of the patient for surgery. The intraservice work in the Mohs micrographic technique involves removal of all gross tumor, surgical excision of tissue specimens, mapping, color coding of specimens, microscopic examination of specimens by the surgeon, and complete histopathologic preparation including the first routine stain (e.g., hematoxylin and eosin, toludine blue).

The tissue technique can be fixed or fresh and up to five specimens per stage. Specimens are cut into tissue blocks, and the number of slides made per block does not affect the code selection. The postservice work includes the discussion of postsurgery wound management

17312 and 17314: These codes correspond to each additional stage after the first stage for their tumor locations. The CPT 17312 corresponds to tumors located on the head, neck, hands, feet, genitalia, any location directly involving muscle, cartilage, bone, tendon, major nerves, or vessels; CPT 17314 corresponds to tumors located on the trunk, arms, and legs, Both of these codes include up to five tissue specimens and represent only the additional surgical work of re-excising positive margins plus the additional pathology work of processing and interpretation of specimens. The RVUs for codes 17312 and 17314 reflect the reduced work done compared to 17311 and 17313.

If additional stains are necessary in any of the stages beyond the first routine stain, then the physician must code each additional stain separately: special stain on frozen section, 88314; immunohistochemistry stain, 88342, or decalcification, 88311. Note that for certain tumors (morpheaform, infiltrative) toludine blue is a special stain when used in addition to the routine hematoxylin and eosin. Other examples include oil red O for sebaceous carcinomas, and various immunostains for melanoma and sarcomas.

17315: This code is used if six or more specimens are required to examine the entire margin in any stage. Code 17305 would be used in addition to the other Mohs codes. Code 17315 is reported for each additional block over five for any layer. (Again, this does not represent the number of tissue slices on the slides or total number of slides prepared.) This code is most commonly used for large tumors

requiring greater than five blocks. This code is used nationally on less than 10% of all tumors treated by Mohs. 17315 is an add-on code that is only reported in conjunction with codes 17311–17314.

Example: A new patient is evaluated and Mohs surgery is performed on two large basal cell carcinomas, the first on the lower left leg and the second on the nasal tip. The first basal cell requires six stages; in addition the first stage requires eight blocks to cover the entire margin. The second basal cell on the nasal tip requires four stages with six blocks on the first stage. After billing the appropriate E/M visit, the Mohs coding for Medicare would be:

> Lower left leg: l7313, 17314 × 5
> Nasal tip: 17311, 17315 × 3
> 17305 × 4: corresponding to 3 blocks on the leg and 1 block on the nasal tip.

Additional Notes on Mohs Surgery: Since the majority of the work for Mohs surgery is intraservice work, little overlap exists in work associated with treating two tumors on the same day. However, some carriers have medical policies regarding multiple procedures during the same encounter. Knowing the specific carrier policy regarding reimbursement of multiple procedures is vital.

If Mohs surgery is performed on one day but carried over to a second day, the first layer on the next day should continue with the next code in the series. It would not be appropriate to start over with 17311 or 17313 on that second day since the initial 17311 or 17313 code includes much work not repeated in subsequent stages such as debulking of the tumor.

The Mohs codes have 0 global days. However, repairs performed after Mohs surgery will have specific global days.

BIOPSIES BEFORE MOHS

A skin biopsy and frozen section may be done to confirm the diagnosis prior to the decision to initiate Mohs surgery. Situations when this should be used include; if a definitive diagnosis is not available, a biopsy report is not available with reasonable effort, the existing pathology report is over 90 days old, or the original biopsy is ambiguous. Another situation when a biopsy and frozen section is useful arises when the original biopsy site is confused. All of this should be documented in the chart. Otherwise, it is not appropriate to report biopsy or frozen section codes to routinely review the histopathologic features of the tumor being treated.

Example of coding a skin biopsy during the same encounter as Mohs surgery: 11100 -59, 88331 -59.

Note: -59 must be appended to both the biopsy and pathology codes to indicate these services are separate procedures and are not a part of the Mohs surgery. 11100 -Biopsy skin, subcutaneous tissue, mucous membrane (including simple closure), single lesion. Use the ICD-9 code describing neoplasm of unknown behavior (238.X). 88331—pathology, frozen section of a single specimen (note a written frozen section pathology report must be generated and in the patient's medical record). Use the appropriate skin cancer diagnosis code (173.X). Note that if the biopsy and frozen section was benign this may also be reported with the appropriate ICD-9 codes (benign skin 216.X).

CODING FOR BENIGN AND MALIGNANT EXCISIONS: 11400–11446, 16000–11646

Excision codes are based on site and excised diameter size. Excision codes are determined by measuring the greatest clinical diameter of the apparent lesion plus the most narrow margin that is required for complete excision. The CPT codes were redefined in 2003 to include the margins of excision. The margins should be added to the total tumor size to determine the excised diameter. The process demonstrating how to measure the excised diameter size is shown in Figure 1.

CODING FOR RECONSTRUCTION

- No repair (second intent)
- Layered closure (simple, intermediate, and complex)
- Adjacent tissue transfer or rearrangement
- Flaps and grafts (split, full, and composite)
- Special sites (lip and lid)
- Combined repairs
- Staged repairs

Simple repair codes (12001–12021) are used for superficial wounds that require simple, one-layered closure/suturing. Reimbursement for anesthesia and cauterization are included in these codes. Simple repairs are coded by site and length (sum of lengths). When more than one simple suture repair is performed in the same anatomical grouping as listed in CPT, only one code is reported based on the sum of the length of the repairs. *Note*: Simple repairs are included in the descriptors for benign and malignant excisions and are not billed separately.

Intermediate repair codes (12031–12057) are used for repair of wounds or defects, which require a layered closure, have deeper layers [subcutaneous tissue and superficial (nonmuscle fascia)], need prolonged support to control tension, or need the obliteration of "dead" space. Again, these repairs are coded by site and length (sum of lengths). It should be noted that single-layer closure for heavily contaminated wounds that require extensive cleaning would also constitute an intermediate repair. However, such circumstances would be unlikely in dermatology.

Complex repair codes (13100–13160) are used for repair of wounds or defects, which require more than a layered closure. For example, wounds that need extensive undermining, stents, retention sutures, or need repair of complicated lacerations or avulsions are considered complex. Again these

Table 4   Complex Closure Codes and Add-Ons

Each additional 5 cm code		Primary code
+13102	Used with	13101 (trunk)
+13122	Used with	13121 (scalp, arms, legs)
+13133	Used with	13132 (forehead, cheeks, chin, mouth, neck, axillae, genitalia, hands, feet)
+13153	Used with	13152 (eyelids, nose, ears, lips)

repairs are coded by site and length (sum of lengths). It is also important to note that there are add-on codes designated by site for complex repairs beyond the first 7.5 cm in length. Each additional 1–5 cm is reported when appropriate. Examples of complex repair codes and their corresponding add-on codes are given in Table 4.

ADJACENT TISSUE TRANSFER OR REARRANGEMENT

Unlike intermediate and complex closure coding, the coding for repair by adjacent tissue transfer or rearrangement also includes the excision (including lesion), if done; the excision is not reported separately. The flap is coded by site and size (square centimeters) including the primary defect of the lesion or excision and secondary defect resulting from the flap design, which is measured by multiplying the longest axis of repair by the widest perpendicular axis. Examples of flap and defect measurements are given in Figures 2 and 3.

Note:

1. If a skin graft is necessary to close the secondary defect, then an additional graft code is billed and is considered an additional procedure to codes 14000–14350.
2. Exceptions exist: The pedicle flap (15740), direct or tubed pedicle (15570–15576), delay of flap and sectioning of flap (15600–15630), and myocutaneous flap (15732–15738) are all based on site and not size.
3. If a physician does a repair of a donor site with a graft or flap, the graft or flap is considered an additional procedure.
4. If a physician does a staged revision, defatting, or rearranging, he/she should bill according to the appropriate reconstructive procedure.

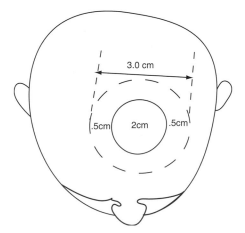

Figure 1   Example of total defect measurement. 2 cm (lesion size) + [(0.5 + 0.5) equals margin] = 3.0 cm total defect size. Remember, the coding for repair by adjacent tissue transfer or rearrangement includes reimbursement for the excision of the original lesion. Thus, only the appropriate adjacent tissue transfer or rearrangement code would be reported.

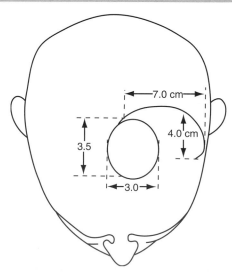

Figure 2   The measurement of a bilobed flap. Primary defect 2.0 × 2.0 = 4.0, secondary defect 4.0 × 4.5 = 18.0, total defect = 22 cm².

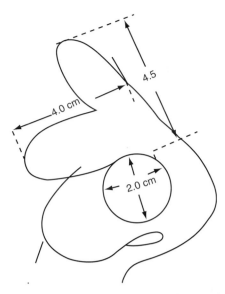

Figure 3 Measurement of a rotation flap. Primary defect 3.5 × 3.0 = 10.5, secondary defect 7.0 × 4.0 = 28.0, total defect = 10.5 + 28.0 = 38.5 cm².

FREE SKIN GRAFTS

Grafts should be coded by identifying the size and location of the defect and the type of graft (full, split, allograft, xenograft, and skin substitute). For full thickness grafts, the code includes the direct closure of the donor site, but if the repair of the donor site requires a graft or local flap, then it is considered an additional procedure. In the case of skin grafts, like for the coding of intermediate and complex repairs, the excision is coded separately. Examples of skin graft codes are given in Table 5.

Notes: When a combination of layered closures, flaps, and/or grafts are necessary, remember to append Modifier -59 to identify separate procedures.

1. Each noted graft described in Table 5 with the exception of the pinch graft has a corresponding add-on code that is not subject to the multiple-procedure reduction rule.
2. Each lower valued procedure is subject to the multiple-procedure reduction rule, -51. The first, and most valuable procedure is not subject to multiple surgery reduction and should be paid at 100%.

LIP RECONSTRUCTION

When reconstruction of the lip is done, the physician has multiple codes to choose from to report the procedure. For example, if a physician removed a basal cell carcinoma on the upper lip and repaired it with a full thickness closure involving over one-half of the vertical height of the lip, the

Table 5 Examples of Free Skin Grafts

15050-pinch grafts (single or multiple)
(15100–15120) split-thickness grafts. Add-on codes- (15101–15121)
(15200–15260) full-thickness grafts. Add-on codes- (15201–15261)
15342- skin substitute/neodermis. Add-on code- 15343
15350- allografts. Add-on code- 15351
15400- xenografts. Add-on code- 15401

Source: From American Medical Association (2005).

Table 6 Codes for Lip Reconstruction

40500-Vermilionectomy (lip shave), with mucosal advancement
40510-Excision of lip; transverse wedge excision with primary closure
40520-V-excision with primary direct linear closure
40650-Repair lip (cheiloplasty), full-thickness; vermilion only
40652-Up to one-half vertical height
40654-Over one-half vertical height, or complex
40525-Excision, full-thickness, reconstruction with local flap (e.g., Estlander or fan)
40527-Excision, full thickness, reconstruction with cross lip flap (Abbe-Estlander)
40812–40816-Excision of lesion of mucosa and submucosa, vestibule of mouth, with simple or complex repair

Source: From American Medical Association (2005).

physician could bill a complex closure (13152, in addition to the appropriate excision code) or a cheiloplasty over one-half vertical height, (40654). Generally the cheiloplasty codes pay slightly more. Remember, the documentation in the medical record must support the codes reported on the claim form. That is, the operative note should say cheiloplasty, not complex closure. Examples of codes for lip reconstruction are given in Table 6.

EYELID RECONSTRUCTION

The same issues involving the lip also apply to the repair and reconstruction of the eyelid. Codes involving reconstruction are given in Table 7.

STAGED REPAIRS AND SCAR REVISION

There are some issues concerning staged repairs and scar revisions, which must be recognized in order to be properly reimbursed for the work performed. For example, if a physician reports the revision as a scar (790.2), with history of skin cancer (V10.83), the work performed may be denied and require an appeal. However, reporting the original tumor diagnosis after the tumor has been treated is not appropriate as per the ICD-9-CM guidelines unless the revision occurs in the 90-day global period. Remember the -58 Modifier is used to indicate a procedure performed during a global period was planned prospectively, more extensive than the original procedure, because the original procedure failed, or for therapeutic effort after the diagnostic procedure. It is very important to know the Carrier's policy regarding such services.

THE REPAIR: COSMETIC VS. RECONSTRUCTIVE?

A repair is reconstructive when the repair is performed to correct the damage resulting from cancer removal, is to "improve function," or to approximate a normal appearance. Medicare's definition says that reconstructive surgery is reimbursable

Table 7 Codes Involving the Eyelid

67930-Suture of recent wound, eyelid, involving lid margin, tarsus and/or palpebral conjunctiva direct closure; partial thickness
67935-Full thickness
67961-Excision and repair of eyelid, involving lid margin, tarsus, conjunctiva, canthus or full thickness, may include preparation for graft or flap; up to one-fourth of lid margin
67966-Over one-fourth of lid margin

Source: From American Medical Association (2005).

when performed on abnormal structures of the body caused by tumors, infections, or disease, and will allow reimbursement to improve function of a malformed body part.

Examples:

1. Delay of flap or section of flap –CPT 15600 (trunk), 15610 (scalp, arms, and legs), 15630 (eyelids, nose, ears, and lips). Example, a physician cuts a flap on the ear of a heavy smoker, but does not transpose it, he bills 15630. The patient returns in three weeks when the flap has matured, and the flap recut and transposed into the defect. The physician bills 14060 with -58 (staged procedure).
2. A flap fails. The physician waits four weeks for demarcation and repeats flap or graft and then reports the new procedure code with modifier -76 (repeat procedure). The proper diagnosis code in this instance is 996.52, which is used for skin graft failure, rejection, or the original skin cancer diagnosis code if with-in the original 90-day period.

BIBLIOGRAPHY

American Medical Association. CPT Assistant. Chicago, Illinois: AMA, 1997:4.

American Medical Association. CPT Assistant. Chicago, Illinois: AMA, 1997.

American Medical Association. CPT Assistant (Winter issue). Chicago, Illinois: AMA, 1992:20.

American Medical Association. CPT Assistant. Chicago, Illinois: AMA, 2003:17.

American Medical Association. CPT Assistant. Chicago, Illinois: AMA, Vol. 14. 2004:7:3.

American Medical Association. CPT Assistant. Chicago, Illinois: AMA, 1997:10.

American Medical Association. CPT Assistant. Chicago, Illinois: AMA, 2003:17.

American Medical Association. CPT (Professional Edition, Appendix A). Chicago, Illinois: AMA, 2005:402.

American Medical Association. CPT Assistant (Fall Edition). Chicago, Illinois: AMA, 1993:7.

American Medical Association. CPT Assistant. Chicago, Illinois: AMA, 2002:5.

American Medical Association. CPT Assistant. Chicago, Illinois: AMA, Vol. 14. 2004:7:3.

American Medical Association. CPT Assistant. Chicago, Illinois: AMA, Vol. 14. 2004:7:2–3.

American Medical Association. CPT Assistant. Chicago, Illinois: AMA, Vol. 14. 2004:7:4.

American Medical Association. CPT Assistant. Chicago, Illinois: AMA, Vol. 14. 2004:7:5.

American Medical Association. CPT (Professional Edition, Appendix A). Chicago, Illinois: AMA, 2005:51–53.

American Medical Association. Medicare RBRVS: The Physicians' Guide. Chicago, Illinois: AMA, 2004:78–80.

American Medical Association. CPT (Professional Edition). Chicago, Illinois: AMA, 2005:54–56.

American Medical Association. CPT (Professional Edition). Chicago, Illinois: AMA, 2005:57.

American Medical Association. CPT Assistant. Chicago, Illinois: AMA, 1999:3.

American Medical Association. CPT Assistant. Chicago, Illinois: AMA, 1999:10.

American Medical Association. CPT (Professional Edition). Chicago, Illinois: AMA, 2005:59.

American Medical Association. CPT (Professional Edition). Chicago, Illinois: AMA, 2005:167.

American Medical Association. CPT (Professional Edition). Chicago, Illinois: AMA, 2005:265.

American Medical Association. CPT (Professional Edition). Chicago, Illinois: AMA, 2005:265.

www.cms.hhs.gov.

14

Skin Biopsy

Bryan C. Schultz

Loyola University Stritch School of Medicine, Maywood, Illinois, U.S.A.

Thomas A. Victor

*Department of Pathology and Laboratory Medicine, Evanston Northwestern Healthcare,
Evanston, Illinois, U.S.A.*

INTRODUCTION

Skin biopsy is a routine diagnostic tool used to evaluate the skin. Ease in sampling of skin has resulted in a large body of information correlating clinical with histopathologic data over more than a century. No other organ in the human body is so easily biopsied for diagnostic purposes. Advances in immunology, molecular biology, electron microscopy, and culturing techniques have contributed greatly to the breadth and depth of knowledge obtained through skin biopsy. Techniques using immunohistochemistry, gene rearrangement, polymerase chain reaction (PCR), human papillomavirus (HPV) typing, DNA flow cytometry, etc., are creating greater demand for skin biopsy to aid in the diagnosis of both cutaneous and systemic disease. Newer techniques that evaluate functional rather than structural microscopic changes will usually require tissue samples obtained via skin biopsy. The quantitative examination of molecular changes after laser surgery and the use of DNA microarrays (gene chips) in functional genomic studies of melanoma are recent examples of these emerging techniques.

The most common circumstances for biopsying the skin are (i) to rule out malignancy, (ii) to evaluate diagnostically a benign tumor, and (iii) to evaluate a dermatosis for histopathologic correlation with clinical data. It is extremely important that the physician consider all possible causes of the condition before performing a skin biopsy. If a nonspecialist who does not have an accurate differential diagnosis is doing the procedure, the dermatopathologist's ability to make the diagnosis may be compromised. It is important that someone with a background in clinical skin disease and its pathologic correlations interpret the biopsy as it relates to the disease.

Surgical principles discussed elsewhere would apply to skin biopsy procedures. General procedures used for skin biopsy will be discussed, as well as considerations that must be taken into account with different diagnoses. Special concerns and preferable techniques in certain body locations are addressed.

GENERAL PROCEDURES AND TECHNIQUE
Skin Preparation

Prepare the skin with 70% isopropyl alcohol or similar agent, including the area to be biopsied and approximately 5 cm surrounding. It is best to let the alcohol dry for a brief period after application. With this skin prep, less than one in 5000 infections occur and infections have never been severe or clinically threatening in the author's experience. In fact, infection or significant pain after biopsy should be considered an unusual event. More complex procedures have been associated with infection rates of approximately 1% to 2.5%. No skin prep can ever prevent infection entirely. Isopropyl alcohol does not discolor or distort clinical borders of the lesions. Povidone-iodine preparations are a favorite of many surgeons but may distort the clinical border of faintly colored or erythematous lesions. Some povidone-iodine solutions have had bacterial contaminants cultured from them. Chlorhexidine compounds are also an acceptable way of cleansing skin. Caution must be used with these agents; they should not be used near the eye or ear canal because of reported problems with corneal clouding and ototoxicity. Both isopropyl alcohol and some chlorhexidine compounds are flammable. The skin should be thoroughly dried before any cautery is used. A rare patient may be allergic to one agent, but would usually tolerate one of the others.

For most small procedures such as skin biopsies a drape is unnecessary. Drapes such as Steridrape® with an adhesive backing and central circular fenestration can be useful. Allergies to this adhesive backing are rare. The adhesive backing also ensures that any blood from the biopsy site will not run under the drape.

Anesthesia

For the vast majority of cases, either 0.5% or 1.0% plain lidocaine may be used. Epinephrine can be used in dilutions of 1:100,000, 1:200,000, or 1:500,000 for hemostasis. A 1:400,000 concentration has been shown to give maximum vasoconstrictive effect, while minimizing the total amount of epinephrine used. Because most biopsies are performed in just a few minutes, it may not be necessary to use epinephrine for prolonged anesthesia. Side effects such as tachycardia and tachyarrhythmia may occur with epinephrine and should be avoided in patients with significant hypertension or vasoconstrictive cardiovascular disease. Severe bradycardia and hypertensive crises have resulted when using this agent in patients receiving a beta-blocker such as propranolol. Although dogma has dictated avoidance of epinephrine in digital anesthesia, a recent literature review disputes this and supports its use with proper technique and careful patient selection. Suspect mastocytosis would be another reason to avoid epinephrine. Low-dose lidocaine with or without epinephrine is considered safe for most biopsies needed during pregnancy.

A 30-gauge needle is used for injecting the anesthetic. Larger gauge needles cause significantly more pain during the injection. A 30-gauge needle with silicone coating will puncture skin smoothly and painlessly. A dental Cook-Waite type syringe with disposable carpules may be used. It is best to obtain the type that allows for aspiration. Carpules are easy to use and preferred by many dentists and some physicians.

Allergy to most local anesthetics is uncommon. Frequently, reactions are due to epinephrine used in the anesthetic. True allergic reactions are usually to the ester group of local anesthetics. The amide group, which includes lidocaine, rarely sensitizes an individual. When sensitization does occur it may be due to the preservative in a multiple-dose vial. In that circumstance, the physician may use a single-dose vial without a preservative, such as the dental carpules mentioned above. Another method of anesthetizing such allergic patients is to use liquid nitrogen or carbon dioxide to freeze the area and then quickly perform the biopsy. Others have used saline infiltration for short anesthesia during biopsy. The benzyl alcohol preservative is the purported anesthetic agent here.

Eutectic mixture of local anesthetics (EMLA) cream, a combination of lidocaine and prilocaine, is quite helpful as an alternative to injection either alone (with occlusion for about 60 minutes) or to minimize the pain of subsequent local anesthetic injection. Over-the-Counter Agents (OTC) agents with plain lidocaine (e.g., LMX-4®) are available now as well. Iontophoresis of lidocaine with or without epinephrine also may be used safely and effectively to avoid injection.

Instrumentation

The standard instrument for skin biopsy is the dermal punch (Keyes' punch). High-quality sterilizable punches in sizes from 1 to 10 mm are available. The convenience, safety and quality of many disposable punches make them appealing for small routine skin biopsies. The most important aspect is the sharpness of the punch. The operator should be able to penetrate the skin with one or two rotations of its axis. A good punch should penetrate the skin like a knife cutting butter. Adequate sharpness not only enables the operator to remove the tissue specimen easily but also

minimizes trauma to the specimen and surrounding tissue. When obtaining subcutaneous tissue, a sharp punch is less likely to cause separation of the dermis from the subcutaneous tissue. Many disposable punches now provide superior cutting quality. They are not only equal to, but in many cases superior to, permanent punches.

PUNCH BIOPSY

Certainly the most common method of performing skin biopsies is the punch biopsy. The Keyes' punch is reminiscent of wood punches used by the carpenter. The instrument is ideal since many skin lesions grow in a radial fashion, resulting in a relatively circular configuration. Any lesion with such a configuration may be considered for punch biopsy. It is also an excellent instrument to obtain tissue for diagnosis of inflammatory processes.

If the punch biopsy is done for small lesions, it also may serve to excise. If the punch is used for total excision, accurate measurement of lesion diameter is important. If the lesion is slightly oval or irregular, the skin man be stretched at the time of biopsy to accommodate the smallest punch. Punches as small as 1 mm are available for dilated pores, while large sizes such as 9 and 10 mm are available for circular excision in nonfacial areas. When choosing a punch, the location of the lesion, and the relative elasticity of the skin in that area will affect the size of circular excision that can be made to allow primary closure without dog ears. As a rule, do not use a punch greater than 5 to 6 mm on the face or 8 to 10 mm on the body. There are exceptions, and trimming of minute dog-ears or conversion to a fusiform shape may be necessary for larger lesions.

It is helpful to outline the area to be biopsied prior to starting. Injection of local anesthetics, especially when epinephrine is used, will blanche the surrounding skin and may make lesional borders less perceptible. This is especially important for lesions that do not have a sharp border or for faintly erythematous dermatoses that may blanche entirely upon injection.

The local anesthetic should be injected into the mid or deep dermis. This provides almost immediate, complete anesthesia. A subcutaneous injection may be used in addition to this, but when used alone results in either delayed or often incomplete anesthesia.

The skin is stretched, with the fingers, perpendicular to skin tension lines so that the wound forms an oval (Fig. 1). In certain areas where tension lines are unclear, such

(A) **(B)**

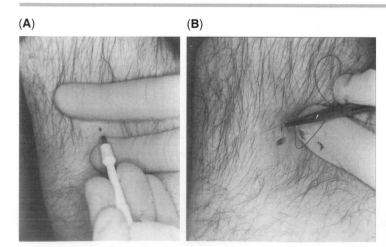

Figure 1 (A) Skin stretched perpendicular to skin tension lines before punch biopsy of small nevus. (B) Placing suture in resulting oval defect.

as the nose, it may be preferable not to stretch the skin. This may give the physician a clue to the direction of closure of that defect. This technique will improve the appearance of the scar.

While holding or stretching the adjacent skin firmly with either the forefinger and thumb or the second and third fingers, gently rotate the punch, cutting to the appropriate depth for that lesion. If sharp punches are used, little pressure is needed to cut through to the subcutaneous tissue. In almost all circumstances, penetration should be at least to the superficial subcutaneous tissue, especially when closed with sutures. If dermis is left at the bottom of the wound and sutured, it may buckle the skin and may cause a gap of the wound edges.

Removal of the biopsy tissue is done with a fine, single-toothed forceps. The tip is placed gently but firmly on dermal tissue, avoiding epidermis and subcutaneous fat. The tissue is gently lifted out until resistance is met, and iris scissors can be used to cut the tissue free at the subcutaneous level. The tissue may also be impaled with a 30-gauge needle used for anesthetic injection. The needle is lifted outward with the specimen and cut with either fine scissors or a number 11 scalpel blade. In many cases, the specimen will be removed easily without cutting, as it is gently, but firmly, pulled from its thin subcutaneous tether.

When penetrating subcutaneous tissue, knowledge of local anatomy, including blood vessel and nerve distribution, is important. Transecting nerves or vessels is an unusual but difficult problem. Examples of such structures would be the angular artery alongside the nose and the spinal accessory nerve beneath the subcutaneous fat of the posterior triangle of the neck.

Suture closure may be helpful for many punch biopsies. This has the advantage of immediately reestablishing a skin barrier to infection. Superficial curet and shave biopsies are best left open to heal by second intention. Other methods to obtain hemostasis in an open punch biopsy wound are Gelfoam, collagen matrix, and Monsel's solution. Mild styptics such as 35% aluminum chloride in 50% to 70% isopropyl alcohol may be used for more superficial procedures when only epidermis and superficial dermis have been removed. They are applied for a few seconds with light pressure and the excess is dried with a small sponge. Any styptic may delay wound healing, but this has been clinically imperceptible for small wounds in my experience.

Without a complete sterile surgical setup, the following technique may be used for sterile placement of two or three sutures (Fig. 2).

1. The wound is prepped with alcohol or povidone-iodine.
2. All instruments are taken from sterile wrappings. Touch only the handles, leaving the tips of the instruments sterile.
3. To sponge, pick up the ends of sterile gauze and use the center only to blot.
4. Suture packs are opened without touching the needles.
5. Grasp the sterile needle in the suture pack with the jaws of the needle holder.
6. The needle is gently pulled from the suture pack so that it maybe passed through skin tissue.
7. After the first pass, the needle is grasped with the sterile needle holder as it exits the skin. It is pulled through the wound until about 3 in. of suture material remain on the initial side.
8. Cut the suture material on the exit side, leaving another 3 in. The needle holder still holds a sterile needle.

9. To reposition the needle holder without touching the sterile needle or the jaws of the needle holder, the end of the remaining suture is grasped with the fingers and the needle is allowed to drop. The needle then may be repositioned on the needle holder. While holding the end of the suture material taut, pass the needle through the wound again.
10. After one to three sutures are placed, go back and tie all sutures that have been placed.

This procedure may be performed with clean, disposable examination gloves. This method enables one to place a few sutures in a sterile fashion without a total sterile field for both operator and assistant. It is not acceptable for larger excisions.

EXCISIONAL BIOPSY

The excisional biopsy may be done with either a punch for smaller lesions or a scalpel for larger lesions. For larger lesions, the excision is done with a scalpel forming elliptical or fusiform wound margins. The length of the excision traditionally is three times the width. A shorter length-to-width ratio can be closed in some areas where skin elasticity is greater.

The primary reason for excisional biopsy is to remove a lesion in toto. A common example would be biopsy of a suspected melanoma. If melanoma is suspected, complete excision of the lesion down to subcutaneous tissue is preferable. This is done to assess accurately the level of invasion and to evaluate the entire breadth of the lesion for atypicality or malignancy; however, incisional or punch biopsy has not been shown to affect adversely the outcome of melanoma. Total excision may not be necessary for most linear pigmented uniform streaks seen in melanoma excisional scars, as these are probably benign. Punch biopsy or theses streaks for assurance may be an acceptable alternative to close observation for a concerned physician and patient.

Excisional biopsy also may be considered for Spitz nevi. Some have considered subtotal excision acceptable if the diagnosis is unequivocal, while others find the term "unequivocal" difficult to use with Spitz nevi. No definitive answer can be given for this dilemma, so evaluation of the clinical and histopathological evidence must still be weighed carefully in choosing treatment.

Excisional biopsy should be considered in larger lesions where a dog-ear effect may result from a punch biopsy. A gently curved fusiform excision will result in a linear scar and superior cosmetic results. Poorly defined tumors or infiltrative dermatoses may be excised to obtain a larger specimen for more accurate pathologic examination. Lesions with deeper pathology in subcutaneous tissue, such as erythema nodosum or panniculitis, may be better biopsied using the excision technique. Deep vascular pathology or ischemic/necrotic lesions (e.g., calciphylaxis) also may be better appreciated with excisional biopsy.

SCISSORS AND SHAVE BIOPSIES

When the pathologic condition is restricted entirely to epidermis or epidermis and superficial dermis (such as a benign pedunculated nevus or fibroepithelial polyp), a scissors, scalpel, or even razor blade shave biopsy may be considered. The lesion may be grasped gently with a small forceps and pulled to cause slight tenting of the epidermis

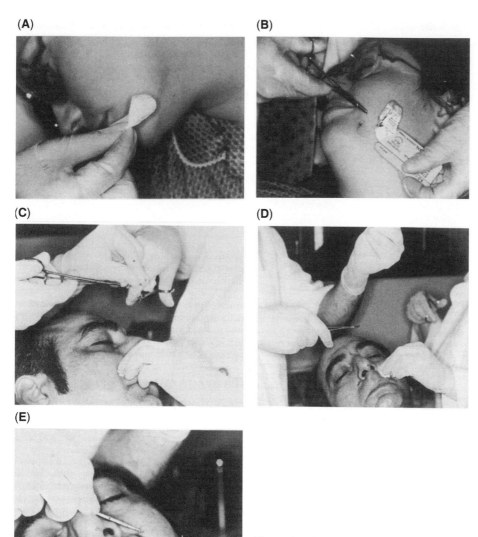

Figure 2 (A) Sponging with sterile center of sponges. (B) Needle holder grasping the needle as it emerges on the opposite side of the wound. (C) Cutting the suture while the needle holder is still grasping the needle. (D) Grasping the free-hanging needle with the sterile jaws of the needle holder while the unsterile hand holds the end of the suture. (E) Passing the needle through the skin for a second suture while holding the suture taut to prevent sagging onto surrounding undraped and unprepped skin. *Source*: From Schultz and McKinney (1985).

and upper dermis. A curved iris scissors with fine points may be used to remove the lesion (Fig. 3). It is preferable to include the superficial dermis to examine for any extension into the dermis (Fig. 4). The base maybe lightly electrodesiccated or a styptic applied. Avoid agents such as Monsel's solution that may pigment or distort histopathologic features on subsequent biopsy or excision. If the lesion is melanocytic (e.g., nevus), it is best to ask the patient to look for any return of color. In experienced hands this rarely will happen, as both clinical assessment of proper depth before and immediately after a transected biopsy/excision can be judged with a significant degree of accuracy. Any unusual pigment pattern or abnormal histopathology would necessitate a deeper and wider excisional biopsy.

CURET BIOPSY

One of the most common skin biopsy techniques is the curet biopsy. A sharp, oval curet is best for most

situations. It provides a wide, flat shearing force at the tip of the instrument. A circular curet is better for scooping out cavities or small pockets of tumor and for smaller lesions. Frequent use and autoclaving will necessitate either sharpening or purchase of new instruments on a regular basis. Disposable curets are available for one-time use.

The sharp shearing force of a curet easily removes epidermal and superficial dermal lesions. A good example is a lesion on firm skin. This provides resistance to the shearing force of the curet. Seborrheic keratoses are ideal lesions for such removal (Fig. 5).

The lesion can be removed with minimal scarring. If the skin is loose or thin, it may be more difficult to stabilize the skin and remove the lesion without tearing normal skin. Apply pressure to the surrounding tissue before curetting. An assistant may help apply pressure for larger lesions. Light electrodesiccation will facilitate curetting if

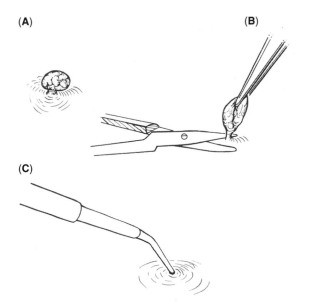

Figure 3 **(A)** Fibroepithelial polyp. **(B)** Grasped with forceps and gently pulled outward. **(C)** Light electrocautery to base. *Source*: From Schultz and McKinney (1985).

material for histologic examination already has been obtained or is not needed. The curet easily removes charred epidermal tissue separated by heat at the epidermal-dermal junction, and scarring is minimal.

Other superficial epidermal lesions that are amenable to curet biopsy include warts, cherry angiomas, and superficial epidermal cysts.

Superficial biopsies such as these leave a wound similar to a superficial abrasion. They may be treated postoperatively with topical petrolatum-based ointments (although allergy is a consideration when using topical antibiotics) or even OTC octyl-2-cyanoacrylates.

Whenever malignancy is considered, the curet should penetrate the dermis to provide an adequate specimen for the pathologist. When curet biopsy of a cutaneous horn reveals squamous cell carcinoma, reexcision must be considered.

Curet biopsy also may be used for basal cell carcinoma. Biopsy of basal cell carcinoma should not penetrate to subcutaneous fat if curettage and electrodesiccation is the planned treatment of choice (Fig. 6). If the biopsy penetrates subcutaneous tissue, it is more difficult to determine the margins of the tumor during treatment with curettage and electrodesiccation.

Basal cell carcinoma that clearly penetrates subcutaneous tissue may be best excised and submitted for pathologic confirmation of tumor-free margins. Mohs surgery may be best for such a deep tumor. A centrally placed deeper punch biopsy may increase the choice of finding invasive histopathological characteristics while avoiding distortion of the wound margin. Curettage also may be used to assess the margins of a basal cell carcinoma prior to excision, but recent evidence has shown a significantly larger wound defect when using this prior to Mohs surgery. The curet is used to debulk or remove the tumor; the area that was curettaged is then excised. This results in an excision that is less likely to leave residual tumor. A delayed excision, after the wound from curettage and electrodesiccation has healed and contracted, may be

chosen as well. This is usually done to improve the cosmetic appearance of the scar.

SKIN BIOPSY IN SPECIAL LOCATIONS
Special considerations should be mentioned when doing skin biopsy in certain locations.

Eyes
An iris scissors with a fine point and slight curve at the tip is helpful for biopsy of epidermal or dermal lesions on the eyelid. The operator can lay the scissors flat on the skin and remove tissue precisely. Gradle scissors with its tapered fine points is ideal as well. To stabilize tissue, a small chalazion clamp is extremely helpful. Protective corneal shields are helpful for some, but not mandatory for all, eyelid work.

Hemostasis may be achieved with light cautery. Topical styptics can be used with extreme caution. A bottle of eyewash should be available. Styptic is applied with a moist (not wet) cotton-tipped applicator. Bottles of chemical styptic should not pass over the patient's eyes to avoid corneal burns from spillage.

Periorbital skin is the most common location for the not uncommon hereditary condition of multiple syringomas. On more than one occasion I have seen this presence reported as a positive margin for excision of a basal cell carcinoma. A recent paper reports subclinical syringomas encountered during Mohs surgery for basal cell carcinoma.

Ears
When a biopsy is performed on the cartilaginous portion of the ear, care is taken to avoid trauma that may result in chondritis. When a large portion of cartilage is exposed, it may be necessary to punch small holes through it to allow granulation tissue to form from skin on the other side.

Forehead and Temples
Knowledge of the superficial anatomy is mandatory. Some vessels and nerves may be transected with punch biopsy. Hemostasis of a large gauge vessel is more difficult through a small punch biopsy defect than larger wounds. On the forehead, the supraorbital and supratrochlear vessels run vertically from the medial third of the eyebrow. The superficial temporal arteries should be palpated laterally before biopsy is performed.

Nose
Before performing a punch biopsy of the nose, the elasticity of the nasal tissue should be evaluated, especially the alae and nasal tip. Curettage may be more acceptable, unless a deeper specimen is needed. Punch biopsies up to 4 mm can easily be closed with 6–0 nylon in these locations with good cosmetic results. Dog-ears can be trimmed with fine scissors.

A biopsy on the rim of the nose may result in notching. The columella presents no particular problem as long as the width of the biopsy is slightly less than the columella. When using very sharp punches, one should be aware of the underlying cartilage and bone to avoid unwanted damage to the support structures. The operator can insert a gloved finger into the nasal airway to help orient the biopsy. Attention should be given to the angular artery as well.

Scalp
Be sure to angle the punch in the direction of the hair shafts and to include subcutaneous tissue to reveal follicular bulbs. The punch should be very sharp to do this properly.

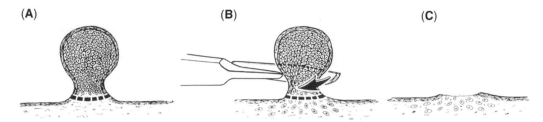

Figure 4 **(A)** Pedunculated nevus with nevus cell at or above the surrounding tissue. **(B)** Pedunculated nevus with some nevus cells penetrating lower into the dermis. **(C)** Shave biopsy may leave nevus cells behind, depending on the level of the shave and the location of the nevus cells. *Source*: From Schultz and McKinney (1985).

Subcutaneous nodules of the scalp should be treated with great respect. The possibility of malignancy and especially of deeply penetrating lesions may prompt radiographic evaluation preoperatively.

When assessing various forms of alopecia, it is helpful to request transverse sectioning of the specimen. Follicular density and diameters, as well as relative telogen counts, can be evaluated with this method of sectioning. For scarring alopecia, two biopsies may be submitted, one each for transverse and vertical sectioning. A third biopsy may be submitted for immunofluorescence processing as well.

Large punch biopsies that are not sutured or deep curet biopsies occasionally form exuberant granulation tissue when healing on the anterior scalp and upper forehead. This tissue may be debulked surgically or with light chemical or electrocautery, but it is best to suture these wounds to avoid this complication and ensure hemostasis in this highly vascularized tissue.

Fingers

Epinephrine traditionally has been considered contraindicated as a vasoconstrictor in the local anesthetic when performing biopsies of the digit. A recent study by Krunic, et al. argues that this caveat need not be absolute with proper patient selection and technique. Hemostasis may be obtained with a brief rubber band tourniquet at the base of the digit. Simple firm pressure with the operator's own finger also is adequate in many circumstances. Thorough knowledge of the anatomy, including digital nerves and vessels, is imperative especially when performing deep or excisional biopsies.

Genital Area

Use of vasoconstrictors should probably be avoided on the penis. Suture closure is preferred if the biopsy is larger than 3 to 4 mm. For smaller superficial biopsies, cautery or light styptic may be used.

Mucous Membranes

Superficial biopsies of mucous membranes heal quite rapidly when a light styptic or chemical (e.g., silver nitrate) is used for hemostasis. Light cautery is acceptable also. For large or deep punch biopsies, closure with plain catgut is preferred. Other synthetic absorbables take too long to dissolve in mucosa. Nonabsorbables such as nylon may be used but may be removed in about three days because these areas heal so rapidly. A chalazion clamp may be used for the lips and the anterior buccal mucosa; it nicely facilitates mobilization of the tissue and provides a virtually bloodless field.

Nails

See Chapter 31.

TECHNICAL CONSIDERATIONS
Proper Locations

In many circumstances, different areas may be biopsied to obtain the pathologic diagnosis. It is most helpful to have a good idea of what pathologic changes you are looking for and where they are best found. For example, in dermatitis herpetiformis, a biopsy of perilesional skin is necessary to demonstrate characteristic histopathologic changes. To identify deposits of Immunoglobulin (Ig) A by direct immunofluorescence; however, normal, intact skin is preferred. A generous portion of fat is required for the diagnosis of erythema nodosum, so biopsying a lesion not directly over the anterior tibial surface would be important. Amyloidosis may be diagnosed by biopsy of rectal mucosa and skin. Papulosquamous disorders should be biopsied in areas where disease is most characteristic and active, such as the volar surface of the lower forearm in lichen planus or thicker plaques on the buttocks for psoriasis.

Proper Depth and Width

Here again it is preferable to anticipate the diagnosis in order to perform the proper biopsy. Histologic diagnosis

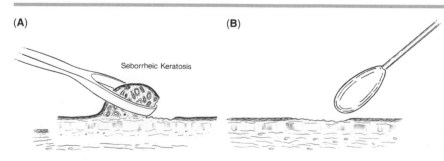

Figure 5 The curet easily removes a seborrheic keratosis with sharp shearing force. Aluminum chloride styptic is applied after removal of the keratosis. *Source*: From Schultz and McKinney (1985).

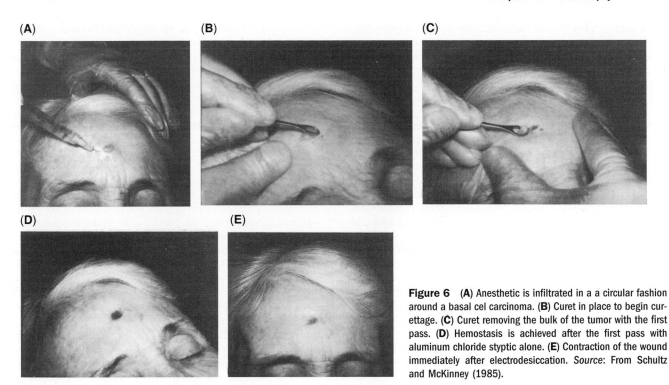

(A)   **(B)**   **(C)**

(D)   **(E)**

Figure 6 **(A)** Anesthetic is infiltrated in a a circular fashion around a basal cel carcinoma. **(B)** Curet in place to begin curettage. **(C)** Curet removing the bulk of the tumor with the first pass. **(D)** Hemostasis is achieved after the first pass with aluminum chloride styptic alone. **(E)** Contraction of the wound immediately after electrodesiccation. *Source*: From Schultz and McKinney (1985).

of lupus panniculitis or erythema nodosum requires a good portion of subcutaneous fat. If a generous amount of fat is present at the chosen location, a punch biopsy frequently will be adequate to visualize both subcutaneous fat and the epidermal-dermal portion of the skin. If there is not a good deal of fat in the area that must be biopsied, an excisional biopsy may be preferable. To assess the follicular bulb in hair disorders, the biopsy also must penetrate to subcutaneous fat. For bullous disorders, an excision or a larger punch biopsy may be preferable to include a part of the bulla and the adjacent uninvolved tissue. The diagnosis of eosinophilic fasciitis requires examination of the superficial fascia and muscle to allow one to see the characteristic pathologic changes. It cannot be overstated that proper clinical diagnosis be used as a guide to obtain a proper specimen with characteristic pathologic appearance.

Multiple Biopsies

Several skin biopsies may be necessary for three reasons. They are as follows:

1. A widespread eruption presents with lesions distinctly different in clinical appearance in different locations. For a better possibility of obtaining the correct diagnosis, several lesions are biopsied, e.g., early cutaneous T-cell lymphoma (CTCL).
2. Some conditions change or develop over time so that nonspecific pathologic changes may later reveal more specific, characteristic changes.
3. Different processing needs for different techniques (e.g., H & E, IMF, electron microscopy, transverse sectioning, etc.).

Erythema multiforme may present in varying stages of development at the same time. Several biopsies over

several months may be required before nonspecific precursor stages of CTCL demonstrate an infiltrate with Pautrier microabscesses or other characteristic features. Conditions such as parapsoriasis and poikiloderma atrophicans vasculare may not show pathologic changes consistent with CTCL for several months or years. Even in fully developed CTCL, some patches may not demonstrate all pathologic characteristics. Conversely, skin biopsy has identified mycosis fungoides in normal appearing pruritic skin, attesting to the remarkable utility of this relatively simple procedure.

One last caveat would be is to avoid using the skin biopsy in place of clinical judgment. A recent paper described three patients with the delayed diagnosis of graft versus host disease. Eosinophils in the biopsy specimen led to the erroneous diagnosis of drug eruption, further delaying appropriate treatment of the graft versus host disease.

A DERMATOPATHOLOGIST'S PERSPECTIVE ON HANDLING AND PROCESSING BIOPSY MATERIAL

An extremely important consideration is how the biopsy is handled. Crush artifact should be avoided, if at all possible. This applies to the punch biopsy where either gentle use of a fine forceps with teeth or a 25-gauge needle or smaller is employed to extricate tissue. This avoids crush artifact in which cells in the biopsy cannot be discerned upon microscopic study as inflammatory or neoplastic.

Once tissue is removed, marking the specimen for special studies such as evaluation of margins in a neoplastic disease becomes important. In larger specimens, sutures to mark apposition to in situ location for margin study are possible. In smaller specimens, this approach is futile and should not be employed as it will be inaccurate and can result in the destruction of the specimen. Use of indelible dyes is more effective and allows more precise localization; these dyes can be seen on histological examination and on gross inspection by the individual submitting the tissue for sectioning. Appropriate additional dyes and special cutting techniques can be employed to assure proper margin study or localization of a particular aspect of a lesion.

Most biopsies sent for routine processing are usually fixed in formalin and stained with hematoxylin and eosin. The best fixative is 10% formalin, usually supplied in vials by the laboratory that is histologically evaluating the specimen. The specimen should be placed immediately in formalin to avoid drying artifact and to obtain the optimal preservation of the tissue. Formalin prepared by commercial laboratories has a limited lifetime because the formaldehyde undergoes polymerization. The expiration date for prepared formalin should be printed on the commercial laboratory's specimen vial label and outdated formalin should not be used.

The amount of fixative in the biopsy container should be several times the volume of the biopsy itself. It is important, especially when it is mailed, that the specimen be completely immersed in fixative and that tight, leak-free caps are used. Usually, specimens are fixed for 24 hours before processing. They then are embedded in paraffin wax and cut with a microtome. Hematoxylin and eosin are the most commonly used stains, but special stains, including immunohistochemistry, can also be performed from these blocks.

Accurate labeling of the specimen is absolutely mandatory. Inadequate attention is often given to this step. Prelabeling or postlabeling of specimen vials both have limitations, but they are necessary to ensure accuracy. The goal should be zero labeling errors. The consequence of an error can be dire. Similar risk management should be employed by the laboratory performing the histological examination to avoid loss of specimens or mix-ups. It should be noted that there are laboratories that do DNA testing to verify the identity of a specimen if a problem should arise.

For more rapid evaluation, frozen sections may be done. The specimen is transported either in liquid nitrogen or saline-moistened gauze. The specimen is frozen and cut in a cryostat. If therapy must be initiated quickly, as in some viral disorders and bullous disease, a frozen section biopsy saline moistened may be very helpful. A second biopsy may be done for formalin-fixed, paraffin-embedded processing, because these slides are generally of better quality. Frozen sections are also helpful when checking the borders of a tumor at the time of excision or Mohs surgery.

It now is possible to get a two-hour processing turnaround time. The laboratory employs microwave technology to achieve this amazing result. Fixation occurs rapidly, avoiding 24-hour liquid routine fixation and processing. The histological detail is identical to conventional processing; there is nucleic acid and protein preservation comparable to formalin fixation. This technology will allow same-day diagnosis in the near future. With internet reporting technology, the report can be in the referring physician's office on the day of specimen biopsy and laboratory reception.

When an infectious process is suspected, culturing and staining of biopsy material may be extremely helpful. A larger biopsy may be obtained and sectioned into segments for permanent processing and for tissue smears and culture. Material for culturing usually is placed in sterile gauze moistened with nonbacteriostatic saline or water in a sterile container. The tissue is homogenized and plated in the laboratory for appropriate cultures. The section for permanent processing may be placed in formalin as usual, and the lab can do special bacterial, acid-fast or fungal stains.

Punch biopsies are done to obtain skin for direct immunofluorescent study. Specimens are transported in liquid nitrogen or dry ice, or an immune-fluorescent transport media such as that described by Michel. Immunofluorescent staining techniques are done to identify IgG, IgM, IgA fibrin, complement and certain infectious antigens such as mycobacterial or viral antigens. Immunochemistry is very useful in identifying the antigens of infectious agents as well, such as Herpes zoster, Herpes simplex, CMV, and *Treponema pallidum*. Electron microscopy most commonly is used for the study of bullous disorders, melanocytic disorders, the identification of abnormal lymphocytic cells such as in mycosis fungoides and Sézary syndrome, and in the identification of viral particles. Although it may be done on paraffin-embedded tissue, glutaraldehyde, kept cold to avoid polymerization, is a better fixative.

To achieve the most accurate histological analysis of a dermatological specimen, the requisition should be filled out accurately and completely. Patient demographics including age, sex, and even skin type in many cases are necessary. A description of the lesion or rash should be given with its duration and other historical facts of importance. Dermatopathology is no less subjective than dermatology and clinical description with a diagnostic impression is necessary. There are many occasions when the histopathology is not specific or classic, but the clinical presentation is characteristic. This information can lead to recognition of a lesion, which has an unusual histological variation. The requisition also provides a venue for giving special instructions such as a rush reading.

Immunohistochemistry

One of the most difficult diagnostic areas, often necessitating additional studies, are the pathologic conditions featuring lymphocytic infiltrates which raise a diagnostic consideration of malignant lymphoma. In this case, immunohistochemical (IHC) studies are required. Antibodies are used in this situation to identify cluster designation (CD) antigens. These stains identify T- and B-cell lymphocytes. Some patterns indicate reactive versus neoplastic cell populations. B- and T-cell gene rearrangement studies may be needed to further clarify the nature of an infiltrate. These studies can be performed on paraffin-embedded tissue using DNA amplification techniques such as PCR. These cases may require fresh tissue in some instances for both flow cytometry and for PCR analysis. In equivocal cases, careful follow-up may be the only course of action to determine the biological nature of a cutaneous lymphocytic infiltrate.

Another situation leading to ancillary IHC studies are spindle cell neoplasms of the skin. The differential diagnosis of such morphologic lesions often includes malignant melanoma, squamous cell carcinoma, leiomyosarcoma, dermatofibrosarcoma protuberans (DFSP), malignant nerve sheath tumor, or atypical fibrous xanthoma (superficial malignant fibrous histiocytoma). Markers for melanocytic differentiation such as Mart 1, HMB 45, or S 100 are frequently used to make a distinction. Cytokeratins are markers used for squamous differentiation. Markers for smooth muscle differentiation include desmin and muscle-specific actin. A positive stain for CD 34 and a negative stain for XIIIa are useful for distinguishing DFSP from a dermatofibroma (CD 34 negative and XIIIa positive).

There are numerous examples of the use of IHC stains to specifically identify primary neoplasms of the skin or neoplasms secondarily involving the skin. This diagnostic activity will only continue to expand as proteomics identifies more useful inflammatory, genetic, and neoplastic disease markers as well as gene expressions that point to effective therapeutic strategies. In general, molecular genetic explanation of skin diseases will constantly expand diagnostic tools to be usefully applied at the cellular and molecular level. These efforts will continuously expand the successful diagnosis and treatment of skin diseases.

BIBLIOGRAPHY

Amin SP, Herman AR, Busam KJ, et al. Multiple subclinical syringomatous proliferations encountered during Mohs surgery for basal cell carcinoma. Dermatol Surg 2004; 30:1420.

Baldwin HE, Berck CM, Lynfield YL. Subcutaneous nodules of the scalp: preoperative management 1991; 25:819–830.

Bolognia JL. I Biopsy techniques for pigmented lesions. Dermatol Surg 2000; 26:89.

Crabb WC. A concentration of 1:5000,000 epinephrine in a local anesthetic solution is sufficient to provide excellent hemostasis. Plast Reconstr Surg 1979; 63:834.

Davis TS, Graham WP, Miller SH. The circular excision. Ann Plast Surg 1980; 4:21.

De Jong RH. Local Anesthetics. 2nd ed. Springfield: Charles C. Thomas, 1977.

deWaard-van der Spek FB, Mulder GH, Oranje AP. Priolocaine/lidocaine patch as a local premedication for skin biopsy in children. J Am Acad Dermatol 1997; 37:418–421.

Dzubow LM, Halpem AC, Leyden JJ, et al. Comparison of preoperative skin preparations for the face. J Am Acad Dermatol 1988; 4:737–741.

Eaglstein WH, Sullivan TP, Giordano PA, Miskin BM. A liquid adhesive bandage for the treatment of minor cuts and abrasions. Derm Surg 2002; 28:1046–1052.

Foster CA, Aston SJ. Propranolol-epinephrine interaction. A potential disaster. Plast Reconstr Surg 1983; 72:74–78.

Harahap M. How to biopsy oral lesions. J Dermatol Surg Oncol 1989; 15:1077–1080.

Harvey DT, Fenske NA. The razor blade biopsy technique. Introduction of the adaptor-designed shave biopsy instrument. Dermatol Surg 1995; 21:482–484.

Ho VC, Sober AJ. Pigmented streaks in melanoma scars. J Dermatol Surg Oncol 1990; 16:663–666.

Huang CC, Boyce S, Northington M, et al. Controlled surgical trial of preoperative tumor curettage of basal cell carcinoma in Mohs micrographic surgery. J Am Acad Dermatol 2004; 51:585–591.

Hudson-Peacock MF, Bishop J, Lawrence CM. Shave excision of benign papular naevocytic naevi. Br J Plast Surg 1995; 48:318–322.

Jacob SE, James WD. Bacitracin after clean surgical procedures may be risky. J Am Acad Dermatol 2004; 51:1036.

Jacob SE, James WD. From road rash to top allergen in a flash: bacitracin. Dermatol Surg 2004; 30:521–524.

Kaye VN, Dehner LP. Spindle epithelioid cell nevus (Spitz nevus): Natural history following biopsy. Arch Dermatol 1990; 126:1582–1583.

Krunic AL, Wang LC, Soltani K, et al. Digital anesthesia with epinephrine: an old myth revisited. J Am Acad Dermatol 2004; 51:755–759.

Kuwahaxa RT, Alexiou JA. Using suture removal kit for punch biopsy. Dermatol Surg 2001; 27:219.

Lees VS, Briggs JC. Effect of initial biopsy procedure on prognosis in Stage I invasive cutaneous malignant melanoma: Review of 1086 patients. Br J Surg 1991; 78:1108–1110.

Madani S, Shapiro J. The scalp biopsy: making it more efficient. Dermatol Surg 1999; 25:537–538.

Marra DE, McKee PH, Nghiem P. Tissue eosinophils and the perils of using skin biopsy specimens to distinguish between drug hypersensitivity and cutaneous graft-versus-host disease. J Am Acad Dermatol 2004; 51:543.

Michel B, Milner Y, David K. Preservation of tissue-fixed immunoglobulins in skin biopsies of patients with lupus erythematosus and bullous diseases-preliminary report. J Invest Dermatol 1972; 5:449–552.

Miller SJ. II. Biopsy techniques for suspected nonmelanoma skin cancers. Dermatol Surg 2000; 26:91.

Olmstead PM, Lund HZ, Leonard DD. Monsel's solution: a histologic nuisance. J Am Acad Dermatol 1980; 492–498.

Orringer JS, Kang S, Johnson TM, et al. Connective tissue remodeling induced by carbon dioxide laser resurfacing of photodamaged human skin. Arch Dermatol 2004; 140:1326–1332.

Pujol RM, Gallardo F, Llistosella E, et al. Invisible mycosis fungoides: a diagnostic challenge. J Am Acad Dermatol 2002; 47:168–171.

Richards KA, Stasko T. Dermatologic surgery and the pregnant patient. Dermatol Surg 2002; 28:248–256.

Robinson JD. Fundamentals of Skin Biopsy. Chicago: Year Book Medical Publishers, 1986:21–22.

Schultz BC, McKinney P. Office Practice of Skin Surgery. Philadelphia: WB Saunders, 1985.

Sinclair R, Jolley D, Mallari R, Magee J. The reliability of horizontally sectioned scalp biopsies in the diagnosis of chronic diffuse telogen hair loss in women. J Am Acad Dermatol 2004; 51:189.

Smack DP, Harrington AC, Dunn C, et al. Infection and allergy reaction in ambulatory surgery patients using white petroleum vs. bacitracin ointment. JAMA 1996; 276:972–977.

Torres A, Seeburger J, Robison D, Glogau R. The reliability of a second biopsy for determining residual tumor. J Am Acad Dermatol 1992; 27:70–73.

Zempsky WT, Parkinson TM. Lidocaine iontophoresis for local anesthesia before shave biopsy. Dermatol Surg. 2003; 29:627.

15

Excision

Mark J. Zalla

Dermatology Associates of Northern Kentucky, Florence, Kentucky, and Department of Dermatology, University of Cincinnati, Cincinnati, Ohio, U.S.A.

R. Steven Padilla

Department of Dermatology, University of New Mexico, Albuquerque, New Mexico, U.S.A.

TECHNIQUE

Preparation

Excision planning and marking should be done with the patient in the upright position, to minimize apparent distortion of the relaxed skin tension lines, and prior to the infiltration of anesthetic, which can distort tension lines and obscure lesion margins. Prior to marking, hair in and around the operative site may be removed using a clipper or scissors, though preoperative shaving should be avoided due to increased risk of wound infection.

After cleaning the skin with 70% isopropyl alcohol, lines of excision may be drawn using a skin-marking pen, fine-tipped permanent marker, or wooden applicator dipped in gentian violet, alcian blue or other marking agent. The surgical site is then anesthetized, including a wide enough margin to allow sufficient undermining, and prepared with an appropriate antibacterial scrub (chloroxylenol, chlorhexidine, povidone-iodine, etc.). One should avoid the use of chlorhexidine around the eyes or ear canal and avoid povidone-iodine in iodine-allergic patients. Following appropriate surgical scrub, universal precautions should be employed, including use of sterile gloves, masks, and eye protection for all operative personnel. The field is then draped with sterile towels and the excision carried out under sterile conditions.

Incisions

Incisions are usually made with a number 15 blade, although some prefer a smaller blade such as the 6700 on a Beaver handle for small excisions or tight locations, and others prefer a number 10 blade for thick skin such as that on the back. The skin is kept taut by an assistant holding two-point tension at the distal end of the incision with the operator's free hand stabilizing the proximal end. The incision is begun at the distal end with the scalpel tip perpendicular to the skin surface (Fig. 1). The blade is then lowered to a 45° angle to carry out the arc of the incision. At the proximal end, the blade is again angled perpendicularly to the surface to avoid incising beyond the tip of the excision. The remaining arc is incised similarly.

The incisions should be made in single, fluid strokes from tip to tip to avoid creating nicks in the skin edge, which may increase scarring. Each stroke should ideally be carried perpendicularly through the dermis into the subcutaneous fat in a single pass to avoid the inadvertent beveling of the wound edge that occurs with multiple passes (Fig. 2). A beveled incision creates a boat-shaped defect in which the deep dermal edges are closer than the epidermal edges; such an incision will leave a gap in the epidermal edge after closure unless closed under excess tension (Fig. 3).

An exception to perpendicular incisions occurs in the scalp or eyebrows, where both arcs are incised parallel to the hair follicles, to avoid transecting follicles and subsequent alopecia along the scar (Fig. 2). On the scalp, these incisions should be carried through the subcutaneous fat and galea to reach the subgaleal plane.

Specimen Removal and Undermining

Following the incisions, the proximal tip of the specimen is gently held with forceps or a skin hook, taking care not to crush the specimen, and the scalpel or scissors is used to remove the specimen in a uniform plane within the subcutaneous tissue. One must be careful not to excise more superficially at the tips than in the center, or the remaining excess tissue may cause "pseudo dog-ears" (Fig. 4).

The level in the subcutis at which the lesion is removed varies depending on the nature of the lesion being excised and according to the anatomic location, considering skin thickness and underlying structures. Following removal, the skin is undermined around the entire defect, including the tips, at the same level as removal of the specimen. Undermining serves to minimize tension on the wound margins, facilitate wound edge eversion, and create a plate-like scar below the wound to ensure an even final contour without dog-ears. Undermining may be done in sharp or blunt fashion. Sharp undermining employs scissors or scalpel to completely cut the overlying skin free of underlying tissue; blunt undermining employs a "spreading motion" with the tips of the scissors to separate the tissue. Sharp undermining is faster and provides more complete separation but causes more bleeding and requires more careful hemostasis. Gentle blunt undermining is slower and may provide less tension relief depending on the extent of undermining but causes less disruption of nerves and blood vessels and lower risk of bleeding.

The extent of undermining necessary depends on the laxity of the surrounding skin. In areas of excess laxity, undermining may be minimal, limited to that amount necessary to facilitate placement of subcutaneous/intradermal sutures. In wounds under significant tension, undermining may extend several centimeters on either side of the defect. Undermining must be carried out beyond the ends of the

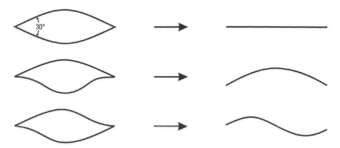

Figure 1 Typical fusiform ellipse allows linear closure (*top*) while variations allow curvilinear (*middle*) and S-plasty (*bottom*).

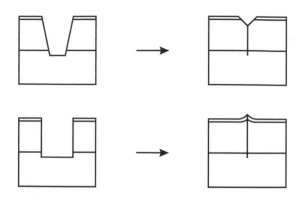

Figure 3 A beveled edge leaves an epidermal gap following closure and makes eversion difficult (*above*) compared to a perpendicular wound edge (*below*).

incision to prevent tissue protrusion after closure (Fig. 5), though the extent of undermining beyond the tips is usually less than that along the sides.

On the face, the plane of undermining is immediately beneath the subdermal plexus in the superficial subcutaneous fat. On the forehead, the plane can be in the superficial subcutaneous fat or subgaleal depending on depth of the defect. On the scalp, undermining is done in the subgaleal plane, which is easily recognized, bloodless, and avoids transection of hair follicles. On the trunk and extremities, undermining is usually done in the mid or deep subcutaneous fat superficial to muscle fascia. Undermining and suturing are best done with a skin hook rather than forceps to avoid unnecessary trauma to wound edges.

Hemostasis

Following undermining, hemostasis is obtained with electrosurgery or suture ligature as needed. Although electrodessication may provide sufficient hemostasis for small excisions, electrocoagulation is more effective and requires the use of a secondary dispersive electrode (ground plate) placed against the skin. Electrocoagulation may be performed using a monopolar probe or bipolar forceps; bipolar coagulation can also be obtained by grasping bleeding points with a forceps and touching the forceps with a monopolar probe. The operative field must be dried to allow effective electrocoagulation. To avoid unnecessary scarring, electrocoagulation should be minimized along the dermal and epidermal edge. Hemostasis of dermal capillaries is usually achieved with sutures at the time of closure. Residual capillary oozing is controlled with pressure for 5 to 10 minutes postoperatively. Although most bleeding can be adequately stopped using electrocoagulation, larger arteries are more reliably treated by suture ligature. Bleeding ends of the vessels may be clamped with a hemostat, around which a

figure-of-eight ligature with absorbable suture can be tied and then the hemostat released (Chapter 8).

Wound Closure

In view of the tension generated by stretching adjacent skin across a defect following excision, prolonged wound support is necessary to minimize risk of dehiscence or scar spreading. Therefore, most excisional wounds are best closed in layered fashion with a buried layer of absorbable subcutaneous/intradermal sutures and a percutaneous layer of suture, tissue adhesive, or adhesive tapes. The subcutaneous/intradermal sutures provide support following removal of percutaneous sutures, when the wound has only 5% of its final tensile strength. The choice of buried suture depends on several factors, including the degree of tension anticipated, the thickness of the dermis, and the length of desired support. For facial wounds and those under little tension, the most commonly employed absorbable sutures include polyglactin 910 (Vicryl®) and polyglecaprone (Monocryl®). Vicryl is a braided suture that retains 50% of its original tensile strength at 21 days and 25% at 28 days, with complete absorption between 56 and 70 days. Undyed Monocryl is a monofilament suture that has 50% to 60% of its original tensile strength at one week, 20% to 30% at two weeks and zero by three weeks. For wounds under greater tension such as those on the back or extensor extremities, especially in young active patients, prolonged dermal support with sutures such as polydioxanone (PDS II®), polyglyconate (Maxon®) or nondissolving clear nylon (Ethicon®) or polypropylene (Prolene®) has been shown

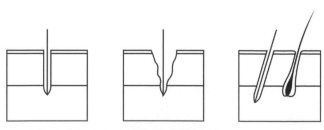

Figure 2 A fluid stroke through the dermis (*left*) leaves a perpendicular wound edge rather than a beveled edge created by multiple passes (*center*), due to retraction of incised dermis. Incisions in hair-bearing skin should follow the direction of the hair shaft (*right*) to avoid transecting follicles.

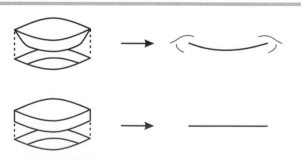

Figure 4 Removal of less tissue at the tips of excision than in the center creates "pseudo dog-ears" (*above*) rather than a uniform flat closure (*below*).

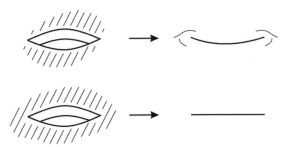

Figure 5 Inadequate undermining of the tips of the excision leaves the ends tethered and protruding after closure (*above*) compared to complete peripheral undermining (*below*).

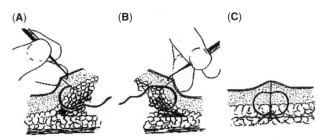

Figure 6 The buried vertical mattress suture provides eversion and prolonged support without causing suture marks. It is important to pivot the skin edge and to place the suture closest to the epidermis at a point 3–4 mm from the skin edge, and deeper in the dermis at the edge. *Source*: From Zitclli JA, Moy RC. The buried vertical mattress suture. *J Dermatol Surg Oncol* 1989:15:17–19. Copyright 1989 by Elsevier Science Publishing Co., Inc.

to better reduce spreading of scars. PDS II and Maxon are monofilament sutures that retain approximately 75% of their original tensile strength at two weeks, 50% at four weeks, and 25% at six weeks, with complete absorption within six months. One must be cautious with the stiffer, long lasting, or permanent sutures to insure placement of knots deeply enough to limit risk of extrusion.

Multiple types of buried sutures have been described, primarily variations of vertical and horizontal mattress sutures, and of running subcuticular/intradermal sutures (Chapter 16). The most commonly employed is the buried vertical mattress suture, which provides support as well as eversion of the wound edges (Fig. 6). Placement of buried sutures is usually guided by the rule of halves, such that each suture bisects the remainder of the unclosed wound. In this way, edges of unequal length can often be approximated without dog-ears. When closing wounds under tension, closure may also begin at either end and progress centrally, decreasing tension on the widest central portion of the defect prior to placement of the central sutures.

Ideally, closure with buried subcutaneous/intradermal sutures should provide excellent approximation of wound edges without percutaneous sutures. The epidermal edges should be free of tension and may then be stabilized with percutaneous sutures, tissue adhesive (e.g., Dermabond®), or adhesive tapes (e.g., Steri-Strips®). If minor adjustment of the epidermal edges is necessary, sutures are most effective. Facial wounds may be closed with simple interrupted 6–0 fast absorbing gut or simple running 6–0 nylon removed at five to seven days. (Fig. 7). Nonabsorbable suture is generally preferred for trunk and extremity excisions, usually 4–0 or 5–0 nylon or Prolene. Wounds requiring percutaneous sutures for more than 10 days may be best closed with running intradermal skin sutures to avoid risk of permanent suture marks.

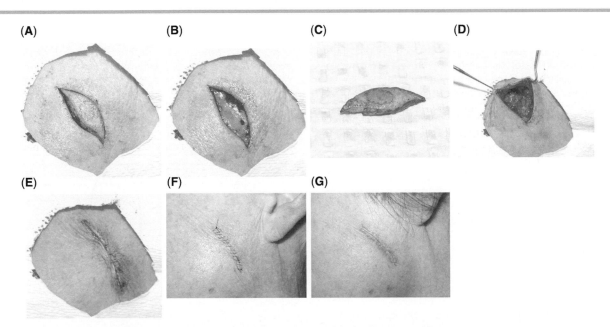

Figure 7 (**A**) Smooth incision from tip-to-tip perpendicularly through the dermis. (**B**) Defect following excision with flat, (**C**) uniformly thick specimen from tip-to-tip. (**D**) Wound undermined laterally and beyond the tips. (**E**) Wound closed with buried vertical mattress sutures. Notice eversion. (**F**) Wound closed with simple running percutaneous sutures (**G**) one-week postoperatively following suture removal. Patients are instructed to wear tape along the incision daily over two weeks following suture removal (e.g., Micropore®).

If no adjustment of epidermal edges is necessary after approximation with buried sutures, adhesive tapes or tissue adhesive may be used in place of percutaneous sutures. Tissue adhesive has been proven faster than sutures and requires no bandage, wound care, or suture removal. Tissue adhesive also has antimicrobial effects and results in less postoperative erythema along the incision line. However, tissue adhesive is significantly more expensive than suture, and one must be careful not to allow adhesive to seep into the wound.

Adhesive tapes may also be used instead of sutures for well-approximated wounds, though they are less secure than tissue adhesive and don't create a complete seal over the wound, which, therefore, still requires routine wound care and bandaging. Security of tape can be improved with the use of liquid adhesive (e.g., Mastisol®) and a semiocclusive dressing (e.g., Tegaderm®), which obviates need for daily wound care. Tapes may also be used with percutaneous sutures for additional support of wound edges if needed.

Wound Dressings and Care

Following closure, for wounds closed without tissue adhesive, a pressure dressing is placed consisting of antibacterial ointment, a nonadherent dry dressing (e.g., Telfa®), gauze, and tape. In areas where a good seal is possible, a waterproof, semiocclusive bandage such as Tegaderm may be applied over the remainder of the dressing, which eliminates the need for wound care. This also allows for showering, swimming, etc., without fear of contaminating the wound. In areas where a complete seal with an occlusive dressing is not possible, wound care begins at 24 hours with b.i.d. tap water cleansing followed by ointment, Telfa, and tape or other suitable bandage. Half-strength peroxide may be used at the first dressing change only, if needed for removal of dried blood. It is suggested that antibiotic ointment such as Polysporin® is used twice daily for the first three days only, thereafter replaced by Vaseline® petroleum jelly. This eliminates the potential for allergic contact dermatitis to the antibiotic and for secondary yeast infections related to prolonged antibiotic use.

Following suture removal, additional support with adhesive tapes or nonsterile flesh-colored paper tape (e.g., Micropore®) is recommended for at least two weeks to minimize potential for spreading of epidermal edges. Such tape may be continued up to several months for wounds under significant tension.

VARIATIONS

Although an excision is a basic procedure, simple modifications by the surgeon can greatly improve the cosmetic result. S-plasties and curvilinear configurations are simple variations that allow reorientation of wound direction, increased length, or improved scar placement along curving skin tension lines (Fig. 8). Other variations of the standard fusiform ellipse allow shortening of scar length or displacement of Burow's triangles when anatomic boundaries or obstructions must be considered. M-plasty and modified M-plasty are methods of shortening the final length of an excision (Fig. 9). For example, when excising a lesion on the temple adjacent to the lateral canthus, the fusiform excision can be converted to an M-plasty that shortens the defect length to spare the canthus. On the dorsal surface of the hand, a 1.0 cm lesion may require an excision 4.0 to 5.0 cm long to avoid dog-ears. Instead of discarding that excess

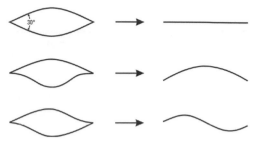

Figure 8 The standard fusiform, "pregnant belly," and S-plasty excisions with resulting closures. *Source*: From Zella (1994).

tissue, a modified M-plasty resembling a bilateral rotation flap can be used to spare the dog-ears that would have been discarded and provide closure with less tension (Fig. 10D).

Likewise, Burow's triangles may be displaced to avoid interference with anatomic structures. Crescentic, single, double, A–T, and A–L advancement flaps are all variations of the fusiform ellipse with displaced Burow's triangles (Fig. 11). For example, a defect on the upper lip can be closed with a crescentic advancement flap which moves and hides the superior Burow's triangle in the alar crease (Fig. 12).

If one is uncertain whether primary closure is possible or about the direction of final closure of a proposed excision, a lesion can be excised in circular fashion and then undermined, to evaluate various closure options. If a linear closure is chosen, once the direction of closure determined, Burow's triangles can then be removed secondarily. Such a "dog-ear repair" is performed by pulling the redundant tissue perpendicular to the direction of closure, incising the first half of the dog-ear and then laying the redundant tissue back across the incision. Excess tissue is then cut off and the wound closed (Fig. 13).

Occasionally, a wound can be excised in circular fashion and closed without removing Burow's triangles. A sutured punch biopsy is a small example of this. Larger lesions can also be excised in such a manner, and, although dog-ears are usually noticeable initially, these will often resolve over time. Some surgeons have recommended this approach to decrease scar length. Although not ideal for most excisions on the face, this approach can be considered for excisions elsewhere and is particularly useful for punch

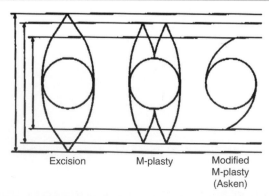

Figure 9 The final wound length of an excision can be shortened considerably with M-plasty or modified M-plasty when removing the same defect.

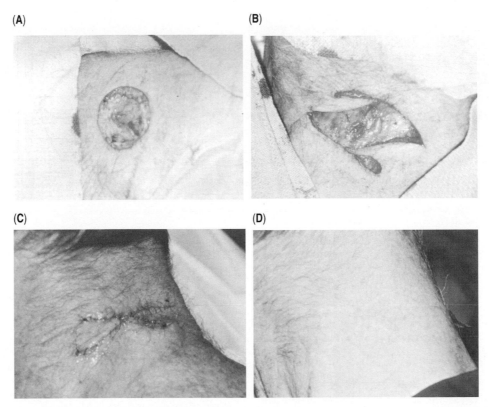

Figure 10 The lesion is removed at the level of the subcutaneous fat. The level of removal in the subcutis and subsequent undermining varies by anatomic location. **(A)** Circular defect. **(B)** Modified M-plasty incised, dog-ears kept in place and rotated into the defect. **(C)** Sutured wound. **(D)** Result 1 year later.

excisions, harvesting full-thickness skin grafts, and excisional biopsies of suspected melanomas.

A "punch excision" can be done for lesions small enough to be completely removed with a punch. For punches 5 mm or greater, the wound may be closed with one or more buried sutures (e.g., 4–0 Vicryl on a P3 needle) which provide complete closure and support over a much longer period than simple interrupted percutaneous sutures. Punch excision sites closed with buried sutures may be dressed with Mastisol, Steri-Strips, ointment, Telfa, and Tegaderm, thereby requiring no wound care or suture removal, and the bandage may be removed at home in

7 to 10 days. This approach is especially useful for excising small atypical nevi or cysts in areas such as the back that are otherwise difficult to reach for wound care (Fig. 14).

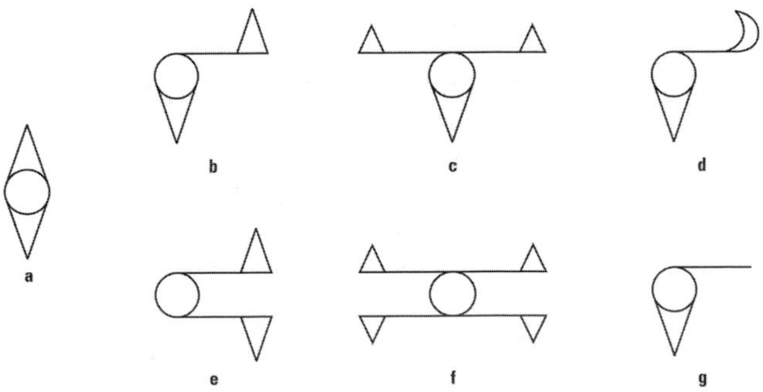

Larger circular excisions can also be performed and closed in layered fashion similar to fusiform excisions or using a pursestring suture. Pursestring sutures are buried sutures that simply "cinch" the defect closed. Wounds may be undermined as needed to facilitate closure. Sutures are wound through the dermis around the defect using absorbable 3–0 or 4–0 sutures such as Vicryl, PDS II, or Maxon, or using 3–0 or 4–0 nylon or prolene removed at two to three weeks. Pursestring sutures create an irregularly puckered wound, which flattens over several months, leaving a small stellate scar. These sutures are rapidly placed and are particularly useful for closure of circular full-thickness skin graft donor sites on the inner upper arm or supraclavicular space (Fig. 15).

Circular excisions are also useful for excisional biopsies of suspected melanomas, when one wants to avoid any additional disruption of surrounding lymphatics by larger excisions, in case of need for sentinel lymph node biopsy following diagnosis. Wounds are not undermined in this case.

COMPLICATIONS

Fusiform excisions routinely heal with excellent results when good planning and technique have been followed. Complications are rare and include bleeding, pain, infection, dehiscence, necrosis, and spread of hypertrophic scars (Chapter 11). Adequate hemostasis, limiting exertion, and avoidance of aspirin, nonsteroidal anti-inflammatory drugs (NSAIDs), Vitamin E, and alcohol—preoperatively

Figure 11 Variations of the fusiform ellipse created by displacing Burow's triangles **(A)**, including A–Z flap **(B)**, A–T flap **(C)**, crescentic advancement flap **(D)**, single **(E)** and double **(F)** advancement flaps. Occasionally one can close a wound without excising Burow's triangles as an A–L flap **(G)**.

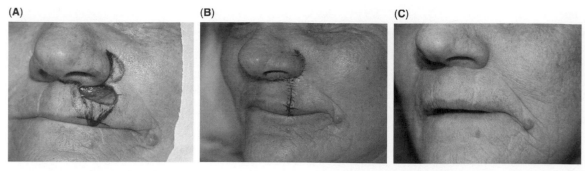

Figure 12 Upper lip defect (**A**), closed with a crescentic advancement flap (**B**) hiding Burow's triangle along the alar crease, and 20 months post-operatively (**C**).

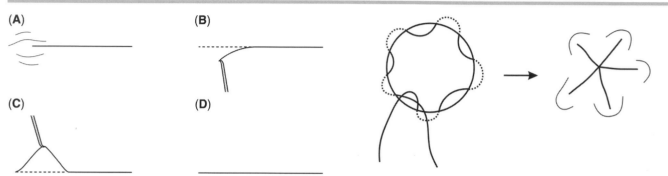

Figure 13 Repair of dog-ear (**A**), performed by retracting excess tissue laterally and incising in the direction of relaxed skin tension lines (**B**), followed by retracting excess tissue across the incision and excising excess (**C**), creating a longer incision without dog-ear (**D**).

Figure 15 Pursestring suture wound through dermis around wound edge closes defect in a puckered, stellate fashion.

and postoperatively (for 48 hours)—will minimize risk of bleeding. Pain is usually minor and can be controlled in most cases with acetaminophen for one to two days postoperatively. Narcotic analgesics can be used if necessary, but nonsteroidal anti-inflammatory agents are discouraged to limit risk of bleeding. Infection occurs in less than 1% of cases, and routine antibiotic prophylaxis is not necessary except in patients with conditions predisposing to endocarditis or in high-risk areas such as the perinasal or perioral areas, where violation of or proximity to mucosa increases risk of bacterial contamination. Dehiscence is rare when subcutaneous/intradermal sutures are used and patients avoid

stress on the wound. Necrosis is also rare when excess tension on the wound edge is avoided and undermining is done below the subdermal plexus. Spread scars can develop with excess tension or with inadequate support from buried sutures. Such spread is invariably narrower than the original width of the defect, and after the wound has matured over four to six months, a spread scar can be reexcised and repaired with less tension and less potential for subsequent spread than the original wound. Hypertrophic scarring is rare on the face and is uncommon elsewhere, though some patients are predisposed to it, especially in wounds under tension. Such scarring may be managed in a variety of ways including reexcision, intralesional, and topical steroids, silicone sheeting, and imiquimod (Aldara®).

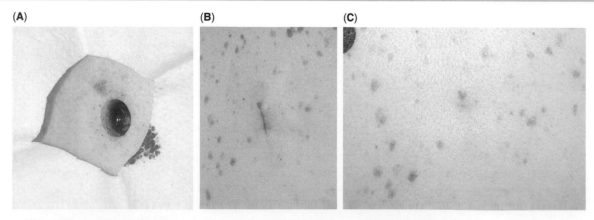

Figure 14 An 8 mm punch excision on the trunk (**A**), closed with buried 4–0 Vicryl suture (**B**), 16 months postoperatively (**C**).

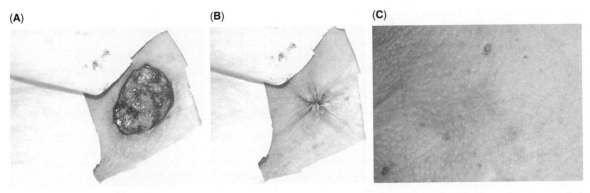

Figure 16 Full-thickness skin graft donor site (**A**), completely closed with pursestring suture of 3-0 Vicryl (**B**), 20 months postoperatively (**C**).

BIBLIOGRAPHY

Alam M, Goldberg LH. Utility of fully buried horizontal mattress sutures. J Am Acad Dermatol 2004; 50:73–76.

Amrein PC, Ellman L, Harris WH. Aspirin induced prolongation of bleeding time and perioperative blood loss. JAMA 1981; 245:1825–1828.

Asken S. A modified M-plasty. J Dermatol Surg Oncol 1986; 12:369–373.

Barnett R, Stranc M. A method of producing improved scars following excision of small lesions of the back. Ann Plast Surg 1979; 3:391–394.

Bennett RG. Cutaneous structure, function, and repair. In: Bennett RG, ed. Fundamentals of Cutaneous Surgery. St. Louis: CV Mosby, 1988:17.

Bennett RG. Basic excisional surgery. In: RG Bennett, ed. Fundamentals of Cutaneous Surgery. St. Louis: CV Mosby, 1988:353–444.

Bernstein G. Surface landmarks for the identification of key anatomic structures of the face and neck. J Dermatol Surg Oncol 1986; 12:722–726.

Bernstein L. Incisions and excisions in elective facial surgery. Arch Otolaryngol 1973; 97:238–246.

Bezwada RS, Jamiolkowski DD, In-Young L, et al. Monocryl® suture, a new ultra-pliable absorbable monofilament suture. Biomaterials 1995; 16:1141–1148.

Blondeel PN, Murphy JW, Debrosse D, et al. Closure of long surgical incisions with a new formulation of 2-octylcyanoacrylate tissue adhesive versus commercially available methods. Am J Surg 2004; 188:307–313.

Borges AF, Alexander JE. Relaxed skin tension lines, Z-plasties on scars, and fusiform excision of lesions. Br J Plast Surg 1962; 15:242–254.

Bourne RB, Bitar H, Andreae PR, et al. An in vivo comparison of four absorbable sutures: Vicryl, Dexon Plus, Maxon, and PDS. Can J Surg 1988; 31:43–45.

Brady JG, Grande DJ, Katz AE. The purse-string suture in facial reconstruction. J Dermatol Surg Oncol 1992; 18:812–816.

Breisch EA, Greenway HT Jr. Cutaneous Surgical Anatomy of the Head and Neck. New York: Churchill Livingstone, 1992.

Breuninger H, Keilbach J, Haaf U. Intracutaneous butterfly suture with absorbable synthetic suture material. Technique, tissue reactions, and results. J Dermatol Surg Oncol 1993; 19:607–610.

Breuninger H. Double butterfly suture for high tension: a broadly anchored, horizontal, buried interrupted suture. Dermatol Surg 2000; 26:215–218.

Breuninger H. Intracutaneous butterfly suture. A horizontal buried interrupted suture for high tension. Comparison of various absorbable suture materials. Eur Plast Surg 1998; 21:415–419.

Chretien-Marquet B, Caillou V, Brasnu DH, et al. Description of cutaneous excision and suture using a mathematical model. Plast Reconstr Surg 1999; 103:145–150.

Collins SC, Whalen JD. Percutaneous buried vertical mattress for the closure of narrow wounds. J Am Acad Dermatol 1999; 41:1025–1026.

Coulthard P, Worthington H, Esposito M, et al. Tissue adhesives for closure of surgical incisions. Cochrane Database Syst Rev 2004; CD004287.

Courtiss EH. The placement of elective skin incisions. Plast Reconstr Surg 1963; 31:31–44.

Cruse PJE, Foord R. The epidemiology of wound infection. A 10-year prospective study of 62,939 wounds. Surg Clin North Am 1980; 60:27–40.

Davis TS, Graham WP III, Miller SH. The circular excision. Ann Plast Surg 1980; 4:21–24.

DuBois JJ. A technique for subcutaneous knot inversion following running subcuticular closures. Mil Med 1992; 157:255.

Eaglstein WH. Occlusive dressings. J Dermatol Surg Oncol 1993; 19:716–720.

Elliot D, Mahaffey PJ. The stretched scar: the benefit of prolonged dermal support. Br J Plast Surg 1989; 42:74–78.

Fleischer W, Reimer K. Povidone-iodine in antisepsis—state of the art. Dermatology 1997; 195(suppl 2):3–9.

Ftaiha Z, Snow SN. The buried running dermal subcutaneous suture technique. J Dermatol Surg Oncol 1989; 15:264–266.

Gennari R, Rotmensz N, Ballardini B, et al. A prospective, randomized, controlled clinical trial of tissue adhesive (2-octylcyanoacrylate) versus standard wound closure in breast surgery. Surgery 2004; 136:593–599.

Giandoni MB, Grabski WJ. Surgical pearl: the dermal buried pulley suture. J Am Acad Dermatol 1994; 30: 1012–1013.

Giddins GE. Experience with knot-free absorbable subcuticular suture. Ann R Coll Surg Engl 1994; 76:405–406.

Goldberg LH, Alam M. Elliptical excisions: variations and the eccentric parallelogram. Arch Dermatol 2004; 140:176–180.

Greenbaum SS, Radonich MA. The purse-string closure. Dermatol Surg 1996; 22:1054–1056.

Guyron B, Vaughan C. Comparison of polydioxanone and polyglactin 910 in intradermal repair. Plast Reconstr Surg 1996; 98:817–820.

Harrington AC, Montemarano A, Welch M, et al. Variations of the pursestring suture in skin cancer reconstruction. Dermatol Surg 1999; 25:277–281.

Harris DR. Healing of the surgical wound. I. Basic considerations. J Am Acad Dermatol 1979; 1:197–207.

Hasson HM. Half-hitch knot for securing the end of continuous sutures. Obstet Gynecol 1992; 80:724–726.

Hicks PD Jr., Stromberg BV. Hemostasis in plastic surgical patients. Clin Plast Surg 1985; 12:17–23.

Hohenleutner U, Egner N, Hohenleutner S, et al. Intradermal buried vertical mattress suture as sole skin closure: evaluation of 149 cases. Acta Derm Venereol 2000; 80:344–347.

Hudson-Peacock MJ, Lawrence CM. Comparison of wound closure by means of dog-ear repair and elliptical excision. J Am Acad Dermatol 1995; 32:627–630.

Hyakusoku H, Ogawa R. A new skin closure technique with running sutures and tissue adhesive. Plast Reconstr Surg 2004; 113:1526–1527.

Jackson IT. Local Flaps in Head and Neck Reconstruction. St. Louis: CV Mosby, 1985.

Katz AR, Mukherjee DP, Kaganov AL, et al. A new synthetic monofilament absorbable suture made from polytrimethylene carbonate. Surg Gynecol Obstet 1985; 161:213–222.

Kneissel CJ. The selection of appropriate lines for elective surgical incisions. Plast Reconstr Surg 1951; 8:1–28.

Kolbusz RU, Bielinski KB. Running vertical mattress sutures. J Dermatol Surg Oncol 1992; 18:500–502.

Kolt JD. Use of adhesive surgical tape with the absorbable continuous subcuticular suture. ANZ J Surg 2003; 73:626–629.

La Padula A. A new technique to secure an entirely buried subcuticular suture. Plast Reconstr Surg 1995; 95:423–424.

Lapins NA. The crescentic ellipse revisited. J Dermatol Surg Oncol 1988; 14:935–936.

Leshin B, McCalmont TH. Preoperative evaluation of the surgical patient. Dermatol Clin 1990; 8:787–794.

Liljestrand KE. The punch and purse-string suture technique. Eur J Surg Suppl 1994; 572:47–50.

MacFie CC, Colville RJ, Reid CA. Back to basics: a new suturing model. Br J Plast Surg 2004; 57:591–592.

Mahabir RC, Christensen B, Blair GK, et al. Avoiding stitch abscesses in subcuticular skin closures: the L-stitch. Can J Surg 2003; 46:223–224.

Mangram AJ, Horan TC, Pearson ML, et al. Guideline for Prevention of Surgical Site Infection, 1999. Centers for Disease Control and Prevention (CDC) Hospital Infection Control Practices Advisory Committee. Am J Infect Control 1999; 27:97–132; discussion 96.

Manstein CH, Manstein ME, Manstein G. Creating a curvilinear scar. Plast Reconstr Surg 1989; 83:914–915.

Marini L. The Haneke-Marini suture; not a "new" technique. Dermatol Surg 1995; 21:819–820.

Matin SF. Prospective randomized trial of skin adhesive versus sutures for closures of 217 laparoscopic port-site incisions. J Am Coll Surg 2003; 196:845–853.

Maw JL, Quinn JV, Wells GA, et al. A prospective comparison of octylcyanoacrylate tissue adhesive and sutures for the closure of head and neck incisions. J Otolaryngol 1997; 26: 26–30.

Morgan JP III, Haug RH, Kosman JW. Antimicrobial skin preparations for the maxillofacial region. J Oral Maxillofac Surg 1996; 54:89–94.

Moy RL, Kaufmann AJ. Clinical comparison of polyglactic acid (Vicryl) and polytrimethylenecarbonate (Maxon) suture material. J Dermatol Surg Oncol 1991; 17:667–669.

Mulliken JB, Rogers GF, Marler JJ. Circular excision of hemangioma and purse-string closure: the smallest possible scar. Plast Reconstr Surg 2002; 15; 109, 1544–1554; discussion 1555.

Paolo B, Stefania R, Massimiliano C, et al. Modified S-plasty: an alternative to the elliptical excision to reduce the length of suture. Dermatol Surg 2003; 29:394–398.

Parell GJ, Becker GD. Comparison of absorbable with nonabsorbable sutures in closure of facial skin wounds. Arch Facial Plast Surg 2003; 5:488–490.

Patel KK, Telfer MR, Southee R. A "round block" purse-string suture in facial reconstruction after operations for skin cancer surgery. Br J Oral Maxillofac Surg 2003; 41:151–156.

Peled IJ, Zagher U, Wexler MR. Purse-string suture for reduction and closure of skin defects. Ann Plast Surg 1985; 14:465–469.

Perry AW, McShane RH. Fine-tuning of the skin edges in the closure of surgical wounds: controlling inversion and eversion with the path of the needle—the right stitch at the right time. J Dermatol Surg Oncol 1981; 7:471–476.

Popkin GL, Gibb RC. Another look at the skin hook. J Dermatol Surg Oncol 1978; 4:366–367.

Quinn J, Wells G, Sutcliffe T, et al. Tissue adhesive versus suture wound repair at 1 year; randomized clinical trial correlating early, 3-month, and 1-year cosmetic outcome. Ann Emerg Med 1998; 645–649.

Ranaboldo C. Simplified method of subcuticular skin closure. Br J Surg 1992; 79:1288.

Randle HW. Modified pursestring suture closure. Dermatol Surg 2004; 30(2 Pt 1):237.

Ray JA, Doddi N, Regula D, et al. A. Polydiaxanone (PDS), a novel monofilament synthetic absorbable suture. Surg Gynecol Obstet 1981; 153:497–503.

Robinson JK. Fundamentals of Skin Biopsy. Chicago: Year Book Medical Publishers, 1982.

Rubio PA. Use of semi-occlusive, transparent film dressings for surgical wound protection: experience in 3637 cases. Int Surg 1991; 76:253–254.

Sadick NS, D'Amelio DL, Weinstein C. The modified buried vertical mattress suture. A new technique of buried absorbable wound closure associated with excellent cosmesis for wounds under tension. J Dermatol Surg Oncol 1994; 20:735–739.

Salasche SJ, Bernstein G, Senkarik M. Surgical Anatomy of the Skin. Norwalk, Connecticut: Appleton & Lange, 1988.

Salasche SJ. Acute surgical complications: cause, prevention, and treatment. J Am Acad Dermatol 1986; 15: 1163–1185.

Salzmann EW. Hemostatic problems in surgical patients. Hemostasis and Thrombosis: Basic Principles and Clinical Practice. 2nd. Philadelphia: Lippincott, 1987:920–925.

Seitz SE, Foley GL, Marretta SM. Evaluation of marking material for cutaneous surgical margins. Am J Vet Res 1995; 56:826–833.

Sharkey I, Brughera-Jones A. Evaluation of potential bleeding problems in dermatologic surgery. J Dermatol Surg 1975; 1:41–44.

Singer AJ, Hollander JE, Valentine SM, et al. Prospective, randomized controlled trial of tissue adhesive (2-octylcyanoacrylate) vs standard wound closure techniques for laceration repair. Acad Emerg Med 1998; 5:94–99.

Singer AJ, Quinn JV, Clark RE, et al. Closure of lacerations and incisions with octylcyanoacrylate: a multicenter randomized trial. Surgery 2002; 131:270–276.

Singh-Ranger D. A simple technique for the retention of a subcuticular suture. Surgeon 2003; 1:149–151.

Smoot EC. Method for securing a subcuticular suture with minimal buried knot. Plast Reconstr Surg 1998; 102: 2447–2449.

Snow SN, Goodman MM, Lemke BN. The short and vertical mattress stitch: a rapid skin everting suture technique. J Dermatol Surg Oncol 1989; 15:379–381.

Sommerlad BC, Creasey JM. The stretched scar: a clinical and histological study. Br J Plast Surg 1978; 31:34.

Sonanis SV, Gholve PA. Continuous oblique mattress suture. Plast Reconstr Surg 2003; 111:2472–2473.

Spicer TE. Techniques of facial lesion excision and closure. J Dermatol Surg Oncol 1982; 8:551–556.

Stegman SJ. Planning closure of a surgical wound. J Dermatol Surg Oncol 1978; 4:390–393.

Stegman SJ. Suturing techniques for dermatologic surgery. J Dermatol Surg Oncol 1978; 4:63–68.

Stiff MA, Snow SN. Running vertical mattress suturing technique. J Dermatol Surg Oncol 1992; 18:916–917.

Swanson NA. Atlas of Cutaneous Surgery. Boston: Little Brown, 1987.

Terracina JR, Wagner RF Jr. Antibiotic use in dermatologic surgery. In: Roenigk RK, Roenigk HH Jr., eds. Surgical Dermatology: Advances in Current Practice. St. Louis: CV Mosby, 1993:31.

Tilleman TR. Direct closure of round skin defects: a four-step technique with multiple subcutaneous and cutaneous "figure-of-8" sutures alleviating dog-ears. Plast Reconstr Surg 2004; 114:1761–1767.

Toriumi DM, O'Grady K, Desai D, et al. Use of octyl-2-cyanoacrylate for skin closure in facial plastic surgery. Plast Reconstr Surg 1998; 102:2209–2219.

van den Ende ED, Vriens PW, Allema JH, et al. Adhesive bonds or percutaneous absorbable suture for closure of surgical wounds in children. Results of a prospective randomized trial. J Pediatr Surg 2004; 39:1249–1251.

Webster R, Smith RC. Cosmetic principles in surgery on the face. J Dermatol Surg Oncol 1978; 4:397–402.

Weisberg NK, Greenbaum SS. Revisiting the purse-string closure: some new methods and modifications. Dermatol Surg 2003; 29:672–676.

Whitaker DC, Grande DJ, Johnson SS. Wound infection rate in dermatologic surgery. J Dermatol Surg Oncol 1988; 14: 525–528.

Wong NL. The running locked intradermal suture: a cosmetically elegant continuous suture for wounds under light tension. J Dermatol Surg Oncol 1993; 19:30–36.

Zalla MJ. Basic cutaneous surgery. Cutis 1994; 53:172–186.

Zitella JA. Wound healing for the clinician. Adv Dermatol 1987; 2:243–267.

Zitelli JA, Moy RL. Buried vertical mattress suture. J Dermatol Surg Oncol 1989; 15:17–19.

Zitelli JA. Tips for a better ellipse. J Am Acad Dermatol 1990; 22:101–103.

16

Scissor Surgery

Roger I. Ceilley

University of Iowa, Iowa City, Iowa, U.S.A.

INTRODUCTION

Scissors are essential instruments for performing dermatologic surgery. They are used for both cutting and blunt dissection because they allow for accurate control. Scissors stabilize tissue between the blades and allow more accurate removal of flaccid tissue than the scalpel. Scissors are designed to make use of three force vectors when cutting: closing, shearing, and torque (Fig. 1). The closing force is transferred from the operator's fingers to the shanks of the scissors, through the fulcrum to the cutting edges. Shearing force occurs when one blade slides against the other. The force that rolls the leading edge of one blade inward to the other is torque. Most scissors are designed so that a gripping motion of the right hand will combine these forces for precise cutting.

TECHNIQUE

Control of direction and accuracy depends on the stability of the tissue between the blades and the security of the operator's grip. The "tripod grip" (Fig. 2) provides the best use of the scissors' design for sharp clean cuts. The tips of the thumb and ring finger are placed through the rings of the scissors and the index finger rests on the fulcrum. This grip provides maximum control of the instrument. The thumb–index finger grip results in two-point control of the scissors and allows the cut to wander. This grip applies less torque and shearing force; therefore, the blades "chew" rather than cut cleanly through the tissue.

The greatest mobility when using scissors is provided when the hand is in the pronated position. For vertical cutting, the forearm is turned midway between pronation and supination. This allows 180° of pronation and 90° of supination.

Scissors can be used for both sharp and blunt dissection (Fig. 3). The scissors can cut flaccid tissue better than a scalpel and provide better control of depth. Flaccid tissue is stabilized between the blades for extra control of direction. This is especially important when dissecting epidermoid cysts or undermining wound edges and flaps. The cleanest, most precise cutting occurs when tissue is cut nearer to the tip of the scissors rather than close to the fulcrum. One should use just enough blade to complete the desired cut. Chewing the tissue can be avoided by taking one large bite rather than several small ones.

Blunt dissection can be performed by pushing the tips of the scissors or by spreading the scissors to separate loose subcutaneous tissue and fascia. The surgeon can alternate between sharp and blunt dissection when using a scissors with blunt tips. The rounded tips of a Metzenbaum or Stevens scissors can be used to probe the wound gently to separate subcutaneous tissue, fascia layers, and scar from normal tissue. Dissection can also be performed with or without direct vision. Blind dissection is safer with scissors than with a scalpel.

SUTURE CUTTING

Suture scissors or Metzenbaum or Gradle scissors are most useful for suture cutting. The scissor blades should be held perpendicular to the suture while the knot is kept in full view between the blades. Also, check the scissor tips to prevent damage to deeper structures. More precise cuts should be done at the outer third of the blade. Do not use fine iris scissors to cut large sutures (especially monofilament) because this may spring the blades and damage the cutting edges. The assistant should bring the scissors into the operative field after the second hitch if three hitches are used to tie the knot. Cut the sutures deliberately and accurately. Jabbing or snapping tends to tear the suture and traumatize the tissue. When cutting sutures deep in a wound, stabilize the scissors with the other hand or on another fixed area. After cutting the suture, discard the suture material so as not to clutter the operative field and leave suture fragments in the wound.

SCISSORS

Proper instrumentation is a key factor in technically successful surgery. There are two main types of scissors: those with a straight blade and those with a curved blade.

Curved

Curved-blade scissors offer more directional mobility, visibility, and cut a smooth curve easily. They have 30% to 40% more mobility than straight scissors and are more useful for undermining or dissecting around epidermal cysts and lipomas.

Straight

Straight-blade scissors have greater mechanical advantage when cutting tougher tissue such as scar or nail plates. Straight scissors may be more precise for straight cutting than curved scissors.

High-quality stainless steel scissors are vital. Handle them carefully, protecting the finely honed surfaces. After use, they should be cleansed and scrubbed manually or with an ultrasonic cleaner. Before sterilizing, the instruments should be dipped in instrument milk for lubrication and to prevent rust. The choice of scissors is dictated by the function they will serve.

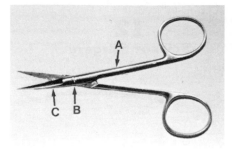
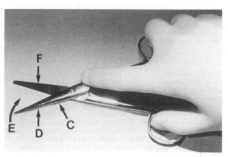

Figure 1   Scissors: (**A**) shank; (**B**) fulcrum; and (**C**) blade. Force vectors: (**D**) closing, (**E**) shearing, and (**F**) torque.

For most procedures performed by dermatologists, small instruments 3½–5 inches long are best. The following scissors should be considered (Figs. 4,5).

1. *Gradle*: 3¾ inches can be used for suture removal or for cutting fine, delicate tissues such as the eyelids.
2. *Stevens tenotomy*: straight or curved, 4½ inches for uses similar to the Gradle.
3. *Iris*: straight and curved, sturdy and delicate, 4½ inches is a little bit heavier than the Stevens tenotomy or Gradle.
4. *Metzenbaum*: small or "baby," 5½ inches is most useful; curved blunt tips are recommended for undermining to prevent puncturing the skin surface. Larger sizes are useful for scalp reduction surgery.
5. *Kilner*: 5½ inches is similar to Metzenbaum but one edge is serrated.
6. *Suture scissors (Spencer Litauer)*: used for removing sutures; do not ruin the edges of your fine tissue scissors by cutting large-caliber monofilament sutures with them.
7. *General operating scissors*: blunt or sharp tips, used for cutting sutures, dressing, and so on.
8. *Bandage scissors*: Lister.
9. *Mayo*: heavy-duty for cutting through thick tissue and sutures.

OFFICE PROCEDURES

Many skin lesions can be readily treated with scissors. Some lesions, such as skin tags, can be removed with sharp iris scissors without anesthesia. A large number of these lesions can be snipped off in a few minutes. Elevated or pedunculated lesions, such as nevi and warts are ideally suited for removal with scissors. Scissors are also important

tools in removing epidermoid cysts, lipomas, punch biopsy specimens, and for excising, trimming, and undermining in more complex surgical procedures. Many nevi, seborrheic keratoses, and acrochordons can be precisely removed level with the skin. The base may then be lightly electrodesiccated or cauterized to provide hemostasis. If aluminum chloride solution is used prior to cautery, less heat is needed and scar formation or hypopigmentation is less likely. In many cases, only local pressure and aluminum chloride or Monsel's solution are required. A slight elevation or irregularity of the margin is easily trimmed away. Scalpel excision with primary wound closure is preferred for active junctional nevi, dysplastic nevi, nevi with terminal hair, or for those lesions in which the diagnosis of malignant melanoma is suspected.

Cysts and Benign Tumors

Small benign lesions, such as papillomas, pyogenic granulomas, fibromas, mucoceles, and small epidermoid cysts can easily be removed with scissors (Figs. 6–9). Hemostasis can be obtained by direct pressure, electrocoagulation, or by a few interrupted sutures. For larger lesions, begin the incision by stabbing one point of the scissors' blades into the edge of the lesion. Larger cysts are best treated by a small ellipse with the scalpel or by punch excision of the overlying pore attached to the skin. Then direct sharp and blunt dissection with curved scissors frees the lesion.

Warts
Filiform

These lesions may be removed with scissors usually without anesthesia. Aluminum chloride or Monsel's solution is applied to the base for hemostasis.

Periungual

Under local anesthesia, the margin between the wart and normal tissue is incised with the curved iris scissors held in the pronated position perpendicular to the skin surface. Overlying nail plate is trimmed away with a heavier scissors and the wart removed with a large-handled dermal curet. Hemostasis is obtained by pressure and application of Monsel's or aluminum chloride solution. Soft wart tissue at the margin is curetted until the gritty feel of normal tissue is obtained. The hyperkeratotic rim is then trimmed with small curved iris scissors.

Palmar and Plantar

Blunt dissection and scissor surgery are very effective for treating these often recalcitrant lesions. If carefully done, blunt dissection may atraumatically separate the wart from the dermis, minimizing the risk of scarring. This technique

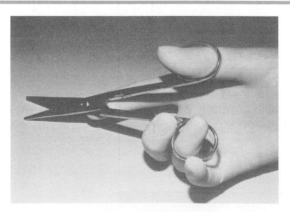

Figure 2   "Tripod grip" for most precise control of scissors.

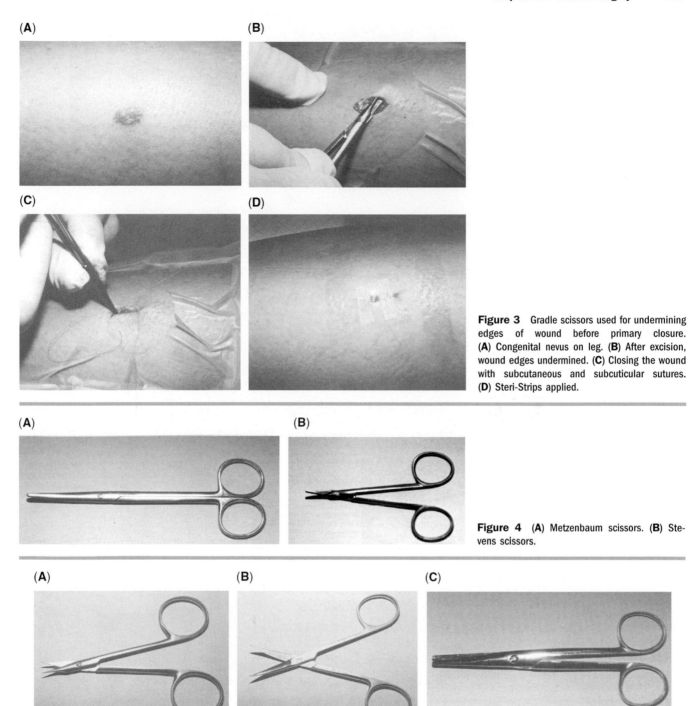

Figure 3 Gradle scissors used for undermining edges of wound before primary closure. **(A)** Congenital nevus on leg. **(B)** After excision, wound edges undermined. **(C)** Closing the wound with subcutaneous and subcuticular sutures. **(D)** Steri-Strips applied.

Figure 4 **(A)** Metzenbaum scissors. **(B)** Stevens scissors.

Figure 5 Types of scissors: **(A)** gradle; **(B)** iris; and **(C)** Mayo.

is most effective for solitary or isolated warts of long duration (over six months) (Figs. 10–13).

Technique. The area is sterilely prepped. If the wart is large or thick, it is helpful to pare the excessive stratum corneum until a sharp margin between the wart and surrounding skin is visualized. The area is then infiltrated with 1% lidocaine using a 25- to 30-gauge needle. Lidocaine with epinephrine 1:300,000 is used on the palms and soles but not on the digits. Avoid passing the needle through the wart to prevent spread along the needle tract. Injecting at an angle almost parallel to the skin instead of directly

perpendicular into the palm is less painful. The needle should be advanced very slowly and gently. The hyperkeratotic skin around the wart is then scored (not in the dermis) with curved scissors. The wart may then be avulsed with a large curet or separated with a nasal septum Freer elevator. Once the base is reached, the wart is carefully separated from the dermal layer. The rete ridges that make the digit dermatoglyphic lines can be seen at this point. A small curet is then used to remove any remaining wart. A dull curet works well for this and ensures minimal damage to the dermis. The calloused margins of the wound are then

(A)

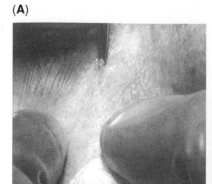

(B)

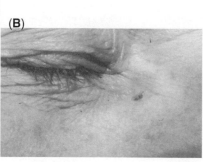

Figure 6   Removal of seborrheic keratosis with iris scissors. (**A**) Removal with curved iris scissors. (**B**) Postoperative appearance.

(A)   **(B)**

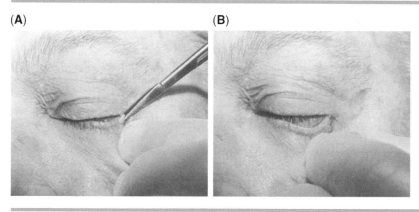

Figure 7   Removal of small epidermoid cyst. (**A**) Completing the cut. (**B**) Postoperative appearance.

(A)   **(B)**   **(C)**

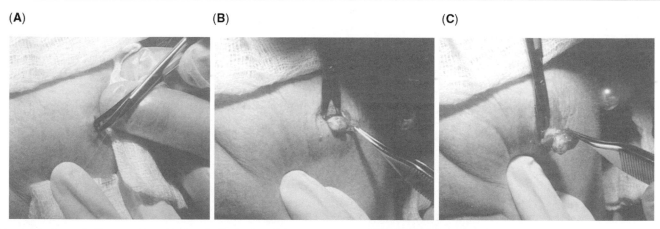

Figure 8   Removal of larger epidermoid cyst. (**A**) Sharp dissection around the cyst. (**B**) Blunt dissection by spreading the scissors. (**C**) Delivering the cyst.

(A)   **(B)**

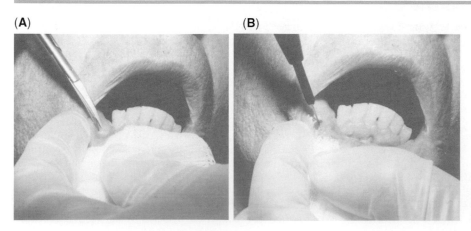

Figure 9   Removal of mucous cyst on the lip. (**A**) After local anesthesia, cyst is sharply dissected off with delicate iris scissors. (**B**) Light electrodesiccation for hemostasis.

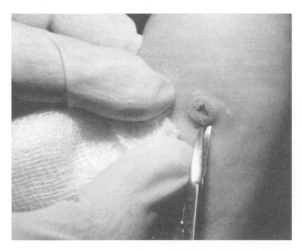

Figure 10 Scoring the surface of a hypertrophic plantar wart with iris scissors.

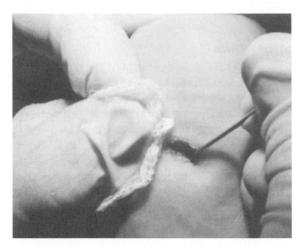

Figure 12 Curetting the margins with a small curet.

trimmed with the scissors, and aluminum chloride or Monsel's solution is used for hemostasis and a pressure dressing is applied. Treatment of the base and margins with a low-powered, defocused beam of the CO_2 laser may also be used as the final step.

Postoperative Care. The pressure dressing is removed in 24 to 48 hours. The wound is cleaned with hydrogen peroxide and an antibiotic ointment applied twice daily. In one week, the calloused edges are trimmed, and in 21 days the wound is checked again. Early recurrences are readily removed with a small curet or frozen with liquid nitrogen. The spread of papillomavirus in patients with hyperhidrosis is well known. It is helpful to treat this to prevent recurrences.

Anogenital

Scissor excision is one of the most useful techniques in the treatment of anogenital condylomata. This technique has been utilized successfully in adults when compared to podophyllin, as reported by Khawaja, and in pediatric groups, as reported by Handley et al.

The wart is infiltrated with 1% lidocaine with epinephrine 1:300,000. This both balloons the tissue, elevating

the wart, and provides hemostasis. Once blanching occurs, the warts are excised at the base with the scissors. Cutting should begin at the upper portion and finish at the most dependent area so that blood does not obscure the operative field. Hemostasis is then obtained by electrocoagulation or by suturing with an absorbant suture. Intra-anal warts can be excised in the same manner using an anal retractor. If the procedure is done under general anesthesia, saline with epinephrine 1:300,000 is used to aid hemostasis. This technique is also used in conjunction with CO_2 laser surgery to "debulk" larger lesions.

SCISSOR SURGERY COMBINED WITH CRYOSURGERY

The removal of warts and nevi with the combined use of cryosurgery and scissor surgery has been reported by Biro and Brand. They recommend freezing the lesion until it is hard and easily removed with flat converse scissors at the junction of the raised portion and the surrounding normal skin. Any raised edges are then trimmed flush and Monsel's or 35% aluminum chloride solution is used for hemostasis. They found that this helps avoid any "delling" that may

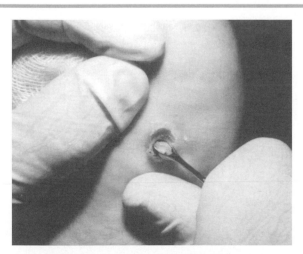

Figure 11 Avulsing the wart with a large curet.

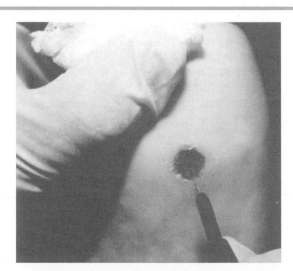

Figure 13 Light electrodesiccation of the margins.

be seen when local anesthesia is used or when using a scalpel or curved scissors.

BIBLIOGRAPHY

Anderson RM, Romf RF. Technique in the Use of Surgical Tools. New York: Appleton-Century Crofts, 1980.

Asarch RG, Ceilley RI. Cold steel surgery. Dermatol Clin 1984; 2:341–351.

Biro L, Brand AJ. Cryosurgery combined with scissor excision. J Dermatol Surg Oncol 1983; 9:185–186.

Ceilley RI. Surgical treatment of warts. In: Epstein E, Epstein E Jr, eds. Skin Surgery. Philadelphia: WB Saunders, 1987:572–579.

Gollock JM, Slatford K, Hunter JM. Scissor excision of anogenital warts. Br J Vener Dis 1982; 58:400–401.

Handley JM, Maw RD, Horner T, et al. Scissor excision plus electrocautery of anogenital warts in prepubertal children. Pediatr Dermatol 1991; 8(3):243–245, 248–249.

Khawaja HT. Podophyllin versus scissor excision in the treatment of perianal condyloma acuminata: a prospective study. Br J Surg 1990; 77(4):474.

Pringle WM, Helms DC. Treatment of plantar warts by blunt dissection. Arch Dermatol 1973; 108:79–82.

Thompson JP, Grace RH. The treatment of perianal and anal condylomata acuminata. J R Soc Med 1978; 71:180–185.

Ulbrich AD. Warts: treatment by total enucleation. Cutis 1974; 14:582–586.

17

Simple Repairs

Jeff Lander and Frederick Fish

Department of Dermatology, University of Minnesota, Minneapolis, Minnesota, U.S.A.

INTRODUCTION

The requirement of any method of skin closure is to hold the skin edges in apposition for sufficient length of time to allow healing that results in the least noticeable scar. Ideally, no movement between skin edges should occur, and excessive tension on wound edges should be avoided. The simple repair can be utilized when a biopsy site or surgical wound can be approximated under little or no tension without undermining, when it is not favorable to place buried suture material in the wound, or in situations such as partial wound closures. The surgeon must know the properties of closure materials (Chapter 3), be able to select the proper suture for a particular use, and know the technique of suture placement (Chapter 18). This chapter will discuss the implementation of simple repairs for a variety of situations including skin biopsies, cyst and lipoma removal, and other surgical situations. When significant undermining is used to increase tissue movement and/or to reduce or distribute tension, or when one or multiple layers of subcuticular sutures are used, the repair may no longer be defined as simple, and it becomes intermediate or complex. In many cases, a small or intermediate sized defect under little or no tension may be repaired with a simple repair using a single layer of skin or intradermal sutures.

GENERAL CONSIDERATIONS

In general, the wound should be closed only when adequate hemostasis has been achieved and the wound margins are easily approximated. It is important to identify natural landmarks (e.g., vermillion border) and ensure they are adequately opposed with a key suture(s). Subsequently, the principle of halving may be useful. A suture is placed in the center of the existing wound, then in the center of the two segments of the wound, and repeated until the wound is closed. In many cases, the simple interrupted suture is the best approach for closure. Natural tension on an ellipse or dead space left by an excised space-occupying lesion will cause the ends to evert and the center to invert. Techniques such as vertical or horizontal mattress sutures can help overcome this tendency.

SIMPLE CLOSURE OF PUNCH BIOPSY DEFECTS

The punch biopsy technique is a fast, easy, inexpensive method for producing a cylinder of tissue from the skin surface to the underlying subcutaneous fat. It may be used to sample both inflammatory dermatoses and tumors, and it yields more information about depth of invasion than the shave biopsy (Chapter 14).

After the area for biopsy is properly cleaned and anesthetized, the skin is drawn taut with the thumb and forefinger of the physician's free hand. The direction of force applied should take advantage of and is usually perpendicular to relaxed skin tension lines (Fig. 1A). This force will cause the eventual defect to be oval rather than round (Fig. 1B). It is important that the orifice of the punch is applied firmly to the skin surface with the handle held perpendicular to the skin, so that the wound edges are at 90° angles to the dermis and subcutaneous tissue.

When the specimen is cut free from the surrounding tissue, the punch is removed. There may be considerable oozing of blood depending on the location. An assistant should apply firm pressure around the perimeter of the defect so that adequate visualization of the base can be obtained. Once the biopsy specimen is lifted up, transected at the base and removed, an oval defect is left. If suture is used to appose the wound edges, no chemical cautery agent is placed in the wound. Proper suture placement will usually stop bleeding. The defect can be closed with a single or several simple interrupted sutures resulting in a closure that is linear (Fig. 1C). Even a 4 mm biopsy is best closed with two simple interrupted sutures (Fig. 2) or a "figure-of-eight" suture to minimize the dog-ear affect that may result with one central suture. The figure-of-eight suture can be performed so that the suture crosses in an X within the skin (Fig. 3A and B) or on top (Fig. 3C and D). Common sutures for closing biopsy sites are those made of nylon or polypropylene. Silk, small diameter nylon (e.g., 7-0 Ethilon), or braided polyester are soft and can be used on or around mucosal sites or eyelids. Braided polyester and nylon incite less tissue reactivity and are easier to remove than silk. Vicryl Rapide is polyglactin 910 that is ionized with gamma rays to speed its absorption. It is completely absorbed in 35 days. It can be used to close biopsy sites when it is not convenient for the patient to return for suture removal (Fig. 4). Gabel et al. compared nylon and polyglactin 910 in the closure of punch biopsy sites and found no statistically significant differences between the two sutures at two weeks and six months with respect to redness, infection, dehiscence, scar hypertrophy, and patient satisfaction. Another option when a biopsy defect is located on the face under low tension and it is inconvenient or unnecessary for the patient to return for suture removal is to use simple interrupted fast-absorbing gut (Fig. 5). Fast-absorbing gut is plain gut that is treated with heat, which results in speedy absorption. It is intended for percutaneous suturing, and the material maintains its tensile strength for only five to seven days. It is completely absorbed within two to four weeks.

(A)   **(B)**

(C)   **(D)**

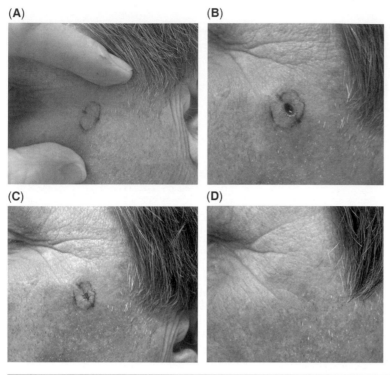

Figure 1 3 mm diagnostic punch biopsy and simple defect repair. **(A)** An erythematous plaque on the malar prominence of a 58-year-old man. The vector of relaxed skin tension line is marked. Tension is applied across the lesion with the thumb and forefinger at right angles to the relaxed skin tension lines. **(B)** As the elastic skin recoils after a 3 mm punch biopsy is performed and the specimen removed, the once circular defect will align itself into an ellipse in an orientation ideal for closure. **(C)** The defect was repaired with two simple interrupted sutures [6-0 polypropylene (Prolene)]. **(D)** The sutures were removed after one week. The biopsy site is barely noticeable at three weeks postbiopsy.

(A)   **(B)**

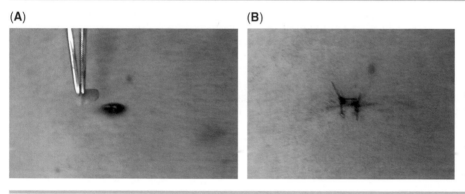

Figure 2 4 mm diagnostic punch biopsy and simple defect repair. **(A)** A papule is biopsied with a 4 mm punch instrument. As in Figure 1, tension was applied across the lesion with the thumb and forefinger at right angles to the relaxed skin tension lines to generate an ellipse in an orientation ideal for closure. **(B)** The defect was repaired with two simple interrupted sutures [4-0 polypropylene (Prolene)] to minimize a dog-ear effect. The sutures were removed after two weeks.

(A)   **(B)**   **(C)**   **(D)**

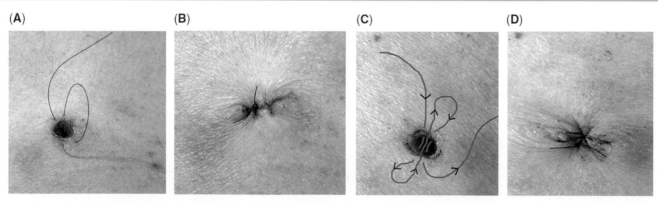

Figure 3 Repair of biopsy defects with two versions of the figure-of-eight suture. **(A)** The needle enters the skin on the top left, exits bottom right, reenters top right, and finally exits bottom left. **(B)** A standard instrument tie is made. The suture crosses in an X configuration within the skin. **(C)** A similar oval defect with lines and arrowheads depicting order of needle throw as entry at top left, exit bottom left, reentry top right, and exit bottom right. **(D)** The suture crosses so that the X configuration is on top. The sutures were removed after two weeks.

In some cases the removal of a 2 to 4 mm circular lesion by the punch technique with suture closure of the wound yields a result comparable to elliptical excision and is much faster to perform (Fig. 4). However, a considerable size round cosmetic defect may result from using a large 5 to 6 mm or greater punch (Fig. 6). Depending on the anatomic site and other factors such as skin elasticity, the cosmetic result may not compare well to that of an elliptical excision. Standing

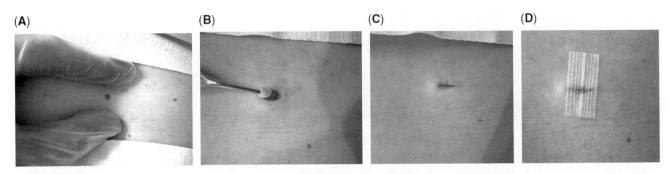

Figure 4 Punch excision and repair of biopsy defect with intradermal fast-absorbing polyglactin 910 (Vicryl Rapide). **(A)** Tension is applied across a papule on the lower abdomen at right angles to the relaxed skin tension lines. **(B)** A 5 mm round punch excision is performed and the specimen is removed, leaving an oval defect. **(C)** The defect is repaired with two intradermal sutures (5-0) rapidly absorbing polyglactin 910 (Vicryl Rapide). **(D)** Steri-strips are applied to closely approximate the wound edge.

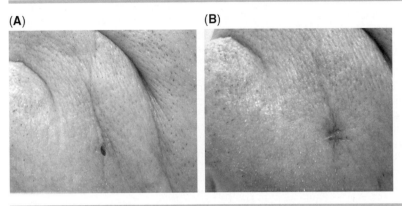

Figure 5 Repair of biopsy defect with fast-absorbing gut suture. **(A)** A dilated pore located on the lateral chin of an elderly man is excised using a 3 mm punch instrument using the techniques illustrated in Figure 1A and B. **(B)** The thin oval defect is repaired with two simple interrupted 5-0 fast-absorbing gut sutures.

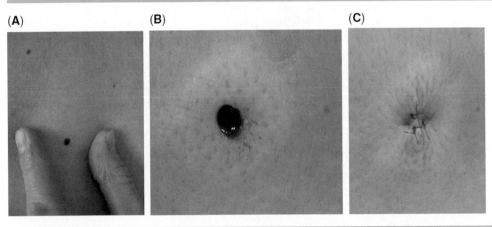

Figure 6 Punch excision of a pigmented lesion and simple repair. **(A)** A 4 mm pigmented lesion located on the lower back. **(B)** A 6 mm round punch is used to excise the lesion in total, leaving an oval defect. **(C)** The defect is repaired by first placing a 4-0 polypropylene vertical mattress suture centrally to bring the defect together and evert the wound edges. This is followed by placing 4-0 polypropylene simple interrupted sutures at each end to complete the approximation of the wound edges. Small redundant cones are situated at each end of the final closure but are cosmetically acceptable. The sutures were removed after two weeks.

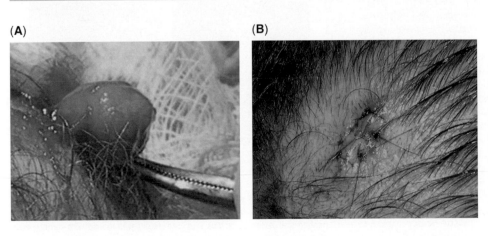

Figure 7 Pilar cyst incision and simple repair. **(A)** A 1 cm pilar cyst of the posterior scalp is removed through a linear incision. **(B)** The defect is repaired by first placing two 4–0 polypropylene vertical mattress sutures centrally to close the dead space, bring the defect together, and evert the wound edges. This is followed by placing simple interrupted sutures at each end to complete the approximation of the wound edges. The sutures were removed after two weeks.

cutaneous cones (dog-ears) commonly result and may be removed at the time of the procedure (Chapter 15). In addition, an absorbable, subcutaneous suture may be placed to approximate wound edges and reduce tension.

CLOSURE OF SMALL INCISIONAL OR FUSIFORM CYST AND LIPOMA EXCISIONS

Closure of small incisional or fusiform excisions may be accomplished by a simple repair if the defect is under no or very low tension. The actual length to width ratio depends on the location of the lesion and the elasticity of the patient's skin (Chapter 15). The recommended ratio achieves a flat, even scar. Small dog-ears usually flatten spontaneously, especially on the extremities, and therefore a small degree of puckering at the tip of a closed excision is often acceptable. If wounds are properly oriented and carefully closed, nearly invisible scars can result. Ideally, the wound should be placed in a natural skin fold or crease, or near an anatomical junction. The most appropriate alignment is to orient the long axis of the excision at right angles to the principle muscle pull and parallel to the natural crease or wrinkle lines. If after careful examination of the patient prior to local anesthesia, the direction of optimal excision is not apparent, the lesion may be excised in a circular manner. Then, fingertips can be used to gently approximate the sides of the defect, which will usually close more easily in one direction than another. The standing cutaneous cones at each end of the defect can subsequently be marked and trimmed (Chapter 15).

Defects after incision or excision of small benign, space-occupying lesions such as lipomas, pilar cysts, epidermal cysts, digital mucous cysts, etc. are often ideally suited for simple epidermal closure or layered closure under little or no tension (Chapters 33 and 34). For example, on the trunk and distal extremities, lipomas usually lie within the fat layer and are surrounded by a loose connective tissue capsule that separates them from surrounding fatty tissue. These lipomas tend to be superficial and are usually removed easily. For small lipomas and epidermal and pilar cysts that are removed easily by an incisional technique, the defect can be closed using absorbable or nonabsorbable suture material (Fig. 7). The large amount of tissue encompassed by vertical mattress sutures aids in the reduction of subcutaneous dead space that is left after a lesion such as cyst or lipoma is removed. If the defect is closed in single layer fashion, a vertical mattress suture placed in the center can bring the wound edges together under tension, evert the wound edges, and help close dead space (Fig. 7). It is placed prior to placing simple interrupted sutures and brings skin borders closer together by combining deep and superficial closure but not tight enough to achieve complete alignment. This should be achieved with simple interrupted sutures. Tying the vertical mattress suture tightly enough to approximate wound edges fully may cause necrosis of wound edges. Vertical mattress sutures can be removed before simple interrupted ones to reduce the possibility of leaving suture marks. When placing the vertical mattress suture, the suture needle selected should allow for a sufficiently wide bite to close dead space and create eversion of the wound edge (e.g., for trunk or scalp, a 4-0 Prolene on a PS-2 3/8 circle reverse cutting needle). To further reduce the subcutaneous dead space, one can pass the deep loop of the vertical mattress suture through the tissue under subcutaneous fat. In addition, if the structure is relatively fixed in position (e.g., periosteum or muscle fascia), this loop may

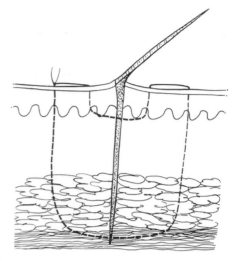

Figure 8 Deep vertical mattress suture. The vertical mattress suture has included deep tissue in the far-far pass to help close dead space. *Source:* From Stasko (1994).

aid in recreating contours and distributing the tension equally between the two sides of the wound (Fig. 8). In some cases when the defect contains only a small amount of residual dead space and is under little or no tension, closure can be achieved with either simple interrupted suture (Fig. 9) or a simple running suture (Fig. 10).

A running suture can be locked on itself to allow the use of a running suture in areas under slightly more tension, or when additional hemostasis is required. The locking is performed by looping the suture through the suture from the previous loop. Disadvantages are that fine edge approximation is difficult to obtain and tension of the suture and loops across the skin surface may result in focal necrosis. Therefore, it is better reserved for closure of areas with limited cosmetic sensitivity or when hemostasis of skin edges is difficult. In cosmetically sensitive areas such as the head and neck, the running horizontal mattress suture is useful for simple repairs of small defects. This suture creates

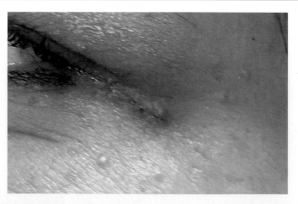

Figure 9 Simple repair at lateral canthus. A simple repair after cyst excision at the lateral canthus is appropriate given the low tension and rapid healing that is typical at this site. The defect was closed with three simple interrupted 6-0 polypropylene (Prolene) sutures. The sutures were removed after one week.

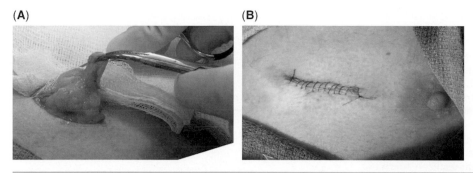

Figure 10 Simple repair after lipoma excision. **(A)** Lipoma on the upper chest removed with a small fusiform excision. There was minimal residual dead space and the wound edges approximated under little tension. **(B)** A 4-0 polypropylene running interrupted suture was placed to align the epidermal wound edges. Sutures were removed after two weeks.

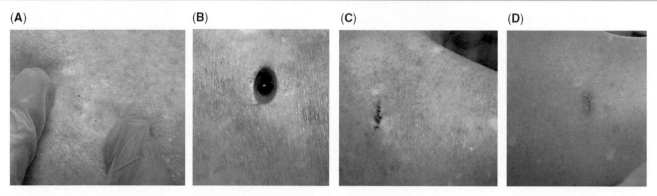

Figure 11 Epidermal cyst excision and simple repair. **(A)** Lateral pressure tangential to relaxed skin tension lines is applied to a small epidermal cyst located on the right upper back. **(B)** The cyst was completely encompassed and excised using an 8 mm punch instrument. **(C)** The defect is repaired by first placing a vertical mattress suture centrally to close the dead space, bring the defect together and evert the wound edges. This is followed by placing two simple interrupted sutures at each end to complete the approximation of the wound edges. **(D)** The sutures were removed after two weeks.

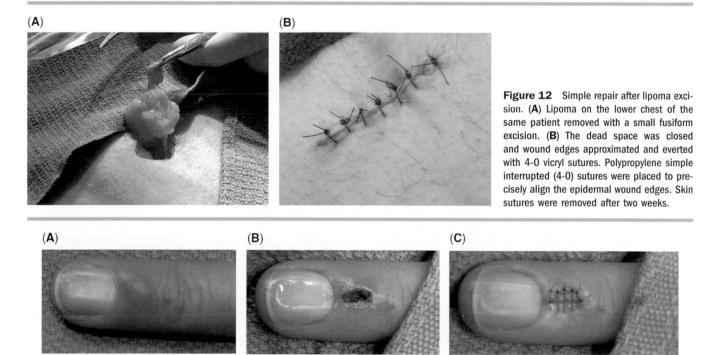

Figure 12 Simple repair after lipoma excision. **(A)** Lipoma on the lower chest of the same patient removed with a small fusiform excision. **(B)** The dead space was closed and wound edges approximated and everted with 4-0 vicryl sutures. Polypropylene simple interrupted (4-0) sutures were placed to precisely align the epidermal wound edges. Skin sutures were removed after two weeks.

Figure 13 Digital mucous cyst excision and simple repair. **(A)** Translucent papule on dorsal distal phalanx causing a depression in the nail plate. **(B)** Defect after triangular excision, expression of gelatinous material, and electrical destruction of base. **(C)** Defect repaired with 6-0 polypropylene (Prolene) simple interrupted sutures. The sutures were removed after two weeks.

slight eversion of the wound edges with added hemostasis by providing adequate wound margin tension.

In some cases, an intermediate layered closure may be preferable if there is a significant dead space left or if there is a depression noted after removing the cyst or lipoma. Likewise, if the cyst or lipoma is removed with a punch instrument or a fusiform excision, a single layer closure aided by vertical mattress sutures can be employed (Fig. 11).

Alternatively, an intermediate repair can be performed using subcuticular interrupted sutures to close the dead space in a layered fashion (Fig. 12).

Simple repairs can be used to close defects after digital mucous cyst excision. These most commonly occur on the dorsal surface of the distal phalanx of the finger. These cysts do not have an epithelial lining and drain clear gelatinous material when punctured. The etiology of digital mucous cyst is controversial, with some authors believing they are degenerative in origin while others believe they extend from the distal interphalangeal joint space. One treatment approach is to (i) make a small triangular excision overlying the cyst, (ii) express the gelatinous contents, and (iii) use electrical destruction at the base of the cyst cavity to cause localized fibrosis and scarring that will disrupt any connection with the adjacent joint space that may exist. The defect is subsequently closed with simple interrupted sutures. These should be placed with a wide bite to allow for approximation of underlying tissues (Fig. 13).

SIMPLE REPAIR WITH PURSESTRING SUTURES

The purpose of the pursestring suture is to reduce the size of the wound and it has been used by many surgical specialties for a diverse range of applications. Brady et al. reported the pursestring closure as adjunct to full-thickness skin grafting for facial reconstruction. Greenbaum and Radonich reported the pursestring closure as a single method for simple closure of round and oval defects. It is particularly useful on the dorsal hand or foot for repairing round defects where preserving optimal mobility and function of the hand/foot and fingers/toes is important. In these areas of high movement and tension, the pursestring (i) allows complete or partial closure of the wound, (ii) distributes tension in all directions, and (iii) lessens or eliminates the need for removing redundant tissue in completing the repair. It can also be used on the head and neck, trunk and extremities.

The traditional pursestring is constructed by running the suture intradermally. With the intradermal pursestring, a suture of appropriately sized polypropylene (Prolene) enters the wound from the skin surface and exits through the mid-dermis. Subcuticular undermining can be used prior to suture placement to enhance tissue movement. Note that on sun-damaged or thin skin, undermining is often not needed. Continuous horizontal loops of intradermal suture are made, with appropriate escape loops placed at intervals around the wound. Near the original entry point, the suture is again passed through the skin surface. Both suture ends are then pulled tightly to reduce the wound size as much as possible without distorting the surrounding tissue (Fig. 14).

A number of variations modifications on the pursestring closure have been reported. For example, a traditional intradermal pursestring can be used to reduce the defect size. The remaining defect can then be closed in side-to-side fashion with a vertical mattress suture, simple interrupted sutures, intradermal vertical mattress sutures, or a combination. Note that in some of these cases (e.g., with multiple layers or extensive undermining), the closure is no longer "simple" and is classified as intermediate. A second simple modification is to use an absorbable 2-0 Monocryl intradermal pursestring to reduce the defect size. This may be followed by side-to-side closure with intradermal buried vertical mattress sutures.

For atrophic skin without significant dermal substance, the tissue may not support the tension of a traditional dermal pursestring. Several modifications can

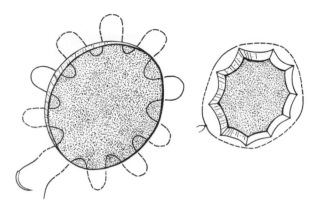

Figure 14 Pursestring suture. To facilitate removal of the pursestring suture, escape loops are placed at appropriate intervals (*left*) so that when the suture is pulled tightly to reduce the overall size of the wound (*right*), it can still be easily removed. *Source*: From Stasko (1994).

be used. One modification can be performed beginning with a 3-0 Monocryl suture at the interior dermal edge of the wound and placing it transversely through the dermis to exit through the epidermis approximately 1 cm back from the wound edge. The suture is then reintroduced through the same epidermal puncture site from which it exits and is woven back through the dermis transversely to exit on the interior of the wound. This technique is continued around the entire perimeter of the wound, with the final knot being tied internal to the wound. Because the suture exits and reenters through the same epidermal site, the final outcome is a fully buried suture with maximal dermal substance to anchor on. The remaining defect can be left to granulate or closed side-to-side with buried vertical mattress sutures (e.g., with 3-0 Monocryl). Initially, wound edge pleating may be substantial, but at several months the wounds are typically well-healed with resolution of the pleating and minimal scar spreading. The pursestring may also be performed in a running interrupted fashion. This is also useful when the dermis is weaker or thin (e.g., sun-damaged skin of the dorsal hand). As with the traditional intradermal pursestring, a suture of appropriately sized polypropylene (Prolene) enters the wound from the skin surface and exits through the deep dermis into the subcutis. Continuous vertical loops of interrupted suture are made. Near the original entry point, the suture is again passed through the skin surface (Fig. 15). Both suture ends are then pulled tightly to reduce the wound size as much as possible without creating excessive tension that could strangulate the tissue. The defect may close completely (Fig. 16). If there is a remaining defect, the wound may be allowed to heal by second intention (Chapter 52) or a full or split thickness skin graft may be used (Chapter 57). If wound edges are closely approximated with the pursestring, subcuticular absorbable interrupted sutures can be added to approximate the wound edges and relieve tension. Simple interrupted sutures can also be used to approximate wound edges (Fig. 15C). The pursestring is left in place for two to three weeks. Initially, for the two modifications used on atrophic skin described above, wound edge pleating may be substantial, but at several months, the wounds are typically well-healed with resolution of the pleating and minimal scar spreading. It should be emphasized, however, that on thick skin in areas of minimal tissue movement (e.g., undamaged skin on upper extremities, trunk) pleating

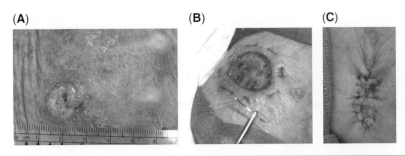

Figure 15 Keratoacanthoma excision and simple repair with pursestring suture. **(A)** Keratoacanthoma situated on the dorsal hand of an elderly man with sun-damaged thin skin. **(B)** After the lesion is excised, a 3–0 polypropylene suture is placed in a running interrupted pursestring fashion. Because the skin was significantly atrophied, the intradermal pursestring technique was not employed. **(C)** After the defect is brought together and the pursestring tied, simple interrupted sutures are placed to finish the closure and approximate wound edges. In this case sutures were removed after three weeks.

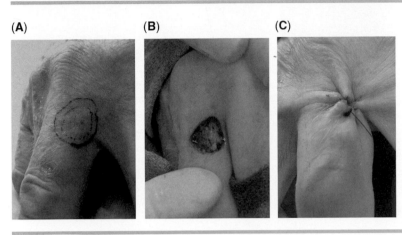

Figure 16 Squamous cell carcinoma excision and simple repair with pursestring suture. **(A)** Invasive squamous cell carcinoma located on the proximal third finger of an elderly man. The tumor is marked and excised with a 3 to 4 mm margin. **(B)** The defect is roughly oval. **(C)** The defect is repaired with a single, 3–0 polypropylene simple interrupted pursestring suture. No redundant tissue was removed. In this case sutures were removed after three weeks.

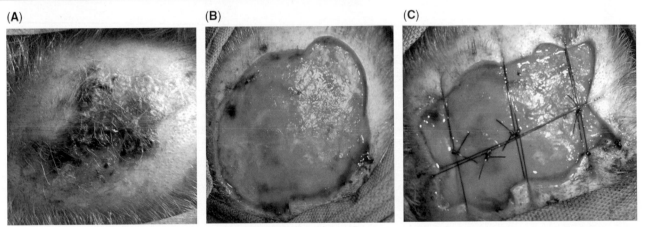

Figure 17 Partial repair of large scalp defect. **(A)** Basal cell carcinoma involving large area of the scalp. **(B)** Defect after Mohs micrographic surgery. **(C)** Defect partially closed with 0 Prolene simple interrupted sutures. The sutures were removed after three weeks.

or rugae may be permanent and leave a scar that is cosmetically unacceptable.

SIMPLE PARTIAL CLOSURES

In some situations, it is not possible, practical, and/or necessary to completely close a surgical defect for a variety of reasons. In 1981 Albright (5) initially reported the concept of guiding sutures to promote wound healing. The placement of guiding sutures across large defects is a fast and simple technique that promotes more optimal wound contraction with significant reduction in defect size. This can improve the final surgical result especially around cosmetically and functionally important structures. Strategically placed sutures may guide the direction of healing, increase laxity in a chosen tissue plane, and counteract unwanted contractile distortion (Chapter 10). Situations when use of simple

partial closures can be helpful include (i) large surgical defects when flap or graft reconstruction is not a preferred or possible option, (ii) aggressive or recurrent tumors when close monitoring of the surgical site is critical, (iii) when delayed grafting is planned, and (iv) when the patient is unable to undergo additional long surgical procedures.

Guiding sutures can be placed across the defect using simple interrupted epidermal sutures of high tensile strength that are removed at two to four weeks, as originally advocated by Albright (Figs. 17 and 18). Alternatively, Walling et al. reported a preference for placing intradermal absorbable sutures that have the advantage of providing ongoing tensile strength without the risk of cross-hatching at the epidermal surface. A combination of intradermal and superficial simple interrupted sutures can also be used, although the closure is then classified as an intermediate partial closure.

(A)   **(B)**

(C)   **(D)**

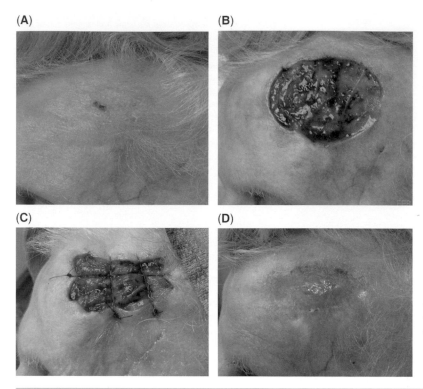

Figure 18 Partial repair of larger defect on the lateral forehead and temple using orienting sutures. **(A)** Recurrent fibrosing basal cell carcinoma on the lateral forehead and temple. **(B)** Defect after Mohs micrographic surgery. **(C)** Defect partially closed in a horizontal orientation with 0 Prolene simple interrupted sutures. **(D)** The sutures were removed after three weeks.

A variety of other suturing techniques can be employed to achieve partial wound closure (see also Chapter 18). These modified sutures provide added mechanical advantage and can be used alone or in combination with simple interrupted, vertical mattress, or pursestring sutures to facilitate partial wound closure (e.g., Fig. 19).

When using a vertical mattress suture to add strength to the wound closure, a small modification may provide a mechanical advantage. After completing, but not tying, the knot of the vertical mattress suture, the suture is looped back through the external loop on the opposite side of the incision and pulled across before being tied normally. This maneuver allows the new loop to function as a pulley that places less tension on each of the other strands (Fig. 20). Another modification that allows for similar mechanical advantage is the "far-near," "near-far" suture. The double loops of suture are produced by placing the first loop of suture 4 to 6 mm from one wound edge, but exiting only 1 to 2 mm on the opposite side. The suture is then looped again across the incision line, and a "near" suture is placed, followed by a "far" suture on the opposite side. This suturing technique also creates a pulley effect as it is tied across the wound (Fig. 21). Both techniques allow greater stretch of the wound edges, but these must not be stretched to the point of vascular compromise. One or two pulley sutures can be placed to begin approximation of the wound.

(A)   **(B)**   **(C)**

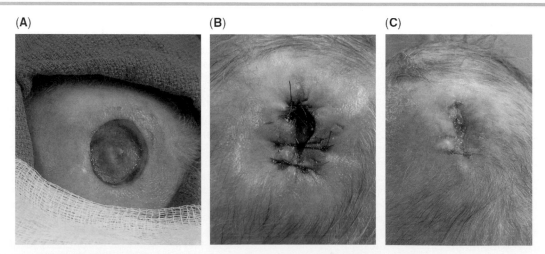

Figure 19 Partial repair of scalp defect. **(A)** Round defect after excision of an ulcerated hemangioma from the vertex scalp of an elderly man. **(B)** Partial closure of the defect under tension using a combination of 2-0 and 3-0 polypropylene pulley sutures, vertical mattress sutures, and simple interrupted sutures. **(C)** Defect after suture removal after two weeks.

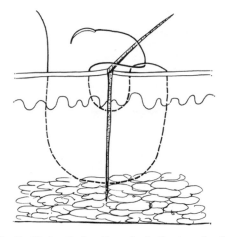

Figure 20 Modified vertical mattress "pulley" suture. A pulley effect is created by looping the suture back through the external loop on the opposite side. *Source*: From Stasko (1994).

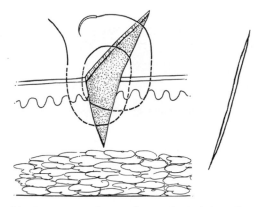

Figure 21 Far-near, near-far, or pulley suturing technique. *Source*: From Stasko (1994).

Skin Tapes

Skin tapes can be used to enhance simple repairs. Microporous surgical adhesive tapes are made of a porous backing coated with a pressure-sensitive adhesive. Some (e.g., Steri-strips, 3M Corp.) are reinforced with polyester filaments for added strength. Sterile skin tapes may be used to complement some wound closures (e.g., Fig. 4D). They are used in conjunction with subcuticular sutures, skin sutures, or glue. By themselves, they stick unreliably and cannot always be depended on for sutureless closure. However, they can decrease the number of sutures needed and can decrease tension on sutured skin in areas of motion. They can be used to tack down the untied ends of a suture or hold them out of a mouth, nose, or eye. While they are easy to apply and leave no skin marks, they do not evert wound edges and may loosen when wet. Prior to application, skin oil and fluid should be removed. When using Steri-strips, it is useful to paint the area with a skin adhesive such as mastisol to facilitate adhesion.

In bearded areas the strips will shed as the hair grows. They may slip with wound bleeding and they can be pulled off accidentally, especially by children. When applied over the full length of a sutured wound, they provide a semiocclusive environment that enhances wound epithelialization in the first 48 to 72 hours. Tapes can be used for wound support after suture removal, allowing earlier removal of skin sutures and providing support to the wound edge while it continues to heal.

Removal of skin tapes should be done carefully by advancing each end of the tape toward the incision line. The two free ends are then pulled directly upward from the wound.

Skin Staples

Staples can be used for simple repairs, especially on the scalp. For example, an ideal situation for skin staples is to close linear incisions under little or no tension after incisional cyst excision on hair-bearing areas of the scalp. Another application is the closure of scalp lacerations. Staples are composed of stainless steel, which has been shown to be less reactive than traditional suturing material. In hair-bearing skin, staples offer the advantage of having no knots to catch hair. Thus it is often not necessary to shave

hair from the surrounding surgical site. Staples can be placed more quickly than sutures, but staples are more expensive than traditional sutures.

Because of the concern over final cosmetic result, skin staples have been used primarily to close scalp wounds. It is worth noting that staples should not be used as a simple repair of wounds that are deep, gaping, or under excessive tension. In these cases, buried sutures are used to take up the tension and approximate the wound before staples can be used. If subcutaneous sutures do not properly oppose the wound edges, skin staples cannot correct this well. Because staples provide tension without completely encircling the wound edge, blood supply is preserved along the wound edges. Removal of staples is generally less painful than removing larger sutures. Staples used on the scalp for simple closures should be removed after two to three weeks.

Glue

For wounds under minimal tension, skin glue can be used for simple repairs. The use of tissue adhesives in dermatologic surgery is still evolving. Use of surgical adhesives can simplify skin closure without the need for local anesthesia, allow patients not to return for suture removal, and can provide cosmetically acceptable results. Several adhesives have been developed to facilitate wound closure. One substance, cyanoacrylate, has been used for 25 years; it easily forms a strong flexible bond. In some forms, it can induce a substantial inflammatory reaction if implanted subcutaneously. If used superficially on the epidermal surface, little problem with inflammation occurs.

There have been reports suggesting acceptable cosmetic outcomes of wounds closed with tissue adhesives in repair of simple lacerations and surgical incisions under low tension. Octyl-2-cyanoacrylate (Dermabond, Ethicon, Somerville, New Jersey, U.S.A.) is the only cyanoacrylate tissue adhesive approved by the U.S. Food and Drug Administration for superficial skin closure. Octyl-2-cyanoacrylate should only be used for superficial skin closure under minimal tension (Fig. 22), and it should not be implanted subcutaneously. For wounds under tension, subcutaneous sutures should be used to take the tension off the skin edges prior to applying the octyl-2-cyanoacrylate. Subcutaneous suture placement will aid in everting the skin edges and minimize the chances of deposition of cyanoacrylate into the

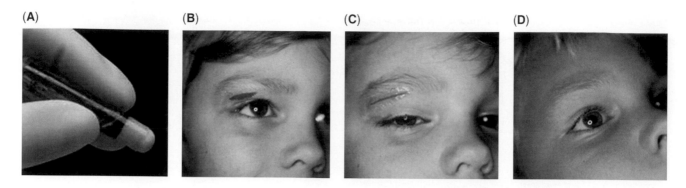

Figure 22 Simple repairs with octyl-2-cyanoacrylate (Dermabond). (**A**) Dermabond topical liquid skin adhesive applicator. (**B**) Laceration to lower eyebrow. (**C**) Closed with Dermabond adhesive. (**D**) Three months after treatment with adhesive. *Source*: From Stasko (1994).

subcutaneous tissues. A study by Bernard et. al. (8) showed that for excisional wounds under tension in children and adolescents, the cosmetic outcome was significantly better in those treated with conventional sutures. A trend toward more hypertrophic scars was seen in the tissue adhesive group. Therefore, the use of octyl-2-cyanoacrylate for closure of wounds under higher tension should be appropriately limited, as octyl-2-cyanoacrylate only just approaches the tensile strength of a 5-0 suture.

REMOVAL OF SKIN SUTURES FOR SIMPLE REPAIRS

The timing of suture removal is important to the final functional and cosmetic result. If done too early, the wound may dehisce. If done too late, suture marks may result. The probability of suture marks is dependent primarily on suture size, tension, and the time left in place. These considerations are particularly important following simple repairs because a single layer of skin sutures provides the majority of tension that holds the defect together. In many instances, it is necessary to remove sutures at longer intervals after simple repairs compared to when layered closures are performed. The surgeon should inspect the wound at an appropriate follow-up interval and remove all or alternate sutures. If ischemia or excessive swelling is occurring in the local area of suture placement, the suture should be removed. Generally, minimizing the time the suture is left in place improves cosmetic result. If sutures are left in place more than seven days, especially on the face, they are apt to leave permanent marks and epithelialized tracks may form around them. However, if extremely small diameter sutures are used under very little or no tension (e.g., 7-0 nylon), they may be left in place longer without adverse cosmetic outcome, For most wounds under minimal tension, at seven days the edges of the incision should be slightly raised in a healing ridge that extends about 1 mm from the incision line. The surgeon can then confidently remove sutures without risk of dehiscence. However, when the defect is closed by simple repair under tension (e.g., pursestring closure or partial wound closure), it is often necessary to leave sutures in place longer (e.g., two to three weeks).

In general, early removal of sutures is possible in those areas of the body with excellent blood supply and more rapid healing of wounds. Wounds under more tension may require that sutures be left in longer to prevent widening of the scar. As noted previously, skin tapes can be used for continued wound support after suture removal.

ACKNOWLEDGMENTS

We wish to thank Steven Q. Wang, M.D. and Jeffrey Squires, M.D. for providing some of the clinical photographs.

BIBLIOGRAPHY

Albright SD 3rd. Placement of guiding sutures to counteract undesirable retraction of tissues in and around functionally and cosmetically important structures. J Dermatol Surg Oncol 1981; 7(6):446–449.

Bennett RG. Fundamentals of Cutaneous Surgery. St. Louis: The C.V. Mosby Company, 1988.

Bernard L, Doyle J, et al. A prospective comparison of octyl cyanoacrylate tissue adhesive (dermabond) and suture for the closure of excisional wounds in children and adolescents. Arch Dermatol 2001; 137(9):1177–1180.

Bernstein G. The far-near/near-far suture. J Dermatol Surg Oncol 1985; 11(5):470.

Brady JG, Grande DJ, et al. The purse-string suture in facial reconstruction. J Dermatol Surg Oncol 1992; 18(9):812–816.

Bruns TB, Worthington JM. Using tissue adhesive for wound repair: a practical guide to dermabond. Am Fam Physician 2000; 61(5):1383–1388.

Coldiron BM. Closure of wounds under tension. The horizontal mattress suture. Arch Dermatol 1989; 125(9):1189–1190.

Fish F. Incisional Surgery. Dermatologic Surgery. Ratz J, ed. Philadelphia: Lippincott-Raven, 1998:127–137.

Gabel EA, Jimenez GP, et al. Performance comparison of nylon and an absorbable suture material (Polyglactin 910) in the closure of punch biopsy sites. Dermatol Surg 2000; 26(8):750–752; discussion 752–753.

Greenbaum SS, Radonich MA. The purse-string closure. Dermatol Surg 1996; 22(12):1054–1056.

Harrington AC, Montemarano A, et al. Variations of the pursestring suture in skin cancer reconstruction. Dermatol Surg 1999; 25(4):277–281.

Monheit G. Wound Closure and Suture Technique. Dermatologic Surgery. Ratz J. Philadelphia: Lippincott-Raven, 1998:117–125.

Peled IJ, Zagher U, et al. Purse-string suture for reduction and closure of skin defects. Ann Plast Surg 1985; 14(5): 465–469.

Robinson J. Fundamentals of Skin Biopsy. Chicago: Year Book Medical Publishers, Inc., 1986.

Romiti R, Randle HW. Complete closure by purse-string suture after Moh's micrographic surgery on thin, sun-damaged skin. Dermatol Surg 2002; 28(11):1070–1072.

Stasko T. Advanced Suturing Techniques and Layered Closures. Cutaneous Surgery. Wheeland R, ed. Philadelphia: WB Saunders, 1994:304–317.

Tremolada C, Blandini D, et al. The round block purse-string suture: a simple method to close skin defects with minimal scarring. Plast Reconstr Surg 1997; 100(1):126–131.

Walling HW, Sniezek PJ, et al. Guiding sutures to promote optimal contraction of a large surgical defect prior to delayed grafting. Dermatol Surg 2005; 31(1):109–111.

Weisberg NK, Greenbaum SS. Revisiting the purse-string closure: some new methods and modifications. Dermatol Surg 2003; 29(6):672–676.

Zachary C. Basic Cutaneous Surgery: A Primer in Technique. New York: Churchill Livingstone, 1991:Inc.

18

Suturing Techniques

Clifford Warren Lober
University of South Florida College of Medicine, Tampa, Florida, U.S.A.

INTRODUCTION

The fundamental purpose of using sutures to close wounds is to provide physical support to tissue during the early phases of wound healing. Sutures are used to eliminate dead space in subcutaneous tissues, to minimize tension that causes wound separation, and to coapt opposing edges of the wound gently. Good suturing technique cannot be substituted for basic surgical technique, such as correct wound placement with respect to relaxed skin tension lines and adequate undermining. Other factors, such as the presence of systemic diseases and the selection of suture material, also influence the ultimate surgical outcome. The surgeon must be aware of alternative methods of wound closure that may be used in conjunction with or as a substitute for sutures, such as the use of staples, tape strips, or laser skin "welding."

The specific technique used to close a given wound will depend upon the force and direction of tensions on the wound, the thickness of the tissues to be opposed, and anatomic considerations, such as the presence of vital structures (e.g., eyes) or landmarks (e.g., vermilion border of the lips). Each wound is unique, and the surgeon must use his or her judgment to determine the most advantageous suture technique for each situation.

SQUARE KNOT

The square knot is the fundamental knot used in cutaneous surgery. When properly placed, it will lie flat on the skin surface and maintain its position without slipping. It is relatively easy to construct and may be placed expediently.

To tie a square knot, the surgeon begins by taking out the slack present in the long end to be tied (that to which the needle is attached). The needle holder is then brought across the wound from the opposing shorter end toward the longer end and, with the needle holder in closed position, is looped twice around the long end of suture. The needle holder is then opened slightly, the short end of suture is grasped and pulled through the two loops, and the surgeon crosses his hands across the wound and teases the double loops onto the cutaneous surface. The loops should be placed on the skin surface gently and should not be under significant tension. The needle holder is then released and, in closed position, looped once around the long end of suture. It is then brought across the wound toward the shorter side of suture, which is subsequently grasped and pulled through the loop. The long end of suture will then be on the opposite side of the wound. The single loop is then teased into position on top of the previously placed double loops. This loop should be placed securely and may be used to adjust the tension of the underlying double loops as needed. The needle holder is then released and a second single loop of suture is constructed exactly as the first single loop was performed, except that the surgeon crosses his hands across the wound so that the second single loop will lie flat. This loop should be placed securely to assure that the knot does not slip. The final configuration of the square knot is shown in Figure 1.

It is occasionally necessary to modify the basic surgical square knot. If, for example, significant tension exists where a square knot is placed, it may be necessary to place another single or double loop of suture to secure the knot. Alternatively, many surgeons elect to use only one single loop of suture instead of two loops to secure the initial double loops into position when closing wounds in areas such as the eyelids or genitalia.

SIMPLE INTERRUPTED SUTURE

The simple interrupted suture is the most fundamental technique of wound closure used in cutaneous surgery. It can be used to approximate large amounts of tissue when it is placed widely and deeply or for relatively fine approximation of tissue when it is placed close to wound edges and more superficially. By altering the depth or angle of the needle on one or both sides of a wound, one can use this technique to coapt wound edges of uneven thickness or make adjustments in tension.

To place a simple interrupted suture properly, the needle enters one side of the wound and penetrates well into the deep dermis or subcutaneous tissue (Fig. 2). As the needle goes deeper into the tissue, it veers slightly away from the wound edge so that it encompasses a larger volume of tissue deeper in the wound. The needle is then passed through the subcutaneous tissue to the opposing side of the wound. As it is passed through the opposing ends of the wound, the needle exits closer to the wound edge so that the final configuration of the suture is flask-shaped. A square knot may then be used to secure the suture on the skin surface.

The principal disadvantage of single interrupted sutures is that they tend to leave a series of crosshatched linear scars on the skin surface that resembles railroad tracks. This is minimized by using proper basic surgical technique (e.g., undermining) and subcutaneous sutures to reduce wound tension. Removing sutures as early as possible further lessens scarring. Epidermal cells begin to migrate down suture tracts approximately five days after sutures have been placed.

Interrupted sutures have a tendency to cause wound inversion if they are not placed correctly. Wound inversion is

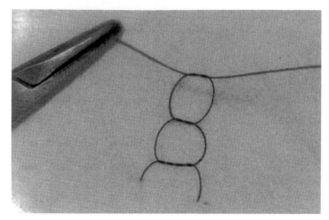

Figure 1 The final configuration of the square knot shows the initial placement of two loops of suture material followed by two single layers of one loop of suture.

usually accentuated when the suture encompasses a larger bulk of tissue close to the epidermis than it does deeper in the dermis (Fig. 3). The suture effectively squeezes the epidermal edges of the wound downward. Wound inversion is minimized by placing suture in the flask-like configuration.

Placing numerous interrupted sutures may be time-consuming when larger wounds are involved. Although small biopsy wounds (2–6 mm) created with circular punches are easily closed with a few interrupted sutures, larger fusiform wounds take significantly longer to close.

VERTICAL MATTRESS SUTURE

Mattress sutures are used to close dead space and provide strong support for wound closure. Vertical mattress suturing is one of the best techniques available to ensure eversion of wound edges and minimize significant wound tension simultaneously. Several vertical mattress sutures can be placed to close dead space, minimize wound tension, and evert the edges of a wound while interrupted sutures are placed in between to ensure finer wound edge approximation and better cosmesis.

Although vertical mattress sutures may be placed anywhere on the body, some surgeons believe that they should not be used on the face, especially when buried sutures are used to close the subcutaneous tissues. Other surgeons avoid the use of buried sutures in the face and favor vertical mattress sutures. Therefore, the use of vertical mattress sutures on the face depends upon the surgeon's preference.

The vertical mattress suture is started 0.5 to 1.0 cm lateral to the wound margin, with the needle inserted toward the depth of the wound to close dead space (Fig. 4). The greater the tension on the wound edge, the wider the insertion of the needle. The needle is then passed through the deep tissue to the opposing wound edge, where it exits the skin on the opposing side equidistant to the insertion. The needle is then reversed in the needle holder, and the skin is penetrated again on the side through which the suture just exited but closer to the wound edge. It is passed more superficially to the opposite side, exiting close to the wound margin. This portion of the vertical mattress suture is usually placed within 1 to 3 mm of the wound edge.

Placing vertical mattress sutures is time-consuming. Both the near and far skin penetrations should be equidistant from opposing wound edges. The wound is then gently teased closed to obliterate dead space and evert the epidermal edges of the wound properly. Improper placement will cause wound inversion, uneven tension, and increasing scarring. Minimal scarring depends primarily on decreased wound tension by using proper surgical technique (e.g., undermining) and removal of the sutures as early as possible, as in the case of single interrupted sutures.

If the wound is under significant tension, it is not always possible to remove vertical mattress sutures early to avoid wound dehiscence. When leaving vertical mattress sutures in the skin for prolonged periods of time, bolsters made of cardboard, rubber, or plastic may be placed between the suture and the skin. This will minimize direct contact of the suture with the epidermis. This contact can cause necrosis when postoperative edema increases pressure on the suture. Sutures can strangulate deeper tissues, especially when under significant tension. Excessive pressure at the depth of the wound may result in ischemic necrosis that is clinically evident as weak points in the healed wound. It is important to emphasize the importance of minimizing wound tension prior to the placement of mattress sutures.

NEAR–FAR VERTICAL MATTRESS SUTURE

The near–far vertical mattress suture is a modification of the standard vertical mattress suture (Fig. 5). Begin near the wound edge (1–3 mm), passing the needle into the deeper aspect of the opposing side, and exit through the epidermis wide to the incision (0.5–1.0 cm). Reverse the needle, and reenter the skin near the wound edge (1–3 mm) of the side just exited, and repeat the same procedure exiting wide to the initial penetration (0.5–1.0 cm). This technique is used primarily when one is trying to elevate the deeper tissues of the wound as well as to evert the epidermis.

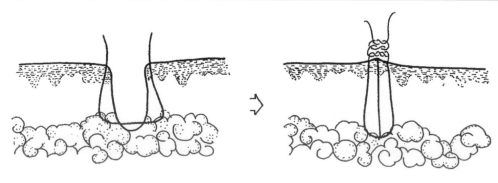

Figure 2 The simple interrupted suture, when properly placed, encompasses a greater bulk of tissue in the depth of the wound than it does more superficially. This results in eversion of the wound edges.

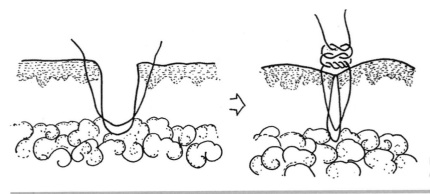

Figure 3 An incorrectly placed simple interrupted suture causes the edges of the wound to invert.

HALF-BURIED VERTICAL MATTRESS SUTURE

This modification of the vertical mattress suture does not cause as much scarring as standard vertical mattress sutures, because it does not penetrate the cutaneous surface on one side of the wound. However, it is also not capable of relieving as much wound tension as a standard vertical mattress suture. Nevertheless, it usually closes more dead space and is stronger than a single interrupted suture. It is particularly useful in areas such as the face and along hairlines where suture marks can be camouflaged by hair.

The placement of a half-buried vertical mattress suture is similar to that of a vertical mattress suture, except that instead of exiting the wound on the opposing side, the needle is passed through the deeper tissue and exits the wound on the side of initial entry only (Fig. 6). Therefore, suture material does not contact the skin surface on one side of the wound.

HORIZONTAL MATTRESS SUTURE

Horizontal mattress sutures are useful for minimizing wound tension, closing dead space, and facilitating wound edge eversion. This may also provide significant hemostasis but should not be used primarily for this purpose. These sutures are quite useful for the initial placement of larger flaps, especially those that may be under a significant amount of tension. The horizontal mattress suture may be placed prior to using interrupted sutures on a wound edge.

To place a horizontal mattress suture, penetrate the skin 5–10 mm from the edge of the wound (Fig. 7). The needle is then passed dermally or subcutaneously toward the opposing wound edge where it enters at the same level in the subcutaneous or dermal tissue. Exit the opposing wound edge through the epidermis equidistant from the insertion. Reenter the skin on the same side at the same distance from the wound edge but several millimeters laterally.

The needle is then passed dermally or subcutaneously to the side of initial penetration.

As in the case of vertical mattress sutures, horizontal mattress sutures may cause strangulation of underlying tissue if they are placed in wounds subject to excessive tension. Tissue hypoxia and necrosis may result in poor wound healing. Protective bolsters are useful to avoid sutures on the skin surface cutting into the skin in the presence of postoperative edema.

TIP STITCH

The tip stitch is a modification of the horizontal mattress suture in which half of the suture is buried. It is used to secure the tip of skin flaps without compressing the epidermal tissue to avoid ischemic necrosis. In the case of a single flap, the skin is initially penetrated on the side of the wound to which the flap is to be attached (Fig. 8). The needle is passed dermally or subcutaneously toward the flap tip. It penetrates the flap tip of the dermis. The flap tip is gently positioned so that the needle can be passed along the same plane, allowing entry and exit at the same level of the dermis. The needle reenters the attachment site of the skin, still in the same dermal plane. It is passed through the skin and tied.

RUNNING SUTURE

Use of the simple running suture is a rapid way to close wounds in which the opposing edges are of approximately equal thickness and in which little or insignificant tension or dead space exists. It is useful on the eyelids, ears, and the dorsa of the hands or may also be used to secure the edges of a full- or split-thickness skin graft. Running suture may be used in conjunction with subcutaneous sutures in other areas of the body. The primary advantage of the running suture is its relative ease and speed of placement.

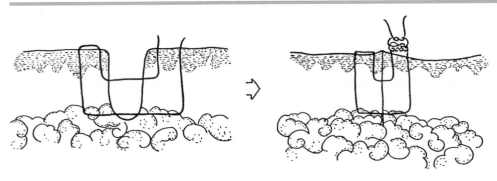

Figure 4 The vertical mattress suture is used to close dead space, thus minimizing wound tension and everting wound edges.

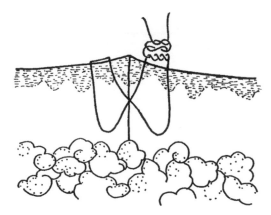

Figure 5 The near–far vertical mattress suture is useful for elevating deeper tissue and closing dead space.

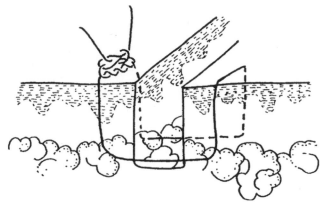

Figure 7 The horizontal mattress suture, like the vertical mattress suture, closes dead space, reduces wound tension, and everts wound edges. *Source: From Swanson (1987).*

The running suture is initiated by placing a simple interrupted suture at one end of the wound. This is tied but not cut. Simple sutures are placed down the length of the wound, repenetrating the epidermis, and passing dermally or subcutaneously (Fig. 9). Tension along the suture must be adjusted continuously so that it is evenly distributed along the length of the wound. It is important to space each interval of the running suture evenly. The suture is terminated by placing a single knot between the suture materials as it exits the skin at the end of the incision with the last loop of suture placed.

Simple running sutures are easily and rapidly placed. However, there is a tendency for the wound to pucker if the skin is thin or excessively loose. Furthermore, it may be difficult to adjust tension using a continuous suture as compared with interrupted sutures.

RUNNING LOCKED SUTURE

This modification of the running suture is useful for wounds closed under a moderate amount of tension or for those with regular thick edges and minimal tendency for inversion. It is particularly useful on the scalp, forehead, and back.

To place the running locked suture, begin in the same manner as for placement of simple running sutures. Instead

of reentering the skin following each loop, the needle is passed through the preceding loop of suture material so that it locks into place (Fig. 10).

The running locked suture is easily and expediently placed. It provides greater strength than the simple running suture but has a greater tendency to cause strangulation of the deeper tissues. It is more difficult to adjust tension along the wound once a locked suture is placed.

RUNNING HORIZONTAL MATTRESS SUTURE

The running horizontal mattress suture enables one to close wounds expediently under a moderate degree of tension. It is basically a modification of the simple running suture. Instead of crossing over the wound prior to reentering the skin, the running horizontal mattress suture is done by reentering the skin on the same side through which the suture material is exited (Fig. 11).

INTERRUPTED SUBCUTANEOUS SUTURE

It is often difficult to avoid closing wounds under significant tension even when proper surgical technique is used. In certain areas of the body, such as the back and lower legs, wounds routinely enlarge due to constant tension on the skin in these areas. It is in these areas that placement of

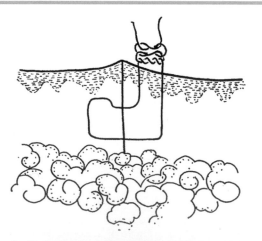

Figure 6 The half-buried vertical mattress suture causes less cutaneous scarring than the standard vertical mattress suture.

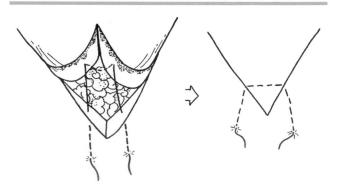

Figure 8 The tip stitch is a modification of the horizontal mattress suture.

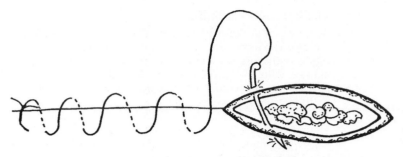

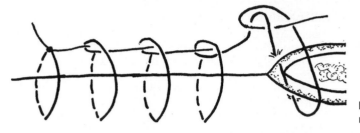

Figure 9 The running suture provides an efficient means of closing wound edges of approximately equal thickness if no significant tension is present.

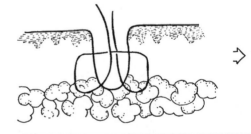

Figure 10 The running locked suture is useful for closing wounds under a moderate amount of tension.

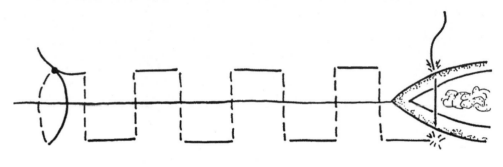

Figure 11 The running horizontal mattress suture is a modification of the horizontal mattress suture.

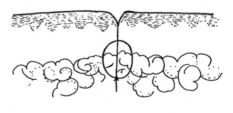

Figure 12 The interrupted subcutaneous suture. It must, almost invariably, be supplemented with cutaneous sutures to approximate and evert the skin surface.

interrupted subcutaneous and dermal sutures is of considerable importance to minimize wound tension.

To place interrupted sutures in the subcutaneous and dermal tissues, the needle is inserted in the undermined wound edges close to the base of the wound (Fig. 12). It is then passed through the dermis and exits the wound edge more superficially. It reenters the opposing side of the wound superficially and is passed to the deeper aspect of the wound at the same level as the opposing side. The suture is tied so that the knot rests in the deepest aspect of the wound. If the knot is present in the upper dermis, the suture material will be absorbed more slowly and there is an increased likelihood that it will be eliminated from the wound (spit).

RUNNING SUBCUTANEOUS SUTURE

Often there is little choice but to place interrupted subcutaneous sutures for large wounds under significant tension. If the wound is relatively narrow and under less tension, a running subcutaneous suture may be sufficient. The primary advantage of a running subcutaneous suture over interrupted sutures is the relatively rapid speed with which it can be placed. The advantage of single interrupted subcutaneous sutures over a running subcutaneous suture is that wound dehiscence following possible suture rupture is less likely.

Begin the running subcutaneous suture similarly to the single interrupted subcutaneous suture. If the wound is deep enough, a running subcutaneous suture may be initiated by placing a single subcutaneous suture with the knot tied towards the wound surface. Instead of the suture being cut, it is looped through the subcutaneous tissue by passing through opposite sides of the wound (Fig. 13). It is tied at the distal aspect of the wound, with the terminal end of the suture to the previous loop placed on the opposing side of the wound.

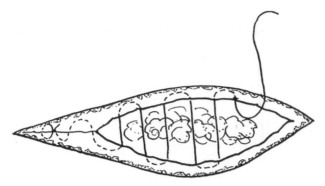

Figure 13 The running subcutaneous suture is used to minimize wound tension and close dead space before cutaneous sutures are placed.

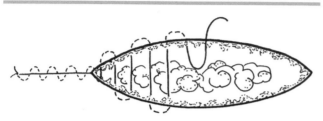

Figure 14 The running subcuticular suture is used to enhance cosmetic results in wounds under virtually no tension.

RUNNING SUBCUTICULAR SUTURE

The running subcuticular suture requires the most finesse. It is used primarily to enhance the cosmetic result and is useful for closing wounds with approximately equal tissue thickness on both sides and in which virtually no tension exists. Generally, the skin edges must already be closely approximated with subcutaneous sutures.

The running subcuticular suture is initiated by placing the needle through one wound edge. The opposite edge may be everted and the needle placed horizontally through the upper dermis.

This is repeated on alternating sides of the wound (Fig. 14). The stitch is terminated similarly to the running subcutaneous suture at the distal end of the wound. Many surgeons, however, prefer to bury the entire suture. If the wound is long, one may elect to bring a loop of the suture through the skin every 1.5 to 2 cm to facilitate suture removal.

One may use either absorbable or nonabsorbable suture material when placing a running subcuticular suture. Absorbable subcuticular sutures may be used in children so that suture removal is avoided. If the sutures are to be left for prolonged periods of time (such as on the back), the surgeon may elect to use a nonabsorbable suture such as nylon.

COMBINATION CLOSURES

Surgeons frequently combine suture techniques to close a wound. The most common example of a combination technique is the use of interrupted or running subcutaneous sutures with interrupted or running sutures on the skin surface. An individual interrupted, vertical, or horizontal mattress suture is particularly useful to adjust tension in one area of a wound or facilitate eversion of a difficult wound edge. Only by becoming familiar with a variety of suture techniques can the cutaneous surgeon achieve optimal functional and cosmetic results.

BIBLIOGRAPHY

Albom MJ. Cutaneous surgery, including Mohs surgery. Moschella SL, Hurley HJ, eds. Dermatology. Philadelphia: WB Saunders, 1992:2314–2402.

Borges AF. Techniques of wound suture. Elective Incisions and Scar Revision. Boston: Little, Brown, 1973:65–76.

Cocke WM Jr., McShane RH, Silverton JS. Suture technique. Essentials of Plastic Surgery. Boston: Little Brown, 1979:17–22.

Converse JM. Plastic surgical technique. In: Reconstructive Plastic Surgery. Philadelphia: WB Saunders, 1977:46–50.

Ethicon, Inc. Suture use. In: Ethicon, Inc., ed. Wound Closure Manual. Sommerville, NJ: Ethicon, Inc., 1985:9–14.

McGregor IA. Technique of wound suture. In: Fundamental Techniques of Plastic Surgery and Their Surgical Applications. New York: Churchill Livingstone, 1975:18–25.

McKinney P, Cunningham BL. Sutures. Handbook of Plastic Surgery. Baltimore: Williams & Wilkins, 1981:19–25.

Nealon TF Jr. Sutures. Fundamental Skills in Surgery. Philadelphia: WB Saunders, 1979:46–54.

Odland PB, Murakami CS. Simple suturing techniques and knot tying. In: Wheeland RG, ed. Cutaneous Surgery. Philadelphia: WB Saunders, 1994:178–188.

Popkin GL, Robins P. Closure of skin wounds. Workshop Manual for Basic Dermatologic Surgery. Kenilworth, NJ: Schering, Inc., 1983:18–36.

Robinson JK. Wound closure by suturing. In: Harahap M, ed. Principles of Dermatologic Plastic Surgery. New York: PMA Publishing Corp., 1988:35–46.

Stegman SJ. Suturing techniques for dermatologic surgery. J Dermatol Surg Oncol 1978; 4:63–68.

Stegman SJ, Tromovitch TA, Glogau RG. Suturing techniques. Basics of Dermatologic Surgery. Chicago: Year Book Medical Publishers, 1982:41–51.

Swanson NA. Atlas of Cutaneous Surgery. Boston, Little, Brown, 1987.

Swanson NA. Basic techniques. Atlas of Cutaneous Surgery. Boston: Little, Brown, 1987:26–49.

Vistnes LM. Basic principles of cutaneous surgery. In: Epstein E, Epstein E Jr., eds. Skin Surgery. Philadelphia: WB Saunders, 1987:51–53.

Zachary CB. Suture techniques. In: Zachary CB, ed. Basic Cutaneous Surgery. New York: Churchill Livingstone, 1991:53–75.

19

Electrosurgery and Electroepilation

Sheldon V. Pollack
University of Toronto, Toronto, Ontario, Canada

Roy C. Grekin
University of California, San Francisco, California, U.S.A.

ELECTROSURGERY

Electrosurgery is one of the most important tools for performing surgery on the skin. This modality provides quick, cost-effective treatment for myriad skin lesions, both benign and malignant. In addition, electrosurgery is used as an adjunct mainly for hemostasis in surgical procedures ranging from simple excision to delicate cosmetic reconstruction.

Simply stated, electrosurgery is the destruction or removal of tissue by electrical energy. This energy, commonly in the form of high-frequency alternating current (AC), is converted to heat as a result of tissue resistance to its passage. The heat generated is passed to the tissue while the active electrode remains "cold" throughout the procedure. This is in marked contrast to electrocautery, in which the tip is heated.

Many electrosurgical devices are available to practitioners, and over the years these have become increasingly sophisticated. A modern electrosurgical unit may generate several different electrical outputs, each with a characteristic waveform for a specific use. Use of the appropriate output allows selective incision, excision, ablation, or coagulation of tissue. If one does not fully understand the capabilities of electrosurgical devices, their efficacy may not be optimized. Moreover, the terminology is often confusing and lacks uniformity.

Historical Aspects

Electrocautery (from the Greek kauterion, branding iron) preceded electrosurgery. For centuries, heated metal was used to cauterize (or burn) tissue to destroy microorganisms and control bleeding. Heating the metal probe was originally accomplished with fire, but later it was done with electricity, thus the term "electrocautery." The metal electrode is heated by resistance to the flow of electric current. Hemostasis can be obtained even in a wet field with electrocautery, but third-degree burns may result, accounting for prolonged healing time and poor scars. It is important to realize that electrocautery with its hot electrode is not considered a form of electrosurgery.

Electrosurgery is performed with a high-frequency current through a cold electrode. Few practitioners actually utilize electrocautery today. Thus, the terms electrocautery and cautery are used inappropriately when referring to modern electrosurgical hemostasis.

In 1892, Arsene d'Arsonval noted that the application of electrical currents with frequencies greater than 10,000 cycles/sec in human subjects failed to cause neuromuscular stimulation and tetanic response. However, heat was produced. In 1899 Oudin, modifying d'Arsonval's equipment, was able to generate tissue sparks that caused superficial tissue destruction. In 1907, deForest developed the triode, a radio tube that amplified and modified electrical output. He was able to make skin incisions when the intensity of the electrical output exceeded 70 W and the frequency surpassed 2 MHz. These innovations paved the way for modern electrosurgery.

Devices

All electrosurgical instruments share certain design features required to produce electrical output suitable for electrosurgery. Power first passes through a transformer that alters the supply voltage. The current then travels through an oscillating circuit that serves to increase the frequency of the current. Finally, it enters the patient circuit.

The major difference between electrosurgical machines is the type of oscillating circuits used. The two main types of oscillating circuits most commonly used employ either a spark gap or solid-state components to increase electrical frequency. Occasionally, thermionic vacuum tubes are used. The output will vary depending on the mode by which it is produced. Some devices, for example, are useful for electrodesiccation but lack cutting current modes.

Older spark gap units such as the Birtcher Hyfrecator, the Sybron Coagulator, the Burton Electricator, and the Cameron-Miller Technicator cannot be used for electrosection. Other units including the Ellman Surgitron, Cameron-Miller 26-0345, Sybron Bantom Bovie, and Birtcher Blentome provide cutting currents by either spark gap or vacuum tube circuits. The Sybron Bovie Specialist, among others, uses solid-state circuitry (in which diodes replace spark gaps and transistors function as vacuum tubes) to produce electrodesiccation, cutting, and coagulating currents.

High-frequency power oscillators used in modern electrosurgical units produce outputs in the low radiofrequency range. They are, in effect, radio transmitters. Electrosurgical circuits differ from radio broadcasting transmitters in that the latter transmit voice- or tone-modified signals. Electrosurgical circuits are not voice-intelligence-modified (modulated). Nonetheless, any radio-frequency transmission has the potential to cause disruptive interference with other radios. Therefore, the frequency range used in electrosurgical units is assigned and regulated in the United States by the Federal Communications Commission and by similar agencies in other countries.

When looking to purchase equipment, one must first decide what function will be required from the electrosurgical unit. In general, the more expensive machines provide a variety of outputs that allow greater flexibility and can perform diverse types of electrosurgery.

How Electrosurgical Devices Work

Spark Gap Units

Electrosurgical devices consist of three major components: (i) the power source (containing one or more transformers), (ii) the oscillating circuit (which increases the frequency), and (iii) the patient circuit (ground plate or handpiece). A transformer consists of two or more coils of wire wound onto or adjacent to each other. Electric current flowing through the first coil will induce the flow of current through the second coil (electromagnetic induction). The voltage (power) of the induced current flowing through the second coil is dependent on the number of loops in the coil. When there are fewer loops of wire on the secondary coil than on the primary coil, the voltage is lowered in direct proportion to the decreased number of turns (step-down transformer). Alternatively, if there are more loops on the secondary coil than the primary coil, the voltage will be raised (step-up transformer). A step-up transformer is used in the spark gap apparatus, while both transformers are used in the tube-type radio-frequency apparatus.

When the voltage has been raised to a suitable level for electrosurgery, it is necessary to increase greatly the frequency (oscillation) of the electric current coming from the wall outlet. This is accomplished by an electric oscillating circuit. A spark gap oscillating circuit consists of condensers (storage areas for electric energy), a small air gap (spark gap), and a transformer (inductance). The condensers (capacitors) become charged by the high-voltage current produced in the secondary coil in the high-voltage transformer. Once fully energized, the condenser releases its electrical energy across the air gap. This has an excitatory effect on the current, causing it to oscillate. Repeated charging and discharging produces a series of damped oscillating wave trains. The current then flows into a transformer (inductance coil) that sustains the oscillations and couples to the patient circuit. A blocking capacitor in the patient circuit prevents the passage of low-frequency utility supply voltage that could result in shock or burn in the event of equipment failure. Radio-frequency voltage to the patient is increased by means of an Oudin step-up transformer in the patient circuit.

Vacuum Tube Units

In vacuum tube units, a thermionic vacuum tube is used to produce oscillations instead of a spark gap. This may be a triode or tetrode tube. To illustrate how vacuum tube units work, the triode tube unit will be used as an example. The triode tube contains a plate (anode), a filament (cathode), and an interposed grid. The power source includes a step-up transformer, a step-down transformer, and a rectifier. The rectifier converts AC to direct current (DC).

Input current is modified, and delivered to both the plate and the filament circuits. In the case of the plate circuit, current first passes through the step-up transformer and rectifier and is delivered as high-voltage, positive direct current. The filament is heated by low-voltage current via the step-down transformer. The high voltage on the plate causes electrons to move toward it. The flow of electrons is

controlled by the grid, which, when negatively charged, prevents this flow in the space between the plate and the filament. A circuit connected between the grid and the filament controls the grid polarity. All of these circuit functions and feedback phenomena combine to generate and sustain high-frequency AC within the oscillating circuit. This current couples into the patient circuit via appropriate capacitive and inductive control elements.

In contrast to spark gap oscillations, the oscillations produced by the vacuum tube circuit are undamped. This is due to the neutralization of internal resistance within the vacuum tube circuit and results in the generation of waves of uniform amplitude. Outputs produced in this manner have qualitative differences from those produced by the spark gap unit and may be modified for electrocoagulation, electrosection, or a combination of both.

Electrosurgical Outputs

Each electrosurgical unit produces its own unique pattern of current flow or waveform. These waveforms can be visualized on the screen of an oscilloscope or traced on an oscillograph (Fig. 1).

Oscillations produced by an electrosurgical apparatus may either be damped or undamped depending on the type of oscillating circuit used. A spark gap generator produces a

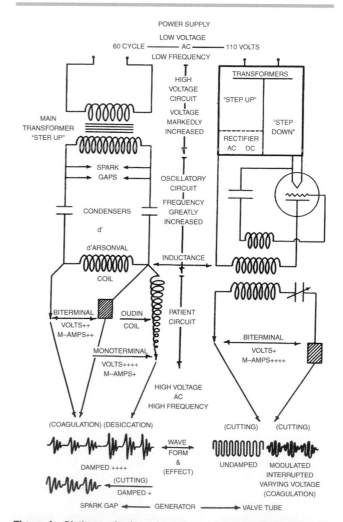

Figure 1   Diathermy circuits and waveforms produced. *Abbreviations*: AC, alternating current; DC, direct current. *Source*: Crumay (1985).

damped wave, which consists of bursts of energy in which successive wave amplitudes gradually return to zero. This is caused by resistance from the gap. As the voltage is lowered, damping decreases and the wave trains occur closer together. Therefore, spark gap generators can be used to provide both damped and relatively undamped output that can be used for a variety of electrosurgical procedures.

Use of a thermionic tube results in a more uniform output. The valve tube circuit is able to neutralize the internal resistance responsible for the damping effect in the spark gap circuit. As a result, the amplitude of the output is unchanged. Depending on the circuitry, the output can be partially rectified (similar to moderately damped) or fully rectified (similar to slightly damped). A filtered, fully rectified output is essentially continuous and uniform, similar to an undamped wave. Different types of waveforms are used for different electrosurgical procedures (Table 1).

Electrosurgical Terminology

Several terms are often misused or poorly understood. The most commonly confused terms are monopolar, bipolar, monoterminal, and biterminal.

Monopolar and Bipolar

Monopolar and bipolar are terms used to denote the number of tissue contact points at the end of the surgical electrode. When the electrode has only one tip projecting from its end, for example, a ball electrode, it is monopolar. If two tips are used with coagulating forceps, the electrode is bipolar.

Monoterminal and Biterminal

Monoterminal and biterminal refer to the number of electrodes used during the procedure. Monoterminal means there is only one connection or electrode from the electrosurgical device delivering current to the patient. Biterminal denotes two connections or electrodes used simultaneously to deliver the current.

When biterminal electrodes are used, the second connection is often an indifferent electrode plugged into the conductive socket of the electrosurgical unit and slipped under the patient. The indifferent electrode is often referred to as a "ground plate." Rather than being a true ground, the indifferent electrode serves to complete an electrical circuit that begins and ends within the electrosurgical unit. The current from the electrosurgical device flows out of the surgical electrode, through the patient, into the indifferent electrode, and directly back to the unit's power generator.

When the indifferent electrode is not used, as in electrodesiccation, the only contact with the patient is with the surgical electrode. This is a monoterminal electrosurgery. Heat energy generated by monoterminal current is concentrated at the site of contact, producing an intense dehydrating effect on tissue. The current may have either a coagulating or volatizing effect on tissue with biterminal electrosurgery.

Clinical Applications

The simplest way to consider clinical applications of electrosurgery is by the three major capabilities of electrosurgical units. These are superficial tissue destruction (electrodesiccation), deep tissue destruction (electrocoagulation), and cutting (electrosection). Most surgical procedures done on the skin require the use of one or more of these three techniques. The objective when destroying or excising skin lesions with electrosurgery is to do so with the least amount of peripheral tissue destruction. Excessive coagulation necrosis will result in increased fibrosis. This is true of electrosurgery as well as cryosurgery or CO_2 laser surgery. Deeper penetration into the skin with a destructive modality will more likely result in an unacceptable scar. Because electrocoagulation destroys tissue more deeply than electrodesiccation, the clinician should know the histologic pathology of the lesion to be removed in order to select the correct current for treatment.

Electrodesiccation

For very superficial lesions, such as those involving the epidermis, electrosurgical destruction by electrodesiccation (from the Latin, desiccare, to dry up) can be done with little, if any, scarring. The damped, high-voltage current generated by spark gap units in a monoterminal (concentrative) fashion is used for electrodesiccation and electrofulguration. Low-amperage output results in superficial damage due to dehydration of the treatment site. If the electrode is held at a slight distance from the tissue, a spark is created from the electrode to the tissue. This technique, termed electrofulguration (from the Latin fulgur, lightning), causes very superficial destruction. This is because carbonized tissue forms an insulating barrier that protects underlying skin.

Electrodesiccation and electrofulguration are the best modalities for superficial tissue destruction. They can be used for the treatment of superficial epidermal lesions such as seborrheic keratoses, actinic keratoses, acrochordons, or plane warts. In addition, it provides hemostasis of small capillary bleeding.

To treat keratoses by this method move the electrode slowly across the surface of smaller lesions or insert it directly into the larger lesions (Fig. 2). At a low-power setting the lesions will bubble after a few seconds as the epidermis separates from the dermis. The lesion is easily removed with a curet or simply by rubbing the site with gauze. Punctate bleeding can usually be controlled with pressure, spot electrocoagulation, or topical hemostatic agents such as aluminum chloride. Extremely small superficial lesions may be treated by fulguration, resulting in minimal adjacent tissue damage.

Local anesthesia (1% or 2% lidocaine) is used, except for small lesions that may be treated without anesthetic. The lesions should be prepared with a nonalcohol-containing skin cleanser such as Hibiclens or povidone-iodine. There is a possibility that alcohol will ignite with electrosurgery.

Table 1 Application of Different Waveforms in Electrosurgery

Modality	Electrodes	Spark gap output	Tube output
Electrodesiccation	Monoterminal	Markedly damped	–
Electrofulguration	Monoterminal	Markedly damped	–
Electrocoagulation	Biterminal	Moderately damped	Partially rectified
Electrosection with coagulation	Biterminal	Slightly damped	Fully rectified
Pure electrosection	Biterminal	Undamped	Filtered, fully rectified

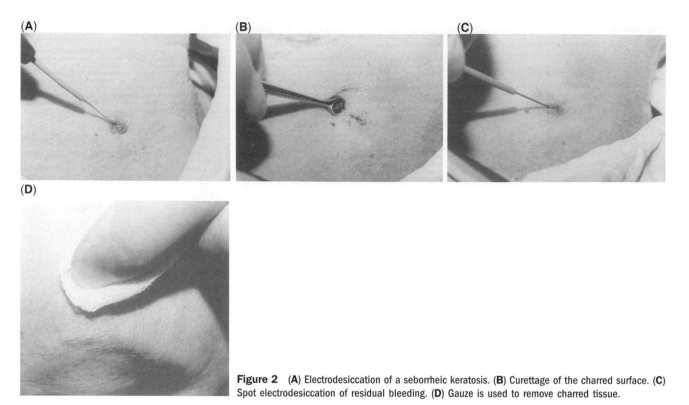

Figure 2 (**A**) Electrodesiccation of a seborrheic keratosis. (**B**) Curettage of the charred surface. (**C**) Spot electrodesiccation of residual bleeding. (**D**) Gauze is used to remove charred tissue.

Standard postoperative wound management is followed. Patients should be warned that delayed bleeding is possible, which can be controlled by constant direct pressure for 20 to 30 minutes. They should also be told that scarring may occur, but this is usually minimal.

Electrocoagulation

Electrocoagulation (from the Latin, coagulare, to curdle) uses a moderately damped (partially rectified) current applied in a biterminal manner with both concentrating and dispersing electrodes. This current has a higher amperage and lower voltage than electrodesiccation. It penetrates more deeply, potentially causing more destruction.

Electrocoagulation is useful for deep tissue destruction and surgical hemostasis. It is used for treating small, primary, uncomplicated basal cell carcinomas and squamous cell carcinomas or benign lesions such as trichoepitheliomas that extend into the dermis. The electrode is applied directly to the tissue and moved slowly across the lesion until it becomes charred. A curet is used to remove the charred tissue. When treating skin cancer, this procedure is repeated three times in an attempt to remove microscopic extensions of the tumor. A small curet is often used during the last pass to remove tiny "roots" of the tumor. Scarring is to be expected and should be considered when discussing therapeutic alternatives with the patient (Fig. 3).

Obtaining hemostasis with electrocoagulation can be achieved with either monopolar or bipolar electrodes. It is important to use a minimal exposure time and the lowest power setting possible because electrosurgical energy may be transmitted several millimeters along the vessel wall; this minimizes delayed bleeding from damaged vessels. Monopolar electrocoagulation can be used by touching the electrode to a hemostat that has been clamped on the severed vessel. For bipolar electrocoagulation, a bipolar forceps may be used to provide more directed, pinpoint hemostasis

(Fig. 4). Electrocoagulating current delivered in this latter manner will cause less adjacent tissue damage but requires a dry operative field to be effective.

Electrosection

Electrosection (cutting) is performed when slightly damped (fully rectified) current is applied in a biterminal fashion. The current has low voltage and high amperage. It vaporizes tissue, causing little lateral heat spread and peripheral tissue damage. Hemostasis and cutting occur simultaneously. The operator may perceive a slight pulsation in the handpiece, denoting a small amount of amplitude variation still present in the waveform. This slightly damped current is responsible for hemostasis.

Pure cutting can be done using an undamped tube current (filtered, fully rectified); this minimizes the amount of lateral heat spread and causes vaporization of tissue without hemostasis. When electrosection is performed using filtered, fully rectified current, spot electrocoagulation can be achieved by changing to the partially rectified current.

Electrosection can be used for electrosurgical excision or incision in an effortless, rapid fashion. Virtually no manual pressure is required by the operator. A narrow straight electrode is used and applied to the tissue in brisk, continuous strokes. The difference between electrosection and an incision with a scalpel is readily apparent. The electrode passes through tissue smoothly, such as a hot knife through butter. If sparking occurs during incision, the power setting is too high; if the electrode drags, the power setting is too low.

Slightly damped currents cause some char at the margins of excised tissue. This can be minimized by the surgeon using smooth, rapid strokes. In addition, vacuum tube units tend to provide outputs that are less destructive to adjacent tissue. However, when a specimen is required for histopathologic analysis, the filtered current should be used

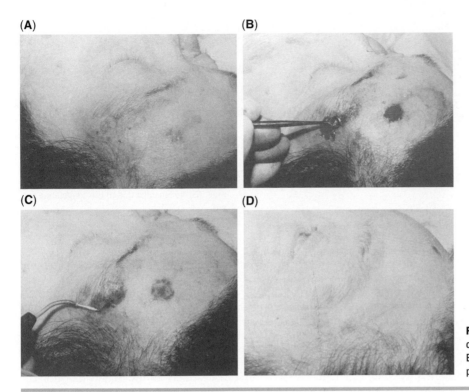

(A) **(B)**

(C) **(D)**

Figure 3 **(A)** Two superficial squamous cell carcinomas on the forehead. **(B)** Curettage. **(C)** Electrocoagulation of treatment sites. **(D)** Hypopigmented scar one-year postoperatively.

because this will not cause significant electrosurgical artifact. The novice in electrosection should develop technical skills by practicing on beefsteak.

The major advantage of electrosection over scalpel surgery is that hemostasis is achieved as the incision is made. However, large-gauge blood vessels (over 2 mm in diameter) may require additional spot electrocoagulation. Training and familiarity with electrosectioning may expand one's use of this technique where scalpel surgery is usually preferred.

Electrosection is extremely useful for relatively bloodless excision of large, bulky lesions such as acne keloidalis

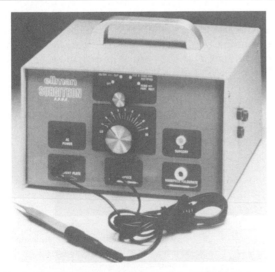

Figure 4 Bipolar forceps attached to the electrosurgical apparatus provides pinpoint hemostasis.

nuchae and rhinophyma, in which the defect is allowed to heal by second intention (Figs. 5 and 6). Electrosurgery has also been used for smaller excisions in which primary closure may be done with no impairment of wound healing. In addition, this modality has been used without complication to create skin flaps, with excellent results.

Potential Hazards of Electrosurgery
Electrosurgery and Cardiac Pacemakers

Fixed rate (asynchronous) pacemakers stimulate the heart at a regular rate, independent of the intrinsic heart rate. They are resistant to external electromagnetic interference such as that caused by electrosurgery. However, in recent years fixed-rate pacemakers have largely been replaced by noncompetitive demand pacemakers, which use a sensor to detect the heart's spontaneous rhythm. Triggered electrical impulses are sent to the heart when the spontaneous rhythm is slower than the preset pacemaker rate. The most commonly used ventricular-inhibited pacemaker is suppressed when impulses from normal ventricular activity are received. If no ventricular activity is detected after a preset interval, it fires at a fixed rate. Because this type of pacemaker is completely inhibited by sensed interference, asystole could occur if a patient has no spontaneous rhythm and electrical interference is prolonged. Because safety factors are built into modern units, including improved shielding and rejection circuits, magnetic and radiofrequency fields rarely cause clinical problems. Nevertheless, electrosurgery is best avoided in particularly unstable cardiac patients and for treatment of skin lesions overlying a pacemaker.

Fire

There is a risk of fire or explosion if electrosurgical procedures are conducted in the presence of alcohol, oxygen, or

(A)

(B)

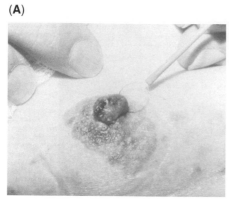
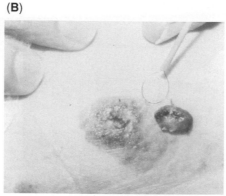

Figure 5 **(A)** Electrosection of an exophytic portion of a seborrheic keratosis with a loop electrode. **(B)** No bleeding due to the coagulating current.

bowel gases (methane). Care should be taken to be certain that the operative site is free of alcohol residue. Oxygen is usually not a problem except in the operating room setting. Bowel gases are highly flammable! Use care in the perianal region.

Microorganism Transmission

The potential exists for transmission of microorganisms either via electrode or via smoke plume inhalation. Neither possibility has been investigated in sufficient depth to yield conclusive results Practitioners should minimize the risk of possible electrode transmission by considering the use of disposable or sterilized electrodes. Adapters are available that allow disposable metal hypodermic needles to be used as electrodes.

With electrosection and extensive electrocoagulation, as with CO_2 laser surgery, a smoke plume is generated. Intact viral particles have been recovered from smoke plumes from both procedures. A smoke evacuator, with the intake held not less than 2 cm from the operative site, is indicated for extensive electrosurgical procedures in which a smoke plume is generated, particularly those involving lesions of viral origin. A variety of smoke evacuation systems are commercially available, and most include viral filters with a filtration to 0.02 μm or less.

ELECTROEPILATION

Dr. C.E. Michel is credited with the first successful use of electricity for the permanent removal of hair. In 1875, he reported the removal of eyelashes in trichiasis using direct (galvanic) current. In the 1920s, Bordier used a high-frequency AC to

remove unwanted hair. This technique was considerably faster and generally replaced galvanic current by the 1940s. Today, depending on the technician and the caliber of hair being treated, either AC or a combination of alternating and DC ("the blend") is used.

The word electrolysis is used by most people as a generic term to mean the electrical destruction of hair, technically, the use of DC for hair removal. Hair destruction with an AC is due to heat and is designated thermolysis. The term "electroepilation" suggested by Richards et al. will be used as the general term for electrical hair removal.

Electroepilation is rarely performed by physicians. However, it remains the most effective modality for permanent removal of unwanted hair. Thus, it is important for the dermatologist to understand electroepilation in order to counsel patients properly.

Electrolysis

Electrolysis is done with DC to create a destructive chemical reaction at the hair root. The negative electrode (anode) is inserted into the hair follicle. The positive electrode (cathode) is a moistened pad held in the patient's hand. When DC is applied, a chemical reaction at the tip of the anode causes the production of sodium hydroxide (lye). The sodium hydroxide acts as a caustic to destroy the hair root. The process is slow and may take from 30 seconds to 1 minute.

Stainless steel needles measuring 0.002–0.005 in. in diameter are used for both electrolysis and thermolysis. The needle tips are rounded to decrease the likelihood of puncturing the hair follicle. Needle length depends on the size of the hair and the area being treated. Insertion of

(A)

(B)

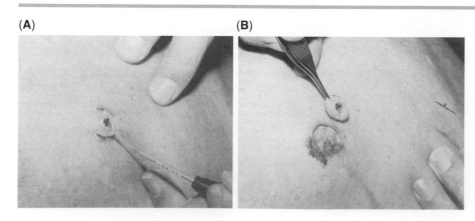

Figure 6 **(A)** Excision of a keratoacanthoma by electrosection. **(B)** The lesion is removed without significant bleeding. There will be some histologic artifact at the base of the lesion due to coagulation.

the needle should be parallel to the hair shaft and is performed under magnification. Excessive force should be avoided so the hair follicle is not punctured. The papilla has been reached when gentle resistance is encountered; the current is then turned on with a foot pedal. Gentle traction is applied to the hair with fine tweezers. When root destruction is complete, the hair may be lifted easily from the follicle.

Electrolysis takes longer than thermolysis. It is said by some technicians to be less painful, less likely to scar, and to result in a higher percentage of permanent hair destruction. However, this is probably technique-dependent and because the technique is so tedious, it has been replaced by thermolysis or the blend.

Thermolysis

Thermolysis relies on heat to cause hair destruction. A high-frequency (13.56 MHz) AC is used. The generated heat is a result of tissue resistance to the flow of current. The current can be applied by the "slow" (manual) technique or the "flash" technique. A lower heat is used over 3 to 10 seconds in the slow technique. Gentle traction of the hair allows the operator to determine when destruction is complete. The flash technique uses a higher heat delivered by a preset timer on the machine for less than one second. Several pulses may be necessary to cause hair root destruction. Theoretically, the flash technique is less painful. Success rates have not been critically evaluated between the two delivery systems.

The technique of needle insertion is the same as for electrolysis. A handheld electrode is not required because the patient is not included in an electrical circuit. The speed of thermolysis allows for treatment of much larger areas over a shorter time period. For this reason, it has replaced electrolysis as the preferred manner of electroepilation.

The Blend

The blend was developed in the 1940s in an attempt to take advantage of attributes of both electrolysis and thermolysis. It was hoped that by combining both currents an apparatus could be developed with the speed of thermolysis and the efficacy of electrolysis. The blend is slower than thermolysis but may offer some advantages in hair root destruction rate, particularly for coarser hairs.

Side Effects

Thermolysis and the blend are more painful than classical electrolysis and the risk of scarring and hair regrowth may be higher. However, highly motivated patients generally tolerate the pain and are treated with 30- to 60-minute sessions once or twice weekly. Recent claims by some manufacturers state that computerization of their electroepilation equipment results in less painful hair removal. A certain amount of energy is required to successfully destroy the hair root, and it is doubtful whether computerized delivery of this energy will lessen the associated pain. Use of Eutectic mixture of local anesthetics (EMLA) topical anesthetic under occlusion for one to two hours pretreatment has decreased the pain in some patients. Some electrologists work with physicians who can perform regional anesthesia for sensitive facial areas.

Scarring is a real risk and is operator-dependent. Generally when this occurs it presents as punctate or icepick-like depressed lesions. In some cases, small hypertrophic papules may be present. Most states do not regulate or certify electrologists. It is, therefore, very important to choose an operator carefully.

Hair regrowth has been reported at between 15% and 50%. This is also technique-dependent. Regrowth may be related in part to the hair cycle. Hairs treated while in telogen phase may not experience root destruction. Some electrologists recommend shaving two days pretreatment so that only actively hairs will be apparent.

There may be varying degrees of erythema and edema shortly after the procedure. Postinflammatory hypo- and hyperpigmentation have been reported. The theoretical risk of infections, both local and systemic, exists, but proper skin cleansing helps prevent this problem. It seems to be idiosyncratic in that some patients are more prone to develop folliculitis than others. Use of an antibacterial cleanser such as chlorhexidine before and after treatment may reduce this risk. Disposable needles are now the norm in the practice of permanent hair removal.

Home Use Devices

Several devices have been marketed for self-electroepilation. Those using tweezers have been found by the Food and Drug Administration to be no more effective than plucking. A handheld electrolysis unit is available. The risk of pitted scarring and pain renders it unsatisfactory as a method of electroepilation, especially when used by unskilled operators.

BIBLIOGRAPHY

Electrosurgery

Bennett RG. Fundamentals of Cutaneous Surgery. Philadelphia: WB Saunders, 1987:553–590.

Blankenship ML. Physical modalities. Electrosurgery, electrocautery, and electrolysis. Int J Dermatol 1979; 18:443–452.

Broughton RS, et al. Electrosurgical fundamentals. J Am Acad Dermatol 1987; 16:862–867.

Crumay HM. Alternating current: electrosurgery. In: Gold-schmidt H, ed. Physical Modalities in Dermatologic Therapy. New York: Springer-Verlag, 1978:203–227.

Crumay HM. Electrosurgery, ultraviolet light therapy, cryosurgery, and hyperbaric oxygen therapy. In: Moschella SL, Hurley HJ, eds. Dermatology. Philadelphia: WB Saunders, 1985.

Jackson R. Basic principles of electrosurgery: a review. Can J Surg 1970; 13:354–361.

Pollack SV. Electrosurgery of the Skin. New York: Churchill-Livingstone, 1991.

Popkin GL. Electrosurgery. In: Epstein E, Epstein E Jr., eds. Skin Surgery. Philadelphia: WB Saunders Co., 1987:164–183.

Sawchuk WS, Weber PJ, Lowy DR, Dzubow LM. Infectious papillomavirus in the vapor of warts treated with carbon dioxide laser or electrocoagulation: detection and protection. J Am Acad Dermatol 1989; 21:41–49.

Sebben JE. Cutaneous Electrosurgery. Chicago: Year Book Medical Publishers Inc., 1989.

Electroepilation

Bordier H. Nouveau traitement de l'hypertrichose par la diathermie. Vie Med (Paris) 1924; 5:561–562.

Hinkel AR, Lind RW. Electrolysis, Thermolysis and the Blend: The Principles and Practice of Permanent Hair Removal. Los Angeles: Arroway Publishers, 1968.

Michel CE. Trichiasis and districhiasis: reflections upon their nature and pathology with a radical method of treatment. St. Louis Cour Med 1879; 1:121–144.

Richards RN, McKenzie MA, Meharg GE. Electroepilation (electrolysis) in hirsutism. J Am Acad Dermatol 1986; 15:693–697.

Wagner RF, Tomich JM, Grande DJ. Electrolysis and thermolysis for permanent hair removal. J Am Acad Dermatol 1985; 12: 441–449.

20

Cryosurgery

Emanuel G. Kuflik
*Department of Medicine, New Jersey Medical School,
Newark, New Jersey, U.S.A.*

INTRODUCTION

Cryosurgery is a versatile method that is used frequently, to one degree or another, by dermatologists for treatment of benign, premalignant, and malignant lesions on all areas of the body. The words cryotherapy and cryosurgery are often used interchangeably; however, the latter is a more accurate description of the destruction that is now attainable with this modality.

The deleterious effects of severe cold on tissue and the benefits from the use of cold as therapy have been well known throughout history. Tissue damage from cold climate conditions was described in ancient manuscripts. This may have led to the well-documented use of cold water and ice application for diverse illnesses and injuries.

Dermatologic cryosurgery began about 100 years ago and has evolved through the use of liquefied air, carbon dioxide, liquid oxygen, nitrous oxide, various refrigerants, and eventually liquid nitrogen (Table 1).

In the early years, eradication of simple cutaneous lesions was all that could be achieved because tissue destruction was limited. The era of modern dermatologic cryosurgery began by the introduction of cryosurgical apparatus that used liquid nitrogen in a closed system. This permitted continuous and rapid extraction of heat from tissue. Two American dermatologists, Douglas Torre and Setrag Zacarian contributed substantially to the further development of cryosurgery. Thus, malignant and benign lesions became amenable to cryosurgical management.

CRYOBIOLOGIC EFFECTS

Cryobiologic alterations are caused by reduction of the tissue temperature and consequent freezing of the tissue. The rate of heat transfer is a function of the temperature difference between the skin and the heat sink (cryogenic agent), resulting in rapid heat flow. The techniques of cryosurgical treatment have evolved from two methods of heat transfer. Boiling heat transfer occurs when the cryogen comes in direct contact with the skin as in the spray and dip-stick techniques. Conduction heat transfer occurs when a cooled metal instrument is applied to the skin.

The mechanisms of injury are related to the direct effects of freezing tissue that results in extracellular and intracellular ice crystal formation, pH changes, thermal shock, and disruption of cell membrane integrity. This is followed by vascular stasis that develops in the tissue after thawing.

The desired destructive effects are achieved by rapid freezing of the target tissue. On the other hand, thawing, or rewarming should proceed slowly. Maximum destructive effects are achieved by repetition of the freeze-thaw cycle. Cryosurgery is capable of relatively selective destruction of tissue by varying the amount of cryogen used, the duration of cooling, and depending on the resistance of particular types of tissues to cold. In benign and shallow lesions, only mild destruction is needed for eradication or improvement. A greater amount of necrosis is required for the successful eradication of malignant lesions, and is achieved by longer duration of freezing and use of deeper temperatures. Predictably, the tissue heals by second intention.

Liquid nitrogen is generally used by dermatologists as it is the coldest cryogenic agent and has the greatest freezing capabilities for all types of lesions. In dermatology, the same hand-held apparatus is used for treatment of benign and malignant lesions (Fig. 1). Depending on the technique chosen, different accessories are available (Fig. 2).

INDICATIONS AND CONTRAINDICATIONS

Cryosurgery can be used as a primary or alternate form of treatment. The indications are related to the nature of the lesion and to the type of patient. There are many lesions and conditions for which it is indicated. While deep cryosurgery can be used for small, medium or large tumors, it is a particularly useful modality for difficult and large tumors. Only lesions with well-delineated margins are indicated for cryosurgery. Several preoperative specimens can be obtained if needed to determine the extent of the tumor. Any area of the body can be treated and the cure rates are high. It is advantageous for patients with a pacemaker, defibrillator, blood coagulopathy, high-risk surgical patient, the very elderly, multiple carcinomas, pregnancy, debilitated patients, those with limited mobility, and for those who are fearful of undergoing surgery. It is suitable when other methods of treatment are impractical or undesirable, and for difficult lesions. Cryosurgery is useful for palliative treatment.

Cryosurgery is safe and simple to perform. It is suitable for office, nursing home, or an out-patient facility and is cost-effective. Depending on the lesion, freezing tissue can be relatively painless. In many instances a local anesthetic is optional. Any discomfort, pain, or stinging is brief and is relieved with analgesics.

Diverse benign and premalignant conditions and lesions are amenable to cryosurgical treatment (Tables 2 and 3). Multiple lesions can be treated either at one or at several visits.

There are few contraindications to the use of cryosurgery. Lesions occurring in high-risk locations, such as the

Table 1 Cryogens Used in Cryosurgery

	Boiling point (°C)
Chlorodifluromethane	−41
Dimethyl ether and propane[a]	−24, −42
Carbon dioxide, solid	−78
Nitrous oxide	−89
Liquid nitrogen	−196

[a]The effective temperatures may vary.

inner canthi and preauricular areas should be examined carefully because of the possibility of deep penetration. Patients with cold sensitivity, cold urticaria, cryofibrinogenemia, or cryoglubulenemia may best be treated by other means. Tumors with indistinct borders are not good candidates for cryosurgery. Deep freezing is generally not recommended for lesions at the margins of the lips, eyebrows, the free margin of the ala nasi, and near the auditory canal as retraction of the tissue can occur. Caution should be observed when treating tumors that overlie nerves that are superficial, such as on the fingers or at the ulnar fossa. Also caution is advisable in patients with darkly pigmented skin. A distinct disadvantage may be a variable degree of hypopigmentation that can be the result of overfreezing or the vagaries of normal tissue response in a particular location or patient. Malignant melanoma is not an indication for cryosurgery. De novo nodular squamous cell carcinoma or other biologically active neoplasms may best be managed by other means.

TECHNIQUES OF TREATMENT

The techniques used fall under the two types of heat transfer that are involved in the use of cryosurgery, namely: boiling heat transfer and conduction heat transfer. The former include the dip-stick, crushed solidified carbon dioxide and acetone, open spray, confined spray, and the closed cone techniques. The latter is the cryoprobe technique that is also known as contact therapy. The selection of the technique to be used rests on the type of lesion and the personal preference of the operator. In general, the spray

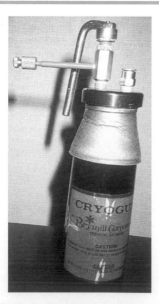

Figure 1 Hand-held cryosurgical unit.

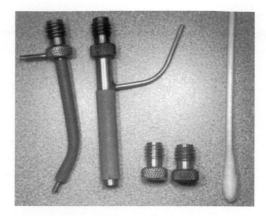

Figure 2 Examples of spray tips, cryoprobes, and cotton-tip applicator.

techniques are more versatile while the cryoprobe has specific indications for use.

Solidified Carbon Dioxide

This is an "old" method; yet, is still effective for acne vulgaris, acne cysts, rosacea, and verrucae planae. It consists of using crushed solidified carbon dioxide, contained in a disposable cloth that is wrapped around a pestle and moistened in acetone. This is then wiped onto the eruption for a light freezing effect. The dry ice can be manufactured in the office by means of the Insta-Ice Dry Ice Machine (Polyfoam Packers Corporation, Wheeling, IL, U.S.A.). This is referred to as a slush treatment, and is effective in reducing the inflammation of comedones, cysts, and erythema as well as reduction of telangiectasia.

Dip Stick

The oldest method is the dip-stick technique and can be used effectively for verrucae, including verruca vulgaris, periungual warts, and filiform warts. This consists of the application of a liquid nitrogen-saturated cotton-tipped swab that is applied to the lesion (Table 4A). The swab can be reinforced by an additional wisp of cotton to provide a reservoir. It is repeatedly dipped into liquid nitrogen, held in a disposable cup, and reapplied until a 2–3-mm ice ball forms around the wart. In the case of filiform warts, it is simply applied to the wart for a few seconds until it turns white; no halo is needed for eradication of the lesion.

The freeze time for verruca vulgaris or periungual warts ranges between 30 and 60 seconds. The development of a blister, sometimes hemorrhagic, is necessary for eradication of the wart and develops after several hours. The blister is caused by separation at the dermal–epidermal junction.

This technique has been used for lentigo, lentigines, and actinic keratoses but is not recommended by the author as the response of the tissue is unreliable and hypopigmentation may result from overfreezing or persistence of the lesion from inadequate freezing.

Spray Techniques

The open-spray method is very versatile and is therefore most frequently used by dermatologists (Table 4B and C). It is suitable for diverse conditions, both benign and malignant. It employs liquid nitrogen, a cryosurgical unit, and spray-tip attachments. The liquid nitrogen is sprayed onto the lesion from a distance of approximately 1–2 cm and the duration of freezing may range between 3 and 60 seconds or longer

Table 2 Benign Conditions Amenable to Cryosurgery

Acne vulgaris, acne cyst	Granuloma annulare	Porokeratosis
Acne keloidalis	Granuloma faciale	Prurigo nodularis
Acquired perforating disorder (Kyrle's disease)	Hemangiomas	Rosacea
Adenoma sebaceum	Keloid	Sarcoidosis
Angiokeratoma	Leishmaniasis	Sebaceous hyperlasia
Cherry angiomas	Lentigines	Seborrheic keratosis
Chondrodermatitis nodularis helices	Lentigo simplex	Syringocystadenoma papilliferum
Chromoblastomycosis	Lichen sclerosus et atrophicus (of vulva)	Syringoma
Clear cell acanthoma	Lupus erythematosus	Trichiasis
Condyloma acuminatum	Lymphangiomas	Trichoepithelioma
Dermatofibroma	Lymphocytoma cutis	Venous lake
Disseminated superficial actinic porokeratosis	Molluscum contagiosum	Verruca vulgaris (including periungual), plantar, plane, filiform
Eccrine poroma	Mucocele	Xanthoma
Elastosis perforans serpiginosa	Myxoid cyst	
Epidermal nevus	Orf	
Erosive adenomatosis of the nipple	Pearly penile papules	

depending on the type, size, and volume of the lesion. Seborrheic keratosis, actinic keratosis, aclinic cheilitis, myxoid cyst, acne cysts, lentigines, verrucae, dermatofibroma, condyloma acuminata, Bowen's disease, basal cell carcinoma, and squamous cell carcinoma are examples of lesions that can be successfully managed. It is particularly useful for superficial, irregular, multiple lesions, and for those on a curved surface.

The confined spray technique employs the liquid nitrogen spray directed into a cone that is held against the skin thereby confining it. The freeze time is similar to the open-spray technique.

The closed cone technique similarly confines the liquid nitrogen spray within a cone that is attached to the unit. It is held against the skin concentrating the liquid nitrogen and rapidly freezing the lesion. The freeze time is approximately one-half of the open-spray technique and therefore should be used cautiously.

The cryoprobe technique, also known as contact therapy, involves the use of a metal probe that is cooled by an internal flow of liquid nitrogen and is firmly applied to the lesion (Table 4D). The probes are available from 1 mm to several centimeters in size. The freeze time can range between 15 and 20 seconds for benign lesions and up to several minutes for malignancies. It is useful for round lesions and those on flat surfaces. Examples of lesions that can be managed advantageously with this technique include venous lake, angioma, dermatofibroma, myxoid cyst, sebaceous hyperplasia, and hemangioma.

TREATMENT FACTORS

In planning treatment, consideration should take into account the characteristics of the lesion, suitability of the treatment, expected outcome, and the esthetic results. In addition, the complexities of the treatment and goals should

Table 3 Premalignant Lesions Amenable to Cryosurgery

Actinic cheilitis
Actinic keratosis
Bowen's disease
Erythroplasia of Quyrat
Keratoacanthoma
Lentigo maligna
Squamous cell carcinoma in situ

be defined. An explanation of the treatment to the patient with the expected response of the tissue, that is, exudation, crusting, reepithelization, and healing time should be given as its course is remarkably different than excision or curettage.

Determination of the adequacy of treatment has been proven through research and experience. When tissue is cooled, surface whiteness and extension of the ice ball is visible but the depth of freezing cannot be visualized. Therefore, the amount of freezing is estimated and this is referred to as the depth dose. The proper depth dose estimation is achieved when the clinical factors coincide for the desired end point. These factors include observation, palpation, freeze time, thaw time, and lateral spread of freeze. The tissue temperature can be monitored through the use of thermocouple-tipped needles inserted into the tissue and registered on a pyrometer (Table 4C). Most tumors do not require monitoring of the tissue temperature as the clinical factors suffice in achieving the depth dose.

Freeze Time

The duration of cooling is referred to as the freeze time. As less necrosis is needed for a benign lesion than for a malignant one, a shorter freeze time suffices. For larger tumors, proportionally longer freeze times are necessary. This can also vary according to the thickness of the lesion and the size of the accessory. The freeze time is longer for the cryoprobe technique than the open spray and shortest with the closed cone technique. The thaw time refers to the duration of thawing of the tissue, which is allowed to occur spontaneously, and is approximately two to three times longer than the freeze time.

The Lateral Spread of Freeze

The lateral spread of freeze refers to the freezing of the tissue beyond the estimated margins of the lesions. For malignancies, it should extend at least 3–5 mm or more beyond the tumor. In the case of verrucae, it should reach 2–3 mm.

Freeze-Thaw Cycle

The actual freezing and subsequent thawing is referred to as a freeze-thaw cycle. A single cycle generally suffices for successful eradication of benign and premalignant

Table 4 Cryosurgical Techniques

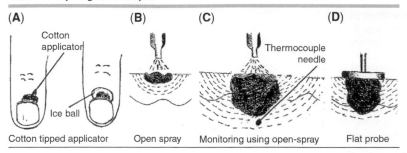

conditions. A double freeze-thaw cycle is recommended for malignant lesions to insure greater lethality.

Tissue Temperature

Measurement of the tissue temperature is used to supplement the clinical factors in the determination of the depth dose. This is used only in the treatment of malignancies, particularly for deeper lesions. It is accomplished by a thermocouple-tipped needle inserted below the base of the tumor. As the temperature recorded is highly localized, several needles can be inserted into a large lesion. The recommended temperature for a malignancy is between $-50°C$ and $-60°C$. It is warmer for benign or premalignant lesions.t

TREATMENT

In general, the actual freezing of the lesion depends on the characteristics, location, desired goals, and the chosen technique. Biopsy of a lesion can be performed prior to treatment for confirmation of the diagnosis. If done immediately before treatment, hemostasis should be obtained before freezing.

BENIGN LESIONS

The techniques of treatment that are used for benign lesions include carbon dioxide slush, the cotton-tipped applicator, the open-spray, the open-cone, and the cryoprobe techniques. Different sized spray tips and probes are available. The duration of freezing will vary and may range between 3 and 60 seconds when the open-spray technique is used. With the cryoprobe the freeze time may be two to three

times longer. A single freeze-thaw cycle is generally sufficient but a second cycle can be administered. During treatment, the clinical factors are monitored both visually and with palpation of the ice ball. A local anesthetic can be injected to alleviate discomfort but mostly is not needed. Lidocaine is sometimes injected for the purpose of lifting a lesion away from underlying tissue or nerves that lie superficially. Examples include the treatment of warts or actinic keratosis on the fingers or hands, and certain malignancies located on the head, neck, and scalp.

Acne

Cryotherapy is beneficial for all types of acne through the use of liquid nitrogen spray or carbon dioxide slush therapy. The carbon dioxide slush, after being dipped in acetone is wiped over all affected areas using slight pressure. The open-spray technique can be similarly used on the face, chest, and back. Comedones and papulopustular lesions are lightly frozen to induce resolution. Treatment is administered at three- to eight-week intervals. Cryotherapy is particularly effective for acne cysts, requiring approximately 5–10 seconds of spray depending on the size of the lesions (Figs. 3A–C). It is useful when treatment with isotretinoin is not desirable because of its teratogenic or other side effects. Acne cysts resolve within approximately two to four weeks. Acne keloids respond to freezing or a combination of freezing and intralesional steroid injections.

Dermatofibroma

For dermatofibroma, either the open-spray or the cryoprobe technique can be used (Figs. 4A–C). A local anesthetic is injected and the lesion is deroofed to facilitate freezing,

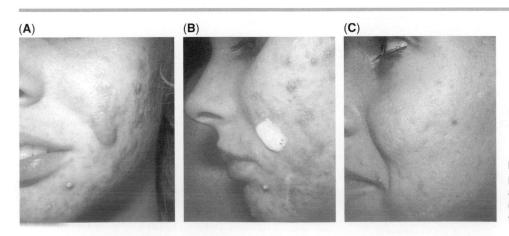

Figure 3 **(A)** Acne cyst on left cheek prior to treatment. **(B)** Acne cyst immediately after treatment with cryosurgery. **(C)** Completely healed 10 months after treatment. (*See color insert.*)

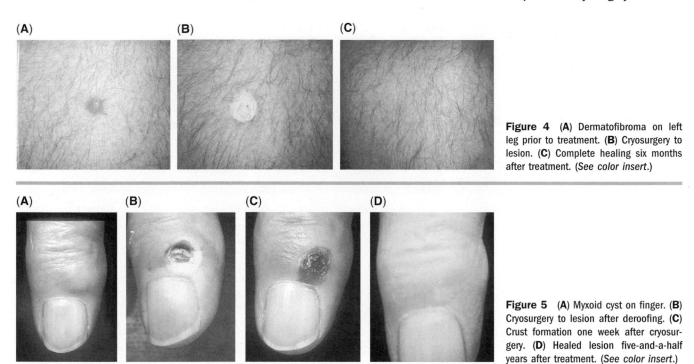

Figure 4 **(A)** Dermatofibroma on left leg prior to treatment. **(B)** Cryosurgery to lesion. **(C)** Complete healing six months after treatment. (*See color insert.*)

Figure 5 **(A)** Myxoid cyst on finger. **(B)** Cryosurgery to lesion after deroofing. **(C)** Crust formation one week after cryosurgery. **(D)** Healed lesion five-and-a-half years after treatment. (*See color insert.*)

while submitting the tissue for a biopsy specimen. The lesion is frozen including a 2–3-mm halo of normal tissue. A crust develops and the healing time is approximately three weeks with excellent results.

Hypertrophic Scar and Keloids
Cryosurgery can be used alone, in combination with surgery or intralesional steroid injections to treat keloids and hypertrophic scars. Either the open-spray, closed-spray, closed cone or cryoprobe technique can be used. The freeze time ranges from 10 to 30 seconds but large keloids require a longer freeze time. More than one treatment is usually needed. In combination therapy, the steroid suspension is injected after thawing of the lesion to prevent freezing of the suspension.

Myxoid Cysts
Myxoid cysts can be easily eradicated yielding excellent cosmetic results (Figs. 5A–D). Following injection of a local anesthetic, the lesion is first deroofed and hemostasis is obtained. Either the open-spray or cryoprobe technique can be used. A single freeze-thaw cycle is sufficient with a

freeze time of 15–20 seconds when using the open-spray technique. Mild edema, bulla formation, and slight pain may occur within 48 hours. The healing time is approximately five weeks. The site heals smoothly and without scarring. In a series of 57 myxoid cysts in 51 patients, the author obtained a cure rate of 76.7%, including several that were retreated.

Venous Lake
The cryoprobe technique is very effective in eradicating venous lakes. An anesthetic is usually not needed. A single-freeze thaw cycle is sufficient, and the freeze time ranges between 15 and 25 seconds. The cosmetic results are excellent, although retreatment can be undertaken if needed (Figs. 6A–C).

Seborrheic Keratoses
The open-spray technique is used and several lesions can easily be treated at one time. Three to ten seconds of freezing is generally effective, although bulky seborrheic keratoses may best be treated by other means to avoid hypopigmentation.

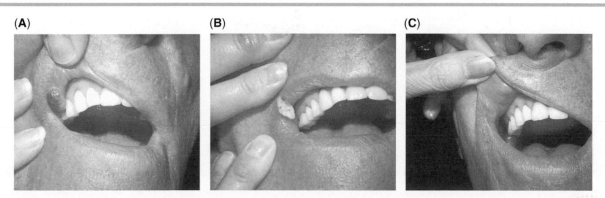

Figure 6 **(A)** Venous lake at right commissure of lips. **(B)** Cryosurgery to lesion. **(C)** Complete healing three-and-a-half weeks after treatment.

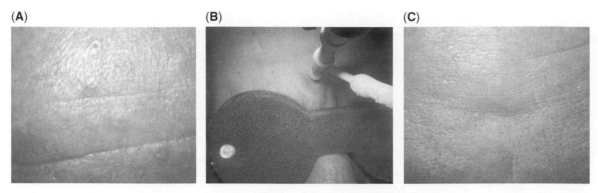

Figure 7   (**A**) Sebaceous hyperplasias on forehead. (**B**) Cryoprobe technique. (**C**) Excellent results nine months after treatment.

Sebaceous Hyperplasia

The cryoprobe technique is very effective in treating sebaceous hyperplasia on the face and no local anesthetic is needed. Small, flat probes are used employing a single freeze-thaw cycle and a freeze time of approximately 10–15 seconds. One treatment usually suffices to flatten the lesions (Figs. 7A–C).

Verrucae and Condyloma Accuminata

Cryosurgery is effective for several types of verrucae and is relatively simple to perform. The dip-stick or the open-spray technique can be used. The author prefers the former for papular verrucae, periungual warts, filiform, and plane warts as this technique enables better control of the lateral spread of freeze and avoids deeper freezing. Formation of a bulla is predictable with the dip-stick technique, which should extend slightly beyond the lesion. Therefore, the lateral spread of freeze should be 2–3 mm beyond the wart

(Figs. 8A–D). The freeze time with the dip-stick technique depends mostly on the size and thickness of the wart but on average is about 45 seconds. The author prefers to have the patient puncture the bulla, which may be hemorrhagic, immediately upon the development of the bulla and again on the following day to relieve discomfort. One treatment generally suffices and healing occurs in approximately three weeks. In the case of recurrence, treatment can be repeated with safety. For large lesions it is best to treat them in sections, with adequate lateral spread of freeze for each section in order to avoid recurrence. Large lesions that encircle the nail are treated in a similar manner; however, caution is advisable against freezing the nail plate (Figs. 9A–D). Warts that extend beneath the nail plate are best treated by other means. Aftercare includes standard washing and analgesics are usually not needed. Healing is generally uneventful and the cosmetic results are excellent. Kuflik reported a cure rate of 97.4% in 80 periungual lesions using the dip-stick technique.

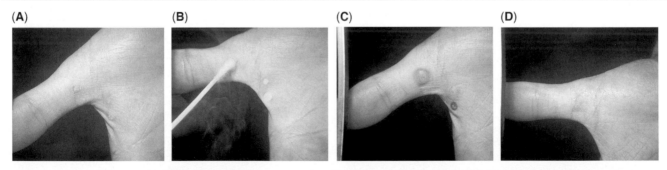

Figure 8   (**A**) Papular wart on thumb. (**B**) Dip-stick technique to several warts. (**C**) Bulla formation after treatment. (**D**) Complete healing four weeks after treatment.

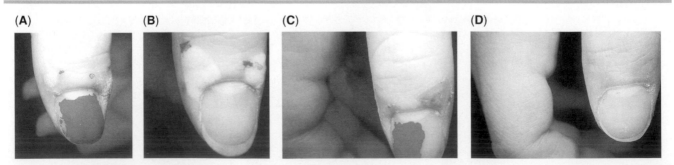

Figure 9   (**A**) Periungual warts prior to treatment. (**B**) Cryosurgery to lesions. (**C**) Healing three weeks after treatment. (**D**) Excellent results four weeks after treatment. (*See color insert*.)

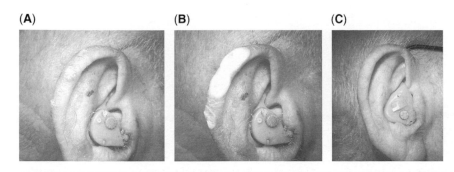

(A) **(B)** **(C)**

Figure 10 **(A)** Actinic keratoses on helix. **(B)** Cryosurgery to lesions. **(C)** Excellent results four years after treatment.

Filiform warts are treated with the cotton-tipped applicator technique without injection of lidocaine. The development of a bulla is to be avoided. The liquid nitrogen is applied to the top of the lesion allowing the freeze to penetrate downward. Removal is not necessary and the cosmetic result is excellent.

Flat warts can be eradicated by light freezing for several seconds with either the cotton-tipped applicator, carbon dioxide slush, or gently with the open-spray technique. Repeated treatments are generally needed. Again, the production of vesicles is to be avoided. The response of treating plantar warts with cryosurgery is not predictable.

Condyloma accuminata can be treated successfully with either the open-spray or the cryoprobe techniques depending on the shape and thickness of the lesion. Periodic freezing is generally needed for large and multiple lesions.

PRECANCEROUS LESIONS
Actinic Keratosis

Eradication of actinic keratosis can be obtained with a single treatment and multiple lesions can be treated (Figs. 10A–C). The open-spray technique is used with a freeze time of four to ten seconds, depending on the size of the lesion, using only a small volume of spray to the lesion. Overfreezing should be avoided to minimize the chance of hypopigmentation. Chiarello reported successful cryopeeling of numerous actinic keratoses and sun-damaged skin of the face and scalp.

Actinic Cheilitis

Cryosurgery is very effective for actinic cheilitis with either the open-spray or closed probe techniques. The freeze time for the former is 15 to 20seconds for an area up to 1 cm, using a single freeze-thaw cycle. Larger lesions are treated in sections. The cosmetic results are excellent (Figs. 11A–C).

Bowen's Disease

The open-spray technique is used with either a single- or double freeze-thaw cycle (Figs. 12A–D). The freeze time can range between 20 to 40 seconds for an area up to 2 cm, and proportionately longer for larger lesions. Lesions can be eradicated in one attempt.

Keratoacanthoma

Cryosurgery is effective for keratoacanthoma and is conducted in a similar manner as for a malignancy.

MALIGNANT LESIONS
Treatment

In the treatment of basal and squamous cell carcinomas, the same volume of tissue should be destroyed that would have been removed by excision if that had been the chosen procedure. This goal is attainable as deep necrosis is possible with cryosurgery. Deep freezing can accomplish destruction of epidermal, dermal, adnexal, and subcutaneous tissue, cartilage, and if needed can be carried into bone. For malignancies, complete destruction should be the goal in one attempt.

Aggressive treatment with one of the spray techniques or cryoprobe technique is used for malignant lesions (Figs. 13–15). The procedure and course of healing should be explained to the patient—especially the tissue response. The target area is cleansed and can be outlined with a skin marker. It is not advisable to drape the site as droplets of liquid nitrogen can accumulate below the drape and may cause inadvertent freezing.

Curettage is often carried out prior to cryosurgery to visualize the extent and depth of the lesion, to obtain a biopsy specimen, or to convert a deep lesion to a shallow one. As a tumor mass can modify the depth of freeze, bulky or fungating lesions can be "debulked" or reduced in size prior to treatment. This facilitates placement of thermocouple needles and freezing can be directed at the invading

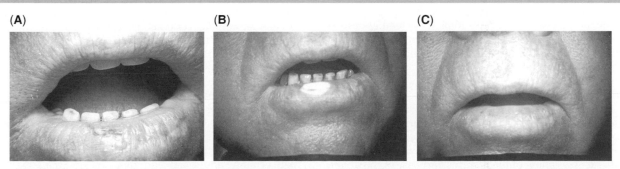

(A) **(B)** **(C)**

Figure 11 **(A)** Small actinic cheilitis on lower lip. **(B)** Cryosurgery to lesion. **(C)** Healed three weeks after treatment. (*See color insert.*)

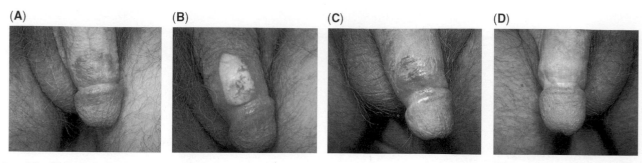

Figure 12 (A) Bowen's disease on penis. (B) Cryosurgery to entire lesion. (C) Healing one week after treatment. (D) Completely healed six months after treatment.

portion or base of the tumor. Hemostasis should be obtained prior to actual freezing.

A local anesthetic can be injected prior to freezing, which can serve two purposes, namely: the anesthetic effect insures that the patient will be comfortable during treatment, and to protect underlying nerves or tissue from the effects of freezing. This is known as "ballooning." Thermocouple needles, if employed, are inserted lateral to the tumor so that the tip of the needle comes to lie beneath the lesion.

The open-spray technique is most frequently used. The spray is emitted from a distance of 1–2 cm from the target site. For the cryoprobe technique, a flat probe is pre-chilled prior to application onto the lesion.

In general, treatment consists of freezing the lesion, allowing it to thaw completely for several minutes, and then subjecting it to a second freeze-thaw cycle. When the depth dose estimation is achieved, freezing of the lesion is halted. The site is allowed to thaw spontaneously without extrinsic warming. When treatment is completed, a dry gauze dressing is applied.

Depth Dose

It is necessary to determine the amount and depth of tissue to be frozen. The depth dose can be estimated clinically whereby the operator palpates the advancement of the ice ball, observes and measures the lateral spread of freeze. This should reach 3–5 mm or greater. The freeze time should be between 45 and 60 seconds with the open-spray technique for a carcinoma measuring up to 1.5 cm. Freezing is undertaken until the proper depth dose is achieved; that is, at the point when the freeze time, lateral spread of freeze, and clinical observations reach the desired end points. Freezing is then halted and the site is permitted to thaw spontaneously for several minutes. A double freeze-thaw cycle is recommended for all malignancies.

To supplement these clinical estimations, one can measure the temperature at the base of the malignancy by use of a thermocouple. The recommended temperature is between $-50°C$ and $-60°C$. As the temperature recorded is highly localized, more than one thermocouple needle may need to be inserted for a large lesion.

Variations in Treatment

A thick or bulky lesion can be reduced to a shallow one with a curette, scissors or electrosurgery, as a tumor mass can modify the depth of freeze (Figs. 16A–F). This is helpful for proper treatment as a tumor mass can hinder the advancement of the ice ball, for assessment of the margins and base of the tumor, and for best placement of thermocouple needles.

A large tumor can be successfully eradicated either by treating it in one session or by dividing it into segments and treating each segment individually. Each section is treated according to its characteristics and depth. Wound healing is not hindered by overlapping treatment at the margins (Figs. 16A–F and 17A–G).

Eyelid tumors are an excellent indication for cryosurgery (Figs. 18A–C). After biopsy, the lesion is treated in the standard manner, although the freeze time might be slightly shorter because of the thinness of the eyelid. The eye should be protected with a shield made of either plastic (Jaeger lid retractor), plastic spoon, or styrofoam. It is advantageous to use cryosurgery for a tumor that lies at the lacrimal punctum because the lacrimal outflow system is not compromised. Shallow lesions at the inner canthi can be treated; however, lesions should be thoroughly examined to determine the depth. Deep lesions or those in which the base is not definable are best treated by other means. Healing of the eyelid occurs within four to five weeks with excellent results. There is little discomfort except for initial periorbital edema. The free margin of the lid heals smoothly with only slight loss of cilia.

Tumors on curved surfaces such as the ears are treated with the open-spray technique (Figs. 19A–D). Attempts should be made to either straighten or evert the site in order to visualize and administer the spray.

Cartilage is rather resistant to freezing. The auditory canal should be protected from inadvertent spray. A lesion on the ear can be "ballooned" with lidocaine and caution should be observed against carrying the freeze into the opposite side of the auricle. Edema of the ear is also to be expected but is temporary.

TISSUE RESPONSE

The response to cryosurgery is predictable but is different for shallow and deep lesions, and for benign and malignant lesions. The reactions that can develop after freezing include erythema, edema, vesiculation, exudation, and sloughing. This is followed by reepitheliazation and healing occurs by second intention.

Shallow lesions require less treatment and therefore there is less tissue reaction, perhaps only slight crusting or vesicle formation. Treatment of deeper lesions will lead to edema, extensive exudation and sloughing, bullae or eschar formation. This also applies to small versus large lesions and whether they are located on the face, trunk, or extremities.

Benign and premalignant lesions generally heal between one-and-a-half and four weeks. Small malignant lesions on the face, eyelids, ears, and neck generally heal

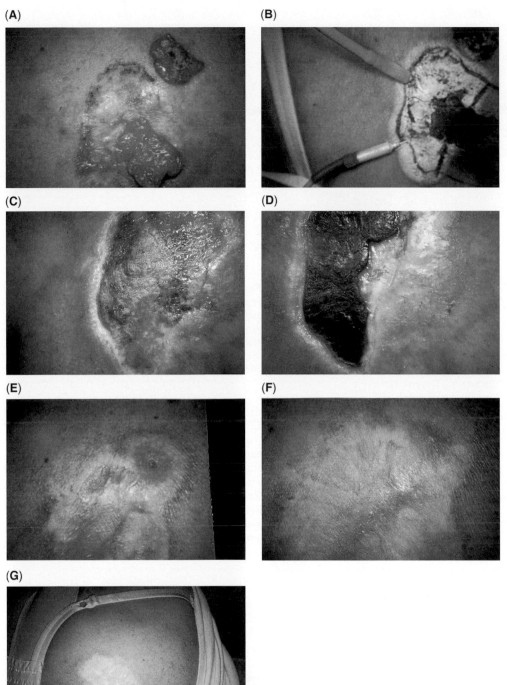

Figure 13 (A) Nine centimeter recurrent basal cell carcinoma on back of 66-year-old woman. (B) Segmental cryosurgery using thermocouple needles. (C) Healing lesions two weeks after treatment. (D) Healing four weeks after treatment. (E) Completely healed nine weeks after treatment. (F) Resolving erythema and hypertrophic scar seven months after treatment. (G) Hypopigmentation two years after treatment. (*See color insert.*)

between four and six weeks. Large tumors and those on the trunk and extremities take longer to heal. As malignant lesions are treated with greater freezing, there is increased tissue reaction that can last up to 14 weeks for complete healing, depending on the size and location of the lesion.

The cosmetic results in some locations are often equal or superior to those achieved by other modalities. There is no keloid formation, and any hypertrophic scarring that may develop improves with time.

AFTERCARE

The postoperative care varies according to the depth of freeze and location. Most benign lesions require little or no aftercare except for normal washing and a dressing. Vesicles formed after treatment of warts can be punctured. For malignancies, washing the site with soap and water four times a day is recommended during the exudative phase. As healing progresses, washing is reduced and light debridment may facilitate healing. One can apply an antibiotic ointment to

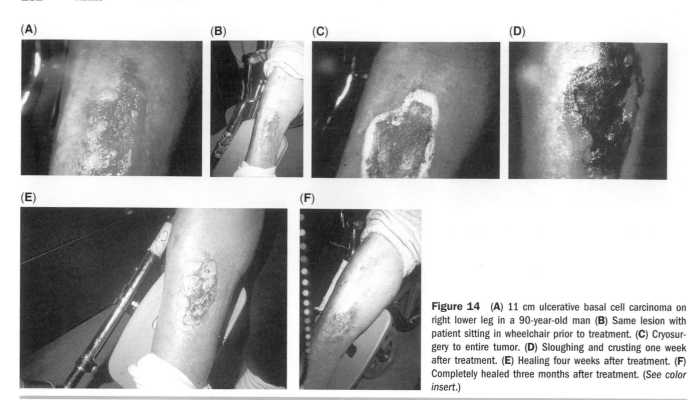

Figure 14 (**A**) 11 cm ulcerative basal cell carcinoma on right lower leg in a 90-year-old man (**B**) Same lesion with patient sitting in wheelchair prior to treatment. (**C**) Cryosurgery to entire tumor. (**D**) Sloughing and crusting one week after treatment. (**E**) Healing four weeks after treatment. (**F**) Completely healed three months after treatment. (*See color insert.*)

reduce eschar formation. Oral antibiotics are beneficial when treating myxoid cysts, ear tumors, and those on the lower legs. A dry gauze dressing is all that is required.

COMPLICATIONS

Complications after cryosurgery are related to the characteristics of the lesion and the depth of freeze, the volume of tissue treated, the technique used, and the experience of the operator. Morbidity is not an actual complication and occurs to a certain degree after freezing tissue. This includes edema, exudation, vesiculation or pain, which are all early reactions (Figs. 20 and 21). Of course, a reaction may be unforeseen or inexplicable. The incidence of true complications after cryosurgery is low. They may arise as an unsatisfactory result, as a greater response to freezing than had been expected, or as an unanticipated event. One should not encounter similar morbidity or complications after treatment of benign lesions as compared with malignant-ones since a lesser amount of freezing is needed to treat benign lesions.

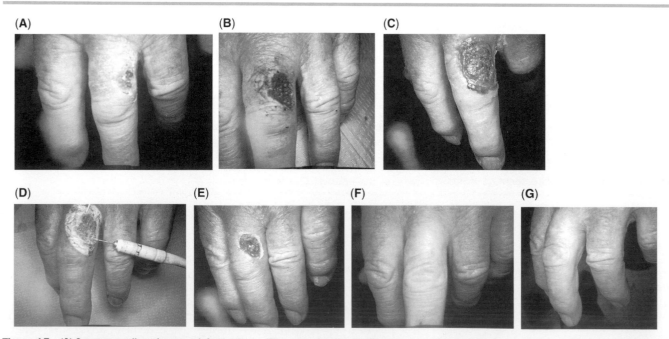

Figure 15 (**A**) Squamous cell carcinoma on left third finger. (**B**) Lesion after biopsy. (**C**) Cryosurgery to lesion with thermocouple needle in place. (**D**) Healing four-and-a-half weeks after treatment. (**E**) Excellent results one year after treatment. (**F**) No evidence of recurrence after five years. (*See color insert.*)

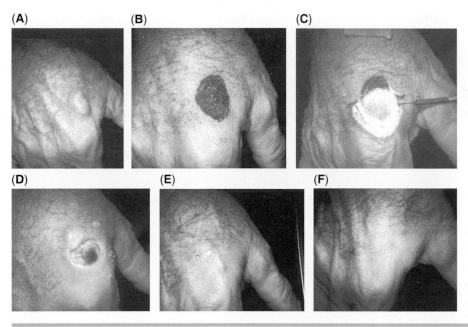

Figure 16 (**A**) Nodular squamous cell carcinoma on dorsum of hand in a 75-year-old man. (**B**) Lesion debulked. (**C**) Cryosurgery to one-half of lesion. (**D**) Healing three weeks after treatment. (**E**) Healed lesion with hypertrophic scar three months after treatment. (**F**) Excellent results one-and-a-half years after treatment.

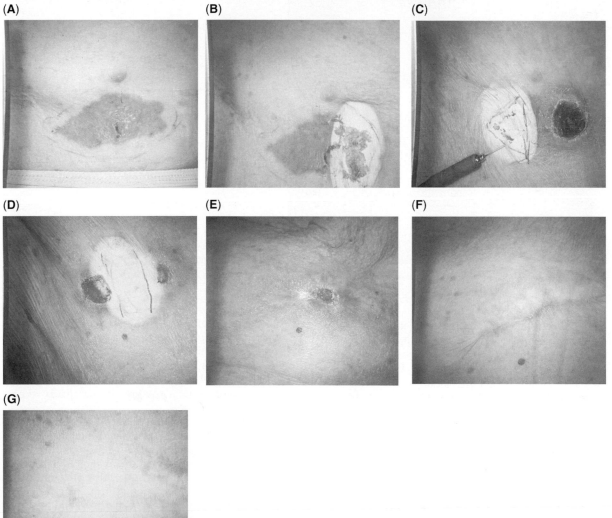

Figure 17 (**A**) Large basal cell carcinoma on abdomen of an 88-year-old woman. (**B**) Cryosurgery to first section of lesion. (**C**) Cryosurgery to second section. Note healing of previously treated site. (**D**) Cryosurgery to third section. (**E**) Healing two months after last treatment. (**F**) Completely healed one year after treatment. (**G**) Excellent results two years after treatment. (*See color insert*.)

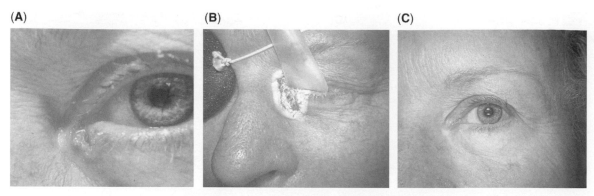

Figure 18 (**A**) Basal cell carcinoma on left lower lid of a 71-year-old woman. (**B**) Cryosurgery to entire lesion. Note protection of eyes. (**C**) Completely healed one year after treatment

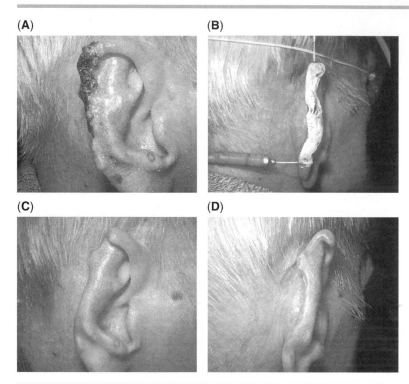

Figure 19 (**A**) Recurrent basal cell carcinoma on ear of an 81-year-old man. (**B**) Cryosurgery to entire lesion with tissue temperature monitoring. (**C, D**) Complete healing two-and-a-half months after treatment.

Temporary Complications

Temporary complications may arise immediately after treatment or after healing, and generally resolve spontaneously. Some may require treatment. One of the common reactions is edema that can occur within 24 hours after treatment. Periorbital edema can be severe and can last for several days (Fig. 22). Open wet compresses, or a short course of prednisone is beneficial. Edema is commonly seen on the hands after treatment of a malignancy and can last up to two weeks. It subsides with compression and soaking.

Bullae can occur at the margins of the treated site and are treated symptomatically (Fig. 23). The bulla that develops after treatment of a wart is to be expected.

A hypertrophic scar may develop after treatment of a large lesion (Fig. 24). It resolves spontaneously during the course of a year although resolution can be hastened through intralesional injection of a steroid suspension. It usually is not seen in association with treatment of small or benign lesions.

Delayed bleeding may sometimes occur during the sloughing phase of healing following treatment of a

malignancy on the nose, temple or forehead, or ear. This is best treated with simple pressure at home or with a hemostyptic solution and a pressure dressing in the office.

Secondary infection is uncommon after cryosurgery. It may develop after treatment of large lesions or those located on the lower part of the legs. Chondritis and edema of the ear may also occur. Systemic antibiotic therapy is recommended in such instances.

Cryosurgery is relatively painless, but discomfort or pain is subjective and also depends on the amount of freezing administered. Mild stinging does occur after spraying a lesion for several seconds but rapidly fades. Treatment of verrucae on the fingers and myxoid cyst can cause moderate pain, which can last for several hours. It can be relieved or avoided by injection of a local anesthetic and mild analgesic medication. In treatment of a malignancy without use of a local anesthetic, pain is limited to the initial freezing process. Rarely, immediate headache or migraine-type pain can develop after treating lesions on the temple, forehead, or scalp.

Other uncommon reactions include syncope, cold urticaria, milia, pyogenic granuloma, nitrogen gas insufflation,

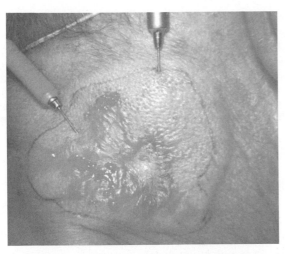

Figure 20 Edema immediately after cryosurgery of a malignancy.

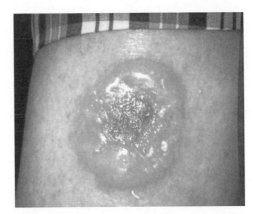

Figure 23 Bulla formation after treatment of a large basal cell carcinoma on the thigh of a 75-year-old man. (*See color insert.*)

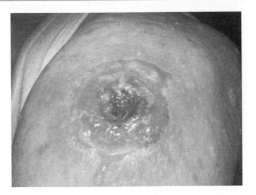

Figure 21 Severe exudative reaction one week after treatment of a squamous cell carcinoma on the left arm of an 88-year-old man.

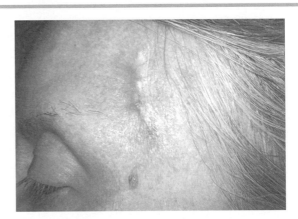

Figure 24 Hypertrophic scar on forehead two months after treatment of a basal cell carcinoma. (*See color insert.*)

hyperpigmentation, paresthesia, and pseudocarcinomatous hyperplasia.

Permanent Complications

A permanent complication is an irreversible tissue response that is generally related to the location of the tumor (Fig. 25). Retraction of tissue can have cosmetic and functional consequences. Examples are lifting of the lips, eyebrows, free margin of the ala nasi, and ectropion of the eyelids (Figs. 26

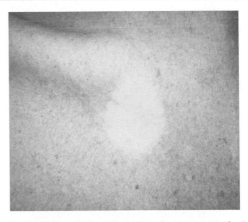

Figure 25 Hypopigmentation 15 months after treatment of a basal cell carcinoma on the chest. (*See color insert.*)

and 27). Slight improvement might develop in an elderly patient because of laxity of the skin.

A tissue defect or indentation can develop on the nose, ears, or eyelids. Overfreezing may be a contributing factor (Fig. 28).

Recurrence following treatment of a benign lesion is not unusual and lesions can be retreated. However, recurrence of a malignancy is serious and appropriate treatment should be undertaken. A selected, small recurrent basal cell carcinoma can be retreated successfully if the lesion is well circumscribed.

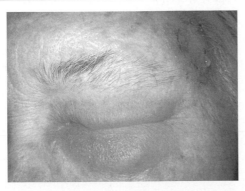

Figure 22 Severe periorbital edema after treatment of a large basal cell carcinoma on the temple on a 67-year-old woman. (*See color insert.*)

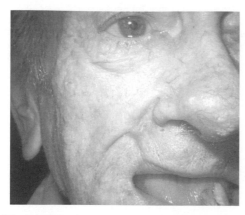

Figure 26 Retraction of upper lip two-and-a-half months after treatment of a basal cell carcinoma.

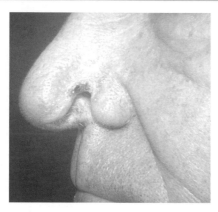

Figure 27 Notching of left ala nasi after treatment of a basal cell carcinoma.

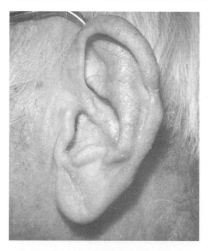

Figure 28 Mild notching on left helix six months after treatment of a basal cell carcinoma.

CURE RATE OF MALIGNANCIES

There are several large series of basal and squamous cell carcinomas treated with cryosurgery that show high cure rates. The author reported treatment of 4406 new and recurrent skin cancers during a 30-year period with an overall cure rate of 96%. The cure rate was remarkably similar in all locations. The latest five-year cure rate by the author was a series of 552 selected cases that yielded a cure rate of 99%.

CONCLUSION

During the past two decades, much progress has been made in dermatologic cryosurgery because of increased clinical experience and greater use of the technique for diverse lesions. For malignancies, the cure rates have increased by the use of aggressive treatment. Cryosurgery may be found to be advantageous for certain difficult and large tumors. Knowledge of the techniques of cryosurgery is well-known worldwide and the indications for its use are widening.

BIBLIOGRAPHY

Elton RF. Complications of cutaneous cryosurgery. J Am Acad Dermatol 1983; 8:513–519.

Gage AA. What temperature is lethal for cells? J Dermatol Surg Oncol 1979; 5:459–464.

Graham GF. Advances in cryosurgery during the past decade. Cutis 1993; 52:365–372.

Kuflik EG. Cryosurgical treatment of periungual warts. J Dermatol Surg Oncol 1984; 10:673–676.

Kuflik EG. Cryosurgery for tumors of the ear. J Dennatol Surg Oncol 1985c; 11:1165–1168.

Kuflik EG. Cryosurgical treatment for large malignancies on the upper extremities. J Dermatol Surg Oncol 1986; 12:575–577.

Kuflik EG. Specific indications for cryosurgery of the nail unit: myxoid cysts and periungual verrucae. J Dermatol Surg Oncol 1992; 18:7.

Kuflik EG. Cryosurgery updated. J Am Acad Dermatol Surg Oncol 1994; 31:925–944.

Kuflik EG. Cryosurgery for cutaneous malignancy: an update. Dermatol Surg 1997; 223:1081–1087.

Kuflik EG. Erosive adenomatosis of the nipple treated with cryosurgery. J Am Acad Dermatol 1998; 38:270–271.

Kuflik EG. Cryosurgery for skin cancer: 30-year experience and cure rates. Dermatol Surg 2004; 30:297–300.

Kuflik EG, Gage AA. Cryosurgical Treatment for Skin Cancer. New York: Igaku-Shoin, 1990.

Kuflik EG, Gage AA. Recurrent basal cell carcinoma treated with cryosurgery. J Am Acad Dermatol 1997; 37:82–4.

Kuflik EG, Webb W. Effects of systemic corticosteroids on post-cryosurgical edema and other manifestations of the inflammatory response. J Dermatol Surg Oncol 1985; 11: 464–468.

Kuflik EG. Cryosurgery for carcinoma of the eyelids: a 12-year experience. J Dermatol Surg Oncol 1985a; 11:243–246.

Kuflik EG. Cryosurgical treatment of large basal cell carcinomas on the trunk. J Dermatol Surg Oncol 1983; 9:226–230.

Kuflik EG. Cryosurgery for palliation. J Dermatol Surg Oncol 1985b; 11:867–869.

Lubritz RR, Smolewski SA. Cryosurgery cure rate of actinic keratosis. J Am Acad Dermatol 1982; 7:631–632.

Nordin P, Stenquist B. Five-year results of curettage-cryosurgery for 100 consecutive auricular non-melanoma skin cancers. J Laryngol Oncol 2002; 116:893–898.

Nordin P, Larko O, Stenquist B. Five year results of curettage-cryosurgery of selected large basal cell carcinomas on the nose: an alternative treatment in a geographical area under served by Mohs surgery. BR J Dermatol 1997; 136:1.

Suhonen R, Kuflik EG. Venous lakes treated by liquid nitrogen cryosurgery. Br J Dermatol 1997; 137:1018–1019.

Suhonen RE, Kuflik EG. Cryosurgical methods for eyelid lesions. J Dermatol Treat 2001; 12:135–139.

Torre D. Cryosurgery of basal cell carcinoma. J Am Acad Dermatol 1986; 15:917–929.

Zacarian SA. Cryosurgery of cutaneous carcinomas: an 18-year study of 3,022 patients with 4,228 carcinomas. J Am Acad Dermatol 1983; 9:947–956.

21

The Scalp

Jerry D. Brewer and Randall K. Roenigk
Mayo Clinic, Rochester, Minnesota, U.S.A.

INTRODUCTION

The scalp is a five-layered soft tissue structure extending from the external occipital protuberance and superior nuchal lines posteriorly, supraorbital margins anteriorly, and zygomatic arches laterally. The tissue of the scalp is composed of many different substances including hair follicles, sebaceous and sweat glands, collagen, elastin, blood vessels, nerve fibers, and lymphatics with mucopolysaccharide ground substance.

A variety of conditions can affect the scalp including multiple benign and malignant tumors, burns, and congenital malformations, making the scalp an anatomical site for medical practice shared by otolaryngological surgery, plastic surgery, neurosurgery, dermatology surgery, and radiation oncology, among others. In addition, the scalp is a frequent site of trauma, with up to 72% of automobile accident victims sustaining head injuries, making the scalp a frequent site of reconstructive efforts.

A working knowledge of scalp anatomy and its innate characteristics is vital to any successful surgical procedure performed on this area of the body.

LAYERS OF THE SCALP

The Skin

The skin of the scalp is hair-bearing, and is the first or the most superficial layer of the scalp (Fig. 1). The hair follicles of the scalp are very close to one another relative to other hair-bearing areas of the body, and extend through the entire thickness of the skin. When viewed in cross-section, the skin of the scalp tends to have a relatively thin epidermis and a variably thicker dermis. The thin epidermis has been found to progressively become thin with age, especially after the age of 80. The thicker dermis is thinnest over the forehead and thickest over the occipital area, being approximately 3- and 8-mm thick in both areas, respectively. Like the epidermis, the dermis has also been shown to become thin with age, most noticeable after the age of 60. The dermal layer contains a rich network of nerves and vascular and lymphatic vessels, mostly derived from the underlying subcutaneous layer. However, with age the vascular network decreases and can adversely impact wound healing. The dermal and epidermal layers of the scalp also contain numerous sebaceous and sweat glands. The increased number of sebaceous glands found in the skin of the scalp results in it being a common site for sebaceous cyst formation.

Subcutaneous Layer

The subcutaneous layer of the scalp is an inelastic fibrous layer containing subcutaneous fat arranged in small compartments via fibrous septae. This layer of the scalp is usually around 4–7-mm thick, being thickest at the vertex. Variations however do exist, with one report existing of a 20-mm thick subcutaneous layer. This layer of the scalp is highly vascularized and well supplied with cutaneous nerves and lymphatics, being in essence the passageway for blood vessels and nerves to the other scalp layers. Many interwoven sheets of connective tissue are found between the fat lobules and vessels in the subcutaneous layer, lending to this layer of the scalp sometimes being referred to as the dense connective tissue layer, superficial fascia layer, or second fibrofatty layer of the scalp. These sheets of connective tissue bind the blood vessels to the dermis and fibrous septae in such a way that vasoconstriction and vasospasms are prevented when a vessel is cut. This is the reason behind the profuse bleeding that can be observed during surgery or following scalp trauma. This concept becomes important, as unconscious patients may potentially bleed to death after receiving traumatic lacerations to the scalp. There are also vertically oriented reticular fibers present that form strong attachments with the dermis above, and galea below. These vertical fibers in essence bind the first three layers of the scalp together. Trauma occurring to the subcutaneous layer of the scalp may result in hemorrhage and edema. When this is because of a difficult vaginal delivery, the resultant edema in this layer of the scalp is called a caput succedaneum.

Galea Aponeurotica

The galea aponeurotica is the third layer of the scalp, and is a strong dense fibrous tendinous sheet, usually 1–2-mm in thickness. This layer has also been called the deep fascial, aponeurotic, tendinous, epicranial aponeurosis, or epicranial muscle layer of the scalp. The galea aponeurotica is better developed in some individuals than others, and can be congenitally absent. Laterally, the galea becomes thinner and continuous with the temporoparietal fascia, which extends over the temporalis muscle. Anteriorly and posteriorly, the galea provides an insertion site for both bellies of the frontalis and occipitalis muscles, respectively. There are blood vessels present in the galea, which extend into the subgaleal layer below, or the superficial vascular plexus of the subcutaneous layer above. Traumatic wounds that extend to the galea will tend to gape open widely and bleed

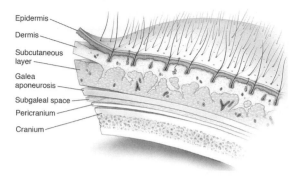

Epidermis

Dermis

Subcutaneous layer

Galea aponeurosis

Subgaleal space

Pericranium

Cranium

Figure 1   Diagram demonstrating the five characteristic layers of the scalp.

profusely. This is because the pull of the frontalis muscle anteriorly, and occipitalis muscle posteriorly will separate the laceration widely. The top of the galea is strongly adherent to the subcutaneous layer, making dissection between these two layers extremely difficult and bloody.

The galea as a dense fibrous sheet is resistant to stretch and is felt by some surgeons to limit one's ability to perform certain scalp resections. Other surgeons however believe the galeas' nonstretchable ability is actually a beneficial quality, and keeps in check the possibility of surgically overstretching manipulated tissue, and the harmful effects this creates. Studies have been undertaken to evaluate the benefit of a galeatomy, or linear galeal transection in efforts to gain more flexibility to scalp tissues before closing defects. This procedure was found to correlate with a mean 40% reduction in closing tension; however, the procedure is also associated with multiple complications, including increased trauma to the subcutaneous tissues, increased bleeding, hematoma formation, and infections rates. By and large, the galeatomy has fallen out of favor and is currently not used much.

Subgaleal Layer or Space

The subgaleal layer or space is the fourth layer of the scalp, bounded by the galea above and the pericranium below. This layer of the scalp is largely avascular and contains a thin layer of loose fibroareolar tissue. The subgaleal layer has been called the loose connective tissue, Merkel gap, innominate fascia, fibrofatty, first fascia, submuscular aponeurotic fascia, loose areolar fascia, and subepicranial fascia layer as well as the subaponeurotic plane. The subgaleal layer is important from a surgical standpoint, and lends itself to easy, avascular dissection during surgical procedures. In addition, the blood supply to the scalp runs in the subcutaneous tissues as noted previously, thus surgical dissection of the subgaleal space does not compromise the blood supply to scalp tissue in any way. There are emissary veins that traverse the subgaleal space connecting the scalp veins to the diploic veins and intracranial venous sinuses. This connection is important as infections in the subgaleal space may dangerously communicate with the surface of the brain via this connection.

The subgaleal space extends beneath the frontalis and occipitalis muscles over the vault of the skull, and is limited posteriorly by the attachment of the occipitalis to the superior nuchal lines, and laterally by the temporal fascia. Anteriorly, the frontalis muscle inserts into the skin and subcutaneous tissue, not bone, allowing this space to extend beneath the orbicularis oculi and into the eyelids and root of the nose. Consequently, injury to the scalp or forehead

may result in the pooling of blood in the upper eyelids and sometimes lower eyelids as well, causing the black eyes that are seen in such injuries. The lateral borders of the subgaleal space are where the galea aponeurotica blends with the temporalis fascia. The portion of the scalp with subgaleal space present has the typical five layers of the scalp. The portion of the scalp lateral to the subgaleal space has only three layers: skin, subcutaneous tissue, and deep fascia (the same fascia that ultimately covers the trapezius and sternocleidomastoid muscles). Generally speaking, wide excisions in areas of the scalp where the subgaleal layer is present are possible; however, excisions over areas with only three layers and no subgaleal space are much more difficult. This property of the scalp is because of the loose fibroareolar tissue present in the subgaleal space, which allows the upper layers of the scalp to essentially slide over the underlying pericranium. Variations of this quality do exist, with some individuals having poorly developed fibroareolar tissue. This causes their scalps to seem tight when attempting to close surgical defects. The extent of a scalp's tightness or fibroareolar tissue in the subgaleal layer may be assessed by the surgeon by simply placing the hands on the scalp, and evaluating the extent of movement over the underlying pericranium preoperatively.

Although the scalp does have five layers, it is sometimes thought of as having two: that which is above the subgaleal space and that which is below it. This is due to the fact that the upper three layers of the scalp are very tightly bound to one another, causing them to act and move in unison during surgical manipulation (Fig. 2).

External Periosteum of the Skull

The external periosteum or pericranium of the skull is the final and fifth layer of the scalp. The thickness of this layer depends on individual variation and location, but the pericranium is usually similar in thickness to the galea aponeurotica, thinner in the frontal areas and slightly thicker on the crown. The pericranium is loosely attached to the galea aponeurotica, and may easily be separated from the galea via the subgaleal space. In anatomy texts, this layer has been described as being tightly bound to the skull especially at the suture lines; however, this layer may be easily dissected away from the outer table of the skull. Dissection of the pericranium from the outer table of the skull is usually bloodless, except for the minimal bleeding experienced because of rare bone perforator vessels. Some reports have suggested that the periosteum ends laterally at the origin of the temporalis muscle, but other descriptions suggest it continues beyond this point. Post-traumatic blood may pool below the periosteum shortly after a difficult birth, forming a cephalohematoma.

The pericranium is a dense membranous or fibrous sheet of connective tissue capable of retaining sutures, and can be incorporated into pericranial flaps of deep wound closures. Some surgeons feel the pericranium to be a very useful tissue, which is often underutilized in reconstructive and cosmetic craniofacial surgery.

MUSCULATURE OF THE SCALP

The musculature of the scalp consists of the frontalis muscle anteriorly, and the occipitalis muscle posteriorly, and the temporoparietalis muscles laterally (Fig. 3). The frontalis and occipitalis muscles are sometimes collectively referred to as the occipitofrontalis muscle.

The frontalis muscle has two bellies, originates from the galea aponeurotica, and inserts into the skin of the

(A)

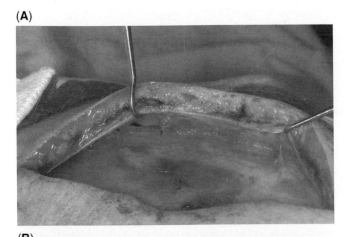

(B)

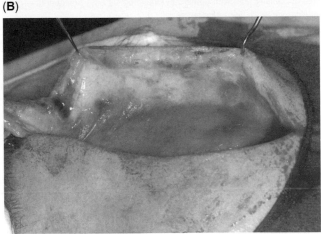

Figure 2 Clinical photos demonstrating the layers of the scalp: **(A)** note the three top layers of the scalp (skin, subcutaneous tissue, and galea) are connected to one another. These three layers have been separated from the periosteum via the subgaleal space. **(B)** Another photo of the forehead demonstrating the three top layers of the scalp separated from the periosteum via the subgaleal space. Note the frontalis muscle seen on cross section. (*See color insert.*)

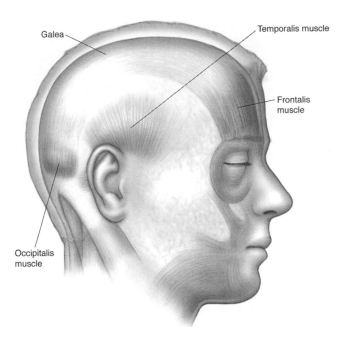

Figure 3 Diagram demonstrating the occipitalis, frontalis, and temporalis muscles of the scalp.

forehead, eyebrows, and upper part of the orbicularis oculi muscle. The action of this muscle is to elevate the eyebrows and skin of the forehead. The frontalis muscle is innervated by the temporal branch of the facial nerve (cranial nerve VII).

The occipitalis muscle also has two bellies. This muscle originates from the lateral three-fourths of the superior nuchal lines and the mastoid processes, and inserts into the galea aponeurotica. The main function of the occipitalis muscles is to anchor the galea, but it may pull the scalp posteriorly in certain individuals. The occipitalis muscle is innervated by the posterior auricular nerve, also a branch of the facial nerve.

The temporoparietalis muscles originate from an aponeurosis common to the auricularis muscles, and insert into the galea aponeurotica. The function of this muscle is mainly to fix the galea, but it can also elevate the ear in some individuals. The temporoparietalis muscles are innervated by the temporal branch of the facial nerve.

VASCULATURE OF THE SCALP
Arteries of the Scalp
A minimal blood supply to the scalp is provided by the bone perforators derived from the meningeal arteries; however, the major blood supply of the scalp is provided by five paired main arteries, two of which derive from

the internal carotid artery, and the remaining three from the external carotid artery. The arteries of the scalp run centripetally, that is the larger trunks of the arteries start laterally, running in a central and medial fashion, becoming smaller as they enter a system of free anastomosis towards the medial aspect of the scalp. As aging occurs, the relative loss of this vascular network adversely impacts wound healing, especially for defects that extend to bone (Fig. 4).

The supratrochlear and supraorbital arteries of the scalp derive from the ophthalmic branch of the internal carotid artery. These arteries accompany their respective nerves and course anteriorly and posteriorly along the midline of the scalp.

The superficial temporal artery is a terminal branch of the external carotid artery. This artery ascends the later aspect of the scalp, beginning anterior to the auricle. The superficial temporal artery mainly supplies the scalp over the temporal region and travels with the auriculotemporal nerve. Distally, the superficial temporal artery divides into anterior and posterior branches.

The posterior auricular artery is a branch of the external carotid artery, and ascends the lateral aspect of the scalp, beginning posterior to the auricle. The posterior auricular artery may run in the general vicinity as the lesser occipital nerve (Fig. 5).

The occipital artery is also a branch of the external carotid artery. This artery ascends the posterior aspect of the scalp running anteriorly along the midline. The occipital artery is accompanied by the greater occipital nerve.

The fact that the scalp does not have musculocutaneous perforators is very important from a surgical prospective, as transection of a peripheral arterial trunk during a surgical flap procedure on the scalp may have dire consequences to the proximal and distal aspects of the flap. As previously mentioned, these arteries supply the scalp via the subcutaneous connective tissue layer of the scalp. These arteries freely anastomose with one another in the second layer of the scalp, providing the rich vascular plexus characteristic of the scalp. Midline anastomoses are rare and diminish with age.

(A)   **(B)**   **(C)**   **(D)**

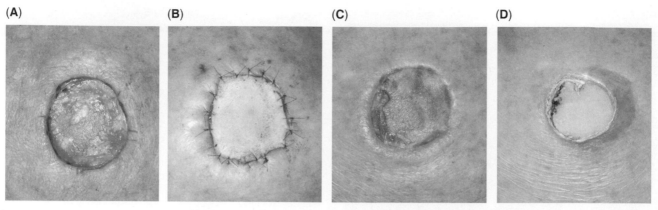

Figure 4 Clinical photos demonstrating the adverse impact that a relative loss of the vascular network can have in defects extending to bone: (**A**) surgical defect extending to the periosteum; (**B**) skin graft placed at the surgical site; (**C**) signs of a failing graft with epidermal sloughing 13 days postoperatively; (**D**) completely failed skin graft with defect extending to bone three months after the original surgery. (*See color insert.*)

The large arteries are held in place by the connective tissue bundles of the subcutaneous layer of the scalp, and send penetrating branches superiorly into the skin, and less frequently inferiorly into the galea and subgaleal layers. Some believe that blood flow may be diminished in areas of male pattern baldness, suggesting that vascularization may play a role in or be a consequence of the pathogenesis of hair loss. This is also an important consideration to keep in mind during hair transplant procedures, and may explain the diminished hair diameters frequently seen post-transplantation, although the genetic characteristics of the donor hair probably plays a more important role.

It has been found that the temporal artery of the scalp is capable of supplying and ensuring the survival of an entire hemisphere of the scalp if need be, which is important information when planning surgical flaps. In contrast, the supratrochlear, supraorbital, and occipital arteries are unable to vascularize other scalp regions when other arteries are sacrificed during surgery.

Veins of the Scalp

The venous drainage of the scalp is mainly via veins closely associated with the previously described arteries, carrying similar names to the artery of their association. These veins usually accompany their respective arteries closely, but may be separated from their artery by as much as 3 cm. Veins of the scalp, similar to the arteries, also freely anastomose with one another and are connected to the diploic veins of the skull and intracranial dural sinuses via emissary veins, which are valveless. The superior sagittal sinus and transverse sinus communicate with the venous drainages system of the scalp via the posterior parietal emissary veins and mastoid veins, respectively.

The supratrochlear and supraorbital veins drain the anterior scalp. These veins begin in the forehead and descend anteriorly, uniting to form the angular vein at the medial angle of the eye. The angular vein continues further as the facial vein.

The superficial temporal vein drains the scalp anterior to the auricle. This vein descends anterior to the auricle and

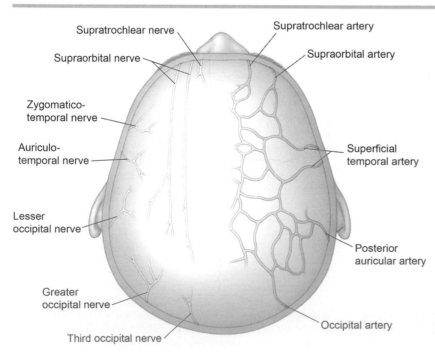

Figure 5 Diagram demonstrating the anatomy of the arteries and nerves of the scalp. The veins of the scalp generally parallel their respective arteries in location and name.

enters the parotid gland joining the maxillary vein to become the retromandibular vein. The anterior division of the retromandibular vein unites with the facial vein to form the common facial vein, which drains into the internal jugular vein. Thus the supratrochlear, supraorbital, and superficial temporal veins all ultimately drain to the internal jugular vein.

The posterior auricular vein drains the scalp posterior to the auricle. The posterior auricular vein often receives a mastoid emissary vein from the sigmoid sinus, and joins the posterior division of the retromandibular vein to form the external jugular vein.

The occipital vein drains the posterior scalp, and terminates in the suboccipital plexus beneath the floor of the superior aspect of the posterior triangle of the neck.

Lymphatic Drainage of the Scalp

The lymphatic drainage system of the scalp is diffuse, contributing to the significant spread of pathology that may be seen in this location. There are no lymph nodes in the scalp, but multiple lymphatic vessels drain the scalp to local-regional lymph node chains. The lymphatic vessels begin initially as lymphatic sinuses of the scalp ($50\,\mu m$) that empty into precollectors ($100\,\mu m$). The precollectors have valves and parallel the surface of the scalp. These precollectors then drain into larger lymphatic channels in the subcutaneous layer of the scalp, which then drain into certain nodal regions. The regional drainage of the scalp is highly variable, with significant individual variation, however, the following patterns are generally observed.

The posterior aspects of the scalp, or regions posterior to the auricle, drain into the posterior auricular (mastoid) and occipital lymph nodes, which then drain into the superficial cervical nodal chains.

The anterior and lateral regions of the scalp, or in other words, regions anterior to the auricle drain into the preauricular and parotid lymph nodes, which further drain into the submandibular and deep cervical nodes.

INNERVATION OF THE SCALP

There are three types of nerves found in the scalp: motor, sensory, and autonomic. The autonomic nerves of the scalp supply glands, smooth muscles, and walls of blood and lymphatic vessels.

The motor innervation of the scalp previously discussed consists of the posterior auricular branch of the facial nerve innervating the occipitalis muscle, the superior zygomatic branch of the facial nerve innervating the frontalis muscle, and the temporal branch of the facial nerve innervating the temporoparietalis muscle.

The temporal branch of the facial nerve lies just below the fascia in the preauricular area. Being superficial, this nerve is vulnerable to being transected during surgery or blocked after the administration of anesthetic in this location, the effect of which would be a ptosis of the frontalis muscle (Fig. 6).

Usually six to seven sensory nerves innervate the scalp, either originating from the trigeminal nerve or the cervical nerve. The sensory innervation of the scalp anterior to the auricles is via all three divisions of the trigeminal nerve (cranial nerve V). Posterior to the auricles, sensory innervation is by spinal cutaneous nerves (C_2 and C_3) (Fig. 5).

The supratrochlear nerve is a branch of the ophthalmic division of the trigeminal nerve (V_1), and supplies the medial plane of the scalp anteriorly to as far as the vertex

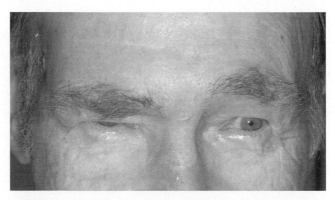

Figure 6 Excision of a skin cancer on the right preauricular area resulted in transection of the temporal branch of the facial nerve. The patient experienced ptosis of the right frontalis muscle and was unable to lift the right eyebrow.

posteriorly. However, anastomosis from nerve twigs of other branches exists. This results in occasional difficulty obtaining anesthesia in the central frontal hairline.

The supraorbital nerve is also a branch of the ophthalmic division of the trigeminal nerve (V_1). This nerve supplies the anterior scalp lateral to the supratrochlear nerve, also extending as far as the vertex. Both the supratrochlear and supraorbital nerves tend to accompany the supratrochlear and supraorbital arteries and veins, respectively.

The zygomaticotemporal nerve is a branch of the maxillary division of the trigeminal nerve (V_2). This nerve supplies the temporal region of the scalp. There is no major artery of the scalp that accompanies the zygomaticotemporal nerve.

The auriculotemporal nerve is a branch of the mandibular division of the trigeminal nerve (V_3), which supplies the skin of the temporal region, and runs with the superficial temporal artery and vein.

The lesser occipital nerve is a branch of the cervical plexus (C_2), which supplies the lateral occipital scalp, and accompanies the posterior auricular artery and vein.

The greater occipital nerve is a branch of the posterior ramus of the second cervical nerve (C_2). This nerve supplies the scalp in the median plane in the posterior or occipital region, as far as the vertex anteriorly. This nerve accompanies the occipital artery and vein.

Finally, there may also be a third occipital nerve (C_3) present supplying the posterior midline of the scalp, medial to the greater occipital nerve.

The sensory nerve supply of the scalp is similar to the arterial supply, in that it is distributed in a centripetal fashion, runs in the second or subcutaneous layer of the scalp, and has similar distributions. Incisions in the peripheral scalp that transect nerve trunks may result in large areas of permanent hypesthesia, a complication that should be avoided if possible. One should be familiar with the anatomical locations of these nerves before performing surgical procedures involving the scalp. In addition, if transection of one of these nerves is likely, the patient should be informed as to the possible outcomes or complications before the procedure is initiated.

Because of the similar distribution and anatomical location of the arteries and nerves of the scalp, an incision in the central scalp results in minimal neurovascular trauma. An incision in this area of the scalp would thus be the preferred choice when this is an option for surgical procedures of the scalp.

(A)   **(B)**   **(C)**   **(D)**

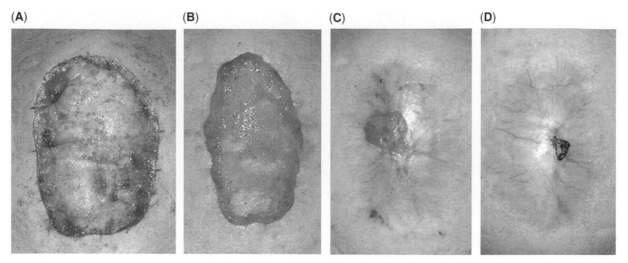

Figure 7   Healing by second intention on the scalp: **(A)** squamous cell carcinoma; **(B)** immediately after resection; **(C)** two months after resection showing healthy granulation tissue; **(D)** one year after resection. (*See color insert.*)

(A)   **(B)**

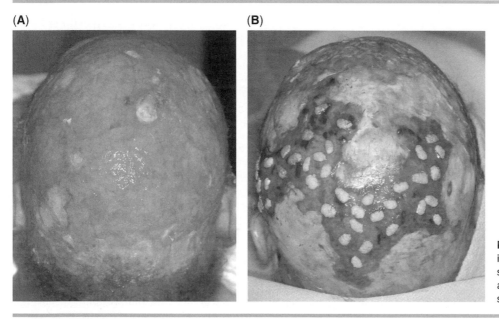

Figure 8 **(A)** Ulcerative sarcoidosis involving the scalp. **(B)** Two sessions of split thickness pinch grafting four months after controlling the disease with immunosuppressive therapy. (*See color insert.*)

(A)   **(B)**

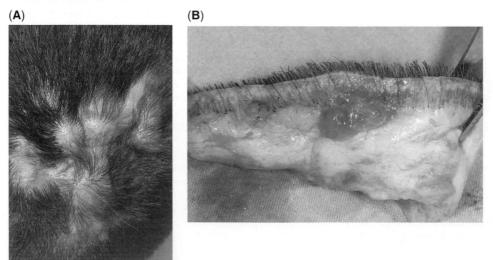

Figure 9 **(A)** Keratosis follicularis spinulosa decalvans resulting in scaring alopecia. **(B)** Gross specimen after resection demonstrates hair, granulation tissue, and scar. (*See color insert.*)

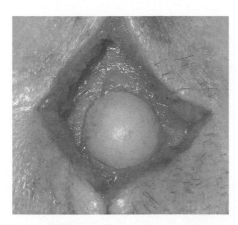

Figure 10 Osteoma demonstrated intraoperatively. (*See color insert.*)

SURGICAL CONSIDERATIONS
Incisions and Excisions of the Scalp
The concept of lines of minimal tension, lines of cleavage, or Langer's lines, was first described by Langer in 1881, and subsequently re-evaluated by Cox in 1941. These lines of minimal tension are thought to correlate with the orientation of collagen bundles in the dermis. If incisions and excisions are performed parallel to these collagen bundles, then the tension of the wound is decreased and scarring is minimized. Although the orientation of dermal collagen bundles are thought to correlate with the lines of minimal tension, this has actually never been proven via electron microscopy. In addition, the direction of elastic fibers is also felt to be important in wound tension and healing. Fortunately, elastic fibers usually parallel collagen bundles, thus incisions that are in parallel to one, will also be parallel to the other.

A correlation exists between skin crease lines and Langer's lines. Where skin crease lines are present, Langer's lines will generally run parallel to these skin creases. Langer's lines tend to be longitudinal on the scalp, supporting the argument that whenever possible incisions on the scalp should be vertical, except for in the occipital area where incisions are best horizontal, paralleling the skin crease lines.

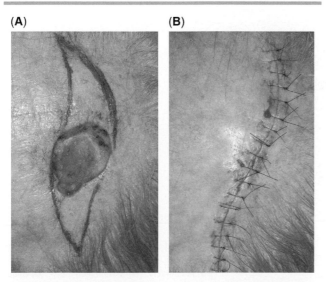

Figure 11 Primary closure of a scalp defect: (**A**) defect after Mohs micrographic surgery; (**B**) primary S-plasty closure. (*See color insert.*)

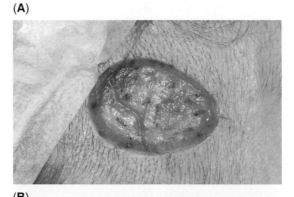

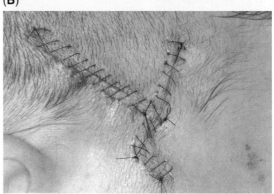

Figure 12 An A-to-T flap: (**A**) surgical defect after Mohs micrographic surgery; (**B**) A-to-T flap with a Burow's triangle inferiorly. (*See color insert.*)

Of equal importance when operating on the scalp, the surgeon should keep in mind the directional orientation of hair follicles. Whenever possible, incisions should be made with the blade at an angle and parallel to the hair follicle directional orientation, thus minimizing hair follicle transection. This practice will avoid localized scarring alopecia.

Scalp Laxity
The extent to which scalp excisions are possible depends upon the scalp laxity. Scalp laxity is the result of two of the scalp's contributing characteristics. The first characteristic of the scalp that contributes to scalp laxity is the ability of the scalp to slide over the pericranium via the loose fibroareolar tissue that makes up the fourth layer of the scalp. As previously mentioned, individual variation exists as to the extent of loose fibroareolar tissue present, or a scalp's ability to slide over the pericranium. Some patients are able to undergo an excision of 5-cm width or more with uncomplicated closure and no undermining necessary, while other patients may undergo an identical excision width, but prove very difficult to close even after extensive undermining. This characteristic does not have anything to do with stretch of the tissue, but more the top layers of the scalps' innate ability to slide over the bottom layer. The second component of scalp laxity is elasticity, or ability of the tissue to stretch. This characteristic is also subject to individual variability, with some scalps having much more elastic tissue than others. Some scalps are able to stretch considerably, even in the setting of a relatively inelastic galea. Langer's lines play a role here, and when incisions are made parallel to Langer's lines, the full capacity of the tissues' ability to stretch can be utilized.

(A)   **(B)**   **(C)**

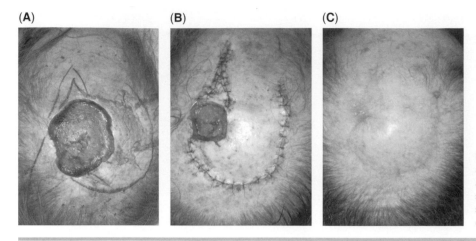

Figure 13 Rotation flap: **(A)** surgical defect after Mohs micrographic surgery; **(B)** closure via a rotation flap inferiorly and an island pedicle flap superiorly, leaving some of the defect to heal by second intention; **(C)** outcome three months postoperatively. (*See color insert.*)

The ability of the tissue to recover from stretch is because of the elastic tissue present. There is, however, a limit to which the tissue may be stretched. When the skin of the scalp is stretched beyond its elastic limit, the elastic fibers rupture and can no longer compensate for stretch. At this point, the tissue will no longer return to its resting state when the force of stretch is removed, resulting in a permanent condition referred to as plasticization or stretch atrophy. Plasticization of scalp tissue is sometimes seen following serial scalp excisions, especially if traction closures have been utilized. Plasticized tissues are not satisfying to work with in subsequent surgeries, and the stretched skin can also attenuate blood vessels, causing tissue ischemia and even necrosis. In addition, the nerves and lymphatics of the scalp will also be stretched in conjunction with the stretched skin. If stretched enough, the nerves and lymphatic vessels can result in pain and edema of the surgical area. This information should be kept in mind when deciding on closures of the scalp, and evaluating the degree of stretch necessary for such closures.

Tissue expansion is a two-staged procedure where silicone or other expandable material is placed under normal skin of the scalp near a defect, or anticipated defect to be closed at a later date. The expandable material under

(A)   **(B)**

(C)   **(D)**

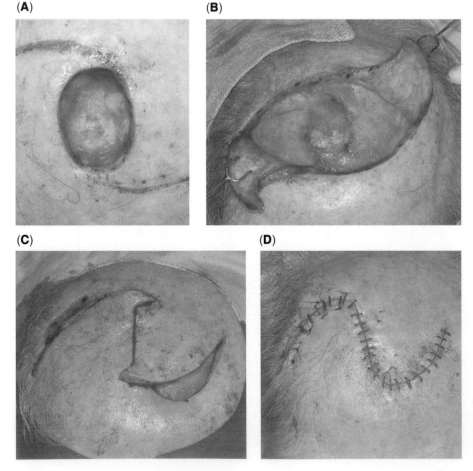

Figure 14 Bilateral rotation flap on the scalp vertex: **(A)** surgical defect after Mohs micrographic surgery; **(B)** undermined flaps; **(C)** initial sutures holding the flaps in place; **(D)** outcome immediately after surgery. (*See color insert.*)

the scalp is expanded over time, gradually stretching the overlying skin. This process ultimately results in expanded tissue that will more easily aid in the closure of larger defects on the scalp. Tissue expansion of the scalp can be utilized in multiple scenarios, including cutaneous malignancy, trauma, or in cicatricial alopecia when the causal agent has resolved. In the later case, tissue expansion-augmented scalp reduction may be very beneficial to some patients who may not be surgical hair transplant candidates.

Undermining

The question of the necessity and/or extent of undermining on scalp defects is regularly debated. Most surgeons would agree that judicial undermining of scalp defects is beneficial and aids in the ideal closure. Extensive undermining, however, especially when done blindly, can be associated with traumatized blood vessels and nerves, increased scaring in the undermined area, and open tissue planes that may increase infection rates. One study recently compared two groups of patients, one group having 1 cm of undermining before closure, and the other group only having 5 cm. In the setting of identical excision widths and procedures, there was no difference found in wounds having stretch-back complications, suggesting that the extra 10 cm of undermining may not have contributed anything to the ultimate outcome.

Second Intention Wound Healing

Because of the rich vascular plexus present in scalp tissue, defects of the scalp tend to heal quickly. This characteristic can be utilized when considering the possibility of wound healing by second intention. Defects of the scalp, especially those in nonhair-bearing areas or in areas easily covered by adjacent hair, may fair better when left to heal by second intention (Fig. 7). It has been our experience that such defects will ultimately have very satisfying outcomes, with much better results than skin grafting. This option should always be considered, especially when alternative closures are complex, and may jeopardize nearby neural or vascular structures unnecessarily.

Special Conditions Involving the Scalp

The scalp can be a unique anatomical site, demonstrating pathology of distinct conditions. Scalp sarcoidosis may have a variety of clinical manifestations, but usually presents as a cicatricial alopecia with erythema, scaling, infiltration and crusting. Sometimes sarcoidal involvement of the scalp can be extensive, causing skin breakdown and ulceration (Fig. 8).

Keratosis follicularis spinulosa decalvans is a rare condition that usually causes a scaring alopecia of the scalp and eyebrows (Fig. 9). Patients with this condition tend to have a genetic predisposition toward follicular hyperkeratosis and subsequent inflammation, ultimately leading to follicular destruction and scarring. The pathogenesis of this acute inflammatory disorder remains unknown, but it is thought to be because of a dysfunction in keratinization.

Cutaneous osteomas represent another condition that may involve the scalp (Fig. 10). Multiple cutaneous osteomas have been demonstrated in female patients with a history of acne. It is not clear whether these lesions are neoplasms or hamartomas, but malignant transformation has never been demonstrated.

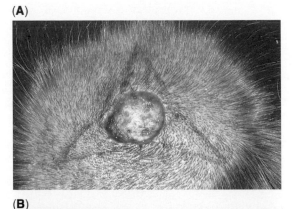

(A)

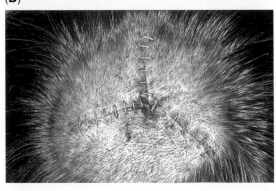

(B)

Figure 15 Mercedes or tripolar advancement flap: **(A)** surgical defect after Mohs micrographic surgery; **(B)** immediate postoperative result. (*See color insert.*)

Closures

As in other areas of the body, defects of the scalp may be closed in multiple fashions. Options to consider when closing a scalp defect include second intention, primary closure, multiple types of flaps (advancement, rotational, transposition, and island pedicle), and skin grafting. In addition, a combination of these options may be used to create the best closure possible for each patient with a scalp defect. The description of closure options is described elsewhere in this text. Figures 11–15 demonstrate some examples of scalp reconstruction performed in our practice.

BIBLIOGRAPHY

Cornell University Automotive Crash Injury Research. The Injury Producing Accident: A Primer of Facts and Figures. New York: Cornell University, 1961.

Field LM. Scalp flaps. Dermatol Surg Oncol 1991; 17:190–199.

Gibson T. Physical properties of the skin. In: Converse JM, ed. Reconstructive Plastic Surgery. 2nd ed. Philadelphia: WB Saunders, 1977:70.

Goh MS, Magee J, Chong AH. Keratosis follicularis spinulosa decalvans and acne keloidalis nuchae. Australas J Dermatol 2005; 46(4):257–260.

Goldminz D, Greenberg RD. Multiple miliary osteoma cutis. J Am Acad Dermatol 1991; 24:878–881.

Goldman B. Transcutaneous pO₂ of the scalp in male pattern baldness: a new piece of the puzzle. Plast Reconstr Surg 1996; 97:1109.

Hayman LA, Shukla V, Ly C, Taber KH. Clinical and imaging anatomy of the scalp. J Comput Assist Tomogr 2003; 27(3):454–459.

Hiatt JL, Gartner LP. Textbook of Head and Neck Anatomy. New York: Appleton-Century-Crofts, 1982.

Katta R, Nelson B, Chen D, Roenigk H. Sarcoidosis of the scalp: a case series and review of the literature. J Am Acad Dermatol 2000; 42:690–692.

Kirolles S, Haikal FA, Saadeh FA, et al. Fascial layers of the scalp: a study of 48 cadaveric dissections. Surg Radiol Anat 1992; 14:331–333.

Klemp P, Peters K, Hanstead Z. Subcutaneous blood flow in male pattern baldness. J Invest Dermatol 1989; 92:725.

Marty F, Montandon D, Gumener R, et al. Subcutaneous tissue in the scalp—anatomical, physiological, and clinical study. Ann Plast Surg 1986; 16:368–376.

Mayer TG, Fleming RW. Aesthetic and Reconstructive Surgery of the Scalp. In: St. Louis: Mosby Year Book, 1991:11–23.

Moore KL, Dalley AF. Clinically Oriented Anatomy. 4th ed. Pennsylvania: Lippincott Williams & Wilkins, 1999.

Rand R, Baden HP. Keratosis follicularis spinulosa decalvans. Report of two cases and literature review. Arch Dermatol 1983; 119:22–26.

Raposio R, Santi L, Nordstrom REA. Serial scalp reductions: a biomedical approach. Dermatol Surg 1999; 25:210–214.

Roenigk RK, Wheeland RG. Tissue expansion in dermatologic surgery. Dermatol Clin 1987a; 5(2):429–436.

Roenigk RK, Wheeland RG. Tissue expansion in cicatricial alopecia. Arch Dermatol 1987b; 123(5):641–646.

Seery GE. Surgical anatomy of the scalp. Dermatol Surg 2002; 28:581–587.

Seery GE. Improved results in scalp surgery by controlling tissue tension vector forces by galea to pericranium fixation sutures. Dermatol Surg 2001; 27:569–574.

Tolhurst DE, Carstens MH, Greco RJ, et al. The surgical anatomy of the scalp. Plast Reconstr Surg 1991; 87:603–612.

Toshitani S, Nakayama J, Yahata F, Yasuda M, Urabae H. A new apparatus for hair growth in male pattern baldness. J Dermatol 1990; 17:240.

Wenzel-Hora BI, Berens von Rautenfeld D, Majewski A, et al. Scanning electron microscopy of the initial lymphatics of the skin after use of the indirect application technique with glutaraldehyde and mercox as compared to clinical findings, part I: the nomenclature and micro topography of the initial lymphatics. Lymphology 1987; 20:126–133.

Yonemoto Y. Studies on measurements of the scalp tissue of the Japanese adult. Okajimas Folia Anat Jpn 1968; 45:83–97.

22

The Ear

Roger I. Ceilley
University of Iowa, Iowa City, Iowa, U.S.A.

The external ear has obvious functional and cosmetic importance. Dermatologic surgeons frequently treat skin cancers and a variety of dermatologic diseases affecting this area. Proper selection of the method(s) of therapy depends upon many factors that include the following:

1. Anatomy of the region
2. Pathology type of the lesion to be treated
3. Skin type and degree of solar damage
4. Age and general health of the patient
5. Surgeon's knowledge of various therapeutic modalities

ANATOMY

The auricle or pinna, formed by skin and cartilage, is dependent upon a complex cartilaginous framework for its contour and support. The auricle contains a number of prominences and depressions. The concha, anthelix and helix, and tragus and antitragus (Fig. 1) are important landmarks. The anterior one-third is attached to the skull and the posterior two-thirds to the scalp only. The skin is intimately attached over the surface of the cartilage except along the helix. The blood and nerve supply is abundant and complex (Fig. 2). The blood supply consists of the anterior auricular artery, a branch of superficial temporal artery supplying the lateral surface, and the posterior auricular artery supplying the medial surface and a small portion of the lateral surface. In addition, the occipital artery gives off a branch supplying the medial surface. The lymphatic drainage consists of superficial, deep cervical nodes and mastoid lymph nodes. The retroauricular area includes the mastoid process behind the ear. The medial area faces the retroauricular area, and the lateral surface is the external auricular surface.

APPLIED ANATOMY FOR LOCAL ANESTHESIA

A review of the anatomy and innervation of the external ear will aid the surgeon in understanding the techniques for local anesthesia in this region. The external ear is formed by the union of tissue from the branchial arches and postbranchial regions. This is reflected in its sensory innervation, which is by branches from cranial nerves V, VII, IX, and X and C2 and C3 of the cervical plexus. There is marked overlap in the sensory distribution of adjacent cutaneous nerves and variation in the contribution from cranial nerves VII and IX.

The mandibular division of the trigeminal nerve innervates the most anterior portion of the auricle through its auriculotemporal branch. It supplies the skin of the tragus, the anterior and superior portion of the external auditory canal, and the anterior portion of the helix and its crus (Fig. 2).

Cranial nerves VII (facial), IX (glossopharyngeal), and X (vagal) contribute to the sensory innervation of the concha on the lateral surface of the auricle and the posterior portion of the external auditory canal (Fig. 3). A small area of skin on the postauricular sulcus and adjacent mastoid is also innervated by these cranial nerves. The auricular branch of the vagus that communicates with the glossopharyngeal and facial nerves emerges from the skull through the tympanomastoid fissure to supply the latter area.

The cervical plexus contributes to the sensory innervation of the auricle by the posterior branch of the greater auricular nerve and the lesser occipital nerve. The greater auricular nerve supplies the major portion of the medial surface of the auricle and posterior portion of the lateral surface of the auricle. There is overlap and communication with fibers from the lesser occipital nerve in the mastoid region. These nerves originate from the second and third cervical nerves (Fig. 2).

LOCAL ANESTHESIA OF THE AURICLE

In very apprehensive patients, intravenous sedation with diazepam and a narcotic may be beneficial. Local anesthesia is induced by field injection of 1% lidocaine with epinephrine 1:100,000 and sodium bicarbonate. The bicarbonate is added to bring up the pH of the mixture, and consequently to decrease the pain associated with the local anesthesia. The epinephrine decreases capillary bleeding by its vasoconstrictor action. The auricle has widespread and profuse vascular plexuses, and there is no danger of necrosis secondary to the use of a vasoconstricting agent in healthy individuals.

Adequate anesthesia may be obtained by a field block of the skin around the periphery of the auricle (Fig. 4). Deep infiltration anteriorly may result in temporary paralysis of the facial nerve (Fig. 5). Local infiltration of the concha and external canal at the bony cartilaginous junction is performed to obtain total anesthesia of the entire auricle and canal. The field block does not anesthetize the canal, which is supplied by cranial nerves. Anesthesia of the localized areas of the auricle may be obtained by regional infiltration. The advantage of a field block is less distortion of tissue and less pain from injection of the anesthetic agent. The major disadvantage is less effective vasoconstriction at the operative site.

METHODS OF SURGICAL TREATMENT

The methods of therapy for carcinoma of the external ear include radiotherapy, conventional excisional surgery,

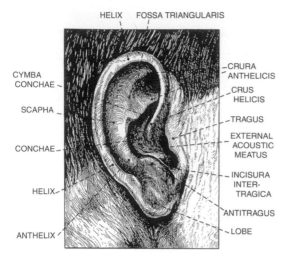

Figure 1 Topographical landmarks of the ear.

HELIX   FOSSA TRIANGULARIS
CYMBA CONCHAE
SCAPHA
CONCHAE
HELIX
ANTHELIX
CRURA ANTHELICIS
CRUS HELICIS
TRAGUS
EXTERNAL ACOUSTIC MEATUS
INCISURA INTER- TRAGICA
ANTITRAGUS
LOBE

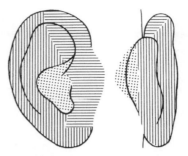

Figure 3 Sensory nerve distribution of the auricle by area. Vertical lines indicate the area supplied by cervical plexus; horizontal lines indicate the area supplied by auriculotemporal nerve; and dots indicate the arc supplied by cranial nerves VII, IX, and X.

electrodesiccation and curettage, cryosurgery, and Mohs micrographic surgery. All would appear to yield acceptable cure rates for primary lesions less than 1 cm in diameter that do not show an aggressive histologic pattern (Figs. 6,7). Mohs surgery should be used for more difficult tumors.

Radiation

The variability in contour of the external ear makes determining the accurate dosage of radiotherapy difficult. Because of the large amount of cartilage in the pinna, the external ear is extremely susceptible to radiation perichondritis. The frequency of recurrence appears to be higher following radiotherapy than following surgical treatment. Recurrent lesions are generally unresponsive to radiotherapy.

Cryosurgery

Cartilage is more resistant to permanent injury from freezing than is the skin. This permits complete freezing of skin lesions of the external ear. Cryosurgery is more effective for lateral lesions rather than the medial on the pinna. However, freezing to lethal temperatures, as is customary elsewhere, can result in necrosis of the full thickness of the external ear. This may result in chondritis and deformity of the auricle.

Elton recently reported on recurrences that follow cryotherapy of large lesions, especially deeply penetrating malignant neoplasms and sclerosing basal cell carcinomas.

They appeared not only at the margins of treated malignancies but also under apparently healthy scars, much in the same way they appear under skin grafts.

Electrodesiccation and Curettage

Electrosurgery is effective for small primary lesions but may result in large areas of exposed cartilage. This heals very slowly because of thermal injury. The incidence of chondritis is greater, as is auricular deformity. Treatment of recurrent lesions with this method is often ineffective because the malignant tissue within the scar is not easily removed with a cruet.

Excision

Pless attempted to define adequate margins for excisional therapy, and he recommended margins of 8–10 mm, respectively, for primary basal cell and squamous cell carcinoma measuring less than 3 cm. Margins of at least 15 mm were recommended for all recurrent lesions and for primary lesions greater than 3 cm. Measurements of the preoperative size of the lesion and the postoperative surgical defect following Mohs surgery suggest that these recommendations fall short of cure in many instances, especially when one is dealing with a recurrent tumor or mor-phea-form basal cell carcinoma.

All lesions should be biopsied prior to excision with primary closure. Local anesthesia may be obtained by regional block or local infiltration of 1% lidocaine with epinephrine 1:100,000. Local infiltration provides better hemostasis than the regional block.

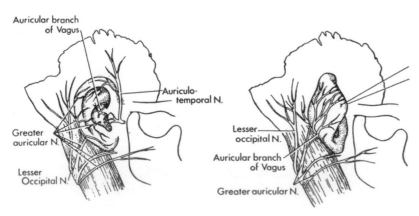

Auricular branch of Vagus
Auriculo-temporal N.
Greater auricular N.
Lesser Occipital N.
Lesser occipital N.
Auricular branch of Vagus
Greater auricular N.

Figure 2 Sensory nerve supply of the auricle.

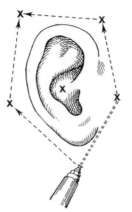

Figure 4 Injection for regional anesthesia of the auricle.

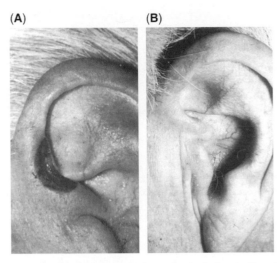

Figure 6 Result after excision and primary closure of a basal cell carcinoma.

The proposed excision margin is outlined with skin marker before local infiltration of anesthesia is performed. A margin of 8–10 mm is suggested for basal cell carcinoma and squamous cell carcinoma. Utilizing margins of this magnitude often prevents a simple wedge excision as marked lateral protrusion of the helix will occur when the incision is closed primarily. To prevent this deformity, a stellate tension-relaxing excision is done (Fig. 8). V-shaped wedges with the long axes perpendicular to the margin of the primary excision are outlined. These are placed near the middle margins of the original wedge and may involve the antihelix. The base of the smaller relaxing wedge is approximately one-third of the base of the primary wedge, while the length is also approximately one-third the length of the primary excision. It is best to make the secondary wedges smaller as they can be easily extended to obtain better closure. Tissue deficiency can be a severe problem.

Tumor and secondary wedges are excised. Skin hooks are used to approximate the margins of the helix to determine if modifications of the secondary wedges are necessary. Hemostasis may be obtained by cautery. Care is taken to minimize cauterization of the auricular cartilage to prevent cartilage necrosis. Subcutaneous absorbable sutures, such as 5-0 vicryl or PDS, are used to approximate the auricular cartilage. These stitches must include the perichondrium, either alone or through cartilage to induce the perichondrium on both sides. Undermining the skin along the margins may be done to facilitate eversion of the skin margin. Care must be taken to remain above the perichondrium while undermining the skin. The skin is closed with interrupted vertical mattress sutures of 6-0 synthetic material for eversion. The incision is covered with an antibiotic ointment and nonadherent gauze. A cotton ball is placed in the concha and a $4'' \times 4''$ piece of gauze is placed in the postauricular region. Then a mild pressure dressing with fluffed gauze and wrapping around the head may be used. The pressure dressing is used primarily where hemostasis is a concern. This can be removed in 24–48 hours. If an open technique is used, the incision is simply covered with an antibiotic ointment.

Oral antibiotics are prescribed for three days. They are initiated the evening prior to surgery. For patients requiring intravenous sedation, it may be administered immediately prior to surgery. Wound care includes cleansing twice on a daily basis with hydrogen peroxide and the application of an antibiotic ointment. This is extremely important to maximize wound healing. It prevents crust formation in the incision, which makes suture removal less traumatic in five to seven days.

An important complication is auricular perichondritis, commonly caused by *Pseudomonas aeruginosa*, which often colonizes the external ear following surgical trauma. Usually within one week postoperatively, the patient will present with a tender erythematous, edematous area surrounding the surgical site. If untreated, the perichondritis can progress into a liquefying chondritis with disfigurement and, in advanced cases, loss of the external ear. Fortunately, this complication in early diagnosis can be easily and

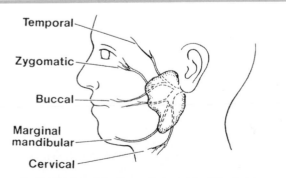

Figure 5 Distribution of the five major branches of the facial nerve.

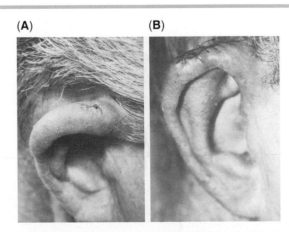

Figure 7 Excision and primary closure of a small basal cell carcinoma.

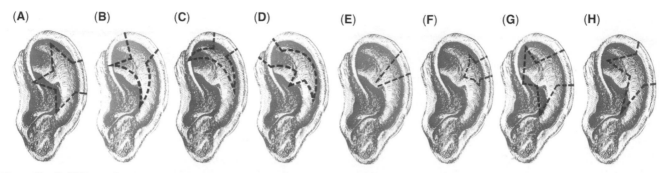

(A)   (B)   (C)   (D)   (E)   (F)   (G)   (H)

Figure 8 (A–H) Types of wedge excisions. A wedge excision can be done for small lesions on the ear. Larger lesions require tension-relaxing incisions or smaller secondary wedges to close the defect with minimal deformity.

successfully treated with norfloxacin 400 mg PO BID for 21 days as reported by Thomas or with ciprofloxacin 750 mg PO BID as reported by Noel.

The primary consideration must always be complete tumor removal, followed by wound closure and cosmesis. The width of these margins should be based on the histologic type of tumor, whether it is primary or recurrent, and the location. No general rule can be given to determine the size of excision margins as the growth patterns and biologic behavior of tumors vary greatly. The typical small nodular basal cell carcinoma (less than 1.0 cm in diameter) usually requires excision margins of 5–7 mm. Smaller squamous cell carcinomas should be excised with 1-cm margins; however, lesions greater than 1 cm in diameter require wider and deeper excision margins of at least 1 cm. In addition, deep excision to the underlying fascia will result in fewer local recurrences. Recurrent tumors and those of longer duration should be more widely excised or treated with Mohs' surgery.

Microscopically Controlled Excision (Mohs Micrographic Surgery)

Mohs technique yields the highest cure rate for all cutaneous malignancies. According to Rowe, for primary squamous cell carcinoma involving the ear, the recurrence rate with non-Mohs modalities is 18.7% compared with 5.3% by Mohs technique and five-year or greater follow-up. The advantages of the fresh tissue technique over the fixed tissue technique are: (i) reduced operative time as several layers can be taken in a single day, (ii) less pain, (iii) more conservation of normal tissue, (iv) less inflammation (less chrondritis in areas where cartilage is present), and (v) possibility of immediate surgical reconstruction. Both techniques provide maximum assurance of complete extirpation of malignancy so that reconstruction may be considered. This reduces operating time as frozen sections are unnecessary at the time of reconstruction. Disadvantages include: (i) requirement of special training to perform the procedure, (ii) a histology laboratory able to make frozen sections readily available, and (iii) increased time required for excision.

Recurrent Tumor

The complete removal of malignant tumors of the external ear is often difficult. Cutaneous neoplasms of the ear tend to infiltrate well beyond the clinically apparent margins of the neoplasm, invading laterally along the perichondrium and deep along the embryonic fusion planes. Special care must be taken for lesions in the anterior and postauricular sulcus as parotid invasion frequently occurs. This may jeopardize the visibility of the facial nerve.

Recurrence, morbidity, and mortality are greater with malignant tumors of the ear than of skin in general. Frederick's 54 cases treated surgically demonstrated a 16.6% recurrence rate. In Blake's series of 146 cases, 16% of tumors treated surgically recurred, and 47% of those treated by radiotherapy recurred with an overall recurrence rate of 25%. There was a 25% recurrence rate in 100 cases reported by Conway and Howell, and 64% of those recurrences had been treated with radiotherapy. Pless recorded 260 cases of carcinoma of the external ear and found an overall recurrence rate of 16% (squamous cell carcinoma, 15%; basal cell carcinoma, 18%). Hansen and Jensen reviewed 1198 cases of carcinoma treated with radiotherapy, and 9.7% of the lesions were on the external ear, but 15.6% of all recurrences were on the auricle.

The complex anatomy and embryonic fusion planes contribute to the high recurrence rate of auricular lesions. The auricle is formed from six knob-like hillocks derived from the first and second branchial arches. These hillocks fuse and form the auricle by the third month of embryonic development. The first hillock becomes the tragus, the second the cms helicis, the third the helix, the fourth the antihelix, the fifth the antitragus, and the sixth the lobule. Recurrent tumors frequently extend anterior along the plane of fusion of the first and second and first and sixth hillocks. It is of interest that this is a common location of preauricular cysts and sinuses.

Pless suggested that the frequency of recurrence is related to increasing tumor size but does not depend on tumor location. Other findings suggest the contrary, with 22 of 29 recurrent lesions located medial to the helix and antihelix reported by Ceilley et al. (1979). A recurrence is most frequently seen when the lesion is located in scar tissue adjacent to but not impinging on the site of the microscopically controlled excision. Because aggressive carcinomas seem to grow in scar tissue in an unpredictable and deceptive fashion, it is best to excise all scar tissue associated with a recurrent carcinoma.

Reconstruction

Indications for immediate surgical reconstruction include: (i) large defects, (ii) defects that have significant amounts of exposed cartilage (Fig. 9), (iii) involvement of more than 180° of external auditory canal, or (iv) functional difficulty for patients who wear glasses. Smaller defects, unable to be closed primarily, are allowed to heal by second intention, and cosmetic results are excellent in four to six weeks.

The type of auricular reconstruction used depends on the degree of certainty of complete tumor removal. A primary

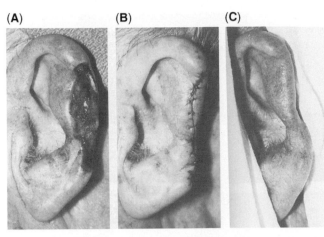

Figure 9 (**A**) A basal cell carcinoma involved the cartilage; therefore, closure is warranted. Simple primary closure advancing postauricular skin (**B**) produces satisfactory results (**C**).

tumor excised with microscopic control may be reconstructed with local flaps or a free skin graft.

Local Flaps

Local flaps usually result in a better cosmetic result than a skin graft. There is better color and texture match while the tissue carries its own blood supply. The disadvantage of local flaps around the ear, as in all locations, is that thicker tissue may prolong detection of recurrent tumors. Recurrent tumors have the capacity to spread widely in the newly created tissue planes before appearing on the skin surface. One indication for a local flap in auricular reconstruction is the patient who wears glasses. If a skin graft is used, pressure from the bows of the glasses may cause tissue necrosis. Local flaps tolerate pressure from the bows of eyeglasses better (Figs. 10,11). The most useful flap for reconstructing the posterior or medial auricular surface would be the transposition or rhomboid flap. Given that the skin on the anterior or lateral auricle is tightly adhered to the underlying cartilage and without much elasticity, a skin graft would be a better choice to repair a defect here if adequate perichondrium provides enough blood supply for grafting. For a large conchal defect, a postauricular revolving door-island flap can be utilized.

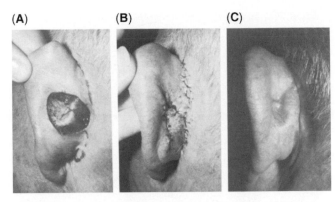

Figure 10 (**A**) Mohs defect after removal of a basal cell carcinoma. (**B**) Inferiorly based transposition flap to repair. (**C**) Satisfactory result.

Skin Grafts

Skin graft survival on cartilage or bone denuded of periosteum or perichondrium is allegedly tenuous. Dermatologic and oncologic surgeons encounter this problem frequently, and often the graft does grow directly on bone or cartilage when small areas of the perichondrium and periosteum have been removed. Split-thickness skin grafts of 0.018–0.021″ were used. If a significant amount of cartilage is exposed, small holes can be made through the cartilage with a 1- to 2-mm dermal punch and the graft delayed until granulation tissue comes through these holes to cover at least half of the exposed cartilage (Fig. 12). This technique has been consistently reproduced with good cosmetic results even for large defects. Bolsters or blasting sutures are always used to hold the graft in place for a minimum of one week.

Meatoplasty

A meatoplasty is indicated after the removal of any tumor that involves 180° or more of the external auditory canal. Skin grafts of this area have a tendency to contract. This is less common with regional flaps.

The meatoplasty is performed by excising a generous amount of conchal cartilage, which forms the posterior portion of the external canal. This opens the ear canal widely, and a skin graft is then placed on the more vascular soft tissue that remains. This technique prevents stenosis of the external auditory canal (Fig. 13).

When evaluating methods of therapy for auricular neoplasms, both the effectiveness and the functional cosmetic

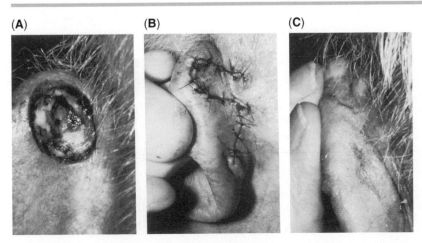

Figure 11 (**A**) Mohs defect. (**B**) Laterally based transposition flap, making it easier for patient to wear glasses (**C**).

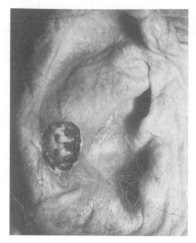

Figure 12 Removal of cartilage by punch excision will allow healing by second intention over exposed cartilage.

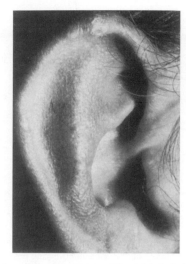

Figure 14 Chondrodermatitis nodularis helicis.

deformity must be considered. Auricular neoplasms, other than primary lesions smaller than 1 cm, are treated best with microscopic control of the surgical margins. Mohs surgery results in higher cure rates and decreases auricular deformity. Tumor recurrence necessitates excision of the lesion and all the adjacent scar tissue. For this reason, the use of local flaps or extensive undermining of adjacent tissue should be avoided in this high-risk location. If conventional surgical excision is used, careful examination of the margins of the specimen should be done at the time of excision. If frozen sections are not readily available, the examination of permanent sections of the entire specimen should be obtained before reconstruction, except for primary lesions that are 1 cm or less.

TREATMENT OF BENIGN LESIONS
Surgical Treatment of Chondrodermatitis Nodularis Chronica Helicis

Chondrodermatitis nodularis chronica helicis is characterized by a painful, red nodule most commonly located on the helix of the ear. Typically, the patient is male and over 40 years of age with a history of outdoor work. Patients

may also report having had frostbite. Nodules on the tragus, antitragus, and antihelix are rare but occur most commonly in women and are often related to trauma. The lesion tends to be oval, inflamed, and fixed to the underlying cartilage (Fig. 14). The cause of this condition is unclear but appears to be related to the unique anatomy of the pinna. The skin here is tightly bound to the underlying cartilage, and the circulation is poor because there is little subcutaneous tissue. Moreover, this area is frequently exposed to mechanical and environmental trauma. These factors get worse with age.

Treatment has included wedge excision and primary closure, intralesional corticosteroids, and curettage or excision allowed to heal by second intention. Recurrence after

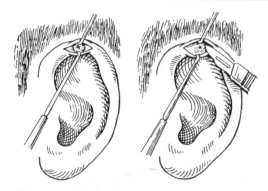

Figure 15 Excision of chondrodermatitis nodularis helicis through the cartilage.

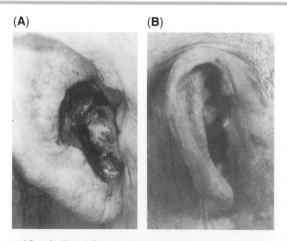

Figure 13 **(A)** This defect involves over 180° of the external auditory canal following microscopically controlled excision of a basal cell carcinoma. **(B)** A patent external auditory canal six months after reconstructive meatoplasty and split thickness skin graft.

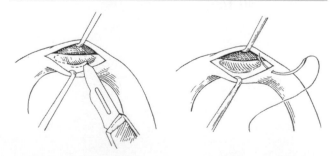

Figure 16 Closure of the defect after the cartilage is smoothed.

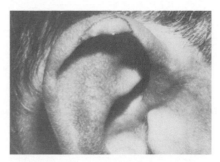

Figure 17 Chondrodermatitis nodularis helices with projections of cartilage through the skin.

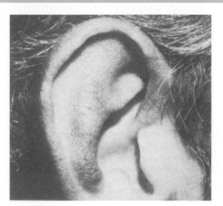

Figure 18 Postoperative results after excision and primary closure.

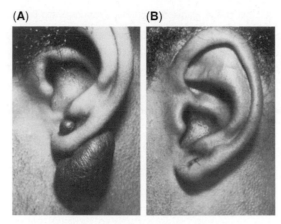

Figure 20 (**A**) Earlobe keloid—preoperative injection of intralesional triamcinolone acetonide; (**B**) postoperative appearance.

simple excision is common, probably because removal of the lesion is incomplete. Projections of damaged cartilaginous tissues may persist, or adjacent cartilage may contain foci of subclinical involvement. Nevertheless, excision is the

most effective treatment because the clinical lesion is removed entirely and pain is relieved by transection of sensory nerves. With sterile technique and local anesthesia, the involved area is excised through a small incision or in an ellipse down to the cartilage (Fig. 15, left). Then the clinically necrotic cartilage is removed (Fig. 15, right). Adjacent cartilage is carefully trimmed so as to contour the defect in the cartilage smoothly, free of sharp edges (Fig. 16, left). The skin is undermined just above the perichondrium, and the wound is closed with fine sutures (5-0 silk or nylon) (Fig. 16, right). The skin on the pinna heals rapidly. Sutures may be removed in four or five days and the tape is applied for a few more days. The preoperative and postoperative results are shown in Figures 17 and 18.

The advantages of this technique are: (i) good visualization of damaged cartilage and adjacent foci of involvement, (ii) contouring of adjacent healthy cartilage, eliminating sharp edges that may produce pain or recurrence later, (iii) improved vascular supply to the overlying skin, (iv) rapid and usually painless healing, and (v) excellent cosmesis. A fine linear scar is hidden within the crease of the helix.

Epidermoid Cysts

The lobule of the auricle is rich in sebaceous glands and is covered with loose skin. Epidermoid cysts commonly

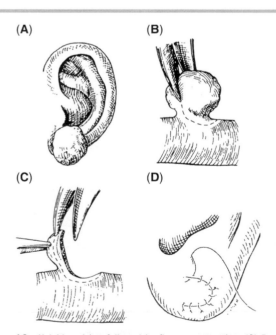

Figure 19 Keloid excision followed by flap reconstruction: (**A**) Preoperative appearance. (**B**) Excision of the bulk of the keloid. Outline a small portion of skin for a flap to cover the defect. (**C**) Dissection with iris scissors of residual keloidal tissue from the skin used as a flap. (**D**) Suture the flap in place without tension.

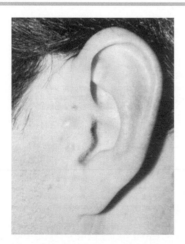

Figure 21 Accessory tragus or preauricular skin tag.

Table 1 Previously Reported Series of Malignancies of the External Ear

Investigator	Basal cell carcinomas	Squamous cell carcinomas	Basosquamous	Other	Total
Mohs (1947)	55	52	0	0	107
Frederick (1956)	25	27	2	0	54
Marfatia (1966)	8	20	0	2	30
Heenan (1966)	46	32	3	2	83
Blake (1974)	51	81	3	11	146
Conway (1957)	51	42	0	7	100
Pless (1976)	79	177	0	4	260
Total	315	431	8	26	780

develop in this area. Other common locations include the concha, floor of the meatus, and the periauricular skin. Clinically they are soft and slightly fluctuant nodules that usually have a point of attachment with an overlying follicular orifice. The lesions recur if simply incised and drained, so it is essential to remove the entire cyst wall and its contents. If the cyst is acutely inflamed, incision and drainage along with systemic antibiotics should be used. Excision is then deferred until after the acute inflammation has resolved.

Keloids

Keloid formation on and around the auricle is common, especially in dark-skinned persons. Keloids often result from trauma, especially after ear piercing. Initial treatment should be pressure, cryosurgery, or intralesional corticosteroids. Larger lesions may be treated by surgical enucleation of the lesion, covering the defect with a flap created from the overlying skin (Figs. 19,20). After excising the lesion, some prefer to immediately give an intralesional triamcinolone injection. Some prefer to excise the lesion followed by 300 R of X-ray.

Preauricular Cysts

A pit-like depression and cyst found anterior to the helix and above the tragus commonly represents embryonic remnants of the first and second branchial arches. The cyst and tracts may extend deeply and are best handled by a head and neck surgeon experienced in their treatment.

Preauricular Tags

Skin tags in this area may or may not contain cartilage (Fig. 21). They are the result of faulty fusion of the hillocks during embryonic development. Removal is indicated only for cosmetic reasons.

Hemangiomas and Venous Lakes

Small lesions are best treated with simple excision or electrosurgery. Larger lesions may be treated by argon laser photocoagulation. Lymphangiomas are best treated with excision, cryosurgery, or carbon dioxide laser vaporization.

Dermoid Cyst

These lesions contain squamous epithelium, hair follicles, sweat glands, and sebaceous glands. They result from faulty embryonic development and should be referred to a head and neck surgeon.

Warts and Seborrheic Keratoses

Shave excision or cryosurgery is most useful. When utilizing cryosurgery, one must be careful in avoiding the damage of the underlying cartilage.

Gouty and Rheumatoid Nodules and Xanthomata

These lesions may be painful and necrotic. Treatment is directed toward the underlying disease.

Nevi

Scalpel excision is the treatment of choice. Other lesions in this area include cholesteatoma of the external auditory canal, osteoma, myomas (rhabdomyoma, leiomyoma), myxoma, and mixed tumors of the salivary gland type. Rare neoplasms include adenocarcinoma, adenoid cystic carcinoma, sarcoma, and malignant melanoma.

TREATMENT OF MALIGNANT TUMORS

Malignant tumors of the external ear (which include the pinna, external auditory meatus, and periauricular structures) constitute approximately 6% of all skin cancers, with reported series ranging from 4.6% to 9.7%. The percentage of basal cell and squamous cell carcinomas varies considerably, while other forms of malignancy of the external ear are rare.

A review of several series totaling 780 patients with malignant ear tumors demonstrated that 55% were squamous cell carcinomas, 40% basal cell carcinomas, and 5% other types of malignancy (Table 1). Malignant melanomas, sarcomas, and carcinomas derived from sudoriferous sebaceous glands and from hair follicles make up most of the remaining malignant tumors that occur as primary tumors on the external ear (Table 2).

Tumors of the external ear often begin as infiltrating growths that spread along the dermis, perichondrium, or embryonic fusion planes rather than becoming discrete and exophytic. Recurrent lesions frequently behave in this manner, often making retreatment with conventional surgical techniques or irradiation ineffective. Therefore, complete removal of malignant tumors of the external ear is often difficult. Many authors believe that the prognosis of squamous cell carcinoma of the auricle is worse than elsewhere on the body surface. Basal cell carcinoma is an unpredictable tumor with varied clinical and histologic manifestations. The sclerosing or morphea form of basal cell carcinoma is particularly resistant to nonsurgical methods of therapy.

In addition to the difficulty in achieving complete tumor removal, the auricle and ear canal play important

Table 2 Uncommon Malignancies on the External Ear

Malignant melanoma	Sarcomas
Endothelioma	Chondrosarcoma
Hemangioendothelioma	Fibrosarcoma
Lymphoendothelioma	Lymphosarcoma
Adenocarcinoma	Myxosarcoma
Adenoid cystic carcinoma	Rhabdomyosarcoma
Atypical fibroxanthoma	Ectopic salivary tissue

cosmetic and functional roles. Methods of reconstruction must be varied depending on the assurance of complete tumor removal and cosmetic and functional considerations. The auricle contains a large amount of cartilage susceptible to the development of perichondritis and chondritis when the overlying skin is excised. This further complicates the therapy and reconstruction of lesions involving the auricle.

BIBLIOGRAPHY

Blake GB, Wilson JSP. Malignant tumors of the ear and their treatment. Br J Plast Surg 1974; 27:67–76.

Bumsted RM, Ceilley RI. Local anesthesia of the auricle. J Dermatol Surg Oncol 1979; 5(6):448–449.

Bumsted RM, Ceilley RI, Panje WR, Crumley RL. Auricular malignant neoplasms: when is chemosurgery (Mohs' technique) necessary? Arch Otolaryngol 1981; 107:721–724.

Ceilley RI, Lillis PJ. Surgical treatment of chondrodermatitis nodularis helicis. J Dermatol Surg Oncol 1979; 5(5):384–387.

Ceilley RI, Bumsted RM, Smith WH. Malignancies on the external ear: ablation and reconstruction of defects. J Dermatol Surg Oncol 1979; 5:762–767.

Conway H, Howell J. Carcinoma of the external ear. Plast Reconstr Surg 1957; 20:45–54.

Davies J. Embryology and anatomy of the face, palate, nose, and paranasal sinuses. In: Paparella MM, Schmurick DA, eds. Otolaryngology. Philadelphia: WB Saunders, 1973:150–178.

Elton RF. Wisdom of subsequent biopsies. J Dermatol Surg Oncol 1977; 3(3):286.

Fredricks S. External ear malignancy. Br J Plast Surg 1956; 9: 136–160.

Gage AA. Cryosurgery for cancer of the ear. J Dermatol Surg Oncol 1977; 3:417–421.

Hansen PB, Jensen MS. Late results following radiotherapy of skin cancer. Acta Radiol (N.S.) 1968; 7:307.

Heenan P, Hueston JT. The distribution of skin tumors on the external ear. Med J Aust 1966; 2:888–889.

Hollinshead WH. Anatomy for Surgeons: The Head and Neck. Vol. 1. 2nd ed. New York: Harper & Row, 1968:213–215, 352–358.

Marfatia PT. Malignant tumors of the ear. Laryngoscope 1966; 76:1591–1601.

Mohs FE. Chemosurgical treatment of cancer of the ear. A microscopically controlled method of excision. Surgery 1947; 21:605–622.

Mohs FE. Chemosurgery for skin cancer. Arch Dermatol 1976; 112:211–215.

Noel SB, Scallon P, Meadors MC et al. Treatment of Pseudomonas aeruginosa auricular perichondritis with oral ciprofloxacin. J Dermatol Surg Oncol 1989; 15:633–637.

Pack GT, Conley J, Oropeza R. Melanoma of the external ear. Arch Otolaryngol 1970; 92:106–113.

Pless J. Carcinoma of the external ear. Scand J Plast Surg 1976; 10:147–151.

Rowe DE, Carroll RJ, Day CL. Prognostic factors for local recurrence, metastasis, and survival rates in squamous cell carcinoma of the skin, ear, and lip. JAAD 1992; 26:976–990.

Shambaugh GE. Developmental anatomy of the ear. In: Surgery of the Ear. Philadelphia: WB Saunders, 1967:5–39.

Shiffman MC. Squamous cell carcinomas of the skin of the pinna. Can J Surg 1975; 18:279–283.

Thomas JM, Swanson NA. Treatment of perichondritis with a quinolone derivative—norfloxacin. J Dermatol Surg Oncol 1988; 14:447–449.

Zimmerman MC. Chondrodermatitis nodularis helicis. In: Epstein E, ed. Skin Surgery. 3rd. Springfield, IL: Charles C Thomas, 1970:641–642.

23

The Eye and Eyelid

June K. Robinson

Department of Dermatology, Northwestern University Feinberg School of Medicine, Chicago, Illinois, U.S.A.

The orbital region presents a challenge to the dermatologic surgeon. Even though basic surgical principles still hold, this area is unique. It is necessary to preserve the function of the eyelid, which include protecting the globe and providing a constant moist environment for the cornea. A thorough knowledge of the anatomy in this region is mandatory prior to performing any surgery. Lesions specific to the orbital region, such as chalazions, hordeola, xanthelasma, and sebaceous carcinoma occur in addition to benign and malignant tumors and diseases seen in other regions. With experience in handling the skin of the eyelid and its special elasticity and properties of motion, the dermatologic surgeon can treat many lesions encountered in this region. For more advanced surgical problems, the dermatologic surgeon may wish to have the patient evaluated preoperatively by an ophthalmologist.

ANATOMY

The orbital area contains the brows and the upper and lower lids. It extends medially to the root of the nose and laterally to the orbital rim. The upper lid is limited above the eyebrows, while the lower merges into the cheek. The configuration of the eye area varies with race, age, and sex. Asymmetry in this region is readily noticed. A series of measures form the points of reference for the ideal proportion of the face. The face divides vertically into fifths, with each segment equal to the width of the eye measured from the medial to the lateral contour. Individual considerations, such as eye size, roundness, and slope; the width between the eyes, close set, or widely spaced, and ptosis are major determinants of the appearance. Ideally, the width of the eye is equal to the distance between the eyes (inner canthal distance); the distance from the lateral canthus to the outer rim of the helix of the ear in a full frontal view, and the width of the nose from the ala to ala. The central facial dimensions are further related by the interpupillary distance being equal to the vertical distance between the medial canthi and the most inferior point of the vermilion of the upper lip. The eyes as the "mirrors of the soul" may be the single most important facial form of expression.

The skin of the eyelids is the thinnest on the body and contains little fat. The palpebral fissures are roughly symmetrical, and the medial and lateral canthi are approximately at the same level horizontally. When the lateral canthus is higher than the medial canthus, this is termed a mongoloid slant. Transverse palpebral creases exist in both the upper and lower lids. The superior palpebral crease, 5–7 mm above the lid margin, marks the superior edge of

the tarsus and is because of the attachment of the levator aponeurosis. The inferior palpebral crease varies considerably. It roughly marks the lower margin of the tarsus and is approximately 5 mm below the lash line. As with any other part of the body, the placement of surgical scars in natural creases will produce good cosmetic results (Fig. 1).

The lid structures can be divided into anterior and posterior lamellae. The anterior lamella consists of skin and orbicularis oculi muscle, while the posterior lamella consists of tarsus and conjunctiva. The lamellae are divided by a fascial plane that extends to the lid margin, where it can be identified as the gray line, a linear change in color along the lid margin that represents the mucocutaneous junction. Anterior to the gray line, the cutaneous surface is hair-bearing up to the level of the orifices of the tarsal glands. Posterior to the gray line, the conjunctiva, a thin transparent mucous membrane, lines the posterior surface of the lids and is reflected forward on the eyeball. The eyelashes are located in the anterior lamella of the lid (Fig. 2).

The orbicularis oculi, with attachments to bone medially and laterally, acts as a sphincter to close the lids and maintain muscle tone. It is divided arbitrarily into orbital and palpebral portions. The palpebral portion is further divided into pretarsal and preseptal parts (Fig. 3). In younger individuals, the skin is firmly adherent to the underlying muscle, while with age the attachment becomes loose, with more folds. The pretarsal portion is firmly attached to the underlying tarsus; the only separation is in the superior portion where the levator aponeurosis attaches the pretarsal muscle at the upper edge of the tarsus (Fig. 2). The upper and lower pretarsal muscles are attached laterally to the lateral orbital tubercle of the malar bone. The upper and lower preseptal fibers fuse over the lateral orbital tubercle laterally at the lateral palpebral raphe. Medially, both the pretarsal and preseptal muscles divide into superficial and deep heads. The superficial heads form the medial canthal tendon, which attaches to the anterior lacrimal crest in the nasal process of the maxilla. The deep heads pass deep to the lacrimal sac and attach to the lacrimal diaphragm and posterior lacrimal crest. Thus, the lacrimal sac is surrounded by muscle, and each blink will help the movement of tears down the lacrimal duct (Fig. 3).

The subcutaneous fascia is immediately posterior to the orbicularis oculi muscle, within which run branches of the facial nerve and the maxillary division of the fifth cranial nerve (Fig. 2). The tarsi are immediately beneath the fascia and are composed of dense fibrous tissue. The upper tarsus is 10 mm in vertical height in the central lid and narrows

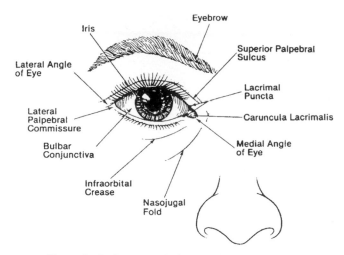

Figure 1 Surface anatomic features of the eyelid region.

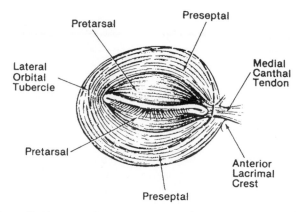

Figure 3 The pretarsal and preseptal parts of the palpebral portion of the orbicularis oculi muscle lie within the dashed line. The orbital portion of the orbicularis oculi muscle is outside the dashed line.

medially and laterally. The lower tarsus is the same length as the upper tarsus, but is only 4–5 mm in vertical height in the central lid. Each tarsus contains meibomian glands arranged in parallel lines, with the meibomian duct orifices in a line along the ciliary border posterior to the gray line. The meibomian glands are specialized sebaceous glands and are responsible for a significant component of the tear film. Adherent to the posterior tarsus is the tarsal portion of the conjunctiva.

The tarsi are attached to the periosteum of the orbital rims above and below by the orbital septum, which lies in the same fascial plane with the tarsi. The tarsi represent thickened portions of the embryologically developed mesodermal layer of the lid (Fig. 2). The septum extends from the

lower lid to the upper lid medially by passing under the attachment of the medial orbicularis muscle and blends in laterally with the lateral canthal tendon. The orbital septum is important in that it keeps the orbital fat in its posterior location (Fig. 4).

The retractors of the eyelids are deep to the orbital fat and their function is to open the eyelids. The upper eyelid is elevated by the levator palpebral superior, which arises as a striated muscle from the apex of the orbit. It passes forward under the roof of the orbit and just under the superior orbital rim, it passes vertically downward and spreads out as a thin, white, glistening tendinous sheet known as the levator aponeurosis. It fuses with the orbital septum inferiorly and attaches anteriorly to the pretarsal orbicularis muscle, where it is marked by the superior palpebral crease

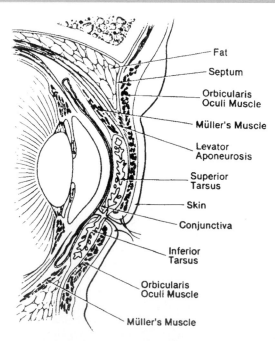

Figure 2 Anterior and posterior lamellae of the lid are separated by a fascial plane, which extends from the gray line at the lid margin to the tarsus, levator aponeurosis, and on up to the septum. This cross-sectional diagram of the lid structures clearly demonstrates the fascial plane of separation of the upper eyelid.

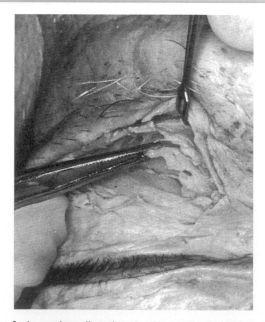

Figure 4 In a cadaver dissection, the skin and the thin orbicularis oculi muscle are elevated under the skin hook, the septum is dissected free, and the levator aponeurosis is held by the forceps. Immediately below the forceps is the superior margin of the upper tarsus. This dissection is performed at the point of fusion of the posterior-lying levator aponeurosis with the septum.

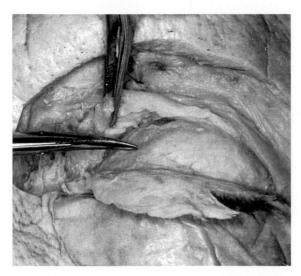

Figure 5 The septum and overlying tissues are removed. The orbital fat is dissected free and held in the clamp. The scissor tip points to the levator aponeurosis where it attaches to the pretarsal orbicularis muscle forming the superior palpebral crease. The thin pretarsal portion of the orbicularis muscle is folded down over the lashes. (Drs. June Robinson and Benjamin Raab performed these dissections.)

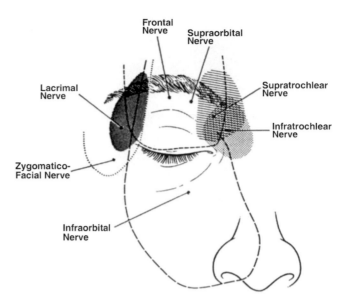

Figure 6 Sensory innervation of the eyelids.

(Fig. 5). On the posterior surface of the levator aponeurosis lies Muller's muscle. This is a thin layer of smooth muscle that originates on the undersurface of the levator and passes down vertically 12–15 mm to insert on the upper border of the tarsus (Fig. 2).

The eyelids receive vascular supply from both the internal and external carotid arterial systems. The ophthalmic artery branches off from the internal carotid artery, whose palpebral branches anastomose with branches from the lacrimal and transverse facial arteries, which come off the external carotid artery. These form the tarsal arcades that run between the tarsus and orbicularis oculi muscle. The good vascular supply to the eyelids promotes rapid healing following surgery. The angular artery lies anterior to the medial palpebral ligament 8 mm nasal to the inner angle of the palpebral fissure. The artery is formed by the anastomosis of the dorsal nasal artery and the facial artery and is easily transected when operating in the medial canthal region.

Sensory innervation of the eyelids is via branches of the first and second divisions of the trigeminal nerve. The first branch gives rise to the supraorbital nerve, arising from the superior orbital fissure and supplying a major portion of the upper lid. It also gives rise to the supratrochlear and infratrochlear nerves, located medial to the eye, which innervate the medial canthal area and the root of the nose, respectively. In addition, the first branch of the trigeminal nerve becomes the lacrimal nerve laterally to the eye, which supplies the lacrimal gland and lateral canthus. The lower lid is supplied by branches of the second division of the trigeminal nerve. The zygomaticofacial nerve innervates the lateral canthal area and the lateral aspect of the lower lid. It exits bone at approximately 1 cm inferior and lateral to the bend where the inferior rim meets the lateral orbital rim. The infraorbital nerve, which exits in the infraorbital foramen, innervates the lower lid, lacrimal sac area, side of the nose, and upper lip (Fig. 6).

The lacrimal apparatus consists of a gland that secretes the tears into the conjunctival sac and lacrimal passages. The lacrimal gland lies beneath the lateral end of the upper eyelid, covered in front by the septum orbitale, orbicularis oculi, and the skin. The gland is a mass of lobules, each about the size of a pinhead. Each lobule consists of a small mass of ramifying tubules branching into the acini of secretory cells. Accessory lacrimal glands are scattered along the conjunctival fornix.

The nasolacrimal system extends on both the upper and lower lids from the medially placed puncta. The upper and lower canaliculi traverse medially deep to the medial canthal tendon and join to form the common internal punctum that connects with the lacrimal sac. The total length of the canaliculi is about 10 mm, with an initial 1–2 mm vertical portion. Tears flow from this into the nasolacrimal duct and into the inferior turbinate of the nose. The lining membrane is continuous with that of the nose. The lacrimal sac lies in the lacrimal fossa surrounded by periosteum. The anatomy of the nasolacrimal system may be best appreciated in passing a probe through the system. The probe should enter the lower punctum and pass initially downward 2 mm, then turn gently toward the nose. The lower lid may be retracted temporally to straighten the canaliculus. When the probe meets a bony resistance, it is in the tear sac and against the lateral wall of the nose (Fig. 7).

The eyebrows are located directly superior to the eye units and tend to extend further both medially and laterally than the eyelids. The medial brow should end at a vertical line passed perpendicularly up from the ala at the nose–cheek junction. The lateral brow should end at a point of intersection with a line passed from the ala–cheek junction to the lateral canthus of the eye. The medial and lateral ends of the brow should lie on a horizontal line. The male brow has less elevation of the arch than the female. In white patients, the hair of the lateral eyebrows slants upward but in Asians these hairs grow downward. While scalp hair grows for 3–10 years, the growing phase of hair in the eyebrow does not exceed six months.

ANESTHESIA

General anesthesia is rarely necessary for eyelid surgery unless it is expected to last many hours and involve

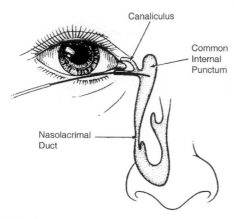

Figure 7 A probe enters the lower punctum and passes into the canaliculus before coming to rest in the lacrimal sac.

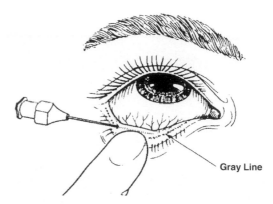

Figure 8 The lid is everted to show the gray line and anesthetic is placed between the conjunctival surface of the lid and the gray line.

extensive manipulation. Even extensive cases can be well managed by local anesthesia. Advantages of local over general anesthesia include: (i) greater safety of local anesthesia especially in elderly patients and those with cardiac, pulmonary, or liver disease; (ii) an awake patient who will cooperate when needed; (iii) a field not obstructed by endotracheal tubes, masks, inhalators, and so on; and (iv) lack of dependence on the anesthesiologist for adequate and prompt anesthesia. The use of local anesthesia by the dermatologic surgeon requires thorough knowledge of the anatomy of the nervous supply to the orbital area.

Local anesthesia can be obtained by infiltration or by nerve block. Infiltration anesthesia is adequate preparation for a small portion of the eyelid. In atrophic tissue in the aged, tissue planes separate from the edema produced by local anesthesia and allow easier identification of structures. However, this can be a liability when landmarks such as palpebral creases need to be preserved. In such cases, the area to be excised and anatomic landmarks can be marked with gentian violet. After injection of local anesthesia, minimal pressure to the area prevents excessive bruising.

When working with local infiltration anesthesia on small eyelid lesions, it may be advantageous to use a chalazion clamp for hemostasis and stability of the lid and to protect the cornea. The application of this clamp puts pressure on the conjunctival surface of the lid. It is necessary to infiltrate both surfaces of the lid. The hair-bearing skin of the lid is injected to the depth of the tarsal plate first. Then the lid is everted and the needle is placed between the conjunctival surface of the lid and the gray line (Fig. 8).

The advantage of nerve block anesthesia is the lack of tissue distortion and the limited volume of anesthesia required. Anesthesia of the upper lid is obtained by palpating the supraorbital notch, located at the junction of the middle and medial third of the upper orbital rim, and injecting 2–3 ml of anesthetic under the orbital rim in this area. This blocks the supraorbital nerve. The needle is then redirected medially and more anesthetic blocks the supratrochlear and infratrochlear nerves, which supply sensation to the medial canthus. The lower lid is anesthetized by palpating the infraorbital foramen, which lies 4–5 mm below the lower orbital margin in a vertical line with the supraorbital notch. The needle is introduced at this point and directed laterally and posteriorly, and about 2 ml of the anesthetic is injected. Finally, the lateral canthal area can be anesthetized by injecting the zygomaticofacial nerve,

which is located 1 cm inferior and temporal to the bend where the inferior orbital rim meets the lateral orbital rim. The lacrimal nerve also supplies the lateral canthus and can be injected by inserting the needle just above the lateral canthal tendon and directing it posteriorly for about 2 mm and then injecting 2–3 ml of the anesthetic.

Lidocaine is the most commonly used agent for local anesthesia. It diffuses well through the tissue and is not irritating. It is available in solutions of 0.5% to 2% with and without epinephrine. The maximum dose that can be safely used is 500 mg; however, this is well beyond the amount required for the eyelid and brow area. Epinephrine acts as a vasoconstrictor that slows the absorption of the lidocaine and prolongs its effect. Lidocaine (1%) with epinephrine in the ratio 1:100,000 are adequate for anesthesia.

Topical anesthetics are necessary when using protective corneal shields and chalazion clamps. Tetracaine can be instilled as drops directly on the cornea and conjunctiva. Its onset of action is within 26 seconds and its duration ranges from 9 to 24 minutes. Most patients initially complain of burning that disappears once the anesthetic effect is established. Some patients require a second installation of drops a few minutes after the first. Because the drug may cause transient punctuate keratopathy in high doses, the 0.5% solution is preferred.

In patients requiring premedication, meperidine (50–75 mg) with promethazine (12.5–25 mg) given intramuscularly at one hour preoperatively is helpful. Tranquilizers are usually not needed; however, in a very anxious patient, 5–10 mg of diazepam by mouth may be used.

SUTURES AND INSTRUMENTS

A variety of suture material is available for use in this region. The commonly used nonabsorbable sutures are silk, nylon, and prolene. Silk has the best tying characteristics and is the most pliable but tends to cause more tissue reaction than nylon or prolene. Braided silk (6-0) is preferred for the delicate thin skin of the eyelids. Because silk softens when moist and lies flat, it will not cause abrasions of the opposing eyelid or the unprotected cornea as may occur with monofilament nylon. However, away from the eyelids, the character of the skin changes and for the thicker skin of the nose and brows 5–0 or 6–0 nylon should be used. Normal lid skin is so thin that subcuticular sutures are rarely indicated. Once beyond the movable lid skin, however, buried sutures are useful. The skin of the brow and zygomatic regions is well suited to subcuticular closure, and 6–0 prolene may be considered for the skin as it tends to slide better than silk or nylon. Ideally, the wound should be closed in layers unless the excision is superficial. For deep absorbable sutures in this area, 4–0 or 5–0 gut sutures are often used.

The preferred needles for this region are the taper and reverse cutting type for skin closure and the spatula needle for suturing the tarsal plate. Skin sutures in this area can be removed between the third and fifth postoperative day. After suture removal, the wound is reinforced with sterile adhesive strips. All periorbital skin sutures should be removed by the seventh postoperative day to minimize the formation of scars or epidermal tracts.

The importance of protecting the cornea with opaque eye shields during orbital surgery cannot be overstated. Corneal shields are placed on the eyeball after topical anesthesia has been obtained. They not only protect the cornea but also bock the patient's view and screen the intense light used by the surgeon. They must be of the appropriate size and not so large that force is necessary to close the lids over them. Another device that protects the globe is the Jaeger plate, the spatula-shaped guard, which may also be used during a shave or punch biopsy of the lower lid. It is placed between the eyeball and the lower lid and functions to support the lid during the procedure and ensures that the orbit is not injured by perforation through the lid.

Two other instruments unique to this area are the chalazion clamp and the lacrimal probe. The chalazion clamp has one jaw with a round open center and another formed of a slightly curved solid plate. The open jaw surrounds the chalazion or lesion and distributes even pressure around it during excision. The back of the solid jaw is lubricated with ointment and rests lightly against the cornea. When the clamp is in place, a small nut is tightened to the desired pressure so that the surgeon can easily manipulate the end with one hand. The clamp is available in a large range of sizes (Fig. 9).

The lacrimal probe is needed when one is operating around the lacrimal duct. Identification and isolation of the lacrimal duct are preformed prior to surgery in this area. A probe, such as the Johnson wire, is rotated into the horizontal plane and passed through the canaliculus to the lacrimal sac. Once surgery has been completed, a silicone stent (Lester Jones tube) can be placed in the lacrimal outflow system. The silicone is left in place until the scar matures and softens. The silicone tubing maintains functional patency during the healing process, which usually takes six to eight months. If lacrimal obstruction was caused by prior surgery,

Table 1 Common Tumors of the Eyelid Region

Benign tumors	Inflammatory lesions
Seborrheic keratoses	Hordeolum (sty)
Actinic keratoses	Chalazion
Verruca vulgaris	*Appendage tumors*
Nevi	Syringoma
Skin tags	Hidrocystoma
Malignant tumors	Trichoepithelioma
Keratoacanthoma	Pilomatricoma
Basal cell carcinoma	Sebaceous adenoma
Squamous cell carcinoma	*Xanthelasma*
Melanoma	

it may be possible to correct the obstruction sufficiently with the Jones tube to improve the epiphora.

EYELID LESIONS

Practically any lesion that may occur elsewhere on the body can occur on the eyelids. In addition, certain lesions are most common in the eyelid region.

Benign Lesions

More than 75% of all eyelid lesions are benign. In addition to common lesions, such as seborrheic keratoses, actinic keratoses, verrucae vulgaris, and nevi, benign tumors that occur more commonly in this region or that may produce diagnostic difficulties with malignant tumors are listed in Table 1 (Fig. 10).

A hordeolum, or sty, is an acute bacterial infection of the meibomian glands or of the accessory glands of the lash follicles. It manifests as a localized erythematous swelling but may spread to involve one or both lids. Treatment is with warm compresses and topical antibiotics. If conservative measures do not suffice, incision and drainage may be necessary (Fig. 11).

A chalazion is a chronic granuloma of a meibomian gland caused by retention of secretion. It tends to increase in size slowly, but after a while it may stabilize. It is usually painless unless secondarily infected, in which case it will clinically resemble a hordeolum, and incision and drainage are required. Noninfectious chalazions are usually removed for cosmetic reasons.

Syringoma is an adenoma of eccrine differentiation. It occurs predominantly in women at puberty or later in life. Although occasionally solitary, syringomas usually are multiple. They are small, skin-colored or slightly yellowish, soft papules usually measuring 1–2 mm. They are usually

(A)   **(B)**   **(C)**

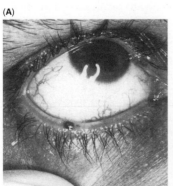 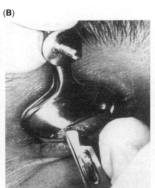 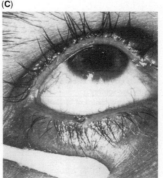

Figure 9 (A) Pigmented lesion of the lower eyelid; (B) chalazion clamp placed on the lower lid protects the eye during the shave removal when the blade is directed toward the eye; (C) immediately after the removal of the pigmented lesion.

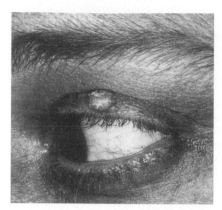

Figure 10   Keratoacanthoma of the upper eyelid.

limited to the lower eyelids but may occur on the cheeks, axillae, abdomen, and vulva. They are entirely benign.

Hidrocystoma is an adenoma that may be of eccrine or apocrine origin. It may be skin-colored or have a bluish hue. Eccrine hidrocystoma (1–3 mm) tends to be smaller than an apocrine hidrocystoma (3–15 mm) (Fig. 12).

Trichoepithelioma is a benign epithelioma of hair follicle differentiation. It is a firm, elevated, flesh-colored nodule usually measuring less than 2 cm. Its onset is in adult life, and it is most commonly seen on the face but may occur elsewhere. Trichoepitheliomas usually occur as multiple lesions, but occasionally are solitary.

Pilomatricoma, or calcifying epithelioma of Malherbe, is a benign epithelioma of hair follicle differentiation. It usually manifests as a firm subcutaneous nodule covered by normal skin. Its size varies from 0.5 to 3 cm, and the face and upper extremities are the most common sites.

Sebaceous adenoma is a rare tumor of the sebaceous gland differentiation and presents as a round, firm elevated papule that may be pedunculated. It is usually solitary and can be located on the face, especially the eyelids, or scalp of adults. The association of sebaceous adenomas of the skin with visceral carcinomas, especially of the colon, is know as Torres's syndrome.

Xanthelasma is a localized infiltrate of lipid-containing histiocytic foam cells in either the upper or lower eyelids. They are yellow, soft macules or slightly elevated papules. Although these xanthomas may suggest underlying hypercholesterolemia when occurring in patients below

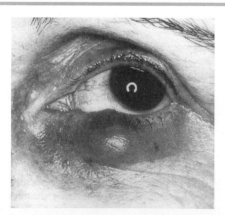

Figure 11   A hordeolum presents as an acute, tender, warm erythematous swelling.

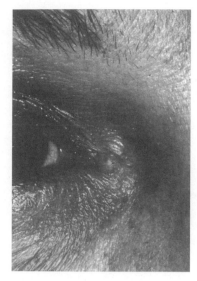

Figure 12   Apocrine hidrocystoma of the medial canthus.

40–50 years of age, less than one-half of the patients have elevated plasma lipid levels. In addition to excision, these can be treated with cryotherapy, electrodesiccation, and application of 25% to 35% of trichloracetic acid.

Malignant Lesions

Basal cell carcinoma is the most common eyelid malignancy, making up more than 90% of all eyelid cancers and nearly 20% of all eyelid tumors (Fig. 13). These tumors most commonly involve the lower lid, followed by the medial canthus, upper lid, and lateral canthus. Although they often invade local tissues, they rarely metastasize. When these tumors arise near the canthi, they tend to infiltrate deeply and may involve the eye or lacrimal drainage system. Because of patient neglect and inadequate early treatment, a mortality rate of 2% was noted in one series. In the same series, enucleation or exenteration was required in 3.6% of the cases.

Surgical excision with histologic control of all margins (Mohs micrographic surgery) is the most effective treatment for basal cell carcinoma in the eyelid area. Histologic examination of the margin is particularly important for morpheaform and metatypical basal cell carcinoma. In treating primary basal cell carcinoma in this area, Mohs micrographic surgery has attained cure rates of 99%. Treatment of basal cell carcinoma of the eyelids by simple excision without histologic control of the margins has a recurrence rate of 10% to 12%. The frequency of recurrence is probably unrelated to the size of the presenting lesion.

Curettage and electrodessications are not effective treatment for lesions on the eyelids, because it is difficult to immobilize the skin. Radiation therapy is effective, but results depend on the type of radiation, size of the irradiated field, duration of the tumor, its location, and the depth of penetration. The recurrence rate with radiation therapy observed by the Skin and Cancer Unit at New York University is 7.9% with a follow-up of five years and 12.6% after 10 years. Finally, while cryosurgical treatment of primary tumors attains cure rates equal to surgical excision as reported by Torre, many variations in the delivery of this modality in practice result in differing cure rates.

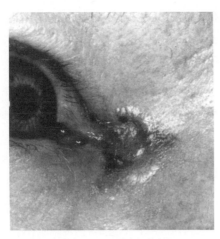

Figure 13 Basal cell carcinoma of the medial canthus with central ulceration and rolled border.

Squamous cell carcinoma, the second most common malignancy of the eyelids, is far less common than the basal cell carcinoma, representing about 5% of the malignant lesions. While any part of the eyelid may be involved, the lower lid is the more common. The mortality from squamous cell carcinoma is higher than that reported with basal cell carcinoma, particularly because it has greater predilection to metastasize to regional lymph nodes. Therefore, in addition to examination of lymph nodes, a wider resection margin is usually required around the tumor than with basal cell carcinoma. Accurate frozen-section examination of margins is mandatory.

Sebaceous gland carcinoma is a rare tumor of the eyelid and adnexa. It usually arises from meibomian glands but can also originate from the glands of Zeis, the sebaceous glands on the cutaneous surface of the eyelids, the sebaceous glands of the eyebrow, and the sebaceous glands located in the caruncle. Sebaceous carcinoma may metastasize and has a high mortality rate (30–40%), probably because of late diagnosis and multicentricity. Many sebaceous carcinomas have a yellow color and cause loss of eyelashes. They may resemble a chalazion and occasionally extend within the conjunctival epithelium by pagetoid spread and mimic blepharoconjunctivitis. Therefore, sebaceous carcinoma should be considered in the differential diagnosis of recurrent or chronic inflammation of the eyelids. Treatment of sebaceous carcinoma consists of wide surgical excision. Because of multicentricity, biopsies from various locations are important to establish the diagnosis. Treatment with Mohs micrographic surgery is the subject of controversy.

Melanoma rarely occurs on the eyelids; however, it may spread to the eyelids from the cheek. The amount of tissue removed is primarily dependent on tumor thickness. An evaluation for metastatic disease is also indicated by tumor thickness.

EXCISIONAL SURGERY OF THE EYELID AND EYEBROW

Surgical treatment depends on the size, location, and anticipated biologic behavior of the malignancy. The main objective of oncologic ophthalmic surgery is to remove the tumor and provide the best functional and cosmetic result

possible. Aesthetic surgery of the eyelid, blepharoplasty, and eyebrow, browlift, may make remarkable improvements in the appearance of the aging face. These procedures are beyond the scope of this chapter.

Providing corneal protection during the procedure with a corneal shield in the eye that is in the surgical field is usually well tolerated by patients. It is helpful to ask the patient if they have claustrophobia prior to inserting the shield. Assuring the claustrophobic patient that the other eye will remain uncovered and the face will not be covered with a drape is usually sufficient. If the patient does not have claustrophobia, it is usually more comfortable to have the eye, which is not in the surgical field, covered with an eye pad.

Simple Elliptical Excision

Elliptical excisions can be performed near the eye by giving consideration to the highly mobile nature of the lower eyelid. To avoid postoperative ectropion, excisions near the eyes should be oriented so that the long axis is perpendicular or slightly oblique to the margin. The tension is then placed lateral to medial and avoids tension directed on the lower lid.

Simple excision leaving an intact tarsus can be done for small tumors that do not cross the gray line. When possible, lid incisions should lie within the natural creases or should parallel the direction of the orbicularis oculi fibers. The defect should be small enough that no ectropion is produced when the defect is closed. Closure should be made with slight eversion of the skin edges to avoid depression when healing takes place. When closed, the edges of the wound should lie together snugly without puckering.

When the tumor lies close to the lid margin, a simple excision parallel to the orbicularis oculi fibers will produce ectropion. In this case, an intramarginal incision is made along the gray line with a #15 blade to free the mass from the tarsal plate. Two curved incisions are made with scissors, starting at the lid margin on each side of the tumor without disturbing the tarsal plate. The lesion is removed, and 6–0 silk sutures are passed horizontally through the skin edges at the ciliary line to approximate the edges of the incision. The orbicularis muscle is sutured with two buried 6–0 chromic catgut sutures, and then the skin is closed with simple interrupted suture of 6–0 silk. Only about 0.5 mm of tissue should be picked up with each bite of the suture. Because of the angled cuts of the incision, the skin closure will slightly overhang the tarsal edge. However, as the scar contracts, the ciliary line is reestablished and the lashes are not distorted.

Chalazion Excision

The chalazion is the most common lid lesion requiring surgical excision. When the lesion presents on the anterior lid, the chalazion clamp is placed around the lesion and a horizontal incision is made over the mass. The cyst is evacuated and fibrous tissue is excised. The skin is closed with 6–0 silk. The horizontal scar blends well with the normal skin crease. When the lesion presents on the posterior lid surface, a chalazion clamp is applied and the lid is everted. A vertical incision is then made over the lesion. The necrotic debris is curetted and fibrosis is excised. Suturing is not necessary and bleeding can be controlled with cautery.

Lower Eyelid Lesions

For small, raised lesions close to the lower lid border and not involving the gray line, a shave excision can be performed.

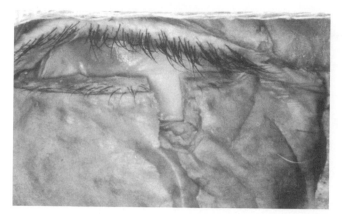

Figure 14 The incision through the lower eyelid is extended to meet in a V (cadaver procedure).

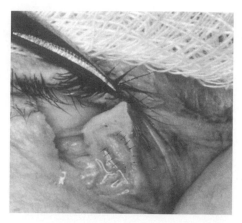

Figure 15 The lateral margin of the incision made in Figure 14 is everted to show the tarsus. Arrows delineate the tarsus (cadaver procedure).

This can be done for biopsy when a lesion is small and not deemed malignant, or when the lesion is not deep or large enough to require an excision. After anesthesia is induced, a guard is inserted down into the inferior fornix. A #15 blade on a Bard-Parker handle or a #67 blade on a Beaver handle is used to shave the tumor at its base, leaving a smooth lid margin. If the lesion is flat, the scalpel is used to perforate the mass at its lateral edge. The incision is carried medially, and the medial end is cut free. The shave excision should be superficial enough to leave the hair bulbs of the eyelashes intact.

If the lesion extends beyond the gray line or if there is a question of malignancy, a full-thickness lid excision is required. After placement of the backguard or eye shield, excision is performed in a perpendicular fashion from the lid margin on both sides of the lesion to the inferior border of the tarsus. The incisions are then extended in a V fashion to meet below the tarsus (Figs. 12, 13, 14 and 15). In older patients, direct closure is useful for central eyelid defects affecting less than 40% of the lid margin. In younger patients, because of less skin laxity, it may be possible to close a defect involving 30% of less of the lid margin.

A three-suture technique of 6–0 silk is commonly used to close a lid margin defect. One end of the suture is passed through the meibomian orifice about 1 mm from the wound margin (Fig. 16). The other end of the suture is passed through an orifice on the opposite wound margin. The lid margin should be in good opposition. A second silk suture is similarly placed posterior to the first at the junction between the skin and the conjunctiva and is secured. The ends of these sutures are left approximately 2-cm long. A third lid margin suture is placed in the lash line. It is important that it should not be placed anterior to the lashes: this will cause the lid margin to invert (ectropion). The long ends of the first two sutures are tied into the knot of the third suture. Three sutures are placed on the free margin of the lid to ensure that tension will be evenly distributed. If one suture ruptures, two others hold the lid in good opposition (Fig. 17).

Two or three interrupted 6–0 chromic gut or vicryl sutures are placed through the tarsus in the vertical incision. Conjunctiva should not be included in these sutures. Closure of the tarsus is the most important aspect of lid repair, and great care should be taken to reapproximate the perpendicular edges precisely. If the tarsus is not closed, a notch in the lid will result. The skin is then closed with interrupted 6–0 or 7–0 silk suture. While some believe that these sutures

should be placed sufficiently deep to engage the severed orbicularis muscle and reapproximate it, others do not place sutures into the muscle and simply allow it to reapproximate itself during would healing (Fig. 18).

If the initial defect is greater than 40% of the original lid margin, a lateral canthotomy will be required to reduce tension on the wound edge. This is done by making a horizontal excision at the lateral canthal angle and extending it approximately 5 mm on the skin surface. The canthotomy should be angled somewhat superiorly. A scalpel or scissors can be used for the incision. Sharp dissection is carried down to the periosteum of the lateral orbital rim, and the lower crus of the lateral canthal tendon is severed from the rim. This will allow mobilization of about 5 mm of the lateral aspect of the lower lid, which can be moved medially. The lid margin is then closed by the three-suture technique, and the skin is closed at the lateral canthus.

Upper Eyelid Lesions

The technique for removing a lesion from the upper eyelid is similar to that described for the lower eyelid. The upper eyelid is not as conducive to shave excision as the lower eyelid, and, therefore, simple excision is often performed. As with the lower eyelid, the incision should extend in a perpendicular fashion from the lid margin to the superior border of the tarsus. At this point, the incision is extended into a V shape.

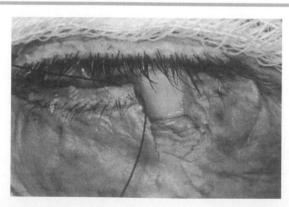

Figure 16 The first suture is placed at the gray line through the meibomian orifice, about 1 mm from the wound margin (cadaver procedure).

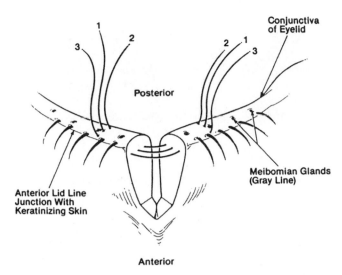

Figure 17 Diagram of the three-suture technique for closure of the lid margin.

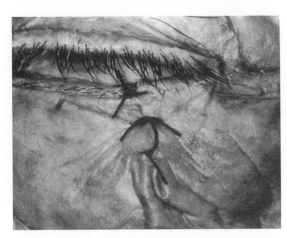

Figure 18 The tarsus is closed and finally the skin is closed (cadaver procedure).

Closure is basically the same as that described for lower eyelids. If the edges cannot be easily approximated, a lateral canthotomy is also performed. However, for upper eyelid defects, the arc of the canthotomy incision curves inferiorly and the upper crus of the lateral canthal tendon is severed. Direct closure of defects up to one-half of the upper lid can be performed using a canthotomy, especially in older patients. The primary defect is closed using the three-suture technique. Reapproximation of the tarsal plate is particularly important.

Medial Canthus

The simplest defect to close in this area is diamond-shaped. Defects should be fashioned in this manner whenever possible. For all types of medial canthal reconstruction, whether second intention, full-thickness skin graft, or glabella flap, the edge of the lid remnants must be attached to the posterior reflection of the medial canthal tendon to restore the normal canthal angle. This is simply done by placing a strong permanent suture, such as 4–0 silky II Polydek, through the tarsal remnant of both upper and lower lids and attaching it to the posterior reflection of the medial-canthal tendon.

In most situations, the best result is obtained by allowing defects of the medial canthus that are equal above and below the caruncle to heal by second intention. The classic teaching of covering exposed periosteum with a flap is not necessary in this location.

Lateral Canthus

In the aging face, redundancy of skin at the lateral canthus creates "crow's feet." If a lesion is benign, less than 3 mm in length, and falls along one of these natural creases, a small simple ellipse may be done. This location is ideal for an M-plasty to reduce the length of the incision.

Malignant primary lesions of the lateral canthus are often deeply invasive when located at the conjunctival margin and will require a resection that disrupts the lateral-canthal tendon and invades the orbit. This should be done with Mohs micrographic surgery. This same principle is true for primary lesions of the medial canthus. Certainly, all recurrent lesions of the eyelids require excision by Mohs micrographic surgery. Similarly, malignancies located along the lid margin near the punctum will migrate along the canaliculus and require the Mohs technique to ensure adequate resection. In these extensive and invasive cases, the Mohs surgeon may work together with an opthalmoplastic reconstructive surgeon.

One needs to consider the morbidity that will result from inadequate resection of eyelid malignancies. The residual tumor often invades deeply and affects vital structures. Recurrent cancer may require orbital exenteration and ablative craniofacial surgery for a potentially life-threatening, recurrent aggressive tumor. It is reasonable to use the technique that provides the best chance of cure as the initial resection.

Skin Graft

When there is insufficient tissue to close a wound primarily without tension, either a skin flap or a graft can be used to provide coverage. If there is a good blood supply and sufficient underlying soft tissue, a full-thickness skin graft may be applied to the base of the defect. The graft should be taken from the tissue that matches closely. For the eyelids, the first choice for a donor site is eyelid skin from the opposite eye. The next choice is retroauricular or preauricular skin. Full-thickness grafts provide better cosmetic result and are less subject to contraction than split-thickness grafts. Split-thickness grafts are more resistant to infection, tolerate poor circulation better, and cause less disfigurement to the donor area. In eyelid repair, a common problem is avoiding ectropion; thus, full-thickness skin grafts are usually chosen (Fig. 19). Contracture may occur under the full-thickness skin graft and ectropion can occur.

If retroauricular skin is used, the thinner skin of the back of the ear is placed along the aspect of the wound closest to the lash line. The thicker skin in the sulcus and nonhair-bearing scalp is oriented in the portion of the defect farthest from the lash line. When taking a full-thickness graft, a template of the shape and size of the graft needed is placed on the donor site. This is used to trace an outline of the defect. The donor area is then anesthetized with lidocaine and epinephrine, excised, undermined, and closed. Subcutaneous tissue should be removed from the graft with scissors. The dermis can be partially removed as well to produce a slightly thinner graft.

(A)

(B)

(C)

(D)

(E)

(F)

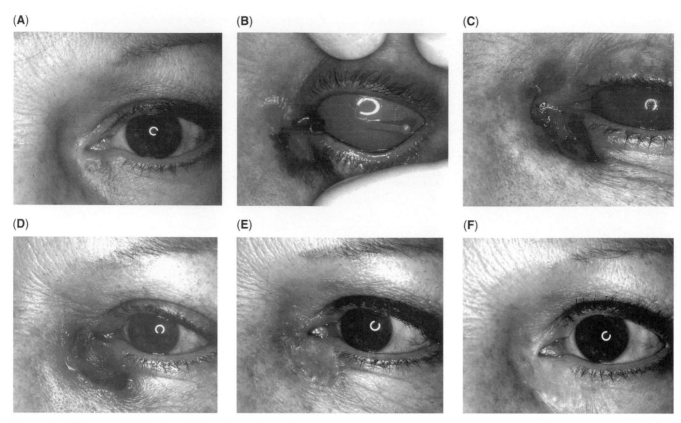

Figure 19   (**A**) Preoperatively, the basal cell carcinoma of the left lower eyelid extends along the lid margin almost to the lacrimal duct. (**B**) After the corneal shield was placed, a Johnson wire was introduced into the lacrimal duct. The area of the tumor is outlined. (**C**) Resection with Mohs surgery preserved the medial canthal tendons and the lacrimal duct system. (**D**) One week after the repair with a full-thickness skin graft and the use of a bolus dressing, the graft has a good take with the expected amount of depression. (**E**) Three weeks after the repair, the graft is elevated and the lid margin is in the proper position. (**F**) One year after surgery, there is a slight epicanthal web and the graft is hypopigmented. There is no epiphora.

The graft is sutured into place on the recipient site with simple interrupted 6–0 silk sutures at the lid margin and 5–0 monofilament nylon sutures at other locations around the perimeter of the graft. Tacking sutures placed through the center of the graft ensure its adherence to the wound bed. The ends of several sutures are left long and lightly tied over a bulky dressing to maintain contact between the graft and the recipient site. The tension on these bolus tie-over sutures is directed away from the lid. The eye area is covered with an eyepad. The bolus tie-over dressing is left in place for three to five days and then removed. When removing the bolus dressing, pressure is applied to the graft with forceps to ensure that it remains flat against the wound bed. Most of the sutures are removed and an antibiotic ointment applied to the surface of the graft under a dressing. This dressing and the remaining sutures are removed seven days after surgery.

Tarsorrhaphy

Apposition of the margins of the two lids may be required either for protection of the cornea and globe or for immobilization of the lids, such as during healing following a graft or flap for lid reconstruction. The lid margin is deepithelialized for the distance necessary to cover the cornea. Vertical mattress sutures of 4–0 or 5–0 silk with curved needles on both ends of the suture are used. The needle enters the skin approximately 3 mm from the ciliary margin of the upper lid and passes directly into the tarsus, exiting at the lid margin posterior to the gray line. The inner lower lid is then entered at a comparable point to pass through the skin below the ciliary margin. The mattress suture is then completed by going completely through the outer lower lid and entering the inner upper lid. The suture is then tied over cotton pledgets. Usually two or three of these sutures are well tolerated for one to two weeks. After suture removal, the lid margins that were deepithelialized are fused.

If a lateral tarsorrhaphy is performed because of permanent loss of the blink reflex and eyelid function due to transaction of the ophthalmic branch of the facial nerve, it is never released. When the lid remnants are opposed after tumor resection and prior to final reconstruction, tarsorrhaphy will only be necessary until the final reconstruction is done. Tarsorrhaphy is also done to stabilize the lid and improve survival of a full-thickness skin graft. It may prevent displacement of the lid margin because of wound contraction following full-thickness skin grafting. In this instance, the tarsorrhaphy may be released four to six months after the grafting procedure.

EYEBROW SURGERY

For lesions on or around the eyebrow, single and double advancement flaps are used. The length of the flap should not move more than three times the width of the base. The lesion is removed in a square or rectangular fashion.

A single-advancement flap is incised and its base widely undermined for forward motion. Burrow's triangles are cut at the base as the flap slides forward. The first suture is placed from the center of the advancing flap to the opposing surface. Then two corner stitches are placed. The Burrow's triangles are cut to accommodate secondary movement. The remainder of the flap is sutured with interrupted or half-buried sutures (Fig. 20).

COMPLICATIONS

An expected consequence of eyelid surgery is postoperative bruising and edema. Bleeding during surgery must be controlled before closure is performed. In addition, an adequate preoperative history must be taken to determine if the patient is taking any medications that will cause excessive bleeding. A variety of medications can affect the clotting mechanism, including aspirin, indomethacin, and anticoagulants. These should be discontinued for at least two weeks before surgery. Nevertheless, postoperative bruising is not uncommon and the patient should be made aware that this may occur.

Eyelid surgery should be done with a plastic non-conducting backguard or corneal shield to prevent abrasion of the cornea. Corneal abrasion can occur whenever an instrument is dragged across the eye when the eyelid is elevated. Inadvertent cautery of the cornea would be disastrous.

Ectropion and entropion refer to eversion and inversion of the eyelid margin, respectively. Ectropion of the lower lid results in epiphora (overflow of tears) and irritation of the skin of the lid by the tears. In addition, corneal exposure may lead to keratitis. Ectropion can occur when a large defect is produced below the lower lid and healing results in contracture. This can be prevented by excising eyelid lesions as described previously and by the use of flaps or full-thickness skin grafts.

Entropion will cause constant irritation resulting in conjunctivitis, keratitis, and corneal ulcers. The occurrence of entropion after eyelid surgery is uncommon as long as the lid margin is reapproximated properly using the three-suture technique and the edges of the tarsus are reapproximated precisely.

Brow ptosis may result from surgery in the temple region. This can be corrected by a browlift procedure on

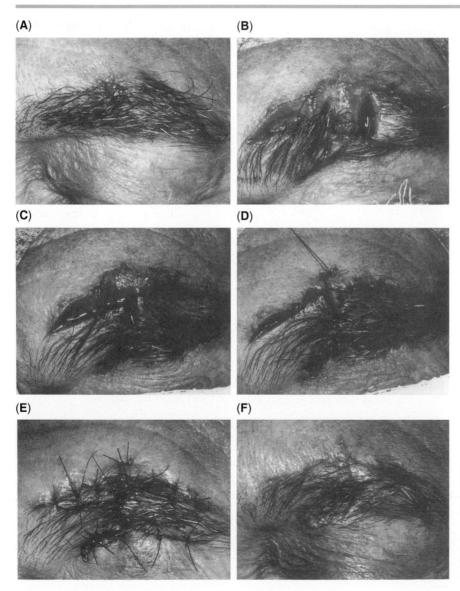

(A)

(B)

(C)

(D)

(E)

(F)

Figure 20 (A) Basal cell carcinoma of the eyebrow. (B) Tumor is excised and the limbs of bilateral advancement flap are incised. (C) Advancement flaps are approximated by subcutaneous sutures. (D) The first corner suture is placed. (E) All incisions are closed with interrupted sutures and two four-point corner sutures. (F) Six weeks after surgery there is no hair loss. Incision lines are slightly erythematous.

the side with loss of frontalis muscle function or botulinum toxin-A injections into the frontalis muscle on the side that is elevated. The toxin is injected into the frontalis muscle approximately 1 cm above the brow. The browlift procedure, which is a permanent way to correct this ptosis is beyond the scope of this chapter.

BIBLIOGRAPHY

Arkel S. Evaluation of platelet aggregation in disorders of hemostasis. Med Clint North Am 1976; 60:881–911.

Bart RS, Kopf AW, Petratos MA. X-ray therapy of skin cancer: evaluation of a "standardized" method for treating basal cell epitheliomas. Proceedings of the 6th National Cancer Conference, 1970:559–569.

Beard C. Observations on the treatment of basal cell carcinoma of the eyelids. Trans Am Acad Ophthalmol Otol 1975; 79:664–670.

Brodkin RH, Kopf AW, Andrade R. Basal cell epithelioma and elastosis: a comparison of distribution. In: Urbach F, ed. The Biologic Effect of Ultraviolet Radiation. London: Pergamon Press, 1969:581–618.

Carruthers A, Carruthers J. Use of Botulinum toxin type A in facial rejuvenation. In: Robinson JK, Hanke CW, Sengelmann RD, Siegel DM, eds. Surgery of the Skin: Procedural Dermatology. Philadelphia: Elsevier Mosby Inc., 2005: 501–510.

Friedman AH, Henkind P. Clinical and pathological features of eyelid and conjunctival tumors. In: Fox SA, ed. Ophthalmic Plastic Surgery. New York: Grune & Stratton, 1976:24–63.

Grove AS Jr. Eyelid tumors, diagnosis and management. In: McCord CD, ed. Oculoplastic Surgery. New York: Raven Press, 1981:151–173.

Iliff CE, Iliff WJ, Iliff NI. Tumors of the ocular adnexa. In: Ilif CE, ed. Oculoplastic Surgery. Philadelphia: WB Saunders, 1979:223–318.

Lim C, Martin P, Benger R, Kourt G, Ghabrail R. Lacrimal canalicular bypass surgery with the Lester Jones tube. Am J Ophthmalol 2004; 137:101–108.

Meltzer MA. Ophthalmic Plastic Surgery for the General Ophthalmologist. Baltimore: Williams & Wilkins, 1979.

Mohs FE. Chemosurgical treatment of cancer of the eyelid: a microscopically controlled method of excision. Arch Ophthalmol 1948; 39:43.

Mohs FE. Chemosurgery: Microscopically Controlled Surgery for Skin Cancer. Springfield, IL: Charles C Thomas, 1978.

Payne JW, Duke JR, Butner R, Eifrig DE. Basal cell carcinoma of the eyelids: a long-term follow-up study. Arch Ophthalmol 1969; 81:553.

Putterman A. Cosmetic Oculoplastic Surgery. New York: Grune & Stratton, 1982.

Robinson JK. Prevention of intraoperative trauma to the lacrimal system. J Dermatol Surg Oncol 1983; 9:802–804.

Torre D. Cryosurgery treatment of eyelid tumors. In: Jakobiec FA, ed. Ocular and Adnexal Tumors. Birmingham, AL: Aesculapius, 1978:517–524.

24

The Nose

Tri H. Nguyen

Department of Dermatology and Otorhinolaryngology, University of Texas
M.D. Anderson Cancer Center, Houston, Texas, U.S.A.

INTRODUCTION

Of all facial subunits, the nose is the most complex in its reconstructive demands. Central and prominent in location, three-dimensional in contour, varied in texture, and functionally critical—the nose fixates our gaze esthetically and dominates the facial landscape. Repair of nasal defects, therefore, requires meticulous attention to both function and form. A firm foundation in nasal anatomy and a thoughtful approach are prerequisite to successful reconstruction.

SURFACE ANATOMY

Nasal skin topography consists of hills and valleys. Planar surfaces of the nose include the nasal dorsum and sidewall. The soft triangles (nasal facet) may be either slightly concave or flat. Convex nasal surfaces include the nasal tip and alar lobules. The alar groove (alar facial sulcus) is a concave curve that extends from the nasal tip medially, the cheek laterally, and to the nostril sill inferiorly. Surface projections of the nose include the lateral ridges of the nasal dorsum and the medial crus of the lower lateral cartilages, which define nasal tip projection.Burget and Menick have popularized two nasal concepts—that of nasal skin zones and subunit repair. Three skin zones of varying thickness and sebaceous texture distinguish the nose (Fig. 1). Zone I is the thin, pliable, and nonsebaceous skin of the nasal root, proximal nasal dorsum, and sidewalls. Zone II is the thicker and more sebaceous skin of the nasal tip and alar lobules. Zone III is also thin and nonsebaceous and consists of the nasal infratip, soft triangles, alar margins, and columella. Unlike Zone I, however, Zone III is not pliable and is fixed to the underlying cartilage structure. As a result, Zone III skin is more prone to distortion from the forces of scar contraction. "Be wary of the nose with sebum" is sage reconstructive advice as traditionally successful techniques become less so on a highly sebaceous nose. Figure 2 illustrates nasal subunits and highlights the concept of subunit repair. A subunit is a region with similar attributes (blood supply, thickness, color, and texture). The tenets of subunit repair dictate the following: (i) repairs confined to the same subunit produce the best reconstructive match in contour, color, and texture, (ii) incisions that cross adjacent regions should be avoided but if needed, be placed between subunit borders for best camouflage, (iii) if 50% or more of a subunit is missing, then whenever possible, the residual skin should be excised so that the entire subunit may be resurfaced. Although important, the subunit repair principle is not inviolate. Incisions may cross subunit regions and the sacrifice of residual tissue is not always needed. Cosmesis may still be excellent by being flexible with these concepts.

STRUCTURAL SUPPORT

The nose is a three-dimensional pyramid, consisting of a bone and cartilage infrastructure that is sandwiched by mucosal lining internally and muscle and skin externally. The nasal bone forms the rigid upper one-third of the nose. From here, the nasal septum and upper lateral cartilages project to form the middle one-third of the nose. The septal cartilage is thick, lies vertically, and divides the nose into two halves. The upper lateral cartilages are thinner and form a slanted roof over the nasal septum. The lower one-third of the nose consists of the caudal end of the upper lateral cartilages and the lower lateral cartilages (a.k.a. alar cartilages). At this junction, the lower lateral cartilages overlap the caudal end of the upper lateral cartilages. This overlapping adherence may be easily dislocated by thoughtless dissection. The lower one-third is most vulnerable to distortion with its free margins (alar rims) and lack of bony support. Functionally, it also contains the internal nasal valve, which is the narrowest cross-section of the air passageway. This internal narrowing is marked superficially by the external nasal valve, which is formed by the confluences of the nasal sidewall, lateral nasal tip, and alar lobule (Fig. 2). Thick flaps overlying this area without cartilage support may compromise the internal nasal valve and result in inspiratory obstruction. The deep superficial musculoaponeurotic system (SMAS) fascia and nasal muscles overlie the nasal cartilages and they are in turn covered by skin. The undermining plane of choice on the nose is the subnasalis space, which is beneath the nasal muscle and SMAS and above the perichondrium. This avascular plane preserves the muscular pedicle above while permitting excellent hemostasis. This cursory discussion of nasal anatomy highlights only the essentials, and more comprehensive references are available.

GENERAL STRATEGY FOR NASAL DEFECTS

Oncologic cure, functional preservation, and esthetic restoration (in that order) are the goals of all reconstruction. For the remainder of this chapter, nasal repairs are discussed in the context of defects from Mohs surgery, the gold standard for negative margin control. With the myriad of repair options, it is critical to approach all nasal defects systematically. Preoperative evaluation must focus on preexisting nasal scars or structural defects (i.e., deviated septum, previous nasal fractures, or rhinoplasty, etc.) that

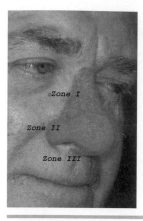

Figure 1 Nasal skin zones: Zone I—thin, nonsebaceous, mobil; Zone II—thick, relatively sebaceous and nonelastic; and Zone III—thin, nonsebaceous, but adherent, not pliable.

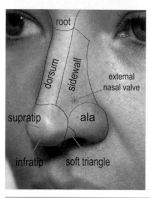

Figure 2 Nasal subunits: nasal tip is subdivided into the supratip and the infratip.

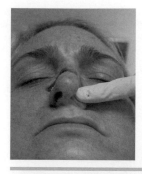

Figure 3 Worm's eye view with nasal valve test in a patient with a deep right sidewall/ala defect—contralateral nostril is occluded and the patient is asked to inspire deeply. Cartilage grafting for nasal valve support is appropriate if there is significant inspiratory obstruction on the defect side.

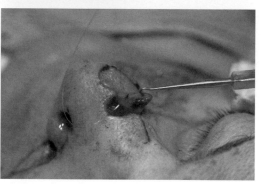

Figure 4 Suture placement on the nose should be placed deeply, between the muscle and dermis.

may compromise tissue mobility or blood supply. Accurate wound assessment is essential and relevant questions are listed in Table 1. Nasal defects should be viewed from all angles and the worm's eye view is often the most revealing for airway collapse and asymmetry (Fig. 3). Reconstruction must address the three nasal layers (the internal mucosal lining, the bony and cartilaginous framework, and the soft-tissue covering) and the three-dimensional nasal topography.

Table 1 Wound Analysis in Nasal Reconstruction

Questions	Relevance
What is missing? Is the breach in skin and soft tissue only, or does it also involve cartilage and mucosal lining?	Full-thickness defects or those that involve nasal lining require complex reconstruction that are often multistaged with cartilage grafting
Is the internal nasal valve adequately supported by existing cartilage, and is additional support required?	Even if native cartilage is not missing, structural grafts may be needed to prevent nasal collapse or support a heavy flap
Where is the wound located?	Shallow wounds in concave or shadow areas such as the alar groove, may heal well with second intention healing. Wounds near free margins may result in distortion from either flap tension or wound contraction
How many subunits does the defect involve?	If possible, repairing within the same subunit is ideal. Incision lines crossing subunits are best placed between their borders for camouflage
Where are the areas of tissue mobility?	Traditional areas of donor skin on the nose include the glabella and forehead, proximal nasal root, nasal sidewall, medial cheek, and lower melolabial fold
How rigid are the cartilaginous structures of the distal nose (nasal tip, alar lobules and margins, and columella)?	By pushing on the nasal tip in a horizontal and vertical direction, one may assess the rigidity of the lower one third of the nose. A nose tip that is easily displaced is one that is prone to distortion even with minimal tension
What is the patient's skin type?	Patients with darker skin types may experience more pronounced hypopigmentation in areas of skin grafting and second-intention healing
How sebaceous is the skin around the defect?	Highly sebaceous skin is predisposed to inflammation, dehiscence, and more visible incision lines. Deeper wounds on sebaceous skin and that heal by second intention will predictably leave a noticeable depression unless the wound edges are tapered
How thick is the sebaceous skin of the nasal tip?	Thick nasal tip skin contributes to nasal tip projection. A defect in this location may require a contour graft to restore form
How prominent is the alar groove?	A deep alar groove is prone to blunting by flaps transgressing this border (i.e., melolabial transposition flap)
Are there relevant comorbidities?	Smoking, rhinophyma, obstructive sleep apnea with continuous positive airway pressure usage, anticoagulation are all factors that may affect reconstructive planning
How sun damage is the remainder of the nasal skin?	The use of actinically damaged skin may result in the transfer of new primary skin cancers to the recipient site
Will this patient tolerate multistage reconstruction?	For some patients, restoration of function is sufficient and multiple complex procedures to achieve esthetic perfection is unnecessary

Table 2 Cartilage Grafts in Nasal Reconstruction

Types of grafts	Function
Restorative	Replacing damaged or resected native cartilage to restore the nasal framework
Structural	Grafts that support existing cartilage. These grafts tend to be long and rectangular in shape and may be harvested from the ear or nasal septum
	Batten grafts
	Placed at the external nasal valve for alar support of an overlying flap and prevent airway collapse
	Placed near the alar margin to prevent rim elevation with scar contraction
	Columellar struts
	Placed between the medial crus of the alar cartilages to give tip support and projection
	Spreader grafts
	Placed between the caudal end of the upper lateral cartilage and the nasal septum to widen the internal nasal valve
Contour	Grafts that are placed to achieve form or projection
	Tip grafts—placed at the nasal tip for projection
	Shield grafts—long graft extending from the columellar base to curve over the supratip
	Cap grafts (Peck grafts)—short grafts that are often layered and secured to the domal aspect of the alar cartilages at the supratip
	Onlay grafts—placed on the nasal dorsum or sidewalls for contour

Table 3 Mucosal Lining Repair Options

Extent of mucosal loss	Technique
<0.5 cm	Second intention, primary closure, full-thickness skin grafts, and bipedicle vestibular advancement flaps
0.5–1 cm	Full-thickness skin grafts, bipedicle vestibular advancement flap, turbinate flaps
1–3 cm	Septal mucoperichondrial hinge flap, composite septal chondromucosal pivotal flap, full-thickness skin grafts when combined with overlying forehead flap
Subtotal mucosal replacement	Inverted forehead flap, microsurgical flaps

The surgeon must resist the first option that comes to mind, and should consider other options after viewing the nose from all angles. The varying skin texture, sebaceousness, color, and contour of the nose are all relevant factors. The traditional options of second-intention healing, primary closure, skin grafting, single-stage flaps, and multiple stage flaps are also applicable to the nose and will be discussed individually. Keeping options simple while preserving function is appropriate for most patients. For any layered closure of the nose, undermining should be in the subnasalis plane. Due to the extensive sebum, all efforts must be made to minimize tissue trauma and inflammation. The suture of choice on the nose for this author is polyglecaprone 25 (Monocryl and Ethicon), due to its low inflammatory nature. Suture placement should be deep on the nose, existing between the deep dermis and muscle interface (Fig. 4). Superficial suture placement (mid-dermis or above) guarantees sebaceous inflammation, which may predispose to more visible incision lines. The number of incision lines is less important than where they are placed or whether they are long and uninterrupted (suboptimal) or short and disrupted (preferred). Also more critical is the restoration of contour and symmetry.

Another reflex to resist is the instinct for "one defect=one flap" or single solution. Incremental closures and considering combination repairs (i.e., flap + graft and flap + flap) is essential. Further, closure of the entire wound is not necessary. Closing the majority of a defect and allowing planned second intention (alar groove and sidewall) is also wise. Finally, not all wounds need immediate closure. Bringing the patient back for a delayed repair when energies are fresh and creativity is greatest may be advantageous to both surgeon and patient.

A key decision in all nasal reconstruction is to determine the need for cartilage grafting. Types of cartilage grafts for the nose are listed in Table 2. In general, cartilage grafts may either restore missing framework, support existing cartilage (to prevent airway collapse), restore or enhance contour, or counteract contractile forces. Cartilage sources may be from the ear, the nose, or the ribs. Auricular cartilage is most familiar to dermatologic surgeons. It is abundant and readily accessible from both the anterior and posterior approach. Cartilage from the ear is appropriate for batten and cap grafts. The thicker septal cartilage is more ideal for shield, spreader, and columellar grafts. The harvesting of nasal septum, however, is technically more difficult and if not properly performed, may weaken the nasal framework.

The subject of mucosal lining repair is beyond the scope of this chapter and may be studied elsewhere. General options are listed in Table 3. Small (<0.5 cm) posterior defects may heal well by second-intention or primary closure. Similar defects more anteriorly (near the alar rim) on the other hand, will cause notching from contraction if not addressed. Simpler mucosal repairs include full-thickness skin grafts (FTSG), bipedicle vestibular advancement flaps, and hinged turnover flaps.

(A)   **(B)**

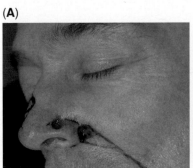
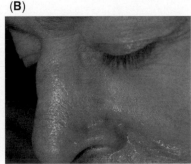

Figure 5 **(A)** Defect at medial ala and **(B)** second intention results at 8 weeks.

(A)

(B)

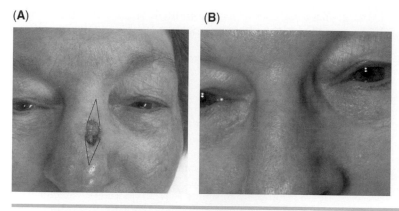

Figure 6 **(A)** Extended elliptical design on the nose and **(B)** result after six months.

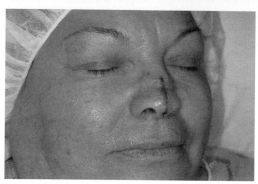

Figure 7 Primary closure at nasal supratip with extension of ellipse onto infratip.

(A) **(B)**

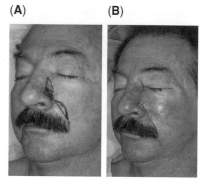

Figure 10 **(A)** Nasal defect straddling ala and sidewall and **(B)** closure with cheek advancement flap for sidewall portion, and full-thickness skin grafts for alar portion.

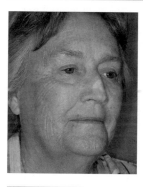

Figure 8 Full-thickness skin graft appearance—note color and contour differences.

diameter of the defect, three to six weeks of healing may be required. The effects of wound contraction on free margins should always be considered and modified if appropriate. A buried guiding suture, for example, will alter the direction of wound contraction and potentially prevent distortion. Another modification involves tapering the wound edges. By doing so, one achieves a gradual transition and a step-off may be minimized for deeper wounds. Contractile distortion is less an issue with thickly sebaceous and rigid noses. For properly selected wounds, cosmesis can be exceptional with less surgical morbidity (less incision and less infection risk) (Fig. 5).

SECOND INTENTION HEALING

Healing by second intention may be ideal if defects are: (i) shallow, (ii) small, and (iii) lie within shadow areas (alar groove and upper sidewall). Depending on the depth and

PRIMARY CLOSURE

A linear closure on the nose is ideal for defects that are relatively midline on the nasal dorsum. The varying thickness

(A) **(B)** **(C)**

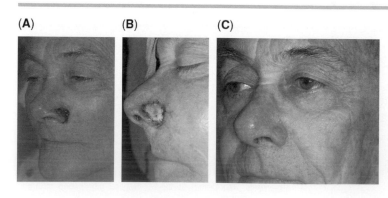

Figure 9 **(A)** Left alar subtotal defect, **(B)** full-thickness skin graft with curettage at periphery for actinic changes, and **(C)** results at four months.

Table 4 Nasal Skin Graft Donor Sites

Two essential questions in selecting graft donor site
Where is the best match for depth, color, and
  texture?
What site will result in the least conspicuous scar
  and donor morbidity?

Donor skin	Advantages	Disadvantages
Preauricular	Easily accessible	Sideburn hair growth in men may limit graft size
	Abundant skin in the elderly	Scar is more visible and then postauricular location
	Well-camouflaged scars	
Postauricular	More sebaceous in quality	More uncomfortable for patients during healing
	May heal by second intention	More difficult access than preauricular
Conchal bowl	Sebaceous pores similar to nose	May not be an option for patients with hearing aids
	May heal by second intention	
	Potentially less contraction than other donor skin	
Melolabial fold	Sebaceous skin closely matches the nose	Hair growth in men may limit graft size
	Donor scar concealed within the melolabial fold	Flattened melolabial fold on the harvested side
Forehead	Sebaceous skin closely matches the nose	Temporary paresthesia may occur at donor site
	Incision lines may be hidden within the forehead creases	Potential bruising and periorbital swelling

and contours of nasal skin are factors that require modifications of the elliptical design. For example, the traditional 3:1 ellipse may still result in a standing cone on the nose and requires lengthening to a 4:1 ratio (Fig. 6). Further, if the ellipse rests on the nasal supratip, then it should be extended to the infratip to again prevent cone formation (Fig. 7). Patients should be warned that the width of their nasal dorsum or nasal tip may be narrowed with a primary closure of a larger defect. A useful maneuver is to reverse bevel the wound edges. The blade angles slightly away from the wound center (reverse bevel) when incising the ellipse.

This facilitates a flush approximation, sealing of the incision edge, and superior cosmesis. Primary closures on the nose are generally oriented vertically but oblique designs near the nasal root or sidewall are also appropriate. Ellipses that cross the nasofrontal angle are prone to tenting due to the abrupt change in topography.

SKIN GRAFTING

For the nose, FTSG will yield a better tissue match and less contraction than split thickness grafts. The cosmesis of skin

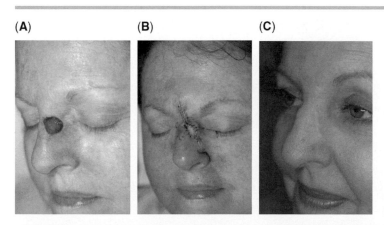

Figure 11 (A) defect at nasal root and sidewall, (B) closure with Burow's full-thickness skin grafts, and (C) long-term results.

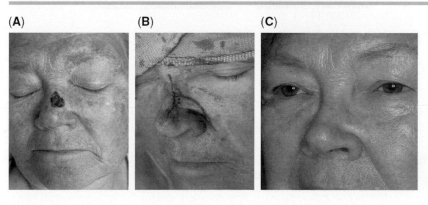

Figure 12 (A) Medium-sized defect at nasal dorsum, (B) Burow's full-thickness skin grafts, and (C) long-term results.

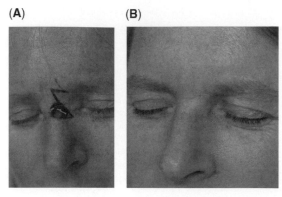

Figure 13 (A) Single transposition flap from glabella to nasal root defect and (B) results at two months.

grafts is superior in women compared to men due to their less sebaceous skin. Zones I and III nasal skin, therefore, receive skin grafts well. Lighter skin color, smoother texture, and a contour mismatch are all potential outcomes of nasal grafts and patients should be so counseled (Figs. 8 and 9). The benefits of nasal skin grafts are: (i) ideal for tumor surveillance, (ii) avoidance of additional surgery at the recipient site, and (iii) potentially excellent cosmesis for the proper defect. Disadvantages of skin grafting include: (i) an additional surgical site for graft harvest with its potential morbidity, (ii) vascular viability is less reliable than flaps, and (iii) potential mismatch in contour, color, and texture. Grafts may be combined with flaps for defects crossing multiple subunits (Fig. 10). A subcutaneous hinge cheek flap

with FTSG is a particularly useful combination for deep, lateral alar defects Donor sites for nasal skin grafts are many and Table 4 highlights the risks and benefits of each location. A Burow's FTSG (BFTSG) is an often neglected option for many nasal defects. By using either the proximal or distal Burow's triangle as the donor skin, the best match in color, texture, and thickness is achieved. Further, the closure of the Burow's triangle results in a smaller wound and therefore, a smaller graft (Fig. 11). Large wounds that would otherwise require flaps may be closed with a BFTSG (Fig. 12). Disadvantages of the BFTSG include a potentially greater incidence of partial graft necrosis. There is a longer delay time between graft harvest and placement due to the need for closure of the contiguous donor site. Further, if the nasal skin is too sebaceous, then the graft may be too thick and be poorly vascularized. Patients should be educated that graft cosmesis is an evolving process. Initial duskiness, partial sloughing, and trapdoor prominence are usually not fatal to a good outcome. Dermabrasion at six to eight weeks postoperatively, steroid injection, and pulse-dye laser are all interventions that optimize final esthetic success. For Zone I type skin, graft esthetics is excellent.

FLAP RECONSTRUCTION

Innumerable options exist for nasal flaps and each has its role. For practicality, flap repairs will be discussed in terms of regional application. The most useful single-stage flaps in this author's hands include: (i) cheek advancement flap (CAF), (ii) island pedicle flap (IPF), (iii) Zitelli's-modified bilobed transposition flap, (iv) Bennett's rhombic transposition with Z-plasty (BRhTZ). Other effective options (but

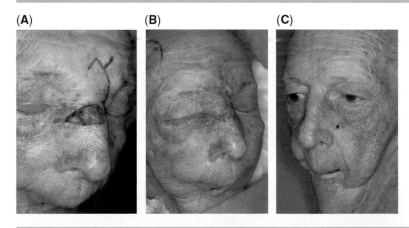

Figure 14 (A) Nasal root defect with glabellar rotation flap (Rieger flap), (B) flap closure, and (C) results at six months.

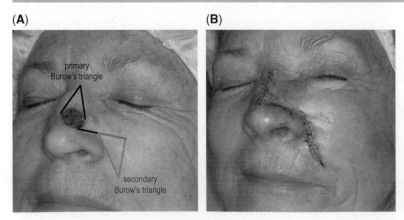

Figure 15 (A) Cheek advancement flap—secondary Burow's triangle is designed larger than primary triangle to facilitate flap mobilization and (B) incision lines are well hidden.

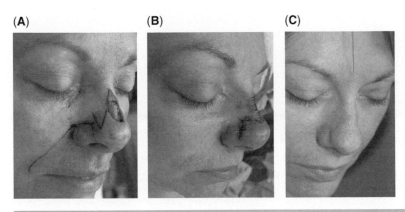

Figure 16 (**A**) Single transposition flap design onto the nasal dorsum, (**B**) flap closure, and (**C**) long-term results.

less used by this author) are the dorsal-nasal rotation flap (Rieger) and melolabial transposition flap (MLTF). The above are applicable to partial thickness defects. Full-thickness defects often require multistage repairs, albeit the turnover nasolabial flap (Spear flap) and hinged turnover flap are noticeable exceptions. Complications of most nasal flaps are due to unanticipated effects of the secondary defect and its tension vectors.

Flap Reconstruction for the Upper One-third of the Nose (Glabella to Rhinion)

The upper one-third of the nose may be defined arbitrarily from the glabella to the rhinion and tissue mobility will be primarily from the glabella. Repairs in this region should consider the medial canthus with its thin, tethered skin, and the nasofrontal angle [depression between the glabella and the nasion (root)]. For smaller defects (< 1 cm), second intention, primary closure, and skin grafts are ideal. Transposition and rotation (dorsal-nasal or Rieger) flaps from the glabella are traditional workhorses for larger defects (Figs. 13 and 14). The glabella has abundant donor skin, excellent vascularity, and depending on the patient, vertical rhytides to conceal incisions. Thinning these flaps is inevitably needed as the glabella is much thicker than the proximal nasal skin. Tacking sutures are also useful at

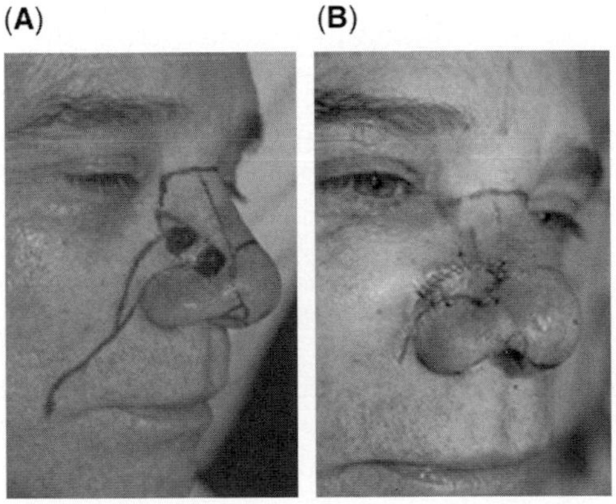

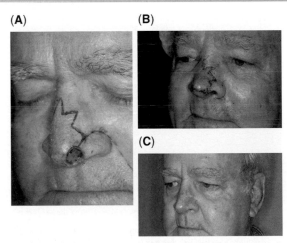

Figure 19 (**A**) Nasal infratip defect with rhombic transposition and Z-plasty design ("trilobe" flap), (**B**) flap closure, and (**C**) results at two months.

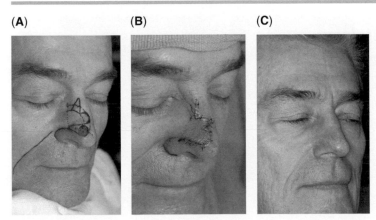

Figure 17 Island pedicle flap combined with superior cone resection repairs two adjacent defects.

Figure 18 (**A**) Zitelli's-modified bilobed transposition flap design, (**B**) flap closure, and (**C**) long-term results.

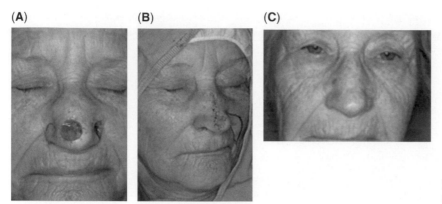

Figure 20 (**A**) Defect at nasal tip, (**B**) Burow's full-thickness skin grafts, and (**C**) long-term results.

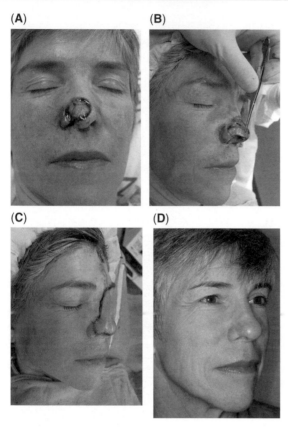

Figure 21 (**A**) Complex defect involving nasal tip, soft triangle, and ala; (**B**) alar cartilage batten graft for flap and alar support; (**C**) forehead flap repair; and (**D**) long-term results.

the nasion to recreate the nasofrontal angle. Webbing at the medial canthus is a potential issue with any glabellar flaps to the nose. This complication may be addressed by thinning the flap at inset, or with Z-plasties for revision.

Flap Reconstruction for the Middle One-Third of the Nose (Rhinion to Proximal Border of Nasal Tip)

More reconstructive versatility is available for this region, as tissue mobility may come from not only the glabella but also the medial cheek. The rich arterial perforators from the nasalis muscles generously perfuse flaps in this area. Large defects on the nasal dorsum are candidates for a CAF, which advances lax cheek skin across the nasofacial sulcus and onto the dorsum. The CAF is essentially a modified Burow's wedge advancement flap that displaces the lower Burow's triangle laterally onto the cheek instead of the nasal tip. Incisions are strategically camouflaged up the superior nasal dorsum, along the shadow areas of the nasal sidewall or alar groove, and down the melolabial fold. Two modifications are useful with a CAF. First, the secondary Burow's triangle is designed wider than the primary triangle (Fig. 15). This wider triangle at the melolabial fold mobilizes the flap more effectively and compensates for the "up the hill" resistance when moving from the sidewall onto the dorsum. Second, a tacking suture (4-0 polyglactin 910) anchoring the flap's underside to the nasofacial sulcus results in further flap movement and recreation of the sulcus. Defects that extend onto the nasal tip yield less predictable results as the tension vectors become less advancement and more

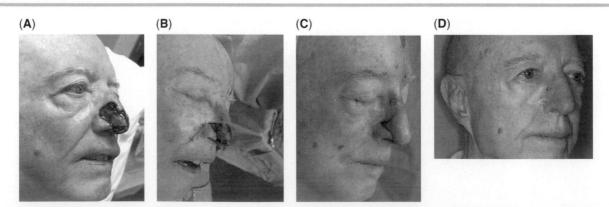

Figure 22 (**A**) Multiple nasal subunit defect, (**B**) cheek advancement to close sidewall portion of defect, (**C**) paramedian forehead flap for remainder of closure, and (**D**) long-term results.

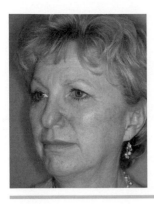

Figure 23 Trapdooring of cheek to nose flap on the lateral nasal tip.

rotational. This results in more torque or twist on the nasal tip and a greater risk for distortion. For patients with a broad nasal base, a Webster design transposition flap from the sidewall onto the dorsum can be especially effective (Fig. 16). Rieger rotation flaps are as applicable to the middle one-third as they are to the proximal one-third. Defects on the lower nasal sidewall (above alar groove and lateral to nasal tip) are candidates for an IPF. The IPF rotates and advances medially from the lax cheek, stays above and preserves the alar facial sulcus, and does not require standing cone revision. Outlining the subunits surrounding a defect often facilitates the conceptualization of repairs (Fig. 17).

Flap Reconstruction for the Lower One-Third of the Nose (Nasal Tip, Infratip, and Alar lobules)

The lower one-third of the nose is functionally (overlies the internal nasal valve) and esthetically the most crucial to successfully repair. However, its reconstruction is more difficult given its inherently sebaceous skin and limited laxity.

Recruitment of nasal dorsum, sidewall, and even the glabella are sometimes necessary for flap movement. The need for cartilage grafting is greatest at the ala and tip.

Nasal Tip

Nasal tip repairs will vary depending on whether the defect is midline or lateral. If the lower lateral cartilages are exposed, one should consider medial crural fixation sutures (MCFS). This is a horizontal mattress or interrupted suture (5-0 or 6-0 polypropylene) between the medial crus of the alar cartilages. The MCFS unifies the medial crus, increases domal tip projection, and facilitates many closures by stabilizing the tip complex. Smaller midline wounds (< 0.5 cm) may be closed primarily or with a FTSG. Medium-sized defects are candidates for the Rieger dorsal-nasal rotation flap or a transposition flap. In general, rotation flaps to the tip are not favored by this author for several reasons: (i) flap recruitment of thicker glabellar skin is often needed (risk of medial canthal webbing unless the flap is thinned), (ii) the incision line is long and uninterrupted (i.e., more visible even if placed along the nasal sidewall), (iii) tissue undermining is extensive for the movement gained, and (iv) better options exist. Similarly, rarely is a single transposition (banner flap) successful without distorting the tip. More reliable are modified transposition flaps, such as Zitelli's bilobed transposition flap (ZBTF), and BRhTZ (Fig. 18). These modified designs displace tension vectors to the more forgiving nasal dorsum and sidewall, thereby minimizing tip displacement. More than other options, these latter two flaps demand meticulous planning and geometric perfection. The BRhTZ may be thought of as a trilobe flap. It will achieve greater tissue movement and possibly better scar camouflage than the ZBTF (Fig. 19). A traditional IPF is not a reliable option for the nasal tip. Modified or "sling" IPF, however, may be more successful. Larger subtotal

(A)   (B)   (C)

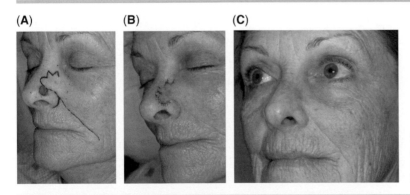

Figure 24 (A) Mohs defect at lateral tip and medial ala with rhombic transposition and Z-plasty design ("Trilobe" flap), (B) flap closure, and (C) results at three months—note camouflage of angulated incision lines.

(A)   (B)   (C)

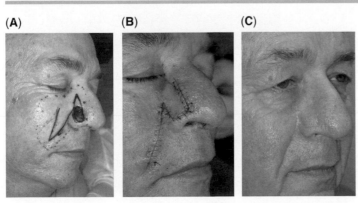

Figure 25 (A) Alar defect with melolabial transposition flap design, (B) flap closure, and (C) predictable blunting of alar facial sulcus.

(A)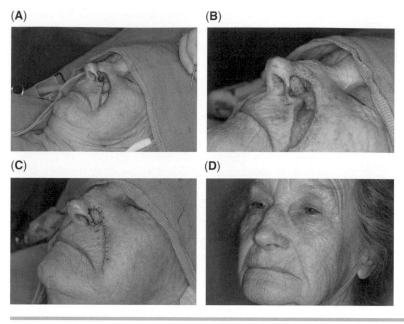

(B)

(C)

(D)

Figure 26 (**A**) Deep lateral alar defect, (**B**) transposition island pedicle flap movement, (**C**) flap closure, and (**D**) results at six months—note preservation of the alar facial sulcus.

(A)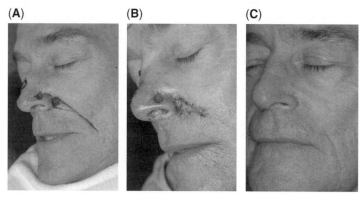

(B)

(C)

Figure 27 (**A**) Lateral alar defect with cutaneous lip extension, (**B**) subunit repair with an island pedicle flap for the lip portion and FTSG for the alar portion, and (**C**) long-term results.

(A)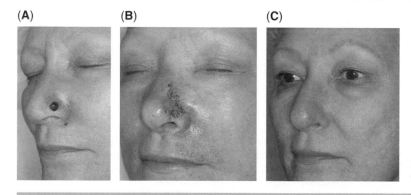

(B)

(C)

Figure 28 (**A**) Medial alar defect, (**B**) medially based bilobed transposition flap, and (**C**) long-term results.

wounds may require a staged repair, such as the paramedian forehead flap although a BFTSG may surprisingly fill the role (Fig. 20). Resection of residual subunit tissue may be helpful but not always necessary in every case. The consideration of a forehead flap should parallel thoughts of cartilage grafting. Even if the native framework is intact, contour grafts may be needed to restore nasal tip projection or stability, given the heavy weight of forehead tissue. This author performs the forehead flap in three stages as first described by Menick. The first stage is flap harvest and inset. Flap thinning during the first stage is limited to the distal 5 mm of the flap edge. Frontalis muscle and fascia are left intact until the second stage. Three weeks later, aggressive thinning occurs in stage II, in which muscle, fascia, and

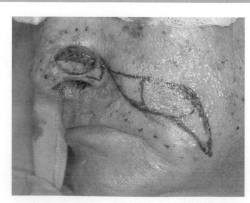

Figure 29 Alar cartilage batten graft prior to a cheek-to-nose staged flap.

(A)   **(B)**   **(C)**

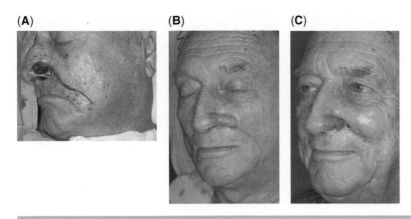

Figure 30 **(A)** Subtotal alar defect, **(B)** cheek-to-nose staged flap supported by an underlying cartilage graft, and **(C)** short-term results.

necessary fat are trimmed. The flap is reset and pedicle division occurs in stage III, now six weeks later. This intermediate stage II offers many advantages: (i) there is less bleeding in stage I, (ii) more aggressive flap contouring is possible, (iii) thinning is easier in stage II—the presence of retained muscle minimizes fibrosis and the fat is softer, more easily sculpted, and (iv) the vascularity of intact muscle permits the use of skin grafts for mucosal lining if needed. If the tip defect involves the nasal facet, then this portion should be allowed to granulate rather than be covered by thick forehead tissue. Second intention at the soft triangle better recreates the planar surface of this area (Fig. 21). The paramedian forehead flap may be combined with other flaps and or grafts for substantial tissue loss (Fig. 22). Comparatively, cheek-to-nose–staged flaps are less ideal for the nasal tip. The cheek skin is softer, more prone to trapdooring, and thus is more suitable for alar reconstruction (Fig. 23).

A diverse repertoire is available for lateral nasal tip defects. FTSG, for example, are more viable options laterally since they are better camouflaged. Smaller lateral tip defects may benefit from the "East West" flap, which essentially is a Burow's advancement flap that is best applied for patients with a broad nasal base. The ZBTF and BRhTZ become favorite options at the lateral tip (Fig. 24). A ZBTF may be laterally based for strictly lateral tip wounds, or medially based for tip and medial alar involvement. Traditional or modified IPF are also viable options. The cheek-to-nose–staged flap is more appropriate for the lateral nasal tip, especially if the alar lobule is also involved.

Ala

The ala is a fibrofatty lobule that is incredibly varied among patients in terms of size, convexity, patency, and rigidity. If poorly reconstructed, this subunit may impair inspiration and become a formless blob. Preserving the alar's patency, convexity, and alar facial sulcus are priorities in its reconstruction. Few single-staged flaps can achieve all objectives. The classic MLTF, for example, often obliterates the alar facial sulcus except in patients who have a flat cheek to alar transition (Fig. 25). One effective distinction among single-staged techniques is the transposed IPF. This versatile flap may resurface both lateral and medial alar defects, and even subtotal wounds. It achieves the same esthetic standards as the multi-stage cheek-to-nose flap with less surgical morbidity (tissue resection and number of procedures) (Fig. 26). Alar wounds that extend onto the cheek or lip are best repaired by subunits (Figs. 10 and 27). Medially based ZBTF or BRhTZ are also excellent alternatives for medial alar wounds (Fig. 28). For deep lateral alar wounds, a hinged turnover fat flap from the cheek followed by an overlying FTSG can be an elegant option.

The cheek-to-nose–staged flap is the gold standard for subtotal alar reconstruction. The soft convexity of cheek skin simulates well the rounded alar lobule. There is a greater need for residual subunit resection for the ala compared to the nasal tip. An alar batten graft is almost prerequisite when performing the cheek-to-nose repair (Fig. 29). The batten graft supports the flap, maintains alar patency, and minimizes rim retraction (Fig. 30).

CONCLUSION

A surgeon's reconstructive skill is maximally tested on the nose. Esthetic nasal restoration requires both technical and artistic dexterity. Tumor-free margins are paramount prior to embarking on any closure. Almost any repair will "plug the hole." Fewer options, however, will achieve both function and form. Reconstructive success begins with a systematic analysis of the tissue loss, followed by a versatile strategy for repair, and finally—meticulous planning and execution. Despite all preparations, secondary revisions are more frequent on the nose than in other facial locations. Usually, the need for revisions may be anticipated and patients so informed. Remarkably, many postoperative distortions self-resolve and interventions should not be premature.

BIBLIOGRAPHY

Adamson DC, Ramsey ML. Graphs and dermatologic surgery: review and update on full and split thickness skin grafts, free cartilage grafts, and composite grafts. Dermatol Surg 2005; 31(S2):1055–1067.

Brodland DG. Paramedian forehead flap reconstruction for nasal defects. Dermatol Surg 2005; 31(8 Part 2):1046–1052.

Burget GC, Menick SJ. The subunit principle in nasal reconstruction. Plast Reconstr Surg 1985; 76:239.

Cook JL. Reconstruction of a full-thickness alar wound with a single operative procedure. Dermatol Surg 2003; 29(9):956–962.

Cook JL. Reconstructive utility of the bilobed flap: lessons from flap successes and failures. Dermatol Surg 2005; 31(8 Part2):1024–1033.

Cook J, Zitelli JA. primary closure for midline defects of the nose: a simple approach for reconstruction. J Am Acad Dermatol 2000; 43(3):508–510.

Fader DJ, Wang TS, Johnson TM. Nasal reconstruction utilizing a muscle hinge flap with overlying full-thickness skin graft. J Am Acad Dermatol 2000; 43(5 part 1):837–840.

Goldberg LH, Alam M. Horizontal advancement flap for symmetric reconstruction of small to medium-sized cutaneous defects of the lateral nasal supratip. J Am Acad Dermatol 2003; 49(4):685–689.

Hairston BR, Nguyen TH. Innovations in the island pedicle flap for cutaneous facial reconstruction. Dermatol Surg 2003; 29:378–385.

Internal lining. In: Baker RS, Naficy S, eds. Principles of Nasal Reconstruction. Mosby, 2002:31–46.

Johnson TM, Baker SR, Brown MD, et al. Utility of the subcutaneous hinge flap in nasal reconstruction. Dermatol Surg 30(3):459–466.

Johnson SC, Bennett RG. Double Z-plasty to enhance rhombic flap mobility. J Dermatol Surg Oncol 1994; 20(2):128–132.

Lee KK, Mehrany K, Swanson NA. Fusiform elliptical Burow's graft: a simple and practical esthetic approach for nasal tip reconstruction. Dermatol Surg 2006; 32(1):91–95.

Lee KK, Gorman AK, Swanson NA. Hinged turnover flap: a one stage reconstruction of a full thickness nasal ala defect. Dermatol Surg 2004; 30(3):479–481.

Menick FJ. A 10 year experience in nasal reconstruction with a three-stage forehead flap. Plast Reconstr Surg 2002; 109(6): 1839–1855.

Mott KJ, Clark DP, Stelljes LS. Regional variation in one contraction of Mohs surgery defects allowed to heal by second intention. Dermatol Surg 2003; 29(7):712–722.

Nguyen TH. Staged cheek-to-nose and auricular interpolation flaps. Dermatol Surg 2005; 31(8 Part 2):1034–1045.

Nose. In: Salasche SJ, Bernstein GE, Senkarik M, eds. Surgical Anatomy of the Skin. Appleton and Lange, 1988: 199–215.

Nose. In: Larrabee WF Jr., Makielski KH, Henderson JL, eds. Surgical Anatomy of the Face. Lippincott Williams and Wilkins, 2004:147–166.

Papodopoulos DJ, Trinei FA. Superiorly based nasalis myocutaneous island pedicle flap with bilevel undermining for nasal tip and supratip reconstruction. Dermatol Surg 1999; 25:530–536.

Secondary tip modification: shaping and positioning the nasal tip using non-destructive techniques. In: Primary Rhinoplasty, a New Approach to the Logic and the Techniques. Mosby, 1998:273–277.

Zitelli JA. Secondary intention healing: an alternative to surgical repair. Clin Dermatol 1984; 2(3):92–106.

25

The Lips and Oral Cavity

Hubert T. Greenway

Scripps Clinic and Research Foundation, La Jolla, California, U.S.A.

SURGERY OF THE LIPS

The lips are graceful structures that symmetrically occupy the lower third of the facial profile we present to others. The lips have been a subject of interest and decoration for societies through the ages. The original tissue expander may well have been a piece of wood inserted into the lower lip, a custom still practiced by the Suya Indian tribe in central Brazil. Once a young man is married, a small light-weight wooden disc is inserted in the lip; with time, the disc is exchanged for larger discs up to three inches in width and three-fourth inch thick. The lip disc in this case signifies masculine self-assertion, while in the Fali tribe of northern Nigeria, women wear the lip disc as ornamentation.

The lips are perfectly symmetric structures, and many attribute certain personality traits based not only on their shape but also their use! Even the slightest movement may convey a subtle emotion, and exaggerated movements such as the protrusion of the lower lip may accentuate strong feelings. The famed smile of the "Mona Lisa" by Leonardo da Vinci has served to convey both simplistic and more complex feelings in the imagination of art lovers since 1503.

The use of lipstick allows one to dramatize the natural shape of the lips. Painting lips appears to be an ancient art practiced by highly developed civilizations for thousands of years. The original lip color, rouge, was a dye of animal or vegetable base, whereas today's formulations use lanolins, alcohols, oils, and waxes.

Anatomy

The lips represent the anterior border of the mouth. In addition to the expression of emotion, they are important for speech, intake of food, and mastication. The topical anatomy of the lips reflect the symmetric nature of all components (Fig. 1). In the midline, the philtrum and Cupid's bow contribute to the delicate symmetry of the upper lip. Laterally, the nasolabial crease denotes the boundary with the cheek. The skin of the lower lip forms a horizontal crease where it contacts the chin. The skin of the lips contains hair, sebaceous glands, and eccrine glands. In the male, the entire upper lip and central portion of the lower lip are hair-bearing.

The vermilion border is the mucocutaneous junction between the skin and the dry mucosa or vermilion of the lip. This border is easily visible and if violated surgically must be precisely reconstructed to preserve normal lip symmetry. The vermilion of the upper and lower lips is red in color because of a lack of keratinization and the underlying capillary plexus. Sebaceous glands are found in normal vermilion tissue 50% of the time, although

normally no hairs are present. The dry vermilion becomes a wet mucous membrane proximally in the oral cavity.

The bulk of the tissue comprising the lips consists of striated muscle, primarily the orbicularis oris (Fig. 2). This is the basic muscle of the lip. The major portion, the orbicularis oris proper, consists of longitudinal fibers arranged in a sphincteric fashion about the mouth. A portion of the sphincteric fibers in the lower lip form a horizontal shelf or protrusion of the vermilion, which can be accentuated in normal expressions. The group of deep anterocaudally oriented fibers provides the compressive movement to force the lips against the teeth. In the philtral area, muscle fibers cross and intersect with vertically oriented fibers present at the philtral columns. The orbicularis oris muscle also decussates at the lateral commissures of the mouth.

Three muscles or muscle groups function in concert with the orbicularis oris muscle. The upper group of muscles, the labial elevators, consists of the zygomaticus major, the zygomaticus minor, the levator labii superioris, the levator labii superioris alaeque nasi, the levator anguli oris, and the risorius muscle. These muscles function in concert as elevators of the lips, contributing with the risorius, to the upward elevation of the corner of the mouth. Additionally, the risorius has been referred to as the "smile" or "unpleasant grin" muscle, as it assists with this function.

The lower group of muscles, the labial depressors, consists of the depressor labii inferioris, the depressor anguli oris or triangularis, and the mentalis. These muscles function in concert as depressors of the lip, acting with the orbicularis oris. The mentalis muscle also functions to force the lower lip against the gum by drawing the skin of the lip upward.

The third muscle group is the singular buccal muscle forming the majority of the muscular substance of the cheek. It arises from the maxilla, the mandible, and the pterygomandibular ligament. The buccinator acts to force the cheek against the teeth, forcing food into the oral cavity.

The commissures of the mouth (Fig. 1) form a complex area with contributions from the orbicularis oris muscle and insertions from the upper elevators, the lower depressors, and the buccinator. Deficiencies in this area may be accentuated by normal actions of the contralateral commissure.

The vasculature of the lips consists mainly of the inferior and superior labial arteries, which are the main branches of the facial artery (Fig. 3). They pass deep to the elevators and depressor muscle groups to run tortuously in the orbicularis oris fibers, at times running superficially between the muscle and mucosa. With age, the tortuosity may increase and with atrophy and thinning of the orbicularis oris these vessels may be more easily palpable.

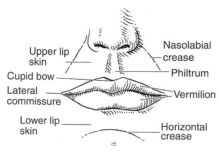

Figure 1 Topical anatomy of the lip.

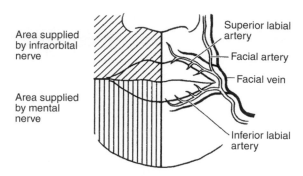

Figure 3 Vascular and nerve supply to the lip and perioral area.

Identification of the labial arteries is important in lip surgery, as ligation of these vessels is often warranted.

Nerve supply to the lips consists of a sensory and a motor portion. The sensory component to the skin and mucosa is via the trigeminal nerve, with the infraorbital nerve supplying the upper lip and the mental nerve (Fig. 3) supplying the lower lip. The facial nerve provides motor innervation to the lips mainly via buccal branches to the orbicularis oris and elevator muscles, while the marginal mandibular branch innervates the depressor muscles of the lips but also contributes to the orbicularis oris fibers. Injury to the branches of the facial nerve in the lip is rare, as innervation of the muscles is from the deep aspect.

Lymphatic drainage of the perioral area is to the submental buccal, mandibular, submandibular, superficial cervical, and upper deep cervical nodal areas. These areas should be evaluated and documented when dealing with squamous cell carcinoma and other tumors that can metastasize to nodal areas. In general, the lateral one-third of the lip drains to the ipsilateral nodes, whereas the central one-third of the lip may drain to nodes on either side.

The nasolabial folds deepen and lengthen with age. The concavity of Cupid's bow flattens, as does the entire upper lip, which is accentuated by the downward and lateral drooping of both lateral commissures. One must take the aging process into account (Fig. 4) as well as the normal anatomy, when performing surgery in this area.

Principles of Lip Surgery

Scars or imperfections after lip surgery can be a distressing problem. The following surgical principles unique to this area should be adhered to:

1. Avoid lip distortion and unsightly scars (once a tumor-free margin is assured in the case of malignant lesions).

Every attempt should be made to retain the normal contours (Fig. 1), with the philtrum and Cupid's bow contributing to the delicate symmetry of the upper lip.
2. Be aware of the underlying anatomy. Undermining may be more difficult in the philtral area and is done superficial to the underlying muscle. Sutures may be required for vascular ligation. Damage to subdermal hair bulbs (upper lip and midline lower lip skin) should be avoided in male patients. Layered anatomic closure (skin, muscle, and mucosa) is important to avoid dead space and restore anatomic function. Underlying architectures, such as the mandible and teeth influence the closure forces and the final result.
3. Incisions should be made at the junction of natural boundaries to hide their placement (i.e., vermilion border, nasolabial fold, and chin horizontal crease). Intraoral incisions should also be considered. Following skin tension lines, the majority of incisions around the lip should be vertical except at the commissures. Incisions crossing the vermilion border should be planned to recreate the border exactly. Marking with 7-0 silk suture prior to administering local anesthesia (Fig. 5) can help identify the border during closure. Marking pens, "nicks" with a #11 scalpel, and careful visual approximation may also be used for this purpose. It may be necessary to close a standard fusiform excision with angles greater than 30° (i.e., 45°) in order to avoid crossing the vermilion border on either the skin or the mucosal side (Fig. 6).
4. Nerve block anesthesia is better tolerated by patients, especially if approached intraorally following the application of topical anesthesia to the mucous membrane. Common nerve blocks performed are of the infraorbital nerve supplying the upper lip and the mental nerve supplying the lower lip. Local infiltration may then be added for hemostasis.
5. In general, defects involving up to one-third of the upper or lower lip can be closed primarily in a layered

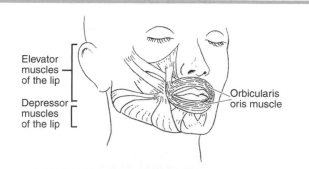

Figure 2 Basic musculature of the lip. The orbicularis oris muscle provides the bulk musculature of the lip proper.

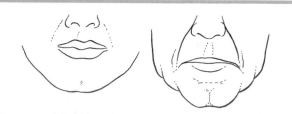

Figure 4 Changes in lip anatomy both topically and structurally with aging. There is flattening of the upper lip and drooping of the commissures.

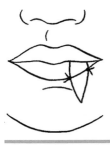

Figure 5 Preanesthesia marking of the vermilion border with 7-0 silk suture prior to local infiltration can allow exact recreation of the border.

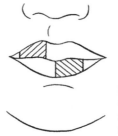

Figure 7 Defects up to one-third of the upper or lower lip (*shaded areas*) can be closed primarily after procedures such as a wedge excision. Larger defects may require flap closure.

fashion (i.e., basic bilateral advancement closure) (Fig. 7). Larger defects may require local or pedicle flap closure. Nasolabial fold, cheek, and neck tissue are commonly utilized for lip reconstruction as well as scalp and forehead tissue via distant flaps. Defects of the commissure require special consideration because of the force of the underlying muscle attachments. Skin grafts may be utilized at times but may offer less acceptable cosmetic results, especially for deeper defects.

6. Stabilizing the lip is critical during surgical procedures and can be achieved with the help of a surgical assistant, tension suture ligatures, chalazian clamps, and dental rolls (or gauze pads), as depicted in Figure 8. These ancillary measures provide greater exposure and patient comfort. On the mucosal surface, soft, braided suture material may be preferable for the patient's comfort, such as 4-0 or 5-0 silk permanent suture or vicryl, dexon, or chromic absorbable suture.

Repair of Superficial Defects

Small superficial lesions around the lip removed by shave excision with a #15 blade heal well by second intention with excellent cosmetic results (Fig. 9). Stabilizing the lip is extremely important. Remember that the labial arteries may be tortuous and superficial in elderly patients.

Small lesions may be removed by excision or punch biopsy and will heal satisfactorily by second intention but may heal more rapidly by simple primary closure. Avoid crossing the vermilion border if possible.

Larger superficial defects may require closure with local rotation or advancement flaps (Fig. 10). Often a portion of the scar can be hidden on the inner moist mucosa, which is not normally visible.

Vermilionectomy of the lower lip may be indicated for severe solar cheilitis. This procedure is done with less frequency today because of excellent results obtained with other destructive modalities, such as carbon dioxide laser vaporization. To perform the vermilionectomy, the area to

be removed is precisely marked so that approximately 1 cm of dry mucosa will be removed. The incision is made with a scalpel and the vermilion excised with scissors. Underlying muscle is left intact. The vestibular wet mucosa is undermined with direct visualization prior to advancement and closure. This procedure often provides good functional and cosmetic results.

Repair of Deep and Full-Thickness Defects of the Lips

Larger defects of skin around the lips can be repaired by local flaps or skin grafts. Defects including loss of underlying muscle or full-thickness defects can often be converted to a wedge excision for primary reconstruction, providing it covers less than one-third of the lip.

Defects of the upper lip skin can often be repaired by a caudally based nasolabial fold transposition flap in which cheek skin is used as the donor area (Fig. 11). At times, a superiorly or cranially based nasolabial fold flap may be considered. Defects of the upper lip may also be closed with a rotation flap from the nasolabial fold area with a Burow's triangle if required (Fig. 12). Avoid distorting the commissure, however. At times, perialar crescent-shaped excisions provide increased donor mobility and improve the cosmetic result. In certain cases, advancement flaps such as an A-to-T flap may be preferred, which normally do not put any upward pull on the lip. Full-thickness skin grafts can be utilized, but there can be problems with graft survival, retraction, and skin matching (i.e., color).

Wedge resection of the lip, performed when the defect is less than one-third of the lip, starts by marking the vermilion border as previously described. The incision or defect lines should cross the vermilion border at 90° angles if possible. On the lower lip, the skin portion of the wedge should not extend below the horizontal chin crease. If necessary, an M- or W-plasty should be done to prevent this. On the mucosal side, the incision should not extend beyond the gingivallabial sulcus.

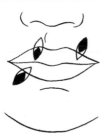

Figure 6 Compromise of the standard 30° angles of fusiform incision may be indicated (*darker areas*) to avoid crossing the vermilion border. Often a 45° angle will close and heal with an acceptable result, especially in older patients.

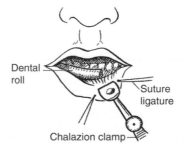

Figure 8 Stabilization of the lip may be achieved with dental rolls (or rolled gauze) between the lip and gums, suture ligatures temporarily placed, or instruments, such as a chalazian clamp.

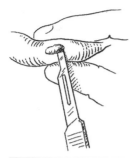

Figure 9 Shave excision of small superficial lip lesions may be allowed to heal by second intention.

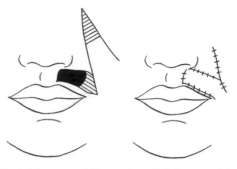

Figure 11 Inferior or caudally based nasolabial transposition flap for upper lip defect reconstruction.

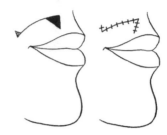

Figure 12 Rotation flap with Burow's triangle to construct upper lip defect in an older patient where a portion of the donor area laterally may be hidden in the nasolabial fold and where, because of age, the commissure is lax and maintains its normal position in spite of the primary and secondary motions of the flap.

Hemostasis must be meticulous with suture ligatures normally used for the labial artery. The mucosal surface can be closed with either absorbable or nonabsorbable sutures. The orbicularis oris muscle must be closed carefully in order to prevent notching, and the anterior shelf protrusion is recreated. Interrupted sutures of 5-0 vicryl or dexon can be used for this. Next, the subcutaneous layer may be closed with absorbable sutures if necessary to remove tension from the surface edges. The skin and dry mucosa are closed first, carefully reapproximating the vermilion border. Monofilament sutures such as 5-0 or 6-0 nylon may be used on the lip skin; however, less irritating sutures such as 6-0 silk should be used on the dry mucosal surface. The mucosal edge may elevate slightly immediately postoperative, but this will resolve (Figs. 13–15).

An Abbe-Estlander flap can be utilized for full-thickness loss where wedge repair is inadequate. The opposing lip acts as the donor area. The pedicle based on the labial artery is divided in three weeks or less.

Repair of the Lip Commissure

The commissure or angle of the mouth has several force rectors acting upon it including the underlying elevator and depressor muscles of the lip. Skin tension lines may vary. Loss of function is more noticeable because of normal function of the contralateral angle. For small defects, primary closure with an M-plasty may provide the best results (Fig. 16). Transposition flaps may be necessary for larger defects of this area in order to prevent distortion (Figs. 17 and 18).

Carcinoma of the Lip

While basal cell carcinoma is the most common cancer of the skin of the lip, squamous cell carcinoma is the most common mucosal lip malignancy. Squamous cell carcinoma of the lip represents 25% of oral cancer tumors, and over 90% of these occur on the lower lip. In the past, this tumor was more common in males but today occurs in both sexes and is most common in the 50- to 70-year-old group.

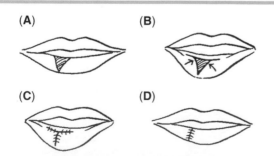

Figure 10 A-to-T closure of a mucosal defect via bilateral advancement/rotation flaps with donor incisions hidden from view. Closure is with interrupted nonirritating sutures, such as 5-0 or 6-0 silk.

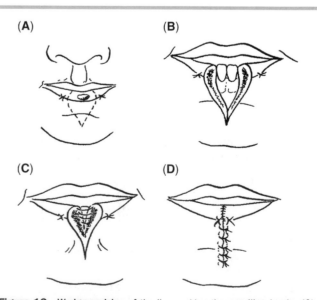

Figure 13 Wedge excision of the lip, marking the vermilion border (**A**), defect with less mucosal surface removal (**B**), closure partially complete with mucosal surface closed and muscle being closed (**C**), and complete closure (**D**).

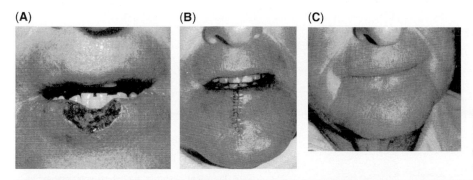

Figure 14 (A) Defect of one-third of the lower lip. (B) Result after completion of layered closure. In this case, the chin horizontal crease was not well defined and could be violated with a V to enhance the result. (C) Final result at two months.

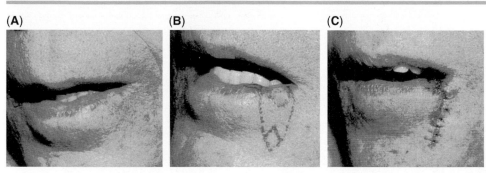

Figure 15 (A) Preoperative squamous cell carcinoma at lower lateral vermilion border after shave biopsy. (B) Wedge resection outlined providing adequate margin and utilizing a W-plasty inferiorly so as not to cross onto the chin. Note small wedge perpendicular triangle on lip proper (medially to defect), which may be of value in decreasing the thickness of the lip in certain cases, (C) W-plasty not performed. However, perpendicular medical wedge resection of adjacent lip proper allowed contouring of remaining margins at closure.

Presenting initially as a readily visible and palpable tumor, it is usually diagnosed early. Treated at an early stage, cure rates are excellent. The two most common risk factors are solar radiation and tobacco. The upright stature of humans and the normal protrusion of the lower lip implicate the lower lip as a recipient of more solar radiation.

In addition to visual examination of suspicious scaly or nodular lesions with or without magnification, palpation allows the surgeon to determine the degree of infiltration and clinical borders. Palpation of the submental, submaxillary, and cervical lymphatics should be performed and documented. Examination of the entire perioral and oral cavity should also be performed. Biopsy confirmation requires an adequate biopsy to provide tissue for histologic examination. In certain cases, radiologic examination of the neck, jaw, sinuses, and chest may be applicable. The tumor node metastasis (TNM) classification of lip cancer categorizes tumors and assists in planning treatment (Table 1).

Treatment of squamous cell carcinoma of the lip requires surgery in most cases. Early tumor (T1 and T2) can be adequately removed and reconstructed as previously described. More extensive tumors may require specialized

reconstructive techniques once the local tumor has been eliminated. Lymph nodes must be evaluated, and a decision on treatment, either surgical, irradiation, or both, must be made. Routine, close follow-up is mandatory to evaluate local and nodal extension of tumor. Cure rates for squamous cell carcinoma of the lip are good overall. As expected, this relates to the size and status of disease at the time of diagnosis. Mohs series of 1448 consecutive patients demonstrated a cure rate of 94.2%. Baker and Krause published statistics of five-year cure rates of over 90% for small tumors, dropping to 80% for more aggressive lesions as indicated by cellular atypia, depletion of lymphocytes, and infiltration into underlying muscle as well as the TNM classification at the time of diagnosis. Evaluation of the tumor for perineural invasion is important. Tumors with perineural spread may extend several centimeters beyond other negative margins. Mohs surgery combined with a course of postoperative radiation may be indicated in tumors with perineural component. Half of the cutaneous squamous cell carcinomas that metastasize have evidence of perineural invasion.

SURGERY OF THE ORAL CAVITY

Anatomy

The interior anatomy of the mouth is divided into two portions: the vestibule and the oral cavity. The vestibule is that space bounded internally by the teeth and gums and externally by the lips and cheeks. Mucous membrane lines the vestibule as well as the oral cavity proper (teeth to oropharynx) (Fig. 19). This mucous membrane must be maintained at the vestibule angle where the alveolar and buccal mucosa meet or the normal sulcus will be obliterated. The tuberculum is that area of the lip proper below the philtrum. The roof of the mouth is formed by the hard and soft palates (Fig. 20). The palatoglossal arch forms the

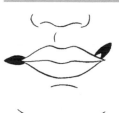

Figure 16 M-plasty closure may provide the best results for small lip commissure defects.

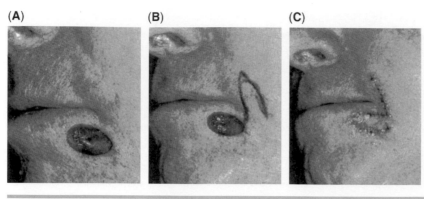

(A)   **(B)**   **(C)**

Figure 17 Defect below the lateral commissure. Reconstruction with transposition flap takes advantage of excess tissue of the nasolabial fold area in order to avoid downward pulling of the lateral commissure.

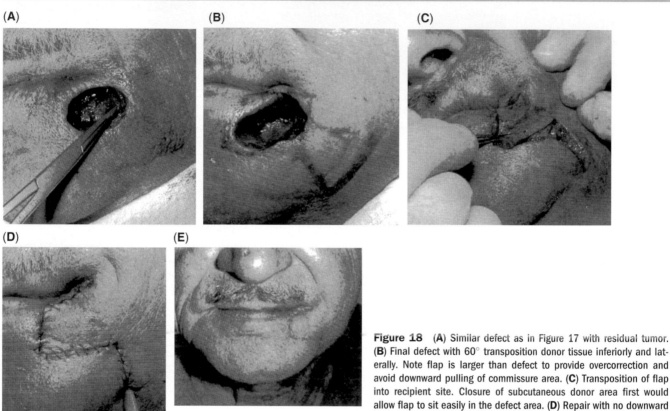

(A)   **(B)**   **(C)**

(D)   **(E)**

Figure 18 (**A**) Similar defect as in Figure 17 with residual tumor. (**B**) Final defect with 60° transposition donor tissue inferiorly and laterally. Note flap is larger than defect to provide overcorrection and avoid downward pulling of commissure area. (**C**) Transposition of flap into recipient site. Closure of subcutaneous donor area first would allow flap to sit easily in the defect area. (**D**) Repair with no downward pulling of lip or commissure. (**E**) Result at one month. Patient is now instructed to massage area to assist in decreasing residual swelling.

boundary between the mouth and oropharynx. The palatine tonsil lies between this and the palatopharyngeal arch. The tongue projects from the mouth floor, and its muscle is covered only with mucous membrane. The lingual frenulum is a vertical fold of mucous membrane connecting the central undersurface of the tongue to the floor of the mouth. Stenson's duct is the opening of the parotid duct into the oral cavity located opposite the upper second molar tooth. Wharten's duct in the anterior floor of the mouth empties the submandibular gland. The orifices of these ducts should be avoided if possible during surgical procedures. Cannulization may allow precise identification during surgery.

The inferior alveolar and lingual nerves provide sensory innervation and can be blocked readily as the two nerves are in close approximation near the mandibular foramen. The infraorbital and mental nerves may also be blocked for procedures involving the mucosa of the lips.

General Principles

1. Airway maintenance is of utmost importance both during and after surgical procedures. Postoperative edema may impair the airway.
2. Direct visualization and exposure is essential and may be different from most cutaneous procedures. Headlights, proper instrumentation, traction sutures, and a suction apparatus must be available.
3. Avoid critical anatomic structures (e.g., ductal orifices) whenever possible.
4. Primary closure can be accomplished in most cases and offers less morbidity than other techniques.

Repair of Surgical Defects

Biopsy or removal of cystic lesions and benign growths as well as malignant growths requires closure in most cases

Table 1 Tumor Node Metastasis Classification for Lip Cancer

Primary tumor (T)	
TIS	Preinvasive carcinoma (carcinoma in situ)
T0	No evidence of primary tumor
T1	Tumor measuring 2 cm or less in its largest dimension, strictly superficial or exophytic
T2	Tumor measuring 2 cm or less in its largest dimension with minimal infiltration in depth
T3	Tumor measuring more than 2 cm in its largest dimension or tumor with deep infiltration, irrespective of size
T4	Tumor involving bone
Regional lymph nodes (N)	
N0	Regional lymph nodes not palpable
N1	Movable homolateral nodes
	N1a: Nodes not considered to contain growth
	N1b: Nodes considered to contain growth
N2	Movable contralateral or bilateral nodes
	N2a: Nodes not considered to contain growth
	N2b: Nodes considered to contain growth
N3	Fixed nodes
Distant metastases (M)	
M0	No evidence of distant metastases
M1	Distant metastases present

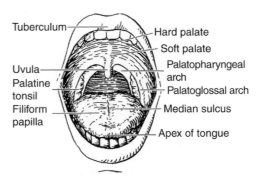

Figure 20 The oral cavity.

except for pedunculated lesions, which may be removed and allowed to heal by second intention. Primary closure can be accomplished with nonirritating sutures, which can be removed in three to five days in most cases.

Figure 21 demonstrates the planning and closure of an ellipse on the tongue. A 3-0 silk (braided) suture is placed in the anterior portion of the tongue to extend and stabilize it in position out of the mouth. Wrapping the tongue in gauze and grasping it with your fingers can be done, but this is less reliable. The ellipse is normally planned so the tip points toward the apex of the tongue.

Removal of oral lesions often causes brisk bleeding from the wound edges because of the excellent vascularization of the mouth. Electrocautery and direct pressure with gauze can be used for hemostasis prior to wound closure. Interrupted 3-0 or 4-0 silk sutures can be used for closure. Interrupted suturing provides a margin of safety over running suture as constant intraoral movement may loosen a suture. Silk is a soft braided material, which is more comfortable to the patient. Alternatively, 3-0 or 4-0 vicryl or chromic can be used, and suture removal is not necessary.

Carcinoma of the Oral Cavity

Carcinoma of the oral cavity develops beause of invasion of malignant epithelial cells. Chronic irritation from tobacco, dentures, sunlight (lips), and other factors may play a role.

Leukoplakia appears as a whitish, painless, shiny patch on the mucous membrane that may undergo malignant change. Biopsy of leukoplakia and, more importantly, biopsy of adjacent erythroplakia is necessary if present.

Clinical staging of carcinoma of the oral cavity is similar to the lip under the tumor nodal metasis (TNM) classification (Table 2). Intraoral squamous cell carcinoma is graded 1, 2, 3, or 4 (well-differentiated, moderately well-differentiated, poorly, or very poorly differentiated). Major initial therapeutic modalities include surgery and irradiation.

Postoperative Management and Care

Airway maintenance is of utmost importance and must not be compromised. In order to prevent bleeding and postoperative edema, stabilization of the surgical area and limitation of motion must be maintained. At times, no dressing or bandage is required (i.e., small lip or intraoral excisions); at other times a large pressure wrap (i.e., Barton's dressing) may be considered.

Infections are rare with minor lip and oral cavity procedures. They must be monitored and treated appropriately, considering the proximity of the sinuses to which the facial vein communicates.

Postoperative care in most cases includes gentle rinsing with mouthwash or saline solution several times a day. Soft diets are encouraged. Hydrogen peroxide is normally not necessary for cleansing oral cavity wounds.

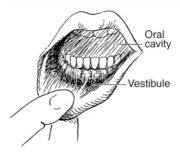

Figure 19 The mouth is divided into two portions: the vestibule and the oral cavity.

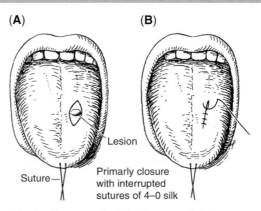

Figure 21 A silk suture through the apex of the tongue provides exposure (**A**). Note the correct method of elliptical excision on the tongue. Closure is accompanied with interrupted 4-0 silk sutures (**B**).

Table 2 Tumor nodal metasis (TNM) Classification for Oral Cavity Carcinoma

Primary tumor (T)

TX   Tumor that cannot be assessed by rules
T0   No evidence of primary tumor
TIS Carcinoma in situ
T1   Tumor 2 cm or less in greatest diameter
T2   Tumor greater than 2 cm but not greater than 4 cm in greatest diameter
T3   Tumor greater than 4 cm in greatest diameter
T4   Massive tumor greater than 4 cm in diameter with deep invasion to involve antrum, pterygoid muscles, roof of tongue, or skin of neck

Nodal involvement (N)

NX   Nodes cannot be assessed
N0   No clinically positive node
N1   Single clinically positive homolateral node less than 3 cm in diameter
N2   Single clinically positive homolateral node 3–6 cm in diameter or multiple clinically positive homolateral nodes, none over 6 cm in diameter
    N2a: Single clinically positive homolateral node, 3–6 cm in diameter
    N2b: Multiple clinically positive homolateral nodes, none over 6 cm in diameter
N3   Massive homolateral node(s), bilateral nodes, or contralateral node(s)
    N3a: Clinically positive homolateral node(s), none over 6 cm in diameter
    N3b: Bilateral clinically positive nodes (in this situation, each side of the neck should be staged separately; that is, N3b: right, N2a: left, N1)
    N3c: Contralateral clinically positive node(s) only

Distant metastasis (M)

MX   Not assessed
M0   No (known) distant metastasis
M1   Distant metastasis present
    Specify site

Abbreviation: TNM, tumor nodal metasis.

The lip and oral areas normally are extremely mobile in daily activity. Movement should be decreased initially to avoid bleeding and wound edge separation. Talking may need to be minimized. The use of dentures may need to be restricted accompanied by dietary management. Dressings should be adherent and moisture-resistant and must not interfere with underlying circulation. Dehiscence and notching of the lip can occur because of the high mobility of the area. If this occurs, conservative management may be all that is necessary; notch formation will require surgical revision. Lip contracture with elevation of the vermilion border may be simply corrected and, if due to scar contracture, may require a Z-plasty. In females, the use of lip color may provide the finishing touch to conceal scars and provide a more pleasing appearance.

BIBLIOGRAPHY

Baker SR, Krause CJ. Cancer of the lip. In: Suen IY, Myers EN, eds. Cancer of the Head and Neck. New York: Churchill Livingstone, 1981:280.

Barrett TL, Greenway HT, Massullo V et al. Treatment of basal cell carcinoma and squamous cell carcinoma with perineural invasion. Advances in Dermatology. Vol. 8. St. Louis: Mosby-Year Book, Inc., 1993.

Beahrs OH, Myers MH. Manual for Staging of Cancer. 2nd ed. Philadelphia: JB Lippincott, 1983.

Breisch EA, Greenway HT. Cutaneous Surgical Anatomy of the Head and Neck. New York: Churchill Livingstone, 1991:1–133.

Calhoun, KH. Am J Otolaryngol 1992; 13:16–22.

Epstein E, Epstein E, Jr. Skin Surgery. 6th ed. Philadelphia: WB Saunders, 1987.

Hollinshead WH. Anatomy for Surgeons. 1. The Head and Neck. 3rd ed. New York: Harper and Row, 1982.

Mohs FE, Snow SN. Microscopically controlled surgical treatment for squamous cell carcinoma of the lower lip. Surg Gynec Obstet 1985; 160:37–41.

Moore Jr. Surgery of the Mouth and Jaws. Oxford: Blackwell Scientific Publications, 1985:728–747.

Schafer ME, ed. Lip surgery. Clin Plast Surg 1984; 11(4).

Trias A et al. Surgical treatment of carcinoma of the lip. J Dermatol Surg Oncol 1982; 8:367–376.

Wheeland RG. Reconstruction of the lower lip and chin using local and random-pattern flaps. J Dermatol Surg Oncol 1991; 17:605–615.

26

The Face (Forehead, Cheeks, and Chin)

Jon G. Meine and Allison J. Moosally

Department of Dermatologic Surgery, Cleveland Clinic Foundation,
Cleveland, Ohio, U.S.A.

BONY LANDMARKS AND SURFACE ANATOMY

The shape and structure of our face is formed by the underlying facial bones (Fig. 1). The forehead is formed primarily by the frontal bone. Several visible and palpable landmarks are notable within the frontal bone. The inferior edge of the frontal bone forms the superciliary arches and the supraorbital margin, which is the superior margin of the orbits and the inferior border of the forehead. The supraorbital notch is a palpable depression along the medial-third of the supraorbital margin in the mid-pupillary line, approximately 2 cm from midline. This serves as the exit point for the supraorbital nerve, a branch of the ophthalmic division (V_1) of the trigeminal nerve [cranial nerve (CN) V] and vessels. The medial border of the supraorbital ridge meets the nasal bone to form the nasion. The lateral border of the orbit ends at the frontal process of the zygomatic bone.

The forehead is framed superiorly by the anterior frontal hairline, inferiorly by the supraorbital margin and the glabella, and laterally by the lateral eyebrow. Forehead creases are horizontal resting skin tension lines (RSTLs), which form perpendicular to the direction of action of underlying frontalis muscle. The lower mid-forehead has vertical lines, which form perpendicular to the underlying corrugator supercilii muscles. The temple lies between the lateral forehead and superior cheek. It is bounded medially by the lateral orbit and laterally by the anterior hairline.

The cheek extends medially from the nose and melolabial fold to the ear, and from the lower eyelid to the edge of the mandible. The superior cheek is supported by the maxilla medially and zygomatic bone laterally. The infraorbital foramen is located in the maxilla, approximately 1 cm below the inferior orbital rim at the mid-pupillary line. The infraorbital nerve, a branch of the maxillary division (V_2) of CN V, and vessels exit from this foramen. The infraorbital nerve can be accessed intraorally when performing a regional nerve block.

The zygomatic bone forms the malar eminence of the cheek, or "cheek bone." The masseter muscle can be palpated between the zygomatic bone and the mandible by clenching the jaw. Immediately anterior to the masseter is the buccal fat pad, which provides fullness to the cheeks. The chin is formed by the anterior process of each mandible joining at the midline. Along each side of the anterior surface of the mandible is the mental foramen from which the mental nerve, a branch of the mandibular division (V_3) of CN V, exits. The foramen is located in the mid-pupillary line approximately 1 cm above the lower edge of the mandible. The ramus of the mandible extends posteriorly to the angle of the mandible. Some individuals have a visible depression in the center of their chin, which is formed by a separation between the left and right mentalis muscles.

COSMETIC SUBUNITS

The face can be subdivided into cosmetic or esthetic units, which are separated by contour lines or anatomic boundaries. Within a given unit, the skin has similar thickness, texture, pigmentation, solar exposure, hair type, and sebaceous gland density. Mobility and elasticity of the skin may vary within an individual unit. The major cosmetic subunits of the face are the forehead, nose, eyes, lips, cheeks, and chin. The junctional lines between these esthetic units serve as good locations to place incision lines to camouflage scars. These include the hairline, eyebrows, alar and melolabial creases, philtrum, vermilion borders, and labiomental crease (Fig. 2).

The forehead can be subdivided into the central forehead, superior eyebrow, and glabella and temporal portions. The horizontal creases of the mid-to-upper forehead and vertical creases of the glabella are excellent sites for creating and hiding incision scars.

The cheek can be subdivided into five units with indistinct boundaries: supramedial (infraorbital), malar (zygomatic), preauricular, inframedial (maxillary and buccal), and lower (mandibular).

Repairing defects within a cosmetic unit generally results in the best cosmetic result because it is the closest matching skin. If needed, recruiting skin from an adjacent cosmetic unit will give the next closest "match" in skin thickness and quality. Incision lines that cross major cosmetic units are more noticeable and should be avoided if possible. Remaining within a cosmetic unit is an important goal in reconstruction.

Certain areas on the face are considered "reservoirs" of skin because of good tissue mobility. These areas include the glabella, temple, preauricular cheek, inferomedial cheek, and inferior cheek or "jowls." Tissue from these areas can be mobilized to create flaps within or adjacent to cosmetic units or used for harvesting a full thickness skin graft. The redundancy and amount of tissue movement depend on the patient's age, skin elasticity, and amount of actinic damage.

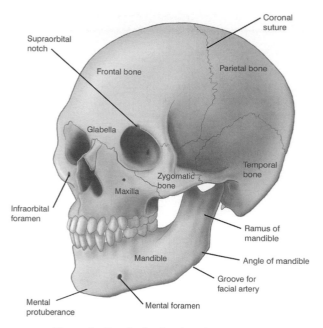

Figure 1   Bony landmarks of the face and skull.

SKIN TENSION LINES

As we age, wrinkles develop on our faces in a predictable pattern. The fine lines that are seen at rest are referred to as RSTLs (Fig. 3). These are the result of many forces weakening the elastic and collagen fibers in the skin. Intrinsic (aging) and extrinsic factors (sun exposure, smoking, and facial movement or expression) all contribute to the formation of these lines. Facial expressions create more prominent lines known as dynamic wrinkles or rhytides. Dynamic rhytides form perpendicular to the axis of the underlying

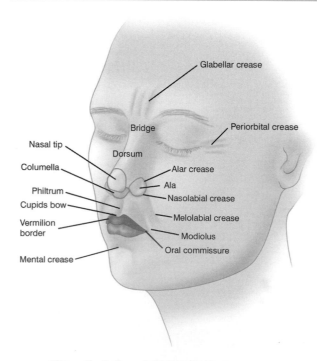

Figure 2   Surface anatomy and cosmetic boundaries.

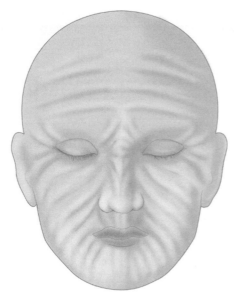

Figure 3   Resting skin tension lines of the face.

muscles of facial expression. Examples include horizontal forehead lines, which are accentuated by contraction of the frontalis muscle in a vertical direction and "crow's feet" in the lateral periorbital areas worsened by contraction of the circumferential orbicularis oculi muscle. Knowledge and understanding of the skin tension lines facilitate planning of incisional surgery and closure of wounds. Placing incisions or closing defects within or parallel to skin tension lines frequently yields the best cosmetic results. In areas where the RSTLs are uncertain, creation of a round defect, such as a punch biopsy, may result in an oval wound because of pulling in the direction of the most prominent local tension forces. Drawing skin tension lines preoperatively with a surgical marker is helpful because local anesthesia and edema can interfere with or distort skin tension lines intraoperatively.

FASCIA

The subcutaneous tissue of the head and neck region is complex and specialized. In the lateral cheeks, a highly organized layer of fibrous tissue lies within the fat between the dermis and deep fascia below. This layer of fibrous tissue has connections to both the dermis above and the underlying facial muscles. This fibromuscular layer was named superficial musculoaponeurotic system (SMAS) by Mitz and Peyronie in 1976.

The SMAS has an important role in transmitting facial expressions. When muscles of facial expression contract, their action is distributed by the SMAS to the skin. Essentially the SMAS assists in modulating and amplifying the contractions of facial muscles, resulting in a large range of facial expressions.

The SMAS stretches over the lateral cheeks from the temporalis and frontalis muscles superiorly to the platysma inferiorly. Anteriorly, it attaches to the orbicularis oculi muscle, and extends posteriorly to the trapezius muscle. The SMAS is thick over the parotid gland and masseter muscle and is attached to the parotid sheath. Medially, the SMAS becomes thin and discontinuous. It is thought to attach at the nasolabial fold, creating a point of fixation. In areas where facial muscles are absent, the SMAS forms a thick, inelastic layer. The galea aponeurotica of the scalp and superficial temporalis fascia are such areas.

The SMAS of the forehead is not continuous with the SMAS below the zygomatic bone. This difference occurs because of different developmental patterns between the upper and lower facial muscle groups. The galea aponeurotica of the scalp and superficial temporalis muscle fascia splits to envelop the frontalis muscle of the forehead. The superior forehead SMAS ends 1 cm below the zygomatic arch.

Most large arteries and nerves on the face are initially found within or deep to the SMAS. Motor nerves course deep to the SMAS, and penetrate muscles of facial expression from their undersurface. Sensory nerves and blood vessels that innervate and supply the face eventually ascend to lie within the SMAS or above the SMAS in the subcutaneous fat. The relatively avascular plane above the SMAS is a good plane of dissection for undermining. Utilizing this plane of dissection helps the dermatologic surgeon to facilitate tissue mobilization and minimize damage to important neurovascular structures.

The subgaleal plane of the scalp, consisting of a layer of loose connective tissue, is an avascular plane, which can be bluntly dissected with ease. This plane extends onto the forehead between the subfrontalis fascia (SMAS) and frontal bone periosteum. When dissecting in this location, one must be aware of the supraorbital and supratrochlear neurovascular bundles, which exit the frontal bone and enter the inferior frontalis muscle.

MUSCLES OF FACIAL EXPRESSION

The muscles of facial expression are located in the central face, and through attachments to the skin (via SMAS) are responsible for facial skin movement and RSTLs (Fig. 4). These muscles arise from the second pharyngeal arch, and are innervated by facial nerve (CN VII). Knowledge of these

muscles and the consequences of damage to their innervation are very important when performing cutaneous surgery on the face.

The forehead has three muscles involved in facial expression. The frontalis muscle begins near the anterior hairline and inserts into the forehead skin near the eyebrow. The frontalis is directly attached superiorly to the galea aponeurotica, which extends over the entire scalp. Posteriorly the galea connects with occipitalis muscle of the posterior scalp. Together, the occipitofrontalis muscle complex pulls the skin of the scalp and forehead, raising the forehead and eyebrows.

The frontalis muscle has two bellies, which are split in the midline. It has connections to the procerus, orbicularis oculi, and the corrugator supercilii muscles. Contraction of the frontalis muscle results in horizontal forehead lines. The frontalis muscle is innervated by the temporal branch of the facial nerve (CN VII). Damage to this nerve results in a flattened forehead and drooped eyebrow on the ipsilateral side. Patients with such damage may also have difficulty in opening their eyes widely.

The corrugator supercilii muscle lies deep to the frontalis muscle. Its origin is the frontal bone close to the nasofrontal suture. It inserts into the skin of the medial eyebrow. Contraction of the corrugator supercilii results in a frown or "scowling" expression by pulling the eyebrows medially and downward. As a result, one or more vertical glabellar rhytides ("frown lines") are formed perpendicular to the vector of the muscle. Injecting this muscle with botulinum toxin temporarily weakens the muscle, and the resulting frown lines diminish or flatten. The corrugator supercilii is also innervated by the temporal branch of the facial nerve (CN VII).

The procerus muscle arises from the upper lateral nasal cartilages and nasal bones, and inserts into the skin of the nasal root. Contraction of this muscle pulls the skin of the forehead down, creating horizontal lines over the root and bridge of the nose. The procerus muscle is typically injected with botulinum toxin when treating the glabellar area. The procerus is innervated by the zygomatic and buccal branches of the facial nerve (CN VII).

The medial cheek contains a group of six muscles that function to elevate the upper lip, and pull the corner of the mouth upward and/or laterally. These muscles are innervated by the buccal branch of the facial nerve (CN VII). The levator labii superioris and levator labii superioris alaeque nasi raise the upper lip. The levator labii superioris originates on the infraorbital maxilla, and extends downward to insert into the orbicularis oris muscle and skin of the lateral upper lip. The levator labii superioris alaeque nasi originates from the medial maxilla and splits as it extends inferiorly. The medial body inserts into the greater alar cartilage and skin at the alar rim. Contraction of this portion results in dilation or flaring of the nares. The lateral body of the levator labii superioris alaeque nasi inserts into the skin of the upper lip and lateral orbicularis oris muscle. The deeper levator anguli oris muscle arises from the maxilla and inserts near the oral commissure. It assists in raising the upper lip.

The zygomaticus minor and major muscles lie lateral and superior to the levator anguli oris muscle. The zygomaticus major originates at the zygomatic bone, and inserts near the oral commissure. It pulls the upper lip and corner of the mouth upward and laterally, and is partially responsible for the formation of the nasolabial fold. The zygomaticus major and minor muscles are the primary muscles involved in smile formation. The risorius muscle

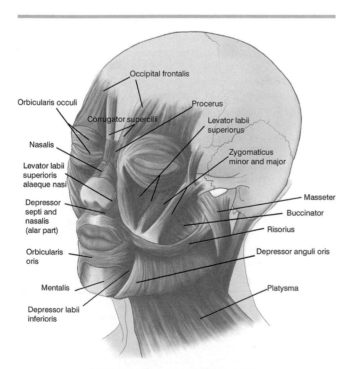

Figure 4 Muscles of facial expression.

originates in subcutaneous tissue over the parotid gland, and runs medially to attach to the skin of the corner of the mouth. It pulls the corner of the mouth laterally.

The buccinator muscle covers a large portion of the cheek. It originates from the posterior maxilla, the pterygomandibular raphe and the medial alveolar surface of the mandible. It runs across the cheek to insert into the orbicularis oris, as well as the lips and oral mucosa. The buccinator muscle is innervated by the buccal branch of the facial nerve (CN VII). The buccinator helps to keep the cheeks flat against the teeth while chewing, and prevents overinflation of the cheeks when high intraoral pressures are produced. The buccinator also works in concert with the orbicularis oris to produce whistling. The facial artery and vein pass over the buccinator, and the parotid duct passes through it to enter the oral cavity near the second maxillary molar. The buccal branch of the facial nerve (CN VII), which innervates the buccinator, emerges at its superior border.

The modiolus is a point of convergence for many of the above mentioned perioral muscles. The modiolus is located approximately 1 cm lateral to the oral commissure. It can be seen as a mass or a "dimple" in some patients. Seven muscles converge at the modiolus: (i) the orbicularis oris, (ii) the levator anguli oris, (iii) the zygomaticus major, (iv) the risorius, (v) the platysma, (vi) the buccinator, and (vii) the depressor anguli oris.

The chin contains three muscles that function as lip depressors and retractors. These muscles are innervated by the marginal mandibular branch of the facial nerve (CN VII). The depressor anguli oris originates from the mandible, and inserts into the skin at the oral commissure and upper portion of the orbicularis oris muscle. Its upper fibers insert into the medial upper lip, helping to form the philtrum. The depressor labii inferioris (quadratus) also arises from the mandible and inserts into the skin and mucosa of the lower lip and the inferior portion of the orbicularis oris. These two depressor muscles pull the corners of the mouth downward and laterally. The mentalis muscle is the third and deepest muscle on the chin. It originates on the mandible, runs downward and medially, and inserts into the skin of the chin. Most individuals have convergence of fibers from both sides in the center of the chin. Patients with a "dimple" in their chin have a space between the two mentalis muscles at their site of attachment, which is a normal variant. Mentalis muscle contraction causes chin elevation and depression, as well as protrusion of the lower lip.

The platysma is a large, thin sheet of muscle in the superficial fascia of the neck. It arises below the clavicle, and ascends through the neck to the mandible. At this point, the more medial fibers insert on the mandible, while the lateral fibers join with muscles around the mouth. The platysma tenses the skin and is innervated by cervical branches of the facial nerve (CN VII).

MOTOR NERVES (FACIAL NERVE)

The muscles of facial expression are innervated by the facial nerve (CN VII) (Fig. 5). Branches of the facial nerve emerge from deep fascia into SMAS before penetrating the underside of facial muscles. Injury to the facial nerve or its branches can have devastating consequences to a patient.

The facial nerve (CN VII) has two major roots. The smaller root provides sensory innervation and taste sensation to the anterior two-thirds of the tongue, and sensory innervation to a portion of the external auditory canal and a small portion of the skin posterior to the ear.

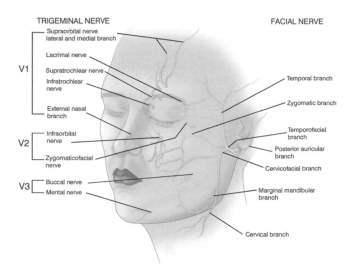

Figure 5 Trigeminal (cranial nerve V) and facial (cranial nerve VII) nerves.

The larger root of the facial nerve (CN VII) exits the skull through the stylomastoid foramen (near the level of the earlobe), anterior and medial to the mastoid process. Its location in children is relatively superficial and subject to injury because they have an incompletely developed mastoid process. Immediately after exiting the foramen, the posterior auricular nerve branches off, providing innervation to the posterior auricular muscle of the ear, the occipitalis muscle, and sensation to the skin posterior to the ear. The facial nerve (CN VII) quickly enters the parotid gland where it bifurcates into the superior temporofacial branch and the inferior cervicofacial branch. The point at which the facial nerve (CN VII) enters the parotid gland is approximately the halfway point between the superior tragus and the angle of the mandible. Within the parotid gland, the temporofacial branch further subdivides into temporal and zygomatic branches of the facial nerve (CN VII), while the cervicofacial branch subdivides into the buccal, marginal mandibular, and cervical branches. These branches course through the parotid gland and become more superficial on their way to penetrating the underside of the muscles of facial expression. Knowledge of the depth and course of these branches will help the surgeon to minimize injury to these nerves.

The temporal branch of the facial nerve (CN VII) runs superiorly across the temple toward the forehead. It innervates the frontalis, corrugator supercilii, and orbicularis oculi muscles, and the anterior and superior muscles of the ear. The temporal branch follows an upward curvature, eventually lying superficial to the SMAS in the mid-temple. Its most superficial point is where it crosses the zygomatic arch approximately 1 cm medial to the tragus. Between the zygomatic arch and the lateral eyebrow, the nerve typically branches into four rami. Near the lateral eyebrow, the nerve "dives" deeper to penetrate the undersurface of the lateral portion of the frontalis muscle. The "danger zone" for the temporal branch of the facial nerve (CN VII) can be approximated by drawing a line from the earlobe to the lateral eyebrow, and a second line from the root of the helix to the uppermost lateral forehead line. In this parallelogram-shaped area, damage to the nerve is most likely. Undermining in this area should be in the superficial subcutaneous fat to avoid damaging the nerve. When undermining from the medial forehead laterally, the subgaleal plane beneath the frontalis muscle is a safe plane for dissection.

Damage to the temporal branch of the facial nerve (CN VII) in this location results in flattening of the forehead and an inability to raise the eyebrow. Closure of the eyelid is weakened. Cross innervation of the orbicularis oculi and corrugator supercilii usually results in functionality of these muscles. If damage occurs, the ipsilateral forehead loses its horizontal lines and the eyebrow droops, leading to eyelid and brow ptosis. The upper visual field may be compromised as a result. Such functional deficits can have significant psychosocial consequences. A brow lift and blepharoplasty may be needed for functional improvement.

The zygomatic branch of the facial nerve (CN VII) branches off the superior division (temporofacial), and innervates the lower orbicularis oculi, buccinator, lip elevators, procerus, and nasal muscles. It runs medially across the cheek with some fibers overlying the parotid (Stenson's) duct. Damage to the zygomatic branch usually results in decreased orbicularis oculi function, which causes inability to close the eyelid tightly. The superior orbicularis oculi is innervated by the temporal branch of the facial nerve (CN VII), therefore complete paralysis of the orbicularis oculi is not likely. Weakness of the nasal muscles and lip elevators can occur but anastomoses with the buccal branch of the facial nerve (CN VII) often results in minimal compromise to these muscles.

The buccal branch of the facial nerve (CN VII) branches off the cervicofacial branch and runs downward on the cheek, inferior to the zygomatic branch. It innervates the zygomaticus muscles, the lip elevators, the orbicularis oris, the buccinator, and the nasal muscles. The buccal and zygomatic branches have anastomoses, which occur in the medial third of the cheek in the majority of patients. In this location, they are most susceptible to damage because of their relatively superficial location in the SMAS overlying muscles. However, limited damage to branches in this location usually does not result in persistent motor weakness because of the cross innervation. Damage to the buccal branch and/or zygomatic can cause buccinator dysfunction, resulting in accumulation of food between the teeth and cheeks while eating. Partial paralysis of perioral muscles may occur resulting in smile asymmetry, defects in lip puckering, lip pursing, drooling, and speech difficulty. Nasal muscle weakness can cause difficulty in wrinkling the nose and flaring the nostril.

The marginal mandibular branch of the facial nerve (CN VII) courses along the inferior border of the mandible and crosses over the ramus of the mandible anterior to the facial artery. The facial artery can be palpated just medial to the masseter muscle along the body of the mandible. The marginal mandibular nerve innervates the orbicularis oris, mentalis, and lip depressors. Its superficial location over the mandible makes it susceptible to damage. This branch typically consists of only one ramus, and it rarely has anastomoses with the buccal branch. Facelift procedures and submental liposuction are procedures in which the nerve is in a precarious location. Damage to the marginal mandibular branch results in an asymmetric smile because of inability to pull the ipsilateral lip down and laterally and evert the vermilion border. These deficits are more noticeable with smiling than at rest.

The cervical branch of the facial nerve (CN VII) emerges from the inferior parotid gland with the marginal mandibular branch and runs inferior to the marginal mandibular ramus toward the neck where it innervates the platysma. Damage to this branch is usually inconsequential but can cause pseudoparalysis of the marginal mandibular branch because the platysma assists in pulling the corner of the mouth downward and laterally.

SENSORY INNERVATION

The trigeminal nerve (CN V) is the primary sensory nerve of the face (Fig. 5). It is the largest CN. In addition to its sensory function, the trigeminal nerve provides motor innervation to the muscles of mastication. The trigeminal nerve divides into three divisions before exiting the skull: The ophthalmic nerve (V_1), the maxillary nerve (V_2), and the mandibular nerve (V_3). Its sensory branches run more superficially than branches of the facial nerve, and therefore are more subject to trauma. Fortunately, damage to these sensory nerves is usually not permanent or debilitating. Regional nerve blocks can be performed by anesthetizing major branches of the trigeminal nerve (CN V) where the branches exit the skull.

The ophthalmic nerve (V_1) splits into three branches before exiting the orbit: the frontal nerve, the nasociliary nerve, and the lacrimal nerve. The frontal branch divides into the supratrochlear and supraorbital nerves. The supratrochlear nerve exists in the skull from the frontal notch, which is located approximately 1 cm lateral to the midline along the supraorbital ridge. The supratrochlear nerve provides sensation to the medial forehead, frontal scalp, and medial upper eyelid. The supraorbital nerve exits from the supraorbital foramen, which can be palpated as a notch along the superior medial orbital rim, approximately 2.5 cm from midline. It provides sensation to the forehead, anterior scalp, and upper eyelids. Both of these nerves send branches upward that course deep to the frontalis muscle and penetrate the muscle in the mid-forehead.

The nasociliary branch of V_1 gives off several branches including the infratrochlear nerve and the anterior ethmoidal nerve, which terminates as the external nasal nerve. The infratrochlear nerve exits in the superior medial canthus, and supplies sensation to the medial canthus and nasal root. The external nasal branch of the anterior ethmoidal nerve emerges between the nasal bones and upper nasal cartilages. It supplies sensation to the dorsum of the nose, nasal tip, and columella. The lacrimal nerve exits at the superior lateral canthus, and provides sensation to the lateral upper eyelid and lateral forehead. Cutaneous involvement of these areas with varicella zoster (shingles) is highly suggestive of ophthalmic nerve (V_1) involvement.

The maxillary nerve (V_2) provides sensation to the mid-face. It divides into three main cutaneous branches: the infraorbital, the zygomaticofacial, and zygomaticotemporal nerves. The infraorbital nerve exits the skull through the infraorbital foramen, which is located in the maxilla 1 cm below the infraorbital rim and 2.5 cm lateral to the midline, along the same vertical line as the supraorbital and mental foramina. It provides sensation to the lower eyelid, medial cheek, upper lip and lateral nasal sidewall, and ala. The infraorbital foramen is close in proximity to the upper gingival sulcus in the oral cavity making an intraoral approach desirable for performing an infraorbital nerve block.

The zygomaticofacial nerve exits the zygomatic bone lateral to the infraorbital foramen on the lateral malar eminence, and innervates the malar eminence and a small portion of the lateral canthal area. The zygomaticotemporal nerve emerges from near the lateral orbital margin.

It innervates the anterior half of the temple and supratemporal scalp.

The mandibular nerve (V₃) is the largest division of the trigeminal nerve. It divides into three branches: the inferior alveolar, buccal, and auriculotemporal nerves. The inferior alveolar nerve courses through the body of the mandible, providing sensation to the lower teeth. It passes through the anterior mandible at the mental foramen where it becomes the mental nerve. The mental neurovascular bundle exits the mental foramen, which is located approximately 2.5 cm lateral to midline and 1 cm superior to the lower edge of the mandible. The mental nerve innervates the chin and lower lip to the angle of the mouth. The mental nerve can be approached via the oral cavity by injecting local anesthetic into the inferior gingival sulcus below the second premolar. The buccal nerve passes through the lower temporalis muscle, courses deep to the parotid, passes over the buccal fat pad and pierces the buccinator muscle to reach the overlying skin. It provides sensation to the mid-cheek, buccal mucosa, and gingiva. The auriculotemporal nerve emerges inferior to the zygomatic arch, near the temporomandibular joint, and courses superiorly anterior to the ear, just deep to the superficial temporal artery. It innervates the posterior temple, temporoparietal scalp, temporomandibular joint, tympanic membrane, and the anterior portion of the external ear and auditory canal.

VASCULAR SUPPLY

The forehead, upper eyelids and upper nose receive arterial supply via the ophthalmic artery, a branch of the internal carotid artery (Fig. 6). The ophthalmic artery gives rise to the supraorbital, supratrochlear, dorsal nasal, and anterior ethmoidal arteries. The supraorbital artery exits its foramen with the supraorbital nerve and runs superiorly on the forehead. It pierces the frontalis muscle on the mid-forehead and courses subcutaneously to the anterior scalp. The supratrochlear artery exits in the superior medial orbit and runs superiorly, supplying the mid-forehead, scalp, and nasal root area. The supratrochlear artery is the axial vessel for the paramedian forehead flap, which is sometimes employed

to repair larger nasal defects. Properly executed this flap has a robust vascular supply. The dorsal nasal artery exits the medial orbit dividing into two terminal branches. One of these branches runs inferiorly to anastomose with the angular artery, a terminal branch of the facial artery, while the other passes along the dorsum of the nose supplying it. A small terminal branch of the anterior ethmoidal artery also exits at the junction of the nasal bone and nasal cartilage to supply the dorsum of the nose.

The lower two-thirds of the face is supplied by branches of the external carotid artery. The superficial temporal and maxillary arteries are the terminal branches of the external carotid artery. The superficial temporal artery arises within or deep to the parotid gland and courses superiorly crossing branches of the facial nerve. Before exiting the parotid gland, the superficial temporal artery gives off the transverse facial artery which runs medially and horizontally, approximately 2 cm below the zygomatic arch. The superficial temporal artery ascends superiorly in the preauricular crease and reaches a subcutaneous plane as it crosses over the zygomatic bone. It can be palpated anterior to the superior root of the helix. Above this point, the superficial temporal artery is located above the plane of the SMAS and splits into an anterior (frontal) branch and posterior (parietal) branch. The anterior branch is commonly visible in elderly patients. The anterior branch supplies the temple, eyebrows, and forehead. The posterior branch supplies the parietal scalp.

The maxillary artery arises from the external carotid artery between the angle of the mandible and the temporomandibular joint, and runs medial or deep to the ramus of the mandible. One of the branches of the maxillary artery, the inferior alveolar artery courses through the mandible and exits the mental foramen as the mental artery. The mental artery supplies the chin along with branches of the facial artery. The infraorbital artery, another branch of the maxillary artery, exits the infraorbital foramen along with the infraorbital nerve. It provides arterial supply to the skin and muscles in the medial cheek. The infraorbital artery anastomoses with branches of the angular artery near the medial infraorbital ridge. Another branch of the maxillary artery, the buccal artery, supplies the buccinator muscle and other muscles of mastication.

The facial artery branches off the external carotid artery and runs deep to the mandible. It crosses the mandible just anterior to the masseter muscle, where it can be palpated. At this point it is deep to the platysma muscle. It courses superior and medially toward the nose. The superior and inferior labial arteries branch off the facial artery. The facial artery becomes the angular artery as it runs alongside the nose, eventually anastomosing with the dorsal nasal artery from the internal carotid system. The facial artery also has branches, which anastomose with the transverse facial artery. These anastomoses provide excellent arterial supply to the face even if distal branches are disrupted during surgery. This robust blood supply is the reason why local flaps and grafts are so viable on the face.

The veins of the face run roughly parallel to their corresponding arteries. The facial vein begins as the angular vein in the medial canthus. Here it has anastomoses to the ophthalmic vein and is directly connected to surrounding structures, such as the forehead, eyelids, and nose. As the facial vein courses inferiorly, it also connects with the infraorbital vein and deep facial vein in the mid-cheek. The deep facial vein parallels the maxillary artery and along with the infraorbital vein, anastomoses with the deep

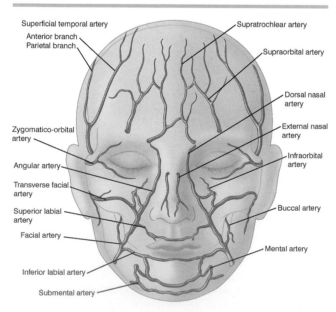

Superficial temporal artery
Anterior branch
Parietal branch
Zygomatico-orbital artery
Angular artery
Transverse facial artery
Superior labial artery
Facial artery
Inferior labial artery
Submental artery

Supratrochlear artery
Supraorbital artery
Dorsal nasal artery
External nasal artery
Infraorbital artery
Buccal artery
Mental artery

Figure 6   Arterial supply of the face.

pterygoid venous plexus. The facial vein runs posterior to the facial artery and deep to most of the facial muscles. It crosses over the mandible and the submandibular glands before draining into the internal jugular vein. The internal jugular vein connects with the external jugular vein via the retromandibular vein.

Unlike veins in the extremities, facial veins lack valves allowing two-way flow of blood. Because of the bidirectional flow, the facial vein has direct connections to the cavernous sinus of the brain via the ophthalmic vein, and to the pterygoid plexus via the infraorbital or deep facial veins. Cutaneous infections in the mid-face area could potentially spread to the cavernous sinus of the brain via these venous connections.

LYMPHATIC DRAINAGE

Lymph nodes of the head and neck filter lymphatic drainage, and trap foreign material from the interstitial fluid. Infection and metastatic tumor cells cause enlargement of regional lymph nodes. It is essential for the cutaneous surgeon to know the location of the principal lymph nodes and drainage patterns in the head and neck. Malignant melanomas and squamous cell carcinomas of the head and neck have a relatively high rate of metastasis. A thorough preoperative exam should include careful examination of the local draining lymph nodes for tumor staging and operative management.

Lymphatic vessels on the face generally course inferiorly and laterally, along the same pathway as the local veins (Fig. 7). They are greater in number than the associated veins. The forehead and temple drain to preauricular and infra-auricular nodes, which are considered part of the parotid nodal basin. The parotid nodes are both intraglandular and extraglandular. The parotid nodes drain inferiorly to the superficial cervical or superior deep cervical nodes and then to the inferior deep cervical nodes. In addition to the lower lip and chin, the submental nodes drain the anterior third of the tongue and floor of the mouth. They are located beneath the platysma under the chin. They are best palpated by having the patient elevate their chin slightly and push their tongue downwards and/or tighten the platysma. In some individuals, the submental nodes drain directly into the internal jugular/lower deep cervical chain rather than into the submandibular nodes.

The submandibular nodes drain structures along the path of the facial artery, as well as gingival and mucous membranes, the tongue, and the teeth. They are best palpated by having the patient relax their neck and lower their chin. The submandibular nodes drain into the superior or inferior deep cervical nodes. Most of the cervical nodes lie deep to the sternocleidomastoid muscle (SCM) and run along with the internal jugular vein. Enlarged nodes in the superior group can sometimes be felt along the anterior–superior border of the SCM. A few of the nodes in the inferior deep cervical group can be palpated along the lower posterior border of the SCM. These are referred to as the transverse cervical lymph nodes. Knowledge of the basic patterns of lymphatic drainage of the head and neck is important for preoperative assessment and staging, especially when dealing with high-risk tumors, such as squamous cell carcinoma and melanoma. There is variability in the drainage patterns from patient to patient. Contralateral lymph node involvement is not uncommon with malignancies; therefore, a thorough bilateral lymph node examination is necessary when evaluating such patients.

ACKNOWLEDGMENTS

Special thanks are due to Elizabeth Halasz for the illustrations and to Dr. Richard Drake for assistance in reviewing this chapter.

BIBLIOGRAPHY

Asarch RG. A review of the lymphatic drainage of the head and neck: use in evaluation of potential metastases. J Dermatol Surg Oncol 1982; 8:869–872.

Bennett R. Anatomy for cutaneous surgery. In: Fundamentals of Cutaneous Surgery. St. Louis: Mosby, 1988:100–135.

de Castro Correia P, Zani R. Surgical anatomy of the facial nerve as related to ancillary operations in rhytidoplasty. Plast Reconstr Surg 1973; 52:549–552.

Drake RL, Vogl W, Mitchell AWM. Head & neck. Gray's Anatomy for Students. 1st ed. Philadelphia: Churchill Livingstone (Elsevier Science), 2005:748–854.

Ellenbogen R. Pseudo-paralysis of the mandibular branch of the facial nerve after platysmal face-lift operation. Plast Reconstr Surg 1979; 63:364–368.

Flowers FP, Zampogna JC. Surgical anatomy of the head and neck. In: Bolognia JL, Jorizzo J, Rapini R, eds. Dermatology. Vol. 2. 1st ed. London: Mosby, 2003:2219–2232.

Furnas DW. Landmarks for the trunk and the temporofacial division of the facial nerve. Br J Surg 1965; 52:694–696.

Mitz V, Peyronie M. The superficial musculo-aponeurotic system (SMAS) in the parotid and cheek area. Plast Reconst Surg 1976; 58:80–88.

Nicolau PJ. The orbicularis oris muscle: a functional approach to its repair in the cleft lip. Br J Plast Surg 1983; 36(2):141–153.

Ozersky D, Baek S, Biller HF. Percutaneous identification of the temporal branch of the facial nerve. Ann Plast Surg 1980; 4:276–280.

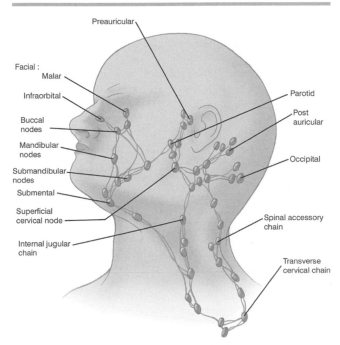

Figure 7 Lymphatic drainage.

Pitanguy I, Ramos AS. The frontal branch of the facial nerve: the importance of its variations in face lifting. Plast Reconstr Surg 1966; 38:352–356.

Salasche SJ, Bernstein G, Senkarik M. Lymphatics of the head and the neck. Surgical Anatomy of the Skin. Norwalk, CT: Appleton & Lange, 1988:141–149.

Stegman SJ, Tromovitch TA, Glogau RG. Planning and designing a surgical excision. In: Basics of Dermatologic Surgery. Chicago: Year Book Medical Publishers, 1982:114–119.

Summers BK, Siegle RJ. Facial cutaneous reconstructive surgery: general anesthetic principles. J Am Acad Dermatol 1993; 29:669–681.

27

The Neck

Allison J. Moosally and Terri McGillis
Department of Dermatologic Surgery, Cleveland Clinic Foundation, Cleveland, Ohio, U.S.A.

INTRODUCTION

The human neck comprises the area between the lower margin of the mandible and the upper surface of the manubrium of the sternum. A great number of vital structures are compressed within this relatively small area, making it a region of vulnerability. Understanding the uniquely complex anatomy of this region is critical to any surgeon or physician involved with tumor diagnosis and management. Additionally, a renewed interest in neck anatomy has accompanied the recent development of esthetic procedures for this area. It is important to understand not only surface anatomy but also the complicated interrelationship and clinical relevance of what lies below.

SURFACE ANATOMY

Clinical evaluation of the neck should begin during initial history taking. Because the neck is exposed, observation for symmetry, mobility, protrusion of neck vessels, and muscular structures can be done while talking with the patient. The natural lines of skin cleavage run in a horizontal direction and it is this direction in which most incisions should be placed. The neck skin is easily observed for rhytids, lesions, discolorations, etc. In a normal erect position, the neck should be supple with full range of motion. The hyoid, larynx, and trachea can be palpated in midline. Upon turning the head, the anterior border of the sternocleidomastoid muscle (SCM) can be easily visualized in the nonobese neck (Fig. 1). This major muscle divides the neck into anterior and posterior triangles.

The thin sheet-like platysmal muscle can be identified by having the patient clinch his or her jaws firmly. This muscle exudes from the jaw, over the clavicle, and onto the anterior chest wall. As the neck ages, linear bands can be visualized and have recently been the focus for injections of Botulinum toxin for cosmetic improvement. The external veins can often be observed crossing over the SCM. Finally, neck evaluation is not complete without palpation of superficial lymph nodes.

The exact position of any mass, growth, or asymmetry should be documented along with relationship to the neck anatomy. These areas will be discussed in more detail.

SKELETON

Posteriorly, the neck is supported by the vertebral column. The hyoid bone is located along the midline just inferior to the chin at the level of C2 or C3 (second or third cervical vertebra) and can usually be palpated. This unique bone has an anterior body and two posterior horns. It is important to document its position when evaluating patients for cosmetic improvement of the neck and jowls. Just below the hyoid bone is the thyroid cartilage, whose prominence gave it the name of Adam's apple. Just below the thyroid cartilage is the cricoid cartilage located at C6. It is between these two cartilages where emergency laryngotomy is performed. The rings of the trachea are located just below the cricoid cartilage. The thyroid gland is located midline at the level of the fourth tracheal ring. These skeletal structures can be visualized on radiologic evaluations and help orient the physician to the surrounding anatomy (Fig. 2).

MUSCLES

The most prominent surface landmark in the neck is the SCM. It is a thick muscle that protects underlying structures. Identifying it sets the stage for understanding neck anatomy. It is a strap-like muscle descending obliquely across the neck. It has two heads, one that originates from the upper portion of the sternum, and one from the medial third of the clavicle. This muscle inserts into the mastoid process of the temporal bone and the lateral aspect of the superior nuchal line of the occipital bone. Both portions of the SCM act to cause flexion of the neck. The SCM rotates the head so that the face looks up and to the opposite side. Innervation of this muscle is by the accessory nerve and the second cervical nerve (Fig. 1). The carotid pulse can be palpated along the anterior edge of the SCM at the level of the sixth cervical vertebra. It divides the neck into two major triangles, the anterior and posterior (Table 1).

Anterior Triangle

The anterior triangle of the neck has three well-defined borders. The posterior border is defined as a line beginning from the anterior edge of the SCM muscle extending from the mastoid process to the sternoclavicular joint. The superior border begins at the mastoid process, runs parallel to the inferior margin of the body of the mandible, ending at the tip of the chin. Lastly, the medial border extends from the tip of the chin inferiorly to the jugular notch (Fig. 3A).

This complex triangle is further divided into four additional triangles by groups of smaller muscles. The four triangles are: the submental, the submandibular (or digastric), the carotid, and the muscular (Fig. 3B).

The submental triangle is bordered by the anterior belly of the digastric muscle laterally, the body of the hyoid bone inferiorly, and the midline. The floor of the triangle is made by the mylohyoid muscle and contains the submental lymph nodes.

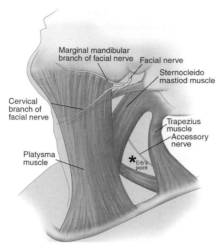

Figure 1 Platysma muscle and its innervation by the cervical branch of the facial nerve.

The submandibular triangle is outlined by the inferior border of the mandible superiorly and the posterior and anterior bellies of the digastric muscles inferiorly. The facial artery, submandibular lymph nodes, and submandibular glands lie within this important triangle. The inferior part of the parotid gland also projects into this triangle.

The carotid triangle is bordered posteriorly by the anterior edge of the SCM, superiorly by the stylohyoid muscle and the posterior belly of the digastric muscle and anteroinferiorly by the superior belly of the omohyoid muscle. The common carotid artery bifurcates into the external and internal carotid arteries within this triangle, hence its name. These vessels along with the internal jugular vein and the vagus nerve lie within the carotid sheath and are thus, all vulnerable to injury at this site.

The *muscular triangle* is formed by the superior belly of the omohyoid muscle and the anterior edge of the SCM laterally, the hyoid bone superiorly, and the midline. This triangle contains the infrahyoid muscles (Table 2).

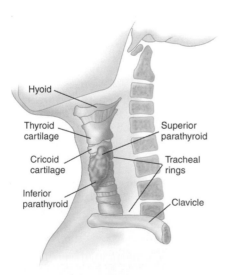

Figure 2 Bony landmarks of the neck.

Posterior Triangle

The posterior triangle of the neck is formed anteriorly by the posterior margin of the SCM, posteriorly by the anterior margin of the trapezius muscle and inferiorly by the clavicle (Fig. 3A). This triangle is additionally divided into *the occipital triangle* and *the subclavian triangles*, respectively (Fig. 3B).

The *occipital triangle* is made up of the posterior edge of the SCM, anterior edge of the trapezius, and the inferior belly of the omohyoid muscle. The *subclavian triangle* is made up of the posterior edge of the SCM, the clavicle, and the inferior belly of the omohyoid muscle.

The brachial plexus as well as the accessory nerve (cranial nerve XI) lie within this posterior triangle. The accessory nerve is of great importance to the cutaneous surgeon performing procedures in this area of the neck. It lies between the superficial fascia and prevertebral layer of the deep cervical fascia, within the investing layer of deep cervical fascia, as it courses diagonally through the posterior triangle. Knowledge of its location is critical to avoiding injury (Table 2).

The platysma muscle is imbedded within the superficial fascia and is the only superficial muscle of the anterior neck. The platysma muscle originates from the fascia of the superior pectoral region inserting upward into the skin of the lower face near the modiolus. The platysma muscle acts to pull the corners of the mouth in a downward direction. When performing surgery in this area, one should be mindful of suturing the platysma carefully as irregularities in this muscle may pull unevenly on a healing scar.

NERVES IN THE NECK

Numerous cranial nerves pass through the neck as they move toward their final destination. These include cranial nerves X (vagus nerve), XI (accessory nerve), and XII (hypoglossal nerve).

The *vagus nerve* is composed of both motor and sensory components. Originating in the medulla oblongata, it leaves the skull via the jugular foramen accompanied by the 9th and 11th cranial nerves. It possesses two sensory ganglia, the superior and inferior, which are located on the nerve within and below the foramen, respectively. The vagus nerve courses down the neck vertically within the carotid sheath. It has the longest course and most extensive distribution of any of the cranial nerves (Fig. 4). This important nerve has many branches which include:

1. A *meningeal branch* supplying the dura mater
2. An *auricular branch* innervating the medial surface of the ear, the external auditory meatus, and a portion of the tympanic membrane
3. A *pharyngeal branch* contributes sensory and motor fibers to the *pharyngeal plexus*. All muscles of the pharynx (except for the stylopharyngeus) and all muscles of the soft palate (except for the tensor veli palatini) are innervated by the vagus nerve through the pharyngeal plexus
4. The *superior laryngeal branch* divides into the internal and external laryngeal nerves. The internal branch provides sensory innervation to the mucosa of the larynx and the vocal cords, and the external branch innervates the cricothyroid muscle
5. *Cardiac branches* of the vagus nerve accompany cardiac branches of the sympathetic trunk as they pass to and innervate the heart
6. The *recurrent laryngeal nerve* at its distal portion runs closely with the thyroid artery. It supplies all muscles of

Table 1 Triangles of the Neck

Anterior triangle—anterior border of SCM, inferior border of mandible, midline
   Submental triangle
      Borders: hyoid bone, mandible, anterior belly of the digastric muscle, midline
   Submandibular triangle
      Borders: anterior and posterior bellies of the digastric muscle, mandible
      Danger zone: facial artery
   Carotid triangle
      Borders: SCM, posterior belly of the digastric muscle, superior belly of the omohyoid muscle, stylohyoid muscle
      Danger zone: internal carotid artery, external carotid artery, internal jugular vein, vagus nerve, hypoglossal nerve
   Muscular triangle
      Borders: hyoid bone, SCM, superior belly of the omohyoid muscle, midline
Posterior triangle
   Borders: SCM, trapezius muscle, clavicle
   Danger zone: spinal accessory nerve, great auricular nerve, lesser occipital nerve, transverse cervical nerve

Abbreviation: SCM, sternocleidomastoid muscle.

the larynx except the cricothyroid. The mucous membrane of the trachea and the mucous membrane below the vocal cords are innervated by this nerve

Perhaps the most important nerve for the dermatologic surgeon to appreciate is cranial nerve XI, the *accessory nerve*. This nerve is a motor nerve that exits the cranial cavity through the jugular foramen as mentioned previously. The accessory nerve passes deep to the SCM, supplying it, and after emerging from its posterior border crosses the posterior triangle of the neck to supply the trapezius muscle (Fig. 1). *Erb's Point* is the site where *the accessory nerve* exits from the SCM to cross the posterior triangle. It is defined by an imaginary line connecting the middle of the angle of the mandible to the mastoid process, intersecting the posterior border of the SCM (Fig. 5).

The main nerves emerging from Erb's Point include not only the accessory nerve, but also the transverse cervical, lesser occipital, and great auricular nerves (Fig. 6). The accessory nerve can also be located by drawing a horizontal line from the thyroid notch to the point of intersection with the posterior border of the SCM. Extreme care must be observed during surgery in the area 2 cm above and below this point to avoid inadvertent nerve injury; for it is here that the nerve becomes relatively superficial. Injury to the accessory nerve results in loss of function of the trapezius

muscle. The patient will develop a shoulder drop and difficulty elevating the arm above the head on the affected side. Patients may also develop chronic shoulder pain and a winged scapula.

The *hypoglossal nerve, cranial nerve XII*, is the motor nerve to the tongue muscles. It supplies all muscles of the tongue except the palatoglossus. Injury to this nerve can cause tongue atrophy on the ipsilateral side. It exits the skull via the hypoglossal canal in the occipital bone (Fig. 6).

While the paths of the cranial nerves through the neck, especially the accessory nerve, are important, it is the more superficial cutaneous nerves that are most familiar to the dermatologic surgeon. The anterior rami of cervical nerves II through IV supply sensation to the skin of the front and sides of the neck. The *lesser occipital nerve* (C2 only) loops around the accessory nerve to supply the medial portion of the ear and the lateral occipital region.

The *great auricular nerve* (C2 and C3) makes its way across the SCM running alongside the external jugular vein. It divides into branches that supply the angle of the mandible, the parotid gland, and lower portions of the ear. It is important to realize that the angle of the jaw is also supplied by this nerve and not by branches of the trigeminal nerve.

The *transverse cervical* nerve emerges behind the posterior border of the SCM, passes across it, and then divides

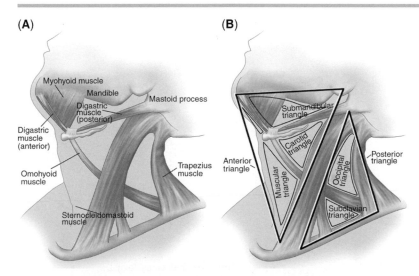

(A)

Myohyoid muscle
Mandible
Digastric muscle (posterior)
Mastoid process
Digastric muscle (anterior)
Omohyoid muscle
Trapezius muscle
Sternocleidomastoid muscle

(B)

Submandibular triangle
Carotid triangle
Anterior triangle
Muscular triangle
Occipital triangle
Posterior triangle
Subclavian triangle

Figure 3 (A) Anterior and (B) posterior triangles of the neck.

Table 2 Midline Defects

Defect	Location
Thyroglossal duct cyst	Midline or just off midline, from posterior tongue to above suprasternal notch
Branchial cleft cyst	Lateral neck, anterior border of the SCM, preauricular, external auditory canal, pinna
Midline cervical clefts	Midline of ventral neck
Congenital cartilaginous rests of the neck (wattles)	Lower half of the SCM (unilateral or bilateral)

Abbreviation: SCM, sternocleidomastoid muscle.

into branches that supply the lateral neck below the mandible. While the *supraclavicular nerves* (C3 and C4) exit from beneath the posterior border of SCM to supply skin overlying the lateral neck, shoulder region, and chest wall.

Finally, the cervical branch of the facial nerve (CN7) supplies motor innervation to the platysma muscle. This is important because skin incisions over the angle of the mandible can distort the mouth if careful observation to muscular innervation is not considered.

Vascular Supply

The three major vessels of the head and neck are the *carotid*, *vertebral*, and *subclavian* arteries (Fig. 7). The right common carotid arises from the brachiocephalic trunk. The left common carotid arises from the aortic arch. These both pass through the carotid sheath, along with the vagus nerve and the internal jugular vein deep to the SCM. The common carotid lies medial to the internal jugular vein and slightly anterior to the vagus nerve. It can be palpated lateral to the thyroid. Bifurcation of the carotids into the external and internal carotid arteries occurs slightly below the level of the hyoid bone at approximately the superior level of the thyroid cartilage. The highest vulnerability of these vessels to surgical trauma is within the carotid triangle of the anterior neck (Fig. 3b).

The external carotid artery and the thyrocervical trunk are the main blood supply to the face and neck. After bifurcating, it runs lateral to the internal carotid giving off three deep branches. The *superior thyroid* is the first branch, at

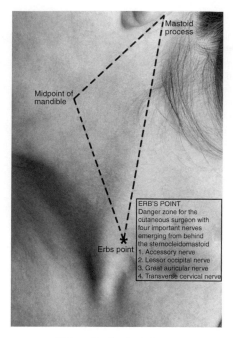

Figure 5 Cervical plexus.

times arising directly from the common carotid. The superior thyroid artery supplies the thyroid, larynx, and the muscles adjacent to these structures. The second branch is the *ascending pharyngeal artery*, which ascends vertically to supply the pharynx, palate, tonsils, tympanic membrane, and the meninges. The third branch is the lingual artery arising at the level of the hyoid bone to supply that area. The other branches include the facial artery, the occipital artery, and the posterior auricular artery. The facial arteries provide many of the branches that will ultimately supply the skin and superficial muscles of the face. They branch from the external carotid just above the lingual arteries. Each courses beneath the posterior belly of the digastric deep to the submandibular gland and crosses the mandible to supply the masseter muscle and superficial muscles and skin. An anastomosis of the facial artery occurs with the ophthalmic branches of the internal carotid at the level of the medial canthal tendon.

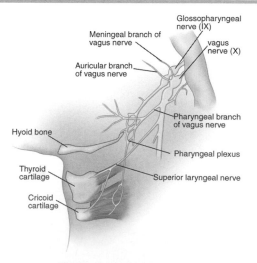

Figure 4 Nerves in the neck.

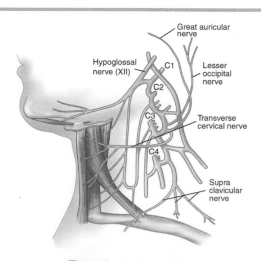

Figure 6 Surface anatomy.

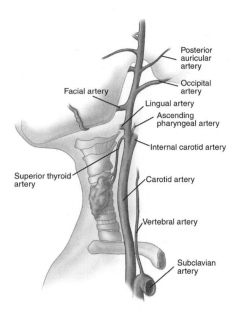

Figure 7   Lateral view of the arterial supply of the neck.

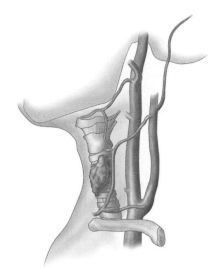

Figure 8   Lateral view of venous drainage of the neck.

The *occipital artery* arises from the posterior surface of the external carotid artery, near the origin of the facial artery, just inferior to the posterior belly of the digastric muscle. It courses superiorly to the posterior scalp, crossing the internal carotid artery and the anterior jugular vein. The occipital artery along with the suprascapular branch of the thyrocervical trunk and the transverse cervical artery supply the skin covering the posterior triangle of the neck.

The posterior *auricular artery* is a small branch arising from the posterior surface of the external carotid at the level of the stylohyoid and the posterior belly of the digastric muscle. It courses deep to the parotid gland providing its blood supply. It also supplies the adjacent muscles, the mastoid air cells, and the posterior aspect of the ear and part of the scalp.

The venous system of the neck includes the *internal jugular veins*, the *external jugular veins*, and the *anterior jugular veins* (Fig. 8). The superficial venous drainage of the anterior neck is located deep to the platysma muscle. The posterior auricular vein joins the posterior division of the retromandibular vein to form the external jugular vein within or just below the parotid gland. The external jugular vein courses inferiorly over the SCM to ultimately drain into the subclavian vein. Submental and submandibular veins join to form the paired anterior jugular veins at the level of the hyoid bone. They course inferiorly near the midline ultimately joining the external jugular vein laterally behind the SCM. The anterior jugular veins communicate across the midline forming a venous arch, which empties into the external jugular and subclavian veins. Often, an anterior communicating vein exists that courses along the anterior border of the SCM connecting the common facial vein with the anterior jugular vein.

LYMPH DRAINAGE

Understanding the anatomy of lymphatic drainage of the head and neck is crucial to locating and working up a suspected malignancy or metastasis. The intricate system of drainage consists of a deep and superficial component. The superficial system can often be evaluated by direct palpation. All superficial lymph channels ultimately drain into deeper cervical nodes. The critical procedure of sentinel lymph node biopsy for managing malignancies is based on an understanding of these complex drainage patterns. Commonly, if metastasis occurs it will be on the ipsilateral side of the primary malignancy.

The lymphatic system starts as a network of small capillaries that merge to form larger lymphatic vessels that drain into the regional lymphatic basin, which filters the lymph fluid before returning it to the venous system. The lymph, derived from the structures of the head and neck, are filtered through a series of regional lymph nodes before emptying into the thoracic duct or right lymphatic duct (Fig. 9).

Superficial Groups

Occipital lymph nodes are found at the apex of the posterior triangle. These small clusters of nodes are located between insertions of the SCM and trapezius. They receive drainage from occipital scalp and nuchal regions and will subsequently drain into the deep cervical lymph nodes.

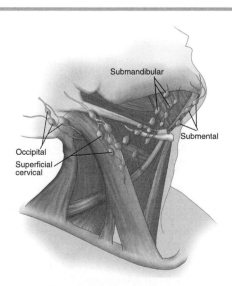

Figure 9   Lymphatic drainage of the neck.

The *submandibular lymph nodes* are considered first line drainage from the nose, upper lip, tongue, teeth (except for incisors), and floor of the mouth, receiving lymph from the submental and facial nodes. These nodes should be palpated when suspecting malignancies in these areas. They are located within the submandibular triangle on the superficial surface of the submandibular salivary gland beneath the cervical fascia. These nodes can often be palpated with an intraoral and external bimanual exam. The lymph draining out of the submandibular gland empties into the jugulodigastric node, and finally into the deep cervical lymph chain.

The *submental lymph nodes* are located in the submental triangle of the anterior neck. They receive lymph from the tip of the tongue, incisor teeth, and center part of the lower lip, chin, and medical cheek. Approximately 25% of the population may have normal palpable nodes in this area.

Superficial cervical nodes run along the course of the external jugular vein. They receive drainage from the parotid gland, lobe of the ear, and angle of the mandible, eventually draining into the deep cervical lymph nodes. This forms the lymphatic drainage system of the anterior neck. The anterior cervical chain likewise receives lymph from skin over the front of the neck.

The posterior triangle of the neck also drains into the superficial cervical lymph nodes. In addition, the posterior triangle drains into the inferior deep cervical lymph nodes, which lie inside the subclavian triangle. The *deeper cervical nodes* parallel the internal jugular vein and are divided into three sections. These include the *spinal accessory* chain, the *transverse cervical* chain, and the *internal jugular* chain. The spinal accessory group of nodes, as its name suggests, runs along the accessory nerve within the posterior triangle. It is here that they can often be palpated. They are often the first point of metastasis from tumors of the nasopharyngeal area. As its name implies, the transverse cervical nodes lie superficial to the transverse cervical vessels.

Finally, deep internal jugular nodes form a chain that runs along the internal jugular vein from the base of the skull to the root of the neck. These nodes are imbedded in the carotid sheath and the adventitia of the internal jugular vein. The internal jugular chain is the major lymph system of the head and neck and ultimately drains into the thoracic duct on the left side and the right lymphatic duct on the right side.

Viscera of the Neck

To fully comprehend the detailed intrarelationship of the neck's anatomy, a brief review of the major visceral structures is included. They can be classified into three groups based on the organ system to which they belong. These may include:

- Endocrine group (thyroid and parathyroid glands)
- Respiratory group (trachea and larynx)
- Digestive group (esophagus and pharynx)

Midline lesions of the neck often derive from persistent embryonic remnants of these structures. They must be well appreciated when evaluating an individual presenting with a midline mass of the anterior neck (Table 2).

Endocrine Group

As the name suggests, the organs in this group are part of the body's hormone secreting system.

Thyroid Gland

The thyroid gland is the largest endocrine gland. It emerges embryologically during the third week as an ectodermal thickening at the midline. This thickening eventually develops into a diverticulum known as the *thyroglossal duct*. This duct eventually becomes a solid cord of cells as the thyroid gland continues to emerge and migrate inferiorly. Persistence of the thyroglossal duct can result in a cyst anywhere along the descending tract. Such cysts are located midline or just off the midline, anywhere from the posterior tongue to the anterior neck just above the suprasternal notch. They typically appear at birth or in the first 10 years of life and should be surgically removed (Table 2). Preoperative evaluation includes a thyroid-stimulating hormone (TSH) and radioisotope scan to evaluate location and function of the thyroid tissue. In other instances, the thyroid fails to descend, resulting in a lingual thyroid gland.

The fully evolved thyroid gland is highly vascular and is surrounded by a sheath, which connects it to the larynx and trachea. The gland itself consists of two lobes connected by an isthmus. The superior and inferior thyroid arteries supply this gland as mentioned previously. They are closely related to the external laryngeal and recurrent laryngeal nerves, respectively, and can be damaged during thyroidectomy surgery.

The clinician should understand that clinically, because the thyroid gland is tethered to the larynx, it would follow the movements of swelling. Neck masses or swelling that rise during swallowing are likely to be fixed to the thyroid gland area.

Parathyroid Glands

The parathyroid glands consist of a pair of superior parathyroid glands and a pair of inferior parathyroid glands. They lie in close proximity to and are intimately involved with the thyroid gland and share its vascular supply. A small portion of individuals may have only two or more than the usual four glands. Inadvertant removal of these glands during surgery can result hypocalcemia and possibly fatal tetany.

Respiratory Group

The visceral structures of this group are involved with respiratory functions of the body.

Trachea

The trachea lies inferior to the larynx. It is a fibrocartilaginous tube that divides into the two main pulmonary bronchi. It is supported by a series of cartilaginous structures known as tracheal rings. It is approximately 2.5 cm in diameter and lies in the midline, posterior to the thyroid gland. If the trachea is seen to deviate from midline on radiographic evaluation, a pathologic process should be suspected. Additionally, patients that develop an upper airway obstruction may require a tracheostomy to establish an airway. This is usually performed between the second and third or third and fourth tracheal rings.

Larynx

This is the organ familiarly known as the "voice box" due to its role in phonation. It also acts as a sphincter to guard air passages during swallowing. It has a complex and varied structure that consists of nine cartilages, the largest of which is the thyroid cartilage. The cartilages may ossify during the aging process.

Digestive Group

The viscera in this group are involved with the alimentary tract and are of minimal concern to the dermatologic surgeon.

Pharynx

The pharynx directs food into the esophagus via constrictor activity. It consists of the oropharynx, the nasopharynx, and the laryngopharynx.

Esophagus

This is a muscular tube with both voluntary and involuntary functions. It lies between the trachea and the vertebral column and conducts food into the stomach. Its lumen expands in size in response to a food bolus. Difficulty in swallowing, or dysphagia, is often the presenting sign of esophageal tumors. Hoarseness can also signify compression of the recurrent laryngeal nerves.

CONCLUSION

The neck serves as an important conduit for many important structures. It has several sites vulnerable to injury during surgery. A complete understanding of anatomical landmarks is imperative for dermatologic surgeons who must often perform surgery in this region. In most instances, surgeries will be limited to the superficial aspects of anatomy. Those managing tumors and masses of the neck must more fully understand the complex interrelationship of structures in this area. By understanding the intricate anatomy of the neck, surgeons will increase their skill and diagnostic acumen while reducing potential adverse outcomes.

ACKNOWLEDGMENTS

We are very grateful for the assistance of Beth Halasz, medical illustrator for the Cleveland Clinic Foundation, and Dr. Richard Drake, anatomist at the Cleveland Clinic Foundation, for their contributions to this chapter.

BIBLIOGRAPHY

Bennet RG. Anatomy of Cutaneous Surgery. In: Fundamentals of Cutaneous Surgery. St Louis, Missouri: C.V. Mosby Company, 1988:100–135.

Bernstein G. Surface landmarks for the identification of key anatomic structures for the face and neck. J Dermatol Surg Oncol 1986; 12:722–726.

Breisch EA, Greenway Jr. HT. Cutaneous Surgical Anatomy of the Head and Neck. 1st ed. New York: Churchill Livingston, 1992:81–107.

Drake RL, Vogl W, Mitchell AWM. Gray's Anatomy for Students. 1st ed. Churchill Livingstone (Elsevier Science), 2005:898–936.

Howard R. Congenital Midline Lesions: Pits and protuberances. Pediatr Ann 1998; 27:150–160.

Moore KL, Dalley AF. Clinically oriented anatomy. 5th ed. Lippincott, Williams and Wilkins, 2005:1046–1122.

Robinson JK, Arndt KA, LeBoit PE, et al. Atlas of Cutaneous Surgery. Philadelphia, Pennsylvania: W.B. Saunders Company, 1996.

Salasche SJ, Bernstein G, Senkirk M. Surgical anatomy of the skin. Appleton and Lange 1988; 141–149, 258–269.

Swanson NA. Atlas of Cutaneous Surgery; 1st ed. Boston, Massachusetts: Little Brown and Company, 1987.

Wiss K. Midline Developmental Defects in Children: Update on diagnosis and management. Adv dermatol 1999; 109–132.

28

The Torso and Appendages

Michael E. Contreras and R. Steven Padilla

Department of Dermatology, University of New Mexico, Albuquerque, New Mexico, U.S.A.

INTRODUCTION

The torso and its appendages are common locations for surgical excisions. Consequently, these sites often pose unique repair considerations for surgeons. In this chapter, we discuss the regional anatomy and special surgical considerations common to the trunk and its extremities.

ANATOMICAL CONSIDERATIONS

The torso, arms, and legs are predominantly convex surfaces owing to their cylindrical nature. As a result, these rounded surfaces create varied forces. These factors contribute to the formation of large dog ears and thus affect the esthetic appearance of the healed wound. The large, mobile joints of the arms and legs create added tensile forces that require careful consideration when closing a wound. In these areas, the nerves and large vessels generally lie deep to the muscle fascia; an exception being the common peroneal nerve which runs superficially in the lateral popliteal fossae. Therefore, superficial blunt dissection and undermining is recommended to avoid damage to vessels and nerves.

EXCISION WITH PRIMARY CLOSURE

As a general rule, wound closure at any site should be kept as simple as possible; keeping in mind that the simplest closure often provides the best result. The use of a flap or graft carries an increased risk of ischemia, necrosis, and distorted excision lines. On the trunk and extremities, where the blood supply is less, compared to the face, this is a particularly important point to remember. In most instances, a primary closure is accomplished by simple elliptical excision with side-to-side closure. Creating a wound edge with minimal tension leads to a better cosmetic result. Less tension also translates into improved blood supply with decreased risk of ischemia, necrosis, and scar spread.

Placing the closure line along the natural lines of force will help reduce wound tension. These relaxed skin tension lines generally run transversely across the trunk and extremity and are oriented perpendicular to the direction of contraction of underlying muscles (Figs. 1–6). This is an important clinical consideration since an incision made parallel to the direction of muscle contraction will be acted on by longitudinal forces, thus contributing to slower wound healing, fibroblast proliferation, and scar formation. In addition, wounds contract to a greater extent along their length than their width. Consequently, mobility over joints is less affected by wound contraction when the relaxed skin tension lines are followed. For example, over the wrists, elbows, knees, shoulders, and anterior neck the incision should be made perpendicular to the primary action of the underlying joint or muscle.

A simple test used to identify skin tension lines is to pinch the skin between your thumb and index finger (pinch test) at the site of the planned excision. If straight lines are produced within the pinch, the pinch is parallel to skin tension lines. If an S-shaped curve results, the pinch is across skin tension lines (Fig. 7). Longer excisions may follow a curved relaxed skin tension line that can be determined by a series of pinches. Use this technique as a guide to planning an excision and repair.

With age, skin demonstrates decreased elasticity, and gravity reorients the tension lines vertically when the patient is upright. Therefore, when performing surgery on the elderly, always plan the incision while the patient is in a sitting or standing position. It is recommended that an excision on a pendulous breast or large abdominal pannus be made parallel to the forces of gravity to minimize wound tension.

When skin tension lines are neutral and not clearly delineated by the pinch test, it is wise to excise the lesion in a circular manner. Evaluation of the wound forces post excision with skin hook traction applied to the wound edges then guides the orientation of the final closure. Wounds requiring this technique are most common on the anterior chest, abdomen, upper arms, and back.

MODIFIED PRIMARY CLOSURES

The following surgical repairs demonstrate modifications of the primary closure that are well suited to surgery of the limbs and torso. The selection of a particular design is dictated by contour of the surgical site, anticipated wound tension, and wound size.

One modification of an end-to-end primary closure is an S-shaped closure. When used over a convex surface, it can minimize wound tension and will help avoid a boat-shaped deformity (Fig. 8).

Bilateral M-plasty repair over a convex surface can similarly correct the boat-shaped deformity. This is particularly useful when trying to minimize the length of the final wound (Fig. 8).

Tissue meshing is another useful technique for repair of large defects under significant tension. The technique is best used for wounds that can be at least two-third covered prior to meshing. The tumor is first removed by elliptical excision and wide undermining is performed. Using a scalpel, 0.5 cm long tension-relaxing incisions are made 0.5 cm apart in a staggered pattern, parallel to the margin of the

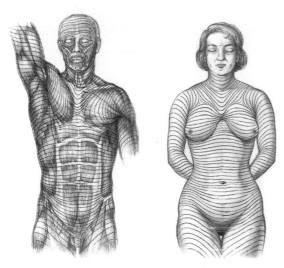

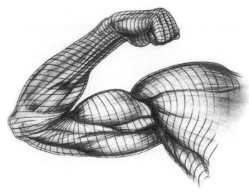

Figure 3   Diagram of the relaxed skin tension lines on the medial aspect of the upper extremity. *Source*: From Kraissl (1951).

Figure 1   Comparative lines on the thorax and abdomen of the male and female. Differences in pattern being due to gravitational action of mammary glands. *Source*: From Kraissl (1951).

wound through the tissue that has been undermined (Fig. 9). This technique was used by Wong to repair six wounds up to 3.5 cm in diameter on the shoulder, shin, scapula, and calf. Each meshed row achieved about a 0.3 cm gain in wound edge movement, in addition to the advantage gained by conventional undermining.

Primary closure can also be achieved with immediate intraoperative tissue expansion using a standard Foley catheter with 10 to 30 cm³ capacity. To expand the tissue, a catheter balloon is inserted into a subcutaneous tunnel formed by undermining 3 to 6 cm on either side of the defect. The catheter is then anchored with towel clips at the wound edge, and the balloon is inflated slowly until the overlying skin blanches and becomes tense. At this point, it

is left in place for three to five minutes. The surgeon then performs a series of three to four cycles of balloon inflation for three to five minutes, each followed by deflation for three to five minutes. Tissue viability at the end of each inflation cycle is confirmed by the presence of dermal bleeding at the wound edge. Using this technique, an additional 0.5 to 2.5 cm of tissue can be gained, depending on the site of expansion. Complications tend to be lowest in the head and neck region (2%) and highest in the lower extremity region (26%) likely secondary to compromise of the blood supply and increased tissue tension in the lower extremities. Inherent to this technique is a risk of circulatory compromise and resultant pain, nerve dysfunction, tissue necrosis, and bone resorption. Meticulous hemostasis minimizes hematoma formation, and perioperative antibiotics limit the risk of infection.

EXCISION WITH SECONDARY REPAIR

Flaps and grafts should be considered when an end-to-end closure is not feasible or would create excessive wound tension or tissue distortion. Compared to primary closure, flaps and grafts are slower to heal and carry an increased risk of ischemia, flap necrosis, and infection.

There are several points to consider in the proper design of a flap on the torso and appendages.

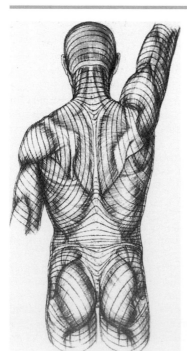

Figure 2   The lines of the back are generally transverse at the neck and waist while the thorax is splinted by the sternum. The muscles approximating the scapulae, latissimus dorsi, and trapezius produce the vertically circular pattern. *Source*: From Kraissl (1951).

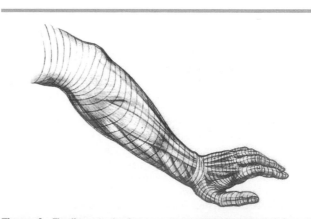

Figure 4   The lines on the forearm extend obliquely downward from the lateral and medial aspect where they join each other over the radius in a rounded fashion. *Source*: From Kraissl (1951).

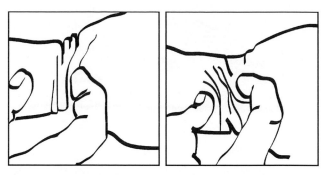

Figure 7 "Pinch test." Straight lines within the pinch indicates orientation along relaxed skin tension lines (**A**). Curved lines indicate that the pinch is not oriented along relaxed skin tension lines (**B**).

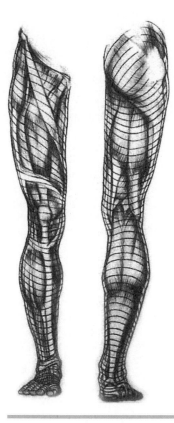

Figure 5 The generally oblique pattern of the anterior thigh changes at the knee were the lines on the medial aspect of the leg extend downward and forward to meet those from the lateral aspect. The posterior aspect is generally transverse. *Source*: From Kraissl (1951).

1. *Blood supply*: On the trunk or extremity where blood supply is relatively poor compared to the face, it is better to maintain a length to base ratio of approximately 1:1. A ratio less than this will compromise the blood supply in an already poorly perfused body region.
2. *Lymphatics*: Maintenance of lymphatic drainage is another feature of proper flap design. This is accomplished by orienting the base of the flap inferiorly whenever possible.

3. *Skin tension lines*: With proper planning, in many cases, the flap margin can be placed within relaxed skin tension lines. The "pinch test" is a useful technique to judge relaxed skin tension lines. This provides minimal tension and improved cosmesis.
4. *Grafting of donor site*: In instances when the donor site cannot be closed primarily, it may be repaired by a full or split thickness skin graft, particularly if healing by second intention is not an option.

In the proper setting, local tissue transfer utilizing a flap on the torso or appendages achieves superior maintenance of surface contour, texture, and color than is possible with a graft. When a graft is used in one of these areas for defect coverage, it often results in a depressed, cosmetically unappealing wound. The inherent advantage of a flap procedure is optimized by moving well-vascularized donor skin, which is low in tension, to a relatively less perfused area. Preserving a 1:1 length to base ratio will maximize the blood flow to the donor skin.

There are many useful flap designs. These designs can be designated transposition, rotation, or advancement flaps. The selection of a particular flap is dictated by defect width and depth and location as assessed within the context of tissue mobility and blood supply. Ideally, flaps are constructed from skin immediately adjacent to the defect with

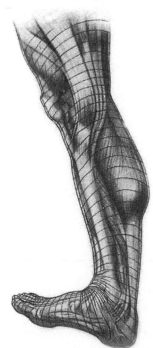

Figure 6 Lines on the medial aspect of the leg. Note the radial effect at the ankle. *Source*: From Kraissl (1951).

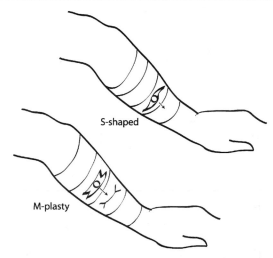

Figure 8 S-shaped closure on dorsal forearm (**A**). M-plasty on dorsal forearm (**B**).

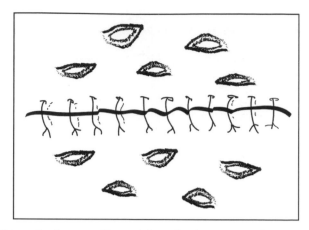

Figure 9 Tissue meshing technique. Resultant wound after tension-relaxing incisions are made 0.5 cm apart in a staggered pattern, parallel to the margin of the wound.

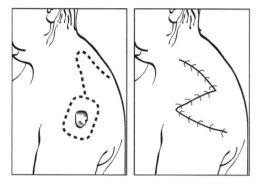

Figure 10 Transposition flap repair for a defect of the upper lateral shoulder. A dorsally based flap is created that respects the skin tension lines over the highly mobile shoulder joint.

created. The laterally oriented closure at the superior and lateral shoulder respects the relaxed tension lines, thereby minimizing risk of contraction and scar spread over this highly mobile joint.

Transposition flaps are excellent for redistribution and redirection of tension vectors. They rely on skin laxity from an adjacent area to fill a defect in an area with little skin laxity. The surgical site is first manipulated with the hand to feel for areas of relative laxity and to predict the effect of various tension vectors on nearby structures. Design the flap transfer so that the donor skin is not required to rotate too far to fill the defect, which could pull too tightly on its pedicle.

Consider this flap in areas where the tight surgical site is adjacent to a well of lax skin. The rhombic flap and the sliding transposition flap are two variations of the basic transposition flap that may also prove useful.

The classic rhombic transposition flap design transfers the tension vectors from those created by primary defect closure to the new secondary defect closure (Fig. 11). It is used when there is insufficient laxity of the surrounding skin to accomplish primary closure, or when tension vectors need to be redirected to prevent distortion of free margins and enhance mobility of a joint. Rhombic flaps are versatile and can be used for a variety of defects. The utility of this design is illustrated by the repair of an axillary defect (Fig. 12). In women, the flap is taken from the anterior axillary fold with a ventral pedicle. In men, a dorsally based flap is taken from the skin above the latissumus dorsi muscle.

A sliding transposition flap is useful in closing poorly vascularized large defects using adjacent well-perfused, mobile skin (Fig. 13). An anterior tibial defect is a typical candidate for this modified transposition flap. Primary closure in this area would create increased tension, further compromising the blood supply, while a graft would have a poor chance of survival. A transposition flap from the mobile, vascular adjacent skin drapes easily over the convex surface with minimal tension at the flap base. However, a graft is often necessary to close the well-vascularized donor site.

A rotation flap involves sliding adjacent skin into the wound without crossing intact skin. The defect is excised as a triangle, and the short edge of the triangle is extended in an arc-shaped incision as shown in Figure 14. Undermining of the pedicle created by the arced incision is followed by rotation of the pedicle into the defect. Removal of a Burrow's triangle removes the laxity created at the pedicle base. Rotation flaps require long incision lines to achieve appropriate flap motion. In addition, they depend on a relatively lax surgical site such as the axilla (Figs. 15 and 16).

similar blood supply, innervation, and sensory qualities as the site of the defect. With any design, it is important to align the wound edges with the relaxed skin tension lines to prevent contractures and scar spread. While performing the procedure, monitor the pallor of the donor skin which is an indicator of tissue perfusion and can indicate potential tissue necrosis.

Transposition flaps involve the movement of the donor tissue across intact skin into the defect. This flap is illustrated in the repair for a defect of the upper lateral shoulder (Fig. 10). The lesion is excised and a dorsally based flap is

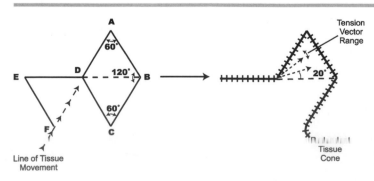

Figure 11 Classic rhombic flap. All sides of the defect and flap are equal length. Line of tissue movement, occurring from point F to D, results in the tension vectors as drawn. The redundant tissue cone is excised away from the flap base to avoid compromising the blood supply to the flap.

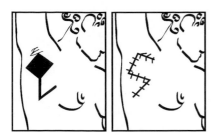
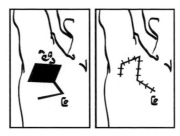

Figure 12 Rhombic flap repair of an axillary defect. In women, the flap is taken from the anterior axillary fold with a ventral pedicle (**A**). In men, a dorsally based flap is taken from the skin above the latissumus dorsi muscle (**B**).

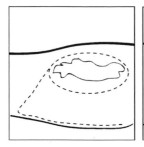
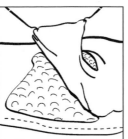
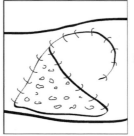

Figure 13 Sliding transposition flap repair of a lower leg defect. The flap (skin plus underlying fascia) is draped over the wound with minimal tension. The donor site is covered with a split thickness skin graft.

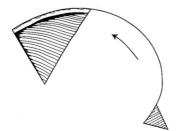

Figure 14 Basic rotation flap. The defect is excised as a triangle, and the short edge of the triangle is extended in an arc-shaped incision. The pedicle is undermined and rotated into the defect, and redundancy at the pedicle base is removed.

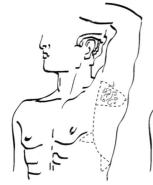
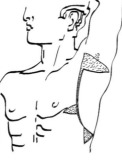
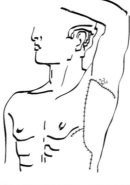

Figure 15 Large rotation flap repair of an axillary defect.

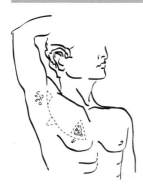
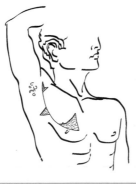
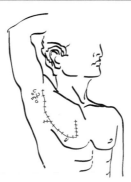

Figure 16 Large rotation flap repair of a chest defect.

The advancement flap entails the movement of adjacent donor tissue in a straight line directly into the wound without rotation around an axis. They are limited by the elasticity of the surrounding skin, and therefore, are not preferred at sites lacking a generous well of donor tissue. The vascular supply is generally less than a rotation flap which, by design, has a broader base. Also, the straight suture lines are sometimes less appealing than the curved

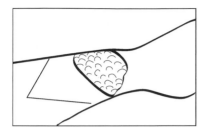
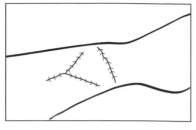

Figure 17   V-Y plasty at the dorsal wrist.

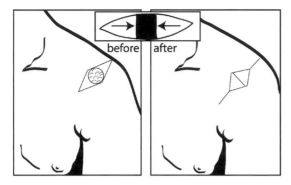

before after

Figure 18   Bilateral island pedicle flap repair of a shoulder defect.

lines achieved with other designs. However, when used appropriately, they are a relatively simple way to reduce wound tension.

A V-Y plasty is a variant of the advancement flap (Fig. 17). The V-shaped incision is placed in an area of increased laxity compared to the original defect. Alternatively, as depicted in the figure, the V-Y plasty is used as a releasing incision to decrease tension over the highly mobile wrist joint. An island pedicle flap is another variation of an advancement flap. It is sometimes referred to as a V-Y flap because the initial incisions have a V-shaped geometry. A bilateral island pedicle flap is useful over the superior

shoulder where maintenance of suture lines along relaxed tension lines is achieved (Fig. 18).

BIBLIOGRAPHY

Borges AF. Relaxed skin tension lines. Dermatol Clin 1989; 7:169–177.

Courtiss EH. The placement of elective incisions. Plast Reconstr Surg 1963; 31:31–44.

Harrison SH, Saad MN. The sliding transposition flap: its application to leg defects. Br J Plast Surg 1977; 30(1):54–58.

Johnson TM, Brown MD, Sullivan MJ, et al. Immediate intraoperative tissue expansion. J Am Acad Dermatol 1990; 22:283–287.

Kolbusz RV, Bielinski KB. Basal cell carcinoma: excision with immediate intraoperative tissue expansion. Cutis 1990; 46(5):419–420.

Kraissl CJ. The selection of appropriate lines for elective surgical incisions. Plast Reconstr Surg 1951; 8:1–19.

Meirson D, Goldberg LH. The influence of age and patient positioning on skin tension lines. J Dermatol Surg Oncol 1993; 19:39–43.

Sasaki GH. Intraoperative sustained limited expansion (ISLE) as an immediate reconstructive technique. Clin Plast Surg 1987; 14:563–573.

Stegman SJ. Guidelines for placement of elective incisions. Cutis 1976: 18(5):723–726.

Wong TW, Sheu HM, Lee JY, et al. Use of tissue meshing technique to facilitate side to side closure of large defects. Dermatol Surg 1998; 24(12):1338–1341.

29

The Hand

John Louis Ratz
Center for Dermatology and Skin Cancer,
Tampa, Florida, U.S.A.

Jefferson J. Kaye
The Ochsner Clinic, New Orleans, Louisiana, U.S.A.

Randall J. Yetman
Cleveland Clinic Foundation, Cleveland, Ohio, U.S.A.

INTRODUCTION

The hand is a unique structure on which dermatologic surgeons often work. Intricate in design and function, its use is vital in our daily lives. Its importance cannot be overstated, and, because of this, any anticipated surgical procedure in this area should be carefully considered with regard to underlying anatomy, innervation, circulation, function, and cosmesis.

A reasonable approach to skin surgery of the hand is discussed here, but it is beyond the scope of the dermatologic surgeon to perform extensive excisional and reconstructive procedures; these are more appropriately left to the hand surgeon. Discussion will be limited here to procedures done with the scalpel. Cryosurgery, electrosurgery, and laser surgery, as they apply to the hand, are discussed in other chapters.

ANATOMY

The anatomy of the hand is complex. Full details of its anatomy are described in appropriate texts on the subject. However, it is not possible to discuss surgery of the hand without understanding some of its important anatomic landmarks.

Surface Anatomy

The surface anatomy of the hand is relatively simple (Fig. 1). There is a dorsal and ventral surface and a radial and ulnar aspect. The five digits are named or numbered, and the fingers are subdivided into distal, middle, and proximal phalanges. Common creases are all named. The volar muscular eminences, which are present proximally, are the thenar radially and hypothenar on the ulnar aspect.

From a surgical standpoint, the anatomy of the dorsal surface of the hand is unique because many of the large veins are superficial due to the relative paucity of subcutaneous fat (Fig. 2). Care should be taken to avoid transecting these vessels during surgery. Punch biopsies can be safely performed in this area by applying pressure only until the instrument has penetrated the skin. Without further downward pressure, a continuous clockwise rotation of the punch will draw up the subcutaneous tissue and minimize the risk of injury to underlying vessels.

Deeper Anatomy

The skeleton of the hand consists of three phalanges for each finger, with the exception of the thumb, which has two. The phalanges are attached to the metacarpals, which, in turn, are attached to the system of carpal bones, each of which is named (Fig. 3). The intrinsic muscles of the hand are the lumbricals and interossei, all of which have their origins and insertions on the skeletal structures of the hand itself (Fig. 4). However, the majority of hand movement is due to muscles in the forearm, and their attachments to the hand are complex. This elaborate system of flexor and extensor tendons and tendon sheaths is demonstrated in Figures 5–7. Further details are available from texts on the subject.

The blood supply of the hand is derived from a superficial and deep palmar arch system that arises jointly from the radial and ulnar arteries (Fig. 8). The digital and interosseous arteries arise from the arch system and form a collateral network about each digit. Patency of both ulnar and radial arteries should be established prior to any surgery to avoid vascular compromise. At no time during surgery on the hand should any vessel be ligated. It is also important that arteries not be entered during administration of local or digital anesthesia. Knowledge of the anatomy for this purpose is important. The syringe plunger should be withdrawn prior to injection of digital anesthesia to ensure that a vessel has not been entered.

It is reasonable to assess motor and sensory status prior to surgery and note any deficits so they cannot be attributed to the procedure. Motor function of most intrinsic muscles of the hand, as well as several of the flexors, is supplied by the ulnar nerve (Fig. 9). The remainder of the intrinsic musculature and flexors receive their innervation from the median nerve (Fig. 10), while all of the extensors are supplied by the radial nerve (Fig. 11). Note that the radial nerve supplies none of the intrinsic musculature of the hand.

Sensory innervation is supplied by a combination of the ulnar, median, and radial nerves (Fig. 12). The radial nerve generally supplies the radial aspect of the dorsal two-thirds of the hand but notably not the distal aspects of the index, middle, or ring fingers. The ulnar third of the dorsal surface is supplied by the ulnar nerve, with the exception of the distal ring and little fingers. The ulnar nerve also

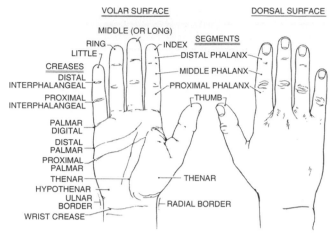

Figure 1   Surface anatomy of the hand.

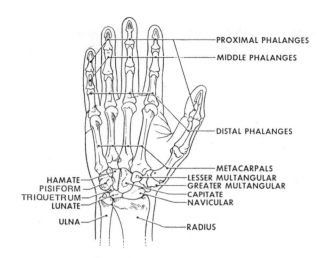

Figure 3   Skeleton of the hand.

supplies the palmar third to the hand on the ulnar aspect. The median nerve is responsible for the remainder of the sensation, most of which is on the palmar aspect of the hand. Knowledge of sensory innervation is important, particularly when regional or digital anesthesia is being considered.

Lines of Tension

An understanding of the skin tension lines is important when one is planning incisions. Naturally occurring tension in the skin of the hand, as well as other parts of the body, is due to elastic fibers in the dermis. These elastic fiber bundles are arranged along "lines of tension." These lines of tension were first noted by Dupuytren in describing wounds of the skin made by penetrating instruments. He noted that when round instruments were used to puncture the skin, the wounds became linear. Langer found that when round incisions of the skin were made, there was a tendency for these wounds to extend along lines of tension. He considered the skin to be less extensible in the direction of the lines of tension than across them.

Experience has shown that incisions heal better when they are made parallel to these naturally occurring skin tension lines. These lines of minimal tension are often at right angles to the long axis of the underlying muscles. An incision parallel to these lines is not subject to the same tension from underlying musculature.

On the hand, these lines of skin tension (Fig. 13) result from the movement of the flexor and extensor muscles. Because flexion and extension take place perpendicular to these tension lines, there is a redundancy of skin parallel to these lines that allows motion to occur. Therefore, skin can be excised parallel to these lines without unduly increasing the amount of tension when the wound is closed.

PLANNING THE PROCEDURE

It is essential to plan the incision carefully. The direction of an elective incision should always be chosen in relation to the lines of minimal tension. A marking pencil is a helpful guide. There are significant differences in the character of the skin

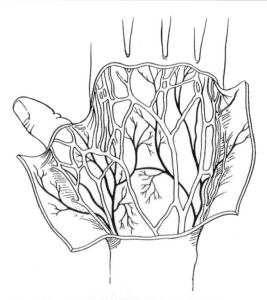

Figure 2   There is very little subcutaneous fat underlying the skin of the dorsal surface of the hand. Large veins in this area are superficial and subject to possible trauma during surgery.

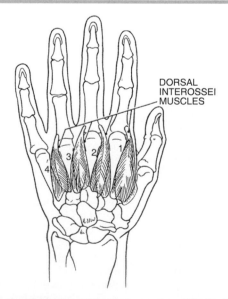

Figure 4   Dorsal interossei: all intrinsic muscles of the hand have their origins and insertions on the skeletal structures of the hand itself.

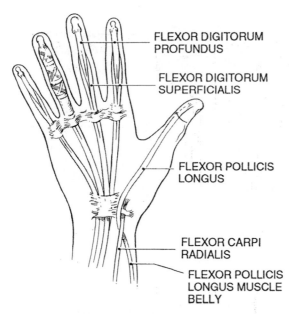

Figure 5 Deep flexor tendon and tendon sheath structures.

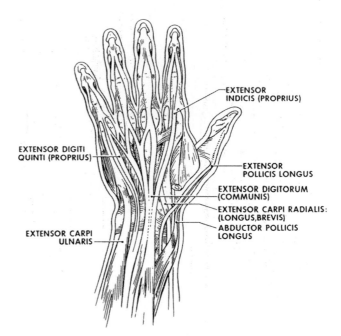

Figure 7 Extensor tendon and tendon sheath structures.

between the dorsal and palmar surfaces of the hand. Incisions, perpendicular to the skin tension lines on the palmar surface of the hand are tolerated much less well than those on the dorsal surface. Scar contracture and functional impairment are common when incisions are made perpendicular to the crease lines on the palmar surface. Incisions must not cross the flexion creases in a perpendicular fashion. Incisions parallel to crease lines are perpendicular to underlying nervous and vascular structures; therefore, care must be taken to avoid injuring these structures.

ANESTHESIA

Detailed knowledge of the anatomy of the hand is essential if one is to administer direct nerve blocks appropriately for anesthesia. Wrist blocks are commonly used to produce

anesthesia. These blocks are simple to perform and provide 20 to 30 minutes of anesthesia.

The median nerve can be blocked at the wrist (Fig. 14), where it lies between the palmaris longus and flexor carpi radialis tendons. Occasionally, the palmaris longus is congenitally absent. A 25-gauge needle is inserted between the two tendons until very light paresthesias are encountered. At that point approximately 5 mL local anesthetic without epinephrine is injected.

In a similar fashion, the ulnar nerve can be blocked at the wrist where it lies just radial to the flexor carpi ulnaris tendon. A 25-gauge needle is inserted just radial to the flexor carpi ulnaris tendon at the level of the proximal wrist crease

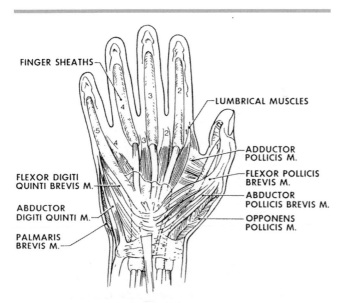

Figure 6 Superficial flexor tendon and tendon sheath structures.

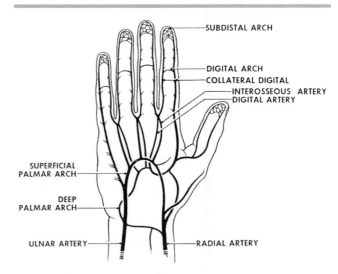

Figure 8 The blood supply of the hand arises jointly from the radial and ulnar arteries through a complex double arch system. The deep arch generally is supplied mostly by the dorsal branch of the radial artery crossing over the radial side of the base of the thumb. The digital and collateral systems, in turn, arise from the superficial and deep palmar arches.

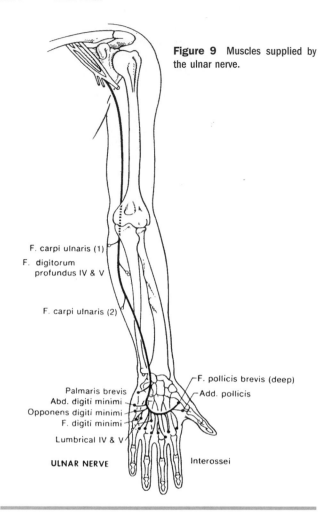

Figure 9 Muscles supplied by the ulnar nerve.

F. carpi ulnaris (1)

F. digitorum profundus IV & V

F. carpi ulnaris (2)

Palmaris brevis
Abd. digiti minimi
Opponens digiti minimi
F. digiti minimi
Lumbrical IV & V

ULNAR NERVE

F. pollicis brevis (deep)
Add. pollicis

Interossei

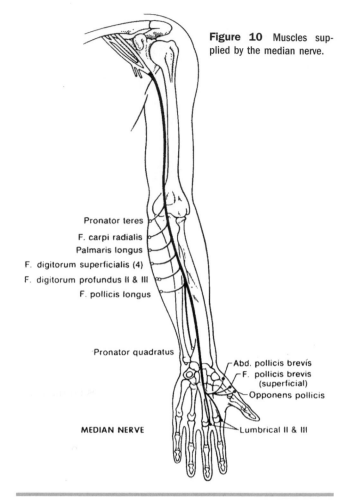

Figure 10 Muscles supplied by the median nerve.

Pronator teres
F. carpi radialis
Palmaris longus
F. digitorum superficialis (4)
F. digitorum profundus II & III
F. pollicis longus

Pronator quadratus

Abd. pollicis brevis
F. pollicis brevis (superficial)
Opponens pollicis

MEDIAN NERVE

Lumbrical II & III

(Fig. 15). When very light paresthesias are elicited, 5 mL local anesthesia without epinephrine is injected.

For anesthesia of one finger only, it is best to use a digital block. The dorsal approach is the preferred method because it is less painful than the palmar approach. This allows block of the dorsal nerves. A 25-gauge needle is inserted just proximal to the web space. A skin wheal is made, and approximately 1 mL anesthetic solution is injected. The needle is advanced in a palmar direction, and another 1 mL local anesthetic is injected. This is repeated in the other web space. Avoid using more than 3 mL on each side to prevent a circumferential pressure increase at the base of the finger, which may result in vascular compromise.

HEMOSTASIS

The hand has a richly endowed vascular supply, and appropriate hemostasis is often important. However, the use of the epinephrine as a hemostatic agent should be avoided. Accidental or inadvertent injection of epinephrine into the arterial circulation could have disastrous results and lead to ischemic necrosis of the digit. A bloodless field is the best means of minimizing potential injury to underlying structures. This can be achieved with the use of a tourniquet. When operating on an individual finger, several methods can be used to obtain hemostasis. The use of a Penrose drain to exsanguinate the finger, in addition to use of the drain as a tourniquet at the base of the finger, allows one to make

incisions safely and efficiently (Fig. 16). Use the minimum pressure needed to achieve hemostasis.

Alternatively, hemostasis of the digit can be achieved by using a rubber band tourniquet at the base of the finger. The rubber band can be looped several times and then tightened further by placing the tip of a hemostat under one of the loops and winding the hemostat. Applying pressure distally to proximally (milking the finger) to create a blanche removes blood that will not return until the tourniquet is released (Fig. 17).

A third method of hemostasis is to fit the patient with a sterile surgical glove in which a small incision is made at the tip of the finger that will be operated on. That portion of the glove can then be rolled down to the base of the finger. This both milks out the blood and provides tourniquet action in one simple maneuver (Fig. 18).

When operating on the palm or dorsum of the hand, a proximal forearm tourniquet is usually necessary. Hemostasis with this tourniquet can be maintained for 25 to 30 minutes. Beyond this, the tourniquet causes significant pain. A general guideline is 100 mm Torr above systolic pressure.

Should bleeding occur during the surgical procedure, electrocautery or chemical cautery can be used. This is most effectively accomplished with a bipolar electrocautery device. Under no circumstance should hemostasis be achieved with ligature. This could result in ischemic necrosis.

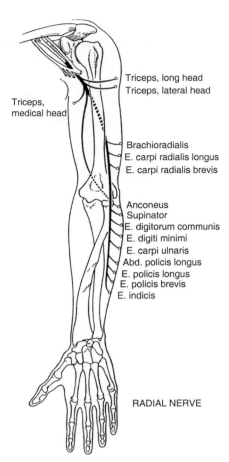

Figure 11   Muscles supplied by the radial nerve. Note that no intrinsic muscles are innervated by the radial nerve.

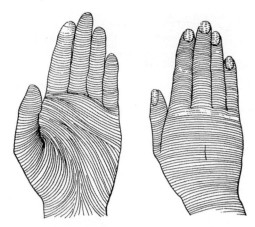

Figure 13   Lines of minimal tension on the hand, as elsewhere, are related to the underlying musculature of its movements.

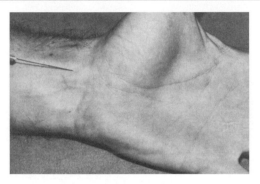

Figure 14   The median nerve block. The nerve can best be approached at the wrist, where it lies between the palmaris longus and flexor carpi radialis tendons.

WOUND CLOSURE

Once an excision is completed, there are various methods of wound closure. Most skin incisions or small excisions can be closed by direct approximation using fine suture material. The use of subcutaneous sutures is generally not necessary on the hand. Wounds should be repaired with fine non-absorbable suture material, such as 5–0 nylon, using a simple everting technique. In general, the sutures are removed on the seventh postoperative day.

If the wound is not amenable to direct suture approximation, a free-skin graft is the method of choice in most situations. When replacing skin on the palmar surface of the hand, it is important to use tissue of similar histologic architecture. It is also important to use a full-thickness graft to maximize the return of sensation to this area.

A convenient source of tissue on the palmar surface is the hypothenar eminence (Figs. 19 and 20). Small defects can be easily replaced with a full-thickness graft from this area. Once the skin graft has been obtained, it is important to remove all subcutaneous tissue to maximize revascularization. Five days of splinting will help revascularization.

In general, use glabrous skin to replace glabrous palmar hand or foot skin, especially in dark-skinned

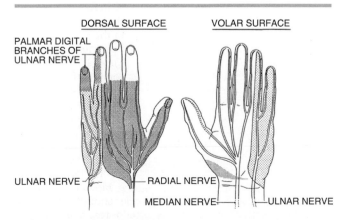

Figure 12   Common pattern of sensory innervation of the hand.

DORSAL SURFACE   VOLAR SURFACE

PALMAR DIGITAL
BRANCHES OF
ULNAR NERVE

ULNAR NERVE   RADIAL NERVE

MEDIAN NERVE   ULNAR NERVE

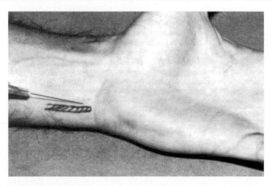

Figure 15   The ulnar nerve can be blocked at the wrist, where it lies radial to the flexor carpi ulnaris tendon.

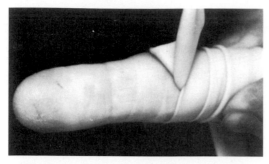

Figure 16 Penrose drain tourniquet: a small Penrose drain is wound tightly around the finger distally to proximally. The drain is unwound beginning at the distal end.

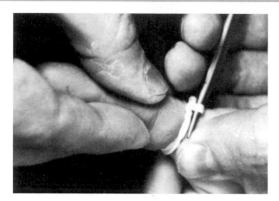

Figure 17 Rubber band tourniquet: a rubber band is looped over the base of the finger and doubled or tripled. A hemostat is placed between the loops and wound to provide the desired minimal tension required.

(A)

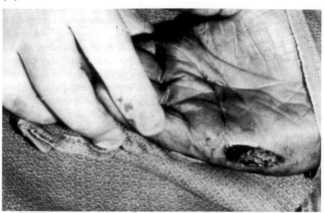

(B)

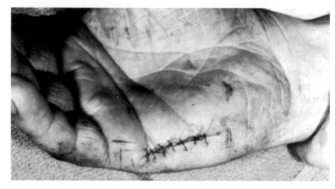

Figure 19 The hypothenar eminence is a convenient source of full-thickness skin graft replacement for other locations on the palmar surface of the hand. Generally, the donor site can be closed primarily with little or no difficulty.

individuals. If the skin is used on the palmar aspect of the hand, significant hyperpigmentation of the graft may result (Fig. 20).

When repairing defects on the dorsum of the hand, either split-thickness or full-thickness grafts can be used. For small defects, full-thickness grafts taken from the antecubital fossa work well but can leave cosmetic defects in that area. For larger defects, a split-thickness skin graft harvested from the groin will cover these wounds. Once the graft is in place with interrupted sutures, the dressing is applied. This is particularly important. Compression must

be applied by the dressing to prevent fluid accumulation between the graft and its underlying bed. A bolus or tie-over dressing is recommended. As long as there is no drainage or sign of infection, the dressing is left undisturbed for approximately one week.

If, after the excisional part of the procedure is completed, bone, blood vessel, or tendon is exposed, and a skin graft is not adequate coverage. A variety of local or regional flaps can be used to achieve coverage for these situations. The V-Y advancement or island pedicle (kite) flap can be

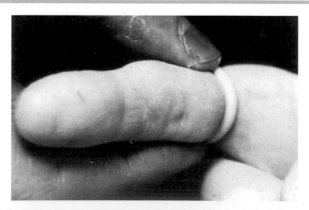

Figure 18 Glove tourniquet: a sterile glove is placed on the hand, and a hole cut in the tip of the finger. The glove finger can be rolled proximally to the base of the digit. Sterility of the entire field can be easily maintained.

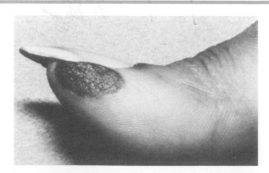

Figure 20 "Nonfingerprint" skin, when used as donor tissue for palmar surface defects, should be avoided, particularly in black individuals. Significant hyperpigmentation of the graft can occur, leaving an unacceptable cosmetic result.

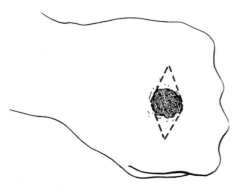

Figure 21 The V-Y advancement or island pedicle (kite) flap is useful in repairing small defects on both the palmar and dorsal aspects of the hand. This is a simple procedure to perform, has a high degree of success, and allows for normal sensation in the area postoperatively.

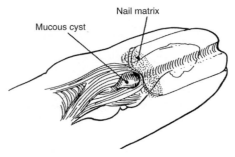

Figure 23 A mucous cyst can cause grooving of the fingernail because of direct pressure on the nail matrix.

used for a number of small defects on both the palmar and dorsal aspects of the hand. These flaps are simple to develop and quite reliable (Figs. 21 and 22). In addition, skin retains its normal sensation.

After wound closure has been achieved, immobilization of the hand is important. The dressing should apply uniform pressure to the entire hand. It should be snug enough to control capillary oozing, but not restrict venous return. Web spaced should be separated to prevent maceration of these areas. A palmar plaster splint may be used to immobilize the hand.

In general, the hand is immobilized in the positions of function. The wrist should be moderate dorsiflexion (30–45°). The metacarpophalangeal joints should be flexed 70°–80°. The interphalangeal joints are only slightly flexed (10° or less). In this position, the collateral ligaments are at almost maximal extension. This will prevent contracture of these important ligaments and subsequent joint stiffness.

COMPLICATIONS

Skin surgery of the hand has attendant risks. Several postoperative complications are possible. The risk of postoperative infection and wound dehiscence is no greater than for any other cutaneous site. However, because of its anatomy and because of the proximity of vascular and nervous elements, several complications more unique to the hand may be encountered.

Ischemia and ischemic necrosis have already been mentioned. These can result from the use of epinephrine as a hemostatic agent, ligation of a functional component of the arterial system, or inadvertent compression of an artery through deep closure, which may have encompassed the vessel. This can be avoided by not using epinephrine and ligature during surgery. Evaluation of the entire hand postoperatively to ensure vascular competence is mandatory.

Decreased or altered mobility is a possible complication of cutaneous hand surgery and can have many causes. The alteration or decrease in mobility may be due to damage to muscle, tendon, or tendon sheath structures. Such damage may be repaired but should only be attempted by a qualified hand surgeon. Damage to a motor nerve can also cause decreased mobility but may be a more difficult situation to remedy, and evaluation by a hand surgeon is suggested. Mobility can be decreased by edema or hemorrhage. These should be relatively easy to detect and appropriate measures undertaken to remedy them. If hemorrhage is the problem, care should be taken when achieving hemostasis to avoid compromising the blood supply to any area of the hand.

Decreased sensation immediately following surgery may be transient and should be evaluated several days after the procedure. Proper evaluation of decreased sensation can only be done if sensation was evaluated preoperatively. Any

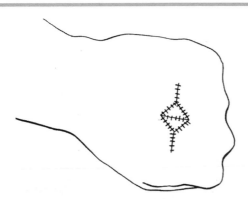

Figure 22 The V-Y advancement or island pedicle (kite) flap is useful in repairing small defects on both the palmar and dorsal aspects of the hand. This is a simple procedure to perform, has a high degree of success, and allows for normal sensation in the area postoperatively.

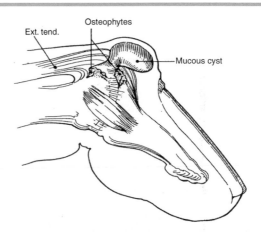

Figure 24 Osteophytes, which commonly accompany mucous cysts, must be excised during the procedure to minimize chances for recurrence.

(A)   **(B)**

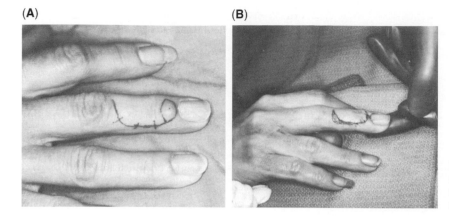

Figure 25 **(A)** A slightly curved incision is a reasonable approach to the mucous cyst. **(B)** Such an incision can usually be closed by means of a rotation flap. Alternatively, a full-thickness skin graft can be used.

sensory deficit present prior to surgery is not likely to have been altered by the surgical procedure. Sensory deficits present several days after the procedure are most likely due to nerve damage and may be irreversible. Digital nerves are approximately 1 mm beneath the skin surfaces at flexion creases of the fingers and are very easily injured during skin closures and surgical procedures unless extreme care is used during the entire surgical procedure.

Because of the flexibility and mobility of the hand, delayed healing is likely, particularly if the procedure is performed over the extensor aspect of a flexing joint. The usual cause of delayed healing is increased mobility and can be remedied by appropriate immobilization measures. Careful preoperative planning is important to avoid tension on lines of closure.

SURGICALLY AMENABLE CONDITIONS SPECIFIC TO THE HAND

Although numerous cutaneous entities can occur on the hand, few are truly peculiar to this location. Common lesions, such as nevi and epidermal cysts are not particularly common on the hand, but when they do occur, they are more likely to be present dorsally rather than on the palmar aspect. Removal of such lesions is generally uncomplicated, and the principles established in this chapter should be followed.

Verruca vulgaris is common on the hand. Its treatment, however, is usually topical, cryosurgical, electrosurgical, or with the use of a laser, and rarely by excisional surgery. Excision of a small wart should follow the parameters already mentioned.

Actinic keratoses, like warts, are common on the hands, and their treatment is usually by other modalities. Squamous cell carcinoma, however, is best removed as an intact specimen so that surgical margins can be evaluated histologically. Mohs micrographic surgery should be considered. Whether excision is done conventionally or by the Mohs technique, the size, location, and orientation of the tumor will dictate the lines of closure. Because complete histologic tumor-free margins are important, it may be difficult to adhere to rules regarding tension lines. Difficult wounds may result, leading to complicated closure or repair techniques.

Vascular lesions, such as glomus tumor and pyogenic granuloma can occur on the hand. All vascular extensions must be removed to avoid recurrence. Occurrence of such lesions subungually or in the nail fold entail special considerations, which are discussed in another chapter.

Of all cutaneous lesions, the most specific to the hand are the ganglion and cutaneous myxoma or mucinous cyst. Although these lesions can occur in other locations, they are most common on the hand and often are attached to deeper structures, which complicates their effective removal. Failure to remove these lesions completely will often result in a recurrence.

A mucous cyst is a small lesion located on or about the distal interphalangeal joint of the finger. It often causes a groove in the adjacent fingernail due to pressure on the nail matrix (Fig. 23). Osteoarthritis in the joint is associated with these cysts. These osteophytes should be excised with the cyst (Fig. 24). If they are not removed with the cyst, recurrence of the cyst is likely.

(A)   **(B)**   **(C)**

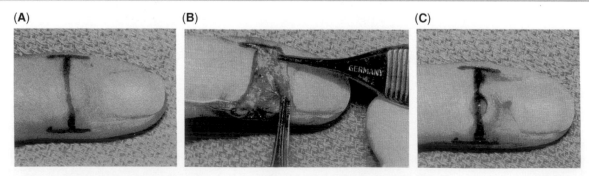

Figure 26 **(A)** Proposed "H"-incision overlying mucinous cyst. **(B)** Excision of mucinous cyst. **(C)** Cyst removal (H-incision) just before closure.

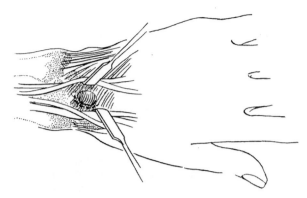

Figure 27 A dorsal wrist ganglion generally has its deepest attachments at its origin on the scapholunate interosseous ligament. An arthrotomy may be required for complete removal.

A slightly curved incision is used (Fig. 25). The cyst is dissected down to its origin on the joint capsule and excised with the joint capsule. The accompanying osteophytes can be removed with fine rongeur. Care must be taken not to injure the extensor mechanism. Skin closure often requires a rotation flap or a full-thickness skin graft (Fig. 26).

Although wrist ganglia appear to be quite superficial, they usually have extensions down to the deeper ligament of the wrist. Simple incision of ganglia is discouraged because there is a high recurrence rate with this procedure. The cyst must be dissected down to its origin on the wrist scapholunate ligament (Fig. 27). Because an arthrotomy is required to excise these ganglia of the wrist properly, this type of surgery should be done by someone with experience in hand surgery. Alternatively, wrist arthroscopy may be used to excise the ganglion yet minimize the size of the scar.

BIBLIOGRAPHY

Angelides AC, Wallace PF. The dorsal ganglion of the wrist. Its pathogenesis, gross and microscopic anatomy and surgical treatment. J Hand Surg 1976; 1:228.

Bauer BS, Vicari FA, Richard ME, Schwed R. Expanded full-thickness skin grafts in children: case selection, planning, and management. Plast Reconstr Surg 1993; 92(1):59–69.

Bean DJ, Rees RS, O'Leary JP, Lynch JB. Carcinoma of the hand: a 20-year experience. South Med J 1984; 77(8):998–1000.

Beasley RW. Local flaps for surgery of the hand. Orthop Clin North Am 1970; 1:219.

Boyes JH. Incisions in the hand. Am J Orthop 1962; 4:308.

Eaton RG, Dobranski AI, Littler JW. Marginal osteophyte excision in treatment of mucous cysts. J Bone Joint Surg 1973; 55A:570.

Heim U, et al. Subungual glomus tumors. Value of the direct dorsal approach. Ann Chir Main 1985; 4(1):51–54.

Hutton K, Podolsky A, Roenigk RK, Wood MB. Regional anesthesia of the hand for dermatologic surgery. J Derm Surg Oncol 1991; 17:881–888.

Langer K. Zur anatomic and physiologic der hant. Z Die Spanning der Cutis SB Akad. Wiss, Wien 1862; 45:133.

LeWinn LR (guest ed.), Perspectives in hand surgery. Clin Plast Surg 1986; 13(2).

Micks JE, Wilson JN. Full-thickness sole skin grafts for resurfacing the hand. J Bone Joint Surg 1967; 49A:1128.

Miller PK, Roenigk RK, Amadio PC. Focal muscinosis (myxoid cyst) surgical therapy. J Derm Surg Oncol 1991; 18:716–719.

Reigstad A, Hetland KR, Bye K, Rokkum M. Free flaps in the reconstruction of hand and distal forearm injuries. J Hand Surg (Br) 1992; 17(2):185–188.

Robotti EB, Edstrom LE. Split-thickness plantar skin grafts for coverage in the hand and digits. J Hand Surg (Am) 1992; 17(1):182.

Salasche SJ. Myxoid cysts of the proximal nail fold: a surgical approach. J Dermatol Surg Oncol 1984; 10(1):35–39.

Salem MZA. Simple finger tourniquet. Br Med J 1973; 1:779.

30

The Foot

Christine Poblete-Lopez and Allison T. Vidimos
*Department of Dermatology, Cleveland Clinic Foundation,
Cleveland, Ohio, U.S.A.*

INTRODUCTION

The human foot is a complex and sensitive structure that is vital in our daily living. Its intricate design has been adapted to perform its two functions: to allow orthograde bipedal stance and locomotion. It is the only part of the body that is in regular contact with the ground.

The skin is the single largest organ of the body. Plantar skin, like palmar skin, significantly differs from the rest of the skin of the body. Plantar skin is unique in several ways. It is markedly thickened, considered glabrous, apocrine and sebaceous glands are absent, and eccrine glands are numerous.

We often encounter lesions/conditions on the foot necessitating a surgical procedure. A good understanding of the anatomy, circulation, innervation, function, and cosmesis is important before performing a surgical procedure.

ANATOMY

The anatomy of the foot is intricate and complex. We refer to review the appropriate textbooks on the foot and ankle for a detailed description of the anatomy. A brief description of the relevant anatomic landmarks, as it pertains to cutaneous surgery, will be discussed.

Surface Anatomy

The surface anatomy of the foot aptly divides it into the dorsal and the plantar aspect. Like the hand, the five toes are numbered and subdivided into distal, middle, and proximal phalanges. Unlike the hand, common creases are not all named. Uniquely so, the skin of the plantar and the dorsal foot vary tremendously, in terms of thickness, and the amount of subcutaneous fat. Therefore, when planning a surgical procedure, be it a punch biopsy or an elliptical excision, care must be taken, as the neurovasculature of the foot is relatively superficial because of the paucity of the subcutaneous fat. Punch biopsies may be easily done with just the appropriate amount of pressure applied while rotating the punch biopsy in a clockwise fashion the subcutaneous fat is released without much damage to the underlying structures.

Bony Anatomy

The foot is comprised of 28 major bones (Figs. 1–4), including the sesamoid bones of the first metatarsophalangeal joint, and 31 major joints, including the ankle joint. The foot can be broken down into the rear foot, midfoot, and forefoot. The rear foot consists of the talus, and the calcaneus; the midfoot consists of the navicular, cuboid, and the three cuneiforms; and the forefoot consists of the metatarsals, and the phalanges. The joints of the foot consist of the distal interphalangeal joints, the proximal interphalangeal (PIP) joints, the hallux interphalangeal joint, the metatarsal phalangeal (MP) joints, the tarsometatarsal joint (Lisfranc's joint), the midtarsal joint (Chopart's joint), the subtalar joint and the ankle joint. All these joints are synovial joints.

Retinacula

In the ankle joint, the tendons of the muscles of the leg are bound down by localized thickenings of the deep fascia, forming retinacular bands that prevent bowstringing of the tendons.

The superior extensor retinaculum, seen in Figures 5–7 is attached laterally to the lower end of the fibula and medially to the tibia. Proximally, it is continuous with the fascia of the leg, and distally, to the inferior extensor retinaculum. It binds down the tendons of tibialis anterior, extensor hallucis longus, extensor digitorum longus and fibular (peroneus) tertius immediately above the anterior aspect of the ankle joint. The inferior extensor retinaculum is a Y-shaped band in front of the ankle joint. The stem of the Y is attached laterally to the calcaneus. Medially, one limb is attached to the medial malleolus, and the other limb to the border of the plantar aponeurosis (Figs. 5–7). It envelops the tendons of extensor hallucis longus, tibialis anterior, extensor digitorum longus, and fibular tertius, and lies superficial to the dorsalis pedis artery and the deep fibular nerve.

The flexor retinaculum (Fig. 7) extends anteriorly from the medial malleolus to the calcaneus posteriorly, and the plantar aponeurosis distally. It converts grooves on the tibia and calcaneus into canals for the tendons, and bridges over the posterior tibial vessels and the tibial nerve. The following tendons enter the sole through the flexor retinaculum, from medial to lateral they are: tibialis posterior, flexor digitorum longus, flexor hallucis longus.

The fibular retinacula (superior and inferior) (Fig. 6) retain the tendons of fibular longus and brevis in position as they curve round the lateral side of the ankle. Anteriorly, the superior fibular retinaculum is attached to the lateral malleolus, and the inferior fibular retinaculum is continuous with the inferior extensor retinaculum. It attaches to the lateral surface of the calcaneus posteriorly.

Tendons

The tendons that cross the ankle joint are all deflected from a straight course and held down by the retinacula as

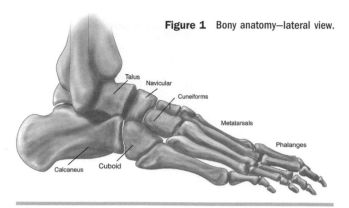

Figure 1 Bony anatomy—lateral view.

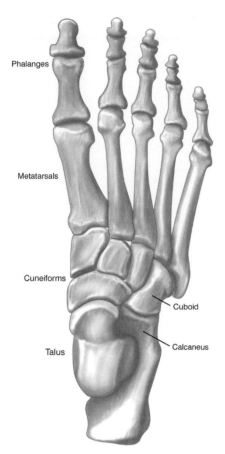

Figure 3 Bony anatomy—dorsal view.

described above. They are enclosed for part of their length in synovial sheaths, which have an almost uniform length. The anterior group (Fig. 5) consists of the tendons of tibialis anterior, extensor digitorum longus and fibular tertius, and extensor hallucis longus. The medial posterior group (Fig. 7) consists of the tendons of tibialis posterior, flexor digitorum longus, flexor hallucis longus tendon, and the Achilles tendon. The lateral posterior group (Fig. 6) consists of the tendons of fibular longus and brevis.

The plantar fascia or aponeurosis is composed of densely compacted collagen fibers oriented mainly longitudinally, but also transversely. Its medial and lateral borders overlie the intrinsic muscles of the great and fifth toe and its dense central part overlies the short and long digital flexors (Fig. 8).

Musculature

A complete musculoskeletal examination consists of assessing the strength and function of the foot. A preoperative assessment will ensure that any preexisting deficits may not be attributed to the surgery. The intrinsic muscles are those contained entirely within the foot, and they follow the primitive limb pattern of dorsal extensors and plantar flexors. The tendons of the extrinsic muscles are associated with them topographically and functionally.

In general, the muscles of the leg (and the foot and ankle) are divided into the anterior group of extensor muscles, a posterior group of flexor muscles, and a lateral group of muscles derived from the extensors.

The anterior compartment contains muscles that dorsiflex the ankle when acting from above, and act from below to pull the body forward on the fixed foot when walking. It consists of the tendons of the tibialis anterior, extensor hallucis longus, and extensor digitorum longus more superficially. These tendons lie inferior to the retinacula to dorsiflex the ankle joint. The latter two extensors also extend the toes, and the tibialis anterior also inverts the foot. The tendon of the fibular tertius lies lateral to the extensor digitorum longus. It often appears to be part of the extensor digitorum longus. It acts with the extensor digitorum longus and tibialis anterior to produce dorsiflexion and eversion of the foot. Deep to these tendons lay the extensor digitorum brevis and extensor hallucis brevis, which are the only muscles that arise from the dorsum of the foot. These short extensors work to extend the middle three phalanges and the proximal phalanx of the great toe (Figs. 5 and 6).

The lateral group consists of the fibular longus and fibular brevis, which lie posterior to the lateral malleolus, in a groove that is shared by the two. They participate in eversion of the foot, and the former, in plantar flexion of the foot (Fig. 6).

The plantar muscles of the foot (Fig. 9) can be divided into medial, lateral, and intermediate groups. The medial and lateral groups consist of the intrinsic muscles of the hallux and minimus, and the intermediate group includes the lumbricals, interossei, and short digital flexors. The extrinsic musculatures in the posterior compartment include the superficial flexors: gastrocnemius, soleus, and plantaris, whose main function is plantar flexion of the foot. Within

Figure 2 Bony anatomy—medial view.

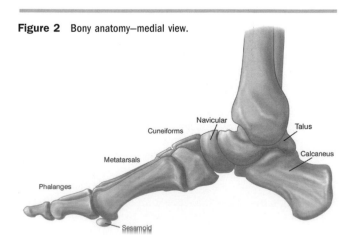

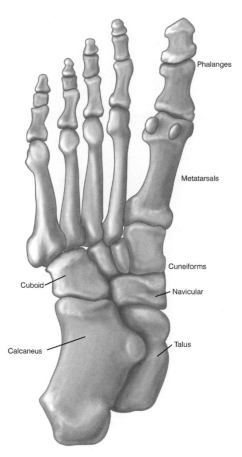

Figure 4 Bony anatomy—ventral view.

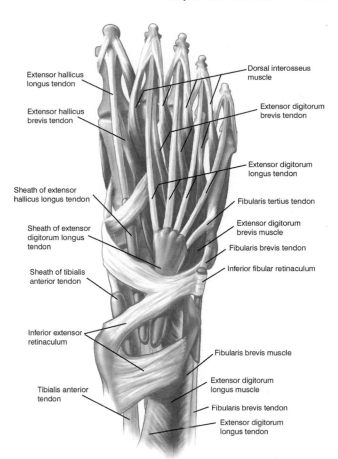

Figure 5 Dorsal view of the foot illustrating the retinacula, tendons and synovial sheaths, and some musculature.

the ankle and foot, the superficial layer includes the abductor hallucis, abductor digiti minimi, and flexor digitorum brevis, whose cut ends are illustrated in Figure 9. All three extend from the heel to the toes and maintain the concavity of the foot. Furthermore, the abductor hallucis abducts the hallux; the flexor digitorum brevis flexes the lesser toes at the PIP joint; and the abductor digiti minimi flexes the little toe at the metatarsophalangeal joint. The second group of intrinsic muscles consists of the quadratus plantae, and four lumbrical muscles. The preterminal tendons of the deep digital flexors, flexor hallucis longus, and flexor digitorum longus, are also intimately associated with them. These deep digital flexors act to flex the distal phalanges of the toes. By pulling on the flexor digitorum longus, the quadratus plantae provides a means of flexing the lateral four toes. The lumbricals, on the other hand, maintain extension of the interphalangeal joints of the toes. The third layer of the foot contains the shorter intrinsic muscles of the flexor hallucis brevis, adductor hallucis, and flexor digiti minimi brevis. The former two muscles jointly flex the proximal phalanx of the hallux and the latter flexes the metatarsophalangeal joint of the little toe. The fourth muscle layer consists of the plantar and dorsal interossei. The dorsal interossei are located between the metatarsal bones. They consist of four bipennate muscles, and abduct the toes about a longitudinal axis through the second metatarsal. The plantar interossei lie below the metatarsal bones, plantar to the dorsal interossei and deep to the muscles of the third layer. The dorsal and plantar interossei flex the metatarsophalangeal joints and extend the interphalangeal joints of the lesser toes.

The tendons of tibialis posterior and fibular longus are also intimately part of this layer. The tibialis posterior is the most deeply placed muscle of the flexor group and is the principal invertor of the foot. It also assists in vigorous plantar flexion.

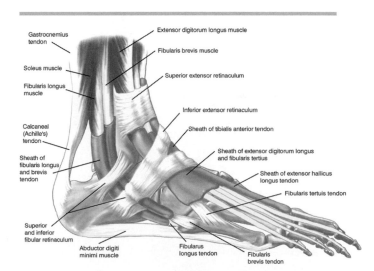

Figure 6 Dorsolateral view of the foot illustrating the retinacula, tendons and synovial sheaths, and some musculature.

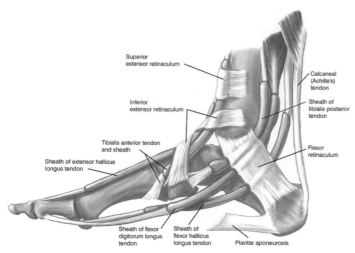

Figure 7 Medial view of the foot illustrating the retinacula, tendons and synovial sheaths, and some musculature.

Vascular Supply

There are two major blood sources of blood supply to the skin: the perforating musculocutaneous arteries and the direct cutaneous blood vessels. As the name implies, the perforating musculocutaneous arteries supply each individual muscle and overlying skin and end in the subdermal plexus. The direct cutaneous vessels travel in the deep layer of the subcutaneous tissue and supply specific and larger areas of the skin. These vessels end in the subdermal plexus. Direct cutaneous arteries are usually accompanied by paired venae

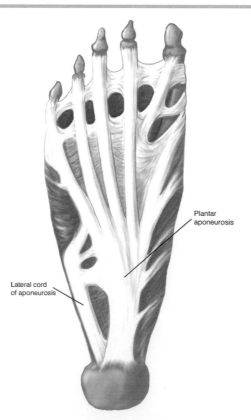

Figure 8 Sole of the foot—the plantar aponeurosis.

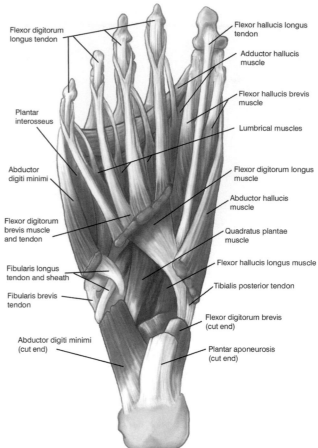

Figure 9 Sole of the foot—deep musculature.

comitantes, while the perforating vessels are not paired with veins. The subdermal arterial plexus (Fig. 10) is the major blood supply to the skin itself, and these are the characteristic "skin bleeders" encountered during a surgical incision. A fine circulatory network is formed as the branches pass through the dermis to supply the appendages (dermal plexus) and end in the papillary dermis (subpapillary plexus). From this subdermal arterial plexus, capillary loops arise and pass to lie within the dermal papillae. The advantage of this dual blood supply to the skin is that any area of skin is not solely dependent on one artery.

Venous drainage begins in the efferent side of the capillary loops and connects in narrow endothelium lined spaces in the superficial papillary dermis. Venous blood drains the entire thickness of the dermis to empty into the subdermal venous plexus. From there, blood drains via the venae comitantes or the superficial venous network within the subcutaneous fascia.

The dorsalis pedis and the plantar arteries provide vascular supply to the foot. The posterior tibial artery (Fig. 11) terminates into the medial and lateral plantar arteries. The plantar arch is a continuation of the lateral plantar artery, and like the palmar arch, is in close relation to the intrinsic muscles of the foot. It is deeply situated and gives off three perforating and four plantar metatarsal branches and numerous other branches that supply the skin, fascia, and muscles of the sole. The dorsalis pedis artery is the dorsal artery of the foot and is the continuation of the anterior tibial artery distal to the ankle (Fig. 12). It gives rise

Knowledge of the vascular anatomy of the foot is crucial when it comes to surgical procedures on the foot. It is important to avoid these vessels during administration of local or digital anesthesia. Withdrawing the syringe plunger prior to injection of digital anesthesia ensures that a vessel has not been entered. Intraoperatively, ligation of these vessels should be avoided, despite the complex network of and numerous perforating arteries that supply the foot.

Plantar digital veins arise from plexuses in the plantar regions of the toes, connecting with dorsal digital veins and uniting into four plantar metatarsal veins. These connect by perforating veins with dorsal veins and continue to form the deep plantar venous arch, which accompanies the plantar arterial arch. From the venous arch, medial and lateral plantar veins run with their corresponding arteries, communicate with the great and small saphenous veins and form the posterior tibial veins behind the medial malleolus.

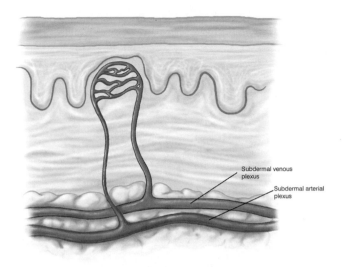

Figure 10   Vascular supply to the skin.

to the arcuate artery (comparable to the plantar arch on the sole), and turns into the sole to complete the plantar arch. Off of the dorsalis pedis artery, branch the four dorsal metatarsal arteries and one proximal perforating artery.

Sensory Innervation

Motor innervation to the foot is supplied by the medial and lateral plantar nerves (S1–3), which are branches of the tibial nerve. Cutaneous innervation is supplied by the superficial peroneal, deep peroneal, saphenous, sural and posterior tibial nerves. The posterior tibial nerve (Fig. 11) gives rise to the medial calcaneal branches (S1, 2), medial plantar

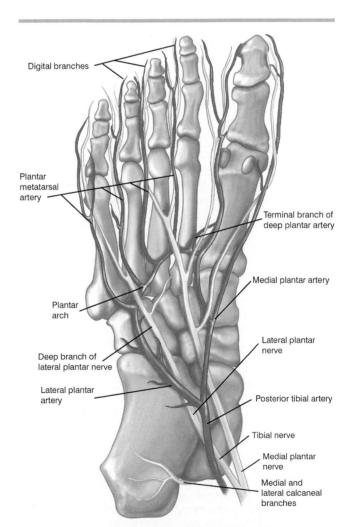

Figure 11   Neurovascular supply to the sole of the foot.

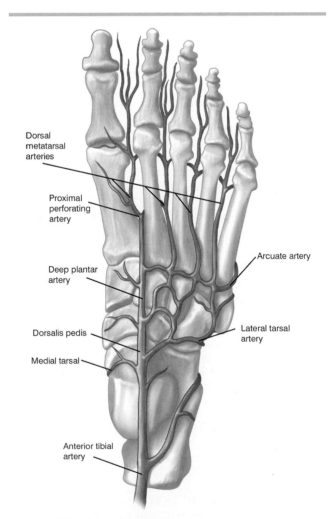

Figure 12   Vascular supply to the dorsum of the foot.

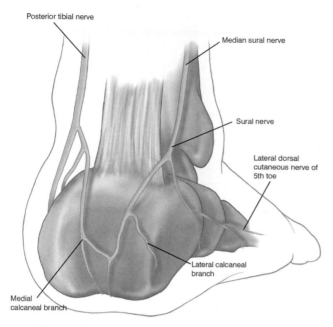

Figure 13 Nerve supply to the lateral aspect of the foot.

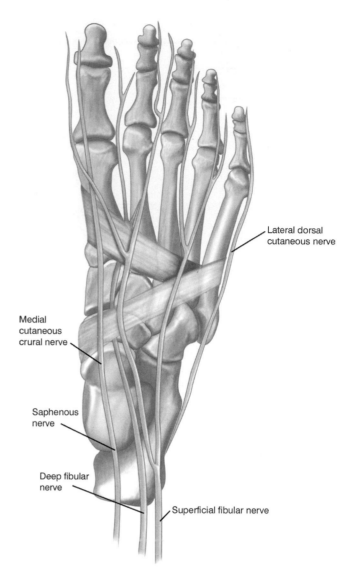

Figure 14 Nerve supply to the dorsum of the foot.

nerve (L4, 5) and lateral plantar nerve (S1, 2) to supply majority of the sole as it terminates via the digital nerves. The sural nerve (S1, 2) (Fig. 13), also a branch of the tibial nerve, supplies the dorsolateral aspect of the foot. It is formed by two proximal branches—the median sural nerve (a branch of the tibial nerve), and an anastomotic branch of the common fibular nerve, gives off one or two calcaneal branches and terminates as the lateral dorsal cutaneous nerve of the fifth toe. The superficial (L4, 5, S1) and deep fibular nerves (S1, 2) (Fig. 14) arise from the common fibular nerve to supply the dorsum of the foot via dorsal cutaneous nerves. The saphenous nerve (L3, 4) (Fig. 14), which is the terminal branch of the femoral nerve, supplies most of the medial midfoot and the area adjacent to the medial malleolus with medial crural cutaneous branches. Knowledge of sensory innervation must be stressed especially when regional or digital anesthesia is being considered (Fig. 15).

PLANNING THE PROCEDURE

The surgical approach to the foot should consider the basic principles of placement of skin incisions, while having a thorough knowledge of the underlying anatomy, and respecting the relaxed skin tension lines. The planned surgical incision should be safe, provide adequate exposure, and result in a cosmetically acceptable and functionally stable scar. Use of a surgical marking pen will aid the surgeon in placing the incision with more accuracy.

RELAXED SKIN TENSION LINES

The inherent tension of the skin in the relaxed position is partially a function of the internal pull of the elastic fibers and partially a function of the external force of gravity. It is an important concept in planning surgical incisions as well as important applications in wound healing. The idea is to have as little tension across an incision as possible, to produce a fine scar.

Creases are usually formed at right angles to the direction of muscle pull. Cleavage lines (or Langer's lines) do not always correspond to elective incision lines, usually due to the direction of the underlying muscle pull. They often run across natural creases and flexion lines, as they are more a function of skin extensibility. Extensibility refers to the ability of the skin to return from the extended or stretched state to its fully relaxed state and is a function of the elastic fiber network. Except for the soles of the feet and the extension aspects of the ankle, crease lines generally coincide with cleavage lines.

The ideal place for an elective incision is within a flexion–extension crease or at right angles to the direction of muscle pull, sometimes going against the lines of cleavage. Curved or oblique incisions can compensate for the resulting scar contraction. Incisions on the lateral surfaces of the toes will allow the scars to bend along with toe movement and heal without much tension. Avoid placing incisions along bony prominences or weight bearing surfaces, where pressure may cause undue pain. If it is necessary, follow skin lines but slightly modify the location of the incision to lessen this adverse reaction (Fig. 16).

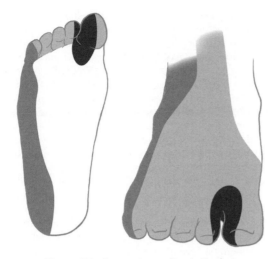

Figure 15 Sensory innervation to the foot.

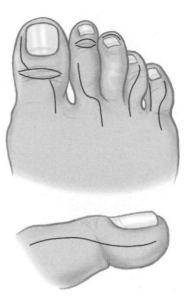

Figure 16 Examples of surgical incision placement.

Some general recommendations may be helpful when planning the surgical incision:

1. Avoid extensive transverse incisions and long incisions;
2. Place incisions to follow nerve pathways in the overlying skin;
3. Avoid extensive undermining of the skin in the foot;
4. Allow enough length to keep retraction from causing skin sloughing;
5. Expose underlying tissue sufficiently to fulfill the goals of operation;
6. Maintain adequate hemostasis;
7. Choose appropriate wound closure materials, and postoperative dressings.

ANESTHESIA

Almost all operative procedures performed by a dermatologic surgeon involving the foot need anesthesia and the choices include: local, digital, and peripheral nerve block. The choice will depend on the specific surgical procedure planned, the duration of the procedure and the amount of time available for the anesthetic to take effect, the cutaneous lesion at hand, and the patient's preference and age.

Digital Block

For toenail or lesser toe surgical procedures, a digital nerve block (Fig. 17) using 1% Lidocaine (without epinephrine) should be adequate. At point A, on the dorsomedial aspect of the toe at its base, a small wheal is raised in the skin. With the needle directed in a vertical direction from the dorsal to the plantar surface of the toe, the anesthetic is infiltrated as the needle is withdrawn into the subcutaneous tissue. The needle is then turned and directed in a horizontal and ventrolateral direction, as well as dorsolateral direction and the anesthetic is infiltrated in the ventral and dorsal aspects of the toe. The dorsomedial and plantar medial sensory nerves are anesthetized in this fashion. The needle is withdrawn and at point B, on the dorsolateral aspect of the base of the toe, another wheal is raised with infiltration of the anesthetic in a vertical direction. Similarly, the needle is turned and directed in a horizontal and ventromedial direction, as well as dorsomedial direction and the anesthetic is infiltrated in the ventral and dorsal aspects of the toe. The dorsolateral and plantar lateral digital nerves are anesthetized in this fashion. For the hallux, 3 to 5 mL of 1% Lidocaine is used for a complete toe block, and

(A)   **(B)**

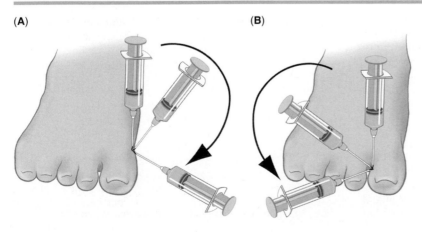

Figure 17 Digital nerve block.

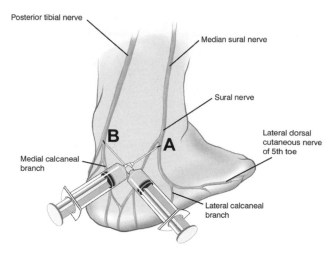

Figure 18   Peripheral nerve block: posterior approach.

relatively less for the lesser toes. The onset of anesthesia is relatively rapid.

Peripheral Nerve Block

A detailed knowledge of the foot anatomy is crucial when planning a nerve block for appropriate anesthesia. One should allot the appropriate amount of time for the peripheral nerve block to take effect before commencing an operative procedure to increase the success of this choice of anesthesia. Generally, it takes 15 to 20 minutes from the time of infiltration to the onset of anesthesia. A 25-gauge $1\frac{1}{2}$ in. needle is used for infiltration with the physicians' choice of 1% lidocaine and/or 0.5% bupivacaine with or without epinephrine. Care should obviously be taken such that intravascular injection of the anesthetic is avoided.

The posterior approach is done with the patient in prone position, and blocks the sural and posterior tibial nerves. The sural nerve provides sensation to the lateral border of the forefoot. It is found 1 to 1.5 cm distal to the tip of the fibula or just adjacent to the peritenon of the Achilles tendon at a distance 7 cm proximal to the tip of the lateral malleolus. At injection point A (Fig. 18), between the Achilles tendon and the lateral malleolus, 3 to 5 mL of the anesthetic agent is injected to block the sural nerve.

The posterior tibial nerve is located at the posteromedial aspect of the tibia at the level of the medial malleolus and provides sensation to the plantar aspect of the foot. At two fingerbreadths proximal to the tip of the medial malleolus, a horizontal line is drawn to mark the level of injection. The posterior tibial nerve is just posterior to the tibial shaft, posterior and lateral to the palpable posterior tibial artery and directly beneath the medial border of the Achilles tendon. At injection point B (Fig. 18), 5 to 10 mL of 0.5% bupivacaine is injected in the region to block the tibial nerve. The images will show that the lateral and plantar aspects of the foot are anesthetized with the sural and tibial nerves, respectively.

The anterior approach is done with the patient in supine position and blocks the superficial and deep fibular nerves, as well as the saphenous nerve. The branches of the superficial fibular nerve are anesthetized in a ring fashion. The needle penetrates the skin at a level two fingerbreadths proximal to the tip of the lateral malleolus, at point A (Fig. 19), just lateral to the extensor hallucis longus. The infiltration is carried out

subcutaneously directed laterally and medially superficial to the long extensor tendons. About 5 to 10 mL of 0.5% bupivacaine is used for the block, and this provides anesthesia to most of the dorsal foot except for the first web space. The deep fibular nerve provides sensation to the first web space. In the interval between the extensor hallucis longus and the extensor digitorum longus on the lateral border of the dorsalis pedis artery, deep to the extensor retinaculum lays the deep fibular nerve. At injection point B (Fig. 19), the needle is advanced to the underlying tarsal bone and withdrawn 2 mm, aspirated to ensure inadvertent vascular injection. About 5 to 10 mL of 0.5% bupivacaine is injected in this region, which provides anesthesia to the first web space. The saphenous nerve provides sensation to the medial midfoot and the area adjacent to the medial malleolus. It is located two fingerbreadths proximal to the tip of the medial malleolus and one fingerbreadth anterior to the medial malleolus, just posterior to the saphenous vein. At point C (Fig. 19), 3 mL of the anesthetic agent is injected into the subcutaneous tissue in a transverse fashion from posterior to anterior to anesthetize the saphenous nerve. It is also often blocked with the ring block of the superficial fibular nerve.

HEMOSTASIS

An extensive vascular network richly supplies the foot. As such, surgery in the foot will require meticulous and adequate hemostasis to keep a bloodless field. This can be achieved with the use of a tourniquet. A Penrose drain is used to exsanguinate the toe, in addition to using the drain at the base of the toe. This way, the surgeon can efficiently and safely make the incision, as well as visualize the field and identify important anatomic landmarks and pathology.

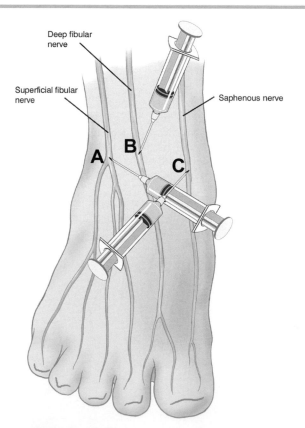

Figure 19   Peripheral nerve block: anterior approach.

Further dissection is through the subcutaneous tissue, just immediately deep to the dermis, where many blood vessels travel. These vessels should be identified, cleanly clamped and electrocauterized as minimally but adequately as possible. Ligation of vascular structures should be avoided as much as possible. There should be little or no undermining or angled dissection until the subcutaneous layer is completely separated. This will preserve as much blood supply to the skin as possible.

WOUND CLOSURE

Small excisions on the foot are frequently conducted with standard fusiform design followed by direct primary approximation of the skin edges, using a simple everting technique. A subcutaneous closure is often not necessary. But if it is, an absorbable buried suture, of a 4–0 or 5–0 caliber is used. The best choice of wound closure material for the epidermis is a fine (4–0 or 5–0) nonabsorbable suture, such as nylon. One should pay particular attention to keeping the articular sutures superficial to avoid inadvertent trapping of underlying structures. Casting or splinting may be necessary. Standard wound care and pressure dressings are employed. Sutures are generally removed in 10 to 14 days.

Larger excisions may require a curvilinear design or a "lazy S" excision, especially over the dorsolateral surfaces of the foot. This is designed as an ellipse with 30° angles at the tips, but the tips are twisted in opposite direction. This design closure more evenly distributes tension and reduces the tissue redundancies at the tips of the excision.

Redundancies at the excisional tips are very common on the dorsal foot, and because these areas remodel well, these redundancies are typically not "chased."

For excisions not amenable to primary closure, skin grafts are preferred over skin flaps. However, for smaller excisions on the dorsal feet, where tension redistribution or redirection is desirable, rhombic transposition or A to T flaps are particularly useful. With regard to skin grafts, split-thickness is preferred over full-thickness grafts because of the higher risk of graft failure in the lower extremity. Split-thickness skin grafts may be harvested elsewhere in the sole or upper inner arm or thigh. Avoiding trauma and weight bearing are crucial for reducing complications such as dehiscence, hematoma, tissue necrosis, and future hypertrophic scarring.

COMPLICATIONS OF FOOT SURGERY

A careful consideration of the natural skin lines, the sensory innervations and vascular supply to the skin helps to minimize some complications unique to the foot. Because of its anatomic function, the foot is predisposed to delayed healing, wound dehiscence, postoperative anesthesia and paresthesia, reaction to suture material, hypertrophic scar or keloid formation, and formation of traumatic neuromas and aneurysms. Therefore, a detailed knowledge of the anatomy of the foot, a carefully planned and meticulous approach to a surgical procedure, and a thorough preoperative counseling and postoperative care are of utmost importance.

31

The Nail

Deborah F. MacFarlane and Nor Chiao
M.D. Anderson Cancer Center, University of Texas, Houston, Texas, U.S.A.

Richard K. Scher
College of Physicians and Surgeons, Columbia University, New York, New York, U.S.A.

INTRODUCTION

As many as 10% of patients seek dermatologic care for a nail disorder and it is essential that a knowledge of nail anatomy be clearly understood. Approximately, half of all nail problems are due to fungal infection and the remainder to psoriasis, lichen planus, tumors, ingrown nails, and a large miscellaneous group. Unlike the skin, where diagnoses are facilitated by changes in color, size, and shape, the spectrum of clinical expression for nail conditions is limited. Consequently, a number of diagnostic procedures must be performed more frequently on the nail than on the skin. It is important therefore that the dermatologist be familiar with nail surgery. In addition, the important functions of the nails must be taken into account when one considers performing nail surgical procedures: protection of the distal digit, facilitation of manual dexterity, and cosmesis.

ANATOMY

A thorough understanding of nail anatomy is crucial for successful nail surgery. The components of the nail unit include the matrix, proximal and lateral folds, plate, bed, hyponychium, four grooves—proximal, distal, and two lateral (Fig. 1).

The most important structure in the nail unit is the nail matrix, which lies deep in the fingertip, below the proximal nail fold, and produces the nail plate. Any defect at this site will be reflected in onychodystrophy of the evolving nail plate. The distal portion of the nail matrix is the lunula, which may be seen in some digits lying beneath the proximal portion of the nail plate distal to the cuticle. The proximal portion of the matrix abuts the bony terminal phalanx. There is no granular layer in the matrix therefore keratohyaline granules are absent. The proximal portion of the matrix produces the upper portion of the nail plate, while the distal portion of the matrix (lunula) produces the underside of the nail plate. Extreme care must be exercised when performing surgery near the proximal nail matrix. A defect will produce a deformed nail plate surface postoperatively. The split nail is an example of such a defect.

The proximal nail fold is a modified extension of the finger that forms a fold over the matrix. It is continuous with the lateral nail fold that forms the side borders of the nail plate. The cuticle is the horny end product of the proximal nail fold which is deposited on the surface of the newly formed nail plate and desquamates shortly thereafter. Unlike the matrix, the nail fold does have a granular layer with keratohyaline granules.

The nail plate extends about 5 mm proximal to the cuticle where it fits into the proximal nail groove, the roof of which is the undersurface of the proximal nail fold; the floor is the matrix. That portion of the nail plate in the proximal groove is often referred to as the nail root. The nail plate fits laterally into the lateral nail grooves formed by the junction of the lateral nail folds to the nail bed.

The nail bed begins at the distal portion of the lunula (matrix) and extends distally to terminate at the hyponychium. The epidermis of the nail bed is arranged in longitudinal grooves and ridges overlying the dermis and contains no granular layer. Splinter hemorrhages occur when a small amount of blood enters a longitudinal groove and is trapped by the overlying adherent nail plate, assuming the longitudinal configuration of this natural trough. The dermis contains both capillaries and glomus bodies.

The hyponychium commences with the termination of the nail bed at a point where the nail plate separates to its free end. A granular layer is present at this site. A transverse groove demarcates the end of the hyponychium. The hyponychium then becomes continuous with the volar epidermis of the digit. This site is often the entry point for fungal organisms that cause the most common fungus infection of the nails: distal subungual onychomycosis. The dermis of the nail appendage is limited by the underlying phalanx upon which it rests. There is no subcutaneous tissue below the nail unit dermis. Consequently, when one cuts through this structure, the underlying periosteum of the distal phalanyx may be exposed. The distance from the surface of the nail plate to the periosteum is only several millimeters. The tendon of extensor digitorum communis inserts onto the proximal dorsal portion of the terminal phalanx, approximately 12 mm proximal to the cuticle, and incisions should be planned to avoid this area.

The blood and nerve supply of the nail unit run approximately the same course. Two lateral digital arteries and nerves on either side of the finger give rise to dorsal branches at the junction of the middle and terminal

Portions of this chapter have been reproduced with permission from the author's contributions to Epstein E, Epstein E Jr, eds. *Techniques in Skin Surgery.* Philadelphia: Lea & Febiger, 1979; Demis DJ, McGuire J, eds. *Clinical Dermatology.* New York: Harper & Row, 1985; Callen JP, Dahl MV, Golitz LE, Rasmussen JE, Stegman SJ, eds. *Advances in Dermatology.* Vol. 1. Chicago: Year Book Medical Publishers, 1986.

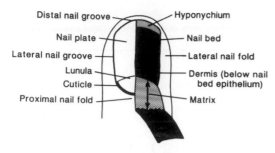

Figure 1 Anatomy of the nail unit.

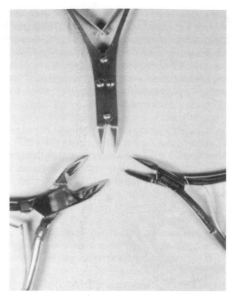

Figure 3 Dual-action nail nipper (*top*); nail clipper (*left*); nail splitter (*right*).

phalanges, which in turn subdivide to form distal and proximal arches with a ramus to both the matrix and the proximal nail fold (Fig. 2). It is important to remember this circulatory and neural pattern when anesthetizing and operating on the nail unit.

PREOPERATIVE CONSIDERATIONS

Prior to the surgical procedure, a careful medical history and physical exam will reduce complication risk. Nail surgery should be avoided, if possible, in those who have peripheral vascular disease, diabetes mellitus, or connective tissue disorders that compromise circulation. This includes Raynaud's phenomenon, particularly when surgery on the toenails is considered. Details of previous surgical procedures, underlying illness, current medications, and allergies should be elicited. Anesthesia may be affected by monoamine oxidase inhibitors, beta-blockers, or phenothiazines. Anticoagulants may prolong bleeding. Systemic or topical steroids may delay healing. Antitetanus immunization status should be ascertained. The risks, benefits, and alternatives to surgery should be discussed in detail with the patient and consent obtained. Preoperative X-rays should be obtained when the condition is suspected to involve the bony phalanx.

If there is evidence of active infection, elective procedures should be deferred until these are treated with antibiotics and soaks for two or more weeks. Nail surgery should be performed only under aseptic conditions. The surgical site should be thoroughly scrubbed with an antiseptic surgical cleanser. Many nail surgeons prefer to administer systemic antimicrobial agents prior to surgery.

Standard surgical instruments are used in procedures on the nail. Several warrant special mention. These include the dual-action nail nipper, which permits close and accurate nail cutting in an atraumatic manner (Fig. 3). This

instrument has a flexible neck that conforms to the patient's nail and allows simple procedures to be performed painlessly without anesthesia. The ordinary nail clipper should only be used for routine nail trimming as it is rigid and requires the patient's nail to conform to the instrument, often producing pain.

The nail splitter is designed for partial longitudinal nail avulsion, with its smooth lower blade for the nail bed and a sharp upper blade for cutting through the nail plate. A nail-pulling forceps (Fig. 4) is practical for gripping the plate prior to avulsion once it has been separated from its attachments. The latter may be accomplished with a dental spatula or Freer elevator. The ingrown nail scissors allow removal of skin-piercing nail spicules from ingrowing toenails with minimal discomfort. A variety of rake retractors are used to retract the proximal nail fold when one is performing matrix surgery.

ANESTHESIA

Adequate anesthesia is vital for successful nail surgery. A plain solution of 1% or 2% lidocaine hydrochloride is most

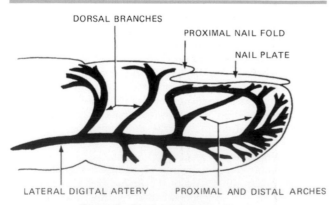

Figure 2 Blood supply to the nail unit.

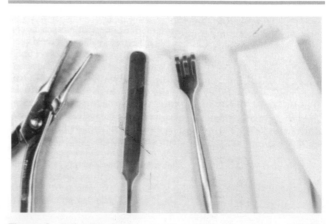

Figure 4 Nail-pulling forceps, dental spatula, rake retractor, and wide Penrose drain (*left to right*).

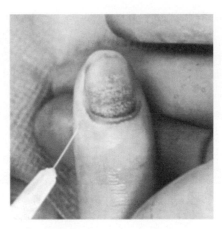

Figure 5 Injection of anesthetic at junction of lateral and proximal nail folds.

commonly used as a local anesthetic. Mepivacaine hydrochloride, 1% or 2%, has also been used as an anesthetic. It may be used in patients sensitive to lidocaine and has the added advantage of longer action and better hemostasis. For more extended anesthesia, bupivacaine is recommended. Tourniquets, digital blocks, and general and regional anesthesia are usually unnecessary for simple nail procedures and should be avoided. Some surgeons use local anesthetic with epinephrine in our opinion, it is rarely required and adds an undesirable element of risk. Digital blocks are preferred by some surgeons; however in most situations, a local block suffices. A tourniquet may be essential for matrix visualization when surgery is performed in this area. A wide Penrose drain should be used to avoid the constricting effect of a rubber band. Keeping in mind the vascular anatomy of the nail unit, simply pinch both digital arteries between the thumb and forefinger to limit bleeding to continue with the procedure. A 30-gauge needle is used to inject at the junction of the proximal and lateral nail fold (Fig. 5). If a cryogen such as ethyl chloride or fluoroethyl is sprayed prior to injection, the pain is diminished.

The injection proceeds distally and inferiorly to include the lateral digital nerve and its branches. The injection then goes across the proximal nail fold to block the transverse nerve branch at this site and then to the other side of the digit (Fig. 6). Place each subsequent injection into a previously anesthetized site. Finally, after anesthesia is complete, additional anesthetic may be injected into the tip of the digit, particularly for procedures on the distal portion of the nail unit. A sufficient quantity of anesthetic may cause moderate blanching, which aids in hemostasis.

If the patient has a history of peripheral vascular disease, is elderly, or has diabetes mellitus, vasospasm because of excess anesthetic must be avoided. To ensure painless nail surgery, a 3- to 5-minute waiting period should precede the procedure.

NAIL AVULSION

As a therapeutic adjunct to various pathologic processes of the nail unit, it is often necessary to perform either chemical avulsion with 40% urea ointment or salicylic acid or surgical avulsion. One indication for surgical avulsion includes the relief of pain from subungual hematoma after failure to evacuate a fresh hematoma by puncture aspiration. In addition, acute bacterial infection and chronic mycotic disease are sometimes indications for nail avulsion. For long-standing onychomycosis of the toenails, removal of the nail may be combined with topical or systemic therapy. Toenail onychomycosis of short duration (less than one year) and fingernail onychomycosis usually do not require avulsion. Other indications for nail avulsion include anatomic abnormalities or excision of nail-unit tumors. Repeated nail avulsion may cause thickening and overcurvature of the nail as well as impaction.

The nail plate is attached to the digit at two locations: the nail bed on its inferior surface and the proximal nail fold on its superior surface. Therefore, the undersurface of the nail plate may be separated with a nail separator or mosquito clamp (Fig. 7).

The same instrument is then used to separate the superior surface of the nail plate from the proximal nail fold (Fig. 8). When using the mosquito clamp (Kelly), the serrated portion of the instrument should abut the nail plate surface rather than the soft tissue. A clamp is then applied to one side of the plate and, with a simple curving motion, it is easily peeled off (Fig. 9). Bleeding is minimal and the patient has little discomfort once the anesthetic has worn off (Fig. 10).

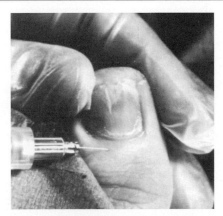

Figure 6 Injection of anesthetic at site of branch of lateral digital nerve in the proximal nail fold.

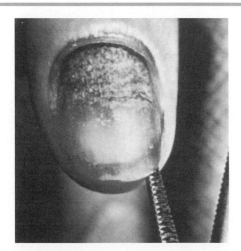

Figure 7 Separation of undersurface of nail palate from nail bed. *Source:* From Scher RK, J Dermatol Surg Oncol 1980b; 6:805–807, with permission.

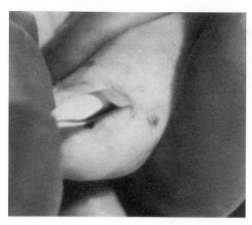

Figure 8   Separation of superior surface of nail plate from proximal nail fold.

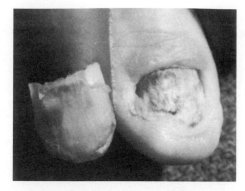

Figure 10   Nail bed after nail avulsion.

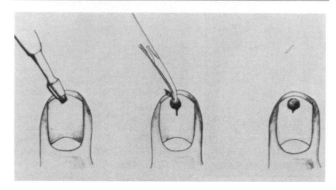

Figure 11   Diagram of nail punch bed biopsy.

PUNCH BIOPSY OF THE NAIL BED

Punch biopsy of the nail bed is the most commonly performed procedure on the nail unit (Fig. 11). A 3- or 4-mm disposable punch is used to bore directly through the nail plate into the nail bed or hyponychium. Disposable punches are preferred because they are sharp, and nail plate penetration is less difficult. The nail plate may damage stainless steel punches that are used for other purposes. Biopsy of the matrix should be avoided to prevent the formation of a permanently dystrophic nail. If matrix tissue is required, an elliptical excision or longitudinal biopsy, which is then sutured, is preferable. The nail plate should not be removed as this may distort the histopathologic appearance. Often, the procedure will dislodge the nail plate, in which case both specimens should be examined by the dermatopathologist. When the punch reaches the underlying periosteum, it is withdrawn. Delicate scissors are then used to remove the specimen (Fig. 12). There is generally little bleeding as the anesthetic bolus tends to compress the arteries in the operative field.

After the specimen is removed (Fig. 13), 35% aluminum chloride in 50% isopropyl alcohol or oxidized cellulose

is applied to the site for hemostasis. Monsel's solution may cause a tattoo effect that can affect pathologic interpretation. Suturing is not necessary as the biopsy site granulates quickly without nail distortion. A small, temporary focus of onycholysis occasionally may result.

A periodic acid-Schiff (PAS) or Gomori methenamine silver stain is required on all nail biopsy specimens. In the presence of onychomycosis, there may be a few fungal elements that can easily be missed if stained only with hematoxylin and eosin.

For narrow (3 mm or less) longitudinal pigmented bands in the nail plate (melanonychia striata in longitudinum), a small punch biopsy from the matrix is acceptable. Care should be taken to avoid bisecting the matrix; a permanently split nail may result.

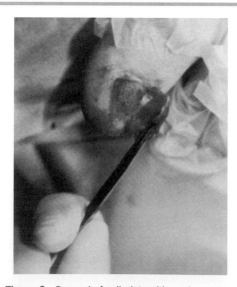

Figure 9   Removal of nail plate with curving motion.

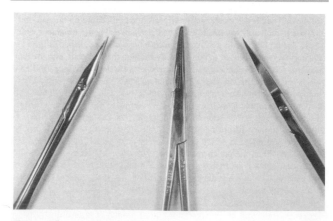

Figure 12   Iris scissors, Kelly clamp, and gradle scissors (*left to right*).

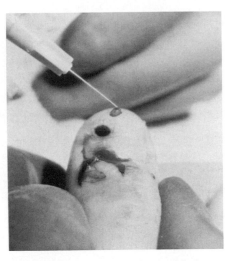

Figure 13   Punch biopsy specimen of the nail bed on needle tip.

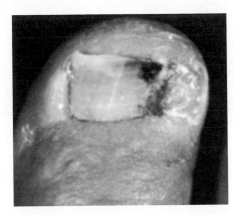

Figure 15   Ingrown toenail: hypertrophy of the lateral nail wall.

INGROWN TOENAIL

Ingrown toenail is a common affliction. Predisposing factors include: (i) hyperhidrosis, a situation most commonly encountered in adolescents, (ii) excess external pressure, because of poor stance and gait, ill-fitting shoes, trauma, (iii) excess internal pressures from subungual growths, malformed phalanges, inflammatory processes, arthropathies, (iv) associated systemic disease, for example, geriatric nail changes (subungual hyperkeratosis, onychauxis), obesity, diabetes mellitus, and (v) incorrectly trimmed nails. Any one or combination of these factors produces one or more of the three features that characterize ingrown toenails: increased transverse overcurvature of the nail plate (Fig. 14), hypertrophy of the lateral nail wall (Fig. 15), perforation of the lateral nail groove epithelium with a spicule of nail plate (onychocryptosis) that results in a foreign body-type reaction.

Prior to corrective surgery for ingrown toenails, simple techniques should be attempted. Removal of skin-piercing nail spicules may be curative. Placing cotton beneath the nail plate allows it to grow out straight. It is advisable to trim the nail plate straight across. Partial or complete avulsion alone may be used, but this may worsen pain when the digit abuts the regrowing nail plate. When conservative measures fail, one method that is successful is longitudinal resection of the lateral nail fold including the adjacent portion of the hyponychium, bed and matrix. Many surgeons prefer to do this in two stages. The first

includes removal of nail spicules with curettage followed by ablation of the hypertrophic granulation tissue from the nail folds (Fig. 16). About one month later, the more definitive resection of the lateral nail fold is performed.

The nail unit is anesthetized and the nail plate partially avulsed. Two longitudinal incisions are made approximately 4 mm apart beginning distally at the hyponychium and proceeding proximally through the bed, proximal fold, and matrix. Following reflection of the proximal nail fold to allow visualization of the matrix, the wedge is removed with delicate scissors and care is taken to include the lateral horn of the matrix.

The nail fold is then returned to its original position and the defect is permitted to heal by secondary intention. The end result is a cosmetically acceptable digit without ingrowth of the nail plate, which is narrower because of partial matrix removal.

Longitudinal resection in an elliptical fashion may be used to include any individual components of the nail unit for biopsy (Fig. 17). This technique is applicable for excision of small neoplasms in the nail bed itself (Fig. 18). After the specimen is removed, the defect is sutured (Fig. 19). Special care is taken to approximate the matrix to avoid a split nail (Fig. 20). In nail surgery, usually 4–0 to 5–0 absorbable suture material is used.

Phenol may also be used for permanent nail matrix destruction either to narrow the nail plate by partial pheno-

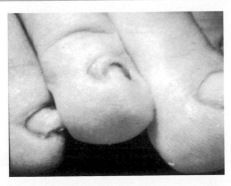

Figure 14   Ingrown toenail: transverse overcurvature of the nail plate.

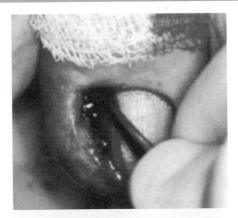

Figure 16   Curettage of lateral nail groove granulation tissue secondary to ingrown toenail.

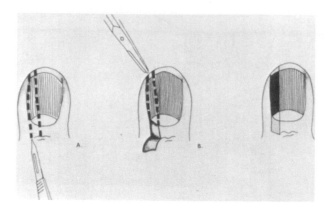

Figure 17 Diagram of longitudinal resection of the nail unit for recalcitrant ingrown toenail.

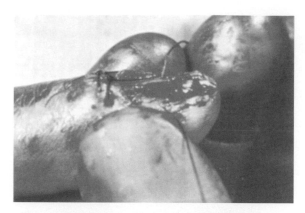

Figure 19 Suturing of nail bed after longitudinal resection.

lization or totally destroy the nail plate with total matrix cauterization. Application of phenol to the nail matrix is simple and may be used in preference to longitudinal resection. After anesthesia and curettage of the lateral nail groove from hyponychium to proximal matrix, a wide tourniquet is applied to dry the wound base and matrix thoroughly (Fig. 21). A supersaturated solution of phenol is next applied to the matrix including the lateral horn. Three 30-second applications of phenol on a Q-tip are all that is required. After the third application, the area is neutralized with alcohol and thoroughly cleansed before a dressing is applied.

PROXIMAL NAIL FOLD SURGERY

Crescent excision of the proximal nail fold and cuticle has been described for the study of patients with connective tissue disorders. This or a modified technique has been used as treatment for intractable chronic paronychia and focal mucinosis (myxoid cyst) of the proximal nail fold. The nail unit is anesthetized as previously described using 1% lidocaine without epinephrine in a local perionychial block fashion. No digital block or tourniquet is necessary. A crescent-shaped area of the cuticle-proximal nail fold is marked with a skin marker. The crescent usually measures 10 × 4 mm. A mosquito hemostat is used to separate the undersurface of the proximal nail fold from the superior surface of the proximal nail plate (nail root). The serrated portion of the instrument must be against the nail plate and not the

nail fold to avoid distortion of the specimen. A dental spatula or Freer elevator may also be used. When the nail fold crescent is separated, it is cut with a scalpel along the outline. Care must be taken not to penetrate title nail plate: this would risk matrix injury and possible permanent nail dystrophy. A dental spatula may be placed beneath the nail fold to prevent this. The excision is completed by removing the tissue with fine scissors and is then sent for histologic study (Fig. 22). Aluminum chloride solution suffices for hemostasis; if needed, hemostatic gauze may be applied. No sutures are required, and the excised area heals by second intention giving an excellent cosmetic result.

When connective tissue disease is present, histopathologic sections reveal the presence of amorphous eosinophilic globules in the cuticle-proximal nail fold area, visible with the PAS stain. Diffuse staining of the ground substance is also noted. Primary Raynaud's disease unassociated with systemic disorders may be differentiated from Raynaud's phenomenon secondary to a connective tissue syndrome, as the former has no deposits. Immunofluorescent studies may also be performed on a portion of the tissue.

Mohs Surgery

Bowen's disease and squamous cell carcinoma are the most common neoplasms affecting the nail unit and the surrounding tissue. Mohs surgery is the treatment of choice once a radiograph has ruled out bony involvement and provides a high cure rate (up to 96% for these types of neoplasms)

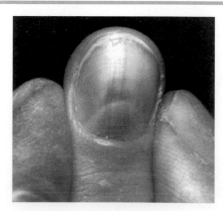

Figure 18 Glomus tumor of the nail bed prior to longitudinal resection.

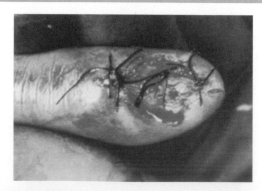

Figure 20 Approximated nail unit after longitudinal resection. *Source:* From Scher RK, J Dermatol Surg Oncol 1980b; 6:805–807, with permission.

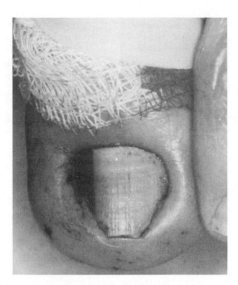

Figure 21 Lateral nail groove thoroughly cleansed and dried prior to phenolization.

while preserving the surrounding healthy tissue. Melanoma involving the nail unit is one of the rarest forms of melanoma, with an incidence of 0.7% to 3.5% of all melanomas. Survival rates are low when compared with melanoma at other sites. Five-year survival rates for Stages I and II diseases have been reported to be from 38% to 61%. A large proportion of nail unit melanomas are amelanotic (15–65%), further contributing to diagnostic difficulty and delay. Amputation has been traditionally recommended as treatment for nail unit melanomas. Mohs surgery has been used to treat such tumors and continued refinements in the use of immunocytochemistry stains will further enhance the use of this technique.

Laser Surgery

Lasers have been used for the treatment of nail conditions since the 1980s. The carbon dioxide (CO_2) laser has been most commonly used for nail unit surgery. A focused-beam CO_2 laser has been used to treat conditions, such as vascular tumors, periungual fibromas, neurofibromas, and hyperkeratotic verrucae vulgaris. Vaporization with an unfocused

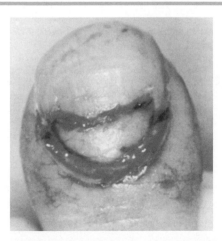

Figure 22 Crescent-shaped excision of cuticle-proximal nail fold for evaluation of connective tissue disease.

beam has been useful for subungual and periungual neoplasms. It has also been used effectively to treat recurrent ingrown toenails. Advantages of the CO_2 laser include: less bleeding, less postoperative pain, and immediate sterilization of infected tissue. Potential complications may result from thermal damage to adjacent tissue.

DRESSINGS

Gelatin sponges or collagen matrix sponges are useful for hemostasis. Minor surgical procedures need cleansing with dilute hydrogen peroxide, an antibiotic ointment and a simple adhesive dressing, which is changed daily. More extensive procedures should be dressed with antibiotic ointment and covered with a Telfa dressing secured by the longitudinal placement of tape. The finger should never be wrapped circumferentially as this may produce vasoconstriction, edema, and vascular compromise. If unusual pain, edema, throbbing, or bluish discoloration is noted, the dressing should be removed at once and the surgeon contacted immediately. A thick and bulbous dressing will absorb external trauma and reduce excessive movement. Where appropriate, use of a sling or orthopedic boot may provide additional protection and immobilization.

BIBLIOGRAPHY

Achten G. Histopathology of the nail. In: Pierre M, ed. The Nail. Edinburgh: Churchill Livingstone, 1981:1.

Baran R, Bureau II. Surgical treatment of recalcitrant chronic paronychias of the fingers. J Dermatol Surg Oncol 1981; 7:106–107.

Boll OF. Surgical correction of ingrowing nails. J Am Podiatr Assoc 1945; 35:8–9.

Brodland DG. The treatment of nail apparatus melanoma with Mohs micrographic surgery. J Am Acad Dermatol 2001; 27:269–273.

Cornelius C, Shelley WE. Pincer nail syndrome. Arch Surg 1968; 96:321.

Crandon JH. Lesser infections of the hand. In: Flynn IE, ed. Hand Surgery. 3rd ed. Baltimore: Williams & Wilkins, 1982:676.

Farber EM, South DA. Urea ointment in nonsurgical avulsion of nail dystrophies. Cutis 1978; 22:689.

Fosnaugh RP. Surgery of the nail. In: Epstein E, Epstein E Jr., eds. Skin Surgery. Vol. 2. 5th ed. Springfield, IL: Charles C Thomas, 1982:981–1007.

Lloyd-Davies RW, Brill GC. The management etiology and outpatient of ingrowing toenails. Br J Surg 1963; 50:592–597.

Maricq HR. Nailfold biopsy in scleroderma and related disorders. Dermatologica 1984; 168:73–77.

Norton LA. Disorders of the nails. In: Moschella SL, Hurley HI, eds. Dermatology. 2nd ed. Philadelphia: WB Saunders, 1985: 1415–1417.

Runne U. Nail surgery: indications and contraindications (translation). Z Hautkr 1982; 58:324–332.

Salasche SJ. Myxoid cysts of the proximal nail fold: a surgical approach. J Dermatol Surg Oncol 1984; 10:35–39.

Samman, PD, Fenton DA. The Nails in Disease. 4th ed. London: Heinemann Medical Books, 1986.

Scher RK. Punch biopsies of nails: a simple, valuable procedure. J Dermatol Surg Oncol 1978; 4:528.

Scher RK. Nail surgery. In: Epstein E, Epstein E Jr., eds. Techniques in Skin Surgery. Philadelphia: Lea & Febiger, 1979:164.

Scher RK. Biopsy of the matrix of a nail. J Dermatol Surg Oncol 1980a; 6:19–21.

Scher RK. Longitudinal resection of nails for purposes of biopsy and treatment. J Dermatol Surg Oncol 1980b; 6:805–807.

Scher RK. Nail surgery. In: Callen JP, Dahl MV, Golitze LE, Rasmussen IE, Stegman SG, eds. Advances in Dermatology. Vol. 1. Chicago: Year Book Medical Publishers, 1986: 191–209.

Scher RK. Nail surgery. J Dermatol Surg Oncol 1992; 18:665–758.

Scher RK, Ackerman AB. The value of nail biopsy for demonstrating fungi not demonstrable by microbiologic techniques. Am J Dermatopathol 1980; 2:55–57.

Scher RK, Daniel CR III. Surgery of the nails. In: Demis DG, McGuire J, eds. Clinical Dermatology. Vol. 1. Sect. 3–15. New York: Harper & Row, 1985:1–10.

Scher RK, Daniel CR III. Nails: Therapy, Diagnosis, Surgery. Philadelphia: W.B. Saunders, 1990.

Scher RK, Tom DWK, Lally EV, et al. The clinical significance of periodic acid-Schiff positive deposits in cuticle-proximal nail fold biopsy specimens. Arch Dermatol 1985; 121:1406–1409.

Schnitzler L, Baran R, Civatte J et al. Biopsy of the proximal nail fold in collagen diseases. J Dermatol Surg Oncol 1976; 2: 313–315.

Siegle RL, Harkness J, Swanson NA. Phenol alcohol technique for permanent matricectomy. Arch Dermatol 1984; 120:348–350.

Thompson RP, Harper PE, Matze JC, et al. Nail fold biopsy in scleroderma and related disorders: correlation of histologic capillaroscopic and clinical data. Arthritis Rheum 1984; 27:97–103.

Zaiac MN, Weiss E. Mohs micrograpliic surgery of the nail unit and squamous cell carcinoma. Dermatol Surg 2001; 27:246–251.

Zaias N. The longitudinal nail biopsy. J Invest Dermatol 1967; 49:406–408.

Zaias N. The Nail in Health and Disease. 2nd ed. Connecticut: Appleton and Lange, 1990.

32

The Genitalia

Rochelle Torgerson
Mayo Clinic, Rochester, Minnesota, U.S.A.

INTRODUCTION

Tumors and diseases of the external genitalia encompass those problems unique to the area as well as those that are part of more generalized processes. To effectively manage tumors and diseases of this region, an understanding of the pertinent anatomy is needed to facilitate safe biopsy, anesthetic delivery, and surgery. Knowledge of the lymphatic drainage of the genitalia is also necessary for appropriate management of malignancies.

Blood supply and drainage of the male external genitalia can be divided into deep and superficial components. Branches of the internal iliac vessels supply and drain the deep structures (Fig. 1). The erectile tissue of the penis is supplied by the dorsal artery, a branch of the internal pudendal artery, and drained by the deep dorsal vein. The deep dorsal vein located beneath the fascia drains the three corporeal bodies into the vesicoprostatic plexus and eventually into the internal iliac vein. The superficial blood supply and drainage of the penis are derived from branches of the external iliac vessels via the femoral and external pudendal vessels (Fig. 2). The superficial external pudendal artery supplies the skin and subcutaneous tissue. The superficial dorsal vein, easily visible beneath the skin, drains the skin and subcutaneous tissue into the superficial external pudendal vein. Just proximal to the glans, is a plexus of small veins that drains into the superficial dorsal vein of the penis. This plexus can be the site of phlebitis of the superficial dorsal vein (Mondor's disease). Possible inciting factors for Mondor's disease include trauma, use of constrictive devices, infection, and intravenous drug injection. This inflammatory process is painful and responds to local infiltration with bupivacaine.

The blood supply and drainage of the external female genitalia occurs mostly via branches of the internal iliac vessels (Fig. 3). The internal pudendal artery, a branch of the internal iliac artery, has four main branches: the posterior labial artery, artery of the vestibular bulb, deep artery of the clitoris, and dorsal artery of the clitoris. These branches anastomose with terminal vessels from the external iliac artery system. Majority of the venous drainage follows the same pattern, terminating in the internal iliac vein. Portions of the anterolateral aspects of the labia majora drain into the external iliac vein.

The lymphatics of the penis drain to both the superficial inguinal lymph nodes and the deep inguinal lymph nodes. Majority of the penis drains through subcutaneous channels and vessels that parallel the dorsal arteries and veins, and empties into the superficial inguinal lymph nodes. However, portions of the distal glans and urethra drain into the deep inguinal nodes. Similarly, the lymphatics of the female genitalia drain to both superficial and deep nodes. The lymphatics from the lower portion of the vagina join those from the vestibule and labia to drain into the superficial inguinal lymph nodes. The perianal region, extending up the anal canal to the dentate line (marker of transition from cutaneous to mucosal epithelium), drains to the superficial femoral nodes. Proximal to the dentate line, drainage is to the deeper pelvic lymph nodes.

ANESTHESIA

Although small procedures on the external genitalia can be performed with local infiltration of anesthetic, larger procedures may require regional blocks. One percent lidocaine injected subcutaneously provides adequate anesthesia for most biopsies. As a rule, it is best to avoid the use of epinephrine when injecting the penis, and in particular, to avoid direct infiltration of the foreskin, as this has resulted in tissue necrosis on occasion. A basic understanding of the innervation of the male and female genitalia is required before attempting a regional block.

The nerve supply of the male external genitalia comes from upper lumbar as well as sacral spinal nerves (Fig. 4). The genital branch of the genitofemeral nerve (L1, L2) and the anterior scrotal branch of the ilioinguinal nerve (L1) innervate the skin of the anterolateral scrotum and base of the penis. The remainder of the penis and scrotum are supplied by the dorsal nerves of the penis and the posterior scrotal nerves, both deep branches of the pudendal nerve (S1, S2, S3). A penile block is achieved by injecting anesthetic in the dermis and subcutaneous tissue circumferentially at the base of the penis. Care should be taken to remain above the penile fascia as cases of impotence following injection below the deep fascia have been reported. If the entire circumference is not meticulously injected, areas of the penis may be left without anesthesia. Because of this difficulty, regional anesthesia in the form of a caudal block can be a consideration depending on the extent of the procedure.

The nerve supply of the female external genitalia also comes from two distinct sources. The ilioinguinal (L1) and genitofemeral (L1, L2) nerves supply the skin and subcutaneous tissue overlying the mons pubis and anterolateral portions of the labia majora. The remainder of the female genitalia is supplied by the pudendal nerve (S2, S3, S4), which reenters the pelvis through the lesser sciatic foramen and accompanies the internal pudendal blood vessels along the lateral wall of the ischiorectal fossa. Branches of the pudendal nerve are the dorsal nerve of the clitoris, the

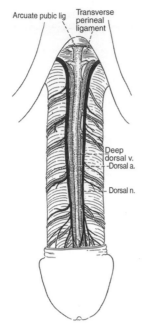

Figure 1   Dorsal view of the penis after removal of the penile fascia.

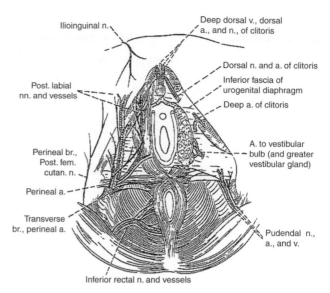

Figure 3   Blood supply and nerves of the female perineum.

perineal nerve, and the inferior rectal or hemorrhoidal nerve. Anesthesia of a significant portion of the female genitalia and distal vagina can be achieved with a pudendal block. A pudendal block is achieved by directing a needle through the wall of the lower vagina towards the ischial spine and depositing anesthesia around the pudendal nerve as it enters the ischiorectal fossa.

Regional blocks can be carried out with either lidocaine (one to three hours) or bupivacaine (three to six hours) depending on the duration of anesthesia required. Regional anesthesia has many benefits but also has greater associated risk than local infiltration, including intravascular injection, ecchymosis formation, and rectal puncture. As such, these techniques should only be performed after adequate training.

BIOPSY

Once adequate anesthesia has been administered, biopsies can be obtained with little or no discomfort to the patient. Most lesions can be adequately sampled using a punch or snip technique. Occasionally, larger excisional biopsies are required. A 4 mm dermal punch biopsy is sufficient in many cases. With this technique, a sharp punch tool combined with adequate tension on the skin and subcutaneous tissue helps ensure the least distortion of the overlying epidermis or mucosa. As with all biopsies, it is important to obtain a specimen of adequate depth, especially when dealing with malignancies. Sutures should be placed perpendicular to the natural skin tension lines. In the penis, this is perpendicular to the long axis to prevent traction during erection. Absorbable sutures are preferable from a patient perspective. Snip excision is a good technique for removal of cystic or papillomatous lesions when histologic examination is desired. With this technique, traction is placed on the lesion

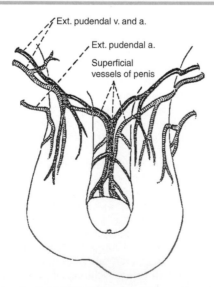

Figure 2   Superficial blood supply of the male genitalia.

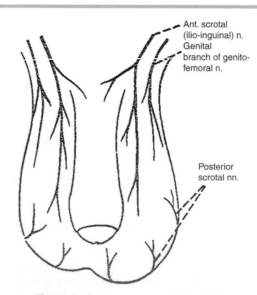

Figure 4   Cutaneous nerves of the scrotum.

with forceps, and scissors is used to gently dissect beneath the lesion. Hemostasis can be achieved with light electrocoagulation, aluminum chloride, or pressure. These superficial wounds typically heal well by second intention. Whichever method of biopsy is employed, attention needs to be placed on wound care. Gentle cleaning with mild soap and water twice a day should be sufficient.

HPV: CONDYLOMATA ACUMINATA, SIN, AND INVASIVE SCC

Human papilloma virus (HPV) is a nonenveloped DNA virus transmitted by direct contact. Basal cells of the epithelium are the target of the virus. To date, over 80 HPV genotypes have been identified, and the number continues to grow. HPV is implicated in genital lesions ranging from benign verrucae to intraepithelial neoplasms and invasive neoplasms. HPV-6 and HPV-11 are considered low-risk and are the most common genotypes found in condylomata acuminata. HPV-16 and HPV-18 are considered high-risk genotypes, and persistent infection is implicated in the pathogenesis of some squamous intraepithelial neoplasia (SIN) and some invasive squamous cell carcinoma (SCC). The importance of HPV lies not only in its broad disease spectrum, but also in its prevalence. As many as 20% to 40% of sexually active young adults are thought to be infected.

Because of a somewhat confusing nomenclature, discussions of HPV-related genital lesions can be burdensome. For ease of organization, the diseases covered will be divided into those lesions associated with low-risk HPV genotypes (most condylomata acuminata and Buschke-Lowenstein tumor) and those associated with high-risk genotypes (some condyloma acuminata, SIN and SCC).

Condylomata Acuminata

Classically, condylomata acuminata are flesh-colored to light brown, veruccal, sessile, or pedunculated papules occurring singly or in agminated plaques. Lesions are often asymptomatic but can become irritated by friction and secondarily impetiginized. More than 90% of the cases are caused by infection with low-risk HPV-6 and HPV-11. Condylomata acuminata often have a multifocal presentation, making evaluation and treatment of patients challenging. Initial evaluation should always include a thorough cutaneous examination. A speculum examination of the vagina and cervix as well as a PAP smear for cytologic evaluation should be done on all female patients presenting with genital condylomata. The importance of this is highlighted by several studies that have shown that vaginal or cervical lesions may be present in approximately 70% of women with vulvar lesions. Depending on sexual practices, anoscopy to evaluate the distal potion of the anal canal and a PAP smear of the anal canal are indicated for both male and female patients. Significant urethral involvement mandates cystoscopy. Visualization of condylomata is often difficult; so pretreatment of the skin with liberal quantities of a low concentration of acetic acid (3–5%) can be helpful. The solution can be swabbed onto the female genitalia, and the penis can be dipped directly into a cup of acetic acid for several minutes. Either a magnifying glass or colposcope can aid in visualization as well. Due to infection field effect, subclinical infection may be present in the skin surrounding the clinically identifiable lesion. This may be accentuated in immunosupressed patients. This phenomenon requires frequent and regular follow-up to ensure adequate therapy.

It is essential to examine the sexual partners of these patients, as treatment must be carried out simultaneously to prevent rapid recurrence. Since condylomata are sexually transmitted, evaluation for concomitant sexually transmitted diseases is advised.

Biopsy is an important, and sometimes overlooked part of the evaluation of condylomata. Given the spectrum of HPV associated disease and the clinical overlap, it is advisable to submit at least one representative lesion for histologic evaluation to rule out SIN or invasive SCC (Fig. 5). Any persistent, changing, or worrisome lesions should be biopsied as well. In situ hybridization (ISH) can be utilized to determine the HPV genotype involved. ISH is commonly available for HPV 6, 11, 16, 18, 31, and 33, and can be performed on paraffin embedded tissue. This information can help stratify lesions into low-risk and high-risk populations.

No specific, antiviral therapies are available for HPV as of yet. Instead, treatment modalities are either aimed at chemical or physical destruction of tissue or immunomodulation. Chemically destructive agents include podophyllin resin, trichloroacetic acid (80–90%), 5-fluorouracil (topical or intralesional), retinoids (topical or intralesional), and bleomycin (intralesional). Topical retinoids are the least effective with a 0% clearance rate. Intralesional bleomycin is the most effective, with a clearance rate of 70% and relapse rate of 0%. However, bleomycin has significant systemic toxicity including fever, malaise, pneumonitis, alopecia, hyperpigmentation, and anorexia. The chemical agent that best balances efficacy and safety is trichloroacetic acid. It causes local discomfort but is safe to use in pregnancy with a 70% to 81% clearance rate and a 36% recurrence rate. Physical destructive agents include cryotherapy, electrosurgery, CO_2 laser, and surgical removal. Cryotherapy, probably the most commonly used, has a clearance rate of 54% to 88% and a recurrence rate of 21% to 55%. Electrosurgery is slightly more efficacious but carries the risk of contamination from the HPV DNA that is dispersed in the plume. Surgery and CO_2 laser ablation are the most promising, with reports of clearance as high as 100% for both and recurrence rates as low as 8% and 4%, respectively. However, there is great variability in results making it greatly operator- or patient-dependent. Immunomodulatory agents include Imiquimod 5% cream and interferon-alpha (topical or intralesional). Imiquimod

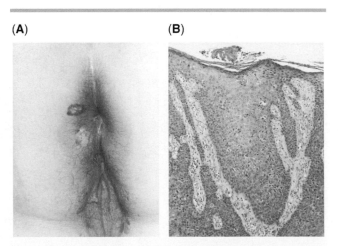

(A)   **(B)**

Figure 5 Squamous cell carcinoma in situ. **(A)** Verrucal papules of the perianal area. **(B)** Extremely irregular, crowded arrangement of the keratinocytes with many atypical mitoses (hematoxylin and eosin, x160).

induces an antiviral effect via tumor necrosis factor, interferon-alpha and other cytokines. It is a cream applied three nights per week for a 16-week course. Side effects are minimal, clearance rates are 35% to 62% and recurrence rates are 13% to 19%, but it is not recommended for use in pregnancy. Each form of treatment has its own limitations. However, in general, destructive modalities can only target clinically evident lesions, requiring repeat treatments and the risk of transmission from residual, nonevident infection. Immunomodulators, in theory, target clinically evident as well as subclinical infection. However, they are more costly and require an intact immune system. Combination therapies, utilizing both a destructive modality and an immunomodulatory agent, provide additional options.

Buschke-Lowenstein tumor (giant condylomata acuminata) was first described in 1925. It is a deep, locally invasive, and destructive tumor associated with HPV-6 and HPV-11. Despite the exophytic and destructive nature, metastases are rare. Because of the possibility of focal malignant transformation and the clinical similarity to (or possible overlap with) verrucous carcinoma, multiple deep biopsy specimens as well as imaging studies should be obtained when evaluating patients. Although histologically benign, the clinical aggressiveness of the tumor warrants early treatment. Recent success has been reported utilizing combined approaches of excision and CO_2 laser ablation as well as imiquimod and CO_2 laser ablation. Long-term intralesional interferon alpha therapy proved successful in a single case report. It remains unanswered as to how HPV-6 and HPV-11 can cause both condylomata acuminata and Buschke-Lowenstein tumor, lesions with such diverse biological behavior. Also controversial is the relationship between Buschke-Lowenstein tumor and verrucous carcinoma.

SIN: Bowen's Disease, Bowenoid Papulosis, Erythroplasia of Queyrat

Although the majority of condylomata are due to infection with low-risk, HPV-6 or HPV-11, a clinically significant portion are due to high-risk HPV-16 or HPV-18. These high-risk condylomata are thought to be part of the clinical and histologic spectrum of lesions progressing from condylomata to SIN and invasive SCC. SIN has atypia confined to the epidermis and is thought to be the precursor of invasive SCC. Because SIN can have several distinct clinical presentations, historically, it has been divided into separate entities.

Whether this historical practice should be continued is a topic of current debate.

Bowen's disease or SCC in situ (SCC IS) is a form of SIN that presents as solitary, well-demarcated, red scaly plaques. Although the squamous atypia in Bowen's disease is by definition confined to the epidermis, there have been cases of nodal metastases. Bowen's disease requires careful examination and multiple biopsies to ensure adequate sampling for histologic evaluation. Due to the high failure rate of treatment with electrodesiccation and curettage, Mohs micrographic surgery or CO_2 laser ablation is recommended for treatment. Preliminary studies with Imiquimod have shown some effectiveness; however, further studies will be needed. Surveillance for systemic malignancies is warranted as up to one-third of patients with Bowen's disease are reported to develop systemic malignancies.

Bowenoid papulosis, a second form of SIN, was first described by Lloyd in 1970 (Fig. 6). It is characterized by multiple, red-brown, verrucal papules or plaques located in the genital area of younger, sexually active men and women. Clinically, these are distinguished from Bowen's disease (SCC IS) by involvement of young adults, multiplicity of smaller lesions, lack of associated symptoms and occurrence in circumcised men. Although cases of bowenoid papulosis have been reported to regress, histologically, these are associated with high-risk HPV-16. Thus, management should include treatment, close follow-up for recurrence, and repeated biopsies.

Erythroplasia of Queyrat, also a form of SIN, is a clinically distinct entity characterized by shiny red velvety plaques that are typically asymptomatic. In men, areas of involvement include the glans, foreskin, and urethral meatus. In women, the glabrous skin of the vulva can be involved. Histologically, these are associated with HPV-16. Once again, although this is an intraepidermal lesion, lymph node metastases have been reported. Successful treatment has been reported with cryotherapy, Mohs micrographic surgery or CO_2 laser ablation.

Because of the clinical and histologic spectrum of lesions progressing from condylomata to SIN and invasive SCC, it is essential to biopsy these lesions when treating these conditions. Because of the tendency to have histologically banal areas with small samples, several punch biopsies are recommended when evaluating SIN. Additionally, close follow-up and repeat biopsies are warranted for lesions that do not resolve or respond to treatment.

(A)   **(B)**

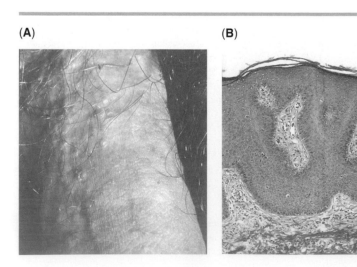

Figure 6 Bowenoid papulosis. **(A)** Small papules on the shaft of the penis. **(B)** Crowded and hyperchromatic nuclei and several mitoses (hematoxylin and eosin, x160).

Invasive SCC

SCC accounts for 95% of penile malignancies and 80% to 90% of vulvar malignancies. Invasive SCC of the genitalia can be divided into three subtypes: basaloid SCC, verrucous SCC, and keratinizing SCC.

The basaloid form is the most prevalent. It tends to occur in younger patients and has a strong association with infection by high-risk HPV. Basaloid SCC is postulated to represent the natural clinical and pathological progression from condylomata to SIN, and eventually to invasive disease. Clinically, lesions range from thickened skin with or without leukoplakia to frank masses. Patients can present with a variety of symptoms including pruritis, burning, bleeding, dysuria, dyspareunia, or discharge. Tragically, because early lesions are often asymptomatic or because of embarrassment, patients often present with metastatic disease.

Verrucous SCC is a less common variant and accounts for only 5% to 16% of penile SCC and a similar fraction of vulvar SCC. Clinically, it presents as a large, exophytic mass, but histologically, there is both exophytic and endophytic growth. The more superficial part of the tumor appears benign, but the deeper portion displays mitoses and pleomorphism. Thus, deep biopsy that includes the base of the lesion is needed for accurate diagnosis. Verrucous carcinoma is slow growing with significant morbidity through local destruction but rare mortality from metastasis. Because of this, some authors consider verrucous carcinoma to be the same entity as Buschke-Lowenstein tumor (giant condylomata acuminata). Others believe that these are unique, Buschke-Lowenstein tumor being associated with HPV and verrucous SCC being associated with poor hygiene and lack of circumcision not HPV. It is an ongoing controversy.

The keratinizing type of SCC is the least prevalent subtype (Fig. 7). It is found in older patients and seems to have an association with the chronic inflammatory disorders, lichen sclerosis, and lichen planus. The complete lack of association with HPV posits the existence of additional pathogenetic mechanisms in this form of SCC.

Surgical excision is the treatment of choice for SCCs of the genitalia, the type and extent of surgery needing to be customized to the extent of disease. Mohs micrographic surgery is an excellent option for those with locally invasive, nonmetastatic disease. In more extensive disease, penectomy and en bloc vulvectomy may be required. These surgeries lead to profound functional and cosmetic morbidity, and

as such, there is obvious interest in tissue sparing, nonsurgical treatments. Modalities including radiotherapy, and oral as well as intralesional chemotherapy may be beneficial. In metastatic disease, radiation and chemotherapy are not sufficient as single modality treatments. Chemoradiation may have a role to shrink lesions prior to surgery. There is a report of a penile verrucous carcinoma being successfully treated with intra-aortic infusion of methotrexate. An additional report communicates success in the form of improvement and control of a verrucous SCC using oral acitretin. No matter what treatment method is used, close follow-up of all genital SCCs is a must. Local recurrences when caught early have not been found to impact morbidity and mortality significantly.

Prevention

Because HPV can be transmitted without clinical evidence of infection, the only current way to truly prevent transmission is abstinence. However, exciting results from a double-blind, placebo-controlled trial with a HPV-16/18 L1 virus-like particle vaccine showed a 93% efficacy against incident infection and a 95% efficacy against persistent infection in an intention-to-treat analysis. There is significant anticipation as potential vaccines progress through clinical trials. Mathematical models of the potential benefit of vaccination indicate a greater than 60% reduction in cervical cancer cases.

PIGMENTED LESIONS

The spectrum of pigmented lesions of the genital area is similar to that occurring elsewhere.

Hyperpigmentation, Lentigines, and Nevi

Simple hyperpigmentation of the genital skin may be due to hormonal fluctuation, injury, or as a result of drugs (including fixed drug reaction, antimalarial use, bismuth intake). Lentigines in the genital area most often present as solitary or multiple, asymptomatic, hyperpigmented macules of uniform color and varying size. In men, the most common location is the glans penis, in women, the labia. Biopsy reveals hyperpigmentation of the basal layer of the epidermis, with varying numbers of dermal melanophages and hyperplasia of melanocytes. A recent report characterizes the dermoscopic patterns seen in 21 genital lentigines, but prospective studies will be needed to establish reliable diagnostic performance. Because of the dearth of information regarding the natural history of pigmented lesions of the genitalia, excision or multiple sampling biopsies are advised. True nevi can also present in the genital area. Once again, biopsy or close observation with photographic documentation is warranted. Because there is often a delay between onset and clinical presentation of pigmented lesions of the genitalia, many believe complete excision is needed due to lack of available history and the challenge of long-term, clinical monitoring. Another argument in support of complete excision is to avoid the histologic challenge faced when recurrence or repigmentation occurs. It is often difficult to histologically distinguish recurrent lesions from melanoma.

Malignant Melanoma

Melanoma of the genital region is rare but of great clinical importance due to its relatively poor prognosis at the time of diagnosis. In men, genital melanomas most often affect the glans or foreskin and account for less than 2% of all

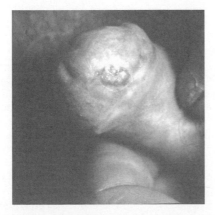

Figure 7 Squamous cell carcinoma. Erosive lesion of the glans on a background of atrophic changes.

malignancies of the penis and 0.2% of the cutaneous melanomas . Vulvar melanoma is more common, and the labia are most often affected (Fig. 8). Melanoma is the second most frequent vulvar malignancy. Although vulvar melanoma comprises less than 2% of all cutaneous melanomas in women, it occurs at a density similar to that of the face and nearly twice that of other body surface areas. Genital melanomas are typically a disease of older patients, presenting in the sixth decade or later. In men, lesions present as enlarging, ulcerated, pigmented tumors. In women, where self-examination is more challenging, presentation is more often prompted by nonspecific symptomatology including bleeding, mass or lump, discharge, pruritis, or pain. Awareness of a changing, pigmented lesion is less common.

Historically, there have been advocates for radical treatments such as pelvic exenteration for melanoma of the genitalia. However, several analyses have shown that there is significant morbidity and no increase in survival with such an approach. One reason for this aggressive approach was the belief that melanomas of the genitalia were more aggressive than other cutaneous melanomas. This impression may have had more to do with the delay in presentation than the disease itself. It is now thought that prognostic factors for genital melanoma are similar to other cutaneous melanomas. Depth, ulceration, and lymph node status are significant prognostic indicators, with lymph node status being the most powerful. Thus, current consensus recommends tailoring the treatment to the depth and extent of the disease. In men with thin (less than 1 mm) melanomas, wide local excision or distal amputation may be sufficient. Most agree that lymph node dissection is not necessary in thin melanomas and appropriate in the setting of palpable adenopathy. The approach is less clear in the setting of deeper melanomas without palpable nodes. One suggestion is to proceed with dissection of the superficial inguinal nodes and continue with radical groin and pelvic node dissection only if the superficial nodes are involved with melanoma. In patients with disseminated disease, nodal dissection is not warranted unless it provides palliation. For patients with penile melanoma less than 1 mm thick, five-year survival rates are greater than 90%. Unfortunately most men present at a later stage, and prognosis is

poor with less than 30% survival at five years. Treatment for women with vulvar melanoma is similarly based on depth and lymph node status. Unfortunately, survival of women is even bleaker ranging from 23% to 63% at five years. In addition to surgery, adjuvant therapies including radiotherapy, interferon-alpha and cytotoxic chemotherapy may play a role in a multimodal approach.

BASAL CELL CARCINOMA

Although basal cell carcinomas usually occur on sun-exposed skin, 10% present in shaded areas including the genitalia. Basal cell carcinomas account for only 2% to 5% of genital cancers and are, therefore, quite rare. Thus, our understanding of presentation, behavior, and response to treatment comes from case reports and small case series. Tumors most often present on the scrotum or labia majora of patients in the sixth, seventh, or eighth decade. Metastases are thought to be rare but were as high as 13% in one retrospective analysis. As with other locations, the clinical lesion can range from a nodule to a superficial plaque or ulceration. If symptoms are present, they range from irritation to pruritis or pain. Location does not alter the classic morphology of nests of basaloid tumor cells with peripheral palisading nuclei. Nodular, morpheaform, adenoid, and metatypical varieties have been described. In two small case series, no evidence of HPV DNA was identified by ISH or PCR. Therefore, viral infection does not seem to be a factor in pathogenesis in the absence of ultraviolet insult. Treatment of basal cell carcinoma of the genitalia with Mohs micrographic surgery or wide local excision is advised.

EXTRAMAMMARY PAGET'S DISEASE

Extramammary Paget's disease (EMPD) is a rare intraepithelial adenocarcinoma of apocrine gland-bearing skin most often affecting the anogenital region (Fig. 9). Clinically it presents as a slowly enlarging, pruritic, erythematous, eczematous patch with serous crust. The clinical similarity to dermatitis often delays accurate diagnosis. Histologically, lesions are characterized by the presence of Paget's cells in the epidermis. Paget's cells are large, round cells, with pale-staining cytoplasm, lacking intercellular bridges. These cells often show a positive reaction with stains for mucopolysaccharides such as Alcian blue, periodic acid-Schiff, or Hale's colloidal iron. Mucin is less abundant than in mammary Paget's disease. Immunohistochemical staining for carcinoembryonic antigen or cytokeratins is recommended. Cytokeratin 7 has become particularly useful, as it does not stain the normal keratinocytes in the epidermis and follicular structures. Once a diagnosis of EMPD has been confirmed histologically, management requires a thorough evaluation to rule out simultaneous or contiguous adenocarcinoma. Twenty percent of patients will have an underlying malignancy, those of the gastrointestinal and urogenital tracts being most common. However, numerous other associated malignancies have been reported (Table 1). Due to the multifocal nature of the disease, many small scouting biopsies may be required to delineate the extent of cutaneous involvement. Treatment with Mohs micrographic surgery has recently been shown to be more efficacious than wide local excision for both primary and recurrent EMPD. Sentinel lymph node biopsy has been shown to be feasible in EMPD, but whether it has a role in evaluation and treatment has not been established. Unfortunately, even with Mohs micrographic surgery, recurrence rates are still as high as 16% for primary disease and 50% for recurrent

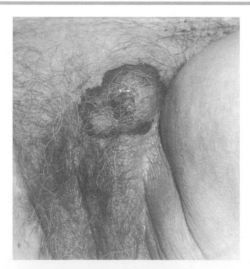

Figure 8 Superficial spreading malignant melanoma. Lesion developed in two months.

(A)   **(B)**

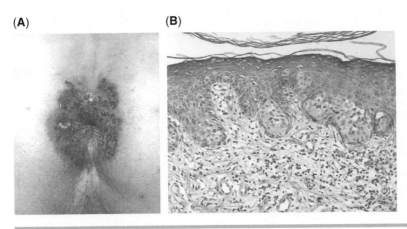

Figure 9 Extramammary Paget's disease. **(A)** Eczematous, eroded, perianal plaque. **(B)** Paget's cells with ample, pale-staining cytoplasm present singly and in groups in the epidermis (hematoxylin and eosin, x160).

disease. Thus, close follow-up with frequent biopsy is warranted. In addition to surgical measures, CO_2 laser ablation, imiquimod 5% cream, photodynamic therapy with 5-aminolevulinic acid, and radiotherapy have all been reported as successful in select cases of either primary or recurrent EMPD.

INFLAMMATORY DISORDERS

Inflammatory dermatoses that affect the genitalia are diagnostically and therapeutically challenging. Not only are they included in the differential diagnosis of SIN and SCC, but patients with some inflammatory dermatoses are at increased risk for developing SIN and SCC.

Lichen Sclerosis

Lichen sclerosus is an inflammatory disease commonly affecting the anogenital region. It has also been termed lichen sclerosus et atrophicus, balanitis xerotica obliterans (in men), and kraurosis vulvae (in women). Prevalence is up to 10 times higher in women than men. Clinically, lesions present as pearly papules that may coalesce into diffuse, shiny, atrophic plaques (Fig. 10). Purpura can result from vessel fragility. Lesions are typically pruritic but rarely can be asymptomatic. In males, the glans is most commonly involved. In females, the vulvar and/or perianal areas can be affected; involvement of both presents as a classic figure-eight pattern. Chronic disease can lead to phimosis in men and architectural effacement of the clitoris, labia, and vestibule in women. The histologic changes of an atrophic epidermis, hyalinized papillary dermis and band of

Table 1 Malignancies Reported in Patients with Extramammary Paget's Disease

Apocrine gland carcinoma
Eccrine gland carcinoma
Carcinoma of Moll's glands
Ceruminal gland carcinoma
Bartholin's gland carcinoma
Perianal gland carcinoma
Adenocarcinoma of the rectum
Carcinoid of the ileum
Adenocarcinoma of the breast
Carcinoma of the ureter, bladder, urethra
Adenocarcinoma of the prostate
Carcinoma of the cervix
Adenocarcinoma of the ovary
Carcinoma of the pancreas

Source: From Powell, Bjonsson, et al. (1985).

middermal inflammation are characteristic and diagnostic. Topical treatment with clobetasol propionate 0.05% is considered first line therapy. Topical tacrolimus has had reported success as well, but initial irritation may be limiting during acute inflammation. Treatment can be expected to control symptoms and improve atrophy, but scarring is not reversible. Surgical intervention is only indicated in the setting of phimosis or marked and symptomatic introital narrowing. Given the well-documented association between lichen sclerosus and vulvar or penile SCC, patients need to be counseled early during their evaluation and followed regularly over the long term. Persistent nodules, ulcers, fissures, or hyperkeratotic crusts require biopsy.

Lichen Planus

Lichen planus is an inflammatory disorder that can affect the skin, hair, nails, and mucous membranes. The classic presentation of purple, polygonal, pruritic, papules and plaques most commonly affects keratinizing surfaces. Hypertrophic and ulcerative variants are seen as well. A similar spectrum of disease occurs on mucosal surfaces. It is estimated that 1% of the population has oral lichen planus. Approximately 25% of women and 4% of men with oral lichen planus have genital involvement. Patients with genital involvement in the setting of generalized lichen planus typically have nonscarring, annular plaques on the shaft and glans of the penis or the labia. The hypertrophic form of lichen planus involves the genitalia much less commonly. The erosive form of lichen planus that involves the mucous membranes of the mouth and genitalia tends to be scarring and affects women more frequently than men. The course can be chronic and debilitating. When the oral and genital mucosal surfaces are involved simultaneously, it is termed the vulvovaginal-gingival syndrome or peno-gingival syndrome. The syndrome is rare in men and the erosions are limited to the glans. In women, erosive plaques with a white, reticulated border can involve the clitoris, labia, introitis, and vagina. As with lichen sclerosis, severe inflammation can lead to scarring and structural effacement. Pruritus and burning, referable to the vulva, and dyspareunia are common presentations. In oral lichen planus, there is strong evidence implicating the role of allergic contact sensitivities to dental metals in the pathophysiologic process. Whether other allergens play a role in genital lichen planus is less clear. Nevertheless, patch testing may have a role in the evaluation of some patients with lichen planus. The histologic features of lichen planus are hypergranulosis, irregular acanthosis and a dense, band-like infiltrate leading

(A)

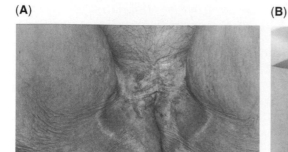

(B)

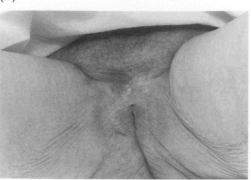

Figure 10   Lichen sclerosis. **(A)** White, reticulated atrophic with effacement of labia. **(B)** Same patient 15 years later with residual scarring and effacement but no active inflammation.

to basal cell vacuolization. Hyperkeratosis is classically seen in skin lesions, but in mucosal lesions of the genitalia, the epidermis is often thinned or eroded. Therapeutic management of lichen planus, particularly the erosive variant, is challenging and often inadequate. The mainstay of treatment is topical corticosteroid ointments, difficult cases requiring clobetasol propionate 0.05%. More recently, there is data from case series that topical tacrolimus is effective. Although frequent irritation occurs with initial application, the long-term safety profile is excellent. Nonspecific measures such as emollients, barrier creams, and 2% lidocaine ointment can reduce discomfort. Erosive disease can be recalcitrant to topical therapies and may require systemic medications. Unfortunately, there are no double-blind, placebo-controlled studies to direct medication choice. Systemic agents with reported benefit include oral prednisone, oral cyclosporine, plaquinil, oral retinoids, methotrexate, Azathioprine, cyclophosphamide, dapsone, and grisioful-van. Because lichen planus can precipitate vulvodynia, tricyclic antidepressants may prove helpful. Because of the chronic nature of genital lichen planus, the benefits of oral agents need to be heavily weighed against the well-known side effects. As with lichen sclerosis, surgical intervention is only indicated in the setting of phimosis or marked and symptomatic introital narrowing. Importantly, lichen planus can keobnerize. There are documented cases of SCC arising in lesions of lichen planus. Possible cofactors in carcinogenesis include HPV and ultraviolet light. As such, patients should be counseled regarding ultraviolet light exposure to the genitalia and consideration should be given to HPV testing. Over the long term, patients should be followed closely and suspicious areas need to be biopsied.

Plasma Cell Balanitis and Vulvitis (Zoon's)

Plasma cell balanitis or vulvitis is an inflammatory condition affecting the glans in uncircumcised men and the vulva in women. It is also known as Zoon's balanitis/vulvitis and balanitis/vulvitis circumscripta plasmacellularis. Its existence as a separate entity in women is questioned by some. Clinically, it is characterized by velvety, erythematous plaques, which rarely erode and bleed. Histologically, there is thinning of the overlying epidermis, with ulceration on occasion. The epidermis is characterized by "lozenge-shaped" keratinocytes and may be separated from the underlying dermis. The infiltrate in the upper dermis contains numerous plasma cells. Treatment by circumcision in men provides excellent results. Thus, poor hygiene and friction are implicated in the pathogenesis. Medical treatment in men and women is unsatisfactory. It is essential to biopsy

this condition to rule out SCC IS or other diseases affecting the genitalia that present similarly.

VASCULAR LESIONS

Vascular lesions may present in the genital region as part of a systematized process or as an isolated phenomenon. Examples of the former include hemangiomas in blue rubber bleb nevus syndrome or angiokeratomas of Fabry's disease. One of the more common vascular lesions of the scrotum and vulva, not part of a systemic process, is the angiokeratoma of Fordyce. These are unilateral or bilateral, red to purple papules that present in midlife (Fig. 11). In some cases, they are thought to be due to increased pressure secondary to varicocele or pregnancy. Histologically, they exhibit acanthosis and ectatic vessels in the papillary dermis, with or without hyperkeratosis. Glomus tumors can affect the genitalia as isolated lesions as well and have been a reported cause of dyspareunia. Kaposi's sarcoma can present in the genital area, especially in patients with acquired immune deficiency. When benign vascular lesions of the genitalia are asymptomatic, observation and follow up are sufficient. If the diagnosis is in question, punch or excisional biopsy is recommended. If benign lesions are symptomatic or cosmetically concerning, destruction with electrocoagulation,

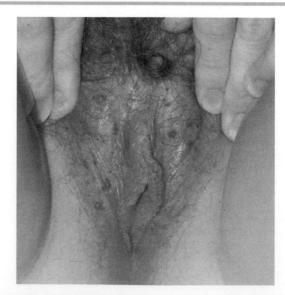

Figure 11   Angiokeratomas. Hyperkeratotic papules on the labia majora.

argon laser, or potassium tritanyl phosphate laser is effective. Lasers may provide better cosmetic and functional results.

Lymphangiomas can also occur on the penis, scrotum, or vulva. When they present as more superficial lesions, they can be mistaken for molluscum contagiosum or verrucca. When they present as subcutaneous swellings involving deeper structures, they can be misdiagnosed as hernias. Most lymphangiomas present before the age of 10 years, but they can present in midlife. Possible complications include fistula formation, infection, chronic leakage of lymph fluid, chronic Lymphedema, and elephantiasis. With chronic lymphedema, one must be aware of the development of angiosarcoma in the edematous structure. These tumors can arise in edematous lesions of congenital origin or those acquired secondary to surgical procedures. Treatment of choice for larger lymphangiomas is surgical excision. However, small lesions can be treated with electrosurgery or carbon dioxide laser ablation.

MISCELLANEOUS BENIGN TUMORS

Cysts

The most common cyst of the genitalia of men and women is the epidermoid cyst. The clinical presentation, histology, and management are similar to those arising outside the genitalia.

The median raphe cyst is one of the most common cystic lesions of the male genitalia. Clinically, it arises in the midline along the genital fold at any point extending from the urethral meatus to the anus. Histologically, it has cystic spaces with no connection to the urethra or overlying epidermis. The epithelium of the cyst is usually of stratified columnar type, but occasionally can be cuboidal or fusiform. Mucin stains of the contents are usually negative, but mucin-containing clear cells can be seen in the cyst wall. The median raphe cyst is postulated to arise from epithelial rests incidental to incomplete closure of the urethral or genital folds or from outgrowths of embryologic epithelium after primary closure of these folds. The treatment of choice is excision with primary closure.

Bartholin's duct cysts occur in women during the reproductive years. Bartholin's glands are paired, located on the poterolateral introitus and drain into the vestibule. Ductal obstruction leads to cyst formation. Speed of growth depends on accumulation of secretions, which depends on sexual stimulation. Excision is not recommended because the function of the gland is lost. Better treatment options include carbon dioxide laser vaporization, marsupialization, and incision with Word catheter placement.

Syringoma

Syringomas are benign tumors of eccrine sweat gland origin. They most commonly occur as flesh-colored, cystic papules on the face, neck, and chest, but they may involve the genitalia. Cases involving the male genitalia are rare, but tend to involve the dorsum and lateral aspects of the penile shaft. Multiple syringomas of the vulva are more common and are associated with pruritis, often exacerbated during the menstrual cycle. Carbon dioxide laser vaporization or excision and primary closure are both effective treatment modalities.

Papillary Hidradenoma

Papillary hidradenoma (hidradenoma papilliferum) is a benign tumor of apocrine sweat gland origin that presents as a flesh-colored to reddish papule or nodule on the vulva.

Twenty percent of papillary hidradenomas occur perianally. The histology shows an apocrine, papillomatous growth in the dermis surrounded by a fibrous pseudocapsule, with no connection to the overlying epidermis in most instances. Treatment consists of excision with primary closure.

Trichoepithelioma

Trichoepitheliomas are adnexal tumors that present as flesh-colored papules and nodules usually located on the face. Rarely, they can occur on the mons pubis or perianal area of men and women. These genital tumors differ from trichoepitheliomas elsewhere in that they are larger and deeper, extending to subcutaneous fat. Only one recurrence has been reported after simple excision.

Leiomyoma

Genital leiomyomas are smooth muscle tumors that arise from the dartos muscle of the scrotum and vulva. They are usually solitary and asymptomatic. Histologically, they are identical to leiomyomas seen elsewhere in the skin and can be highlighted with a Masson-trichrome stain. Treatment, if needed, consists of excision with primary closure.

Calcinosis

Idiopathic calcinosis cutis can affect the scrotum or vulva, but scrotal involvement is much more frequently reported. Lesions can be single or multiple. They are often asymptomatic but may be pruritic or discharge chalky material. The classic histologic appearance is of a calcified dermal nodule without epithelial lining. However, multiple authors have identified keratin fragments or cystic remnants. This supports the theory that the nodules are not idiopathic, but instead dystrophic calcification of ruptured cysts. Excision provides definitive treatment.

Endometriosis

Ectopic endometrial tissue can occur on the skin of women. It is believed to arise after accidental implantation during a surgical procedure. The hormonally responsive tissue can present as a cyclically enlarging and painful mass. Excision is the treatment of choice.

BIBLIOGRAPHY

Al Aboud K, Al Hawsawi K, et al. Vulval lymphangiomata mimicking genital warts. J Eur Acad Dermatol Venereol 2003; 17(6):684–685.

Asarch RG, Golitz LE, et al. Median raphe cysts of the penis. Arch Dermatol 1979; 115(9):1084–1086.

Assmann T, Becker-Wegerich P, et al. Tacrolimus ointment for the treatment of vulvar lichen sclerosus. J Am Acad Dermatol 2003; 48(6):935–937.

Ault KA, Giuliano AR, et al. A phase I study to evaluate a human papillomavirus (HPV) type 18 L1 VLP vaccine. Vaccine 2004; 22(23–24):3004–3007.

Azzan BB. Bartholin's cyst and abscess. A review of treatment of 53 cases. Br J Clin Pract 1978; 32(4):101–102.

Bain L, Geronemus R. The association of lichen planus of the penis with squamous cell carcinoma in situ and with verrucous squamous carcinoma. J Dermatol Surg Oncol 1989; 15(4):413–417.

Balch CM, Soong SJ, et al. Prognostic factors analysis of 17,600 melanoma patients: validation of the American Joint Committee on Cancer melanoma staging system. J Clin Oncol 2001; 19(16):3622–3634.

Barnhill RL, Albert LS, et al. Genital lentiginosis: a clinical and histopathologic study. J Am Acad Dermatol 1990; 22(3):453–460.

Bechara FG, Altmeyer P, et al. Unilateral angiokeratoma scroti: a rare manifestation of a vascular tumor. J Dermatol 2004; 31(1):39–41.

Beck S, Cotton DW. Recurrent solitary giant trichoepithelioma located in the perianal area; a case report. Br J Dermatol 1988; 118(4):563–566.

Begun FP, Grossman HB, et al. Malignant melanoma of the penis and male urethra. J Urol 1984; 132(1):123–125.

Berman B, Spencer J, et al. Successful treatment of extramammary Paget's disease of the scrotum with imiquimod 5% cream. Clin Exp Dermatol 2003; 1(suppl 28):36–38.

Bernardo BD, Huettner PC, et al. Idiopathic calcinosis cutis presenting as labial lesions in children: report of two cases with literature review. J Pediatr Adolesc Gynecol 1999; 12(3):157–160.

Bezerra AL, Lopes A, et al. Clinicopathologic features and human papillomavirus DNA prevalence of warty and squamous cell carcinoma of the penis. Am J Surg Pathol 2001; 25(5):673–678.

Bohm M, Frieling U, et al. Successful treatment of anogenital lichen sclerosus with topical tacrolimus. Arch Dermatol 2003; 139(7):922–924.

Boyd AS, Neldner KH. Lichen planus. J Am Acad Dermatol 1991; 25(4):593–619.

Bradgate MG, Rollason TP, et al. Malignant melanoma of the vulva: a clinicopathological study of 50 women. Br J Obstet Gynaecol 1990; 97(2):124–133.

Brown MD, Zachary CB, et al. Penile tumors: their management by Mohs micrographic surgery. J Dermatol Surg Oncol 1987; 13(11):1163–1167.

Busund B, Stray-Pedersen S, et al. Blue rubber bleb nevus syndrome with manifestations in the vulva. Acta Obstet Gynecol Scand 1993; 72(4):310–313.

Byrd JA, Davis MD, et al. Recalcitrant symptomatic vulvar lichen planus: response to topical tacrolimus. Arch Dermatol 2004; 140(6):715–720.

Carlson JA, Ambros R, et al. Vulvar lichen sclerosus and squamous cell carcinoma: a cohort, case control, and investigational study with historical perspective; implications for chronic inflammation and sclerosis in the development of neoplasia. Hum Pathol 1998; 29(9):932–948.

Cerri A, Gianni C, et al. Lymphangiosarcoma of the pubic region: a rare complication arising in congenital non-hereditary lymphedema. Eur J Dermatol 1998; 8(7):511–514.

Cohen PR, Young AW Jr., et al. Angiokeratoma of the vulva: diagnosis and review of the literature. Obstet Gynecol Surv 1989; 44(5):339–346.

Cox NH. Squamous cell carcinoma arising in lichen planus of the penis during topical cyclosporin therapy. Clin Exp Dermatol 1996; 21(4):323–324.

Cribier B, Ndiaye I, et al. Peno-gingival syndrome. A male equivalent of vulvo-vagino-gingival syndrome? Rev Stomatol Chir Maxillofac 1993; 94(3):148–151.

Crowther ME, Lowe DG, et al. Verrucous carcinoma of the female genital tract: a review. Obstet Gynecol Surv 1988; 43(5):263–280.

Cubilla AL, Barreto J, et al. Pathologic features of epidermoid carcinoma of the penis. A prospective study of 66 cases. Am J Surg Pathol 1993; 17(8):753–763.

Curtis JM. Marsupialisation technique for Bartholin's cyst. Aust Fam Physician 1993; 22(3):369.

Dalziel KL, Millard PR, et al. The treatment of vulval lichen sclerosus with a very potent topical steroid (clobetasol propionate 0.05%) cream. Br J Dermatol 1991; 124(5):461–464.

Davis GD. Management of Bartholin duct cysts with the carbon dioxide laser. Obstet Gynecol 1985; 65(2):279–280.

Davis G, Wentworth J, et al. Self-administered topical imiquimod treatment of vulvar intraepithelial neoplasia. A report of four cases. J Reprod Med 2000; 45(8):619–623.

DeMatos P, Tyler D, et al. Mucosal melanoma of the female genitalia: a clinicopathologic study of forty-three cases at Duke University Medical Center. Surgery 1998; 124(1):38–48.

Diaz-Arrastia C, Arany I, et al. Clinical and molecular responses in high-grade intraepithelial neoplasia treated with topical imiquimod 5%. Clin Cancer Res 2001; 7(10):3031–3033.

Dini M, Colafranceschi M. Should scrotal calcinosis still be termed idiopathic? Am J Dermatopathol 1998; 20(4):399–402.

Dwyer CM, Kerr RE, et al. Squamous carcinoma following lichen planus of the vulva. Clin Exp Dermatol 1995; 20(2):171–172.

Edwards L. Vulvar lichen planus. Arch Dermatol 1989; 125(12):1677–1680.

Eilber KS, Raz S. Benign cystic lesions of the vagina: a literature review. J Urol 2003; 170(3):717–722.

Eisen D. The evaluation of cutaneous, genital, scalp, nail, esophageal, and ocular involvement in patients with oral lichen planus. Oral Surg Oral Med Oral Pathol Oral Radiol Endod 1999; 88(4):431–436.

Eisen D. The vulvovaginal-gingival syndrome of lichen planus. The clinical characteristics of 22 patients. Arch Dermatol 1994; 130(11):1379–1382.

Finan MA, Barre G. Bartholin's gland carcinoma, malignant melanoma and other rare tumours of the vulva. Best Pract Res Clin Obstet Gynaecol 2003; 17(4):609–633.

Flores JT, Apfelberg DB, et al. Angiokeratoma of Fordyce: successful treatment with the argon laser. Plast Reconstr Surg 1984; 74(6):835–838.

Franck JM, Young AW Jr. Squamous cell carcinoma in situ arising within lichen planus of the vulva. Dermatol Surg 1995; 21(10):890–894.

Gerdsen R, Wenzel J, et al. Periodic genital pruritus caused by syringoma of the vulva. Acta Obstet Gynecol Scand 2002; 81(4):369–370.

Golitz LE, Robin M. Median raphe canals of the penis. Cutis 1981; 27(2):170–172.

Gorse SJ, James W, et al. Successful treatment of angiokeratoma with potassium tritanyl phosphate laser. Br J Dermatol 2004; 150(3):620–622.

Gualco M, Bonin S, et al. Morphologic and biologic studies on ten cases of verrucous carcinoma of the vulva supporting the theory of a discrete clinico-pathologic entity. Int J Gynecol Cancer 2003; 13(3):317–324.

Haley JC, Mirowski GW, et al. Benign vulvar tumors. Semin Cutan Med Surg 1998; 17(3):196–204.

Handa Y, Yamanaka N, et al. Large ulcerated perianal hidradenoma papilliferum in a young female. Dermatol Surg 2003; 29(7):790–792.

Harper DM, Franco EL, et al. Efficacy of a bivalent L1 virus-like particle vaccine in prevention of infection with human papillomavirus types 16 and 18 in young women: a randomised controlled trial. Lancet 2004; 364(9447):1757–1765.

Harwood CA, Mortimer PS. Acquired vulval lymphangiomata mimicking genital warts. Br J Dermatol 1993; 129(3):334–336.

Hatta N, Morita R, et al. Sentinel lymph node biopsy in patients with extramammary Paget's disease. Dermatol Surg 2004; 30(10):1329–1334.

Heah J. Methods of treatment for cysts and abscesses of Bartholin's gland. Br J Obstet Gynaecol 1988; 95(4):321–322.

Hendi A, Brodland DG, et al. Extramammary Paget's disease: surgical treatment with Mohs micrographic surgery. J Am Acad Dermatol 2004; 51(5):767–773.

Hood AF, Lumadue J. Benign vulvar tumors. Dermatol Clin 1992; 10(2):371–385.

Hopkins JA, Hudson PB. Kaposi's sarcoma; penile and scrotal lesions. Br J Urol 1953; 25(3):233–236.

Hording U, Junge J, et al. Vulvar squamous cell carcinoma and papillomaviruses: indications for two different etiologies. Gynecol Oncol 1994; 52(2):241–246.

Huang YH, Chuang YH, et al. Vulvar syringoma: a clinico-pathologic and immunohistologic study of 18 patients and results of treatment. J Am Acad Dermatol 2003; 48(5):735–739.

Kanik AB, Lee J, et al. Penile verrucous carcinoma in a 37-year-old circumcised man. J Am Acad Dermatol 1997; 37(2 Pt 2): 329–331.

Kaufmann T, Pawl NO, et al. Cystic papillary hidradenoma of the vulva: case report and review of the literature. Gynecol Oncol 1987; 26(2):240–245.

Kirtschig G, Van Der Meulen AJ, et al. Successful treatment of erosive vulvovaginal lichen planus with topical tacrolimus. Br J Dermatol 2002; 147(3):625–626.

Koch P, Bahmer FA. Oral lesions and symptoms related to metals used in dental restorations: a clinical, allergological, and histologic study. J Am Acad Dermatol 1999; 41(3 Pt 1):422–430.

Kopf AW, Bart RS. Tumor conference #38. Lymphangioma of the scrotum and penis. J Dermatol Surg Oncol 1981; 7(11): 870–872.

Kunstfeld R, Kirnbauer R, et al. Successful treatment of vulvar lichen sclerosus with topical tacrolimus. Arch Dermatol 2003; 139(7):850–852.

Kurzl RG. Paget's disease. Semin Dermatol 1996; 15(1):60–66.

Laeijendecker R, Dekker SK, et al. Oral lichen planus and allergy to dental amalgam restorations. Arch Dermatol 2004; 140(12):1434–1438.

Lapins J, Emtestam L, et al. Angiokeratomas in Fabry's disease and Fordyce's disease: successful treatment with copper vapour laser. Acta Derm Venereol 1993; 73(2):133–135.

Leal-Khouri S, Hruza GJ. Squamous cell carcinoma developing within lichen planus of the penis. Treatment with Mohs micrographic surgery. J Dermatol Surg Oncol 1994; 20(4): 272–276.

Leicht S, Youngberg G, et al. Atypical pigmented penile macules. Arch Dermatol 1988; 124(8):1267–1270.

Lewis FM, Harrington CI. Squamous cell carcinoma arising in vulval lichen planus. Br J Dermatol 1994; 131(5):703–705.

Livne PM, Nobel M, et al. Leiomyoma of the scrotum. Arch Dermatol 1983; 119(4):358–359.

Luk NM, Yu KH, et al. Extramammary Paget's disease: outcome of radiotherapy with curative intent. Clin Exp Dermatol 2003; 28(4):360–363.

Mandal AK, Bhatnagar R. Solitary trichoepithelioma of mons pubis. Indian J Pathol Microbiol 1987; 30(4):401–402.

Mannone F, De Giorgi V, et al. Dermoscopic features of mucosal melanosis. Dermatol Surg 2004; 30(8):1118–1123.

Mansur CP. Human papillomaviruses. In: Tyring SK, ed. Mucocutaneous Manifestations of Viral Diseases. New York: Marcel Dekker, Inc., 2002:247–294.

McCance D. Papillomaviruses. In: Zuckerman AJ, Banatvala JE, Pattison JR, Griffiths PD, Schoub BD, eds. Principles and Practice of Clinical Virology. West Sussex: John Wiley & Sons Ltd, 2004:661–674.

Mehta RK, Rytina E, et al. Treatment of verrucous carcinoma of vulva with acitretin. Br J Dermatol 2000; 142(6):1195–1198.

Mohs FE, Sahl WJ. Chemosurgery for verrucous carcinoma. J Dermatol Surg Oncol 1979; 5(4):302–306.

Moodley, 2004 #40.

Moyal-Barracco M, Edwards L. Diagnosis and therapy of anogenital lichen planus. Dermatol Ther 2004; 17(1):38–46.

Nagore E, Sanchez-Motilla JM, et al. Median raphe cysts of the penis: a report of five cases. Pediatr Dermatol 1998; 15(3):191–193.

Nahass GT, Blauvelt A, et al. Basal cell carcinoma of the scrotum. Report of three cases and review of the literature. J Am Acad Dermatol 1992; 26(4):574–578.

Nasca MR, Innocenzi D, et al. Penile cancer among patients with genital lichen sclerosus. J Am Acad Dermatol 1999; 41(6):911–914.

Nascimento AF, Granter SR, et al. Vulvar acanthosis with altered differentiation: a precursor to verrucous carcinoma? Am J Surg Pathol 2004; 28(5):638–643.

National Institutes of Health consensus development conference statement on diagnosis and treatment of early melanoma, January 27–29, 1992. Am J Dermatopathol 1993; 15(1):34–43; discussion 46–51.

Nehal KS, Levine VJ, et al. Basal cell carcinoma of the genitalia. Dermatol Surg 1998; 24(12):1361–1363.

O'Connor WJ, Lim KK, et al. Comparison of Mohs micrographic surgery and wide excision for extramammary Paget's disease. Dermatol Surg 2003; 29(7):723–727.

Occella C, Bleidl D, et al. Argon laser treatment of cutaneous multiple angiokeratomas. Dermatol Surg 1995; 21(2):170–172.

Ohnishi T, Watanabe S. The use of cytokeratins 7 and 20 in the diagnosis of primary and secondary extramammary Paget's disease. Br J Dermatol 2000; 142(2):243–247.

Ohtake N, Maeda S, et al. Leiomyoma of the scrotum. Dermatology 1997; 194(3):299–301.

Oonk MH, de Hullu JA, et al. The value of routine follow-up in patients treated for carcinoma of the vulva. Cancer 2003; 98(12):2624–2629.

Ozcelik B, Serin IS, et al. Idiopathic calcinosis cutis of the vulva in an elderly woman. A case report. J Reprod Med 2002; 47(7):597–599.

Pandher BS, Rustin MH, et al. Treatment of balanitis xerotica obliterans with topical tacrolimus. J Urol 2003; 170(3):923.

Partridge EE, Murad T, et al. Verrucous lesions of the female genitalia. II. Verrucous carcinoma. Am J Obstet Gynecol 1980; 137(4):419–424.

Patrizi A, Neri I, et al. Syringoma: a review of twenty-nine cases. Acta Derm Venereol 1998; 78(6):460–462.

Pelisse M, Leibowitch M, et al. A new vulvovaginogingival syndrome. Plurimucous erosive lichen planus. Ann Dermatol Venereol 1982; 109(9):797–798.

Penna C, Fambrini M, et al. CO(2) laser treatment for Bartholin's gland cyst. Int J Gynaecol Obstet 2002; 76(1):79–80.

Phillips GL, Bundy BN, et al. Malignant melanoma of the vulva treated by radical hemivulvectomy. A prospective study of the Gynecologic Oncology Group. Cancer 1994; 73(10): 2626–2632.

Powell FC, Bjornsson J, et al. Genital Paget's disease and urinary tract malignancy. J Am Acad Dermatol 1985; 13(1):84–90.

Ragnarsson-Olding BK. Primary malignant melanoma of the vulva—an aggressive tumor for modeling the genesis of non-UV light-associated melanomas. Acta Oncol 2004; 43(5):421–435.

Ragnarsson-Olding BK, Nilsson BR, et al. Malignant melanoma of the vulva in a nationwide, 25-year study of 219 Swedish females: predictors of survival. Cancer 1999; 86(7): 1285–1293.

Rogers RS 3rd, Eisen D. Erosive oral lichen planus with genital lesions: the vulvovaginal-gingival syndrome and the peno-gingival syndrome. Dermatol Clin 2003; 21(1):91–98, vi–vii.

Rogers RS 3rd, Bruce AJ. Lichenoid contact stomatitis: is inorganic mercury the culprit? Arch Dermatol 2004; 140(12): 1524–1525.

Rojansky N, Anteby SO. Gynecological neoplasias in the patient with HIV infection. Obstet Gynecol Surv 1996; 51(11): 679–683.

Ruiz-Genao DP, Rios-Buceta L, et al. Massive scrotal calcinosis. Dermatol Surg 2002; 28(8):745–747.

Scott PM. Draining a cyst or abscess in a Bartholin's gland with a word catheter. JAAPA 2003; 16(12):51–52.

Sheen MC, Sheu HM, et al. Penile verrucous carcinoma successfully treated by intra-aortic infusion with methotrexate. Urology 2003; 61(6):1216–1220.

Shieh S, Dee AS, et al. Photodynamic therapy for the treatment of extramammary Paget's disease. Br J Dermatol 2002; 146(6):1000–1005.

Smith KJ, Tuur S, et al. Cytokeratin 7 staining in mammary and extramammary Paget's disease. Mod Pathol 1997; 10(11): 1069–1074.

Song DH, Lee KH, et al. Idiopathic calcinosis of the scrotum: histopathologic observations of fifty-one nodules. J Am Acad Dermatol 1988; 19(6):1095–1101.

Sonobe H, Ro JY, et al. Glomus tumor of the female external genitalia: a report of two cases. Int J Gynecol Pathol 1994; 13(4):359–364.

Stillwell TJ, Zincke H, et al. Malignant melanoma of the penis. J Urol 1988; 140(1):72–75.

Taira AV. Evaluating human papillomavirus vaccination programs. Emerg Infect Dis 2004; 10(11):1915–1923.

Tatnall FM, Jones EW. Giant solitary trichoepitheliomas located in the perianal area: a report of three cases. Br J Dermatol 1986; 115(1):91–99.

Ting PT, Dytoc MT. Therapy of external anogenital warts and molluscum contagiosum: a literature review. Dermatol Ther 2004; 17(1):68–101.

Trimble EL, Lewis JL Jr., et al. Management of vulvar melanoma. Gynecol Oncol 1992; 45(3):254–258.

Tyring SK. Vulvar squamous cell carcinoma: guidelines for early diagnosis and treatment. Am J Obstet Gynecol 2003; 189(3 suppl):S17–S23.

Vapnek JM, Quivey JM, et al. Acquired immunodeficiency syndrome-related Kaposi's sarcoma of the male genitalia: management with radiation therapy. J Urol 1991; 146(2):333–336.

Velazquez EF, Barreto JE, et al. Limitations in the interpretation of biopsies in patients with penile squamous cell carcinoma. Int J Surg Pathol 2004; 12(2):139–146.

Velazquez EF, Cubilla AL. Lichen sclerosus in 68 patients with squamous cell carcinoma of the penis: frequent atypias and correlation with special carcinoma variants suggests a precancerous role. Am J Surg Pathol 2003; 27(11): 1448–1453.

Vente C, Reich K, et al. Erosive mucosal lichen planus: response to topical treatment with tacrolimus. Br J Dermatol 1999; 140(2):338–342.

Verschraegen CF, Benjapibal M, et al. Vulvar melanoma at the MD Anderson Cancer Center:25 years later. Int J Gynecol Cancer 2001; 11(5):359–364.

Wang LC, Blanchard A, et al. Successful treatment of recurrent extramammary Paget's disease of the vulva with topical imiquimod 5% cream. J Am Acad Dermatol 2003; 49(4):769–772.

Wechter ME, Gruber SB, et al. Vulvar melanoma: a report of 20 cases and review of the literature. J Am Acad Dermatol 2004; 50(4):554–562.

Wedel DJ, Horlocker TT. Nerve blocks. In: Miller RD, ed. Miller's Anesthesia. Orlando: W.B. Saunders Company, 2005: 1685–1715.

Weedon D. Skin Pathology. London: Elsevier Science Limited, 2002.

Woodworth H Jr., Dockerty MB, et al. Papillary hidradenoma of the vulva: a clinicopathologic study of 69 cases. Am J Obstet Gynecol 1971; 110(4):501–508.

Yamazaki M, Hiruma M, et al. Angiokeratoma of the clitoris: a subtype of angiokeratoma vulvae. J Dermatol 1992; 19(9):553–555.

Yiannias JA, el-Azhary RA, et al. Relevant contact sensitivities in patients with the diagnosis of oral lichen planus. J Am Acad Dermatol 2000; 42(2 Pt 1):177–182.

Zampogna JC, Flowers FP, et al. Treatment of primary limited cutaneous extramammary Paget's disease with topical imiquimod monotherapy: two case reports. J Am Acad Dermatol 2002; 47(suppl 4):S229–S235.

Zawislak AA, McCarron PA, et al. Successful photodynamic therapy of vulval Paget's disease using a novel patch-based delivery system containing 5-aminolevulinic acid. BJOG 2004; 111(10):1143–1145.

33

Epidermal Tumors

Glenn Kolansky
Advanced Dermatology Surgery Center, Tinton Falls, New Jersey, U.S.A.

Christopher Tignanelli
*University of Medicine and Dentistry of New Jersey, New Jersey Medical School,
Newark, New Jersey, U.S.A.*

Barry Leshin
The Skin Surgery Center, Winston-Salem, North Carolina, U.S.A.

Duane C. Whitaker
University of Arizona, Tucson, Arizona, U.S.A.

INTRODUCTION

There is a wide clinicopathologic spectrum of epidermal tumors. Some, such as seborrheic keratoses, have a characteristic appearance that can be easily recognized. Others, such as the dermatitic appearance of extramammary Paget disease, can be more difficult. There is also great histologic variability expressed by these epidermal growths. The keratin-filled sac of an epidermoid cyst is diagnosed at low power with a rapid glance. However, the proliferation of atypical keratinizing squamous epithelium can make differentiation of a keratoacanthoma (KA) from a squamous cell carcinoma more subtle.

The biologic spectrum of epidermal tumors is also vast. The explosive onset of inflammatory seborrheic keratoses, or the sign of Leser-Trélat, may signal the presence of an occult malignancy. Bowen's disease of the penis is a potentially invasive, life-threatening squamous cell carcinoma. Extramammary Paget disease may be a cutaneous marker of underlying carcinoma.

Just as the clinical, histologic, and biologic nature of epidermal tumors varies, treatment options for these tumors are similarly varied. Simple electrodesiccation and curettage or cryosurgery may be sufficient in many cases, while wide excision and work-up for internal disease may be indicated for others.

SEBORRHEIC KERATOSIS

Seborrheic keratosis are benign epidermal tumors that occur on the skin of middle-aged and older individuals. Clinically the lesions appear as one or more exophytic light brown to brown-black plaques with slightly raised and sharply demarcated borders. They are verrucous papules with a characteristic "stuck-on" appearance with dirty, friable scale. Close inspection may show keratotic follicular plugging of the surface (Fig. 1). A variant termed dermatosis papulosa nigra is frequently seen in blacks and Asians. These lesions consist of multiple small, heavily pigmented papules that

usually develop on the face, especially on the upper cheeks and orbital areas, usually arising in adolescence. They are primarily of cosmetic importance and are asymptomatic unless the lesions are irritated. Malignant melanoma, basal cell carcinoma, and squamous cell carcinomas have been reported to arise within a seborrheic keratosis. In a prospective study of 4310 tumors clinically diagnosed as seborrheic keratosis, 60 (1.4%) proved to be squamous carcinoma in situ. The majority of these were on sun-exposed areas of the head and neck.

Occasionally, a deeply pigmented seborrheic keratosis is clinically indistinguishable from malignant melanoma. This warrants removal by excisional biopsy. In other cases where cosmetic factors might warrant surgery, it can be treated by such measures as curettage, cryosurgery, electrodessication, or chemical destruction. The sudden eruptive appearance of multiple seborrheic keratosis, known as the sign of Leser-Trélat, may suggest an internal malignancy. Traditionally, the sign of Leser-Trélat is associated with adenocarcinomas of the stomach. However, hematopoietic malignancies as well as several cases of patients with mycosis fungoides and Sézary syndrome have been described.

Histologically, seborrheic keratoses are benign epithelial growths with no malignant potential. Although recent research has showed that in few cases malignant melanomas can be found There are five histologic types: acanthotic, hyperkeratotic, adenoidal (reticulated), clonal, and inflamed (irritated or inverted follicular).. A few cases of seborrhic keratosis with focal acantholysis have been reported. Separation of intraepidermal epithelioma (IE) and the clonal type of seborrheic keratosis is based on histological grounds, with IE showing atypical nests of keratinocytes, nuclear pleomorphism, atypia, malignant dyskeratosis, and mitosis within the epidermis. These lesions are regarded as premalignant—about 9% may invade the underlying dermis and subcutaneous tissue—whereas the clonal variant of seborrheic keratosis is benign.

These common tumors are primarily of cosmetic importance. When histologic confirmation is not required, these lesions are easily removed in several ways.

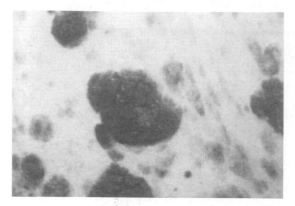

Figure 1 Seborrheic keratosis on back.

Liquid Nitrogen Cryotherapy

Depending on the size of the lesion, either a spray apparatus or a cotton-tipped applicator may be used. The entire lesion with a 1- to 2-mm halo of surrounding skin is treated with a 30- to 45-second freeze-thaw cycle. Several lesions can be treated at a time without anesthesia. Lesions will persist if inadequately frozen, and thick lesions may require additional treatment. However, deeper freezes my result in hypopigmentation or scar. The patient feels a burning sensation initially, which increases in intensity as the area thaws. Instructions for local wound care are given, and the area heals with minimal to no scarring. Curettage is an effective supplement to cryotherapy. After freezing lightly with liquid nitrogen or skin refrigerants (Frigiderm), the seborrheic keratosis can be easily curetted off the underlying normal skin.

The fast curette method consists of holding the skin taut and with a firm grasp of the instrument, sweeping the lesion off the skin with a single motion. Pedunculated lesions can be removed with a small scissor. These small lesions may shrink down and char quickly when touched by the hyfrecator tip. This is followed by curettage. As many of these patients have dark skin, avoidance of cryotherapy decreases the risk of hypopigmentation.

Electrodesiccation and Electrofulguration Plus Curettage

The acanthotic epidermis of a seborrheic keratosis can be ablated by electrosurgery. Electro-desiccation and electrofulguration cause the most superficial type of tissue destruction. This type of treatment usually requires local anesthesia. For electrodesiccation, touch the lesion gently and move the electrode across the lesion with low power current. Thicker lesions may require direct insertion of the electrode into multiple points for 1 to 2 seconds. The destroyed tissue is easily removed with a piece of gauze or a curette for adherent lesions. Punctate bleeding is controlled with spot electrocoagulation, pressure, or aluminum chloride solution. Use of Monsel's solution on the face is avoided because of the risk of permanent brown staining. Extremely small lesions can be treated with electrofulguration, during which the electrode does not touch the lesion. A few sparks are dispersed across the lesion, minimizing the extent of adjacent tissue damage.

Shave Excision

Seborrheic keratoses can be easily removed with a superficial shave excision. This technique is particularly effective and offers the advantage of a specimen for histologic examination, should the clinical diagnosis be in doubt. Shave excision should not be used when melanoma is in the differential diagnosis. In this instance, a full-thickness excision is the treatment of choice to provide a specimen for complete histological examination and measurement of depth if melanoma is discovered. Shave excision requires the use of local anesthesia and has the potential for scar ring.

Dermabrasion and Chemical Peel

Superficial dermabrasion can be used for the treatment of giant seborrheic keratosis and for patients with multiple lesions. Mild hypertrophic scarring without evidence of recurrence has been described. Trichloroacetic acid (25–50%) can be used as a treatment by carefully painting the surface of the lesion with acid and repeating the application at a later date if necessary.

Alexandrite Laser

Recent studies have shown that the usage of an Alexandrite Laser can produce excellent results in the removal of seborrheic keratosis. This laser was originally approved by the FDA for usage with hair removal. It should be noted that this procedure is purely for cosmetic purposes.

SEBACEOUS HYPERPLASIA

Sebaceous hyperplasia is a common disorder, occurring in adults with increasing frequency with age. These lesions usually occur in middle age, however, lesions arising at puberty have been well documented. The lesions are cream- to yellow-colored papules with a central area of umbilication and are 2 to 6 mm in size located on the forehead, cheeks, lower eyelids, and nose.

Histologically, numerous sebaceous glands are arranged around a central follicle. There are clearly too many normal glands for the central, single follicle.

Treatment is often performed for cosmetic reasons. When basal cell carcinoma cannot be ruled out, excision is the treatment of choice. Excision, deep curettage, or hot cautery are effective but may leave a visible scar. Trichloroacetic acid 50% or 1% bichloroacetic acid is applied directly to the lesion with a cotton tip or pointed wooded applicator for a few seconds, until the lesion turns white. This is followed with antibiotic ointment for one week.

Cryosurgery with a cotton-tipped applicator for a freezing time of 10 to 15 seconds with a 1-mm frost halo around the lesion results in resolution without discernible scarring. Systemic administration of isotretinoin has been reported as successful, however, lesions returned three weeks after discontinuation of therapy. Treatment with lasers (pulse-dye, CO_2, 1450 nm) might be effective in the treatment of sebaceous hyperplasia.

EPIDERMOID CYSTS

Epidermoid cysts arise from implantation and proliferation of the epidermis within the dermis or subcutaneous tissue. They commonly occur on the face, scalp, neck, or trunk and range from 1 to 5 cm. Uncommon cases of a giant epidermoid cyst on the chest as well as an epidermoid cyst arising on the sole of the foot have been reported. They may arise from occlusion of pilosebaceous follicles or from implantation of epidermal cells into the dermis following penetrating injury. Clinically they appear as spherically shaped, slowly enlarging firm to fluctuant nodules. A small central punctum connecting to the cyst cavity representing the plugged orifice of the pilosebacous unit can often be observed. Malodorous, cheesy-white keratinous material may be expressed from this punctum. Lesions are asymptomatic unless they become inflamed after rupture of the cyst wall or become infected. Clinically, infected epidermoid cysts exhibit bacterial growth predominantly with *Staphylococcus aureus*. The presence of human papillomavirus (HPV) antigen has been reported, but the association between the virus and the epidermoid cyst remains obscure. Rare instances of cyst-derived Bowen's disease, basal cell carcinoma, and squamous cell carcinoma have been reported. The cyst is lined by a stratified squamous epithelium with a well-formed granular layer. Within the cyst, a thick, compact, keratinous material is organized into laminated layers. Foreign-body reaction with giant cells may occur due to trauma or infection in response to spillage of cyst contents to the surrounding dermis (Fig. 2).

The removal of epidermoid cysts is a common problem. Procedures for the treatment of epidermoid cysts include different modes of surgical excision, incision, and drainage, and some have suggested electrocautery, cryosurgery, and the injection of chemical irritants. We favor incision and thorough drainage or surgical excision.

Excision

Noninflamed, uninfected cysts are easily removed. To prevent recurrence, the complete removal or destruction of the cyst wall is necessary. Before cyst removal, simple palpation is used to define the dimensions of the cyst and to determine how freely mobile the cyst is. The area is prepared in a surgical manner, and the surgical site is marked with gentian violet. The skin overlying the cyst and the surrounding skin needs to be anesthetized. Anesthesia is injected between the skin and around the cyst wall in a ringlike manner, taking care to avoid injection into the cyst itself, as this will increase the likelihood of rupture. Supplemental injections may be required into the surrounding tissue and deep to the cyst. It is recommended that the dermatologic surgeon wear a protective cap and protective eyewear to shield the eyes from the occasional "eruption" of cyst contents.

Minimal Surgery Technique

A small to medium-sized cyst may be excised by making a single 2- to 3-mm linear excision over the cyst. Pressure is applied to the base of the cyst for delivery of the contents. The cyst wall may evert as the cyst contents are expressed or extracted with a hemostat. It is then identified and completely removed. The wound is carefully inspected to ensure

complete removal of the capsule and irrigated with sterile saline to remove any retained fragments of the wall to prevent cyst recurrence. The surgical wound is closed with suture, and hemostasis is with electrocautery.

After palpation, a freely movable cyst with little attachment to its surroundings can be excised with a #15 scalpel blade. The top of the cyst is incised along the maximal skin tension lines to the level of the glistening white capsule wall. This incision should be through the punctum or directly to the side of it. A small amount of tissue enclosing the punctum is removed with it. Continue as above, removing cyst contents and then the capsule.

Elliptical excision should include the punctum overlying the cyst. A small ellipse overlying the cyst is excised up to the capsule overlying the cyst with a #15 scalpel blade. The epidermis attached to the cyst can be elevated with an Allis clamp and using blunt-tipped dissection scissors (tenotomy scissors or baby Metzenbaum scissors) or hemostat, carefully dissect around the cyst, and the cyst can usually be delivered intact. The standard elliptical excision is closed in the usual manner; if the defect left by the cyst is small, skin sutures of only 4.0 to 6.0 monofilament nylon may be necessary. Vertical mattress sutures assist in opposing wound edges and decreasing dead space. For a large defect, buried absorbable 4.0 or 5.0 suture is used.

Substituting a biopsy punch for a scalpel provides a simple, rapid method for removal of epithelial cysts. The cyst is anesthetized with a needle inserted superficially into the opening of the cyst and then deeply into the cyst itself. Squeezing the base of the cyst firmly, a 2- to 4-mm biopsy punch is inserted perpendicular to the cyst over the visible pore until it penetrates the cyst wall. The contents of the cyst are squeezed out with firm pressure through the hole until no more of the contents appear. Then a curet or a small scissor is inserted to dislodge the wall from the surrounding stroma, and it is grasped with a small hemostat and removed. To reduce wound care requirements and afford a superior cosmetic result, the wound is closed with suture only if the surgeon is confident that the cyst wall is completely removed. If there are any retained contents, the wound is not closed and the wound heals by secondary intention aided by moist warm compresses. It should be emphasized that this method works well for small cysts of the face and is not to be used for severely inflamed or fibrosed cysts.

An epidermoid cyst can be easily removed unless the cyst wall has become fibrosed to the adjacent tissue from trauma or infection. Acutely inflamed cysts should be allowed to "cool down." Treatment is with an oral antibiotic that provides good Staphylococcus coverage, such as dicloxacillin, azithromycin, or a cephalosporin, followed by a small amount of intralesional triamcinolone (5–10 mg/ mL) into the cyst cavity can be employed. The cyst may contract in three to four weeks and then it can be excised.

Fluctuant cysts are treated with a central stab incision to drain the cyst contents, followed by gauze packing. Local anesthesia may be necessary, and the walls of the cyst can then be curetted to assist in removing contents and breaking up tabulations. Before packing the defect, generously place antibiotic ointment inside the cavity for local antibacterial effect and to allow easy removal of the gauze packing without adhesion. The packing is removed slowly at 24 to 72 hours and an appropriate antibiotic is prescribed. If the area is acutely inflamed, a modest amount of intralesional triamcinolone can be injected into the surrounding area. Excision can be performed in four to six weeks.

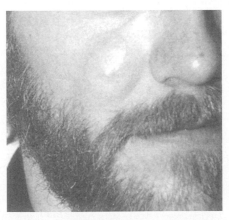

Figure 2 Epidermoid cyst on cheek. Note puncta.

TRICHILEMMAL CYSTS (PILAR CYSTS)

Trichilemmal cysts occur most commonly on the scalp and are often referred to as a "wen" or sebaceous cyst. Clinically they are similar to epidermoid cysts, however, trichilemmal cysts occur on the scalp 90% of the time, comprising 15% of surgically excised cysts. There is an autosomal dominant genetic disposition. They are produced from budding off of the external root sheath in the region of the follicular isthmus. Individual cysts enlarge, and some of the central keratin may disintegrate to produce a pseudo-calcareous mass. True calcification is found in 25% of cysts. There is a tendency for trichilemmal cysts to recur after excision, when only the parent cyst is removed and one or more daughter cysts are left behind. Budding of new cysts occurs de novo from the cyst wall or directly around areas of calcification.

Histologically trichilemmal cysts are rarely connected to the epidermis. The cyst wall is composed of stratified squamous epithelium with a palisaded outer layer resembling the outer root sheath of the hair follicle. The inner layer of pale-staining cells keratinizes without a granular layer, consequently without keratohyalin granules in contradistinction to an epidermoid cyst. The keratin lining the cyst is dense, pink, and homogeneous, in contrast to the delicate loose keratin of an epidermoid cyst. Calcium is displayed in 24% and cholesterol clefts in 92% of cysts.

Excision of trichilemmal cysts is similar to epidermoid cysts. The wall of the cyst is firmer and more likely to remain intact. A shallow incision is made over the cyst, scissors are used to dissect surrounding tissue bluntly, and the cyst is expressed easily intact If the cyst wall is incompletely removed, recent research shows there is a significant chance of reoccurrence.

Moderate-sized cysts may be removed using the punch excision method. After obtaining superficial anesthesia, a 4- to 5-mm punch of skin is removed to the depth of the capsule. Anesthetic is injected deeper around the cyst. Pressure is applied around the punch site until the cyst is visible. The cyst is then grasped by a small hemostat and dissected out intact. The defect is closed by simple wound closure.

This can often be accomplished on the scalp without hair removal, since the hair can be taped with paper tape or clipped with hair clips out of the operative field. Wound care consists of moist sterile compresses twice daily followed by antibiotic ointment dressing.

PROLIFERATING TRICHILEMMAL TUMOR

Proliferating trichilemmal tumor is an uncommon variant of trichilemmal cysts. It is usually a solitary lesion occurring on the scalp of elderly women. However, this tumor has occurred in individuals in their twenties and thirties. They may arise from trauma or inflammation of common trichilemmal cysts. The possibility of malignant transformation should be considered in longstanding cystic and nodular scalp lesions that show rapid growth or exophytic enlargement.

Histologically the tumor represents a proliferation of the outer root sheath epithelium composed of irregularly shaped, well-circumscribed lobules of squamous epithelium in a palisading pattern. Trichilemmal keratinization without a granular layer, foci of calcification may be present in areas of amorphous keratin, and squamous epithelium may contain squamous pearls and eddies. In some tumors' foci of cytological atypia, nuclear pleomorphism and numerous mitoses can produce a picture difficult to distinguish from squamous cell carcinomas.

The tumor should be excised with a margin of normal tissue to prevent recurrence. Routine follow-up of patients is recommended, especially in tumors with a malignant appearance.

MILIA

Milia are small, 1- to 3-mm, white papular lesions. Primary lesions occur on the face and are seen in adults or children. Secondary lesions occur in diseases associated with subepidermal bullae such as porphyria cutanea tarda, epidermolysis bullosa, bullous pemphigoid, bullous lichen planus, and lichen sclerosis et atrophicus. Histologically both forms resemble tiny epidermoid cysts. Milia may connect to the epidermis or to an eccrine sweat duct or to a hair follicle.

Milia commonly appear during the healing phase of dermabrasion, chemical peel, or incisional surgery, and may result from fragments of detached epidermis that continue to keratinize. The incidence of milia may be reduced by scrubbing the face after dermabrasion with a "gauze pad with copious amounts of saline."

Milia are treated by incising the overlying dermis with the tip of a #15 blade, a 25 needle, or surgical lancet. The contents are expressed by simple finger pressure or a comedone extractor. Electrocautery or electrosurgery with an epilating needle set at low current touched lightly to the top of the milia for a fraction of a second will break the cyst sac. The contents may boil out or be removed as above.

KERATOACANTHOMAS

KA is a proliferation of squamous epidermis characterized clinically by dome-shaped nodules 1 to 2.5 cm in diameter with a keratotic plug in the center. KAs usually arise on sun-exposed, hair-bearing skin, although their etiology remains unclear. This is usually followed by a slow involution over three to six months without metastases. The appearance of KAs can be divided into three stages: proliferative, fully developed, and involuting.

In the early proliferative stage, a horn-filled invagination of the epidermis arises from contiguous hair follicles, from which epidermal strands may extend into the dermis. The lesion shows mild hyperkeratosis, acanthosis, and premature keratinization with atypical mitotic cells (Figs. 3 and 4).

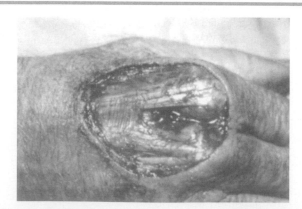

Figure 3 Surgical defect following Mohs micrographic surgery. Deep extent of tumor necessitated removal of peritenon overlying extensor tendons.

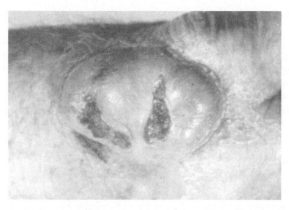

Figure 4 Keratoacanthoma, recurrent after excision. Unresponsive to intralesional fluorouracil.

A fully developed lesion shows a crateriform nodule with a central depression filled with keratin. The epidermis buttresses over the sides of the crater. Irregular epidermal proliferations extend upward into the crater and downward below its base. These epidermal proliferations may appear atypical but less so than during the initial stage. Keratinization of the squamous cells is marked, producing an eosinophilic glassy appearance. Horn pearls are present, and the base in mature lesions appears regular and well demarcated and usually does not extend below the level of the sweat glands.

In the involuting stage, proliferation has concluded and most of the cells at the base of the lesion have undergone keratinization. A mixed dermal infiltrate with granulation tissue may be present with fibrosis. The lesion flattens and finally disappears, leaving an atropic scar in its place.

KAs have characteristic histologic features that are best observed in a section cut through the center of a mature lesion. Although the histologic diagnosis is usually possible when an adequate and properly oriented biopsy specimen includes the lateral and lower margins of the lesion, the final diagnosis must be based on clinicopathologic correlation. A rapidly growing lesion exhibiting features of a well-differentiated squamous cell carcinoma is likely to be a KA, whereas a slowly enlarging tumor with similar histologic features but without regression is likely to be a squamous cell carcinoma.

Although a solitary lesion that occurs spontaneously and regresses is the classic prototype of KA, there are other clinical variants of the tumor that follow an unconventional clinical behavior. The Ferguson-Smith or self-healing lesion begins in adolescence or early adult life with hundreds of lesions on exposed and nonexposed areas. These familial lesions persist throughout the patient's life, suddenly appearing, fading and recurring, tending to be deeper and more destructive. Eruptive or Grzybowski lesions occur after the fourth decade of life and are characterized by hundreds to thousands of small pruritic papules on exposed and nonexposed areas.

KAs may be extremely aggressive, causing local tissue destruction, or may disappear spontaneously, leaving scarring that may have adverse effects. A tumor such as on the upper eyelid or an invasive giant KA variant greater than 3 cm occurring on the middle face requires active intervention. It is critical to recognize KAs that behave in an atypical manner. These must be differentiated from squamous cell carcinoma. Cases have been reported that were initially diagnosed as KA, but recurred after conservative therapy with rapidly spreading metastatic cutaneous lesions resulting in death.

In practice, it is often difficult to pathologically differentiate a well-differentiated squamous cell carcinoma from a KA. Keratocanthomas usually have intraepithelial elastic fibers, eosinophilic, ground glass cytoplasm with glycogen in a cup-shaped lesion with a well-defined border along with microabscesses—features that assist in differentiation.

Excision is the treatment of choice because it removes the specimen in its entirety. Complete excision including the deep margin allows the pathologist to evaluate the architectural pattern of the tumor to distinguish it from a squamous cell carcinoma. When differentiation between them cannot be made with certainty, an assessment of surgical margins is made to assess the adequacy of resection. The scar resulting from an excisional biopsy is more acceptable than that resulting from ablative techniques or the atrophic scar that can follow spontaneous resolution. A razor blade excision, starting a few millimeters outside the lesion and down to mid-dermis centrally, creates a convex defect. This simple technique provides material for histopathologic examination with minimal scarring.

Incisional biopsy is a limited procedure that is useful for a large KA or one that is in a location that would make excision technically difficult. Incisional biopsy frequently triggers spontaneous involution. To ensure adequate sampling, the incisional biopsy specimen should be large enough that the architecture of the tumor can be assessed. A proper biopsy specimen may be obtained by performing a wedge or an elliptical incisional biopsy through the center of the lesion, making certain to include the deep margin of the lesion. A punch biopsy does not allow evaluation of the overall configuration of the tumor.

Mohs Micrographic Surgery

KAs arising at sites of functional or cosmetic importance, particularly the nasal bridge, canthi, and periauricular regions, are appropriately treated by Mohs surgery. Giant KA threatening critical underlying structures is best treated by this technique as well. In a series of 43 treated lesions by Mohs surgery, there was only one recurrence after a follow-up period of six months to two years.

Destructive Procedures

Destructive procedures such as curettage and electrodesiccation or cryotherapy do not provide a specimen for histologic analysis and margin determination. Such therapy applied to a squamous cell carcinoma with a KA-like appearance might result in the local recurrence of a problematic tumor and allow an interval time for tumor invasion. Finally, the scars resulting from these procedures are often depressed and hypopigmented, which are no more desirable than the scar resulting from spontaneous involution.

Radiotherapy

A KA may be treated with radiotherapy in a dosage and fractionation similar to that used to treat squamous cell carcinoma. Radiotherapy may afford effective therapy in the elderly patient or in a patient with general poor health. Skin changes with radiation include telangiectasia and atrophy. These must be weighed against the disfiguring appearance and/or sequelae of an aggressive lesion. Lesions should be treated before they damage underlying cartilage, creating a less favorable cosmetic defect. Radiotherapy is useful for treating KAs not amenable to conventional treatment. However, there is a risk of developing a malignant lesion within the treatment field in later years.

Intralesional Chemotherapy

Surgical excision can result in functional and cosmetic defects when large or strategically located lesions are treated. A nonsurgical approach may be desirable in these cases.

Intralesional fluorouracil has displayed effectiveness in the treatment of KAs. Intralesional injection of 0.1 to 0.2 mL of 50 mg/mL 5-fluorouracil using a 27 to 30 gauge needle in a series of weekly injections for five to nine weeks was effective for small KAs. Large KAs treated with 1 to 2 mL at one- to four-week intervals for two to six treatments responded favorably without recurrence of lesions. However, intralesional 5-fluorouracil may be effective only in rapidly proliferating lesions. Topical 5% 5-fluorouracil has also been effective.

Intralesional interferon-a injected into the borders and into the base of large KAs (>2 cm) was successful in five out of six patients treated. The starting treatment was 3 × 3 million units per week increased to 3 × 6 M units per week for four to seven weeks. The main side effects were pain during injection and transitory fever, which responded to acetaminophen. Regression was obtained with good cosmetic results.

Treatment with intralesional methotrexate, infiltrated into the shoulder of the KA, into four quadrants at a depth of 2 to 8 mm with a 30 gauge needle in a way to blanch the entire rim of the lesion has been reported to be successful in the treatment of KAs. The dose was 0.4 to 1.5 mL of 12.5 or 25 mg/mL of methotrexate and was repeated in two weeks at follow-up if any portion of the lesion remained. The lesions responded with complete resolution after one or two injections with minimal scarring. No side effects were noted, and discomfort with injection was minimal with or without lidocaine. Intralesional therapy may be considered in patients with multiple lesions, relatively inaccessible locations, large lesions on the head and neck, and in cosmetically sensitive areas for lesions with histories and morphologies characteristic of KA.

Retinoids

Retinoids have been used in the treatment of KAs. Although the exact mechanism of action is unknown, these agents may act by regulating gene expression. Retinoids have been shown to be modulators of epithelial cell differentiation and can suppress carcinogenesis in a variety of epithelial tissues.

A few case reports have documented successful treatment of KA with oral retinoids. Etretinate has been used to treat patients with multiple KAs of the Ferguson-Smith type. Dosages of 1 mg/kg/day resulted in resolution of lesions, but new papular lesions reappeared when the dose was titrated down to 0.25 mg/kg/day. A maintenance dose of 0.75 mg/kg/every other day resulted in complete resolution of lesions. In a patient with eruptive KAs, etretinate 40 mg/day titrated down to 10 mg/day resulted in a gradual decrease in lesions over one month. Maintenance therapy of 10 mg/day was stopped, and a few lesions reappeared. Isotretinoin (13-*cis* retinoic acid) for solitary and multiple KAs has been documented in doses ranging from 0.5 to 1.0 mg/kg/day for 4 to 12 weeks with resolution of lesions. Also, a dosage of 1.5 mg/kg/day followed by a lower maintenance therapy resulted in clearing of lesions and prevention of new lesions.

Retinoid therapy is associated with multiple dose-related side effects. Mucocutaneous side effects, arthralgias, and elevation of serum cholesterol, triglycerides, and elevation of liver enzymes may occur. Retinoid therapy may be indicated for patients with multiple lesions, aggressive lesions, and in those cases where surgery would result in severe disfigurement. It may also be used as adjunctive therapy to maintain remission.

The single disadvantage of retinoid therapy and intralesional therapy is the lack of histological confirmation of the lesion before treatment. Therefore, it would be best to reserve this treatment for lesions verified by biopsy or for those that remain or recur postoperatively. A complete excision of the lesion should not be delayed if a response is not obtained promptly.

EPIDERMAL NEVUS

The epidermal nevus is an uncommon epidermal hamartoma present at birth or arising during childhood. It consists of wartlike and scaling overgrowths of the epidermis without nevus cells. It is often characterized by light brown, closely set hyperkeratotic papules in a linear distribution. Lesions tend to occur on the trunk and extremities. There is substantial clinical variation in the form of ichthyosis hystrix, nevus unius lateris, nevus verrucous, inflammatory linear verrucous nevus, and epidermal nevus syndrome. Extensive lesions may be associated with skeletal deformities, seizures, mental retardation, and neural deafness. In the epidermal nevus syndrome, there are associated abnormalities of the central nervous, vascular, and musculoskeletal systems. Malignant degeneration of epidermal nevi is unusual and usually consists of a basal cell carcinoma. KA has been reported to develop in some lesions, while in others malignant transformation beginning as Bowen's disease and becoming an invasive, well-differentiated squamous cell carcinoma has been described. Usually, cutaneous lesions occur without associated abnormalities, but they become a substantial cosmetic problem when located in exposed areas. Histologic patterns vary, displaying epidermal hyperplasia and papillomatous thickening, hypertrophy of the granular and cornified layers, with spotty areas of parakeratosis. Normal or abnormal appendages may appear or be distinctively inflammatory and psoriasiform or may show epidermolytic hyperkeratosis.

The variety of reported treatments for epidermal nevi are evidence of the adversity encountered treating these lesions. The treatment of epidermal nevi is often unsatisfactory, and treated lesions tend to recur within weeks to months. There are a collection of treatment case reports describing effective therapy in a very limited group of patients.

Nonsurgical treatments have consisted of keratolytics, topical or intralesional steroids, and topically applied tars. Steroid ointments as well as Dermojet injections have produced remission or pruritus and cutaneous lesions, but after a few months the lesions recur. Weekly application of 0.125% to 75% podophyllin ointment under occlusion for nine months resulted in a complete cure during a three-month follow-up period in one case report. However, the application of podophyllin ointment over a large area of skin or in areas of maceration may lead to systemic absorption and is associated with central nervous system toxicity, renal damage, thrombocytopenia, and death. For these reasons, treatment with topical podophyllin is not recommended (Figs. 5–7). Topical steroids can result in decreased erythema and inflammation; however, these results are only temporary.

Excision

Surgical excision has been cited as the treatment of choice. However, to avoid recurrence, a full-thickness excision is necessary and may be impractical for large lesions and also can lead to problematic scarring.

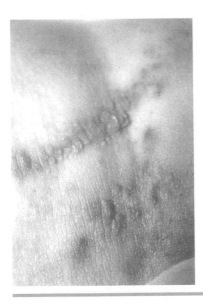

Figure 5 Epidermal nevus involving the medial thigh of a 30-year-old woman.

Dermabrasion

The treatment of epidermal nevi by dermabrasion is effective in removal of epidermal nevus lesions but usually produces scarring. Recurrence of lesions after dermabrasion has been reported. Success depends on complete removal of the epidermis and dermal component. Scarring depends on the depth of the lesion's involvement in the dermis.

Cryosurgery

Cryosurgery employing a freeze-thaw cycle of 1 to 2 minutes thawing time and repeating this cycle one time has been described as effective. Local anesthetic is necessary because a deep freeze with liquid nitrogen produces a significant amount of discomfort. Scarring results, and it is often more prominent than scarring resulting from carbon dioxide laser vaporization. There is also some limitation on the amount of nevus treated by cryotherapy in a single session.

Carbon Dioxide Laser

The carbon dioxide laser is used at low wattage in the defocused mode to vaporize the abnormal epidermis. Two to three passes over the treatment area are necessary before normal-appearing dermis is achieved. The CO_2 laser offers many advantages over topical and excision methods for

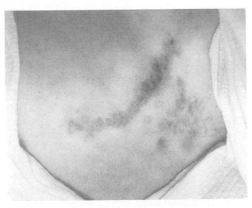

Figure 6 Epidermal nevus immediately following vaporization by carbon dioxide laser.

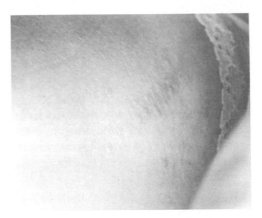

Figure 7 Scar six months following carbon dioxide laser ablation of epidermal nevus.

treating Epidermal Nevi. New advances in CO_2 lasers allow for proper tissue ablation. The A curet is useful between passes to help define a normal dermal plane. Residual epidermal nevus has a characteristically darker appearance than adjacent, uninvolved tissue. It is often beneficial to treat large lesions in segments at six-week intervals. This may minimize the risk of hypertrophic scar formation. Even with laser surgery, some degree of scarring, yet this can be minimized with the latest short-pulsed systems, because of controlled tissue heating, may result. Treatment of verrucous nevi with argon laser requires multiple treatments and may result in hypopigmentation.

Surgical excision, dermabrasion, cryotherapy, CO_2 laser, and argon laser may produce acceptable cosmetic results in some patients, but there is the risk of recurrence. When a surgical procedure is selected, it should be the one that will afford the highest chance of success with the least amount of morbidity for the patient.

Recently a linear verrucous epidermal nevus was treated using a combination of topical tretinoin 0.1% and 5% 5-fluorouracil for 3–6 months twice a day under occlusion. The lesions resolved with minimal postinflammatory hyperpigmentation. Recurrence of the lesions after three to four weeks prompted reinitiation of therapy on a twice-weekly basis, with apparent good results.

WARTS (VERRUCA)

Warts are benign epidermal tumors of the skin occurring in adults and children. They are induced by the HPV. The HPV is a double-stranded DNA virus enclosed in an icosahedral capsid. Clinical lesions of warts include common warts (verruca vulgaris), filiform warts, flat warts (verruca plana), plantar warts (including myrmecia and mosaic types), anogenital warts, and bowenoid papulosis. Extracutaneous lesions occur on mucous membranes and include oral common warts, oral condylomata acuminata, focal epithelial hyperplasia, oral florid papillomatosis, nasal papillomas, conjunctival papillomas, laryngeal papillomatosis, and cervical warts.

Common warts are rough keratotic papules that occur on the dorsal hands, fingers, or knees of children. Butcher's warts are commonly caused by HPV-7 and are found on the hands and fingers of meat cutters. Flat warts are slightly elevated flesh-colored to gray or brown smooth papules. The Koebner phenomenon is common in flat warts. Plantar warts are covered with a thick hyperkeratotic surface with punctate black dots or thrombosed capillaries. A mosaic wart is the result of multiple warts coalescing into a large plaque. Condyloma acuminatum or anogenital warts consist of hyperplastic, verrucous papules, which may coalesce into cauliflowerlike lesions.

Small, macular, and slightly elevated lesions have been defected on normal-appearing penile skin after the application of 5% acetic acid. Bowenoid papulosis consists of multiple, small, velvety pigmented papules in the anogenital region. HPV-16 and HPV-18 virus have been demonstrated in lesions of bowenoid papulosis.

Histologic features of common warts are acanthosis, papillomatosis, hyperkeratosis, and parakeratosis with acanthotic rete ridges. There are foci of vacuolated cells, referred to as koilocytes, and foci of clumped keratohyalin granules. Plantar warts (myrmecia) contain large eosinophilic inclusions within the cytoplasm of keratinocytes. Flat warts have a diffuse zone of vacuolated cells in the upper stratum corneum but, unlike verrucae vulgaris, have no papillomatosis or areas of parakeratosis. Anogenital warts show considerable acanthosis, with thickening and elongation of the rete ridges. Bowenoid papulosis shows changes of carcinoma in situ of Bowen's disease with an irregular, "wind-blown" arrangement of nuclei.

Although warts are often of cosmetic importance, they can also be painful or even disabling. They are common in immunosuppressed patients. There are many effective treatments for warts. The treatment choice should be based on the size and location of lesions, patient compliance, effectiveness of previous treatments, and cost factors. Common treatment of warts involves physically destroying the cells infected with virus. Pulse Dye Laser has also been shown to produce excellent results in treatment of warts. Keratolytic agents such as salicylic, lactic, and trichloroacetic acids cause simple destruction of the epithelial cells infected with papilloma virus. Destruction of the wart can be accomplished by cryosurgery, curettage, or electrocautery. However, to be effective, any form of therapy must remove the entire wart and eradicate all of the virus, otherwise recurrences are common. Chemotherapeutic agents such as podophyllin, bleomycin, and 5-fluorouracil are reported to be effective. When traditional forms of therapy prove to be ineffective, surgical removal with the carbon dioxide laser is often performed.

Salicylic Acid

Salicyclic acid is topically applied in concentrations of 15% to 40%. It is usually a simple first-line treatment with few complications. Patients are instructed to soak the wart in warm water for approximately five minutes and to remove any loose tissue with a pumice stone or an emery board. The salicylic acid is then applied to the wart surface, which may be covered with an adhesive bandage. The procedure is repeated once or twice daily as tolerated. Vaseline may be placed around the wart to minimize irritation to unaffected tissue. Hand warts treated with salicylic acid or liquid nitrogen alone had similar cure rates, whereas combination therapy showed higher cure rates. However, keratolytic agents applied every second day under occlusive dressing proved to be more beneficial than daily application alone.

Cryotherapy

One of the most common office procedures for the treatment of warts is cryosurgery. Liquid nitrogen is applied to the wart surface with a cotton-tipped applicator or with a liquid nitrogen spray. Before treatment, excessive keratin is removed with a #15 scalpel blade, as this acts as an insulator. This is necessary for plantar warts, but plane warts and anogenital warts with scant keratin freeze more readily. The liquid nitrogen is applied to the wart until a 1- to 2-mm halo surrounds the wart base, indicating that the full depth has been frozen. Usually two freeze-thaw cycles are performed. The interval between treatments should be no longer than three weeks, and less if response is not obtained. A salicylic acid preparation may be applied between treatments. Patients experience a burning sensation while warts are being frozen and may have throbbing pain afterwards. Patients with a low pain threshold can be helped by taking an analgesic one-half hour before treatment or at bedtime if the throbbing persists. There are generally few complications with cryosurgery. However, side effects include edema, necrosis, blister formation, hypopigmentation, and a slight risk of superficial nerve damage. Periungual verrucae using a cotton-tipped applicator should encompass the lesion plus a small rim of normal tissue. The intent of freezing is necrosis with the development of a bulla, usually hemorrhagic because of the dermal-epidermal separation. Large or multiple warts that encircle the nail should be treated in sections. Healing occurs without scarring, but retraction of the nail can rarely occur. Recalcitrant warts or those that extend beneath the nail plate are not good candidates for cryosurgery.

Caustic Acids

The application of acids, such as trichloroacetic acid 50%, destroys cellular protein, which causes inflammation and cell death. It is applied to the wart surface after excessive keratin is removed. Therapy is repeated at weekly intervals until the wart resolves.

Glutaraldehyde

Glutaraldehyde is used topically as a freshly prepared buffered solution. It fixes keratin and has a success rate analogous to topical salicylic acid. Side effects are drying and fissuring of the skin, possible sensitization to glutaraldehyde, and brown staining of skin.

Surgery

Simple surgical excision of warts may be effective when few warts are present. The area is infiltrated with local anesthetic. The wart is dissected away from the surrounding tissue, and any remaining wart is removed by curettage. The base and the sides of the wound are treated with electrodesiccation to stop the bleeding, and a dry dressing is applied. However, there is still a significant risk of recurrence with surgery and the potential risk of scarring.

Bleomycin

Intralesional bleomycin has been used in the treatment of recalcitrant warts. Bleomycin inhibits DNA synthesis and repair causing tissue necrosis and a hemorrhagic scar. The agent is diluted with 0.9% sodium chloride to 1 U/mL. Small amounts of 0.05 to 0.1 mL are injected into individual warts. The solution is stable for four months under refrigeration. However, James et al. found that bleomycin 1 mg/mL stored at -20°C in glass containers led to no significant loss of immunore-activity in 27 months. The use of intralesional bleomycin in the treatment of warts may result in systemic drug exposure and this treatment should be avoided in pregnant women or women of childbearing age. However, intralesional bleomycin has not been associated with any systemic toxicity.

A dose of 0.1 to 0.2 mL is injected into the wart with a 30-gauge syringe to achieve blanching. In one study the cure rate was 77% for warts on the extremities, 71.4% for periungual warts, and 47.6% for plantar warts after one or two treatments.

The multiple puncture technique using a bifurcated vaccination needle resulted in elimination of 92% of warts after a single treatment. The wart is soaked for 10 minutes in warm water to hydrate the keratin, and plain lidocaine is injected. Bleomycin solution (l U/mL) is dropped onto the wart surface with a tuberculin syringe. The wart surface is punctured 40 times per 5 mm of wart surface and the needle must penetrate to the wart base. A dry dressing is applied, and patients may experience local pain.

The bifurcated needle technique uses less than one-tenth of the amount of bleomycin than the intralesional technique. Therefore, it may introduce bleomycin more uniformly into the wart and lead to lower peak blood levels. Intralesional bleomycin is associated with moderate to severe pain and may require prior local anesthesia. Tenderness or pain at the treatment site can occur from one to seven days after injection. Patients may need to take aspirin or acetaminophen, and some patients may require a codeine-containing analgesic for a day or two. Extreme caution is necessary when treating periungual warts, since loss of nails or permanent nail dystrophy may occur. Scarring or local urticaria has been reported. It is judicious to refrain from treating patients with symptoms of unusual sensitivity to cold suggestive of Raynaud's disease, as isolated reports of Raynaud's phenomenon developing after intralesional injection of finger warts have been described.

Interferon Therapy

Interferons are a family of proteins and glycoproteins, which occur naturally in the body and are now able to be produced by recombinant biotechnology. These naturally occurring hormones have antiviral, antiproliferative, antitumor, and immunomodulatory activities.

Interferon (1 million units) injected into genital warts (condylomata acuminata) three times a week for three weeks cleared 36% of patients and produced a reduction in mean wart area of 39.9%. The most common adverse effects of recombinant interferon-α therapy for warts are fever, chills, headache, myalgia, and pain at the injection site. These effects are usually mild, with decreasing intensity during treatment, and rarely interfere with daily routines. Interferon-α injected with a Dermo-Jet twice a week produced clearance of hand and plantar warts. This method enhances patient acceptance by significantly reducing local pain at the injection site. While some studies have shown promising results for condyloma acuminata, plantar warts have displayed no response in some reports. The role of interferon in the treatment of verruca remains to be elucidated, although recent studies have shown complete cure of recalcitrant and extensive periungual and subungual warts after IFN– treatment.

Podophyllotoxin

Genital warts have been successfully treated using a 0.5% solution of podophyllotoxin. The solution is applied twice a day by the patient for three days for a cycle of three weeks. This preparation can be applied by the patient and has a greater safety profile than the resin. Side effects are generally well tolerated and consist of mild erythema, burning, and tenderness.

Carbon Dioxide Laser

Carbon dioxide laser is a therapeutic technique reserved for the treatment of recalcitrant warts. In the defocused mode, the CO_2 laser can vaporize tissue in a relatively bloodless field. Local anesthesia is injected into the area being treated. A power setting of 3 to 10 W, depending on the thickness of the tissue, is used. After each pass, the resultant charred tissue is removed with a curette or gauze pad. The laser beam is moved slowly over the wart surface in a series of passes. The first pass should include a 5-mm border beyond the visible edge of the wart, as papillomavirus has been demonstrated in apparently normal tissue. Three to four passes are continued until all visible signs of warts tissue are removed. The cessation of treatment is based on clinical judgment. The patient is advised to perform local wound care until reepithelialization takes place. Healing may take four to eight weeks to occur. During the procedure, the patient and the staff should wear protective goggles, and safety masks, and the immediate perioperative area should be protected by moist surgical drapes. The smoke and vapor plume should be extracted with a vacuum system. This is necessary to minimize hazard to both patient and staff, as papillomavirus has been detected in the vapor of warts treated with carbon dioxide laser and electrocoagulation.

Carbon dioxide laser treatment may eradicate recalcitrant warts after other therapeutic methods have failed. Cure rates of 56% for hand and foot warts that have failed prior treatments and cure rates of 71% for periungual warts with one or two treatments have been reported. In another study 81% of recalcitrant hand and foot warts were cured during a six-month follow-up with one treatment, 15% required a second treatment, and 4% three treatments.

Side effects include postoperative pain after laser treatment, scarring, and loss of function. Pain can vary from mild to moderate in severity. In the treatment of periungual warts, there was significant pain in some patients as well as changes such as distal onycholysis, nail thickening, nail curvature, and grooves.

The reappearance of warts can occur after any treatment. This may be due to incomplete treatment, latent infection in normal-appearing tissue, or reexposure to the papillomavirus.

Pulse Dye Laser

A pulse dye laser can be used to destroy wart capillaries, since the oxyhemoglobin contained in such vessels absorbs yellow light. Post-treatment the wart can become dry and darkened with minimal post-operative pain.

Immune Response Modulators

Aldara an Immune Response Modulator is now used commonly for the treatment of warts. It is a topical lotion which is rubbed around the wart. While Aldara does not exhibit any antiviral ability of its own, it works by stimulating surrounding white blood cells to respond to the warts. However, this medication is only currently FDA approved for genital warts. It is believed that Aldara might work via the induction of cytokines for example Alpha-interaction (a complex found in the body which has antiviral activity).

BIBLIOGRAPHY

Altaian J, Mehregan AH. Inflammatory linear verrucose epidermal nevus. Arch Dermatol 1971; 104:385–389.

Amer M, Diab N, Ramadan A, Galal A, et al. Therapeutic evaluation for intralesional injection of bleomycin ulfate in 143 resistant warts. J Am Acad Dermatol 1991; 17:234–236.

Barrasso R, DeBrux J, Croissant O, et al. High prevalence of papillomavirus-associated penile intraepithelial eoplasia in sexual partners of women with cervical intraepithelial neoplasia. TV Engl J Med 1987; 317: 916–923.

Benoldi D, Alinovi A. Multiple persistant keratoacanthomas: Treatment with oral etretinate. J Am Acad Dermatol 1984; 10:1035–1038.

Bolognia JL. Biopsy techniques for pigmented lesions. ASDS J 2000; 26:89–91.

Boyce, Sarah, Alster, Tina. CO2 laser treatment of epidermal nevi: long-term success. ASDS J 2002; 28:611–614.

Brook I. Microbiology of infected epidermoid cysts. Arch Dermatol 1989; 125:1658.

Bunney MH, Nolan MW, Williams DA. An assessment of methods of treating viral warts by comparative treatment trials based on a standard design. Br J Dermatol 1976; 94: 667–676.

Bunney MH. Viral Warts: Their Biology and Treatment. Oxford, : Oxford University Press, 1982.

Burgdorf WHC. Tumors of sebaceous gland differentiation in Pathology of the Skin. Farmer ER, Hood AF, eds. Norwalk, CT, : Appleton and Lange, 1990, :p. 617.

Burton CS, Sawchuk WS. Premature sebaceous gland hyperplasia: successful treatment with isotretinoin. J Am Acad Dermatol 1985; 12:182–184.

Cassidy DE, et al. Podophyllin toxicity: Report of a fatal case and review of literature. J Toxicol Clin Toxicol 1982; 19:35–44.

Cohen BH. Prevention of postdermabrasion milia (letter). J Dermatol Surg Oncol 1988; 14(ll):1301.

Cohen JH., Lessin SR. Vowels BR, et al. The sign of Leser-Trélat in associated with Sezary syndrome: simultaneous disappearance of seborrheic keratosis and malignant T-cell clone during combined therapy with photopheresis and interferon alpha. Arch Dermatol 1993; 129:1213–1215.

Cox, Sue Ellan. Rapid development of keratoacanthomas after a body peel. ASDS J 2003; 29:201–203.

De Villez RL, Roberts LC. Premature sebaceous gland hyperplasia. J Am Acad Dermatol 1982; 6:933–935.

Donohe B, Cooper JS, Rush S. Treatment of aggressive keratoacanthomas by radiotherapy. J Am Acad Dermatol 1990; 23: 489–493.

Duque MI et al. Frequency of seborrheic keratosis in the United States: a benchmark of skin lesion care quality and cost effectiveness. ASDS J 2003; 29:796–801.

Epstein E. Intralesional bleomycin and Raynaud's phenomenon (letter). J Am Acad Dermatol 1991; 24:785–786.

Epstein W, Kligman AM. The pathogenesis of milia and benign tumors of the skin. J Invest Dermatol 1956; 26:1–11.

Eron LJ, Judson F, Tucker S, Prawer S, et al. Interferon therapy for conylomata acuminata. N Engl J Med 1986; 315:1059–1064.

Eubanks SW, Gentry RH, Patterson JW, May DL. Treatment of multiple keratoacanthomas with intralesional fluorouracil. J Am Acad Dermatol 1982; 7:126–129.

Fisher BK, Macpherson M. Epidermoid cyst of the sole. J Am Acad Dermatol 1986; 15:1127–1129.

Fox BJ, Lapins NA. Comparison of treatment modalities for epidermal nevus: a case report and review. Dermatol Surg Oncol 1983; 9(ll):879–885.

Garb J. Nevus verrucosus unilateris cured with podophyllin ointment. Arch Dermatol 1960; 81:606–609.

Gewirtzman, Aron. Eruptive keratoacanthamos following carbon dioxide laser. ASDS J 1999; 25:666–668.

Golitz LE, Western WL. Inflammatory linear verrucous epidermal nevus associated with epidermal nevus syndrome. Arch Dermatol 1979; 115:1208–1209.

Golitz LE, Poomeechaiwong S. Cysts. In Pathology of the Skin. Farmer ER, Hood AF, eds. Norwalk, CT, : Appleton & Lange, 1990, pp. :516–517.

Goldberg LH, Rosen T, Becker J, Knauss A. Treatment of solitary keratoacanthomas with isotretinoin. J Am Acad Dermatol 1990; 23:934–936.

Grob JJ, Suzini F, Weiller RM, et al. Large keratoacanthomas treated with intralesional interferon alfa-2a. J Am Acad Dermatol 1993; 29:237–241.

Hayes ME, O''Keefe EJ. Reduced dose of Bleomycin in the treatment of recalcitrant warts. J Am Acad Dermatol 1986; 15:1002–1006.

Hodak E, Jones RE, Ackerman AB, et al. Controversies in dermatology. Solitary keratoacanthoma is a squamous cell carcinoma: three examples with metastasis. Am J Dermatopathol 1993; 15:332–352.

Hodge SJ, Barr JM, Owen LG. Inflammatory linear verrucose epidermal nevus. Arch Dermatol 1978; 114:436–438.

Holdiness MR. On the classification of the sign of Leser-Trélat. J Am Acad Dermatol 1988; 19:754–757.

Hong WK, Lippman SM, Itri LM, et al. Prevention of second primary tumors with isotretinoin in squamous-cell carcinoma of the head and neck. N Engl J Med 1990; 323:795–801.

Hurwitz S. Epidermal nevi and tumors of epidermal origin. Ped Clin North Am 1983; 30:483–494.

James MP, Collier PM, Aherne W, Hardcastle A. Histologic, pharmacologic and immunocytochemical effect of injection of bleomycin into viral warts. J Am Acad Dermatol 1993; 28:933–937.

Johannesson A. Razor blade surgery of keratoacanthoma. J Dermatol Surg Oncol 1986; 12:1056–1057.

Kao GF. Benign tumors of the epidermis. In Pathology of the Skin, Farmer ER, Hood AF, eds. Norwalk, CT, : Appleton & Lange, 1990, pp. :537–546.

Kettler AH, Goldberg LH. Seborrheic keratosis. Am Fam Phys 1986; 34(2):147–152.

Klin Baruch, Ashkenazi. Sebaceous cyst excision with minimal surgery. Am Fam Phys 1990; 41(6): 1746–1748.

Kopf AW. Keratoacanthoma. In Cancer of the Skin. Andrade R, Gumport SL, Popkin GL, Rees TD, eds. Philadelphia,: W.B. Saunders Co, 1976, pp. :755–781.

Kuflik EG. Specific indications for cryosurgery of the nail unit. J Dermatol Surg Oncol 1992; 18:702–706.

Laing V, Knipe RC, Flowers FP, Stoer CB, Ramos-Caro FA. Proliferating trichilemmal tumor: report of a case and review of the literature. J Dermatol Surg Oncol 1991; 17:295–298.

Landthaler M, Haina D, Waidelich W, et al. Argon laser therapy of verrucous nevi. Plast Reconstr Surg 1984; 74:108–111.

Larson PO. Keratoacanthomas treated with Mohs micrographic surgery (chemosurgery): a review of forty cases. J Am Acad Dermatol 1987; 16:1040–1044.

Leppard BJ, Sanderson KV. The natural history of trichilemmal cyst. BJD 1976; 94:379–389.

Lever WF, Schaumburg-Lever G, eds. Histopathology of the Skin. Philadelphia,: JB Lippincott, 1990, pp. :411–418, 535–536.

Lieblich LM, Geronemus RG, Gibbs RC. Use of a punch for removal of epithelial cyst. J Dermatol Surg Oncol 1982; 8(12):1059–1062.

Logan RA, Zachary CB. Outcome of carbon dioxide laser therapy for persistent cutaneous viral warts. Br J Dermatol 1989; 121:99–95.

Maeda M,. Mori Shunji M. Seborrheic keratosis with focal acatholysisacantholysis. J Dermatol 1989; 16:79–81.

Mahler D, Ben-yaker, Rosenberg L. Linear verrucous nevus. J Dermatol Surg Oncol 1981; 7:262–265.

Manz LA, Pelachyk JM. Bleomycin-lidocaine mixture reduces pain of intralesional injection in the treatment of recalcitrant verrucae. J Am Acad Dermatol 1991; 25:524–526.

Martin H, Strong E, Spiro RH. Radiation-induced skin cancer of the head and neck. Cancer 1970; 2:61–71.

McBurney, El, Rosen DA. Carbon dioxide laser treatment of verrucae vulgares. J Dermatol Surg Oncol 1984; 10:145–148.

McGavran MN, Binnington B. Keratinous cysts of the skin. Identification and differentiation of pilar cyst from epidermal cysts. Arch Dermatol 1966; 94:499–508.

Mehregan AH, Lee KC. Malignant proliferating trichilemmal tumors—report of three cases. J Dermatol Surg Oncol 1987; 13(12):1339–1342.

Mehrabi, Don, Brodell RT. Use of the alexandrite laser for treatment of seborrheic keratosis. ASDS J 2002; 28:437–439.

Mehrabi D, leonhardt JM, Brodell RT. Removal of keratinous and pilar cysts with a punch incision. ASDS J 2002; 28:673–677.

Melton JL, Nelson BR, Stough DB, Brown MD, Swanson NA, Johnson TM. Treatment of keratoacanthomas with intralesional methotrexate. J Am Acad Dermatol 1991; 25: 1017–1023.

Morag C, Metzker A. Inflammatory linear verrucous epidermal nevus: report of seven new cases and review of the literature. Pediatr Dermatol 1985; 3:15–18.

Morison WL. Viral warts, herpes simplex and herpes zoster in patients with secondary immune deficiencies and neoplasms. Br J Dermatol 1975; 92:625.

Naples SP, Brodell RT. Verruca vulgaris. Arch Dermatol 1993; 129:698–700.

Nelson BR, Kolansky G, Gillard M, et al. Management of linear epidermal nevus treated with topical 5-fluo-rouracil 5% and tretinoin. J Am Acad Dermatol 1994; 30:287–288.

No D, McClaren M, Chotzen V, Kilmer SL. Sebaceous hyperplasia treated with a 1450-nm diode laser. ASDS J 2004; 30:382–384.

Oliveira AS, Picoto AS, Verde SF, Martins O. A simple method of excising tricholemmal cysts from the scalp. J Dennatal Surg Oncol 1979; 5(8):625–627.

Orth G, Jablonska S. Favre M, et al. Identification of papillomavirus in butcher's warts. J Invest Dermatol 1981; 76:97–102.

Parker CM, Hanke CW. Large keratoacanthomas in difficult locations treated with intralesional 5-fluorouracil. J Am Acad Dermatol 1986; 14:770–777.

Pepper E. Dermabrasion for the treatment of a giant seborrheic keratosis. J Dermatol Surg Oncol 1985; 11(6):646–647.

Pollack SV. Electrosurgery of the Skin; Electrodesiccation and Electrofulguration. New York,: Churchill Livingstone, 1991, pp. :31–35.

Popkin GL, Brodie SJ, Hyman AB, Andrade R, Kopf AW. A technique of biopsy recommended for keratoacanthomas. Arch Dermatol 1966; 94:191–193.

Rapaport J. Giant keratoacanthoma of the nose. Arch Dermatol 1975; 111:73–75.

Ratz JL, Bailin PL, Wheeland RG. Carbon dioxide laser treatment of epidermal nevi. J Dermatol Surg Oncol 1986; 12:567–570.

Requena L, Romero E, Sanchez M, Ambrojo P, Yus ES. Aggressive keratoacanthoma of the eyelid: "malignant" keratoacanthoma or squamous cell carcinoma. J Dermatol Surg Oncol 1990; 16:564–568.

Rios, AS, Ocampo CJ. Giant epidermoid cyst: clinical aspect and surgical management. J Dermatol Surg Oncol 1986; 12(7): 734–736.

Rosen T. Keratoacanthomas arising within a linear epidermal nevus. J Dermatol Surg Oncol 1982; 8:878–880.

Rosian R, Goslen JB, Brodell RT. The treatment of benign sebaceous hyperplasia with the topical application of bichloracetic acid. J Dermatol Surg Oncol 1991; 17:876–879.

Ross BS et al. Pulse dye laser treatment of warts: an update. ASDS J 1999; 25:377–380.

Sawchuk WS, Weber PJ, Lowry DR, Dzubow LM. Infectious papillomavirus in the vapor of warts treated with carbon dioxide laser of electrocoagulation: detection and protection. J Am Acad Dermatol 1989; 21:41–49.

Schwartz RA. The keratoacanthoma: a review. J Surg Oncol 1979; 12:305–317.

Shaw JC, White CR. Treatment of multiple keratoacanthomas with oral isotretinoin. J Am Acad Dermatol 1986; 15:1079–1082.

Shelley WB, Shelly D. Intralesional bleomycin sulfate therapy for warts. Arch Dermatol 1991; 25:524–526.

Sloan JB, Jawoesky, C. Clinical misdiagnosis of squamous cell carcinoma in situ as seborrheic keratosis, a prospective study. J Dermatol Surg Oncol 1993; 17:413–416.

Solomon LM, Fretzin DF, Dewald RL. The epidermal nevus syndrome. Arch Dermatol 1968; 97:273–285.

Stadler R, Mayer da Silva, Bratzke B, et al. Interferons in dermatology. J Am Acad Dermatol 1989; 20:650–656.

Stegman SJ, Tromovitch TA, Glogau RG, Cosmetic Dermatologic Surgery; 2nd ed. Chicago: Year Book Medical Publishers, 1990, pp. :20–21.

Stegman SJ, Tromovitch TA, Glogau RG. Benign facial lesions. In Cosmetic Dermatologic Surgery. 2nd ed., Chicago, : Year Book Medical Publishers, 1990, p. :26.

Street ML, Roenigk RK. Recalcitrant periungual verrucae: the role of carbon dioxide vaporization. J Am Acad Dermatol 1990; 23:115–120.

Strong EW. Treatment of head and neck cancers. J Dermatol Surg Oncol 1983; 19:644–646.

Swint RB, Klaus SN. Malignant degeneration of an epithelial nevus. Arch Dermatol 1970; 101:56–58.

Thomas I, Kihiczak NI, Rothenberg J, et al. Melanoma within the seborrheic keratosis. ASDS J 2004; 30:559–561.

Tosti, Antonella, Piraccini BM. Warts of the nail unit: surgical and nonsurgical approaches. ASDS J 2001; 27:235–239.

Vance JC, Bart BJ, Hansen RC, Reichman RC. Intralesional recombinant alpha-2 interferon for the treatment of patients with condyloma acuminatum or verruca plantaris. Arch Dermatol 1986; 122:272–277.

Veien NK, Madsen SM, Avrach W, et al. The treatment of plantar warts with a keratolytic agent and occlusion. J Dermatol Treat 1991; 2:59–61.

Wheeland RG, Wiley MD. Q-tip cryosurgery for the treatment of senile sebaceous hyperplasia. J Dermatol Surg OncoZl 1987; 13:729–730.

Winkelmann RK, Brown J. Generalized eruptive keratoacanthoma. Arch Dermatol 1968; 97:615–623.

Winer LH, Levin GH. Pigmented basal cell epitheliomas arising in a linear nevus. Arch Dermatol 1961; 83:114–118.

Yoshikawa K, Hirano S, Kato T, Mizuno N. A case of eruptive keratoacanthoma treated by oral etretinate. Br J Dermatol 1985; 112:579–583.

34

Benign Soft Tissue Tumors

Richard M. Rubenstein and Kevin Spohr

Dermal and Subcutaneous Tumors, Wellington Regional Medical Center, Wellington, Florida, U.S.A.

DERMATOFIBROMAS

Dermatofibromas are benign dermal tumors that usually present as a papule or nodule on the lower extremities (Fig. 1). They are generally solitary, although multiple lesions do occur. Women are affected more frequently than men, and often there is a history of trauma or insect bite.

The typical lesion is a 0.5 to 1 cm dome-shaped, firm brown nodule attached to the overlying skin, but freely movable, and unattached to the subcutaneous tissues. Lateral compression on the tumor produces a depression or characteristic dimple sign. These tumors may grow rapidly in a short period, then reach a maximal size and persist. Regression occurs uncommonly.

Histologically, dermatofibromas are composed of fibroblasts, mature collagen, capillaries, and histiocytes. They may appear fibrous if they are composed mainly of fibroblasts and collagen or cellular if histiocytes predominate. The epidermis is spared, but the tumor can involve much of the dermis and extend into the subcutis.

Treatment of dermatofibromas is not necessary. Reassuring the patient of the benign nature of the lesion is frequently all that is required. If treatment is requested, surgical excision is the method of choice. Since the tumor can extend into the deep layers of the subcutis, a deep elliptical excision is recommended with removal of all tissue to the fascial layer. The lateral margins need only encompass the nodule itself. It is important, however, to distinguish this entity from dermatofibrosarcoma protuberans, as the latter entity is an aggressive recurring tumor. Adequate deep surgical specimens will help in this regard. The defect created is usually not large and can be closed after careful undermining with subcutaneous and skin sutures. Because these lesions are usually on the lower extremity, risks inherent to that location, such as wound separation, infection, or slower healing, must be considered during the postoperative care. Alternatively, superficial lesions may be treated with a #15 blade shave excision, allowing the wound to heal by secondary intention. Cryotherapy has also been reported to be effective in selected cases, with some risk of hypopigmentation. It is important to inform patients that the ultimate cosmetic outcome of dermatofibroma treatment on the lower extremities may be far from optimal. Recurrence is less than 5% and is probably related to the incomplete removal of the deepest layers.

KELOIDS

Hypertrophic scars, or keloids, are proliferations of fibrous tissue, usually occurring in sites of tissue injury. By definition, a hypertrophic scar remains in the boundary of the site of initial trauma, while keloids grow beyond this area. Keloids are firm, slightly tender or pruritic, hyperpigmented nodules or tumors (Fig. 2). They tend to occur in areas where skin tension from underlying musculature pulls across the wound, such as the deltoid region or on the anterior chest. Then, there is a rapid growth phase lasting several weeks or months after the inciting event, followed by a more stable period of growth. There is a genetic predilection, especially in black patients. Histologically, there is a fibroblastic proliferation, with formation of new collagen bundles.

Both hypertrophic scars and keloids have increased cellularity compared to normal dermis. There is an abundance of extracellular material, primarily chondroitin 4-sulfate. Collagen synthesis is both increased and abnormal while collagen degradation may also be altered.

The treatment of keloids includes the combination of surgery and intralesional corticosteroids. There is a high risk of recurrence with most forms of therapy, which is sometimes greater than the risk from the original lesion. Smaller keloids may be excised entirely, but it is important that the wound be closed without tension. This is done with wide undermining and closure in skin-tension lines. Larger keloids may be shaved with the scalpel and allowed to heal by second intention. Hemostasis is obtained with pressure, using as little cautery as possible to avoid damage to the dermis and subsequent fibroblast proliferation. The base of the wound is injected with intralesional corticosteroids at the time of surgery and at two-week intervals. The dose of triamcinolone acetonide is diluted with physiologic saline to concentrations of 5 to 40 mg/ml. A 30-gauge needle is used for injections. Intradermal or intralesional injections through the base of the lesion should result in significant blanching. Larger-gauge needles are required for thick, fibrous lesions. The concentration of glucocortoid is titrated with the clinical response. Adverse effects may include pain, atrophy, and hypopigmentation. Recurrence of keloid may occur up to two years after treatment.

Cryotherapy has been used in the treatment of keloids. Repeated vigorous freezes at two- to three-week intervals may be helpful, but will probably not result in complete resolution. Cryotherapy preceding intralesional steroids may yield better results. Edema following a freeze–thaw cycle of cryotherapy may make intralesional injections easier. Concern for hypopigmentation in darker skin individuals should be considered.

Pressure is useful to prevent recurrences of keloids after surgical excision. The mechanism of action may be related to

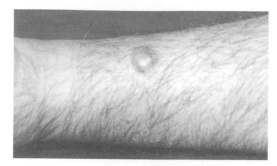

Figure 1 Dermatofibroma.

tissue ischemia and increased collagenase activity. Pressure must be maintained for six months or more, and can be in the form of elastic garments, corsets, or adhesive wraps. A spring pressure device has been reported to be effective to prevent recurrences of ear-lobe keloids. Unfortunately, the pressure devices must be worn up to 18 hours a day, and can be cumbersome to the patient. Older keloids are less likely to respond.

Laser therapy has brought significant advances in the treatment of keloids. The use of carbon dioxide, argon, and Nd:YAG lasers did not prove to offer advantages over scalpel surgery, as high rates of recurrence were noted, as well as unacceptable side effects, including pigment changes and atrophy. Pulse dye laser (PDL) has shown excellent responses in the treatment of keloids. The mechanism of action of PDL involves the targeting of the vascular component of the keloid. Other theories include laser-induced hypoxia, destruction of disulfide bonds, and collagenolysis.

Topical anesthesia with lidocaine-type products such as Elamax (Ferndale) or EMLA (Astra Pharmaceuticals) may be applied 30 to 60 minutes with or without occlusion to the affected area to prevent local discomfort. It is useful to moisten hair-bearing areas with saline to slow thermal conduction. Treatment with PDL is begun at low fluences, and generally will require multiple sessions. Higher fluences may be used at subsequent sessions, or in thicker or darker keloids. The patient will frequently experience postoperative purpura after PDL treatment, lasting seven to 14 days. Hyperpigmentation is also common and may be treated with hydroquinone-type bleaching creams. If hyperpigmentation occurs, follow-up sessions may be delayed to avoid the pigment acting as a competing chromophore. If postoperative crusting or edema is significant, lower fluences should be used in later sessions. Avoidance of overlapping pulses may also be helpful. Generally, side effects from PDL treatment of keloids are temporary and well tolerated.

In general, multiple PDL sessions are required to treat keloids. Thicker keloids will require the most sessions, with slower improvement in scar texture, erythema, and associated symptomatology. Combination therapy with intralesional corticosteroids may show added benefit. Overall PDL therapy has been a major advance in the treatment of keloids.

Silicon gel sheeting has been shown to improve the appearance of hypertrophic scars and keloids. Topical gel sheets or liquid must be worn over the affected area 12 hours daily for several months. The mechanism of action has not been fully elucidated, but may involve alterations of hydration, subsequently affecting fibroblasts. There are many over the counter silicone products which have been used to both prevent and treat keloids. As with any of these modalities, it may be best to combine silicon with PDL or intralesional corticosteroids.

Other therapies used to treat keloids include interferon injections, though results have been conflicting. Intralesional flourouracil has shown improvement in the size and appearance of keloids, both alone and in combination with PDL and intralesional corticosteroids. Radiation therapy has been occasionally used in combination with surgical excision for treatment of keloids. Recurrence rates have ranged from 10% to 20% in the ear-lobe area. This modality is quite expensive and the benefits of using radiation for a benign condition must be carefully weighed.

Cryotherapy has been used in the treatment of keloids. Repeated vigorous freezes at two- to three-week intervals may be helpful, but will probably not result in complete resolution. Cryotherapy preceding intralesional steroids may yield better results. Edema following a freeze–thaw cycle of cryotherapy may make intralesional injections easier. Pressure is useful to prevent recurrences of keloids after surgical excision. Pressure must be maintained for four to six months, and can be in the form of elastic garments, corsets, or adhesive wraps. A spring pressure device has been reported to be effective to prevent recurrences of ear-lobe keloids.

The most promising new advance in the treatment of keloids involves imiquimod 5% cream. This immune response modifier induces interferon alpha, which may explain the mechanism of action. Application of imiquimod immediately after surgical excision of keloids by Berman showed no recurrence in 10 patients after 24 weeks of topical therapy. If these results are repeated, it would represent a major advance in the management of keloids. Further studies are indicated to determine the efficacy of combination therapy with imiquimod, PDL, and intralesional corticosteroids.

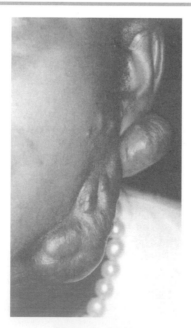

Figure 2 Keloid.

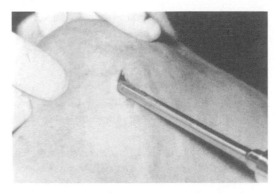

Figure 3 Lipoma, treated by liposuction.

LIPOMAS

Lipomas are benign tumors of adipose tissue, usually solitary and encapsulated. They occur commonly on the trunk, nape of the neck, and forearms. They most frequently arise in subcutaneous tissue, but can occur in deeper soft tissue. Histologically, lipomas are surrounded by a connective tissue capsule, but the fat cells contained within are indistinguishable from normal adipose tissue.

Angiolipomas are a variant of lipoma consisting of adipose tissue and clusters of thin-walled vessels. These tumors are often painful, and there may be several. Liposarcomas are pleomorphic neoplasms that infiltrate surrounding tissues. Atypical lipoblasts are found histologically.

The standard treatment for lipomas is excision. The length of the incision needed is one-fourth to one-half of the tumor itself and should be made the full thickness of the skin and upper subcutis. Gentle but firm pressure around the lipoma will express the tumor through the incision, often intact. Blunt dissection with scissors is usually needed to separate the lipoma from both the underlying fat and fascia. There can be a significant dead space after excision of larger lipomas. Hemostasis must be obtained to avoid a hematoma or seroma. The dead space should be closed with subcutaneous sutures. If the overlying epidermis is atrophic and redundant, it can be trimmed.

Large lipomas can be treated with liposuction (Figs. 3 and 4). The lipoma is infiltrated with dilute lidocaine and epinephrine and the skin injected only at the insertion of the cannula. A 1 cm incision is made in the base of the tumor. A standard liposuction cannula and suction machine are passed into the body of the tumor, with the openings in the cannula directed *away* from the skin to avoid injury to epidermal structures. Manual pressure with the operator's free hand is necessary at the periphery of the tumor to facilitate suctioning. Scissors and forceps may also be necessary to free fatty tissue from the surrounding stroma. This method is useful for giant lipomas (> 8 cm), for which a large surgical excision has greater risk of hematoma and requires an extensive multilayered closure. While some fat cells may remain, the tumor can be considerably reduced, giving an excellent cosmetic result with little chance of recurrence.

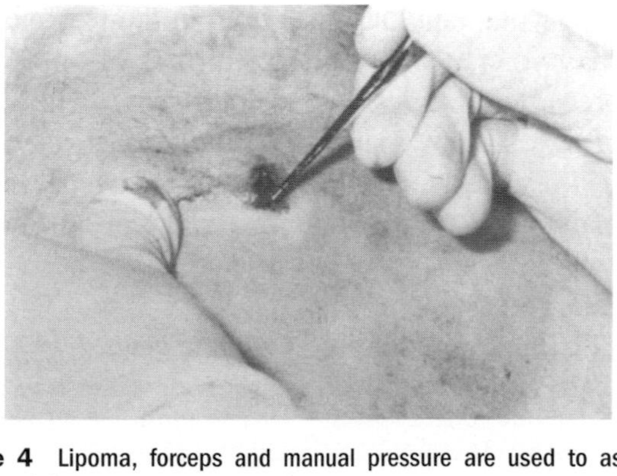

Vascular Tumors

Vascular tumors comprise a range of lesions including pyogenic granulomas, hemangiomas, cherry angiomas, and angiokeratomas.

Pyogenic Granulomas

Pyogenic granulomas are solitary, slightly pedunculated soft nodules with a dull red color (Fig. 5). They usually grow rapidly for a short period of time and then stabilize. The surface may be smooth, but often there is crusting or ulceration due to the tendency to bleed easily. Pyogenic granulomas occur at sites of trauma or mechanical irritation and are usually found on the fingers or face. There is a slightly increased incidence during pregnancy. Histologically, these lesions show a proliferation of capillaries embedded in an edematous stroma. The lesion is neither pyogenic nor a granuloma, but this misnomer has persisted.

A simple method of removal is shave excision to the deep dermis. Only the visible borders of the lesion need to be removed. Alternatively, the lesion can be shelled out with a curet. Since these tumors are vascular, brisk bleeding should be anticipated. On the finger, a tourniquet may be applied to minimize bleeding and provide a dry field for electrocautery. Vigorous manual pressure for 5 to 10 minutes may still be required to control bleeding adequately. The wound can then heal by second intention.

The entire lesion can be excised and closed primarily. Cryosurgery may be attempted in difficult areas such as beneath the nail plate, or in young children. Freezing is less reliable, however, especially in larger lesions, and does not provide tissue to confirm the diagnosis histopathologically. Although the argon and carbon dioxide laser have been used successfully, PDL is the most specific laser treatment. No

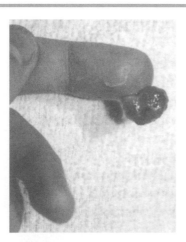

Figure 4 Lipoma, forceps and manual pressure are used to assist in removal of fat.

Figure 5 Pyogenic granuloma.

Table 1   Hemangiomas

Elevated
Capillary
Cavernous
Mixed
Nevus flammeus
Flat
Nevus flammeus (port-wine stain)

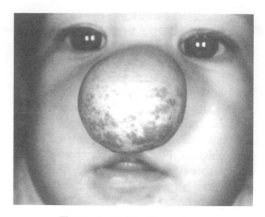

Figure 7   Capillary hemangioma.

anesthesia is required, though topical lidocaine preparations (LMX or EMLA) are helpful. Multiple treatments are occasionally required, but complications are rare. Intense pulsed light is also effective for PG.

Recurrent pyogenic granuloma may occur with satellite lesions in rare cases which usually resolve with or without treatment in months.

Hemangiomas

Hemangiomas are vascular anomalies that occur sporadically but can be associated with widespread cutaneous or systemic disease. They can be either flat or raised. The elevated variety includes capillary (65%), cavernous (15%), and mixed lesions (20%) (Table 1). Flat lesions such as the nevus flammeus or port-wine stain (Fig. 6) are sharply demarcated as pink, red, or purple patches present at birth. Blanching on diascopy suggests lesion is thin with minimal deep dermal involvement. Lesions generally persist into adult life. The most common hemangioma is the asymptomatic, rarely noticed, "Stork bite." These usually occur on the nape of the neck and are covered by the patient's hair.

A common hemangioma of infancy is the capillary hemangioma (Fig. 7). These may become quite large, occasionally obstructing such vital functions as vision or smell when in these vital areas. These hemangiomas undergo a rapid growth phase followed by spontaneous involution over several years.

Surgery is best avoided unless the lesion persists into puberty or obstructs vital function; however, controversy over when to treat persists.

Hemangiomas undergo a rapid growth phase followed by spontaneous involution over several years. Cavernous hemangiomas are a variant of the capillary type, with predominance of dilated blood vessels and less tendency for resolution. The combined lesions have features of both.

Oral prednisone may be of value during active growth phases. Dosages begin at 1 mg/kg, with gradual tapering as

the growth phase slows or stops. Intralesional corticosteroids are also effective for small hemangiomas in the facial area. Low doses of triamcinolone (2.5–5 mg/kg) are injected monthly for up to five months. Response rates are variable but may be as effective as systemic corticosteroids. Caution is advised in the periocular area, as cases of blindness have been reported. Topical clobetasol under occlusion has also been used with reduction in the size of the hemangioma. Cryotherapy and sclerosing agents have been tried with varying rates of success.

Surgical resections are indicated in the treatment of large hemangiomas if they interfere with vital structures such as the eyes, mouth, or ears. Large cavernous hemangiomas may cause extensive regional tissue destruction. Surgical procedures in early childhood should be attempted only in special situations including ulceration and bleeding as the risks of morbidity and scarring are quite high. Many of these lesions are now amenable to laser therapy (see below). Since many vascular lesions of childhood naturally involute, it is prudent to wait until the child is eight to 10 years old before considering elective surgery. Consideration should be given to the psychosocial status of the patient. When surgery is performed, preoperative arteriography helps to evaluate the extent of these lesions. Selective embolization of feeder vessels significantly aids in surgery. These procedures are best performed by physicians with extensive experience in these areas.

Port-wine stains, when small, can be treated by excision and direct closer. Large areas may require serial excisions, flaps, and grafting. Again, laser therapy has diminished the need for many surgical procedures. Dermabrasion has been used when the port-wine stain is limited to the superficial dermis, as demonstrated by blanching with diascopy. A biopsy may also help determine the depth of the lesion.

Lasers have revolutionized the treatment of hemangiomas. Laser therapy has tremendous selectivity in targeting blood vessels, allowing for greater efficacy with much fewer side effects than any of the prior treatments. Originally, the 694 nm ruby laser was used for vascular lesions. This less selective laser had a significant side effect profile. The argon laser which emits light at 488 and 514 nm is more selectively absorbed by hemoglobin in the blood vessel. Although the argon laser was effective in many cases, its side effect profile was at times unacceptable with scarring, textural, and pigment changes among the complications.

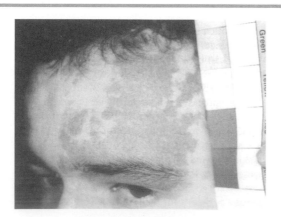

Figure 6   Nevus flammeus.

The PDL has become the treatment of choice for port-wine stains and hemangiomas. The 585 nm wavelength has been shown to coincide with the absorption of oxyhemoglobin, the so-called selective photothermolysis. This allows for preferential destruction of blood vessels with sparing of surrounding tissue. Just as important as the wavelength is the pulse duration. Optimally, the hemoglobin is absorbed by the laser light with the heat remaining in the blood vessel. Pulse durations (400 μs) have been modified to be shorter than the thermal relaxation times of small vessels. This allows the PDL to selectively injure vessels without damaging adjacent structures. Darker skin types may be treated with lower risk of pigmentary disturbances.

Cooling systems have been developed to minimize the risk of epidermal damage and to increase patient comfort during the procedure. PDL is usually described as a rubber band-snapping sensation. Pain during the procedure is well tolerated. Higher energies may be associated with greater pain, and treatment areas such as the face and digits can be more sensitive, requiring topical lidocaine preparations prior to treatment. PDL can use fluences ranging from 2 to 10 J/cm^2 with minimal pulse overlap. Spot size and fluence can be adjusted depending on the depth of penetration needed. Multiple sessions are generally needed. Postoperative purpura is expected and will last seven to 10 days. Longer wavelengths (595 and 600 nm) are now also used to treat vascular lesions. These systems use higher fluences (5–15 J/cm^2) with longer pulse durations (1.5–40 milliseconds). This allows for deeper penetration with less purpura, but comparable results. With proper training and experience, postoperative complications can be minimized. PDL treatment is most effective in the telangiectatic type of hemangioma. Deeper or proliferative lesions do not respond as well.

Cherry Angiomas

These common lesions, also called senile hemangiomas or cherry red spots, are small persistent red papules that present on the trunk, neck, and face of middle-aged patients (Fig. 8). Often dozens of these occur. Histologically, they are a variant of capillary hemangiomas with fewer vascular spaces and more abundant stroma.

Treatment is unnecessary except for cosmetic purposes. Superficial electrodesiccation or cryotherapy is generally adequate. Another method is fluoroethyl refrigerant spray

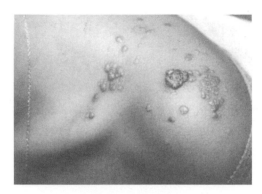

Figure 9 Angiokeratoma.

followed by curettage with a firm brush stroke. Several lesions can be removed with minimum discomfort.

Alternatively, shave excision with local anesthesia and light electrodesiccation will remove lesions with minimal scarring. The PDL is also very effective in the treatment of these lesions.

Angiokeratomas

These are round, elevated, purplish papules, which may become hypekeratonic (Fig. 9). There are six clinically recognizable types (Table 2). The solitary angiokeratoma is present in childhood, often on the arms or legs. Angiokeratoma circumscriptum is present at birth as a warty growth in bands or streaks. Angiokeratoma of Mibelli occurs as hemorrhagic keratotic papules in adolescence. Angiokeratoma of Fordyce present as multiple red-purple papules is seen primarily on the scrotum. The last two types of angiokeratomas are associated with enzyme deficiencies. In fucosidosis, multiple angiokeratomas appear on the trunk and legs in association with mental retardation. In Fabry's disease (angiokeratoma corporis diffusum), the lesions are also on the trunk, in association with defective function of the enzyme galactosidase A. Histologic examination reveals dilated capillaries surrounded by a thickened epidermis. Lipid stains can detect deposits associated with Fabry's disease. No treatment is necessary for angiokeratomas, but punch excision, shave biopsy, electrodesiccation, cryotherapy, Krypton, and PDL will also give acceptable results.

Xanthelasma

Xanthelasma are soft, yellow-orange plaques on the eyelids, and are the most common form of xanthomas (Fig. 10). They start as small growths but may become large nodules. They are generally present in the fourth to fifth decade of life, and approximately 50% will result from an underlying serum lipoprotein disorder. Histologic examination reveals collections of lipid-laden histiocytes in the upper levels of the dermis.

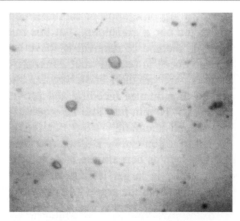

Figure 8 Cherry hemangioma.

Table 2 Angiokeratoma

Solitary
Angiokeratoma circumscription
Angiokeratoma of Mibelli
Angiokeratoma of Fordyce
Fucosidosis
Angiokeratoma corporis diffusum (Fabry's disease)

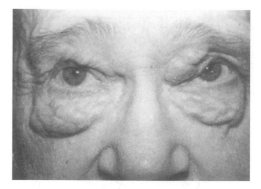

Figure 10   Xanthelasma.

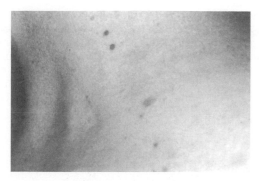

Figure 12   Acrochordon.

The treatment of xanthelasma is essentially cosmetic. Small lesions can be excised and the wound closed with fare, nonabsorbable sutures, which are removed after three to four days. Alternatively, these may be treated with light electrodesiccation and curettage to remove the viscous fatty material. Cryosurgery can also be used. CO_2 or argon lasers are also effective. Low energies are used to minimize scarring.

Other methods include trichloroacetic acid applied directly to the lesions. Start with a 20% to 25% solution and increase to 50% as needed. The acid is applied for approximately 30 seconds and a white frost is noted. The solution is then removed with moist cotton gauze or alcohol.

Sebaceous Hyperplasia

Sebaceous hyperplasia is a benign condition occurring on the forehead and cheeks of middle-aged patients. It presents as elevated, soft, yellowish papules 2 to 3 mm in diameter (Fig. 11). This must be differentiated from basal cell carcinoma, which can look similar. The histologic examination of sebaceous hyperplasia reveals a greatly enlarged sebaceous gland with numerous lobules grouped around a wide duct.

The surgical treatment is essentially cosmetic, and any superficial destructive method can be used. One or two lesions may be removed by shave or circular pouch excision. Larger areas can be treated with cryotherapy, or light electrodesiccation, and curretage. A linear incision allows easier curettage. These areas heal in several weeks with minimal scarring. CO_2, argon, or PDLs are also effective treatments for sebaceous hyperplasia. Recently, leuvulan has been used in conjunction with various light sources including blue light to treat sebaceous hyperplasia. Results have been promising, though multiple treatments are required.

Acrochordons

Acrochordons, or skin tags, are benign flesh-colored pedunculated tumors that occur in several forms. The most common is the 1- to 2-mm soft furrowed papule that occurs on the trunk, axila, and face coalesced in body folds (Fig. 12). Acrochordons are also present as single or multiple filiform growths, usually measuring 2 to 5 mm. The large solitary pedunculated tags may be 1 cm or larger.

Histologically, these lesions are composed of loose collagen fibers and dilated capillaries, with varying degrees of fatty tissue. The epidermis ranges from flattened to acanthotic.

Small skin tags are easily removed with sharp carved scissors cut flush to skin level, often without local anesthesia. The minor bleeding is controlled with pressure, chemical cautery, or light electrodesiccation. Larger skin tags require local anesthesia and can be shaved with a #15 blade.

Alternative methods include light electrocautery or liquid nitrogen. The lesions will usually fall off within several days.

ACKNOWLEDGMENT

A special thanks to Dr. Jerome Garden for supplying the clinical photographs.

BIBLIOGRAPHY

Alster TS. Laser scar revision: comparison study of 585 nm pulsed dye laser with and without intralesional corticosteroids. Dermatol Surg 2003; 29:25–29.

Alster TS, Tanzi EL. Hypertrophic scars and keloids. Am J Clin Dermatol 2003; 4:1–9.

Alster TS, Tanzi EL. Photodynamic therapy with topical aminolevulinic acid and pulsed dye laser irradiation for sebaceous hyperplasia. J Drugs Dermatol 2003; 2:501–504.

Alster TS, Williams CM. Treatment of keloid sternotomy scars with 585 nm flashlamp-pumped pulsed-dye laser. Lancet 1995; 345:1198–1200.

Aversa AI, Miller OF III. Cryo-curettage of cherry angiomas. J Dermatol Surg Oncol 1983; 9:930–931.

Bader RS, Scarborough DA. Surgical pearl: intralesional electrodesiccation of sebaceous hyperplasia. J Am Acad Dermatol 2000; 42(l Part 1):127–128.

Bailin PL. Lasers in dermatology-1985. J Dermatol Surg Cited 1985; 11:328–334.

Berman B, Kapoor S. Keloid and hypertrophic scar. eMedicine 2001; 2:l–12. (Available at: www.emedicine.com).

Berman B, Villa A. Imiquimod 5% cream for keloid management. Am Soc Derm Surgery 2003; 29:1050–1051.

Brent B. The role of pressure therapy in management of earlobe keloids. Ann Plast Surg 1978; 1:579–581.

Ceilley RI, Babin RW. The combined use of cryosurgery and intralesional injections of suspensions of fluorinated

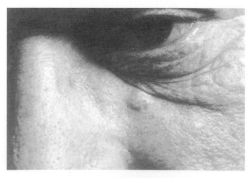

Figure 11   Sebaceous hyperplasia.

adrenocorticosteroids for reducing keloids and hypertrophic scars. J Dermatol Surg Oncol 1979; 5:54–56.

Christenson L, Patterson J, Davis D. Surgical pearl: use of the cutaneous punch for the removal of lipomas. J Am Acad Dermatol 2000; 42:675–676.

English RS, Shenefelt PD. Keloids and hypertrophic scars. Dermatol Surg 1999; 25:631–638.

Fitzpatrick RE. Treatment of inflamed hypertrophic scars using intralesional 5-FU. Dermatol Surg 1999; 25:224–232.

Fulton JE. Silicone gel sheeting for the prevention and management of evolving hypertrophic and keloid scars. Dermatol Surg 1995; 21:947–951.

Garden JM, Bakus AD. Clinical efficacy of the pulsed dye laser in the treatment of vascular lesions. J Dermatol Surg Oncol 1993; 19:321–326.

Gonzalez S, Vibnagool C, Falo LD Jr, Momtaz KT, Grevelink J, Gonzalez E. Treatment of pyogenic granulomas with the 585 am pulsed dye laser. J Am Acad Dermatol 1996; 35(3 Part 1):428–431.

Granstein RD, Rook A, Flotte TJ, et al. A controlled trial of intralesional recombinant interferon-gamma in the treatment of keloidal scarring. Clinical and histologic findings. Arch Dermatol 1990; 126:1295–1302.

Griffith BH, Monroe CW, McKinney P. A follow up study on the treatment of keloids with triamcinolone acetonide. Plant Reconstr Surg 1970; 46:145–150.

Henderson DL, Cromwell TA, Mes LG. Argon and carbon dioxide laser treatment of hypertrophic and keloid scars. Lasers Surg Med 1984; 3:271–277.

Hoffman SJ, Walsh P, Morelli JG. Treatment of angiofibroma with the pulsed tunable dye laser. J Am Acad Dermatol 1993; 29(5 Part l):790–791.

Hruza GJ, Geronemus RG, Dover IS, Arndt KA. Lasers in dermatology-1993. Arch Dermatol 1994; 129:1026–1035.

Kantor GR, Wheeland RG, Bailin PL, et al. Treatment of earlobe keloids with carbondioxide laser excision: a report of 16 cases. J Dermatol Surg Oncol 19S5; 11:1063–1067.

Levy DS, Salter MM, Roth RE. Postoperative irradiation in the prevention of keloids. Am J Roentgenol 1976; 127:509–510.

Lupton JR, Alster TS. Laser scar revision. Dermatol Clin 2002; 20(1):55–65.

Mercer NGS. Silicone gel in the treatment of keloid scars. Br J Plastic Surg 1989; 42:83–87.

Pariser RJ. Benign neoplasms of the skin. Med Clin North Am 1998; 82:1285–1307.

Poochareon VN, Berman B. New therapies for the management of keloids. J Cranialfacial Surg 2003; 14:654–657.

Ragoowansi R, Glees JP. Ear-lobe keloids: treatment by a protocol of surgical excision and immediate postoperative adjuvant radiotherapy. Br J Plast Surg 2001; 54:504–508.

Rosian R, Goslen JB, Brodell RT. The treatment of benign sebaceous hyperplasia with the topical application of bichloracetic acid. J Dermatol Surg Oncol 1991; 17:876–879.

Rubenstein R, Roenigk HH Jr., Garden JM, et al. Liposuction for lipomas. J Dermatol Surg Oncol 1985; 11:1070–1074.

Sclafani AP, et al. Prevention of earlobe keloid recurrence with postoperative corticosteroid injections versus radiation therapy: a randomized, prospective study and review of the literature. Dermatol Surg 1996; 22:569–574.

Stern JC, Lucente FE. Carbon dioxide laser excision of earlobe keloids. A prospective study and critical analysis of existing data. Arch Otolaryngol Head Neck Surg 1989; 115:1107–1111.

Tanzi EL, Lupton JR, Alster TS. Lasers in dermatology: four decades of progress. J Am Acad Dermatology 2003; 49:1–31.

Wong TW, Chiu HC, Yip KM. Intralesional interferon Alfa 2b has no effect in the treatment of keloids. Br J Dermatol 1994; 130:683–685.

35

Benign Pigmented Lesions

Melanie Warycha, Robert J. Friedman, and Darrell S. Rigel
*Department of Dermatology, New York University School of Medicine,
New York, New York, U.S.A.*

INTRODUCTION

Patients with problems related to pigmented lesion disorders are among the most commonly evaluated for dermatologic surgery. The vast majority of these lesions do not require surgical intervention. However, recent data suggest that some of these lesions may be both markers for and precursors to malignant melanoma. It is, therefore, important that patients with pigmented lesions be carefully evaluated and treated appropriately.

"DYSPLASTIC NEVUS SYNDROME"

The management of patients with dysplastic nevus syndrome remains a controversial topic in dermatology. The concept of dysplastic nevi was first documented in two melanoma-prone families over 20 years ago by Clark et al. The term "B-K mole syndrome" was used to refer to these two family members with multiple atypical nevi, who had an increased risk of developing malignant melanoma. Since then, this clinicopathologic entity has also been known as atypical mole syndrome and familial atypical multiple mole melanoma (FAMM) syndrome. Recognition of the dysplastic nevus syndrome in the nonfamilial setting was later noted. In 1992, the National Institutes of Health held a consensus conference to establish unifying concepts concerning the validity of this lesion in addition to its diagnosis and treatment. The panel recommended that the term "dysplastic nevus" be replaced with atypical mole, and that the syndrome for melanoma-prone families be called FAMM syndrome. They defined the FAMM syndrome as (i) the occurrence of malignant melanoma in one or more first- or second-degree relatives; (ii) a large number of melanocytic nevi, often more than 50, some of which are atypical (Figs. 1–6) and often variable in size; and (iii) melanocytic nevi that demonstrate certain histologic features (Fig. 7). In addition, they proposed renaming lesions histologically as "nevus with architectural disorder" and recommended commenting on the degree of cytologic atypia. Despite their recommendations, the term dysplastic nevus continues to be used widely among the medical community.

Dysplastic nevi are considered distinct lesions on the continuum between banal nevi and melanoma. Their presence is not an uncommon occurrence in the population. The estimated incidence of dysplastic nevi has been reported to be between 2% and 53%, the wide range being a result of discrepancies in the clinical or histologic definitions of dysplastic nevi. A more realistic calculation of the incidence is believed to be below 10% of the population, however. It has been surmised that sun exposure in addition to genetic susceptibility can influence the development of dysplastic nevi, thus adding to the difficulty in approximating their prevalence. There is an increased incidence of dysplastic nevi in the fairer skin types (I–II) compared with the darker types (III–IV), which may explain the increased risk that these individuals have for subsequently developing malignant melanoma.

DYSPLASTIC NEVI AND MELANOMA

When it comes to the issue of whether dysplastic nevi function as markers of increased risk for melanoma, the evidence set forth in the literature is overwhelming. The frequency of clinically atypical nevi among patients with a history of melanoma has been reported to range from 34% to 59%. Patients with atypical nevi and two or more family members with melanoma seem to be at the highest risk of melanoma, with relative risks ranging from 85 to 1269 according to various reports. Following the same principle, it has been shown that patients with a family history of melanoma but the absence of atypical nevi have only an average risk. Thus, a patient's risk of developing melanoma becomes more worrisome as the number of nevi and the degree of atypia rise.

Clinically, dysplastic nevi have been documented to progress to melanoma. Studies have also associated dysplastic nevi with melanoma through histologic means, with reports ranging from 0.5% to 46%. The noted variation may arise from differing criteria used by histopathologists. Melanomas of the trunk and proximal extremities seem to be the most common anatomic sites associated with nevi.

Despite these reports and the documented increased risk of melanoma in patients with dysplastic nevi, it is important to emphasize that the vast majority of dysplastic nevi are biologically benign and do not themselves progress to melanoma. The large majority remains stable in appearance over time but should be closely monitored for any changes.

Clinical Features

One of the most striking features of dysplastic nevi is their heterogeneity. Most lesions differ significantly from one another by marked variations in size, shape, and color. However, several critical clues can be used regularly to differentiate dysplastic nevi from common acquired nevi. In general, dysplastic nevi tend to be more oval than acquired nevi. They are at least 5 mm in diameter and have blurred and irregular borders that blend gradually into the surrounding skin. They tend to be macular or slightly elevated,

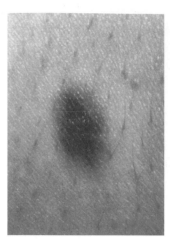

Figure 1 Typical dysplastic nevus showing oval shape, gradual peripheral "diffusing" of pigmented with poorly circumscribed margins.

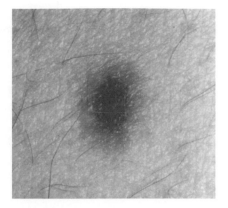

Figure 3 Dysplastic nevus: dark target, centrally elevated type. Note the raised dark center with trailing lighter peripheral pigment.

and have variable shades of tan and brown. In addition, they may have a background of erythema. They typically appear in adolescence and early adulthood but have been documented to develop in older individuals. Dysplastic nevi may be multiple or solitary, and can develop in patients with or without a family history of dysplastic nevi.

Friedman et al. classified dysplastic nevi into eight clinical types (Table 1). The most common clinical variant of dysplastic nevus is the dark target/centrally elevated type. This is characterized by a darkly pigmented papular central component surrounded by a lighter, tan-brown, macular periphery. The macular-pigmented halo gradually diffuses into the surrounding normal skin. The second most prevalent type of dysplastic nevus is the dark target/macular variety. This is similar to the dark target/centrally elevated variety but lacks the central papular component.

Next in prevalence is the mammillated variety. This lesion is slightly elevated with a barely perceptible macular

"shoulder." The surface of the lesion is best described as "cobblestoned," and, with careful observation, occasional tiny "milia-like" structures may be seen. The halo is minimal.

A less common variant is the erythematous type, which is characterized by a prominent red-orange component. There is also the light target variety. This lesion is characterized by a more deeply pigmented light to dark brown macular periphery and a less pigmented, centrally located, tan to light brown papular component. This type of nevus may also have a central macular area.

The least common varieties include the lentiginous type and melanoma simulant. The lentiginous type has clinical features similar to simple lentigo. However, it is generally larger and often has a more striking reticulated pigment pattern. The melanoma simulant has many of the early features of a malignant melanoma. However, these features are not as striking as would be seen in a clinically apparent early malignant melanoma.

Dysplastic nevi are predominantly distributed on the trunk and upper extremities in addition to arising on intermittently sun-exposed areas. It has been suggested that dysplastic nevi are larger and more numerous on relatively sun-exposed sites compared to sun-protected sites. Atypical nevi may evolve from normal appearing nevi or they may appear dysplastic from the onset. The majority, however, have been shown to remain stable or regress over time. The role that sun exposure plays in the dynamic nature of nevi continues to be explored.

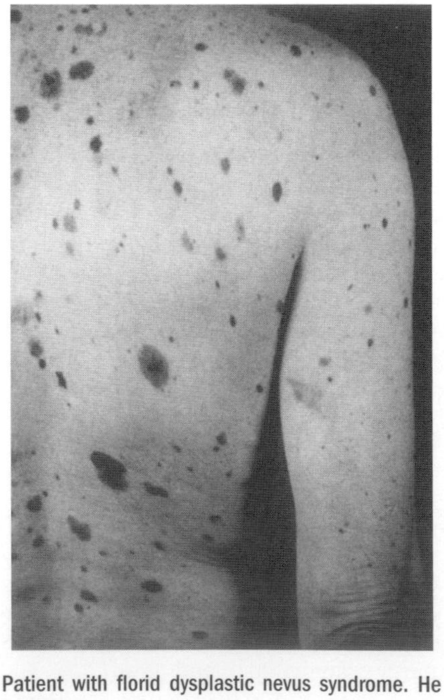

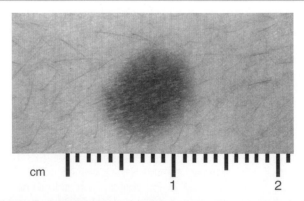

Figure 4 Dysplastic nevus: mamillated variety. Note prominent center with fine mamallation and minimal shoulder.

Figure 2 Patient with florid dysplastic nevus syndrome. He has already had two melanomas.

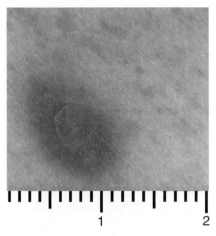

Figure 5 Dysplastic nevus: erythematous variety. The superior one-third of the lesion had an erythematous/orange component.

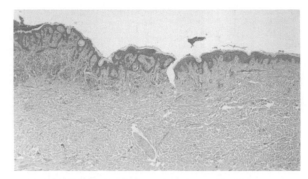

Figure 7 Photomicrograph of dysplastic nevus shows nests of nevus cells in the center with a trailing off of the nests to the periphery at the dermal-epidermal junction (×100).

Although it has been suggested that dysplastic nevi can be clinically identified as a specific entity, it is not always a simple task to differentiate them from early melanoma. Dermoscopy has been shown to increase the clinical accuracy of detecting malignant melanoma, and thus can serve as an aid in distinguishing between the two. While there can be overlap between the dermoscopic structures of dysplastic nevi and malignant melanoma, a few pathognomonic features raise the suspicion for melanoma, such as the presence of a pigment network with an abrupt margin, four or more colors, and a whitish veil.

Histologic Features

The National Institutes of Health Consensus Conference on Diagnosis and Treatment of Early Melanoma listed the histologic criteria for atypical nevi as follows (Figs. 7, 8A and B): Architectural disorder with asymmetry, subepidermal fibroplasia, and lentiginous melanocytic hyperplasia with spindle or epitheliod melanocytes aggregating in nests of variable size and forming bridges between adjacent rete ridges. Variable degrees of melanocytic atypia may occur in addition to dermal infiltrates of lymphocytes or intraepidermal melanocytes extending singly or in nests beyond the main dermal component. Despite the recommendations set

forth by the NIH, there continues to be a lack of consensus regarding the histologic criteria needed to diagnose dysplastic nevi. Many of the histologic features are not specific to dysplastic nevi, but can in fact be observed in common and congenital nevi. Studies on intraobserver and interobserver reliability among dermatopathologists concerning the histologic diagnosis of dysplastic nevi have been variable. One report noted intraobserver concordances of 67% to 87% and interobserver concordances of 45% to 75%, pointing to discrepancies in this diagnosis both within and across pathologists. However, Clemente et al. and de Wit et al. noted a high degree of agreement on the diagnosis of dysplastic nevi. Because of the continuing controversy, many dermatologists do not require biopsy confirmation of atypical moles.

Management

The main objective in the treatment of dysplastic nevi is the early detection of melanoma. The establishment of specific guidelines has been hampered by the continued debate over clinical and histologic criteria of dysplastic nevi. An additional complicating factor is the affect that the presence of additional risk factors for melanoma will have on management. Ascertaining whether or not the patient has a family history of melanoma or whether other family members have dysplastic nevi is of utmost importance. Most dermatologists can successfully manage the majority of dysplastic nevus syndrome patients; however, referral to a pigmented lesion clinic or specialist may be warranted if total body photography, digital imaging analysis, and dermoscopy are not available locally.

Regular dermatologic examinations of the entire skin surface, including scalp and eyes, should begin in adolescence. The recommended frequency of examinations

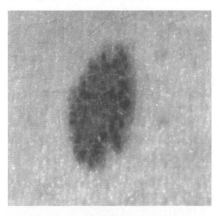

Figure 6 Dysplastic nevus: light target variety. Note the central light brown area with an irregularly marginated darker periphery.

Table 1 Clinical Types of Dysplastic Nevi

Most common
Dark target/centrally elevated
Dark target/macular
Papillated/mammillated
Erythematous
Less common
Light target/centrally elevated
Light target/macular
Lentiginous
Melanoma stimulant

(A)

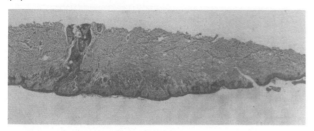

(B)

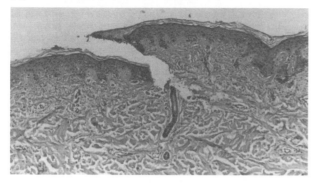

Figure 8 **(A)** Dysplastic nevus shows central aggregation of nevus cells with surgical etching at clinically apparent margin (×100). **(B)** Higher-power view (×400) shows nests of nevus cells extending lateral to clinically etched margin.

techniques, however, has found that saucerization or deep shave biopsy provided adequate tissue for making a histologic diagnosis. Shave biopsies were 88% accurate in determining tumor thickness as compared to measurements obtained through local wide excision specimens. Despite this report, excisional or deep saucerization techniques are still preferred, although the surgical margins utilized to ensure an optimal specimen vary by dermatologist. In a survey conducted by Tripp et al., 75% of dermatologists used margins of 2 mm or less, 17% use margins of 2 to 3 mm, and 3% use margins of 4 to 5 mm. At times, pathologists recommend reexcision if melanocytes extend to or are in close proximity to the surgical margin of the specimen. NIH has suggested reexcision with 0.2 to 0.5 mm margins in such circumstances. Cohen et al. examined the utility in reexcision considering the fact that most dysplastic nevi do not progress into melanoma. Of the 189 lesions recommended for reexcision, only one demonstrated melanoma, which calculated to a frequency of missed diagnosis of only 0.5%. Thus, the utility of reexcision remains controversial.

All patients with dysplastic nevi should be educated about the dangers of the sun and the importance of broad-spectrum sunscreen, and should be encouraged to avoid sun exposure between the hours of 10.00 AM. to 4.00 PM. The consistent use of sunscreen in children can prevent the development of nevi. Patients should also get into the habit of self-examination of the skin, paying particular attention to warning signs of melanoma: asymmetry, border irregularity, color variation, and a diameter greater than 6 mm.

depends on both personal and family history of melanoma in addition to the number of atypical moles, but typically ranges from every 3 to 12 months. For patients with dysplastic nevi and a family history of melanoma, follow-up examinations generally are recommended every three to six months. Once the moles appear stable, the interval period between follow-ups can be extended. Screening should continue indefinitely as the risk of developing malignant melanoma does not diminish. Total body photography can enhance melanoma surveillance, allowing one to evaluate the stability or changes in nevi over time, facilitating the detection of early melanoma. Dermoscopy has also proven useful in the differentiation of benign verses malignant pigmented lesions. Patients may also be at increased risk of developing intraocular melanoma; therefore, a baseline ophthalmologic examination should be conducted. If a family history of melanoma is elicited, then efforts should be made to examine first-degree relatives.

Most dermatologists would not recommend prophylactic excision for lesions diagnosed clinically as dysplastic nevi since excision does not reduce the overall risk of melanoma. The probability that a single nevus will develop into melanoma is very low, and the patient would still be at increased risk for de novo development of melanoma in clinically normal skin. In a prospective study by Kelly et al., 13 of 20 detected melanomas arose from new lesions, and only three from preexisting nevi. They surmised that prophylactic excision of dysplastic nevi would not provide significant risk reduction to justify the cost and morbidity associated with this procedure. However, if the dermatologist believes that melanoma cannot be ruled out or if a documented change (according to "ABCDE" rule for melanoma) is noted, then total excision with a 2 mm margin has been traditionally recommended. A review of biopsy

CONGENITAL NEVI

A congenital nevus is a melanocytic nevus present at birth. Not all pigmented lesions present at birth represent melanocytic nevi. Some congenital melanocytic nevi do not become apparent until months to years after birth because they have not yet acquired sufficient pigment to make them clinically visible. These nevi have been termed "congenital-nevus–like nevi". Most of these are believed to be true congenital melanocytic nevi; however, the distinction is complicated by the histologic overlap between the two. Congenital nevi have been classified into three groups according to the size they are anticipated to attain in adulthood: (i) small (<1.5 cm in diameter); (ii) medium (1.5–20 cm in diameter); and (iii) large (greater than 20 cm in diameter). The size of the lesion has different implications for diagnosis, treatment, and prognosis. Recently, support has surfaced for the belief that speckled lentiginous nevi (nevi spili) are a subset of congenital nevi.

It is estimated that congenital melanocytic nevi are present in approximately 1% of newborns, while the incidence of congenital-nevus–like nevi has been reported between 2% and 6%. Large congenital melanocytic nevi are quite rare, developing in about one in 20,000 births.

The importance of congenital melanocytic nevi lies in their potential for malignant transformation. In addition, the psychosocial effects of a cosmetically disfiguring lesion need to be taken into account when choosing between treatment options.

Clinical Appearance

The clinical appearance of congenital nevi is variable and somewhat dependent on their size. Typically, medium to large congenital melanocytic nevi (Fig. 9A and B) present as well-circumscribed, round, homogeneous to multipigmented brown lesions, often with irregular surfaces, hypertrichosis, and with or without coarse dark hairs. Some lesions,

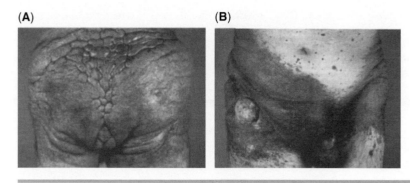

Figure 9 (A) Giant "bathing trunk" congenital nevus. (B) Note melanoma arising on right lateral thigh. *Source*: Courtesy of NYU Skin and Cancer Clinic.

however, may mimic melanoma by displaying asymmetry with irregular borders. A subset of these lesions occupies a major portion of the body surface and are called giant congenital, bathing trunk, or garment nevi.

Small congenital nevi typically have a smooth surface, more uniform pigmentation, and lack hair. They may be difficult to distinguish from acquired nevocytic nevi if they are not present at birth due to their clinical similarity.

With time, many lesions become lighter, rather than darker, in color, with increased hair growth and nodularity. Benign proliferative nodules that tend to regress spontaneously have also been documented to occur within congenital nevi at birth. Most nodules develop early in life, with one report citing the majority presenting before two years of age. In addition, erosions and ulcerations have been reported within some giant congenital melanocytic nevi during the neonatal period, most likely a result of trauma to the epidermis during birth. Satellite nevi have also been associated with large congenital melanocytic nevi up to 74% to 80%.

Dermoscopic features of congenital melanocytic nevi include a globular pattern with cobblestone arrangement. In addition, the presence of milia-like cysts and terminal hairs are diagnostic clues to the presence of congenital melanocytic nevi.

Histologic Features

The classic histologic description of congenital nevi includes nevus cells in the lower two-thirds of the dermis, occasionally extending into the subcutis; between collagen bundles distributed as single cells, or cells in single file, or both; and on the lower two-thirds of the reticular dermis or subcutis associated with appendages, nerves, and vessels. However, many congenital nevi do not have these microscopic features. In addition, there is considerable histologic overlap between acquired nevi and congenital nevi, making a diagnosis based on these criteria difficult.

Management

Giant Congenital Melanocytic Nevi

The increased risk of malignant transformation within a large congenital melanocytic nevus has been well established in the literature, with lifetime risks ranging from 4.5% to 8.5% in various studies. The development of melanoma in patients with large congenital nevi is most common in the first decade of life, with the majority occurring within the first five years. Large congenital nevi of the extremities have a reported lower risk of malignant transformation than those in an axial location. No melanoma has been reported to have had developed within a satellite nevus.

Although melanomas have been documented to arise within giant nevi, numerous instances of malignant transformation in extracutaneous sites have been reported, including neurocutaneous melanosis, rhabdomyosarcoma, liposarcoma, and malignant peripheral nerve sheath tumor.

Neurocutaneous melanosis (NCM) is characterized by the presence of benign and/or malignant pigment cell tumors of the central nervous system (CNS) in association with a large congenital melanocytic nevus or three or more smaller congenital nevi. In a report by DeDavid et al., 12% of the patients followed developed NCM . Large congenital melanocytic nevi (LCMN) of the scalp and posterior midline may be associated with leptomeningeal melanocytosis. In a study by DeDavid et al., those patients with LCMN and satellite nevi posed the greatest risk for development of NCM. CNS involvement can lead to increased cerebrospinal fluid pressure and hydrocephalus, with subsequent risk of developing seizures, ataxia, aphasia, or gait disturbances. magnetic resonance imaging (MRI) findings suggestive of NCM include T1, and in some cases T2, shortening of the brain parenchyma, primarily in the temporal lobes, without meningeal enhancement. In a study by Frieden et al., it was shown that 45% of neurologically asymptomatic patients with large congenital melanocytic nevi had abnormal findings on MRI; however there does not appear to be any correlation between evidence of melanosis by MRI and development of symptomatic neurologic disease. The prognosis for patients with symptomatic NCM is poor, with most patients dying within three years of initial presentation. Prophylactic surgical excision of LCMN in patients with symptomatic NCM is often not advocated because of its relatively poor prognosis.

Indications for the treatment of congenital melanocytic nevi include prophylactic reduction in the risk of malignant changes in addition to cosmetic and psychosocial considerations. Although surgical removal is believed to lower the risk of developing melanoma, this has not been established in any controlled studies. Despite this, early surgical excision remains the standard of care. The extent of resection needs to take into account the availability of reconstructive options. Complete excision is often impossible because nevus cells can reside in deep subcutaneous structures such as appendages, nerves, vessels, and muscles. One must also take into consideration the disfigurement and scarring that may result from surgery. Reconstructive techniques include tissue-expanded flaps or grafts, serial excisions, and either full-thickness or split-thickness skin grafts. Tissue expansion is recommended for lesions involving the head, neck, or torso, with skin grafts recommended for lesions involving the extremities distal to the knee or elbow joint. Complete removal may be compromised by the lack of available donor tissue for reconstruction because of presence of satellite nevi.

Other approaches to the treatment of congenital melanocytic nevi have been utilized, including curettage, dermabrasion, and lasers. The success of lasers has been variable in the literature. Goldberg et al. found marked improvement in two of four patients treated; however, Waldorf et al. saw partial repigmentation in all patients subsequent to the discontinuation of therapy. Side effects of laser treatment have been limited to transient erythema and hypopigmentation in darker-skinned patients. Application of lasers remains controversial as the effect it will have on the malignant potential of remaining cells is unknown. In a study of 215 patients treated with dermabrasion, 33.8% had "good" removal of pigmentation, while reduction of pigmentation was "satisfactory" in 29.7%. Success was dependent on size of the nevus and timing of the procedure, with best results with treatment of large nevi in the newborn period. The use of these modalities continues to be explored.

One must keep in mind that lightening pigmented large congenital nevi may make it more difficult to monitor the remaining lesion for signs of malignant transformation. Ongoing observation of residual nevi, scars, and satellite nevi is thus prudent.

Medium and Small Congenital Melanocytic Nevi

Due to the lack of universally applicable recommendations, the management of medium to small congenital melanocytic nevi must be determined on an individual basis. While the risk of developing melanoma in association with large congenital nevi is well documented, the malignant potential of small and medium sized melanocytic nevi remains controversial. Lifetime risks for small congenital melanocytic nevi have been reported between 0% and 4.9%. It also appears that the risk of melanoma arising in medium-sized congenital melanocytic nevi is small, with two reports failing to identify any malignant transformation in these lesions. One difference between the malignant transformation between large and small nevi is that melanoma appears predominantly at or after puberty in small nevi, whereas it occurs earlier in large congenital nevi. In addition, melanomas arising from smaller nevi tend to develop in the dermoepidermal junction.

There is insufficient evidence at present to recommend prophylactic excision of all congenital nevi. If the lesion is homogenous, with a smooth texture, absent of nodules, and light in color, then it may be appropriate to clinically follow the lesion for any changes. Periodic evaluation should utilize photography, dermoscopy, and educating the patient about the warning signs of melanoma, including any changes in color, borders, texture, or size. However, if the lesion is more deeply pigmented with an uneven texture, or a significant alteration in the nevus has occurred, then surgical excision may be considered. Of critical importance is the consideration of additional risk factors, including the presence of acquired or atypical nevi or a family history of melanoma.

Common Acquired Nevi

One of the most common requests made of the dermatologist is to remove a common acquired nevus. Estimates of the prevalence of common acquired nevi have been variable, with reports ranging from the presence of at least one nevus in virtually all adults, to a study citing that 55% of adults have between 10 to 45 nevi greater than 2 mm in diameter. Although common acquired nevi may enlarge and increase

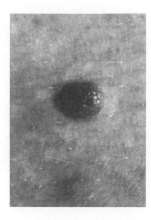

Figure 10 Common acquired nevus showing uniform color, round shape, and crisp border demarcation.

in frequency throughout childhood and puberty, most remain less than 5 mm in diameter (Fig. 10).

Despite the low risk of an acquired nevus evolving into melanoma, there is overwhelming evidence in the literature, which indicates that patients with an increased number of benign melanocytic nevi have an increased risk for the development of melanoma. One study found that patients with 50 to 100 nevi had a risk for the development of melanoma 3.2 times that of patients with none to four nevi, while patients with more than 100 nevi had a relative risk of 7.7. Thus, patients with large numbers of acquired nevi should be evaluated more closely than average to allow detection of melanomas as early as possible.

Treatment of nevi is usually not warranted other than for cosmetic concerns or an inability to rule out melanoma. In most cases, the lesion can be removed by shave excision with closure by second intention. Often these lesions will partially recur after treatment as a hyperpigmented macule or papule. Repeat biopsy may yield atypical features shared with melanoma, so-called "pseudomelanoma," histologically. Therefore, it is important to warn the patient of this possibility. A deeper excision closed primarily with sutures usually results in a more definitive removal. The cosmetic result is as good but the procedure takes longer and is slightly more expensive.

BIBLIOGRAPHY

Augustsson A, Stierner U, Rosdahl I, Suurkula M. Common and dysplastic naevi as risk factors for cutaneous malignant melanoma in a Swedish population. Acta Derm Venereol 1991; 71:518–524.

Barkovich AJ, Frieden IJ, Williams ML. MR of neurocutaneous melanosis. Am J Neuroradiol 1994; 15:859–867.

Bataille V, Grulich A, Sasieni P, et al. The association between naevi and melanoma in populations with different levels of sun exposure: a joint case-control study of melanoma in the UK and Australia. Br J Cancer 1998; 77:505–510.

Bataille V, Bishop JA, Sasieni P, et al. Risks of cutaneous melanoma in relation to the numbers, types, and sites of naevi: a case-control study. Br J Cancer 1996; 73:1605–1611.

Betti R, Inselvini E, Vergani R, et al. Small congenital nevi associated with melanoma: case reports and considerations. J Dermatol 2000; 27:583–590.

Borbujo J, Jara M, Cortes L, Sanchez de Leon L. A newborn with nodular ulcerated lesion on a giant congenital nevus. Pediatr Dermatol 2000; 17:299–301.

Byrd SE, Darling CF, Tomita T, Chou P, de Leon G, Radkowski MA. MR imaging of symptomatic neurocutaneous melanosis in children. Pediatr Radiol 1997; 27:39.

Castilla EE, da Graca Dutra M, Orioli-Parreiras IM. Epidemiology of congenital pigmented naevi: I. incidence rates and relative frequencies. Br J Dermatol 1981; 104:307–315.

Clark WH Jr., Reimer RR, Greene M, et al. Origin of familial malignant melanomas from heritable melanocytic lesions. 'The B-K mole syndrome'. Arch Dermatol 1978; 114: 732–738.

Clemente C, Cochran AJ, Elder DE, et al. Histopathologic diagnosis of dysplastic nevi: concordance among pathologists convened by the World Health Organization Melanoma Programme. Hum Pathol 1991; 22:313–319.

Cohen LM, Hodge SJ, Owen LG, et al. Atypical melanocytic nevi. Clinical and histopathologic predictors of residual tumor at reexcision. J Am Acad Dermatol 1992; 27:701–706.

Consensus Statement. Diagnosis and treatment of early melanoma. NIH Consensus Development Conference, Jan 27–29, 1992.

Consensus Development Conference of the National Institutes of Health: precursors to malignant melanoma. JAMA 1984; 251:1864–1866.

Crutcher WA, Sagebiel RW. Prevalence of dysplastic naevi in a community practice. Lancet 1984; 1(8379):729.

DeDavid M, Orlow SJ, Provost N, et al. Neurocutaneous melanosis: clinical features of large congenital melanocytic nevi in patients with manifest central nervous system melanosis. J Am Acad Dermatol 1996; 35:529–538.

DeDavid M, Orlow SJ, Provost N, et al. A study of large congenital melanocytic nevi and associated malignant melanomas: review of cases in the New York University Registry and the world literature. J Am Acad Dermatol 1997; 36:409–416.

Duray PH, Ernstoff MS. Dysplastic nevus in histologic contiguity with acquired nonfamilial melanoma: clinicopathologic experience in a 100-bed hospital. Arch Dermatol 1987; 123:80–84.

de Wit PE, van't Hof-Grootenboer B, Ruiter DJ, et al. Validity of the histopathological criteria used for diagnosing dysplastic naevi: an interobserver study by the pathology subgroup of the EORTC Malignant Melanoma Cooperative Group. Eur J Cancer 1993; 29A:831–839.

Egan CL, Oliveria SA, Elenitsas R, et al. Cutaneous melanoma risk and phenotypic changes in large congenital nevi: a follow-up study of 46 patients. J Am Acad Derm 1998; 39(6):923–932.

Frieden IJ, Williams ML, Barkovich AJ. Giant congenital melanocytic nevi: brain magnetic resonance findings in neurologically asymptomatic children. J Am Acad Dermatol 1994; 31:423–429.

Gallagher RP, Rivers JK, Lee TK, et al. Broad-spectrum sunscreen use and the development of new nevi in white children: a randomized controlled trial. JAMA 2000; 283:2955–2960.

Giam YC, Williams ML, Leboit PE, et al. Neonatal erosions and ulcerations in giant congenital melanocytic nevi. Pediatr Dermatol 1999; 16:354–358.

Goldberg DJ, Stampien T. Q-switched ruby laser treatment of congenital nevi. Arch Dermatol 1995; 131:621–623.

Gosain AK, Santoro TD, Larson DL, Gingrass RP. Giant congenital nevi: a 20-year experience and an algorithm for their management. Plast Reconst Surg 2001; 108:622.

Greene MH, Clark WH, Tucker MA, et al. Acquired precursors of cutaneous malignant melanoma: the familial dysplastic nevus syndrome. N Eng J Med 1985; 312:91–97.

Grob JJ, Gouvernet J, Aymar D, et al. Count of benign melanocytic nevi as a major indicator of risk for nonfamilial nodular and superficial spreading melanoma. Cancer 1990; 66:387–395.

Halpern AC, Guerry D IV, Elder DE, et al. Natural history of dysplastic nevi. J Am Acad Dermatol 1993; 29:51–57.

Halpern AC, Guerry D IV, Elder DE, et al. A cohort study of melanoma in patients with dysplastic nevi. J Invest Dermatol 1993; 100:346S–349S.

Hendrickson MR, Ross JC. Neoplasms arising in congenital giant nevi. Morphologic study of seven cases and a review of the literature. Am J Surg Pathol 1981; 5:109–135.

Hoang MP, Sinkre P, Albores-Saavedra J. Rhabdomyosarcoma arising in a congenital melanocytic nevus. Am J Dermatopathol 2002; 24:26–29.

Holly EA, Kelly JW, Shpall SN, Chiu SH. Number of melanocytic nevi as a major risk factor for malignant melanoma. J Am Acad Dermatol 1987; 17:459–468.

Illig C, Weidener F, Hundeiker H, et al. Congenital nevi less than or equal to 10 cm as precursors to melanoma: 52 cases, a review, and a new conception. Arch Dermatol 1985; 121:1274–1281.

Kadonaga JN, Frieden IJ. Neurocutaneous melanosis: definition and review of the literature. J Am Acad Dermatol 1991; 24:747–755.

Kaplan EN. The risk of malignancy in large congenital nevi. Plast Reconstr Surg 1974; 53:421–428.

Kelly JW, Yeatman JM, Regalia C, Mason G, Henham AP. A high incidence of melanoma found in patients with multiple dysplastic naevi by photographic surveillance. Med J Aust 1997; 167:191–194.

Kopf AW, Levine LJ, Rigel DS, et al. Prevalence of congenital nevus-like nevi, nevi spili, and café au lait spots. Arch Dermatol 1985; 121:766–769.

Kopf AW, Bart RS, Hennessey P. Congenital nevocytic nevi and malignant melanomas. Arch Dermatol 1979; 115:123–130.

Kopf AW, Levine LJ, Rigel DS, et al. Congenital-nevus-like nevi, nevi spili, and café-au-lait spots in patients with malignant melanoma. J Dermatol Surg Oncol 1985; 11(3):275–280.

Kraemer KH, Greene MH. Dysplastic nevus syndrome: familial and sporadic precursors of cutaneous melanoma. Dermatol Clin 1985; 3:225–237.

Lee G, Massa MC, Welykyj S, et al. Yield from total skin examination and effectiveness of skin cancer awareness program: findings in 874 new dermatology patients. Cancer 1991; 67:202–205.

Lynch HT, Frichot BC III, Lynch JF. Familial atypical multiple mole-melanoma syndrome. J Med Genet 1978; 15:352–356.

Makkar HS, Frieden IJ. Congenital melanocytic nevi: an update for the pediatrician. Curr Opin Pediatr 2002; 14:397–403.

Marghoob AA, Schoenbach SP, Kopf AW, et al. Large congenital melanocytic nevi and the risk of developing malignant melanoma: a prospective study and review of the world literature. J Invest Dermatol 1995; 104:563.

Marks R, Dorevitch AP, Mason G. Do all melanomas come from "moles"? A study of the histological association between melanocytic naevi and melanoma. Australas J Dermatol 1990; 31:77–80.

Marghoob AA. Congenital melanocytic nevi: evaluation and management. Dermatol Clin 2002; 20:607–616.

Nelson JS, Kelly KM. Q-switched laser treatment of a congenital melanocytic nevus. Dermatol Surg 1999; 25:274–276.

Ng PC, Barzilai DA, Ismail SA, et al. Evaluating invasive cutaneous melanoma: is the initial biopsy representative of the final depth? J Am Acad Derm 2003; 48(3):420–424.

Nordlund JJ, Kirkwood J, Forget BM, et al. Demographic study of clinically atypical (dysplastic) nevi in patients with melanoma and comparison subjects. Cancer Res 1985; 45(4):1855–1861.

Piepkorn MW, Barnhill RL, Cannon-Albright LA, et al. A multiobserver, population-based analysis of histologic dysplasia in melanocytic nevi. J Am Acad Dermatol 1994; 30:707–714.

Piepkorn M, Meyer LJ, Goldgar D, et al. The dysplastic melanocytic nevus: a prevalent lesion that correlates poorly with clinical phenotype. J Am Acad Derm 1989; 20:407–415.

Reintgen DS, Vollmer R, Seigler HF. Juvenile malignant melanoma. Surg Gynecol Obstet 1989; 168:249–253.

Rhodes AR, Sober AJ, Day CL, et al. The malignant potential of small congenital nevocellular nevi. J Am Acad Dermatol 1982; 6:230–241.

Rhodes AR, Harrist TJ, Day CL, et al. Dysplastic melanocytic nevi in histologic association with 234 primary malignant melanomas. J Am Acad Dermatol 1983; 9:563–574.

Rhodes AR, Weinstock MA, Fitzpatrick TB, Mihm MC, Sober AJ. Risk factors for cutaneous melanoma. JAMA 1987; 258:3146–154.

Rhodes AR, Melski JW. Small congenital nevocellular nevi and the risk of cutaneous melanoma. J Pediatr 1982; 100:219–224.

Rhodes AR, Wood WC, Sober AJ, et al. Nonepidermal origin of malignant melanoma associated with giant congenital nevocellular nevus. Plast Reconstr Surg 1981; 67:782–790.

Rivers JK, Kopf AW, Vinokur AF, et al. Clinical characteristics of malignant melanomas developing in persons with dysplastic nevi. Cancer 1990; 65:1232–1236.

Rompel R, Moser M, Petres J. Dermabrasion of congenital nevocellular nevi: experience in 215 patients. Dermatology 1997; 194:261.

Ruiz-Maldonado R, Tamayo L, Laterza AM, Duran C. Giant pigmented nevi: clinical, histopathologic, and therapeutic considerations. J Pediatr. 1992; 120:906–911.

Sagebiel RW. Melanocytic nevi in histologic association with primary cutaneous melanoma of superficial spreading and nodular types: effect of tumour thickness. J Invest Dermatol 1993; 100(suppl):322S–325S.

Sahin S, Levin L, Kopf A, et al. Risk of melanoma in medium-sized congenital melanocytic nevi: a follow-up study. J Am Acad Dermatol 1998; 39:428–433.

Salopek TG, Kopf AW, Stefanato CM, Vossaert K, Silverman M, Yadav S. Differentiation of atypical moles (dysplastic nevi) from early melanomas by dermoscopy. Dermatol Clin 2001; 19(2):337–345.

Sanders C, Tschochohei H, Hagedorn M. Epidemiology of dysplastic nevus. Hautarzt 1989; 40(12):758–760.

Schaffer JV, Orlow SJ, Lazova R, et al. Speckled lentiginous nevus: within the spectrum of congenital melanocytic nevi. Arch Dermatol 2001; 137:172–178.

Skender-Kalnenas TM, English DR, Heenan PJ. Benign melanocytic lesions: risk markers or precursors of cutaneous melanoma? J Am Acad Dermatol 1995; 33:1000–1007.

Swerdlow AJ, English JS, Qiao Z. The risk of melanoma in patients with congenital nevi: a cohort study. J Am Acad Dermatol 1995; 32:595–599.

Tripp JM, Kopf AW, Marghoob AA, Bart RS. Management of dysplastic nevi: a survey of fellows of the American Academy of Dermatology. J Am Acad Dermatol 2002; 46:674–682.

Tucker MA, Goldstein AM. Melanoma etiology: where are we? Oncogene 2003; 22:3042–3052.

Tucker MA, Halpern A, Holly EA, et al. Clinically recognized dysplastic nevi: a central risk factor for cutaneous melanoma. JAMA 1997; 277:1439–1444.

Tucker MA, Fraser MC, Goldstein AM, et al. Risk of melanoma and other cancers in melanoma-prone families. J Invest Dermatol 1993; 100:350S–355S.

Waldorf HA, Kauvar AN, Geronemus RG. Treatment of small and medium congenital nevi with the Q-switched Ruby Laser. Arch Dermatol 1996; 132:301–304.

Williams ML, Pennella R. Melanoma, melanocyte nevi and other melanoma risk factors in children. J Pediatr 1994; 124:833–845.

36

Noninvasive Intraepidermal Neoplasia
(Premalignant Lesions)

Jeffry A. Goldes

Associated Dermatology of Helena, Helena, Montana, U.S.A.

Wynn H. Kao

Department of Dermatology, University of Puerto Rico Medical Center,
San Juan, Puerto Rico

Grace F. Kao

Department of Pathology and Laboratory Medicine, Baltimore VA Medical Center,
Baltimore, Maryland, and George Washington University,
Washington, D.C., U.S.A.

INTRODUCTION

Invasive malignant neoplasms of epithelial and melanocytic histogenesis may arise from preexisting noninvasive intraepidermal or in situ malignant lesions. These lesions have been known as premalignant lesions or precancers. The concept of skin precancers has been revisited recently. The controversy lies primarily in whether the lesions that had been previously recognized both clinically and microscopically as noninvasive tumors should be regarded as early invasive cancers and treated accordingly, due to their potential to develop invasion into the underlying or adjacent dermal stroma, if left untreated. It is widely accepted that in situ (noninvasive) malignant neoplasms are curable by early detection and complete excision, whereas invasive tumors require more aggressive and destructive chemotherapy as well as radiation. Although de novo invasive carcinomas do exist, the majority of epithelial and melanocytic tumors undergoes cytologic evolution (malignant transformation) under the influence of chemical carcinogens and other carcinogenic factors, through intraepithelial nuclear DNA alterations, and eventually breaks through the epithelial–stromal junctional zone, to become an invasive lesion capable of metastasis.

The term "noninvasive intraepidermal neoplasia of the skin" is emerging, alongside noninvasive intraepithelial lesions seen in other organs, such as uterine cervix (cervical intraepithelial neoplasia or CIN), vagina (vaginal intraepithelial neoplasia, or VaIN), prostate (prostatic intraepithelial neoplasia, or PIN), and pancreas (pancreatic intraepithelial neoplasia, or Pan IN). Early detection and treatment of lesions with epithelial nuclear atypia prior to invasion into the surrounding structures can arrest aggressive cancers. With the aid of immunohistochemistry, such as actin, P63, and Tenascin, differentiation between noninvasive and early invasive lesions is even more promising.

Several skin disorders commonly affecting sun-exposed skin and mucocutaneous junctions exhibit a natural history resulting in the development of invasive carcinoma and malignant melanoma. Invasive neoplasms arising in association with underlying noninvasive premalignant lesions are discussed. Solar (actinic) keratosis, actinic cheilitis, radiation keratosis, Bowen's disease, and arsenical keratosis all show microscopic features of noninvasive squamous carcinoma (SCC) in situ. These lesions affect the epidermis, the pilosebaceous adnexal structures, or both. Arsenical keratosis is discussed with Bowen's disease, because they share similar clinical and histopathologic features. Lentigo maligna (LM) and acquired melanosis are discussed together, because both lesions demonstrate atypical melanocytic proliferation at the dermo–epidermal junction (DEJ).

Each noninvasive premalignant tumor has characteristic clinicopathologic features, and progresses into an invasive malignant neoplasm in a significant percentage of patients. The diagnosis of invasive malignant disease is made based on evidence of cytologic atypia and invasion through the dermo–epidermal basement membrane zone or surrounding stroma of each tumor. Recognition of noninvasive premalignant disease of the skin is important, because these lesions can be treated less aggressively at the in situ stage. Early clinical detection and microscopic examination of noninvasive lesions are important for preventing and arresting aggressive invasive malignant neoplasms.

SOLAR (ACTINIC) KERATOSIS AND ACTINIC CHEILITIS

Symptoms for these conditions include: actinic keratosis, solar precancerosis, senile keratosis, senile keratoma, and solar cheilitis.

Clinical Features and Gross Pathologic Appearance

Actinic keratoses (AKs) are one of the top three, most common reasons for patients to consult a physician. In the fair-skinned population of the United States and Australia, the incidence ranges from 11% to 26%, and the prevalence of AKs is estimated as high as 40% to 50% in the population

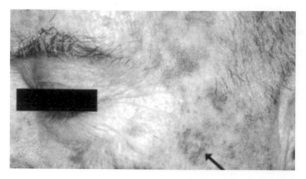

Figure 1 Erythematous to yellow papules and plaques of actinic keratosis, with adjacent scale crust on the zygomatic area (*arrow*) of the cheek in a 60-year-old man with severe sun damage. (*See color insert.*)

40 years and older. Among Caucasians, the rate is less than 10% in the third decade and greater than 80% in the seventh decade of life.

Solar (actinic) keratoses develop in sun-exposed, aging skin, which is often dry, wrinkled, and atrophic, with irregular, mottled hyperpigmentation (actinic melanosis). Lesions are discrete, flat or slightly elevated, rough, round, or irregularly shaped papules and plaques with adherent scales, and are usually less than 1 cm (3 mm to 1–2 cm) in diameter. Their color varies from red to yellow (Fig. 1), or gray–brown. They slowly enlarge with time, and may show exuberant hyperkeratosis and form a nodular or warty configuration, resembling a cutaneous horn. The term "cutaneous horn" should be used descriptively, not as a diagnostic term, because in addition to solar keratosis and SCC, other epidermal neoplasms, such as seborrheic keratosis, inverted follicular keratosis, trichilemmoma, and basal cell carcinoma, may present as a cutaneous horn.

Solar keratoses are more often multiple than single, and are usually located on the face, particularly on the forehead, cheeks (Fig. 2), nose, and sideburns, as well as on other sun-exposed areas, such as the ear, neck, dorsum of the hands, forearms, anterior chest, back, and bald scalp. The lesions may be symptomatic. Pruritus, burning, or a splinter-like sensation in the involved skin has been recorded. The average patient is in his early 60's when first diagnosed. In recent years, with more leisure-time sun exposure, young people are developing solar keratoses. Solar keratoses occur in both sexes, but affect primarily fair-complexioned individuals (Types I and II) who have had significant sun exposure over many years.

Patients with solar keratoses may also have other mucocutaneous premalignant lesions, such as actinic cheilitis (Fig. 2), or malignant lesions, such as SCC, basal cell carcinoma, LM, or malignant melanoma. Solar keratosis is also often associated with other cutaneous sun damage, such as solar elastosis of the dermal collagen and solar lentigo. Within 5 to 10 years of onset, solar keratoses and actinic cheilitis tend to spread peripherally, with loss of skin markings. Spontaneous bleeding and induration signal progression to invasive SCC.

Prolonged ultraviolet (UV) B radiation (wavelengths 290–320 nm) damages nuclear DNA of the basal epidermal keratinocytes, which leads to mutations. The tumor-suppressor gene protein p53, located on chromosome 17p132, and/or ras proto-oncogene protein mutations, are most likely responsible for the development of AKs. Immunostains have shown that the p53 mutation is present in 53% of AKs and in 70% to 90% of invasive SCC arising in AKs.

Immunosuppressed patients tend to show accelerated evolution of AKs to invasive SCC. In addition, malignancy in these patients tends to behave more aggressively, with frequent metastases. Patients with xeroderma pigmentosum develop solar keratoses in the first year of life. The incidence of solar keratoses and invasive SCC increases in patients after prolonged psoralen/UVA (PUVA) treatment.

Actinic cheilitis is similar to solar keratoses, but involves the sun-exposed mucous membranes and the mucocutaneous junction of the lips, particularly the lower lip margin (Fig. 3). The lesions are scaly and fissured. Invasive SCC of the lip has a higher incidence of metastases than that of the skin.

Microscopic Features

Five histologic types of solar keratosis and actinic cheilitis are recognized: hypertrophic, atrophic, bowenoid, acantholytic (Fig. 2), and pigmented. The epidermis and mucous membrane epithelium show hyperkeratosis, parakeratosis, hypergranulosis, frequent irregular acanthosis, and sometimes atrophy. The palisaded basal layer of the epidermis and the pilar epithelium above the sebaceous gland level are replaced by small buds and broad or elongated rete ridges containing atypical keratinocytes, sometimes associated

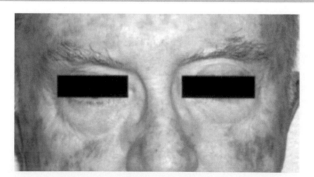

Figure 2 Multiple erythematous plaques of actinic keratosis on the bridge of nose and the cheek of the same patient shown in Figure 1. (*See color insert.*)

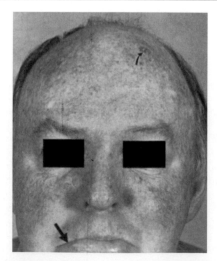

Figure 3 Flat erythematous to brown, scaly papule of actinic keratosis (*curved arrow*) on the forehead of a middle-aged man. Note also a scaly, fissured actinic cheilitis on the right lower lip margin (*straight arrow*).

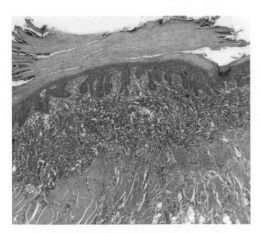

Figure 4 Low-power view of an actinic keratosis, showing small buds and diffuse basal epidermal atypical keratinocytes. Note a dense upper dermal lymphocytic infiltrate and underlying severe solar elastosis of the dermal collagen (hematoxylin and eosin, X100). (*See color insert.*)

with liquefaction degeneration or acantholysis. The atypical keratinocytes are characterized by enlarged, pleomorphic, hyperchromatic nuclei, with loss of nuclear polarity, disordered maturation (Fig. 4), prominent nucleoli, vacuolated cytoplasm, malignant dyskeratosis, multinucleated giant cells, and abundant mitoses. On cytologic grounds alone, lesions of AK and invasive SCC are indistinguishable. Indications for biopsy of AKs include rapid growth, bleeding, induration, or pain suggesting progression to invasive SCC.

In the hypertrophic type of solar keratosis, papillomatosis is prominent, and sometimes forms a cutaneous horn (Fig. 5). Atrophic solar keratoses exhibit thinned, atrophic epidermis, with liquefaction degeneration of the DEJ. The bowenoid type shows a windblown pattern of atypical keratinocytes and frequent clumped nuclei. Similarly to lesions of Bowen's disease, atypical keratinocytic proliferation in bowenoid solar keratosis frequently extends along the outer root sheath of the hair follicle; however, unlike Bowen's disease, bowenoid actinic keratosis displays surface epidermal maturation, i.e., the atypical keratinocytes involve the mid and lower Malpighian layers. There is no full-thickness epidermal atypia in bowenoid actinic keratosis, as in

Bowen's disease. The basal epidermis in acantholytic solar keratosis shows prominent acantholysis, with suprabasal lacunae containing malignant dyskeratotic cells. Pigmented solar keratosis (actinic melanosis) contains prominent pigmented melanocytes in the epidermis and melanophages in the dermis. In all types of solar keratosis, there is evidence of solar damage: moderate-to-severe elastosis of dermal collagen, and a dense, chronic inflammatory infiltrate composed of lymphocytes, histiocytes, and plasma cells. In some instances, the infiltrate lies near the base of the lesion, and shows a lichenoid pattern.

Solar (Actinic) Keratosis and Actinic Cheilitis with Invasive Squamous Cell Carcinoma (Solar Carcinoma)

Without treatment, approximately 10% to 20% of patients with solar keratoses develop one or more lesions that invade the dermis as invasive SCC. The invasive lesions appear as flesh-colored, pink, red, or brown keratotic papules, or nodules with scale and elevated pearly, crusted margins (Fig. 6). Patients complain about nonhealing, indurated, enlarging lesions that bleed with trauma and are pruritic, sometimes painful. Microscopically, these lesions are seen to invade the DEJ with atypical keratinocytes that extend into the dermis at various depths (Fig. 7A and B). Adenoid SCC arising in the acantholytic type of solar keratosis demonstrates a pseudoglandular pattern (Fig. 8). Hypertrophic AK involving the dorsum of hand, wrist, or forearm have been shown to have a high rate (50% in Caucasians) of developing invasive SCC. The risk of metastasis for cutaneous invasive SCC is related to tumor thickness or depth of invasion. Adenoid (acantholytic) SCC may metastasize when the tumor is larger than 2.5 cm.

SCC arising in actinic cheilitis has been associated with a higher rate of metastasis (10%–30%). Therefore, excision with microscopically controlled margins (Mohs' micrographic surgery) and evaluation for lymph node metastasis are indicated.

Differential Diagnosis

The clinical variation among AKs gives rise to a broad differential diagnosis. Given that the characteristic clinical features

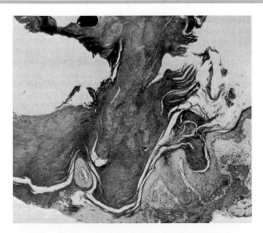

Figure 5 A hypertrophic type of actinic keratosis with cutaneous horn formation (hematoxylin and eosin, X25).

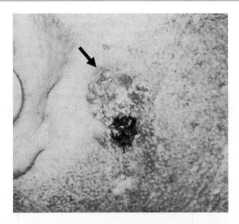

Figure 6 Crusting, hyperkeratotic nodules of invasive squamous cell carcinoma, arising in an actinic keratosis on the antihelix skin of an elderly man. The clinical differential diagnosis of this lesion includes an amelanotic malignant melanoma and atypical fibroxanthoma.

(A)   (B)   (C)

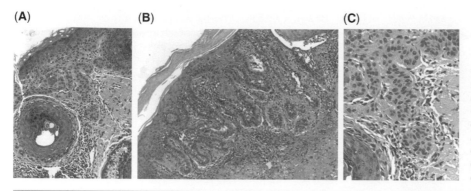

Figure 7 Photomicrographs of invasive squamous cell carcinoma arising in actinic keratosis, displaying various depths of dermal invasion by carcinoma cells, branching down from the dermo–epidermal junction (**A** and **B**) (hematoxylin and eosin, X60, X25). Higher magnification of (**A**) depicts dermal irregular strands of invasive tumor cells (**C**) (hematoxylin and eosin, X125). (*See color insert.*)

of AK include irregularly sized, shiny pink–red macules, with varying degrees of pigmentation and keratotic thickening, to verrucous plaques on sun-exposed skin, the differential diagnosis includes noninfectious inflammatory dermatoses, such as discoid lupus erythematosus; and papulosquamous lesions, including guttate psoriasis, lichen planus, and sometimes seborrheic dermatitis. Indeed, these conditions often coexist with lesions of actinic keratosis.

Clinical differentiation of AK from other neoplastic lesions mainly involves seborrheic keratosis, solar lentigo, and LM (melanoma in situ), particularly the pigmented AK. In more infiltrative plaques of AK, an invasive SCC or basal cell carcinoma must be ruled out. Infectious dermatoses such as tinea infection, and sometimes deep fungal infections as well as parasitic infestation such as cutaneous leishmaniasis, may also mimic lesions of AK.

The distinction of solar keratosis from seborrheic keratosis can usually be made clinically. The latter is more discrete and elevated from the surrounding epidermis. It has a typical stuck-on appearance with comedonal openings of the skin surface.

The hypertrophic type of solar keratosis should be distinguished from verruca vulgaris, invasive SCC arising in solar keratosis, the de novo type of invasive SCC, and "keratoacanthoma." Because of the clinical similarity of these lesions, a biopsy should include lateral margins, and determine whether invasion into the underlying dermis or submucosa is present. Invasive SCC lacking the marginal changes of solar keratosis should be classified as the de novo type. A superficial multicentric type of basal cell

carcinoma may resemble solar keratosis clinically; but a rolled, translucent, telangiectatic edge characterizes the basal cell carcinoma. An atrophic solar keratosis may be mistaken for discoid lupus erythematosus, but lupus usually contains follicular plugging, and has easily detachable scale. The microscopic absence of atypical keratinocytes, prominent liquefaction degeneration of the DEJ, and a patchy peri-appendageal lymphocytic infiltrate, are features that favor discoid lupus erythematosus. Localized forms of poikiloderma, atrophic lichen planus, and lichenoid drug eruption, should also be considered in the microscopic differential diagnosis of atrophic solar keratoses. These lesions, however, do not show atypia or pleomorphism of the keratinocytes.

Unlike bowenoid solar keratoses, Bowen's disease on sun-exposed areas usually has a more irregular contour and a red base. Microscopic examination shows full-thickness involvement of epidermis and pilar epithelium, with atypical keratinocytes.

The acantholytic type of solar keratosis must be distinguished from the following diseases microscopically: isolated dyskeratosis follicularis (warty dyskeratoma), keratosis follicularis (Darier's disease), familial benign chronic pemphigus (Hailey-Hailey disease), transient acantholytic dermatosis, and pemphigus vulgaris. Cellular pleomorphism, disorderly arrangement of keratinocytes, malignant dyskeratosis, and absence of corps ronds and grains, characterize acantholytic solar keratosis.

A pigmented solar keratosis may resemble LM (melanotic freckle of Hutchinson), an acquired precancerous pigmented melanosis that frequently degenerates into LM melanoma or sometimes into desmoplastic or neurotropic malignant melanoma. In LM, there is more flattening of the epidermis than in pigmented solar keratoses, and more importantly, atypical melanocytic cells, not keratinocytes, are present at the DEJ.

Benign lichenoid keratosis may be mistaken for solar keratosis or actinic cheilitis on low-power examination. However, it does not exhibit keratinocyte atypia.

Treatment

The treatment of patients with solar keratoses and related invasive SCC should be conservative. Complete ablation is the treatment of choice, with cure rates of 75% to 95% or higher. Several modalities are available, depending on the size, number, and anatomic location of the lesions. All AKs should be treated in order to prevent their progression to invasive SCC.

Cryosurgery utilizing liquid nitrogen (−195.8°C) is the most common method of treating scattered solitary lesions (usually fewer than 15 lesions) of AKs in the United States.

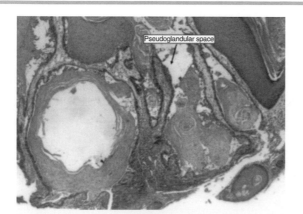

Pseudoglandular space

Figure 8 Adenoid squamous cell carcinoma arising in an acantholytic type of actinic keratosis, showing prominent acantholysis with pseudoglandular spaces (hematoxylin and eosin, X60).

(A)   **(B)**

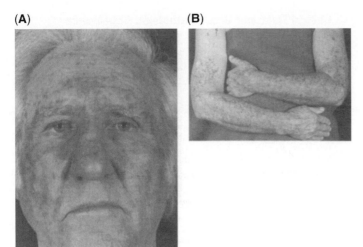

Figure 9 Actinic keratoses of the (**A**) face and (**B**) arms of a fair-skinned, middle-aged man, showing redness and prominence of the plaques, two weeks after 5% 5-fluorouracil cream application.

A cotton tipped applicator or cryostat spray is used to freeze both the cutaneous and mucosal lesions and a thin rim of surrounding skin for 5 to 15 seconds repeated two to three times; this procedure suffices to ablate these lesions. Pain and discomfort when the liquid nitrogen is applied to the forehead and scalp areas is mild-to-moderate, and local anesthesia is not needed. The most common side effect is hypopigmentation. Bullae followed by an exudative crust may supervene; healing occurs in one to three weeks. Complications may include scarring, secondary infection, especially if the wound is occluded without proper dressing changes, and change of skin texture.

Excision, as well as curettage and electrodessication, is used to treat hypertrophic AKs and lesions suspicious for invasive SCC. It is useful to obtain a biopsy to assess dermal invasion before ablating the lesion with curettage and electrodessication. This procedure offers high cure rates for hypertrophic AKs on the forearms, hands, scalp, and ears, also for cutaneous horns. It is also performed on lesions that have resisted other forms of treatment and, especially after a biopsy. This therapeutic method usually requires local anesthesia, and is usually well tolerated. Scar tissue associated with the procedure is usually not conspicuous.

Topical applications of 1% to 5% 5-fluorouracil (5-FU) cream or solution twice daily is especially indicated in patients with multiple lesions, and can be used effectively on the face, scalp, hands, and forearms. Five percent 5-FU is the standard concentration used; however, lower concentrations have been advocated by some, for patients with more sensitive facial skin. This treatment causes clinical and subclinical lesions to be more pronounced (Fig. 9A and B), and culminate in acute erythema and tender erosions after one to four weeks. Symptoms are improved by the application of 1% hydrocortisone cream (Fig. 10A and B). The time span for this mode of therapy averages six weeks. Topical 5-FU interferes with DNA and RNA synthesis, and the cure rates are up to 93%. Scarring is a rare complication, unless secondary infection has supervened. Injection of 5-FU (50 mg/mL) at 0.1 to 0.5 mL/plaque has been advocated for larger lesions of AKs and associated invasive SCC. However, recurrences are common. Other disadvantages of this treatment include the duration and the

(A)   **(B)**

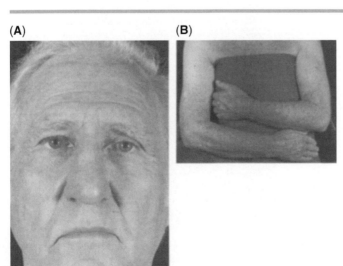

Figure 10 Dramatic improvement of actinic keratoses (**A**) on the face and (**B**) on the arms of the patient illustrated in Figure 9, observed four weeks after initiation of treatment. The therapy consisted of two weeks of 1% hydrocortisone cream twice daily following two weeks of 5% 5-fluorouracil.

unsightly appearance as well as discomfort that the patient must endure.

A relatively new topical agent, a nonsteroidal anti-inflammatory drug, 3% *diclofenac* in a 2.5% hyaluronan gel, is available for the treatment of AKs. It is applied twice daily for two to three months. A 50% total clearance rate one month after completion of treatment has been reported. The treatment is well-tolerated, with mild-to-moderate itching noted.

Approval for dermatologic use of 5% *imiquimod cream* was recently granted by the Food and Drug Administration (FDA). This is an agent that acts on the immune system. It was previously approved for the treatment of genital warts. For lesions of AKs, application of 5% imiquimod three times weekly results in clinical clearing of treated lesions in nearly 85% of patients. However, side effects include irritation, scabbing, blister formation, and ulceration. About 10% of patients develop a recurrence one year afterwards.

Salicylic acid and alpha-hydroxyl acids may remove atypical cells by their exfoliant characteristics. Topical reti- noids have been found to reduce the number and size of AKs.

Dermabrasion, removing the top layer of the skin by sanding or using a wire brush, is a popular alternative to 5-FU for treating groups of multiple solar keratoses. Wound healing is rapid, generally within two weeks. Furthermore, recurrences are less frequent, and make this alternative treatment more cost-effective. Chemical peel with trichloro- acetic acid has also been described.

The defocused CO_2 laser is used to vaporize cutaneous neoplasms and verrucae, and is especially successful for the treatment of actinic cheilitis. Retinoids (Acutane and Tegison) may be used to prevent the develop- ment of new solar keratoses and invasive SCC's, but are not effective for treating well-established lesions. Radiation therapy is reserved for established neoplasms, and is not used for solar keratosis. Further radiation damage to solar- damaged skin is counterproductive.

Prognosis and Prevention

The prognosis of solar-keratosis–derived invasive SCC is excellent. The biologic potential for metastasis is rare, with the exception of the adenoid (acantholytic) subtype, in which about 2% to 3% of patients with tumors larger than 2 cm develop metastasis.

Sunscreens are available, to prevent sun damage of the skin. The best protection is offered by agents that contain para-aminobenzoic acid and benzophenones. Water- resistant formulations are available, that require less frequent application when swimming. Sun protection factor (SPF) is defined as that amount of protection required to prevent ery- thema after a minimal erythema dose (MED) of sunlight on a sunscreen-treated site. Each factor unit protects for one MED, so that SPF-15 protects for 15 MEDs, and is generally adequate for a full day of erythemogenic sun exposure. A high SPF combined with protective clothing constitutes effec- tive sunscreening, in conjunction with avoidance of the midday sun, which contains the highest proportion of UVB. Opaque sunscreens with zinc oxide ointment and red petrolatum are an effective block, but they are difficult to apply over large areas, and are cosmetically unappealing.

RADIATION KERATOSIS

Symptoms for this condition include X-ray keratosis, postir- radiation keratosis, irradiation dermatitis, X-ray burns, X-ray dermatitis, radiation atypia, and roentgen dermatitis.

Clinical Data and Gross Pathologic Appearance

Radiation keratosis may occur in a scar following radiation therapy or excessive fluoroscopy. People at high risk, such as radiologists, radiotherapists, dentists, surgeons, and patients exposed to radiation for a variety of disorders, including acne, basal cell carcinoma, and SCC, may be exposed to small doses of X-ray, and develop postirradiation keratoses. Such cases are now becoming rare. Chronic radi- ation dermatitis and radiation keratosis may occur several months to many years after the exposure. The skin is atrophic, with telangiectasia and irregular hyperpigmenta- tion and hypopigmentation. Ulceration and foci of hyperkeratotic scale may be seen in areas of atrophy. Cutaneous malignancy frequently develops in these areas.

Microscopic Features

The epidermis is irregular, showing both atrophy and vari- able hyperplasia. There is hyperkeratosis, and the squamous cells show disorderly maturation, pleomorphism with indi- vidual cell keratinization, and atypia (Fig. 11). Degeneration of the cells in the stratum malpighii and scant lymphocytic exocytosis may be present. In the dermis, the collagen bun- dles are enlarged, and often show hyalinization; and there are scattered, enlarged, atypical fibroblasts, sometimes with bizarre hyperchromatic nuclei. The deep dermal blood ves- sels often show fibrous thickening of their walls. Some of the vessels show thrombosis and recanalization. In contrast, the upper dermal vessels may be dilated. Lymphedema in the subepidermal region may be seen. Pilosebaceous units and sweat glands are usually preserved.

Carcinoma Arising in Radiation Keratosis (Radiation Carcinoma)

SCC and basal cell carcinoma are the most common malig- nancies attributed to irradiation. In most cases, the tumor develops either within hyperkeratotic areas of chronic radiodermatitis or in a persistent ulcer. There is a long latent period between irradiation and carcinoma, varying from 4 to 39 years, with a median of 7 to 12 years. Before 1940, most reported cases of radiation carcinoma were SCC, occurring

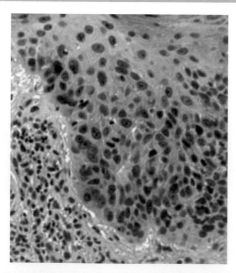

Figure 11 A radiation keratosis on the skin of the chest at the site of a radiation port in a patient with esophageal carcinoma, displays disorderly, atypical keratinocytes, with pleomorphic and hyperchromatic nuclei involving the basal epidermis (hematoxylin and eosin, X200). (*See color insert.*)

on the hands, feet, and, occasionally, on the face. An increasing number of basal cell carcinomas have been reported since 1951. In cases of radiation dermatitis, basal cell carcinoma develops almost exclusively on the head and neck; while in all other areas, SCC is more common. Many cases of radiation carcinoma seen in recent years have been due to the treatment of acne or other benign disorders. Due to a general awareness of the potential dangers of repeated low-dose X-ray irradiation, it can be expected that the incidence of radiation carcinoma will decrease.

SCC arising in radiation keratosis is frequently of the spindle cell type. Large columns of atypical keratinocytes are connected to the overlying epidermis, and interlacing spindle-shaped cells with hyperchromatic nuclei, frequent mitoses, and abundant eosinophilic, sometimes vacuolated, cytoplasm are present. The dermal changes are similar to those seen in chronic radiodermatitis or radiation keratosis. Histologic differential diagnoses of spindle cell SCC should include spindle cell amelanotic malignant melanoma, desmoplastic malignant melanoma, LM melanoma, and atypical fibroxanthoma. Immunoperoxidase staining for high-molecular weight keratin (CK903) is usually positive, and electron microscopic demonstration of intercellular desmosomes and cytoplasmic tonofilaments confirms the diagnosis.

Treatment

Radiation keratoses should be treated in the same way as solar keratoses. Radical surgical extirpation with skin grafting was the standard treatment for radiation carcinoma in the past. Topical treatment with 5-FU has been effective for superficial tumors. Cryosurgery and Mohs' micrographic surgery should be considered. Prevention or minimization of chronic X-ray exposure remains of paramount importance.

BOWEN'S DISEASE

Symptoms for this condition include Bowen's dermatosis, epithelioma of Bowen, precancerous dermatosis of Bowen, dyskeratose lenticulaire et en disque (Darier), SCIC, and vulvar intraepithelial neoplasia (VIN), bowenoid dysplasia.

Clinical Data and Gross Pathologic Appearance

Bowen's disease occurs in both sexes, but predominantly in fair-complexioned men; only one-fifth of patients are women. Sun-sensitive, predominantly older persons are affected most often. Bowen's disease is relatively uncommon. It is estimated to occur in less than 1% of the population. The average age at onset is 48 years. About one-third of cases involve the head and neck, particularly the face.

Bowen's disease is a slowly enlarging, reddish-brown, annular or polycyclic, scaly, fissured, crusty, eroded plaque (Fig. 12). The lesions are devoid of hair, and are sharply demarcated from normal skin. Areas of normal-appearing skin may occur within the boundaries of larger plaques. The average duration to diagnosis is 6.4 years. Lesions of short duration appear as small, scaly, nonelevated keratoses. In the anogenital area, they are often verrucous and pigmented.

The criteria for referring to Bowen's disease as a precancerous lesion are based on microscopic SCC in situ involving the epidermis and the pilosebaceous epithelium. The association with extracutaneous malignancy has been a controversy since Bowen first reported that a patient died of gastric carcinoma after having had Bowen's disease for

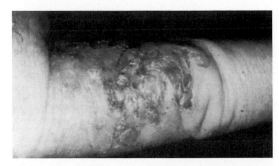

Figure 12 Focally pigmented, scaly plaque of Bowen's disease (squamous carcinoma in situ) is sharply demarcated from the surrounding normal skin.

34 years. Similar observations have been made by several others. Recent studies, however, have shown no direct cause and effect relationship between Bowen's disease and internal malignancy.

Microscopic Features

The typical microscopic features of Bowen's disease are hyperkeratosis, parakeratosis, hypergranulosis, acanthosis, and a chronic inflammatory infiltrate in the upper corium. The epidermis exhibits total or focal loss of normal polarity and progression of keratinocyte maturation. The loss of normal epidermal architecture is characterized by a windblown appearance of atypical keratinocytes, hyperchromatism, vacuolated cells, multinucleated cells, malignant dyskeratosis, and abnormal mitoses (Fig. 13). These changes occur at all epidermal levels (Fig. 13A), but may be focal, and are confined by an intact dermo–epidermal basement membrane. Examination of lesions from hair-bearing areas shows involvement of the pilar acrotrichium, infundibulum, and sebaceous gland. The atypical cellular proliferation involves all levels of the outer root sheath, and eventually replaces the sebaceous gland cells. In some lesions, the majority of the atypical epithelial cells appear vacuolated. Hyperchromatic, undifferentiated keratinocytes replace the epidermal

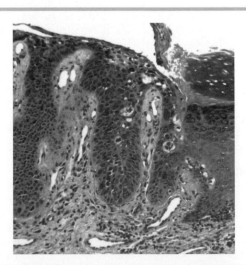

Figure 13 Plaque-like lesion of Bowen's disease showing hyperkeratosis, and atypical keratinocytes replacing the entire thickness of the epidermis, absent normal keratinocytic maturation and marked nuclear atypia with abnormal mitoses (hematoxylin and eosin, X250). (*See color insert.*)

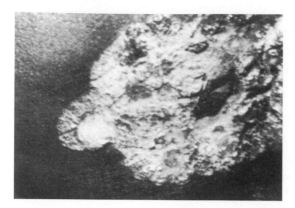

Figure 14 Large, exophytic tumor arising in a long-standing plaque of Bowen's disease on the back of an African man.

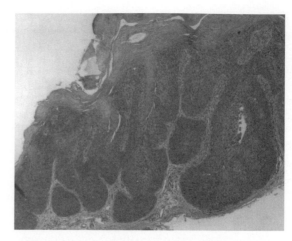

Figure 15 Invasive adnexal carcinoma arising in Bowen's disease shows prominent basaloid and squamoid differentiation. Note marked nuclear anaplasia (hematoxylin and eosin, X100). (*See color insert.*)

basal layer and the pilar outer root sheath. This gives the appearance of cellular nesting. The acrosyringium generally is not involved. The inflammatory infiltrate of lymphocytes, histiocytes, and sometimes plasma cells is seen in the upper corium. In the upper dermis, there is capillary endothelial proliferation and some ectatic small vessels. Lesions located on the sun-exposed areas of the body show prominent solar elastosis. The atypical vacuolated keratinocytes are routinely negative for cytoplasmic mucin; however, some contain glycogen. Melanin is present in the atypical cells in most lesions. The abnormal keratinizing cells are intensely reactive with glucose-6-phosphatase dehydrogenase. Ultrastructural changes include abnormal cell division of dyskeratotic cells, abnormal mitotic figures, and an increase in tonofilament-desmosomal attachments, absence of keratohyalin, and aggregate tonofilaments and nuclear substances.

Bowen's Disease and Invasive Adnexal Carcinoma

Without treatment, about 3% to 5% of patients with Bowen's disease develop invasive carcinoma. This invasive carcinoma presents as a rapidly growing, ulcerating, or nodular tumor in a preexisting patch of many years' duration (Fig. 14). In a study of 100 such cases from the Armed Forces Institute of Pathology, the patients ranged in age from 29 to 91 years, with a male–female ratio of 3:1 and a white–black ratio of 20:1. The extremities, face, and anogenital areas were common sites of involvement. The size of the tumor varied from 1 to 12 cm. Histopathologic evidence of Bowen's disease was identified in all cases. The cytologic changes of invasive adnexal carcinoma showed basaloid, squamoid (Fig. 15), pilar, pilosebaceous, and occasionally glandular differentiation, favoring interpretation of the invasive lesion as a form of adnexal carcinoma. Mitoses and malignant dyskeratosis are commonly seen.

Differential Diagnosis

Bowenoid solar keratosis differs from Bowen's disease. The former is usually smaller, occurring almost exclusively on sun-exposed areas. On microscopic examination, the atypical squamous keratinocytes do not involve the entire thickness of the epidermis or pilar epithelium, as seen in Bowen's disease. Mammary and extramammary Paget's disease may share with Bowen's disease the presence of vacuolated cells, but in contrast, there is no dyskeratosis. In addition, the cytoplasm of Paget's cells often contains sialomucin. The material in vacuolated cells of Bowen's disease is glycogen. The

cellular nesting of vacuolated pagetoid cells in some lesions of Bowen's disease can cause confusion with malignant melanoma and intraepidermal epithelioma.

Bowenoid papulosis shares some histologic similarity to Bowen's disease, particularly the presence of keratinocytic atypia and mitoses. Therefore, Bowen's disease involving the genitalia must be differentiated from bowenoid papulosis, which shows an orderly background with scattered dysplastic, dyskeratotic cells, and mitotic figures, in a salt-and-pepper fashion (Fig. 16). Atypical keratinocytes are seen in full thickness in the epidermis, pilosebaceous epithelium, and mucosal epithelium in Bowen's disease and carcinoma in situ but not in bowenoid papulosis. Plasma cells are rare in the dermal and submucosal infiltrate in bowenoid papulosis, in contrast to Bowen's disease.

The clinical presentation of bowenoid papulosis is quite different from that of Bowen's disease. Bowenoid papuloses predominantly affect patients under the age of 46 years, and are typically small, dome-shaped papules or plaques located on the external genitalia (Fig. 17). Bowenoid papulosis is considered benign, and spontaneous regression is common. Condyloma acuminatum with epithelial atypia

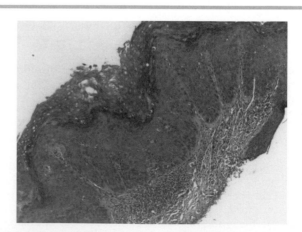

Figure 16 A section of vulvar bowenoid papulosis, showing mild hyperkeratosis, acanthosis, and scattered dysplastic and dyskeratotic keratinocytes (hematoxylin and eosin, X160). (*See color insert.*)

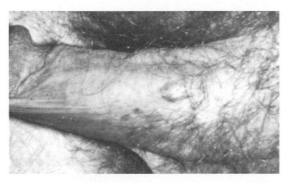

Figure 17 Flesh-colored, grouped papules of bowenoid papulosis on the penile shaft of young individual.

may sometimes be mistaken for Bowen's disease. Superficial keratinocyte maturation and prominent koilocytotic atypia with vacuolated cells in the parakeratotic layer typify condylomata. The role of human papillomavirus in all these lesions as a precursor of malignancy has yet to be clarified.

Treatment

The origin of Bowen's disease from pilar outer root sheath cells at the sebaceous gland level helps explain the high recurrence rate after treatment with superficial X-ray, curettage and desiccation, and topical 5-FU. Mohs' micrographic surgery should be considered. Liquid nitrogen cryotherapy and topical chemotherapy with 5-FU are less effective. Ionizing radiation using soft X-rays is suitable for elderly patients who are poor candidates for surgery. CO_2 laser vaporization has been used, but is limited because of the lack of histologic margin control.

ARSENICAL KERATOSIS AND ARSENICAL CARCINOMA

Arsenical keratoses frequently present as horn-like, punctate papules on the extremities, characteristically affecting the palms and soles (Fig. 18). The microscopic features and subsequent carcinoma are indistinguishable from Bowen's disease and subsequent adnexal carcinoma. Intake of arsenic in small amounts for long periods produces a general neoplastic tendency. It is possible that arsenic is a cause of

Bowen's disease. There is an affinity of arsenic for keratinizing epithelium.

Differential Diagnosis

Arsenical keratoses must be differentiated from punctate keratoderma, Darier's disease, and lichen planus. Plantar warts are more papillomatous, and are easily differentiated microscopically.

Treatment

The multiplicity of the lesions makes radical treatment and complete removal impractical. Frequent monitoring for clinical evidence of carcinoma is important. Keratolytics, such as salicylic acid, urea, and lactic acid, as well as physical debridement, are helpful.

ERYTHROPLASIA OF QUEYRAT

Symptoms include carcinoma in situ and Bowen's disease of the glans penis.

Clinical Data and Gross Pathologic Appearance

Erythroplasia of Queyrat is a distinct clinicopathologic entity: carcinoma in situ involving the penile skin, mucosa, and mucocutaneous junction of the glans penis. The clinical and histologic features of erythroplasia of Queyrat are similar to those of Bowen's disease, particularly involving the vulva. The disease occurs almost exclusively in uncircumcised men. It typically manifests as an asymptomatic, well-demarcated, red, velvety plaque with yellow-crusted flecks on the glans penis, in the coronal sulcus (Fig. 19), or on the inner surface of the prepuce. Ulceration, crusting, and erosion are sometimes observed. The disease more commonly affects middle-aged and older men. The average duration to diagnosis is about three years, and the median size of lesions is 1.0 cm.

Microscopic Features

Erythroplasia of Queyrat shows thickening of the epidermis and mucosa with increased cellularity, hypokeratosis, and focal erosion. The normal keratinocytes are entirely replaced by nonkeratinizing basaloid cells with mild nuclear hyperchromatism and pleomorphism. The microscopic features are those of carcinoma in situ.

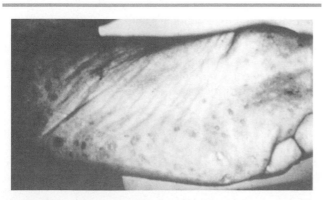

Figure 18 Horn-like, punctuate, arsenical keratosis on the soles of a patient with a history of chronic arsenism.

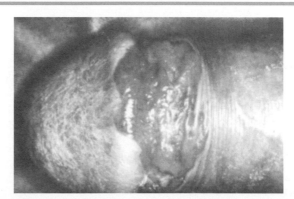

Figure 19 Well-demarcated, focally eroded plaque of erythroplasia of Queyrat involving the penile skin, mucosa of the glans penis, and corona sulcus.

Adnexal Carcinoma Arising in Erythroplasia of Queyrat

Without adequate treatment, up to 30% of patients may develop invasive carcinoma. Squamous, basaloid, and ductal differentiation are frequently observed. About 20% of those with invasive carcinoma develop metastasis.

Treatment

Surgical excision is the treatment of choice. Electrodessication and curettage and topical 5-FU are effective. About 1% to 2% 5-FU cream is applied. If no reaction occurs with twice-daily application after one week, 5% 5-FU should be used. Application under occlusion may be more effective. Phallectomy with inguinal lymph node dissection is reserved for cases of invasive carcinoma. When ionizing irradiation is used as the only treatment, a high recurrence rate (up to 80%) has been noted. Mohs' micrographic surgery may be the best approach.

INTRAEPIDERMAL EPITHELIOMA

Symptoms for this condition include: intraepidermal epithelioma of Borst-Jadassohn, intraepidermal basal cell epithelioma, combined intraepidermal basosquamous carcinoma, intraepidermal acanthoma, intraepidermal nevus, hidroacanthoma simplex, eccrine poroepithelioma, and intraepidermal eccrine poroma.

Clinical Data and Gross Pathologic Appearance

Intraepidermal epithelioma occurs as a single gray to tan-brown, keratotic, scaly, flat, sometimes verrucous, round to irregularly shaped papule, plaque, or nodule varying from 0.5 to 10 cm in diameter. The plaque usually is sharply demarcated from the adjacent skin. Differentiation from seborrheic keratosis requires microscopic examination. Papillary lesions are uncommon, and erosion and ulceration sometimes occur. Lesions occur on all parts of the body except the palms and soles. About 25% occur on the head and neck, particularly the face (17%), 46% on the lower extremities, and the rest on other parts of the body; in decreasing order of frequency: the buttocks, chest, back, upper extremity, abdomen, and feet. They predominantly occur in white patients aged 40 to 79 years, and more commonly in women than men. The duration to diagnosis varies from less than one month to more than 30 years, but more than half are present for less than three years.

There is controversy about the cell of origin. Some conclude that the lesion represents a benign epidermal proliferation. The cells of origin are acrosyringeal keratinocytes or multipluripotential adnexal cells. When the dermo–epidermal basement membrane is disrupted and atypical keratinocytes invade the corium, intraepidermal epithelioma is considered to represent an adnexal eccrine carcinoma. Support for eccrine histogenesis is based on histopathologic features and immunohistochemical studies, particularly evidence of carcinoembryonic antigen and enzyme reactivity of discrete cell nests. Intraepidermal epithelioma may represent the premalignant counterpart of eccrine porocarcinoma. Long-term follow-up shows that 15% of patients develop local recurrences, in most cases due to incomplete removal.

Microscopic Features

Intraepidermal epithelioma is characterized by hyperkeratosis, spotted parakeratosis, hypergranulosis, occasional horn cysts, and plaque-like acanthosis, with discrete nests of uniform and dysplastic keratinocytes, composed of basaloid or squamoid cell types within the stratum malpighii (Fig. 17). Some lesions show prominent papillomatosis and verrucous acanthosis. Spindle-shaped, pigmented cells are sometimes present. Some keratinocytes form squamous eddies reminiscent of inflamed seborrheic keratosis, inverted follicular keratosis, and epidermal nevus. The pigmented lesions have melanin pigment associated with discrete nests of keratinocytes. Capillary-endothelial proliferation, vascular ectasia, and fibrosis are present in the upper dermis of most lesions. The dermo–epidermal basement membrane remains intact for long periods of time in most cases.

Intraepidermal Epithelioma and Invasive Carcinoma

Eight percent of patients show clinical and microscopic evidence of invasive carcinoma in the primary lesion. In general, these lesions are larger, and appear papillary, with areas of erosion and ulceration (Fig. 18). There are intraepidermal cell nests with marked cellular atypia, pleomorphism, malignant dyskeratosis, vacuolated cells, mitotic figures, and occasionally multinucleated cells and disruption of the dermo–epidermal basement membrane with atypical keratinocytes invading the dermis. The tumor cells infiltrating the dermis and those at metastatic sites show some tendency toward nesting, as seen in the epidermis. This tumor should be regarded as a form of adnexal carcinoma. Metastasis occurs in 6% of patients. The potential for distant metastasis requires consideration of intraepidermal epithelioma along with other cutaneous premalignant neoplasms.

Differential Diagnosis

Cutaneous epithelial neoplasms with cellular nesting can be confused with intraepidermal epithelioma; these include seborrheic keratosis, epidermal nevus, inverted follicular keratosis, lichenoid benign keratosis, Bowen's disease, mammary and extramammary Paget's disease, spindle cell nevus, and precancerous-acquired melanosis (melanoma in situ). Epidermal nevi demonstrate squamous eddy formation when inflamed, and are often confused with intraepidermal epithelioma.

Treatment

Excision, curettage, and desiccation are acceptable methods of treatment for lesions of carcinoma arising in intraepidermal epithelioma.

PRECANCEROUS ACQUIRED PIGMENTED MELANOSIS

Symptoms for this condition include melanotic freckle of Hutchinson, premalignant melanosis, premalignant melanocytic dysplasia, atypical melanocytic hyperplasia, malignant melanoma in situ, precancerous melanosis of the compound nevus type, malignant melanoma, Clark's level I, and pagetoid melanocytic proliferation.

Clinical Data and Gross Pathologic Appearance

The noninvasive malignant melanomas exhibit two clinical forms. Precancerous melanosis and LM are melanocytic disorders of the epidermal melanocytes. The clinical features of the two forms are similar. The clinical location, however, includes both sun-exposed and nonexposed skin. Lesions of LM commonly affect facial sun-exposed skin in elderly men. The brown-pigmented macule slowly extends laterally,

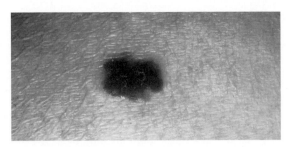

Figure 20 An irregularly bordered, enlarging pigmented lesion of malignant melanoma in situ (precancerous melanosis) present on the arm of a 32-year-old-man. (*See color insert.*)

with an irregular border and variegated pigmentation (Fig. 20). The color varies from dark-brown to gray or black. The adjacent skin is usually unremarkable. The patients with noninvasive melanomas are middle-aged or older. Without treatment, lesions progress to become pigmented nodules and increase in size, which are signs of invasive malignant melanoma. They vary in size from a few millimeters to 2 to 3 cm. An adequate excisional biopsy specimen for histologic evaluation is essential for accurate diagnosis, particularly for distinction from invasive melanoma.

Microscopic Features

The histologic findings include nests, theques, or individual atypical, frequently pigmented melanocytes present either at the DEJ or scattered in all layers of the epidermis (Fig. 21). The junctional change is extensive, and frequently extends into the pilar epithelium. Nuclear pleomorphism, with large epithelioid cells, spindle-shaped atypical melanocytes, and mitoses, is characteristic. Dyskeratotic cells and eosinophilic bodies (apoptotic cells, Kamino bodies) are sometimes seen. Preexisting benign nevocellular nevus cells can be identified in about one-third of lesions.

Prognosis and Treatment

The prognosis of in situ melanomas is excellent with complete surgical removal. Precancerous melanosis is treated by complete surgical excision. The lesions will recur following incomplete excision. Lack of treatment will eventually result in invasion into the dermis by the atypical melanocytes. The current recommended regimen of treatment is listed under LM treatment.

LENTIGO MALIGNA (MELANOTIC FRECKLE OF HUTCHINSON)

Symptoms for this condition include senile freckle, lentigo malign des velars, Milanese circumscribe precancerous, premalignant lentigo, malignant freckle, precancerous melanosis, malignant melanoma in situ of the LM type and acquired melanosis.

Clinical Data and Gross Pathologic Appearance

LM or melanotic freckle of Hutchinson is a multicentric, melanocytic disorder of the epidermal melanocytes, the clinical features of which were described by Hutchinson in the early 1890's. It begins as a small brown-pigmented macule, which slowly extends in an irregular fashion. The lesion is composed of small spots and lines of pigment. The color varies, producing a variegated pigmented macule. Individual lesions are light- to dark-brown or gray and black. The clinical appearance of the surrounding skin is unremarkable; however, elderly patients with LM on sun-exposed skin occasionally have other sun-induced lesions in the vicinity. LM occurs exclusively in whites, while men and women are equally affected. It is predominantly a disease of the middle-aged and elderly; patients' ages average 57 years. Only 10% of cases are found in patients younger than 40 years. The average duration is 14 years. The most common location is the head, particularly the face (over 50%) and neck, but other areas, including the back, upper extremity, chest, and abdomen, are also affected. The size varies from 1 to 3 cm. Larger lesions, particularly those greater than 4 cm, are more likely to develop LM melanoma.

Microscopic Features

A single layer of pleomorphic, hyperchromatic, frequently spindle-shaped, atypical melanocytes replaces the DEJ (Fig. 20, left). The junctional change is extensive, and frequently extends along the outer root sheath of the hair follicle. Nests and theques of similar cells are sometimes present. The atypical melanocytes are often vacuolated, with clear cytoplasm and irregular, hyperchromatic nuclei resembling Paget's cells. Spindle cell forms of typical melanocytes (Fig. 22) are common; however, multinucleated cells and mitoses are rare. A band-like inflammatory infiltrate in the upper dermis is usually present.

Treatment

The cornerstone of treatment for primary noninvasive (in situ) melanomas is excisional surgery with adequate

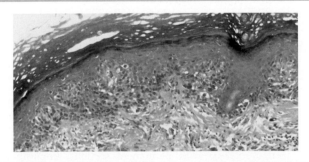

Figure 21 A malignant melanoma in situ showing contiguous atypical melanocytic proliferation at the dermo-epidermal junction, with occasional intraepidermal pagetoid spread (hematoxylin and eosin, X200). (*See color insert.*)

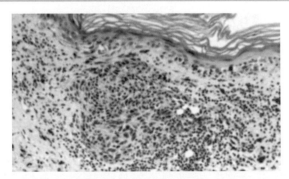

Figure 22 Photomicrographs of a lentigo maligna melanoma illustrates extensive dermo-epidermal junction involvement by contiguous atypical melanocytes, with focal upper dermal invasion. Note spindle-shaped tumor cells (hematoxylin and eosin, X250). (*See color insert.*)

margins. The in situ tumor is classified as Stage 0 by the American Joint Commission on Cancer (AJCC) staging system. A 0.5 to 1.0 cm. (5.0–10.0 mm) uninvolved surgical margin is recommended for these tumors. A recent publication assessing the standard recommendation of 5-mm margins of resection of LM showed that it is adequate in only less than 50% of cases (Agarwal-Antal, Bowen, Gerwis, 2002). Margins may be modified to accommodate individual anatomic or cosmetic considerations. The preferred treatment for LM is complete surgical removal. However, the large size of some of these lesions, coupled with common occurrence on the face in elderly patients, warrant consideration of radiation therapy, cryotherapy, topical chemotherapy, or observation in some cases. Topical imiquimod 5% cream has been reported effective for treating LM. Complete resolution after seven months of daily application to an initial (the most pigmented) test area inside the lesion, followed by three months of application over the entire affected area is recommended (Ahmed and Berth-Jones, 2000). More recent studies by Naylor, Crowson, et al. in 2003 shows that imiquimod 5% cream is a highly effective therapy for LM (in situ melanoma). In long-term follow-up of patients with LM beyond the 5-mm clinical margin, imiquimod may represent a nonsurgical alternative in treating such lesions, with excellent therapeutic and cosmetic results. Systemic chemotherapy is not required for patients with in situ lesions. Lifelong follow-up at least annually should be carried out.

The complete treatment regimen for all types of invasive melanomas is discussed in the chapter dealing with malignant melanomas.

LENTIGO MALIGNA MELANOMA AND INVASIVE MELANOMA, ARISING IN LENTIGO MALIGNA AND MELANOMA IN SITU

In lesions of LM and melanoma in situ, after a period of intraepidermal proliferation of atypical melanocytes, there is often invasion of the papillary dermis by the atypical cells, either in single units or as small nests that become invasive LM melanoma or invasive malignant melanoma. These tumors are usually pigmented with a history of recent enlargement or change in color (Fig. 23). The invasive tumors can be detected using the classic A, B, C, D clinical signs of a

malignant melanoma: A for *asymmetry*, B for irregular *border*, C for varying shades of *color*, and D for greater than 6.0 mm in *diameter*. However, microinvasive melanomas may be difficult to recognize, due to prominent host response in the papillary dermis, typically a dense cellular infiltrate consisting of lymphocytes, monocytes, and melanophages. Furthermore, the invasive melanoma cells are frequently spindle-shaped, especially in LM melanoma (Fig. 22). The spindle-shaped tumor cells may be indistinguishable from activated dermal fibrocytes, without immunostains using a monoclonal melanoma cell marker, i.e., HMB-45.

Differential Diagnosis

In the sun-damaged skin, diffuse benign intraepidermal melanocytic proliferation (IEMP) with atypia may be mistaken for malignant melanoma in situ. The former shows prominent junctional melanocytic proliferation along the DEJ, and sometimes often extending into the pilar outer root sheath, with frequent skipped areas of uninvolved basal epidermal keratinocytes. In areas with IEMP there is no intraepidermal pagetoid spread or mitoses. The in situ melanoma, in contrast, displays contiguous proliferation of atypical melanocytes along the DEJ and the pilar adnexal epithelium, with frequent pagetoid intraepidermal spread and mitotic activity. The morphologic changes of benign IEMP are also commonly encountered in scar tissue and areas adjacent to a melanoma. In the areas of a recently excised melanoma, when observing changes of benign IEMP, care must be taken not to over diagnose IEMP as melanoma in situ, and thus lead to unnecessary additional surgery on the sun-exposed skin, especially in cosmetically critical locations.

ERYTHEMA AB IGNE

Erythema ab igne is a form of postinflammatory hyperpigmentation due to chronic heat exposure. Invasive SCC may rarely develop from this type of lesion. The condition was typically found in the world in which heating was inadequate, and sitting close to fires or furnaces was necessary to keep warm. The lesions can be seen in older individuals, in the areas of skin with prolonged exposure to heating pads or hot water bottles. The lower legs are most common site of involvement. These lesions are reported in the developing and sometimes developed world, where the heat from laptop is a new cause.

ACKNOWLEDGMENT

The authors wish to acknowledge the editorial assistance by G. William Moore, M.D., Ph.D., of the Department of Pathology and Laboratory Medicine, Baltimore VA Medical Center, Baltimore, Maryland U.S.A.

BIBLIOGRAPHY

Ackerman AB, Godomski J. Neurotropic malignant melanoma and other neurotropic neoplasms in the skin. Am J Dermatopathol 1984; 6:63–80.

Ackerman AB. Histopathologists can diagnose malignant melanoma in situ correctly and consistently. Am J Dermatopathol 1984; 6:103–107.

Agarwal-Antal N, Bowen G, Gerwis J. Histologic evaluation of lentigo maligna with permanent sections: implications regarding current guidelines. J Am Acad Dermatol 2002; 47:743–748.

Ahmed I, Berth-Jones J. Imiquimod: a novel treatment for lentigo maligna. Br J Dermatol 2000; 143:843–845.

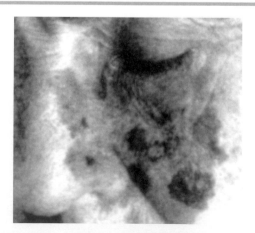

Figure 23 A large, pigmented lesion of LM melanoma on the cheek-temporal area of an 83-year-old fair-skinned individual. These tumors are characterized by a flat (macular) lesion with a prolonged radial growth phase, and developed invading tumor with pigmented nodule formation. (*See color insert.*)

Anderson NP, Anderson HE. Development of basal cell epithelioma as a consequence of radiodermatitis. Arch Dermatol Syphilol 1951; 63:586.

Arbesman H, Ransohoff DF. Is Bowen's disease a predictor for the development of internal malignancy? A methodological critique of the literature. JAMA 1987; 257:516–518.

Berger P, Baughman R. Intraepidermal epithelioma. Br J Dermatol 1979; 9:343.

Bettley FR, O'Shea JA. The absorption of arsenic and its relation to carcinoma. Br J Dermatol 1975; 92:563.

Berger TG, Graham JH, Goette DK. Lichenoid benign keratosis. J Am Acad Dermatol 1984; 11:635–638.

Bowen JT. Precancerous dermatoses: The further course of 2 cases previously reported. Arch Dermatol Syphilol 1920; 1:23.

Braverman IM. Skin Signs of Systemic Disease. 2nd. Philadelphia: WB Saunders, 1981:67–77.

Brownstein MH, Rabinowitz AD. The precursors of cutaneous squamous cell carcinoma. Mt J Dermatol 1979; 18:1.

Callen JP, Headington J. Bowen's and non-Bowen's squamous intraepidermal neoplasia of the skin. Arch Dermatol 1980; 116:422.

Callen JP. Cutaneous Aspects of Internal Disease. Chicago: Year Book Medical Publishers, 1981:209–212.

Clark WH, Mihm MC. Lentigo maligna and lentigo maligna melanoma. Am J Pathol 1969; 55:39.

Clark WH, From L, Bernardino EA, Mihm MC. Histogenesis and biologic behavior of primary human malignant melanomas of the skin. Cancer Res 1969; 29:705–727.

Cook MG, Ridgway HA. The intraepidermal epithelioma of Jadassohn: a distinct entity. Br J Dermatol 1979; 101:659.

Conley J, Lattes R, Orr W. Desmoplastic malignant melanoma (a rare variant of spindle cell melanoma). Cancer 1971; 28:914.

Committee on Guidelines of Care for Actinic Keratosis. The American Academy of Dermatology. Guidelines of care for actinic keratoses. J Am Acad Dermatol 1995; 32:95–98.

Cox FH, Becker FF. Metastatic potential of biologic variants of skin squamous cell carcinoma. J Fla Med Assoc 1982; 69:516.

Cockerell CJ. Pathology and pathophysiology of the actinic (solar) keratosis. Br J Dermatol 2003; 149(suppl 66):34–36.

Costello MJ, Fisher SB, DeFeo CP. Melanotic freckle-lentigo maligna. Arch Dermatol 1959; 80:753.

Davis DA, Donahue JP, Bost JE, et al. The diagnostic concordance of actinic keratosis and squamous cell carcinoma. J Cutan Pathol 2005; 32:546–551.

Dinehart SM, Nelson-adesokan P, Cockerell C, et al. Metastatic cutaneous squamous cell carcinoma derived from actinic keratosis. Cancer 1997; 79:920–923.

Dubrench MW. Lentigo maim des vieillards. Bull Soc Fr Der, natol Syphiligr 1984; 460.

Flaxman BA. Actinic keratoses- malignant or not? Ackerman AB. Response. J Am Acad Dermatol 2001; 45:466–469.

Fulton J Jr. Actinic Keratosis. http://www.emedicine.com/erm/topic 9.htm. Updated November 12, 2003.

Fu W, Cockerell CJ. The actinic (solar) keratosis: a 21st-century perspective. Arch Dermatol 2003; 139:66–70.

Goette DK. Erythroplasia of Queyrat. Arch Dermatol 1974; 110: 271–273.

Goette DK. Topical chemotherapy with 5-fluorouradil. J Am Acad Dermatol 1981; 4:633–649.

Goltz RW, Fusaro RM, Sweitzer SE. Borst-Jadassohn epithelioma. Arch Dermatol 1957; 75:117.

Graham JH. Is Bowen's disease a marker of internal cancer? In: E Epstein, ed. Controversies in Dermatology. Philadelphia: WB Saunders, 1984:86–95.

Graham JH. Selected precancerous skin and mucocutaneous lesions. In: Neoplasms of the Skin and Malignant Mela-

noma. Chicago: Year Book Medical Publishers, 1976:86–99, 118–121.

Grimaitre M, Etienne A, Fathi M, et al. Topical colchicine therapy for actinic keratoses. Dermatology 2000; 200:346–348.

Graham JH, Helwig EB. Erythroplasia of Queyrat. A clinicopathologic and histochemical study. Cancer 1973; 32:1396–1414.

Haber H. Intraepidermal epithelioma (Borst-Jadassohn). Trans St. Johns Hosp Dermatol Soc 1954; 33:46.

Haber H. Intraepidermal acanthoma. Dermatologica 1958; 117:304.

Haber H, Seville RH. Borst-Jadassohn intraepidermal epithelioma. Proc R Soc Med 1953; 46:171.

Heaphy MR, Ackerman AB. The nature of solar keratosis: a critical review in historical perspective. J Am Acad Dermatol 2000; 43:138–150.

Holman CD, Armstrong BK, Evans PR, et al. Relationship of solar keratosis and history of skin cancer to objective measures of actinic skin damage. Br J Dermatol 1984; 110:129–138.

Houghton A, Coit D, Bloomer W, et al. NCCN melanoma practice guidelines. Natl Compr Network Oncol (Huntingt) 1998; 12:153–177.

Holubar K, Wolff K. Intraepidermal eccrine poroma. Cancer 1969; 23:626.

Huang CL, Halpern AC. Management of patient with melanoma. In: Rigel DS et al., eds. Cancer of the Skin. Philadelphia, Edinburgh, London: Elsevier Saunders, 2005:265–274.

Ikenberg H, Gissmann L, Gross G, Grussendorf-Conen EI, zur Hausen H. Human papillomavirus type 16 related DNA in genital Bowen's disease and in bowenoid papulosis. Int J Cancer 1983; 32:563–565.

Ishikawa K. Malignant hidroacanthoma simplex. Arch Dermatol 1971; 104:529.

Jackson R, Williamson GS, Beattie WG. Lentigo maligna and malignant melanoma. Can Med Assoc J 1966; 95:846.

Kao GF. Carcinoma arising in Bowen's disease (editorial). Arch Dermatol 1986; 122:1124–1126.

Kao GF, Graham JH. Premalignant cutaneous disorders of the head and neck. In: English GM, ed. Otolaryngology. 5. Vol. Philadelphia: Harper & Row. Philadelphia: Harper & Row, 1987:581–20.

Kamino H, Ackerman AB. Malignant melanoma in situ. The evolution of malignant melanoma within the epidermis. In: Ackerman AB, ed. Pathology of Malignant Melanoma. New York: Masson, 1981:59–91.

King CM, Yates YM, Dave VK. Multicentric pigmented Bowen's disease of the genitalia associated with carcinoma in situ of the cervix. Br J Vener Dis 1984; 60:406–408.

Lane CW. Senile freckle. Arch Dermatol 1930; 21:494.

Lever WF, Schaumburg-Lever G. Tumors and cysts of the epidermis. In: Lever WF, Schaumburg-Lever G, eds. Histopathology of the Skin. Philadelphia: JB Lippincott, 1983: 489–493, 498.

Maiorana A, Nigrisoli B, Papotti M. Immunohistochemical markers of sweat gland tumors. J Cutan Pathol 1986; 13: 187–196.

Mehregan AH, Levson DN. Hidroacanthoma simplex. Arch Dermatol 1969; 100:303.

Mehregan AH, Pinkus H. Intraepidermal epithelioma: a critical study. Cancer 1964; 17:609.

Mitchell RE. Squamous cell carcinoma developing in the Jadassohn phenomenon: a case report. Australas J Dermatol 1975; 16:79.

Mishima Y. Epitheliomatous differentiation of the intraepidermal eccrine sweat duct. J Invest Dermatol 1969; 52:233.

Mikhail GR. Cancers, precancers and pseudocancers on the male genitalia. J Dermatol Surg Oncol 1980; 6: 1027–1035.

Miki Y, Kawatsu T, Matsuda K, et al. Cutaneous and pulmonary cancers associated with Bowen's disease. J Am Acad Dermatol 1982; 6:26.

Ollstein RN, Kaplan HS, Crikelair GF, et al. Is there a malignant freckle? Cancer 1966; 19:767.

Patterson JW, Kao GF, Graham JH, Helwig EB. Bowenoid papulosis. A clinicopathologic study with ultrastructural observations. Cancer 1986; 57:823–836.

Penneys NS, Nadji M, Morales A. Carcinoembryonic antigen in benign sweat gland tumors. Arch Dermatol 1982; 118:225.

Pinkus H. Keratosis senilis. Am J Clin Pathol 1958; 29:193.

Reese AB. Precancerous melanosis and the resulting malignant melanoma (cancerous melanosis) of the conjunctiva and lids. Arch Ophthalmol 1943; 29:737.

Reed RJ, Clark WH Jr., Mihm MC. Premalignant melanocytic dysplasias. In: Ackerman AB, ed. Pathology of Malignant Melanoma. New York: Masson, 1981:178.

Reese AB. Precancerous and cancerous melanosis. Am J Ophthalmol 1966; 61:1272.

Reed RI, Leonard DD. Neurotropic melanoma: a variant of desmoplastic melanoma. Am J Surg Pathol 1979; 3:301–311.

Rywlin AM. Malignant melanoma in situ, precancerous melanosis, or atypical intraepidermal melanocytic proliferation. Am J Dermatopathol 1984; 6:97–100.

Salasche SJ, Levine N, Morrison L. Cycle therapy of actinic keratoses on the face and scalp with 5% topical imiquimod cream. An open-label trial. J Am Acad Dermatol 2002; 47:571–577.

Sachs W. Intraepidermal nevus. Arch Dermatol 1952; 65:110.

Sagebiel RW. Histopathology of borderline and early malignant melanomas. Am J Surg Pathol 1979; 3:543–552.

Saunders TS, Montgomery H. Chronic roentgen and radium dermatitis. JAMA 1938; 110:23.

Sims CF, Parker RL. Intraepidermai basal cell epithelioma. Arch Dermatol 1949; 59:45.

Siegel JM. Intraepidemial epithelioma of Jadassohn. Arch Dermatol 1974; 110:478.

Smith JLS, Cobum JG. Hidroacanthoma simplex. Br J Dermatol 956; 68:400.

Sturm HM. Bowen's disease and 5-fluorouracil. J Am Acad Dermatol 1979; 1:513–522.

Stanley RI, Roenigk RK. Actinic cheiitis: treatment with the carbon dioxide laser. Mayo Clin Proc 1988; 63:230–235.

Steffen C, Ackerman AB. Intraepidermal epithelioma of Borst-Jadassohn. Am J Dermatopathol 1985; 7:5–24.

Stockfleth E, Meyer T, Benninghoff B, et al. A randomized, double-blind, vehicle-controlled study to assess 5% imiquimod cream for the treatment of multiple actinic keratoses. Arch Dermatol 2002; 138:1498–1502.

Subrt P, Jorizzo JL, Apisarnthanarax P, et al. Spreading pigmented actinic keratosis. J Am Acad Dermatol 1983; 8:63–67.

Urback F. Reactions to physical agents. In: Moschella SL, Pillsbury DM, Hurley HJ Jr., eds. Dermatology. Vol. 2. Philadelphia: WB Saunders, 1975:1452–1455.

Wayte DM, Helwig EB. Melanotic freckle of Hutchinson. Cancer 1968; 21:893.

Wade TR, Ackerman AB. The many faces of solar keratoses. J Dermatol Surg Oncol 1978; 4:730–734.

Winton GB, Salasche SJ. Dermabrasion of the scalp as a treatment for actinic damage. J Am Acad Dermatol 1986; 14:661–667.

Yeh S. Cancer in chronic arsenicism. Hum Pathol 1973; 4:469–485.

37

Basal Cell Carcinoma

Adam I. Rubin
University of Pennsylvania, Philadelphia, Pennsylvania, U.S.A.

Elbert H. Chen
Department of Dermatology, Columbia University, New York, New York, U.S.A.

Donald J. Grande
Department of Dermatology, Boston University School of Medicine, Stoneham, Massachusetts, U.S.A.

Désirée Ratner
Department of Dermatology, Columbia University, New York, New York, U.S.A.

INTRODUCTION

Basal cell carcinoma (BCC) is the most common malignancy in humans. According to the American Cancer Society, there will be more than one million new cases of skin cancer this year. Eighty percent of the cases of nonmelanoma skin cancers are BCC. While nevoid BCC syndrome left evidence of its existence in mummified Egyptian skeletons nearly 4000 years ago, BCC was not described as a unique entity until 1827. Other names for BCC include Jacob's ulcer, rodent ulcer, trichoma, and basalioma.

EPIDEMIOLOGY

As opposed to most other human cancers, nonmelanoma skin cancer is not regularly recorded in cancer registries. Therefore, it can be difficult to determine incidence rates over large populations. There is also great variability in the incidence of BCC between various locations in the world. The highest incidence of BCC in the world occurs in Australia, where up to 2074 BCCs/100,000 population have been recorded. A recent study from the German Schleswig-Holstein Cancer Registry showed European age-standardized incidence rates of 80.8 BCC/100,000 population for men and 63.3 BCC/100,000 population for women. In the United States, age-standardized incidence rates in Caucasian patients range from 159 to 407 BCC/100,000 population for men and 87 to 212 BCC/100,000 population for women.

Many factors, including skin type, heredity, sun exposure, exposure to ionizing radiation, and arsenic exposure, play a role in the development of BCC. Although this slowly growing tumor tends to appear most often in elderly patients, BCCs are developing in increasing numbers in younger patients in their 20s and 30s. Recently, an increasing incidence of BCC in young women has been recognized.

BCC is most typically found on sun-exposed areas of fair-skinned individuals. The prevalence of BCC is highest in sun-exposed areas. Nevertheless, correlation with sun exposure is not perfect, because up to one-third of all BCCs occur in relatively sun-protected areas of the face, including the medial canthal and postauricular areas. BCCs have also been reported in other sun-protected sites including the axillae, breast, genitalia and sole of the foot. The most common predisposing factor for the development of BCC is a prior history of BCC development. Marcil and Stern showed in a meta-analysis that after a patient had developed one BCC, there was at least a 10 fold increased incidence of developing a second BCC, as compared to patients who had not previously developed BCC.

BCC may also result from exposure to other external carcinogens, such as ionizing radiation. In the past, patients were treated with irradiation for benign dermatoses, such as eczema, psoriasis, acne vulgaris, and tinea capitis. These patients are at increased risk of developing BCC in the treated areas. Lichter et al. showed that patients treated with irradiation for acne have a significantly higher risk of developing BCC as compared to patients treated for other indications. Trivalent inorganic arsenic, once commonly used as an insecticide and medicinal ingredient (Fowler's solution), is also recognized as a predisposing factor. Most BCCs associated with chronic arsenic exposure are of the superficial type. Exposure to psolaren and ultraviolet A (PUVA) has also been linked to an increased incidence of BCC. Several chronic cutaneous conditions have been associated with the development of BCC, including burn scars, chronic ulcers, and nonhealing wounds.

BCC develops more frequently in a number of inherited genetic syndromes (Table 1). It may also arise within or in proximity to other cutaneous tumors, such as epidermal nevi, linear unilateral basal cell nevus with comedones, nevus sebaceous of Jadassohn (organoid nevus), seborrheic keratosis, dermatofibroma, and melanocytic nevi. BCC may also occur in scars secondary to blunt trauma, sharp trauma, and vaccination.

As its incidence increases, the distribution of BCC may be changing. Rates of increase are highest in areas of the body not continuously exposed to the sun. Associations among age, gender, site distribution, and histology suggest

Table 1 Syndromes Associated with Basl Cell Carcinoma

Syndrome	Gene defect	Inheritance	OMIM# (39)	Findings
NBBCS (Gorlin's syndrome)	PTCH1	AD	109400	Pitting of palms and soles Odontogenic keratocysts Bifid ribs Hypertelorism CNS defects
Albinism (OCA1)	TYR	AR	203100	Reduced or absent melanin formation
(OCA2)	P gene		203200	Squamous cell carcinoma
(OCA3)	TRYP1		203290	Visual disturbances
(OCA4)	MATP		606574	
Xeroderma pigmentosum	XPA	AR	278700	Sun sensitivity
	XPB		133510	Photophobia
	XPC		278720	Freckling
	XPD		278730	Abnormal DNA repair
	XPE		278740	Other neoplasm
	XPF		278760	
	XPG		278780	
	XPV		278750	
Rombo	NI	AD	180730	Vermiculate atrophoderma Milia Hypotrichosis Trichoepithelioma Peripheral vasodilatation with cyanosis
Bazex–Dupré–Christol (Bazex's syndrome)	NI	XLD	301845	Follicular atrophoderma Localized anhidrosis Hypotrichosis

Abbreviations: AD, autosomal dominant; AR, autosomal recessive; MATP, membrance-associated transporter protein; NBCCS, nevoid basal cell carcinoma syndrome; NI, not identified; OCA, oculocutaneous albinism; OMIM, online mendelian inheritance in man; TYR, tyrosinase; TRYP1, tryosinase-related protein-1; XLD, X-linked dominant; CNS, central nervous system.

distinct mechanisms of development for different subsets of BCCs. Superficial BCC occurs more often in younger patients, more frequently in women than in men, and more often on the trunk and extremities. Nodular BCC occurs most often on the head and neck of older men.

PATHOGENESIS

Derangements in the normal functioning of the hedgehog molecular signaling pathway have been shown to be an important cause for the development of BCC. The end result of this pathway is to transmit a proliferation signal to the cell nucleus. When functioning correctly, at baseline, the protein product of the patched gene (PTCH1) is a transmembrane receptor that blocks the hedgehog signal transduction pathway by binding the protein smoothened (SMO). The downstream targets of SMO are the nuclear transcription factors CI and GLI. When functioning normally, the protein sonic hedgehog, present in the extracellular space, will bind to the patched receptor, thereby releasing SMO and allowing it to exert its effect on the downstream transcription factors, thereby promoting nuclear activation. In BCC, mutations in the PTCH1 gene can cause constitutive activation, with the patched receptor losing its ability to bind SMO, resulting in unchecked cellular signaling. Each of the other components of the hedgehog signaling pathway (sonic hedgehog, SMO, and GLI) can also mutate, thereby causing activation of this signal transduction pathway. As noted in Table 1, mutations in the PTCH1 gene are present in the nevoid BCC syndrome, an autosomal dominant genodermatosis with one characteristic being the production of numerous BCCs. Mutations in the tumor suppressor gene p53 have been found in sporadic BCCs, and these mutated genes have shown ultraviolet B exposure signature mutations.

CLINICAL FEATURES

BCC can present with many different clinical appearances, and a high index of suspicion must be maintained. Features common to many BCCs include scaling with erosion or ulceration, surrounding erythema with telangiectases, and slow but relentless growth. Any chronic, nonhealing ulceration should be evaluated by skin biopsy to exclude the possibility of BCC. A variety of presentations of BCC exist, as detailed below.

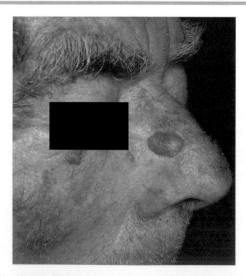

Figure 1 Nodular BCC present on the nasal sidewall. Note the exophytic nature of the tumor with the characteristic pearly quality and overlying telangiectasias. (*See color insert.*)

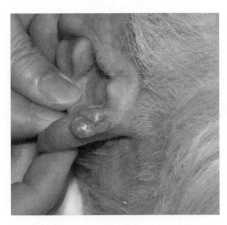

Figure 2 Nodular BCC present on the superior helix of the ear. Sun-exposed sites such as the face and ear are common locations for BCC. (*See color insert.*)

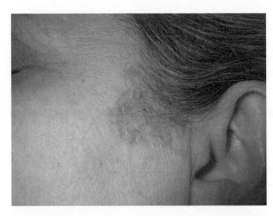

Figure 4 Superficial pattern BCC on the cheek. Note its presentation as an erythematous, scaly patch. The appearance is similar to that of benign processes such as psoriasis, seborrheic dermatitis, or eczematous dermatitis such as atopic dermatitis or allergic contact dermatitis. (*See color insert.*)

Nodular BCC

Nodular BCC is the most common clinical form of BCC, and presents as a translucent papule or nodule with surface telangiectases. The borders may become rolled or pearly (Figs. 1–3). The size of a nodular BCC is quite variable. While most nodular BCCs are small, they can grow to large sizes if neglected. Local invasion and destruction of tissue ensue if the lesion is not treated. Ulceration is common, and if present, may be considered a noduloulcerative type of BCC. Patients will often give a history of persistent bleeding and crusting, which eventually causes them to seek evaluation.

Superficial BCC

Superficial BCC presents as an erythematous, scaly, slightly indurated plaque, which may contain telangiectases at its border. (Fig. 4) Crusting and ulceration are common features. Portions of a superficial BCC may evolve into nodular BCC over time. Most often, superficial BCC occurs on the shoulders, back, or chest, and multiple lesions may be present. Because of its similarity in appearance to other inflammatory dermatoses such as psoriasis or eczema, one

should consider the diagnosis of superficial BCC when confronted with a persistent erythematous, scaly patch.

Pigmented BCC

Pigmented BCC occurs when melanin pigment is mixed within the tumor mass. Most commonly, pigmented BCC occurs because of melanin deposition in nodular BCC (Fig. 5). Because of its appearance, pigmented BCC may not be the initial diagnosis of the examining physician, and it may be mistaken for a seborrheic keratosis, melanocytic nevus, or melanoma.

Morpheaform BCC

Morpheaform BCC is often not recognized by patients because of its subtle appearance. It presents as a flat or a slightly depressed plaque that may be indurated and can resemble a scar (Figs. 6–8). Ulceration may occur in long-standing lesions. For patients who have a scar or scar-like lesion without a previous history of trauma or surgery, a skin biopsy should be performed to rule out the possibility of a morpheaform BCC. Other desmoplastic tumors should also be considered in the differential diagnosis.

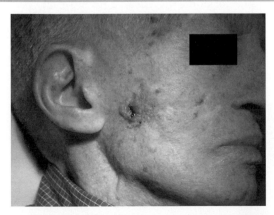

Figure 3 Nodular pattern BCC of the face appearing decades after radiation therapy. Note the extensive ulceration of the tumor. This patient has evidence of multiple prior surgical procedures for cutaneous malignancies. Patients who were treated with irradiation for benign dermatoses such as acne vulgaris and tinea capitis are prone to developing BCC in the treated areas. (*See color insert.*)

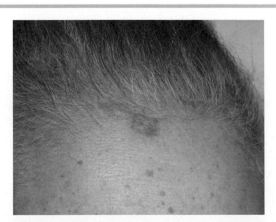

Figure 5 Pigmented BCC on the forehead. Note the hyperpigmented nature of this lesion, which might be confused with a seborrheic keratosis, melanocytic nevus, or melanoma. (*See color insert.*)

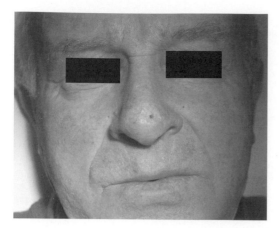

Figure 6   Morpheaform pattern BCC present on the lateral nasal tip. Note its scar-like indented appearance. These tumors can be easily overlooked by patients because of their banal appearance. (*See color insert.*)

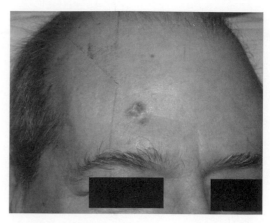

Figure 9   Mixed pattern BCC located on the forehead. Portions of this tumor are ulcerated and crusted, while other areas resemble white scars. (*See color insert.*)

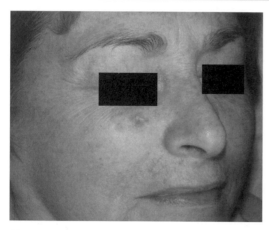

Figure 7   Morpheaform pattern BCC located in the periorbital area. This tumor appears as an atrophic, indurated plaque. Minute telangectasias can be seen within the plaque on close observation. (*See color insert.*)

HISTOPATHOLOGIC FINDINGS

Confirmation of clinically suspected BCC is accomplished by skin biopsy. A variety of biopsy methods are acceptable, including shave, punch, and excisional biopsy, as BCC can generally be demonstrated in the superficial portion of a biopsy specimen. It is important to include some portion of the dermis to differentiate between superficial BCC and other invasive subtypes. Multiple subtypes of BCC are recognized. The value in classifying BCC histopathologically lies in the fact that certain BCC subtypes demonstrate a more aggressive clinical course with respect to recurrence after treatment.

An extensive study by Sexton et al. examined the frequency of a variety of histologic BCC subtypes in a sample of 1039 BCC specimens. The most common presentation was mixed—meaning more than one subtype was present. This pattern occurred in 38.6% of the specimens. The most common mixed pattern was that of nodular–micronodular (21.8%). The frequency of occurrence of other growth patterns, in the order of decreasing frequency, are nodular (21.0%), superficial (17.4%), micronodular (14.5%), infiltrative (7.4%), and morpheaform (1.1%). Those BCC subtypes that have a higher recurrence rate after therapy include the morpheaform, micronodular, infiltrative, and basosquamous BCC subtypes. In general, the nodular and superficial BCC subtypes do not have as high a rate of recurrence as

Other BCC Presentations

Correlation between other clinical and histologic subtypes is more difficult for mixed subtype BCCs (Fig. 9) and infiltrative subtype BCCs (Figs. 10 and 11). BCC may present as an enlarged pore.

(A)

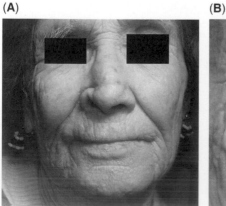

(B)

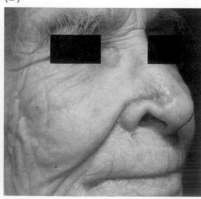

Figure 8   (A and B) Morpheaform pattern BCC involving the lower nose. Note the extensive elevation of alar rim as a result of involvement with BCC. Treatment for complicated lesions located in a cosmetically sensitive area can be challenging and may require a multidisciplinary team of physicians.

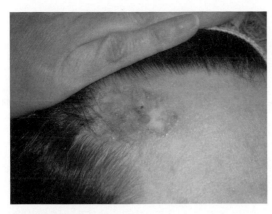

Figure 10 Infiltrative pattern BCC located on the upper forehead. The destructive nature of this tumor is demonstrated by alopecia due to tumor invasion at the hairline. (*See color insert.*)

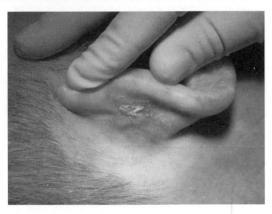

Figure 11 Infiltrative pattern BCC of posterior ear. Note the indistinct clinical margins and waxy appearance. (*See color insert.*)

are nonanaplastic, lacking evidence of cellular atypia or mitotic activity. Retraction artifact between the tumor mass and its surrounding stroma can often be seen. Mucin deposition is usually present within the tumor as well. Tumor necrosis and ulceration are variably noted. The surrounding stroma shows increased numbers of fibroblasts, as well as an increased amount of collagen. Searching a histologic slide for the characteristic features at the periphery of a sample can be useful for tumors that may initially present with a confusing picture.

The nodular BCC subtype displays rounded, relatively large masses of tumor cells with peripheral palisading of nuclei at the tumor borders. Tumor nodules can be seen attached to the overlying epidermis as well as in the dermis. The superficial BCC subtype shows small buds of basaloid cells descending from the epidermis (Fig. 12). To qualify as superficial, the tumor masses are limited to those attached to the epidermis. Dermal invasion is not seen. The micronodular BCC subtype shows histologic features similar to those of the nodular subtype, except that the tumor is composed of multiple smaller nodules (Fig. 13). The infiltrative BCC subtype is composed of irregularly sized and shaped islands of basaloid cells (Fig. 14). The morpheaform (or sclerosing) BCC subtype is composed of thin strands of basaloid cells that invade the dermis. The adenoid BCC subtype shows tumor strands forming gland-like structures. The keratotic BCC subtype contains horn cysts in association with typical basaloid tumor cells without evidence of squamous differentiation. Basosquamous or metatypical BCC shows features of both BCC and squamous cell carcinoma and is considered to be an aggressive histologic variant. The exact nature of this lesion is controversial. Pigmented BCC results from the presence of melanocytes and melanin admixed with the tumor cells. Other rare types of BCC include clear cell BCC, in which a portion of tumor cells contain glycogen-filled cytoplasmic vacuoles and granular BCC, in which cells are present, which show granular cytoplasmic changes. BCC may show tumor cells with sebaceous or matrical differentiation.

The fibroepithelioma of Pinkus, initially described in 1953, is visualized histologically as anastomosing strands and aggregates of tumor cells surrounded by a fibrous stroma. The nature of this lesion is controversial, with some authors considering it as a variant of BCC, and others categorizing it as a trichoblastoma.

The histologic differential diagnosis for the nodular, micronodular, or infiltrative subtypes may include trichoepithelioma or trichoblastoma. For the morpheaform BCC

those aggressive BCC subtypes. Oram et al. showed that in immunocompromised patients, there was a higher percentage of infiltrative pattern BCC as compared to immunocompetent patients. In this series, the nodular BCC pattern was most common among all patients.

The histologic feature seen in all BCC is the characteristic basaloid cell. These small, tightly packed polymorphic cells are composed of a basophilic nucleus without a discernible nucleolus and scanty cytoplasm. In general, they

(A)

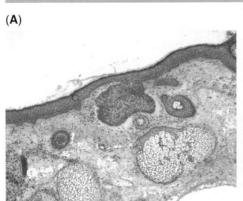

(B)

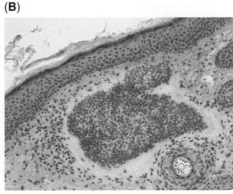

Figure 12 (A) Low-power photomicrograph demonstrating the superficial subtype of BCC. A bud of basaloid cells connects to the epidermis. (B) High-power view of a separate section of the same tumor. Note the retraction artifact and peripheral palisading of cell nuclei. There is no intervening stroma in the tumor nodule. (*See color insert.*)

(A)

(B)

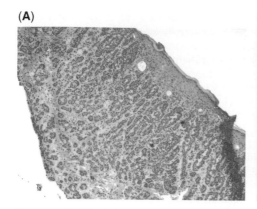

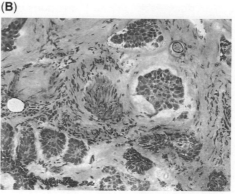

Figure 13 **(A)** Low-power photomicrograph demonstrating the micronodular subtype of BCC. Small islands of basaloid cells are present in the dermis. Note the connection of the tumor cells to the epidermis in areas of this specimen. **(B)** High-power photomicrograph of a micronodular subtype BCC shows characteristic peripheral palisading of tumor cell nuclei and retraction artifact. (*See color insert.*)

subtype, one should also consider desmoplastic trichoepithelioma, microcystic adnexal carcinoma, or metastatic lesions in the histologic differential diagnosis.

RECURRENT BCC

While the majority of BCCs are small, low-risk tumors that are easily treated, there is a high-risk population of tumors that must be treated more carefully, due to their greater risk of recurrence. These high-risk BCCs have the potential to exhibit extensive subclinical extension beyond the visually apparent tumor, resulting in impressive local tissue destruction. They may invade into parotid gland, cartilage, bone, and occasionally even the central nervous system through involvement of peripheral nerves. High-risk BCCs include tumors that are recurrent, located in anatomic sites with a high rate of recurrence (such as the eyelid, lip, or nose), have an aggressive or morpheaform pattern of growth on biopsy, are clinically characterized by ill-defined borders or multicentricity, or develop in sites previously exposed to radiation, are large (i.e., >2 cm), or exhibit perineural invasion (Fig. 15).

METASTATIC BCC

While a rare event, it is also possible for BCC to metastasize, with metastatic rates ranging from 0.0028% to 0.5% of cases. Tumor characteristics seen in recurrent BCC are those that

are also associated with metastasis of BCC. Metastatic BCC most often results from tumors with aggressive histologic subtypes, recurrent tumors, or a history of previous exposure to radiation. It has been reported that the mean interval from presentation of the initial BCC to discovery of metastasis is nine years. Most tumors that have metastasized originate from the head and neck region. The most common sites of metastasis include the regional lymph nodes, bone, lung, liver and skin, although involvement of salivary glands, brain, and spine has also been reported. Recently, Saladi et al. have shown that a monoclonal antibody directed against the Ber-EP4 protein may be useful in confirming the diagnosis of metastatic BCC. The prognosis of metastatic BCC is poor, with mean survival times ranging from 8 months to 3.6 years.

TREATMENT

Many factors should be evaluated before determining the most appropriate treatment method. Beyond the tumor characteristics listed above, patient considerations include general medical condition and individual needs, psychosocial factors, and the ability to return for multiple treatments. The cure rate of the treatment modality, the physician's experience and training, and cost should also be weighed. The goal of treatment is to eradicate the tumor such that the likelihood of recurrence is as low as possible.

Figure 14 Low-power photomicrograph demonstrating the infiltrative subtype of BCC. Tumor islands with irregular borders are present in the dermis. (*See color insert.*)

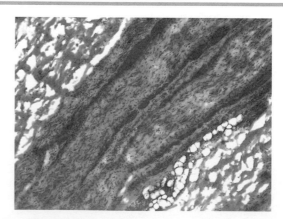

Figure 15 High-power photomicrograph demonstrating intraneural involvement with BCC. BCC tracking along nerves can travel far from the initial tumor presentation site and can be challenging to treat. (*See color insert.*)

When evaluating the literature regarding treatment modalities for BCC, it is essential to note the duration of follow-up for treated lesions. Rowe examined the recurrence rates of BCC in published studies over a 40-year time period and found that only 50% of recurrences occurred within two years after treatment. Five years after treatment, 82% of recurrences had appeared. Rowe therefore recommended considering data with a minimum of five years of follow-up in order to accurately compare treatment modalities. This comprehensive tabulation showed that five-year recurrence rates for primary BCC by treatment modality was 10.1% for surgical excision, 7.7% for curettage and electrodesiccation, 8.7% for radiation therapy, and 7.5% for cryotherapy. Overall, all non-Mohs modalities had a recurrence rate of 8.7%. Mohs micrographic surgery had the lowest recurrence rate of all treatment modalities with a 1.0% rate. For recurrent BCC, five-year recurrence rates were 17.4% for surgical excision, 40% for curettage and electrodesiccation, and 9.8% for radiation therapy. Overall, the non-Mohs modalities had a recurrence rate for recurrent BCC of 19.9%. Mohs micrographic surgery again had the lowest recurrence rate, 5.6%, for recurrent BCC.

More recently, Thissen et al. performed a systematic review of treatment modalities and recurrence rates for primary BCC. While 298 studies were identified, only 18 satisfied identified criteria for analysis. Their calculations show that after five years, the lowest recurrence rates were obtained with Mohs micrographic surgery followed by surgical excision, cryosurgery, and curettage and electrodesiccation.

Curettage and electrodesiccation and cryosurgery cure rates are highly dependent on experience, technique, and tumor selection. Efficacy of cryosurgery is increased with additional freeze–thaw cycles and preoperative curettage to define tumor margins, with some authors reporting cure rates greater than 90% in high-risk locations.

Topical 5-fluorouracil cream is an Food and Drug Administration (FDA)-approved treatment for superficial pattern BCC. However, many of the available studies fail to document long-term follow-up, and the technique for using 5-fluorouracil is inconsistent. A study of 25% fluorouracil paste under occlusion for three weeks documented a 21% five-year recurrence rate for thin BCC and a 6% five-year recurrence rate when preceded by light curettage. Injectable fluorouracil/epinephrine gel demonstrated a 91% clearance rate in a series of 122 patients, which included 84 nodular pattern BCCs.

Tazarotene is a synthetic retinoid selective for the retinoic acid receptor-β and -γ isotypes, which has activity in acne, psoriasis, and photoaging. A recent study demonstrated complete or partial regression in 70.8% of a mixed group of BCCs treated with tazarotene 0.1% gel applied once daily for 24 weeks.

Intralesional interferon alpha-2b is another investigational therapy that has not attained widespread use. Intralesional interferon 1.5 million IU three times per week for three weeks demonstrated 86% clearance rate of a mixed group of BCCs. Using a similar protocol, only 27% of aggressive BCCs were cleared histologically.

Imiquimod was approved by the Food and Drug Administration in 2004 for the treatment of biopsy-proven, small, primary, superficial BCC located on the trunk, neck, or extremities. The exact mechanism of action is unknown. Imiquimod binds to Toll-like receptor 7 and has been shown to stimulate an immune response via the production of proinflammatory cytokines such as interferon alpha, interleukin 12, and tumor necrosis factor alpha. Using imiquimod once daily five days per week for six weeks resulted in a 75% composite clearance rate of superficial BCC at 12 weeks. The histologic clearance rate for small nodular BCC treated with imiquimod ranges from 42% to 76%.

Photodynamic therapy (PDT) is a treatment for BCC, in which an applied photosensitizing agent is activated with visible light to selectively destroy superficial tumors. PDT using 5-aminolevulinate is highly effective for the treatment of superficial BCC. Complete response rates range from 79% to 100%. PDT employing methyl aminolevulinate has achieved up to 91% clearance of nodular BCC. Short-term recurrence rates when using PDT for the treatment of BCC range from 6% to 44%.

CONCLUSIONS

BCC will be encountered by almost every physician, and its frequency is increasing. Knowledge of the clinical and histological presentation of this tumor, as well as the current status of its known molecular derangements, is useful to the practitioner. Current information on the usefulness of medical and surgical treatments for this tumor will help to increase cure rates for this common malignancy and reduce the likelihood of morbidity from this largely preventable disease.

BIBLIOGRAPHY

Ackerman AB, Gottlieb GJ. Fibroepithelial tumor of pinkus is trichoblastic (basal-cell) carcinoma. Am J Dermatopathol 2005; 27(2):155–159.

Akasaka T, Kon S. Two cases of basal cell carcinoma arising in seborrheic keratosis. J Dermatol 1997; 24(5):322–327.

American Cancer Society Cancer Facts and Figures 2003.

Barnadas MA, Freeman RG. Clear cell basal cell epithelioma: light and electron microscopic study of an unusual variant. J Cutan Pathol 1988; 15(1):1–7.

Betti R, Menni S, Cerri A, et al. Seborrheic keratosis with compound nevus, junctional nevus and basal cell carcinoma in the same lesion. Dermatology 2001, 203 (3), 265–267.

Bianchi L, Orlandi A, Campione E, et al. Topical treatment of basal cell carcinoma with tazarotene: a clinicopathological study on a large series of cases. Br J Dermatol 2004; 151(1):148–156.

Boonchai W, Green A, Ng J, et al. Basal cell carcinoma in chronic arsenicism occurring in Queensland, Australia, after ingestion of an asthma medication. J Am Acad Dermatol 2000; 43(4):664–669.

Bowen AR, LeBoit PE. Fibroepithelioma of pinkus is a fenestrated trichoblastoma. Am J Dermatopathol 2005; 27(2):149–154.

Bowman PH, Ratz JL, Knoepp TG, et al. Basosquamous carcinoma. Dermatol Surg 2003; 29(8):830–832; discussion 833.

Boyd AS, Shyr Y, King LE Jr. Basal cell carcinoma in young women: an evaluation of the association of tanning bed use and smoking. J Am Acad Dermatol 2002; 46(5):706–709.

Ceylan C, Ozdemir F, Ozturk G, et al. A case of basal cell carcinoma arising in epidermal nevus. Int J Dermatol 2002; 41(12):926–927.

Chave TA, Finch TM. The scrotum: an unusual site for basal cell carcinoma. Clin Exp Dermatol 2002; 27(1):68.

Cornell RC, Greenway HT, Tucker SB, et al. Intralesional interferon therapy for basal cell carcinoma. J Am Acad Dermatol 1990; 23(4 Pt 1):694–700.

Cribier B, Scrivener Y, Grosshans E. Tumors arising in nevus sebaceus: A study of 596 cases. J Am Acad Dermatol 2000; 42(2 Pt 1):263–268.

de Vries E, Louwman M, Bastiaens M, et al. Rapid and continuous increases in incidence rates of basal cell carcinoma in the southeast Netherlands since 1973. J Invest Dermatol 2004; 123(4):634–638.

Diepgen TL, Mahler V. The epidemiology of skin cancer. Br J Dermatol 2002; 146(Suppl 61):1–6.

Dundr P, Stork J, Povysil C, et al. Granular cell basal cell carcinoma. Australas J Dermatol 2004; 45(1):70–72.

Epstein E. Fluorouracil paste treatment of thin basal cell carcinomas. Arch Dermatol 1985; 121(2):207–213.

Fink-Puches R, Soyer HP, Hofer A, et al. Long-term follow-up and histological changes of superficial nonmelanoma skin cancers treated with topical delta-aminolevulinic acid photodynamic therapy. Arch Dermatol 1998; 134(7): 821–826.

Gardner ES, Goldberg LH. Axillary basal cell carcinoma: literature survey and case report. Dermatol Surg 2001; 27(11):966–968.

Geisse J, Caro I, Lindholm J, et al. Imiquimod 5% cream for the treatment of superficial basal cell carcinoma: results from two phase III, randomized, vehicle-controlled studies. J Am Acad Dermatol 2004; 50(5):722–733.

Green A, Battistutta D, Hart V, et al. Skin cancer in a subtropical Australian population: incidence and lack of association with occupation. The Nambour Study Group. Am J Epidemiol 1996; 144(11):1034–1040.

Guo HR, Yu HS, Hu H, et al. Arsenic in drinking water and skin cancers: cell-type specificity (Taiwan, ROC). Cancer Causes Control 2001; 12(10):909–916.

Haskell HD, Haynes HA, McKee PH, et al. Basal cell carcinoma with matrical differentiation: a case study with analysis of beta-catenin. J Cutan Pathol 2005; 32(3):245–250.

Horn M, Wolf P, Wulf HC, et al. Topical methyl aminolaevulinate photodynamic therapy in patients with basal cell carcinoma prone to complications and poor cosmetic outcome with conventional treatment. Br J Dermatol 2003; 149(6):1242–1249.

Jacob A. Observations respecting an ulcer of peculiar character which attacks eyelids and other parts of the face. Dubl Hosp Reprs 1827; 4:231–239.

Jaramillo-Ayerbe F. Cryosurgery in difficult to treat basal cell carcinoma. Int J Dermatol 2000; 39(3):223–229.

Jih MH. Linear unilateral basal-cell nevus syndrome with comedones. Dermatol Online J 2002; 8(2):12.

Katalinic A, Kunze U, Schafer T. Epidemiology of cutaneous melanoma and non-melanoma skin cancer in Schleswig-Holstein, Germany: incidence, clinical subtypes, tumour stages and localization (epidemiology of skin cancer). Br J Dermatol 2003; 149(6):1200–1206.

Kennedy C, Bajdik CD, Willemze R, et al. Chemical exposures other than arsenic are probably not important risk factors for squamous cell carcinoma, basal cell carcinoma and malignant melanoma of the skin. Br J Dermatol 2005; 152(1):194–197.

Kinoshita R, Yamamoto O, Yasuda H, et al. Basal cell carcinoma of the scrotum with lymph node metastasis: report of a case and review of the literature. Int J Dermatol 2005; 44(1):54–56.

Koga Y, Sawada Y. Basal cell carcinoma developing on a burn scar. Burns 1997; 23(1):75–77.

Kokoszka A, Scheinfeld N. Evidence-based review of the use of cryosurgery in treatment of basal cell carcinoma. Dermatol Surg 2003; 29(6):566–571.

Kowal-Vern A, Criswell BK. Burn scar neoplasms: a literature review and statistical analysis. Burns 2005; 31(4):403–413.

LeSueur BW, DiCaudo DJ, Connolly SM. Axillary basal cell carcinoma. Dermatol Surg 2003; 29(11):1105–1108.

Lear JT, Tan BB, Smith AG, et al. Risk factors for basal cell carcinoma in the UK: case-control study in 806 patients. J R Soc Med 1997; 90(7):371–374.

Lichter MD, Karagas MR, Mott LA, et al. Therapeutic ionizing radiation and the incidence of basal cell carcinoma and squamous cell carcinoma. The New Hampshire Skin Cancer Study Group. Arch Dermatol 2000; 136(8):1007–1011.

Lovatt TJ, Lear JT, Bastrilles J, et al. Associations between UVR exposure and basal cell carcinoma site and histology. Cancer Lett 2004; 216(2):191–197.

Maalej M, Frikha H, Kochbati L, et al. Radio-induced malignancies of the scalp about 98 patients with 150 lesions and literature review. Cancer Radiother 2004; 8(2):81–87.

Maloney ML. What is basosquamous carcinoma? Dermatol Surg 2000; 26(5):505–506.

Malone JP, Fedok FG, Belchis DA, et al. Basal cell carcinoma metastatic to the parotid: report of a new case and review of the literature. Ear Nose Throat J 2000; 79(7):511–515, 518–519.

Maloney ME, Jones DB, Sexton FM. Pigmented basal cell carcinoma: investigation of 70 cases. J Am Acad Dermatol 1992; 27(1):74–78.

Marcil I, Stern RS. Risk of developing a subsequent nonmelanoma skin cancer in patients with a history of nonmelanoma skin cancer: a critical review of the literature and meta-analysis. Arch Dermatol 2000; 136(12):1524–1530.

McKenna KE, Somerville JE, Walsh MY, et al. Basal cell carcinoma occurring in association with dermatofibroma. Dermatology 1993; 187(1):54–57.

Michaelsson G, Olsson E, Westermark P. The Rombo syndrome: a familial disorder with vermiculate atrophoderma, milia, hypotrichosis, trichoepitheliomas, basal cell carcinomas and peripheral vasodilation with cyanosis. Acta Derm Venereol 1981; 61(6):497–503.

Miller BH, Shavin JS, Cognetta A, et al. Nonsurgical treatment of basal cell carcinomas with intralesional 5-fluorouracil/epinephrine injectable gel. J Am Acad Dermatol 1997; 36(1): 72–77.

Miller DL, Weinstock MA. Nonmelanoma skin cancer in the United States: incidence. J Am Acad Dermatol 1994; 30(5 Pt 1):774–778.

Misago N, Suse T, Uemura T, et al. Basal cell carcinoma with sebaceous differentiation. Am J Dermatopathol 2004; 26(4):298–303.

Misago N, Satoh T, Narisawa Y. Cornification (keratinization) in basal cell carcinoma: a histopathological and immunohistochemical study of 16 cases. J Dermatol 2004; 31(8):637–650.

Morton CA, Whitehurst C, McColl JH, et al. Photodynamic therapy for large or multiple patches of Bowen disease and basal cell carcinoma. Arch Dermatol 2001; 137(3): 319–324.

Nagpal S, Chandraratna RA. Recent developments in receptor-selective retinoids. Curr Pharm Des 2000; 6(9):919–931.

Naldi L, DiLandro A, D'Avanzo B, et al. Host-related and environmental risk factors for cutaneous basal cell carcinoma: evidence from an Italian case-control study. J Am Acad Dermatol 2000; 42(3):446–452.

Nehal KS, Levine VJ, Ashinoff R. Basal cell carcinoma of the genitalia. Dermatol Surg 1998; 24(12):1361–1363.

Nijsten TE, Stern RS. The increased risk of skin cancer is persistent after discontinuation of psoralen ultraviolet A: a cohort study. J Invest Dermatol 2003; 121(2):252–258.

Noodleman FR, Pollack SV. Trauma as a possible etiologic factor in basal cell carcinoma. J Dermatol Surg Oncol 1986; 12(8): 841–846.

Nordin P, Larko O, Stenquist B. Five-year results of curettage-cryosurgery of selected large primary basal cell carcinomas on the nose: an alternative treatment in a geographical area underserved by Mohs' surgery. Br J Dermatol 1997; 136(2):180–183.

Online Mendelian Inheritance in Man OT. McKusick-Nathans Institute for Genetic Medicine, Johns Hopkins University (Baltimore, MD) and National Center for Biotechnology Information, National Library of Medicine (Bethesda, MD); 2000.

Oram Y, Orengo I, Griego RD, et al. Histologic patterns of basal cell carcinoma based upon patient immunostatus. Dermatol Surg 1995; 21(7):611–614.

Pastorino L, Cusano R, Nasti S, et al. Molecular characterization of Italian nevoid basal cell carcinoma syndrome patients. Hum Mutat 2005; 25(3):322–323.

Peng Q, Warloe T, Berg K, et al. 5-Aminolevulinic acid-based photodynamic therapy. Clinical research and future challenges. Cancer 1997; 79(12):2282–2308.

Pinkus H. Premalignant fibroepithelial tumors of skin. Arch Dermatol Syphil 1953; 67:598–615.

Ramos J, Villa J, Ruiz A, et al. UV dose determines key characteristics of nonmelanoma skin cancer. Cancer Epidemiol Biomarkers Prev 2004; 13(12):2006–2011.

Raszewski RL, Guyuron B. Long-term survival following nodal metastases from basal cell carcinoma. Ann Plast Surg 1990; 24(2):170–175.

Rhodes LE, de Rie M, Enstrom Y, et al. Photodynamic therapy using topical methyl aminolevulinate vs surgery for nodular basal cell carcinoma: results of a multicenter randomized prospective trial. Arch Dermatol 2004; 140(1):17–23.

Rosen N, Muhn CY, Bernstein SC. A common tumor, an uncommon location: basal cell carcinoma of the nipple and areola in a 49-year-old woman. Dermatol Surg 2005; 31(4):480–483.

Roth MJ, Stern JB, Haupt HM, et al. Basal cell carcinoma of the sole. J Cutan Pathol 1995; 22(4):349–353.

Rowe DE. Comparison of treatment modalities for basal cell carcinoma. Clin Dermatol 1995; 13(6):617–620.

Saladi RN, Singh F, Wei H, et al. Use of Ber-EP4 protein in recurrent metastatic basal cell carcinoma: a case report and review of the literature. Int J Dermatol 2004; 43(8):600–603.

Satinoff MI, Wells C. Multiple basal cell naevus syndrome in ancient Egypt. Med Hist 1969; 13(3):294–297.

Schwarze HP, Loche F, Gorguet MC, et al. Basal cell carcinoma associated with chronic venous leg ulcer. Int J Dermatol 2000; 39(1):78–79.

Serrano H, Scotto J, Shornick G, et al. Incidence of nonmelanoma skin cancer in New Hampshire and Vermont. J Am Acad Dermatol 1991; 24(4):574–579.

Sexton M, Jones DB, Maloney ME. Histologic pattern analysis of basal cell carcinoma. Study of a series of 1039 consecutive neoplasms. J Am Acad Dermatol 1990; 23(6 Pt 1):1118–1126.

Shore RE, Moseson M, Xue X, et al. Skin cancer after X-ray treatment for scalp ringworm. Radiat Res 2002; 157(4):410–418.

Shumack S, Robinson J, Kossard S, et al. Efficacy of topical 5% imiquimod cream for the treatment of nodular basal cell carcinoma: comparison of dosing regimens. Arch Dermatol 2002; 138(9):1165–1171.

Silverman MK, Kopf AW, Grin CM, et al. Recurrence rates of treated basal cell carcinomas. Part 2: Curettage-electrodesiccation. J Dermatol Surg Oncol 1991; 17(9):720–726.

Somoano B, Niendorf KB, Tsao H. Hereditary cancer syndromes of the skin. Clin Dermatol 2005; 23(1):85–106.

Spitz JL. Genodermatoses: A Clinical Guide To Genetic Skin Disorders. 2nd ed. Lippincott Williams & WilkinsPhiladelphia 2005.

Stanley MA. Imiquimod and the imidazoquinolones: mechanism of action and therapeutic potential. Clin Exp Dermatol 2002; 27(7):571–577.

Stenquist B, Wennberg AM, Gisslen H, et al. Treatment of aggressive basal cell carcinoma with intralesional interferon: evaluation of efficacy by Mohs surgery. J Am Acad Dermatol 1992; 27(1):65–69.

Sterry W, Ruzicka T, Herrera E, et al. Imiquimod 5% cream for the treatment of superficial and nodular basal cell carcinoma: randomized studies comparing low-frequency dosing with and without occlusion. Br J Dermatol 2002; 147(6):1227–1236.

Stern RS, Liebman EJ, Vakeva L. Oral psoralen and ultraviolet-A light (PUVA) treatment of psoriasis and persistent risk of nonmelanoma skin cancer. PUVA Follow-up Study. J Natl Cancer Inst 1998; 90(17):1278–1284.

Taipale J, Beachy PA. The Hedgehog and Wnt signalling pathways in cancer. Nature 2001; 411(6835):349–354.

Thissen MR, Neumann MH, Schouten LJ. A systematic review of treatment modalities for primary basal cell carcinomas. Arch Dermatol 1999; 135(10):1177–1183.

Vabres P, Lacombe D, Rabinowitz LG, et al. The gene for Bazex-Dupre-Christol syndrome maps to chromosome Xq. J Invest Dermatol 1995; 105(1):87–91.

van Dam RM, Huang Z, Rimm EB, et al. Risk factors for basal cell carcinoma of the skin in men: results from the health professionals follow-up study. Am J Epidemiol 1999; 150(5):459–468.

Vinciullo C, Elliott T, Francis D, et al. Photodynamic therapy with topical methyl aminolaevulinate for 'difficult-to-treat' basal cell carcinoma. Br J Dermatol 2005; 152(4):765–772.

von Domarus H, Stevens PJ. Metastatic basal cell carcinoma. Report of five cases and review of 170 cases in the literature. J Am Acad Dermatol 1984; 10(6):1043–1060.

Walling HW, Fosko SW, Geraminejad PA, et al. Aggressive basal cell carcinoma: presentation, pathogenesis, and management. Cancer Metastasis Rev 2004; 23(3–4):389–402.

Weihrauch M, Bader M, Lehnert G, et al. Carcinogen-specific mutation pattern in the p53 tumour suppressor gene in UV radiation-induced basal cell carcinoma. Int Arch Occup Environ Health 2002; 75(4):272–276.

Xie J, Murone M, Luoh SM, et al. Activating Smoothened mutations in sporadic basal-cell carcinoma. Nature 1998; 391(6662):90–92.

Zhu YI, Ratner D. Basal cell carcinoma of the nipple: a case report and review of the literature. Dermatol Surg 2001; 27(11):971–974.

38

Squamous Cell Carcinoma

J. Barton Sterling
Spring Lake, New Jersey, U.S.A.

Jeffrey L. Melton
Department of Dermatology, University of Illinois at Chicago, Chicago, Illinois, U.S.A.

C. William Hanke
Laser and Skin Surgery Center of Indiana, Carmel, Indiana, U.S.A.

INTRODUCTION

Squamous cell carcinoma (SCC) affects approximately 140,000 patients in the United States each year and represents about 20% of skin cancers treated by dermatologists. Approximately 2500 patients die of SCC metastasis per year. The number of patients afflicted with SCC is growing, in part due to longer life spans, increased recreational sun exposure, and prolonged survival of immunosuppressed patients who are prone to develop SCC more than any other type of skin cancer.

METASTATIC SPREAD

The metastatic rate of SCC is controversial and a wide range of metastatic rates (0.5–31%) appear in the literature. Because the survival of patients with metastatic SCC is only about 25%, it is important to identify those patients at high risk for metastasis and treat them aggressively. In 1992, Rowe et al. identified eight factors associated with metastatic SCC:

- Size 2 cm or greater in diameter
- Depth 4 mm or greater
- Aggressive histology
- Perineural invasion
- Anatomic location
- Etiology
- Immunosuppression
- Recurrence after prior treatment

The larger the clinical size of the tumor, the more likely it is to metastasize. In Rowe's review, only 9% of lesions smaller than 2 cm in diameter metastasized, whereas 30% of lesions larger than 2 cm metastasized.

Like melanoma, histologic depth of SCC is also predictive of metastasis, with lesions 4 mm or greater or penetrating to the reticular dermis (Clark's level IV or V) being much more likely to metastasize.

The degree of histological differentiation is also predictive of metastasis. Poorly differentiated SCC is more likely to metastasize. In studies reporting the degree of differentiation, the metastatic rate was 9% for well-differentiated tumors versus 33% for poorly differentiated tumors.

Perineural invasion is another indicator of poor prognosis. The branches of the trigeminal and facial nerves are particularly susceptible to neurotropic invasion and spread. Direct intracranial extension may occur along these nerves. Occasionally, patients with neurotropic invasion will experience symptoms of pain, paresthesia, or motor paralysis. Perineural invasion seen histologically requires an aggressive surgical effort to clear the tumor from proximal portions of the nerve.

SCC arising in certain anatomic locations is more likely to metastasize. The most notable example is SCC of the lip, which has an 11% metastatic rate (Fig. 1). Eyelid, ear, oral mucous membrane, glans penis, and vulva are other high-risk sites for metastasis. SCC arising in sites of chronic injury or scars also has notably high rate of metastasis. For example, 31% of SCC arising in foci of chrome osteomyelitis metastasizes (Fig. 2). Similarly, 20% of SCC resulting from radiation injury and 18% of SCC arising in old scars will metastasize (Figs. 3–5).

SCC occurs more frequently and is more aggressive in immunosuppressed patients. In immunosuppressed patients, SCC is more prevalent than basal cell carcinoma. It has been estimated that SCC occurs 18 times more frequently in renal transplant patients than in the general population. In a significant number of these tumors, human papillomavirus (HPV)-5 or HPV-8 can be detected. Evidence suggests that cardiothoracic transplant patients have an even higher rate of developing aggressive SCC than renal transplant patients. This may be due to their greater immune suppression. SCC represents a major cause of morbidity in transplant patients. Reduction of immune suppression and the oral retinoid therapy have been shown to decrease the rate of development of new SCC.

Previously treated SCC has a higher rate of metastasis than primary SCC, ranging from 25% to 45%, depending upon the site of the lesion.

In 2002, Basil et al. reviewed 200 cases of invasive SCC and found a 12.5% metastatic rate. Metastatic risk was strongly correlated with size, Clark's level, the degree of differentiation, the presence of small tumor nests, infiltrative tumor strands, single-cell infiltration, perineural invasion, acantholysis, and recurrence after treatment. In their series, location, ulceration, inflammation, and Breslow depth

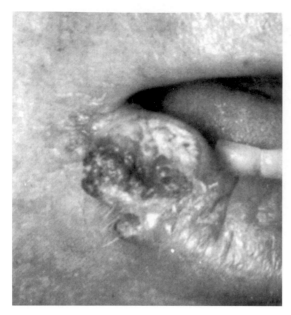

Figure 1 Ulcerated nodule on the lower lip. This is a common presentation of squamous cell carcinoma.

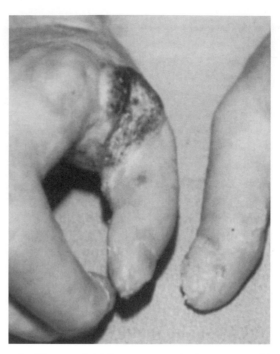

Figure 3 After superficial X-ray treatment for hand eczema 30 years previously, the patient now has an infiltrating recurrent squamous cell carcinoma involving the right metacarpal head and proximal thumb.

did not correlate with metastasis. The authors attribute the lack of correlation between Breslow depth and metastasis to the inability to determine Breslow depth in a number of specimens.

CAUSE AND PATHOGENESIS

Ultraviolet (UV) radiation is the most important cause of SCC of the skin. Other etiologic factors include HPV infection, chronic wounds, arsenic, coal tar, radiation therapy, and hydrocarbons.

UV Light Carcinogenesis

UV radiation, especially UVB (290–320 nm), causes photochemical alterations in DNA, resulting in abnormal nucleotide pairing and carcinogenesis. UV exposure also induces immunologic defects in skin and in lymphocytes, which may predisposes to malignancy. Animals exposed to high-dose UV radiation develop SCC almost at the exclusion of all other types of skin cancer.

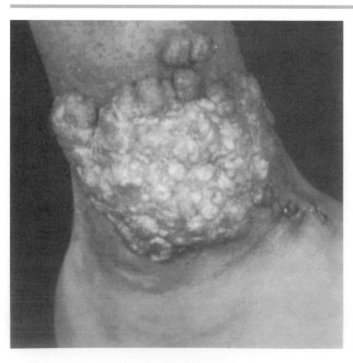

Figure 2 A draining sinus in a patient with chronic osteomyelitis. An exophytic squamous cell carcinoma developed after several years.

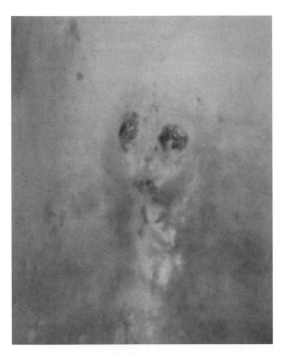

Figure 4 An ulcerated squamous cell carcinoma in an old burn scar on the leg.

Nearly all SCCs occur on sun-exposed areas, whereas only two-thirds of all basal cell carcinomas are similarly distributed. Common areas include the head, neck, dorsal hands, and forearms (Figs. 6 and 7). Ears and scalp (in balding men) are also particularly susceptible (Fig. 8).

Sun exposure was first implicated as a carcinogen during the late 1800s. In 1906, Hyde observed that some people had a greater sensitivity to sunlight than others. He recognized that skin pigmentation provided some protection from the sun's effects.

Skin type and color are the most important factors affecting the frequency of skin cancer. SCC occurs most commonly in people with fair skin, who sunburn easily and do not tan well (Fitzpatrick's skin types I and II). These individuals usually have blue eyes and red or blond hair. Irish, Scottish, and English ancestry is associated with an especially high risk of SCC as well as other forms of skin cancer.

The intensity of UV light that reaches the skin is determined in part by latitude. Ratzer and Strong found that each 3°45′ latitude closer to the equator doubled the frequency of skin cancer. In the United States, the incidence of SCC in the skin is much higher in the south than in the north.

Altitude, air pollution, meteorologic conditions, and the stratospheric ozone layer also affect the intensity of UV radiation. The ozone layer has been damaged by pollutants and is not as effective barrier as it once was.

Occupation and leisure activity influence the amount of UV exposure that the skin receives. Unna observed changes in sailor's skin due to excessive sun exposure. People who work outdoors, such as farmers, sailors, construction workers, and some professional athletes, have a higher incidence of skin cancer than people who work indoors. PUVA treatment also puts patients at increased risk for SCC.

CHEMICAL CARCINOGENESIS

SCC of the skin may also result from contact with chemical carcinogens. Arsenic and organic hydrocarbons are the most common offenders. Exposure is frequently occupational. The cancers are produced by the direct action of the chemical on the skin. The incidence of chemically induced skin cancer is proportional to the duration of exposure to the carcinogen.

The Englishman Percivall Pott was the first to describe chemical carcinogenesis. In 1755, he reported that the high frequency of scrotal cancer in chimney sweeps was due to chronic exposure to soot. Since then, other environmental

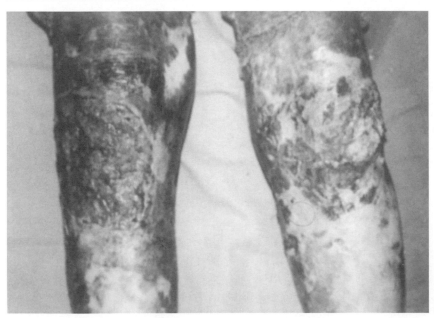

Figure 5 Extensive scarring due to epidermolysis bullosa dystrophia. Large squamous cell carcinomas developed below the knees.

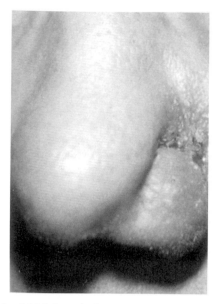

Figure 6   A painful, indurated subcutaneous nodule in the nasofacial sulcus due to poorly differentiated squamous cell carcinoma.

carcinogens have been identified, including coal tar, paraffin oil, shale oil, creosote oil, petroleum oil, and asphalt (Fig. 9).

Arsenic is another chemical carcinogen. Industrial exposure occurs in the smelting of metal ores and the manufacturing and agricultural use of insecticides. Carcinogenic amounts of arsenic can be found in drinking water in several parts of the world. During the 19th and 20th centuries, arsenic was used medicinally. Fowler's solution (As_2O_3), Donovan's solution (AsI_3 plus HgI_2), and Asiatic pills (As_2O_3) are arsenic-containing medications previously used to treat many common diseases.

Cigarette smoking has been shown to increase the risk of developing cutaneous SCC by twofold, but not BCC.

Ionizing Radiation Carcinogenesis

Ionizing radiation may produce SCC of the skin as a result of fractionated, small doses of radiation. The cancers appear following a lag period of 10 to 30 years. Occupational groups exposed to radiation include physicians, dentists, nurses, technicians, and engineers. Radiation used to treat malignancies as well as the prior practice of treating benign conditions such as acne, hirsutism, and hemangiomas is associated with SCC (Fig. 10).

Friehen first reported roentgen-radiation–induced SCC in 1902 soon after the discovery of X rays. He reported SCC in people working with roentgen machines. Shortly thereafter, cutaneous carcinoma was observed in patients who had received roentgen radiation therapeutically.

Today, ionizing radiation is rarely responsible for cutaneous carcinoma. The treatment of benign skin conditions with radiation has largely been abandoned, and occupational and industrial exposure is better controlled. Radiation therapy for malignancy has advanced and the technology improved to minimize this adverse effect.

Human Papillomavirus

HPV induces the development of cervical and some forms of cutaneous SCC. Most cervical and penile SCC contains HPV DNA. DNA of HPV type 16 is the HPV type most strongly associated with malignancy. Moy et al. first reported the presence of HPV-16 in nongenital SCC. HPV16 was present in five of seven cases of SCC of the finger. HPV DNA has also been demonstrated in keratoacanthomas. HPV is much less likely, however, to be present or involved in SCC of nongenital, nonperiungal sites. One exception is the disease epidermodysplasia verruciformis, where patients have an immune defect against HPV. These patients develop multiple low-grade SCC, mostly on sun-exposed areas. HPV type 5 as well as many other HPV types is implicated in the pathogenesis of SCC in these patients. The exact mechanism of HPV-induced oncogenesis is currently the subject of much investigation.

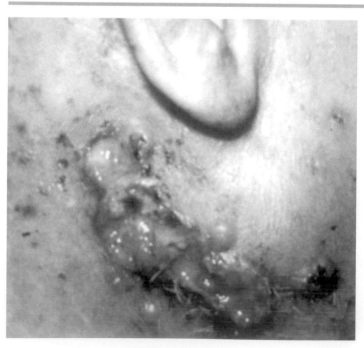

Figure 7   Squamous cell carcinoma of the neck.

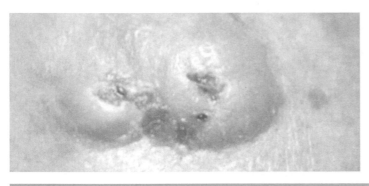

Figure 8 A nodular squamous cell carcinoma on the bald scalp of a 70-year-old man.

PREMALIGNANT FORMS OF SCC

SCC has premalignant forms (actinic/solar keratosis and its analogs, radiation keratosis, actinic cheilitis, arsenical keratosis, thermal keratosis, and hydrocarbon keratosis) and in situ forms (SCC in situ, Bowen's disease, and Erythroplasia of Queyrat) (Fig. 11).

Ackerman has championed the viewpoint that actinic keratoses (AK) are not premalignancies but rather early expressions of SCC. AKs display similar cytologic characteristics and contain many of the same gene mutations as invasive SCC, including p53 mutations. Further, when a large number of AKs are present in an area, the potential for the development of invasive SCC is increased (Fig. 12). The rate of transformation of an individual AK to invasive SCC, however, is very low, varying widely depending on the study. Therefore, while labeling all AKs "SCC" maybe theoretically appealing; this terminology may alarm and confuse patients and clinicians who receive this diagnosis.

If AKs are in fact considered SCC, then SCC is the most common skin cancer in humans, more common than basal cell carcinomas.

Bowen's Disease

Bowen's disease presents clinically as a sharply circumscribed, scaling, erythematous plaque that is generally larger than the usual AK (Fig. 13). The plaque may mimic eczema or psoriasis. Most cases of Bowen's disease are on sunexposed sites and may be related to solar exposure. Bowen's disease on non-sun-exposed areas may be caused by inorganic arsenic exposure. Bowen's disease in blacks occurs three times more frequently on non-sun-exposed areas.

Some dermatopathologists use the term "Bowen's disease" histologically to denote SCC in situ, which also involves the hair follicles. This alerts the clinician that a more aggressive modality of treatment may be necessary.

Erythroplasia of Queyrat

"Erythroplasia of Queyrat" is a clinical term for SCC in situ localized to the glans penis. This lesion occurs more commonly in uncircumcised men. Clinically, it is characterized as a well-defined, shiny, red plaque (Fig. 14). The histopathologic appearance is identical to mat of SCC in situ.

CLINICAL FEATURES OF SCC

The clinical features of SCC vary. Commonly, SCC appears as an ulcerated nodule or a superficial ulceration on the skin or lower lip (Fig. 15). Another common presentation is a verrucous papule or plaque with a thick cornified layer. Less commonly, a large verrucous nodule may develop. The typically rolled pearly border with overlying telangiectases seen in basal cell carcinoma easily differentiates this from SCC. When a rolled border is present in SCC, it usually does not have overlying telangiectasia. The peripheral margins of the SCC are not well defined, as in basal cell carcinoma. The tumor may fix to deeper structures as it invades.

HISTOPATHOLOGIC FINDINGS

SCC consists of nests of squamous epidermal cells, which extend into the dermis. The most malignant varieties of SCC contain a larger proportion of atypical cells.

Well-differentiated SCC is composed of large polygonal cells with intercellular bridges, round nuclei, and eosinophilic cytoplasm (Fig. 16). Horn pearls are common, composed of concentric layers of keratin and characterized by incomplete keratinization in the center. Poorly differentiated SCC is characterized by nuclear atypia and mitotic figures (Fig. 17). Tumor cells vary in shape from polygonal to stellate or fusiform (i.e., spindle cells).

Histologically, SCC can be graded based on cytologic characteristics. Broders' classification of the degree of malignancy of SCC is based on the proportion of differentiated squamous cells to undifferentiated squamous cells. SCC grade I contains greater than 75% well-differentiated cells; grade II, 50% to 75%; grade III, 25% to 49%; grade IV, less than 25%. Most dermatopathologists grade SCC on a more subjective basis calling them "well," "moderately," or

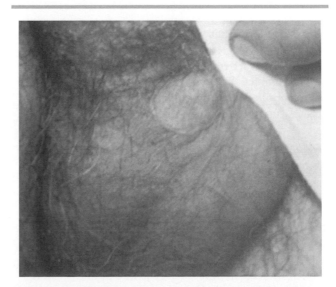

Figure 9 Chronic exposure to oils. Squamous cell carcinoma of the scrotum in a textile worker.

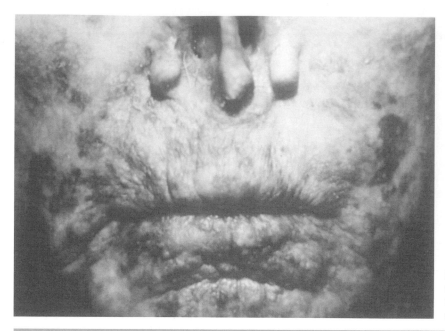

Figure 10 Chronic radiodermatitis secondary to superficial X-ray treatment for facial acne. The patient now has pigment changes as well as multiple basal cell and squamous cell carcinomas in this area.

"poorly" differentiated, rather than use Broders' classification. Well-differentiated SCC has a good prognosis, while, at the other end of the spectrum, poorly differentiated SCC has a worse prognosis. The majority of SCCs are low-grade with a high degree of cellular differentiation and a superficial depth of invasion.

Another feature that affects prognosis off SCC is depth of invasion. Invasion depth is predictive of metastasis, with lesions 4 mm or greater or penetrating to the reticular dermis (Clark's level IV or V) being much more likely to metastasize.

Perineural invasion is uncommon but is an ominous sign when it occurs (Figs. 18–20). Perineural invasion is more likely to be seen in deeply invasive tumors.

The adenoid or pseudoglandular variant of SCC occurs predominantly on sun-exposed areas in elderly patients. Clinically, it is impossible to distinguish from other types of SCC. Metastases occur only rarely. Several layers of tumor cells line tubular lumina and alveolar formations (Fig. 21). The luminal spaces are filled with acantholytic cells, some of which are keratinized. The process of acantholysis in adenoid SCC is similar to that seen in acantholytic AKs. An additional feature of acantholytic SCC is a proliferation of sweat duct epithelium induced by the inflammatory infiltrates surrounding the tumor.

Spindle cell SCC occurs largely on sun-damaged or radiation-damaged skin. The cells are spindle-shaped and sometimes difficult to differentiate from malignant melanoma, atypical fibroxanthoma, and fibrosarcoma. Differentiation is more difficult when there is no evidence of keratinization, intercellular bridges, or epidermal connection. Immunoperoxidase staining with antikeratin antibodies and electron microscopy may be necessary.

KERATOACANTHOMA

Although considered a benign entity by some, keratoacanthoma is considered by most to be a variant of SCC. It is often difficult to differentiate between the two clinically or histopathologically. Both entities occur on sun-exposed skin of older patients. HPV-16 DNA has been found in

keratoacanthomas as well as in classical SCC. Immunocompromised patients have a higher incidence of both keratoacanthomas and classical SCC. Multiple lesions are common in this clinical setting.

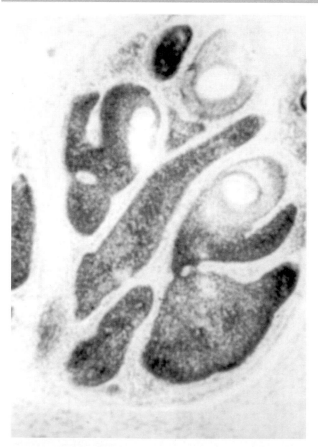

Figure 11 Bowen's disease involving the hair follicle epithelium deep in the scalp (hemotoxylin & eosin, ×200).

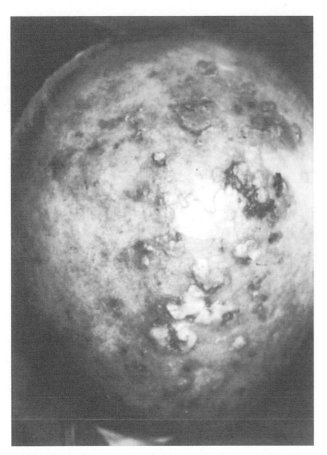

Figure 12 Multiple hypertrophic actinic keratoses on the bald scalp of a 75-year-old man.

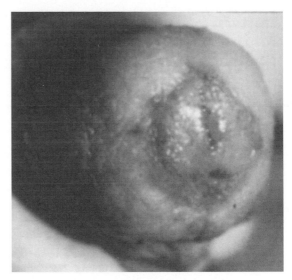

Figure 14 Erythroplasia of Queyrat in an uncircumcised man. Surgical resection revealed involvement of the distal third of the urethra.

may continue to grow rapidly and become quite large. Considerable deformity and destruction of tissue may occur, particularly when keratoacanthomas occur in the nasal area (Fig. 22). A keratoacanthoma may also remain static for several years, followed by renewed rapid growth. Metastasis has been reported.

An excisional biopsy of the entire lesion provides the best material for histopathologic diagnosis. Alternatively, a pie-shaped wedge biopsy may be helpful if taken to adequate depth. Intracytoplasmic glycogen and intraepithelial elastic fibers are more abundant in keratoacanthoma than in SCC. Immunohistochemical stains have not been helpful in differentiating keratoacanthoma from SCC. Resolution of the lesion, either spontaneously or in response to intralesional chemotherapy, is perhaps the most reliable diagnostic criterion, albeit a retrospective one. Both 5-fluorouracil and methotrexate have been successfully used as intralesional agents. Two to four injections are usually

Keratoacanthomas appear as a dome-shaped verrucous nodule with a central, keratin-filled crater. Characteristically, keratoacanthomas are faster growing than most SCCs. The key feature that differentiates keratoacanthoma from SCC is its tendency to involute and resolve spontaneously. Regression usually occurs over a six-month period. However, keratoacanthomas do not always follow the prototypical course. They

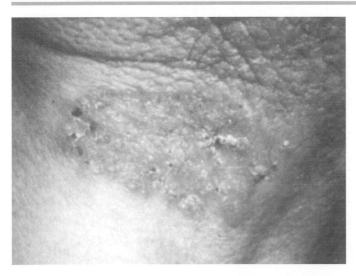

Figure 13 Bowen's disease.

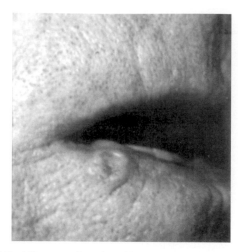

Figure 15 A biopsy specimen from this nodule on the Nermilion border of the lip demonstrated a well-differentiated squamous cell carcinoma.

required. Careful follow-up is important if intralesional treatment is used. If there is any question regarding the diagnosis, the lesion should he treated as if it were SCC.

VERRUCOUS CARCINOMA

Verrucous carcinoma is a low-grade SCC that occurs in the oral cavity, anogenital region, and on the plantar surface of the foot. It appears as an exophytic verrucous mass that grows slowly (Fig. 23). The diagnosis is made both on clinical and on microscopic grounds.

In the oral cavity, verrucous carcinoma is also called oral florid papillomatosis. Large areas of the oral mucosa are involved with white cauliflower-like vegetations. In the anogenital region, it is called giant condyloma of

Buschke and Loewenstein. Papillomatous vegetations most commonly occur on the glans penis of uncircumcised men, and the urethra may also be involved. On the plantar aspect of the foot, verrucous carcinoma is also called epithelioma cuniculatum and may be confused with a large plantar wart. Deep crypts develop on the tumor surface as it enlarges. In late stages, the plantar fascia and metatarsal bones may be involved.

A large excisional biopsy is important for diagnosis. Features of verrucous carcinoma in common with warts include hyperkeratosis, parakeratosis, and acanthosis. Some portions of verrucous carcinoma demonstrate blunted, broad proliferations of well-differentiated keratinocytes and keratin-containing cysts that compress normal collagen. Nuclear atypia is absent even at the depth of the tumor. HPV viral particles have been identified by DNA hybridization techniques in some patients with plantar verrucous carcinoma.

Verrucous carcinoma can penetrate deeply into local tissues, but metastasis rarely occurs. It has been suggested that radiation therapy for verrucous carcinoma may increase metastatic potential. The first case of verrucous carcinoma from the foot with extranodal metastases was reported by Mckee et al. One patient with plantar verrucous carcinoma seen by the senior author (CWH) had not received radiation yet developed regional lymph node metastases.

TREATMENT

Treatment of SCC is based on several factors including size, location, and degree of histologic differentiation, as well as the age and health of the patient. Preoperative biopsy is essential to determine the degree of cellular differentiation and depth of penetration. These facts aid in the selection of the proper treatment.

Mohs micrographic surgery (MMS), standard surgical excision, radiation, curettage and electrodesiccation (C & E), and cryosurgery are methods of primary treatment. MMS is best-suited for tumors in critical anatomic sites and for recurrent tumors. Further, when SCC demonstrates an infiltrating pattern with narrow microscopic strands of tumor cells, MMS is the best alternative.

When metastases develop, wide excision is usually indicated (Fig. 24). Radiation may be given as the primary treatment or following surgery to increase the cure rate. Radiation and chemotherapy are useful as palliative measures.

Mohs Micrographic Surgery

MMS is the most precise method of tumor removal. MMS involves surgical excision of tumors in thin layers that are color-coded, mapped, and prepared for microscopic horizontal frozen section examination of deep and peripheral margins. MMS requires that the surgeon also act as the dermatopathologist. The Mohs surgeon excises and reexcises cancerous tissue until no residual tumor remains microscopically.

Compared to standard surgical excision where approximately 0.1% of the peripheral tumor margins are examined, in MMS 100% of the tumor margins are examined. The advantage of this method includes the highest cure rates, maximum conservation of normal tissue, and preservation of important anatomic structures.

MMS is indicated for tumors that may require disfiguring surgery (periorbital, perinasal, preauricular, and perioral), recurrent tumors, tumors with a high likelihood of recurrence, tumors with indistinct margins, and tumors where tissue preservation is imperative (fingers and

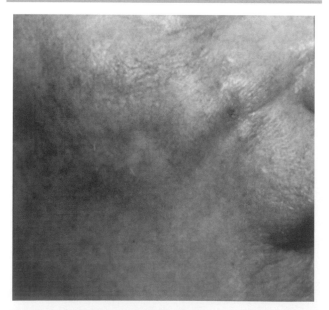

Figure 16 Preoperative photograph of a squamous cell carcinoma (with extensive perineural invasion) on the central right cheek that had recurred many times.

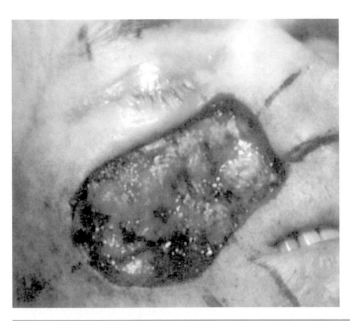

Figure 17 Extensive perineural invasion was evident after three stages of Mohs micrographic surgery. This is the immediate postoperative wound. The tumor ultimately invaded the brainstem and caused the patient's death (same patient shown in Fig. 16).

genitals) (Figs. 25 and 26). MMS is also cost-effective because it markedly reduces the likelihood of future treatment of the same tumor.

The cure rate for difficult SCC with MMS is more than 94%. Dzubow et al. reported a 93.3% five-year cure rate in a series of 414 primary SCCs treated with MMS. Risk factors for local recurrence include male patients less than 50 years old, tumors requiring more than five tissue layers, and patients with SCC on the lower extremity. SCCs larger than 5 cm are more likely to recur than smaller tumors.

In a retrospective review by Rowe et al., recurrent rates for Mohs versus non-Mohs modalities were as follows: 3.1% versus 10.9% for all areas of the skin and lip, 5.3% versus 18.7% for ears, 10% versus 23.3% for locally recurrent SCC, 0% versus 47% for perineural SCC, 25.2% versus 41.7% for SCC greater than 2 cm, 32.6% versus 53.6% for poorly differentiated SCC.

Surgical Excision

The efficiency and simplicity of surgical excision are distinct advantages for the patient and physician. Like MMS, standard surgical excision can be performed under local anesthesia on an outpatient basis. Disadvantages to standard surgical excision compared to MMS include lack of precise margin control, need for larger surgical margins, and higher recurrence rates.

Based upon a prospective study of subclinical tumor extension, Brodland and Zitelli have proposed guidelines for surgical margins for excision of SCC. Four-millimeter margins were proposed for all but high-risk SCC, for which

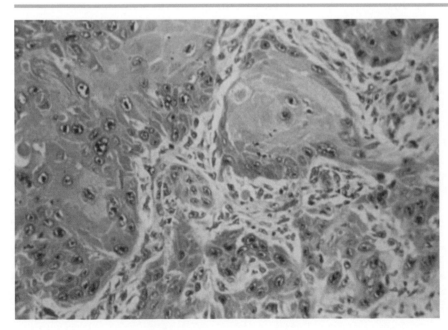

Figure 18 Well-differentiated squamous cell carcinoma with horn pearls (hemotoxylin & eosin, ×200).

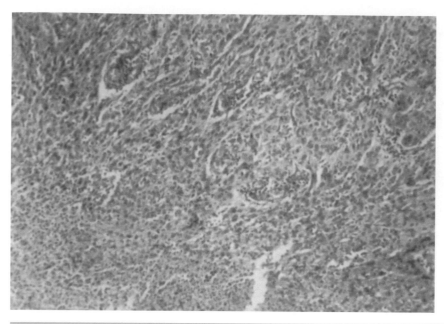

Figure 19 Poorly differentiated squamous cell carcinoma with sheets of anaplastic cells without horn pearl formation (hemotoxylin & eosin, ×200).

a minimum margin of 6 mm was recommended. High-risk features associated with greater risk of subclinical extension included size of 2 cm or larger, Broders' histologic grade 2 or higher, invasion of subcutaneous tissue, and location in high-risk areas.

For recurrence of large, aggressive SCC, reconstruction of the defect should not be done until there is confirmation of clear margins. A split-thickness skin graft or healing by second intention may be a better alternative. Delayed closure should be considered when the risk of recurrence is high. Recurrent tumor after complete reconstruction may be camouflaged.

C&E

C&E is useful for in situ tumors or tumors less than 1 cm in diameter that do not extend to the subcutaneous fat. The

procedure is quick and simple, it avoids suturing, and scars are usually acceptable.

A disadvantage of C&E compared to surgical excision is that no pathology specimen is sent for margin examination. However, the cure rates for C&E indicate that this is not significant when the appropriate tumors are selected for treatment. The cure rate for uncomplicated superficial SCC with C&E is greater than 90%. Physicians have the skill and experience with this method and obtain significantly higher cure rates than physicians in training. Curettage is not recommended for recurrent, fibrosing, or deeply invasive tumors.

Cryosurgery

Cryosurgery with liquid nitrogen (−196°C) is commonly used to destroy AK and may also be used in some clinical

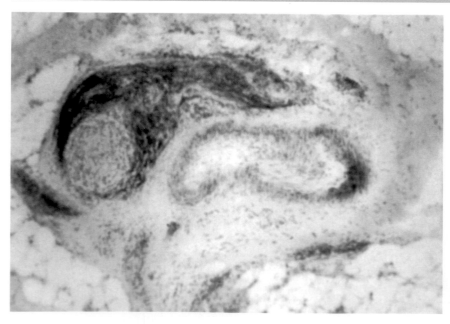

Figure 20 Chronic inflammation and tumor cells surrounding cutaneous nerves (hemotoxylin & eosin, ×300).

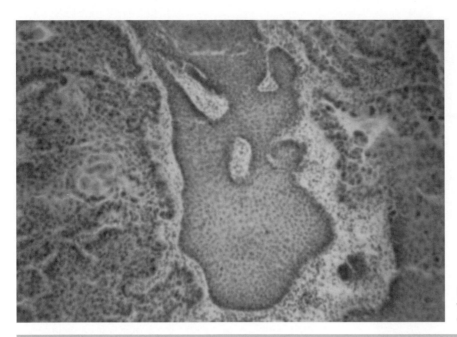

Figure 21 An adenoid squamous cell carcinoma with atypical cells and clefts containing acantholytic cells (hemotoxylin & eosin, ×200).

situations to treat SCC. Like C&E, the procedure is quick and simple, and suturing is unnecessary.

Also similar to C&E, a disadvantage of using cryosurgery for SCC is that no specimen is sent for margin examination. The clinical limits of the tumor are determined visually, and a 2- to 5-mm margin of normal skin is treated. The liquid nitrogen spray is directed at close range to the central portion of the tumor. The spray is continued until the ice ball spreads to the desired margin and then for an additional 15–45 seconds. More precise monitoring of the depth of the freeze can be done with thermocouple needles inserted at the margin of the tumor. A temperature of –40°C should be obtained at the depth of the tumor. The treatment site will require 90–120 seconds to thaw, if freezing has been

adequate. A slow thaw is more damaging to tumor cells than a rapid thaw. A second freeze–thaw cycle creates more tissue damage and may be associated with a higher cure rate.

Cure rates greater than 90% are reported with cryosurgery, although rates vary widely in the literature. The cure rate for cancer of the scalp is less, due to the rich vascular supply that thaws the ice ball. Cryosurgical treatment of cancers on the legs or thighs is avoided because of prolonged wound healing time (six months). Finally, melanocytes are very sensitive to freezing, and cryosurgery can lead to marked depigmentation.

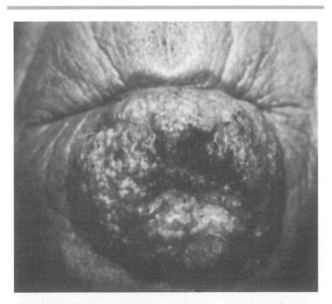

Figure 22 A giant keratoacanthoma rapidly enlarged over 6 weeks.

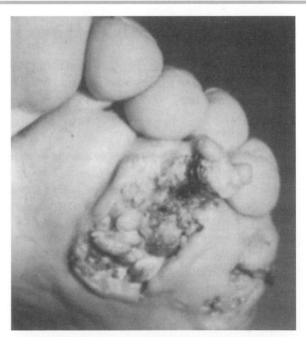

Figure 23 Verrucous carcinoma of the plantar surface.

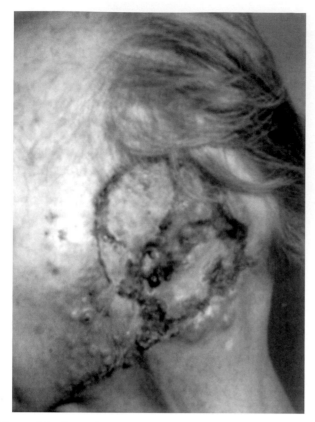

Figure 24 Metastatic nodules around a skin graft six weeks after excision of squamous cell carcinoma from the auricle.

Radiation

Radiation may be a good alternative to surgery for primary SCC, especially in elderly patients with several medical problems. The cure rate for primary, well-defined SCC is approximately 90%. This is similar to cure rates for primary BCC treated with radiation. Large exophytic SCCs on the ears and nose in elderly patients may be treated without a significant deformity. Radiation may also be recommended adjunctively for tumors with perineural involvement, when lymph nodes are involved, and for palliation of unresectable tumors. With radiation, local anesthetic injections are avoided.

Smaller SCC may be clinically well defined and can be treated with 3- to 5-mm margins. For larger or infiltrative tumors, margins may reach 2–3 cm. Once the area to be treated has been determined, a lead cutout is prepared to protect surrounding skin and is taped in place during each treatment session.

Large SCC is often treated with surgical removal of as much tumor as possible followed by postoperative radiation. The effectiveness of postoperative radiation is improved by the surgical debulking of gross tumor.

Radiation is given in fractional doses over several days or weeks. Radiation given in a single dose will not allow the tissue to recover adequately. This results in poor healing and a lower cure rate. SCCs less than 10 mm in diameter may be treated with a single dose of 2200 rads. Larger lesions may require up to 6000 rads in fractionated doses. Proper fractionation reduces the potential for osteonecrosis, chondronecrosis, and unnecessary damage to the dermis and other structures. The best results are achieved with 10 fractions for lesions up to 20 mm and 15 fractions when lesions are larger.

If an SCC involves an area immediately adjacent to a regional lymph node group, the group can be included in the radiation field. This is easily accomplished in the parotid, preauricular, and postauricular areas. The radiation field is also enlarged when perineural invasion is present. These patients must be followed carefully for paresthesias, which can indicate recurrence.

Various types of radiation have been used to treat SCC, including electron beam, radionucleotide implants, superficial X-ray therapy (photon beam), and contact X-ray therapy. Contact X-ray therapy is ideal for lesions less than 35 mm in diameter and less than 5 mm in thickness. This method allows a minimal number of fractions and leaves minimal radiation change in the skin. Deeper SCC is treated with more penetrating orthovoltage or megavoltage radiation.

Electron beam therapy is used for the control of extensive SCC when surgery may be unsuitable. Electron beam (3–18 MV) therapy has the advantage of a high-surface dose with a rapid reduction in dose several millimeters into the dermis.

Implants of radium, cesium, tantalum, or iridium are used when other forms of radiation cannot be given. Implant treatment is complex and usually requires hospitalization. Approximately 1000 rads are given daily, to a total dose of 6000 to 7000 rads.

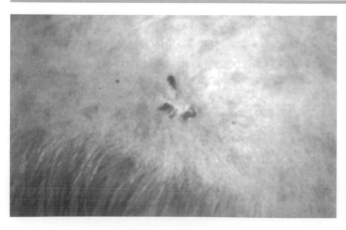

Figure 25 Recurrent squamous cell carcinoma presenting as a superficial ulceration on the scalp.

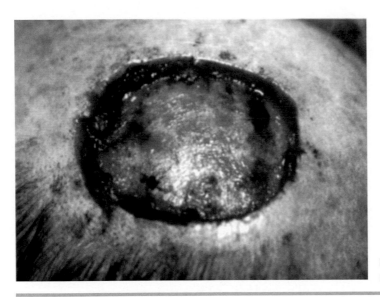

Figure 26 The tumor-free defect following Mohs surgery for the patient in Fig. 25. The galea was involved but not the periosteum.

In contradistinction to scars that occur following excisional surgery, scars that develop in areas of radiation treatment worsen with time. If patients are 65 years or older when treated, this may not be a practical concern.

Radiation is not the treatment of choice for cancers of the lips and eyelids. Considerable morbidity can occur on the eyelids due to conjunctival keratinization following radiation. Excisional surgery is a better alternative.

SCC in hair-bearing areas is best treated with methods other than radiation because permanent hair loss can result. SCC that arises in chronic sinuses or scars is usually treated surgically because of poor tolerance to radiation in these areas. Similarly, radiation is not th e preferred treatment for SCC of the penis and anogenital area.

Tumors invading bone are not well suited to radiation because of the potential for necrosis of the bone. Devitalized bone must be removed surgically to allow the area to heal. When SCC occurs in an area of previous radiation damage, a modality other than radiation is usually chosen. Skin can tolerate a finite amount of radiation before ulcers and necrosis develops.

Chemotherapy

Partial and complete remissions have been obtained in three patients with extensive SCC receiving chemotherapy with cisplatin and doxorubicin. An 83-year-old woman with multiple keratoacanthomas and SCC on the legs was treated successfully with oral isotretinoin, with complete regression over six months. Partial response has been reported after the treatment of SCC and actinic keratosis with oral retinoids. Four of fourteen patients with advanced SCC have been reported to undergo complete remission following treatment with systemic retinoids. Twenty-eight patients with advanced inoperable cutaneous SCC were treated with. 13 *cis*-retinoic acid and interferon-alpha-2a. Sixty-eight percent responded, and seven (25%) had a complete response. Response rates were better with advanced local disease (93%) than with regional disease (67%) or distant metastasis (25% response rate).

In organ transplant patients, oral retinoids have been shown to decrease the number of new AK and SCC. Side effects often limit the usefulness of this treatment modality, and patients need to be maintained on the lowest retinoid dose possible. The preventive effect of retinoids rapidly reverses when therapy is discontinued.

BIBLIOGRAPHY

Ackerman LV. Verrucous carcinoma of the oral cavity. Surgery 1948; 23:670.

Anderson SLC, Nielsen A, Reymann F. Relationship between Bowen disease and internalmalignant tumors. Arch Dermatol 1973; 108:367.

Arhelger SW, Kremen AJ. Arsenical epitheliomas of medicinal orgin. Surgery 1951; 30:977.

Arons MS, Lynch JB, Lewis SR, et al. Scar tissue carcinoma. I. A clinical study with special reference to burn scar carcinoma. Ann Surg 1965; 161:170.

Barn RJ, Wueker RB, Graham JH. Ultrastructure of atypical fiboxanthoma. Cancer 1977; 40:736.

Bernstein SC, Lim KEC, Brodland DG, et al. The many faces of squamous cell carcinoma. Dermatol Surg 1996; 22:243–254.

Blau S, Hyman AB. Eryrnroplasia of Queyrat. Acta Derm Venereol (Stockh) 1955; 35:341.

Borelli D. Aspetti pseudoglandolari nell'epithdioma discheratosicoas: "Adenoacanathoma of sweat glands" Lever. Dermatologica 1948; 97:193.

Borders AC. Squamous cell epithelioma of the skin. Ann Surg 1921; 73:141.

Brodland DG, Zitelli JA. Surgical margins for excision of primary cutaneous squamous cell carcinoma. J Am Acad Demtatol 1992; 27(2 Pt 1):241.

Callen JP, Headington J. Bowen's and non-Bowen's squamous intraepidermal neoplasia of the skin. Arch Dermatol 1980; 116:422.

Canfield PJ, Greenoak GE, Mascasaet EN, et al. The characterization of squamous cell carcinoma induced by ultraviolet irradiation in hairless mice. Pathology 1988; 20:109–117.

Cherpelis B, Marcusen C, Lang P. Prognostic factors for metastasis in squamous cell carcinoma in the skin. Dermatol Surg 2002; 28:268–273.

Chuang TY, Heinrick LA, Schultz MD, et al. PUVA and skin cancer. The historical cohort study on 492 patients. J Am Acad Dermatol 1992; 26(2 Pt 1):173–177.

Cottel WI. Moh's surgery for carcinoma of the skin. Dallas Med J 1977; 63:176.

Cottel WI. Perineural invasion by squamous cell carcinoma. J Dermatol Surg Oncol 1982; 8:589.

Cottel WI, Proper S. Mohs surgery, fresh-tissue technique: our technique with a review. J Dermatol Surg Oncol 1982; 8:576.

Craven N, Griffiths C. Retinoids in the management of non-melanoma skin cancer and melanoma. Cane Surv 1996; 26:267–288.

Crum CP, Mitao M, Levine RU, et al. Cervical papillomaviruses segregate within morphologically distinct precancerous lesions. J Virol 1985; 54:675.

Dawson DF, Duckworth JK, Bernhard H, et al. Giant condyloma and verrucous carcinoma of the genital area. Arch Pathol 1965; 79:225.

DeHertog SAE, Wensveen CAH, Bostioens MT, et al. Relation between smoking and skin cancer. J Clin Oncol 2001; 19:231–238.

Delacretaz J, Madjedi AS, Loretan R. Epithelioma spinocellulare segregans. Uber die sogennannten "Adenocanome der Schweissdruen" (lever). Hautartz 1957; 8:512.

DiLuca DR, Pilotti S, Stanfanon B, et al. Human papillomavirus type 16 in genital tumors: a pathological and molecular analysis. J Gen Virol 1986; 67:583–589.

Dzubow LM, Rigel DS, Robins P. Risk factors for local recurrences of primary cutaneous squamous cell carcinomas. Arch Dermatol 1982; 118:900.

Elierzri YD, Silverstein SI, Nuovo GJ. Occurrence of human papillomavirus type 16 DNA in cutaneous squamous and basal cell neoplasms. J Am Acad Dermatol 1990; 23:836.

Elliot JA, Welton DG. Epithelioma: report on 1742 treated patients. Arch Dermatol Syphilol 1946; 53:307.

Epstein EE, Epstein NN, Bragg K, et al. Metastases from squamous cell carcinoma of the skin. Arch Dermatol 1968; 97:245.

Epstein E. Malignant sun-induced squamous-cell carcinoma of the skin. J Dermatol Sug Oncol 1983; 9:505–506.

Evans HL, Smith JL. Spindle cell squamous carcinomas and sarcoma-like tumors of the skin. Cancer 1980; 45:2687.

Forman AB, Roenigk HH, Caro WA. Long-term follow-up of skin cancer in PUVA-48 cooperative study. Arch Dermatol 1989; 125:515.

Frieben A. Carcoid des rechten Handruckens nach langdauernder Einwirkung von Rotgenstrahlen. Fortschr Roentgenstr 1902; 6:106.

Ghadially FN. The role of the hair follicle in the origin and evolution of some cutaneous neoplasms of man and experimental animals. Cancer 1961; 14:801.

Graham JH, Helwig EB. Bowen's disease and its relationship to systemic cancer. Arch Dermatol 1959; 80:133.

Graham JH, Helwig EB. Erythroplasia of Queyrat. In: Graham JH, Johnson WC, Helwig EB, eds. Dermal Pathology. Hagerstown, MD: Harper & Row, 1972:597–606.

Grier WRN. Squamous cell carcinoma of the body and extremities. In: Andrade R et al., eds. Cancer of the Skin. Vol.2. Philadelphia: W B Saunders, 1976:916–932.

Grinspan D, Abulafia J. Oral florid papillomatosis (verrucous carcinoma). Int J Dermatol 1979; 18:608.

Grupper CH, Beretti B. Cutaneous neoplasia and etretinate. In: Spitzy KH, Karrer K, eds. Proceedings of the 13th International Congress of Chemotherapy. Vienna, Egermann VH, 1983:204–207.

Guthrie TH Jr, McElveen LJ, Porubsky ES, et al. Cisplatin and doxorubicin. Cancer 1985; 55:1629.

Hanke CW, Zollinger TA, O'Brien JJ, Bianco L. Skin cancer in professional and amateur women golfers. Phys Sportsmed 1985; 13(8):51.

Haynes HA, Mead KW, Goldwyn RM. Cancers of the skin. In: DeVita Jr VT, Hellman S, Rosenberg SA, eds. Cancer Principles and Practice of Oncology. 2nd ed. Philadelphia: JB Lippincott, 1985.

Hodak E, Jones RE, Ackerman AB. Solitary keratoacanthoma is a squamous cell carcinoma: three examples with metastasis. Am J Dermpathol 1993; 15(4):332.

Honigsman H, Wolff K, Gschnalt F, et al. Keratosis and nonmelanoma skin tumors in long-term photochemotherapy (PUVA). J Am Acad Dermatol 1980; 3:406.

Hoxtell EO, Mandel JS, Murray SS, et al. Incidence of skin carcinoma after renal transplantation. Arch Dermatol 1977; 113:436.

Hueper WC. Occupational Tumors and Allied Diseases. In: Springfield. IL: Charles C Thomas, 1942.

Hyde JN. On the influence of light in the production of cancer of the skin. Am J Med Sci 1906; 131:l.

Immerman SC, Scanlon EF, Christ M, et al. Recurrent squamous cell carcinoma of the skin. Cancer 1983; 51:1537.

Johnson WC, Helwig EB. Adenoid squamous cell carcinoma (adenocarcinoma). Cancer 1966; 19:1639.

King DF, Barr RJ. Intraepithelial elastic fibers and intracytoplasmic glycogen: aids in differentiating keratoacanthomas from squamous cell carcinoma. J Cutan Pathol 1980; 7:140.

Kingston T, Gaskell S, Marks R. The effects of a novel potent oral retinoid (R013–6298) in the treatment of multiple solar keratosis and squamous cell epithelioma. Eur J Cancer Clin Oncol 983; 19:1201.

Kochevar IE, Pathak MA, Parrish JA. Photophysics, photochemistry, and photobiology. In: Fitzpatrick TB et al., eds. Dermatology in General Medicine. 3rd ed. New York: McGraw-Hill, 1987.

Kripke ML, Fisher MS. Immunologic parameters of ultraviolet carcinogenisis. J Natl Cancer Inst 1976; 57:211.

Kripke ML. Ultraviolet radiation and tumor immunity. J Reticuloendothel Soc 1977; 22:217.

Lever WF. Adenocanthomas of sweat glands. Arch Dermatol Syphilol 1947; 56:157.

Levine H, Bailin P, Wood B, et al. Tissue conservation in the treatment of cutaneous neoplasms of the head and neck. Arch Otolaryngol 1979; 105:140.

Levine N, Miller RC, Meyskens FL. Oral isotretinoin therapy. Arch Dermatol 1984; 120:1215.

Lippman SM, Meyskens FL. Treatment of advanced squamous cell carcinoma of the skin with isotretinoin. Ann Intern Med 1987; 107:499.

Lippman SM, Parkinson DR, et al. 13-cis-Retinoic acid and interferon-2A: effective combination therapy for advanced squamous cell carcinoma of the skin. J NatI Cancer Inst 1992; 84(4):235.

Lund HZ. How often does squamous cell carcinoma of the skin metastasize? Arch Dermatol 1965; 92:635.

MacDonald EJ. The epidemiology of skin cancer. J Invest Dermatol 1959; 32:379.

Magee KL, Rapini RP, Duvic M. Human papillomavirus associated with keratoacanthoma. Arch Dermatol 1989; 125:1587.

Martin HT, Strong E, Spiro RH. Radiation-induced skin cancer of the head and neck. Cancer 1970; 25:61.

McKee PH, Wilkinson JD, Black MM, et al. Carcinoma (epithelioma) cuniculatum. Histopathology 1981; 5:425.

McKee PH, Wilkinson JD, Corbett MF, Davey A, Sauven P, Black MM. Carcinoma cuniculatum: a case metastasizing to skin and lymph nodes. Clin Exp Dermatol 1981; 6:613.

McKenna D, Murphy G. Skin cancer chemoprophylaxis in renal transplant recipients: 5 years experience using low-dose acitretin. Br J Dermatol 1999; 140:656–660.

Melton JL, Nelson BR, Stough DB, et al. Treatment of keratoacanthomas with intralesional methotrexate. J Am Acad Dermatol 199l; 25:1017.

Meyskens FL, Gilmartin E, Alberts DS, et al. Activity of isotretinoin against squamous cell cancers and preneoplastic lesions. Cancer'Treat Rep 1982; 66:1315.

Mikhail GR. Chemosurgery in the treatment of skin cancer. Int Dermatol 1975; 14:33.

Mikhail GR. Cancers, precancers, and pseudocancers on the male genitalia. J Dermatol Surg Oncol 1980; 6:1027.

Miller RA, Spittle MF. Electron beam therapy for difficult cutaneous basal and squamous cell carcinoma. Br J Dermatol 1982; l06:429.

Miller DL, Weinstock MD. Nommelanoma skin cancer in the United States: incidence. J Am Acad Dermatol 1994; 30:774.

Mohs FE. Chemosurgery: microscopically controlled surgery for skin cancer: past, present, and future. J Dermatol Surg Oncol 1978; 4:41.

Mohs FE. Chemosurgery: Microscopically Controlled Surgery for Skin Cancer. Springfield, IL: Charles C Thomas, 1978.

Mohs FE. Chemosurgery for the microscopically controlled excision of cutaneous cancer. Head Neck Surg 1978; l:150.

Moller R, Reymann F, Hou-Jensen K. Metastases in dermatological patients with squamous cell carcinoma. Arch Dermatol 1979; 115:703.

Mora RG, Perniciaro C. Cancer of the skin in blacks. I. A review of 163 black patients with cutaneous squamous cell carcinoma. J Am Acad Dermatol 1981; 5:535.

Mora RG, Perniciaro C, Lee B. Cancer of the skin in blacks. III. A review of nineteen black patients with Bowens disease. J Am Acad Dermatol 1984; 11:557.

Muller SA, Wilhelmj CM Jr, Harrison EG Jr, et al. Adenoid squamous cell carcinoma (adenoacanthomas of Lever). Arch Dermatol 1964; 89:589.

Monograph 5, Chapter 7, DOT-TST-75–55. Washington, DC. Department Transportation, 1975.

National Academy of Sciences. Protection Against Depletion of Stratospheric Ozone by Chloroflourocarbons, Washington, DC, 1979.

Nikolowski W. Zur Problematic des Keratoacanthomas. Dematol Monatsschr 1970; 156:148.

Ong CS, Keogh AM, Kossard S, et al. Skin cancer in Australian heart transplant recipients and different long-term immunosuppressive therapy regimens. J Am Acad Dermatol 1999; 40:27–34.

Parker CM, Hanke CW. Large keratoacanthomas in difficult locations treated with intralesional 5-fluorouracil. J Am Acad Dermatol 1986; 14(5):770.

Perez CA, Kraus FT, Evans JC, et al. Anaplastic transformation in verrucous carcinoma of the oral cavity after radiation therapy. Radiology 1966; 86:108.

Potter M. Percivall Pott's contribution to cancer research. Natl Cancer Inst Monogr 1963; 10:1.

Ratzer ER, Strong EW. Squamous Cell carcinoma of the scalp. Am J Sutg 1967; 114:570.

Robins P. Chemosurgery: my 15 years of experience. J Dermatol Surg Oncol 1981; 7:179.

Robins P, Dzubow LM, Rigel DS. Squamous cell carcinoma treated by Mohs surgery. J Dermatol Surg Oncol 1981; 7:800.

Roenigk HH Jr, Caro WA. Skin cancer in the PUVA-48 cooperative study. J Am Acad Dermatol 1981; 4:319.

Rowe DE, Carroll RJ, Day CL. Prognostic factors for local recurrence, metastasis, and survival rate in squamous call carcinoma of the skin, ear, and lip. J Am Acad Dermatol 1992; 26:976.

Rundel RD, Nachtwey DS. Projections of increased nonmelanoma skin cancer incidence due to ozone depletion. Pbotochem Pbotobiol 1983; 38:517.

Rundel RD. Promotional effects of ultraviolet radiation on human basal and squamous cell carcinoma. Photochem Photobiol 1983; 38:569.

Sage HH, Casson PR. Squamous cell carcinoma of the scalp face, and neck. In: Andrade R et al., eds. Cancer of the Skin. Vol. 2. Philadelphia: W B Saunders, 1976.

Schoelch S, Barrett T, Greenway H. Recognition and management of high risk cutaneous tumors. Dermatology Clinics 1999; 17:93–111.

Sedlin ED, Fleming JL. Epidermal carcinoma arising in chrome osteomyelitic foci. J Bone Joint Surg (Am) 1963; 43:827.

Sheild AM. A remarkable case of multiple growths of the skin caused by exposure to the sun. Lancet 1899; 1:22.

Sommers SC, McManus RG. Multiple arsenical cancers of skin and internal organs. Cancer 1953; 6:347.

Stern RS, Laird N, Melski J, et al. Cutaneous squamous cell carcinoma in patients treated with PUVA. N Engl J Med 1984; 310:1156.

Stern RS, Thibodeau LA, Kleinerman RA, et al. Risk of cutaneous carcinoma in patients treated with oral methoxsalen photochemotherapy for psoriasis. N Engl J Med 1970; 300:809.

Stoll HL Jr, Schwartz RA. Squamous cell carcinoma. In: Fitzpatrick TB, ed. Dermatology in General Medicine. 3rd ed. New York: McGraw-Hill, 1987.

Sullivan JJ, Donoghue MF, Kynaston B, et al. Multiple keratoacanthomas. Australas J Dermatol 1980; 21:16.

Ten Seldam. Skin cancer in Australia. J Natl Cancer Inst Monogr 1963; 10:153.

Traenkle HL. X ray induced skin cancer in man. J Natl Cancer Inst Monogr 1963; 10:423.

Turner JE, Callen JP. Aggressive behavior with squamous cell carcinoma in a patient with preceding lymphocytic lymphoma. J Am Acad Dermatol 1981; 4:446.

Unna PG. Die Histopathologie der Hautkrenkheiten. Berlin: Hirschwald, 1984.

Urbach F, Epstein JH, Forbes RD. Ultraviolet carcinogenesis: experimental, global, and genetic aspects. In: Fitzpatrick TB, ed. Sunlight and Man. Tokyo: University of Tokyo Press, 1974:249.

Urbach F. Ultraviolet radiation carcinogenesis. In J Dermatol Surg Oncol 1983; 9:597.

Urbach F, Forbes PD. Photocarcinogenesis. In: Fitzpatrick TB et al., eds. Dermatology in General Medicine. 3rd ed. New York: McGraw-Hill, 1987:1477.

Van der Leun JC, Daniels F Jr. Biologic effects of stratospheric ozone decreases: a critical review of assessments. In: Grobecker AJ, ed. Impacts of Climatic Change on the Biosphere. CIAP.

Veness MJ, Quinn DI, Ong CS et al. Aggressive cutaneous malignancies following cardiothoracic transplantation. The Australian experience. Cancer 1999; 85:1758–1764.

Von Essen CF. Roentgen therapy of skin and lip carcinoma: factors influencing success and failure. Am J Roentgenol 1960; 83:556.

Weidner N, Foucar E. Adenosquamous carcinoma of the skin. Arch Dermatol 1985; 121:775.

39

Keratoacanthoma

Robert A. Schwartz

New Jersey Medical School, Newark, New Jersey, U.S.A.

INTRODUCTION

Keratoacanthoma (KA) is a common and distinctive epidermal neoplasm that often demonstrates a growth pattern of rapid enlargement combined with histology often indistinguishable from that of an ordinary cutaneous squamous cell carcinoma (SCC). For this reason, it has been viewed as a cutaneous pseudomalignancy. Alternatively, KA may rarely be clinically aggressive, so perhaps it is safer to use Kwittken's designation, keratocarcinoma. The diagnosis of KA requires that the clinician rule out the highly malignant de novo type of SCC. The solitary KA usually appears on sun-exposed regions of light-complexioned persons of middle age or older. I regard it as an aborted cancer that only rarely progresses into an aggressive SCC. Nevertheless, KA is quite unique in many ways, mandating a management approach that is often different from that of SCC.

HISTORICAL ASPECTS

In 1889, the renowned British surgeon Sir Jonathan Hutchinson made the first description of KA, labeling it as "The 'crateriform ulcer of the face,' a form of acute epithelial cancer." He illustrated the tumor in an atlas a year earlier and described its histologic features a few years later. Hutchinson wrote, "It is a disease of very rapid growth ... I have for many years been in the habit of calling it the 'crateriform ulcer,' a name more or less appropriate on account of its taking on the form of a large elevated boil (or beehive), and then breaking down into a deep hollow in the center. Microscopic examination, which has been made in at least four cases, has always revealed conditions considered characteristic of epithelial cancer..." He noted "... it occurs on the same parts and under very similar conditions as does the rodent ulcer." All eight of his patients had KA excised without recurrence; he did not mention spontaneous resolution. Similar descriptions followed, notably by Dupont and by Gourgerot. Shaw Dunn and Ferguson Smith in 1934 called the solitary KA a "self-healing primary SCC of the skin." A report on the morphologic and biologic behavior of KA by MacCormac and Scarff in 1936 refocused attention. KA "develops rapidly to its maximum in four to six weeks and remains stationary." They described 10 patients, each with a solitary KA, usually on the middle of the face. They named it molluscum sebaceum, as they thought the KA's "microscopic architecture bears a resemblance to molluscum contagiosum." Freudenthal is credited with suggesting the name "keratoacanthoma," observing that sebaceous glands were not usually involved, and one of the tumor's most impressive histological changes are acanthosis. Rook and Whimster used this designation in their 1950 report of 29 cases. Synonyms for KA include kyste sébacé atypique, molluscum pseudocarcinomatosum, verrucome avec adénite, self-healing primary squamous carcinoma, tumor-like keratosis, multiple self-healing epithelioma, familial primary self-healing squamous epithelioma of title skin, and keratocarcinoma.

Although most early descriptions emphasized the solitary KA, others recognized multiple KAs. Poth in 1939 described multiple "tumor-like keratoses" on the dorsal hand of a man after severe sunburn. The multiple-familial types of KAs were described by the British dermatologist and long-time head of dermatology at the Glasgow Royal Infirmary, John Ferguson Smith in 1934. The generalized eruptive type of KAs was described by the Polish patriot Marian Grzybowski in 1950. By the time of this publication, Grzybowski, professor and head of dermatology at Warsaw University since 1931, who had risked his life to teach dermatology during German occupation, had already been murdered as a part of a notorious Stalinist action, the General Tartar Purge of 1949. An expanding massive tumor form, KA centrifugum, was described in 1962 by the Polish dermatology professors Franciszek Miedziński (professor and head of dermatology at the Medical Academy in Gdańsk and Grzybowski's former student) and Jerzy Kozakiewicz. In 1959, Dąbska and Madejczykowa studied the histopathology of 60 KAs, emphasizing the need for representative skin biopsies for diagnosis, with specimen taken by incisional biopsy to include peripheral and central tumor.

Historically, KA has sometimes been diagnosed as a clinically aggressive SCC, resulting at times in inappropriate therapy. The KA does share clinical and histological features with an aggressive type of SCC, especially an initial period of rapid growth. The best test of distinction is often spontaneous resolution. However, this would require anxiety-filled months of waiting and often a cosmetically unacceptable final result due to an atrophic and even disfiguring scar.

CLINICAL FEATURES

KA occurs mainly on sun-exposed areas of the skin of elderly persons. Actinic skin damage is often evident, including solar elastosis, actinic keratoses, solar lentigines, and at times sun-induced cutaneous cancers such as basal cell carcinomas or ordinary SCCs. KA is best considered an abortive malignancy that only rarely progresses into an invasive SCC. Its peak incidence is between 50 and 69 years of age. Most KAs occur on the face, the forearms and hands. Baer and Kopf noted a predilection to sites where resting hair is found, such as the upper cheeks, nose, ears, forehead, eyelids, temples, forearms, and dorsa of hands and wrists. KAs of the hand occur more commonly in men, and KAs of the calf and anterior tibial area are more frequent in women (and are very uncommon in men). However, KA may develop on any cutaneous surface, including the male nipple. It is more frequent in light-complexioned persons and much less so in more darkly pigmented individuals. Several studies indicate that the incidence of KA is about one-third that of SCC. Jackson and Williamson found KA to be much less common, with only 355 cutaneous SCCs as against only nine KAs in their series from Ottawa, Canada. Yet a South African study found KA to be 1.8 times more frequent. Because the KA is either often presumptively or mistakenly treated as an SCC, its true incidence is often unavailable or difficult to determine. A recent study from Kauai, Hawaii showed an incidence among whites of 104 per 100,000 residents, virtually the same as that of SCC in that population. The incidence of KA has been said to plateau after the age of 55 years, although a recent report suggests it increases with advancing age. The familial type of multiple KAs often has its onset in adolescence. Most studies of solitary KAs have shown that men are affected more often, up to three times more frequently as women. Baer and Kopf observed both sexes to be affected equally. Beare found a higher incidence in women. A Belgian study by Piérard-Franchimont and Piérard showed an overall men-to-women ratio of 1.1:1, with the rate of estimated prevalence increasing steadily in women but not men over the age of 70 years, so that KA was more common in women than men over the age of 80 years. Multiple eruptive KAs of Ferguson Smith have a three to one male predominance, with generalized eruptive KAs of Grzybowski of roughly equal incidence in men and women.

There are three clinical stages in the natural history of the KA: proliferative, mature, and resolving (Figs. 1–4). The proliferative stage produces a firm hemispheric, smooth, enlarging papule that grows rapidly for two to four weeks, often achieving a size of 2 cm or greater. The border is skin-colored or slightly erythematous. Fine telangiectasias may be evident. The mature form is a bud-shaped, dome-shaped or berry-shaped, skin-colored or erythematous nodule with a central, often umbilicated, keratinous core (Figs. 1,2 and 4). It is firm, but without induration at its base or fixation to underlying structures. If the keratotic core is partially removed, KA may appear crateriform. Involution tends to take place after a few months with tumor resorption and expulsion of the central keratotic plug, leaving a typical slightly depressed puckered, often hypopigmented unattractive looking scar. Some lesions persist for a year or more. In its resolving phase, it appears as a keratotic necrotic nodule (Fig. 3). The keratotic debris gradually becomes detached, healing with scar formation. The entire process from origin to spontaneous resolution usually takes about four to six months.

The morphologic features of the mature KA are distinctive. Ghadially's studies classified the KA into three clinicopathologic types: type-1, or bud-shaped; type-2, or dome-shaped; and type-3, or berry-shaped. He considered the latter two patterns to represent lower follicular origin and the former, upper follicular derivation. Histologically, typical KAs, that are bud-shaped or berry-shaped are encountered in practice, which resemble a hypertrophic actinic keratosis, a digitate verruca vulgaris or at times even a seborrheic keratosis.

TYPES OF KERATOACANTHOMA

KA is usually solitary. In one report from the private referral practice of a distinguished dermatology professor, Kingman

and Callen found that 84 of 90 patients had a solitary lesion. However, multiple lesions may be present (Table 2). In fact, two solitary KAs in that study were seen in each of four patients; two patients had more than two KAs, and could be classified as having the Ferguson Smith type of multiple KAs. The KA may have many morphologic forms. In some, no central core is evident clinically. Rarely, the hyperkeratosis is massive so that KA resembles a cutaneous horn. There are, in addition, several special morphologic or syndromic types.

Agglomerated KAs: This type, originally described by Stevanović, is composed of several nodules that coalesce to form a large keratotic tumorous plaque. These plaques persist for almost six months and then spontaneously involute. Some show ulceration before healing. Stevanović coined the name, KA dyskeratoticum et segregans, based upon the histologic findings in his one patient.

KA centrifugum: This form of KA exhibits peripheral growth up to 20 cm in diameter with concurrent central healing. A small KA of 1 cm or less may expand to more than 5 cm in diameter. New KAs may form peripherally. There may be no spontaneous resolution, or it may heal in 6 to 12 months rather than the two to six months for the common KA. It affects men and women of middle age or older (range 41–92 years) and involves the face, trunk, or extremities. Only about 25 cases have been reported. This variant has been reported as aggregated KA, coral-reef KA, nodulo-vegetating KA, multinodular KA, KA centrifugum marginatum, and KA centrifugum of Miedziński and Kozakiewicz. It was first described by Miedziński and Kozakiewicz, who coined the term "keratoacanthoma centrifugum." Puente Duany had described a similar case earlier.

Giant KA: The tumor may grow to 9 cm or larger. Although the KA usually does not invade below the level of the eccrine sweat glands, in some giant KAs, there may be destruction of underlying tissue and cartilage. Some of these patients might be better viewed as having a verrucous carcinoma. KA centrifugum is, in a sense, a giant KA, but its growth characteristics and morphologic features distinguish it.

Subungual KA can be persistent, painful, and locally destructive to underlying bone: It originates in the nail

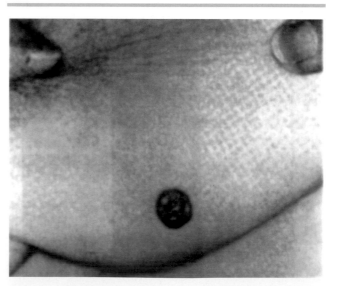

Figure 1   Fully developed crateriform keratoacanthoma in a patient with florid cutaneous papillomatosis and gastric adenocarcinoma. *Source:* From Schwartz (1979).

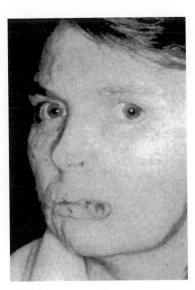

Figure 2 Mature bud-shaped keratoacanthoma, lower lip, in an adolescent with xeroderma pigmentosum. *Source*: From Schwartz (1979).

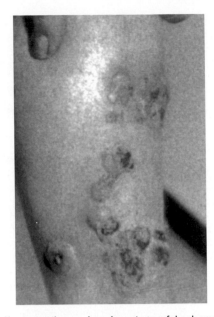

Figure 4 Keratoacanthomas, in various stages of development on the leg of a patient with multiple persistent keratoacanthomas. Solitary dome-shaped nodule on the left is an early proliferative lesion. To its right are mature and resolving keratoacanthomas, adjacent to a large skin graft site. *Source*: From Schwartz (1979).

bed, growing at times to destroy the distal phalanx. Twenty-three subungual KAs in 19 patients have been reported, 80% of who were men, usually between the third and seventh decade of life (average age, 49 years). The thumb or little finger was involved in 70% of the cases. There is one report of an interdigital KA with osteolysis of the proximal and middle phalanges. Shatkin and associated reported two siblings with both subungual KA and incontinentia pigmenti. McKee et al. considered that the infiltrating nature and other findings suggest many of these cases may be better classified as verrucous carcinoma (epithelioma cuniculatum).

Intraoral and other mucous membrane KAs: KA can occur on the hard palate, lips, and other oral sites, and also on the bulbar conjunctiva, nasal mucosa, and genitalia.

Because there are no hair follicles in the oral mucosa, KA may develop from ectopic sebaceous glands. A rare type of KA, generalized eruptive KAs of Grzybowski, has a tendency to involve the mucosal surfaces. Solitary ones with localization on the lips and nose are most often derived from skin rather than mucosa.

Multiple eruptive KAs of Ferguson Smith type: This disorder, also called familial primary self-healing squamous epithelioma of the skin, is characterized by several to many KAs that suddenly erupt, slowly involute and periodically reappear for many years. Each lesion starts as an erythematous macule, becomes papular, and then grows rapidly into an ordinary solitary KA. The number of KAs varies from only a few to hundreds; they may heal with deep unsightly scars, especially on the face, unless each lesion is treated at an early stage. They usually begin in childhood, adolescence, or early adulthood. They may even begin in infancy. The mean age of onset in women is 25.5 years (standard deviation 11.1 years); and in men the mean age of onset is 26.9 years (standard deviation 12.4 years). They persist throughout life, mainly on sun-exposed areas, but the scalp and external genitalia may be involved. It affects both sexes with equal severity, but its distribution differs in men and women because of differences in sun-exposure patterns. They also tend to develop at sites of trauma such as the edge of a donor site of a graft or in a fingertip puncture site. Multiple KAs remained unilateral in three patients who had involvement of the face and upper extremities. One patient had a moderate elevation of the T-helper/T-suppressor ratio. This disorder appears to be inherited in an autosomal dominant manner. One patient with Ferguson Smith type of eruptive KAs was reported by Weber et al. to have an adenocarcinoma of the Fallopian tube plus stem cell leukemia. In another patient an eruption of over a dozen typical KAs was associated with a poorly differentiated laryngeal SCC.

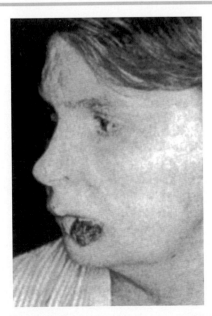

Figure 3 Resolving keratoacanthoma of the lower lip showing abundant green–black keratotic debris in this adolescent with xeroderma pigmentosum. *Source*: From Schwartz (1979).

Multiple persistent KAs are slow healing and nonfamilial: The conjunctivae, palms, soles, and penis have been
involved (Fig. 4). In one possible case, the KAs continued
to develop for 35 years, becoming a painful mass that
extended around the underlying tendon.

Generalized eruptive KAs of Grzybowski: Literally,
thousands of tiny disseminated, 2 to 3 mm KAs, are present.
Grzybowksi observed the lesions to be "varying in size from
a nearly invisible point to the size of a bean." Jaber et al. calculated that the 22 patients reported, tended to be middle
aged or older, with an age of onset ranging from 32 to 84
years (mean age, 57 years). Of these, 13 were woman and 9
were men. No familial pattern has been shown, with the
cases being sporadic. Most patients are white, but it has been
described in one black American and two Japanese. Individual lesions resolve spontaneously with scarring in about six
months. Pruritus is common, as is ectropion, caused by KAs
of the eyelids. Corrective blepharoplasty may be required to
prevent a serious keratopathy. The face may become so
involved as to produce a masked facies. Individual nodules
may coalesce to become tumors cherry-sized or larger. Köb-
nerization may be evident. An unexplained hepatomegaly
may be noted. KAs may appear as multiple papulonodules
on the palms and soles, oral mucosa and palate, larynx, and
glans penis. Snider and Benjamin have reported adenocarcinoma of the ovary in one patient with generalized eruptive
KAs. Another patient was reported to have a lymphoma.

KA in Muir-Torre syndrome: An eruption of KAs may
appear in association with sebaceous neoplasms and one or
more low-grade visceral cancers usually of gastrointestinal
or urogenital origin. The association of KAs and sebaceous
neoplasms may be explained by their common derivation
from pilosebaceous glands. Almost half the patients with
this syndrome have at least one KA. The KAs tend to be
0.5 to 1.0 cm in diameter, 3 to 10 in number, and scattered
on the head and trunk. Patients may have one or multiple
KAs, no sebaceous tumors, and an internal cancer, possibly,
in at least some of them, a manifestation of this syndrome.
However, Kingman and Callen found that patients with a
solitary KA (and no sebaceous tumors) do not have an
increased risk of concurrent or subsequent internal cancer. I
believe that every patient with multiple KAs should be evaluated for the presence of sebaceous neoplasms, the absence
of which still requires consideration of this syndrome. It is
inherited as an autosomal dominant trait.

KA in xeroderma pigmentosum: This defect of DNA
repair is associated with development, at an early age, of
basal cell carcinomas, SCCs, melanomas, and KAs on sun-
exposed sites (Figs. 2 and 3). KA in a child may be suggestive of this syndrome. A three-year old Bantu child with
probable xeroderma pigmentosum had KA.

KA in florid cutaneous papillomatosis and an underlying cancer: Multiple papillomas and a KA were noted in
the original report. This disorder is believed to be caused
by a malignancy-secreted growth factor.

KA in nevus sebaceus of Jadassohn: This type of epidermal nevus tends to occur on the scalp in infants, proliferate at puberty, and contains a wide variety of neoplasms
within it. Most are a basal cell epitheliomas or benign appendageal tumors such as a syringocytostadenoma papilliferum, but occasionally a KA or SCC develops. One series
of 150 cases had 52 tumors, four of which in adults were
KA. KA can also occur in childhood within a nevus sebaceus.
KA may also occur with an ordinary linear epidermal nevus.

Pseudorecidive KA: Pseudorecidives are defined as
pseudoepitheliomatous reactions that occasionally develop

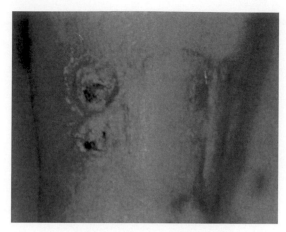

Figure 5   Multiple keratoacanthomas developing at the site of a previous
excision and graft. *Source*: From Schwartz (1979).

after radiotherapy for skin and other cancers. These are a rap-
idly-developing early sequella of radiation therapy that may
be confused with a recurrence of the original skin cancer,
hence the name "pseudorecidive." They occur when the
initial radiation reaction is subsiding and evolve rapidly,
sometimes in a few days, at other times in a few weeks. They
tend to appear granulomatous or wart-like. Their histologic
pattern varies from acanthomatous (wart-like) to closely
resemble or be indistinguishable from KA. Pseudorecidives
may lack the typical central keratotic plug of the KA, and their
exact categorization is still unclear. Lesions with both clinical
and histologic features considered "classical" for KAs have
been described, that developed in cutaneous radiotherapy
sites several years after treatment of a basal cell carcinoma.

Reactive KAs: KAs have been noted to appear at the
site of scar formation (Fig. 5), recently healing herpes zoster
sites, in hypertrophic lichen planus, in discoid lupus erythematosus, and in other benign inflammatory disorders,
including psoriasis, pemphigus foliaceus, and epidermolysis
bullosa dystrophica. Some of these KAs may have been associated with the underlying therapy used, such as tar, or body
peel. Just as crops of KAs may occur after an outbreak of dermatitis, multiple KAs were reported to suddenly appear
three weeks after a thermal burn from a gasoline explosion.
With multiple eruptive KAs of the Ferguson Smith type, KAs
tend to develop at sites of trauma.

Chemical induced (mainly tar) KAs: In man as well as
in animals, contact with tar or pitch enhances the chance of
KA formation. There is a significantly increased incidence of
KAs in tar and pitch workers. Often the occupational
exposure occurs in machinists such as chronic contact with
machine oil. Typical KA has been described after topical
podophyllin therapy.

The KA in an immunosuppressed patient: The
immunocompromised patient may be at increased risk of
KAs as well as skin cancers. There seems to be no significantly increased incidence of KAs with the use of cyclosporine. At least some skin neoplasms and possibly KA may
show increased aggressive potential in immunosuppressed
patients. Eruptive KAs in an immunosuppressed transplantation recipient has been described.

HISTOGENESIS

The probable derivation of KAs from hair follicles has been
well documented in humans and in animals by Ghadially

and others. In fact, the pioneer study in chemical carcinogenesis by Yamagiwa and Ichikawa in 1918 produced a number of growths that these investigators labeled folliculoepitheliomas. Many were undoubtedly KAs. They observed the histologic evolution of these tumors as follows: "The epithelium, and especially that at the periphery of the hair follicles, gradually undergoes hyperplasia; (i) each layer increases considerably in thickness; (ii) many symmetrical mitoses are found in its basal layer; (iii) the hair follicles become cystic; (iv) the basal layer grows irregular in outline owing to the projection of processes, which ramify in the surrounding subcutaneous tissues."

The role of hair follicles and epidermis in the origin and evolution of cutaneous tumors in man and animals has been elucidated and summarized by Ghadially. Rigdon found a chemical induced KA-like lesion arising from a feather follicle in a white Pekin duck. Ghadially noted that the usual description of most benign cutaneous growths produced during experimental carcinogenesis has been a "papilloma," an inadequate term for a variety of tumors. He illustrated diagrammatically and histologically how some of these benign neoplasms are of sebaceous gland origin, and others of epidermal or hair follicle origin. The latter began as striking cellular growth and keratinization in the upper part of the hair follicle and evolved into a KA. He also described a type of KA derived from the hair follicle below the attachment of the erector pili muscle. Although this lower hair follicle histogenesis is not universally accepted, it serves as a model for the histogenesis of the three distinct morphologic types of KAs. These deeper types of KAs displayed a consistent and rapid resolution, and were derived from the cyclically evanescent hair germ rather than the permanent upper portion of the hair follicle.

ETIOLOGY

The etiology of KA is uncertain. Its usual occurrence on sun-exposed areas in elderly persons suggests that ultraviolet light (UVL) may be of etiologic significance in the common solitary type of KA. In England and Australia, the incidence of both KA and SCC show parallel increases with increased sun-exposure. The occurrence of KAs in patients with xeroderma pigmentosum is also consistent with solar induction (Figs. 2 and 3). The defective deoxyribonucleic acid repair in xeroderma pigmentosum after UVL injury has been well characterized. KA production in the autosomal dominant Muir-Torre syndrome appears closely associated with a defect in one of the DNA repair systems, the mismatch DNA repair system, as a result of a defective DNA mismatch repair gene. However, microsatellite instability and loss of heterozygosity appear to be significant factors in KA development only in people with this syndrome. The role of higher electromagnetic frequencies in tumorigenesis is suggested by the possible induction of KAs by cutaneous X-ray therapy.

Chemical tumorigenesis has been documented in KAs in several animal models (rabbit, rat, hamster, mouse, hedgehog, duck, and chicken) by painting the skin with tar derivatives. KAs induced in rabbit skin in this way and human KAs both show a relatively high frequency of an activated H-ras oncogene. Human KAs were shown to display p53 oncoprotein expression in 16 of 20 (80%) of KAs examined by Kerschmann and associates. In animal studies, two main types of tumors have been noted, papillomas derived from surface epithelium and KAs of hair follicle origin. The latter were both clinically and histologically indistinguishable from the KA of humans. A somewhat greater tendency for continued local growth was observed in mice and hamsters than in rabbits. In humans a study of 250 KAs in 238 patients showed a significantly increased incidence of these tumors among pitch and tar workers than in matched controls. A larger proportion of the 238 patients were smokers than would be anticipated in the control group. There have also been a number of patients who worked as machinists in constant contact with oil. Crude coal tar, which enhances UVL carcinogenesis in animals, has been used in conjunction with UVL to treat psoriatic patients for many years. The development of multiple KAs in six psoriatic patients has been reported, although this is rather unusual. There is also a description of two psoriatic patients with multiple KAs possibly induced by oral psoralens and ultraviolet light (PUVA). However, the risk of developing a KA after PUVA therapy is less than a SCC or basal cell carcinoma.

A viral etiology for KA has been postulated by Koziorowska and Dux, and by many others. This idea is suggested by the fact that Shope virus-induced tumors of rabbits are similar to KA. In 1961, viral-like particles were observed within the nucleus of 40% to 60% of KA tumor cells; however, others believe these intranuclear particles are nonviral in origin, and inoculation experiments, including those by Koziorowska and Dux, have been negative. Using PCR, cutaneous HPV of no predominating type was found by Florslund and associates in 51% of 72 KAs. Thus, the role of HPV in the development of KA remains unclear. A study among renal transplant recipients by Euvrard and associates found benign and oncogenic human papilloviruses within KAs.

It is possible that there is an interaction between genetic predisposition and other cofactors such as UVL, infrared radiation, X rays, chemical agents, and viral infections together with trauma or immunosuppression in the pathogenesis of KA. Clearly, trauma plays a role because KAs tend to occur at or near skin graft sites. Ghadially's experiments demonstrated that trauma to the chemically pretreated experimental animal produced KAs. The appearance of KAs after bone marrow transplantation or during cyclosporine therapy suggests the possibility of immunosuppression as a contributory factor.

Genetics is also important in a number of ways. A light-complexioned person has a relatively high risk of UVL-induced tumors, including KA. One study of 43 cases of solitary KAs claimed an increased incidence of HLA-B16 and HLA-B18 antigens. The Ferguson Smith type of multiple KAs was studied in 62 persons from 11 Scottish families. It seemed probable that these were the result of a single mutation occurring before 1790. The same mutation was probably responsible for some cases in Canada and the United States, as members of affected families immigrated to North America.

HISTOPATHOLOGIC FINDINGS

The histologic appearance of KA has been reviewed by many including Kwittken, Lever and Schaumburg-Lever, Dąbska and Madejczykowa, Milewski and Chorzelski, Ghadially and Ghadially, and Ackerman and associates. It can be divided into three stages: proliferative, fully developed, and involuting.

Proliferative Stage

In the early, rapidly growing phase there is a horn-filled invagination of the epidermis arising from contiguous hair follicles, from which epidermal strands may extend into

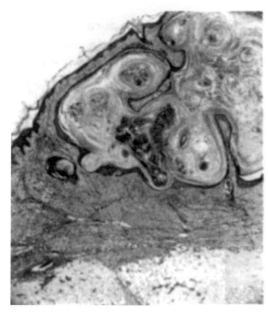

Figure 6 Early development of a keratoacanthoma, displaying keratin-filled invagination of the epidermis and a few epidermal stands extruding into the dermis (hematoxylin-eosin, original magnification ×30). *Source*: From Schwartz (1979).

the dermis (Figs. 6 and 7). This incipient lesion shows mild hyperkeratosis, acanthosis, and premature keratinization, characterized by enlarged cells of the lower portion of the malpighian layer reportedly often with a thick granular layer with prominent keratohyalin granules. There may or may not be a central depression. The hyperkeratosis forms a crenulated border with the acanthotic epidermis. The epidermal strands may be carcinoma-like, containing atypical-appearing squamous cells with multiple mitotic figures as the KA enlarges and extends downward toward the level of the eccrine sweat glands (Fig. 7). Some of these mitotic

figures may appear atypical. Tripolar mitosis was described by Giltman; Ghadially and Ghadially believe that abnormal mitoses, in general, and tripolar ones, in particular, strongly indicate a carcinoma. Some tumor regions may show pronounced keratinization with the abundant and pale staining cytoplasm producing an eosinophilic "glassy" appearance. Eosinophils and neutrophils may be present, probably causing some of the keratinocytes to be come necrotic and others to disassociate as evidenced by acantholysis. One variant, KA dyskeratoticum et segregans, was named for its marked dyskeratosis and acantholysis. Collagen and elastin fiber fragments may be trapped within the expanding tumor. A sparse dermal inflammatory infiltrate may be present at the tumor interface with the dermis. Perineural invasion may occasionally be seen at this stage and should not be interpreted as a sign of malignancy. Likewise, intravascular extension and deep invasion below the eccrine glands can be present, but are considered benign phenomena. Nests of squamous cells can be seen in medium size veins. However, deep invasion below the level of the eccrine glands is considered by this author to be an ominous sign.

Fully Developed Stage

The fully developed dome-shaped crateriform nodule contains a central depression composed of a keratotic central core (Fig. 8). The epidermis extends around the crater sides, forming a lip. Irregular epidermal proliferations protrude both into the crater and below its base. In the mature KA, the individual squamous cells may appear somewhat atypical; but atypia is more pronounced in the rapidly growing stage. However, carcinoma-like foci appear either focally or diffusely in almost three-fourths of established KAs, and are more common in them than in early or regressing lesions. Keratinization of these squamous cells is marked, producing an eosinophilic and glassy appearance. Many keratinocytes have undergone necrosis. Microabscesses may be evident, composed of neutrophils and often eosinophils. Horn pearls, also characteristic of cutaneous SCC, are present (Fig. 9).

These are concentric layers of squamous cells with central keratinization that increases centripetally. Lateral tumor strands projecting between collagen bundles can also be seen. There is a focally dense mixed dermal infiltrate composed of lymphocytes, histiocytes, eosinophils, neutrophils, and plasma cells. In carcinoma-like foci, the infiltrate is prominent at its advancing margins but does not infiltrate the tumor. Atypical eccrine sweat duct hyperplasia may be present.

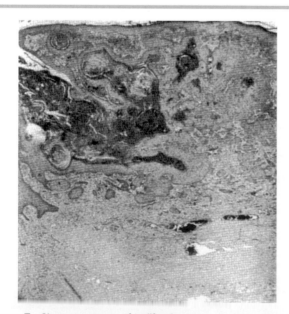

Figure 7 Glassy appearance of proliferating keratoacanthoma (hematoxylin-eosin, original magnification ×30). *Source*: From Schwartz (1979).

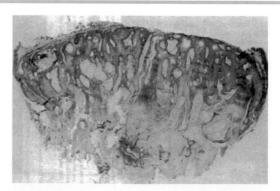

Figure 8 Mature keratoacanthoma with large keratin filled core, epidermal lip, and tumor cells extending into dermis (hematoxylin-eosin, original magnification ×25). *Source*: From Schwartz (1979).

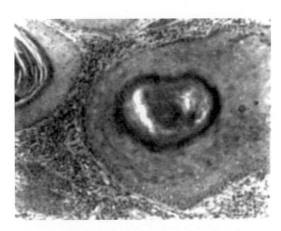

Figure 9 Keratoacanthoma, showing somewhat glassy appearance of keratinocytes, that are arranged in concentric layers with increasing keratinization centrally. Note collection of neutrophils (hematoxylin-eosin stain; ×160). *Source*: From Schwartz (1979).

Involutional Stage

During involution, the lesion becomes flattened and less crateriform, as most cells at the crater base have become keratinized. There may be shrunken cells staining intensely with eosin adjacent to tumor cells nearby and within the stroma. A mixed dermal infiltrate is usually evident, sometimes containing multinucleated histiocytes, probably best considered a foreign body granuloma to keratin. Beneath the KA, granulation tissue may be evident, with fibrosis at its base. Fibroblasts at the KA base proliferate, with resultant fibrosis pushing the neoplastic remnants through the crater to the surface. A lichenoid reaction may be seen at the epidermal-dermal interface lining the regressing crater. The crater slowly becomes flat and heals with the formation of an irregularly shaped atrophic scar.

Ultrastructural Pathology

Electron microscopic analysis of the KA has been performed on both human KAs and experimental animal tumors. There appears to be an increased number of desmosomes in KA than in normal skin. They may be seen within abnormally keratinized cells. Intranuclear inclusions may sometimes be evident; these virus-like particles may actually be perichromatin granules and nuclear bodies. The main morphologic features distinguishing KA from SCC are the desmosomes and the intercellular space. In both, the number and surface density of desmosomes are lower than in normal skin; in well-differentiated SCC, these are significantly lower than in KA. The intercellular space, a reflection of keratinocyte cohesiveness, is significantly larger in SCC than in KA.

Cellular and Basement Membrane Features

There are two important pathologic features commonly used to separate benignity from malignancy that require consideration for KAs. These are individual cell cytology and invasiveness below the basement membrane. Premalignant tumors can usually be distinguished from malignant tumors by the invasion or otherwise of the tumor below the basement membrane. However, a number of exceptions, as in the case of the verrucous carcinoma, have reduced the value of this generalization. Immunologic, histochemical, and electron microscopic studies of KA have shown conflicting

results. The other point is that the degree of cellular atypia may be useful in separating benign from malignant neoplasms. Studies demonstrated aneuploidy in some KAs, although to a lesser extent than in well-differentiated SCC. The majority of both were diploid. One DNA image cytometry study showed a significant difference in peak DNA index and highest DNA content between KA and SCC.

DIFFERENTIAL DIAGNOSIS

The most frequent consideration in the clinical and histological differential diagnosis of KA is SCC. Clinically, the rapid tumor growth may suggest a de novo cutaneous SCC, a relatively rare, aggressive tumor that produces regional or distant metastases in at least 8% of the patients. A series of four such patients illustrated this point. Each de novo SCC was initially diagnosed as KA, but each had an early recurrence after conservative therapy. In three of the four patients, rapidly spreading metastatic cutaneous SCC occurred, resulting in the death of two. Other examples exist. Occasionally, an unusual type of cutaneous SCC, verrucous carcinoma, requires distinction. This slow growing tumor may produce a bulky locally destructive mass that may necessitate distinction from a giant KA or from a subungual KA. However, our main discussion focuses on the differences between the ordinary type of SCC and its de novo form.

Fortunately, the morphologic features and growth pattern of KA are sufficiently distinctive to be diagnostic in most cases. In short, the diagnosis of KA is based upon its architecture rather than its cytologic features. Although the cellular characteristics of KA and SCC are similar, the tumor architecture usually provides the distinction. Thus, as Dąbska and Madejczykowa pointed out, it is important to obtain a representative tissue specimen. It is done with a biopsy specimen down to subcutaneous fat, achieved either by total excision or by a fusiform partial excision through the entire KA to include its center and both sides. In this way both the tumor architecture and the presence or absence of tumor invasiveness into underlying tissue can be analyzed. Incision through KA is not associated with an increased risk of aggressive behavior. The presence of deep invasion necessitates therapy for SCC.

In distinction from SCC, KAs tend to be both exophytic and endophytic with a central keratin-filled crater, whereas most cutaneous SCCs are mainly endophytic, with ulceration often present. The crater is surrounded by overhanging epithelial "lips" that are absent in SCC. Intraepidermal abscesses are common in KA and rarely seen in SCC. In KA, acantholytic cells and polymorphonuclear leukocytes are present in these abscesses; when abscesses occur in cutaneous SCCs, there are few, if any, inflammatory cells. KAs have abundant pale-staining keratinocyte cytoplasm; less is seen in the SCC. Resolving KAs often show fibrosis at their-base; in SCCs fibrosis, when present, is of the desmoplastic type.

There are a number of features that help to distinguish KA from SCC, but none is absolute. The most valuable method may be that described by Phillips and Helm, who found the distribution of proliferating cell nuclear antigen positive cells important in distinguishing KA from SCC. In KA it occurred mainly in the periphery of squamous cell nests rather than as the diffuse staining pattern seen throughout the squamous cell nests in SCC. In addition, atypical eccrine duct hyperplasia is more common in KA, as are actinically damaged elastic fibers and an increased content of intracytoplasmic glycogen within the epidermis of KA. Likewise, a relatively homogeneous staining pattern for involucrin favors KA. Other potential aids in distinction include morphometry on ultrastructural sections, DNA cytometry and content, staining for peanut agglutinin lectin, quantitation of Langerhans cells, nucleolar organizer regions, filaggrin, stromelysin 3, blood group antigens, transforming growth factor-alpha, and expression of angiotensin type-1 receptor, oncostatin M, syndecan-1 expression, and a variety of oncogenes. Loss of expression of the light chain part of HLA, beta-2 microglobulin, was not found to be a reliable feature in distinguishing KA from SCC.

The diagnosis of KA relies more upon architecture than cytologic features. Although the cellular characteristics of both KA and SCC are similar, their architecture usually allows distinction. No sufficiently sensitive and specific criterion has been established to distinguish KA from SCC. The five most relevant ones are epithelial lipping and sharp demarcation between tumor and stroma favoring KA and ulceration, numerous mitoses and marked pleomorphism/anaplasia favoring SCC. Yet, even the combination of these five did may not be of value in difficult cases, as Cribier and associated observed in analyzing 296 specimens. In practice, it is sometimes necessary to give a histologic diagnosis "probable KA; SCC cannot be ruled out." SCC resembling KA may be seen in many settings, including within a fibroepitheliomatous polyp. Many times a well-differentiated SCC and pseudoepitheliomatosis hyperplasia overlying certain granulomatoses can be difficult to distinguish from KA without a clinical history.

A KA may be associated with other lesions, with or without a transition between the two. KA has been reported to arise from a preexistent basal cell carcinoma or superficial spreading malignant melanoma or vice versa; however, this author views the situation as, more likely, a matter of histologic collision between two sun-induced tumors. However, when elements of sebaceous adenoma and KA occur in the same lesion presumably caused by joint pilosebaceous proliferation, the lesion may be classified as a "seboacanthoma," reflecting the strong possibility of the Muir-Torre syndrome. These lesions show converging follicular and sebaceous proliferation often with an epidermal buttress or collarette.

The clinical differential diagnosis besides ordinary SCC, de novo type SCC, and verrucous carcinoma include hypertrophic actinic keratosis, other causes of cutaneous horns, inverted follicular keratosis, warty dyskeratoma, giant molluscum contagiosum, verruca vulgaris, metastatic cancer, deep fungal infections such as chromoblastomycosis or North American blastomycosis, other pseudopitheliomatous hyperplasias, syphilis, histoid lepromas, and seborrheic keratosis. Small KAs as seen in generalized eruptive KA of Grzybowski may resemble Darier's disease. Giant molluscum contagiosum has become more common because of an increased incidence in patients with AIDS. Some sebaceous neoplasms in the Muir-Torre syndrome may clinically mimic a KA, with sudden appearance, rapid growth, a central plug, and a heaped-up border.

MALIGNANT TRANSFORMATION

The KA may be viewed as an "abortive malignancy, which only rarely progresses into an invasive SCC." The presence of aneuploidy in KAs has been found indistinguishable from that of many cutaneous SCCs, supporting the idea that the KA is a true neoplasm rather than a reactive hyperplasia. KAs progressing to SCCs or KA-like SCCs are rare.

A study of 39 KAs in 35 patients by Janecka et al. is noteworthy. Careful histologic examination revealed six with perineural invasion and one with vascular invasion. During a follow-up period ranging from four to eight years, none of these histologically disturbing findings was associated with metastases. However, adequate surgical excision was apparently used in these six patients. Even invasion of medium-sized veins does not suggest malignant transformation. The progression of a KA into SCC in a patient with Hodgkin's disease receiving polychemotherapy has been reported; this raises the question whether the transformation into SCC may have resulted from a mutagenic effect of chemotherapy. Immunosuppression associated with Hodgkin's disease or chemotherapy has been postulated to account for the lack of tumor rejection (i.e., regression) and its progression into SCC. However, there is evidence that factors other than immunologic are responsible for KA regression in man. In Ramselaar and van der Meer's study of cell-mediated immunity in 11 patients with a solitary KA, no delayed hypersensitivity reaction was observed after intradermal injection of tumor extract. An unconfirmed electron microscopic study some years ago suggested that certain, probably nonviral intranuclear particles correlated with malignant degeneration. However, no clinical or histologic finding has been convincingly linked with "malignant transformation." An alternative viewpoint is that malignant transformation does not occur, but rather such a tumor is SCC from its inception, possibly as a malignantly altered clone of keratinocytes initiating proliferation by the same histogenic mechanism as KA.

IMMUNOLOGY OF KERATOACANTHOMA

Few nonimmunocompromised patients with KAs have deficient humoral or cellular immunity; most have an intact humoral and cellular immune system. Some KAs display altered expression of class II antigen expression (HLA-DR). An analysis of the lymphocytic infiltrate around KAs casts doubt on a possible major role played by natural killer cells in KA regression. In immunosuppressed patients, there may be an increased incidence of KAs as there is of cutaneous SCCs, and to a lesser extent, of basal cell carcinomas. It is possible that lepromatous leprosy patients may also fit within this category. In one patient with multiple KAs treated successfully with etretinate, there were notable increases in both interleukin-2 production and mitogen-induced lymphocyte proliferation during therapy. An analysis by Morita and Sagami of lymphocyte subpopulations in KA was interpreted as displaying a meaningful infiltration of killer T-cells and OKT-6 positive dendritic cells. The role of immunity in spontaneous tumor regression has been argued, noting the following: a halo of erythema around some regressing KAs, tumor regression during febrile illness, increased incidence with advancing age or immunosuppression, dense mononuclear infiltrate, and fibroblastic tissue reaction associated with regressing tumors, variable presence of Langerhans cells, and detection of an anti-squamous antibody. Nevertheless, there is growing evidence that the regression of human KAs is not immunologically mediated, implying that it is similar to the pattern of natural regression seen within a normal hair follicle.

KERATOACANTHOMA AS A MARKER FOR INTERNAL MALIGNANCY

There have been several reports linking KAs with internal malignancy; these have been summarized by Kingman and Callen, who concluded that there is no evidence linking the solitary type KA with internal malignancy in a greater than chance association.

However, multiple KAs may serve as a marker for the Muir-Torre syndrome, an important autosomal dominant familial cancer syndrome resulting from a defective DNA mismatch repair gene. As noted previously, very few patients have had either Ferguson Smith multiple eruptive KAs or Grzybowski generalized eruptive KAs and an underlying tumor. A solitary KA too may occur as part of a generalized eruption such as florid cutaneous papillomatosis or the Muir-Torre syndrome, both of which are markers for internal malignancy. The KA may also occur with xeroderma pigmentosum.

TREATMENT

Although KA usually involutes spontaneously, biopsy and treatment are undertaken for several important reasons. Biopsy establishes the diagnosis and serves to rule out SCC. Treatment provides hastened resolution or cure, prevention of rapid enlargement or impingement on important structures, and improvement in overall cosmetic result. Solitary KAs should usually receive complete conservative excision, which also provides an optimal biopsy specimen and in most patients a greater likelihood of a favorable cosmetic outcome than one would anticipate with spontaneous resolution. One recent analysis by Griffiths observed a mean time of 27 weeks (range, 12–64 weeks) for resolution from the time of appearance, for solitary KAs, with no scar revision being needed.

A fusiform partial excision cut symmetrically through the center so as to include normal lateral tissue and underlying normal fat, also provides an adequate specimen to distinguish SCC from KA. If this is done, it is important that the pathologist is informed, so that appropriate sections showing the lateral aspects as well as deep margins of the lesions can be visualized microscopically. Although the fusiform partial excisional biopsy was initially thought to possibly hasten resolution of KA, time has not shown this observation to be valid in my experience. Shave and incisional punch biopsy specimens are not acceptable forms of biopsy when one is considering the diagnosis of KA. Excision of a subungual KA may require amputation of a digit when underlying bone is involved and other options fail. Micrographic surgery may be used to preserve a maximum of normal tissue in selected patients. With the Smith Ferguson type of multiple eruptive KA, limited surgical excision, cryosurgery, curettage, or other options should be considered for use on early lesions, to avoid the disfigurement that may ensue with spontaneous resolution.

Simple curettage may be employed, as may blunt dissection. Curettage is usually used together with electrodesiccation. An 8% recurrence rate was found for solitary KA treated mostly in this manner. Radiotherapy with superficial X ray, orthovoltage radiation, or electron beam may be used primarily, or after the recurrence of KA following excision or curettage and electrodesiccation. The same tumoricidal doses as employed for SCC should be used. Large facial KAs may be treated by radiotherapy with acceptable cosmesis. Laser surgery has also been employed with good success for small solitary KAs in difficult-to-treat locations. Kuflik and Kuflik recommend cryosurgery with liquid nitrogen is of value, especially for small early KAs. For larger ones, it is usually used as adjunctive therapy to the base after the KA has been removed by excisional biopsy or curettage. The base is frozen completely with at least a 3 mm halo of healthy tissue after hemostatis is achieved. Topical podophyllin has been used alone, in combination with curettage and electrodesiccation, or in combination with radiotherapy. Curiously, topical podophyllin may also produce KA formation. Topical treatment with imiquimod may induce regression of facial KA.

Intralesional and topical 5-fluorouracil (5-FU) for KAs, was introduced by Klein and associates in 1962. It may be administered by either daily or every other day focal injections of 0.1 mL of a 5% solution directly into the base of the KA or by topical application of 5-FU cream or ointment up to five times daily, with or without occlusion. Therapy is continued for about 2.5 weeks. Others used 50 mg/mL of 5-FU injected with a 27- or 30-gauge needle inserted tangentially into the slopes of the KA in three or four sites and 0.1 to 0.3 mL injected circumferentially and 0.1 to 0.2 mL sublesionally. This approach was performed weekly until the KA size was decreased by 60% to 80%. It took up to eight weeks, with an average of three weeks, for each KA to resolve. Only one of 26 KAs in 14 patients did not respond. This modality provides an excellent therapeutic result and has proven valuable for large KAs in difficult-to-treat locations. It may be ineffective in the KA that is not rapidly proliferating. Intralesional bleomycin may also be used instead of 5-FU. Intralesional injection of oil bleomycin, with a depot effect, has also been suggested. Intralesional methotrexate may also be employed. Systemic chemotherapy including methotrexate has been used for multiple KAs.

Other therapies may have value in treating KAs. Intralesional injections of triamcinolone have also been utilized. Intralesional interferon alpha may also be of value for selected KAs. Transfer factor was found effective in two patients with the Ferguson Smith type of familial multiple eruptive KAs. Etretinate, 1 mg/kg/day for two months, may be valuable for multiple KAs, including the eruptive type Ferguson Smith, and for the generalized eruptive type of Grzybowski. With the latter, no therapy seems to give persistent regression of eruptive KAs, nor affects the natural course of the disease with its spontaneous regression within one to two months of single KAs and reappearance of new ones.

KERATOACANTHOMA—AN OVERVIEW

KA is a common skin tumor that tends to occur on sun-exposed sites in light-skinned persons of middle age or older. It is best viewed as an aborted SCC that only rarely evolves into a progressively invasive SCC. Sometimes labeled a typical pseudomalignancy, KA may paradoxically merit the alternative designation as pseudobenignity. It is most likely derived from hair follicle cells. Its etiology is unknown, although UVL, viruses, and chemical carcinogens have been considered. Its diagnosis should be made by complete conservative excision or by a properly performed fusiform partial excision designed to provide an adequate biopsy specimen to distinguish KA from SCC. The Ferguson Smith type of multiple eruptive KAs is particularly important to recognize and treat, to avoid natural healing, which can lead to disfigurement.

BIBLIOGRAPHY

Ackerman AB, Ragaz A. The lives of lesions. In: Chronology in Dermatopathology. New York: Masson Publishing USA, 1984:102–109.

Agarwal M, Chander R, Karmakar S, Walia R. Multiple familial keratoacanthoma of Witten and Zak – a report of three siblings. Dermatology (Basel) 1999; 198:396–399.

Ahmed AR, Sofen H, Saxon A. Detection of an antisquamous antibody in multiple keratoacanthoma. Clin Immunol Immunopathol 1982; 22:20–31.

Akiyama M, Hata Y, Nishikawa T. Keratoacathoma with glandular proliferation. J Dermatol (Tokyo) 1993; 20:109–113.

Andreassi A, Pianigiani E, Taddeucci P, et al. Keratoacanthoma treated with intralesional bleomycin. Eur J Dematol 1999:403–405.

Baer RL, Kopf AW. Keratoacanthoma. In: Year Book of Dermatology (1962–1963 series). Chicago: Year Book Medical Publishers, 1963:7–41.

Baer RL, Kopf AW. Complications of therapy for basal cell epitheliomas (based on 1,000 histologically verified cases). In: Year Book of Dermatology (1964–1965 series). Chicago: Year Book Medical Publishers, 1965:7–26.

Beare JM. Molluscum sebaceum. Br J Surg 1953; 41:167–172.

Belisario JC. Brief review of keratoacanthomas and description of keratoacanthoma centrifugum marginatum, another variety of keratoacanthoma. Austral J Dermatol 1965; 8:65–72.

Benest L, Kaplan RP, Salit R, et al. Keratoacanthoma centrifugum marginatum of the lower extremity treated with Mohs micrographic surgery. J Am Acad Dermatol 1994; 31:501–502.

Benoldi D, Alinovi A. Multiple persistent keratoacanthomas: treatment with oral etretinate. J Am Acad Dermatol 1984; 10:1035–1038.

Berenblum I, Haran-Ghera N, Trainin N. An experimental analysis of the "hair cycle effect" in mouse skin carcinogenesis. Br J Cancer 1958; 12:402–413.

Beer GM, Widder W, Cierpka K, et al. Malignant tumors associated with nevus sebaceous: therapeutic consequences. Aesthetic Plast Surg 1999; 23:224–227.

Bhatia N. Imiquimod as a possible treatment for keratoacanthoma. J Drugs Dermatol 2004; 3:71–74.

Binkley GW, Johnson HH Jr. Keratoacanthoma (molluscum sebaceum). AMA Arch Dermatol Syphilol 1954; 71:66–72.

Blohmé I, Larkö O. No difference in skin cancer incidence with or without cyclosporin—a 5-year perspective. Transplant Proc 1992; 24:313.

Blitstein-Willinger E, Haas N, Nurnberger F, et al. Immunological findings during treatment of multiple keratoacanthoma with etretinate. Br J Dermatol 1986; 114:109–116.

Bönniger F, Burg G. Multiple keratokanthome. Hautarzt 1979; 30:92–94.

Borum K. The role of the mouse hair cycle in epidermal carcinogenesis. Acta Pathol Microbiol Scand 1954; 34:542–553.

Bonnetblanc JM, Gualde N, Bonnetblanc F. Hypocomplementemia in keratoacanthoma. Arch Dermatol Res 1981; 270: 189–191.

Bogdanowski T, Rubisz-Brzezińska J, Macura-Gina M, et al. Ocena chirurgicznego leczenia rogowiaka kolczystokomòrkowego. Przegl Dermatol 1990; 77:29–33.

Brothers WS, New WN, Nickel WR. Keratoacanthoma. A review of histopathological specimens previously diagnosed as keratoacanthomas or as squamous cell carcinoma of the skin. AMA Arch Dermatol 1960; 81:369–372.

Bryant J. Basal cell carcinoma associated with keratoacanthoma. J Dermatol Surg Oncol 1985; 11:1230–1231.

Burgdorf WHC, Pitha J, Fahmy A. Muir-Torre syndrome: histologic spectrum of sebaceous proliferations. Am J Dermatopathol 1986; 8:202–208.

Buescher L, DeSpain JD, Diaz-Arias AA, et al. Keratoacanthoma arising in an organoid nevus during childhood: case report and literature review. Pediatr Dermatol 1991; 8:117–119.

Calonje E, Wilson Jones E. Intravascular spread of keratoacanthoma. An alarming but benign phenomenon. Am J Dermatopathol 1992; 14:414–417.

Cabotin PP, Vignon-Pennamen MD, Miclea JM, et al. Kérato–acanthomes multiples éruptifs révélateurs d'un lymphome. Ann Dermatol Venereol (Paris) 1989; 116:860–862.

Chapman RS, Finn OA. Carcinoma of the larynx in two patients with keratoacanthoma. Br J Dermatol 1974; 90:685–688.

Chuang TY, Reizner GT, Elpern DJ, et al. Keratoacanthoma in Kauai, Hawaii. The first documented incidence in a defined population. Arch Dermatol 1993; 129:317–319.

Cipollaro VA. The use of podophyllin in the treatment of keratoacanthoma. Intern J Dermatol 1983; 22:436–440.

Claudy A, Thivolet J. Multiple keratoacanthomas: association with deficient cell mediated immunity. Br J Dermatol 1975; 93:593–595.

Clausen OPF, Beigi M, Bolund L, et al. Keratoacanthomas frequently show chromosomal aberrations as assessed by comparative genomic hybridization. J Invest Dermatol 2002; 119:1367–1372.

Cox S. Rapid development of keratoacanthomas after a body peel. Dermatol Surg 2003; 29:201–203.

Cockerell CJ. Cutaneous manifestations of HIV infection other than Kaposi's sarcoma: clinical and histologic aspects. J Am Acad Dermatol 1990; 22:1260–1269.

Cooper PH, Wolfe JT III. Perioral keratoacanthoma with extensive perineural invasion and intravascular growth. Arch Dermatol 1988; 124:1397–1401.

Corominas M, Sloan SR, Leon J, et al. Ras activation in human tumors and in animal model systems. Environ Health Perspect 1991; 93:19–25.

Corominas M, Leon J, Kamino H, et al. Oncogene involvement in tumor regression: H-ras activation in the rabbit model. Oncogene 1991; 6:645–651.

Cribier B, Asch P, Grosshans E. Differentiating squamous cell carcinoma from keratoacanthoma using histopathological criteria. Is it possible? A study of 296 cases. Dermatology (Basel) 1999; 199:208–212.

Currie AR, Ferguson Smith J. Multiple primary spontaneous-healing squamous-cell carcinomata of the skin. J Pathol Bacteriol 1952; 64:827–839.

Dąbska M, Madejczykowa A. Rogowiak kolczastokomórkowy – keratoacanthoma (molluscum sebaceum, molluscum psuedocarcinomatosum). Studium patologiczno-kliniczne. Nowotwory 1959; 9:1–23.

De Moragas JM, Montgomery H, McDonald JR. Keratoacanthoma versus squamous-cell carcinoma. AMA Arch Dermatol 1958; 77:390–395.

De Moragas JM. Multiple keratoacanthomas. Relation to Jamarsan therapy for pemphigus foliaceus. Arch Dermatol 1966; 93:679–683.

Donahue B, Cooper JS, Rush S. Treatment of aggressive keratoacanthoma by radiotherapy. J Am Acad Dermatol 1990; 23: 489–493.

Dogliotti M, Caro I. Keratoacanthoma in a Bantu child. Intern J Dermatol 1976; 15:524.

Drut R. Solitary keratoacanthoma of the nipple in a male. Case report. J Cutan Pathol 1976; 3:195–198.

Dupont A. Kyste sébacé atypique. Bull So Beige Dermatol Syphiligr 1930: :177–179.

Eliezri YD, Libow L. Multinodular keratoacanthoma. J Am Acad Dermatol 1988; 19:826–830.

Ereaux LP, Schopf-Locher P, Fournier CJ. Keratoacanthomata. AMA Arch Dermatol 1955; 71:73–83; with abstract of discussion by Winer LH, Becker FT, Weidman FD, et al.

Ereaux LP, Schopflocher P. Familial primary self-healing squamous epithelioma of skin: Ferguson-Smith type. Arch Dermatol 1965; 91:589–594; with abstract of discussion by Piper WN, Epstein NN, Belisario JC, et al.

Euvrard S, Chardonnet Y, Pouteil-Noble C, et al. Association of skin malignancies with various and multiple carcinogenic and noncarcinogenic human papillomaviruses in renal transplant patients. Cancer 1993; 72:2198–2206.

Fathizadeh A, Medenica MM, Soltani K, et al. Aggressive keratoacanthoma and internal malignant neoplasm. Arch Dermatol 1982; 118:112–114.

Fanti PA, Tosti A, Peluso AM, Bonelli U. Multiple keratoacanthoma in discoid lupus erythematosus. J Am Acad Dermatol 1989; 21:809–810.

Ferguson Smith J. Multiple primary, self-healing squamous cell carcinomas of the skin. Br J Dermatol Syphil 1948; 60: 315–318.

Ferguson-Smith MA, Wallace DC, James ZH, Renwick JH. Multiple self-healing squamous epithelioma. In: Bergsma D, ed. Birth Defects: Original Article Series. The Third Conference on the Clinical Delineation of Birth Defects. Part XII: Skin and nails. Baltimore: Williams and Wilkins, 7(8); 1971:157–163.

Ferguson Smith J. A case of multiple primary squamous-celled carcinomata of the skin in a young man, with spontaneous healing. Br J Dermatol Syph 1934; 46:267–272.

Fisher AA. Subungual keratoacanthoma: possible relationship to exposure to steel wool. Cutis 1990; 46:26–28.

Fisher ER, McCoy MM II, Wechsler HL. Analysis of histopathological and electron microscopic determinants of keratoacanthoma and squamous cell carcinoma. Cancer 1972; 29:1387–1397.

Fléchet ML, Barba L, Beltzer-Garelly E, et al. Kerato-acanthomes multiples sous-unguéaux. Ann Dermatol Venereol (Paris) 1989; 116:862–864.

Flannery GR, Muller HK. Immune response to human keratoacanthoma. Br J Dermatol 1979; 101:625–632.

Foschini MP, Magnani P, Marconi F, et al. Multiple keratoacanthomas: a case report with evidence of regression with thymic hormone. Br J Dermatol 1991; 124:479–482.

Forslund O, DeAngelis PM, Beigi M, Scholberg AR, Clausen OP. Identification of human papillomavirus in keratoacanthomas. J Cutan Pathol 2003; 30:423–429.

Friedman RP, Morales A, Burnham TK. Multiple cutaneous and conjunctival keratoacanthomata. Arch Dermatol 1965; 92: 162–165.

Furukawa M, Hamada T, Shibata H, et al. Keratoacanthoma ensuing from bone marrow transplantation for chronic myeloid leukemia. Osaka City Med J 1992; 38:83–88.

Gheeraert P, Goens J, Schwartz RA, et al. Florid cutaneous papillomatosis, malignant acanthosis nigricans, and pulmonary squamous cell carcinoma. Intern J Dermatol 1991; 30: 193–197.

Ghadially FN, Barton BW, Kerridge DF. The etiology of keratoacanthoma. Cancer 1963; 16:603–611.

Ghadially FN. A comparative morphological study of keratoacanthoma of man and similar experimentally produced lesions in rabbit. J Pathol Bacteriol 1958; 75:441–453.

Ghadially FN. The experimental production of kerato-acanthomas in the hamster and the mouse. J Pathol Bacteriol 1959; 77:277–282.

Ghadially FN. The role of the hair follicle in the origin and evolution of some cutaneous neoplasms of man and experimental animals. Cancer 1961; 14:801–816.

Ghadially FN. A Text and Atlas of Physiological and Pathological Alterations in the Fine Structure of Cellular and Extracellular Components. In: Ultrastructural pathology of the cell and matrix. 3rd. London: Butterworths, 1988:66–68, 1110.

Ghadially R, Ghadially FN. Keratoacanthoma. In: Fitzpatrick TB, Eisen AZ, Wolff K, et al., eds. Dermatology in General Medicine. 4th ed. New York: McGraw Hill, 1993:848–855.

Giltman LI. Tripolar mitosis in a keratoacanthoma. Acta Derm Venereol (Stockh) 1981; 61:362–363.

Giesecke LM, Reid CM, James CL, Huilgol SC. Giant keratoacanthoma arising in hypertrophic lichen planus. Australas J Dermatol 2003; 44:267–269.

Goldschmidt H, Sherwin WK. Radiation therapy of giant aggressive keratoacanthomas. Arch Dermatol 1993; 129:1162–1165.

Godbolt AM, Sullivan JJ, Weedon D. Keratoacanthoma with perineural invasion: a report of 40 cases. Australas J Dermatol 2001; 42:168–171.

Goldberg LH, Silapunt S, Beyau KK, Peterson SR, Friedman PM, Alam M. Keratoacanthoma as a postoperative complication of skin cancer excision. J Am Acad Dermatol 2004; 50:753–758.

Gougerot H. Verrucome avec adénite, à structure épithéliomatifome, curable par le 914. Arch Dermato-Syphililigr Clin Saint-Louis 1929; 1:374–385.

Graham JH. Selected precancerous skin and mucocutaneous lesions. In: Neoplasms of the Skin and Malignant Melanoma. Chicago: Year Book Medical Publishers, 1976:69–121.

Graham RM, MacFarlane AW, Curley RK, et al. Beta 2 microglobulin expression in keratoacanthoma and squamous cell carcinoma. Br J Dermatol 1987; 117:441–449.

Green WS, Underwood LJ, Green R. Multiple keratoacanthomas on upper extremities. Arch Dermatol 1977; 113:512–513.

Griffiths RW. Keratoacanthoma observed. Br J Plastic Surg 2004; 57:485–501.

Grinspan D, Abulafia J. Idiopathic cutaneous pseudoepitheliomatous hyperplasia. Verrugoma (Gougerot), molluscum sebaceum (MacCormac and Scarff), self-healing, primary, squamous-cell carcinoma (Ferguson Smith), and keratoacathoma (Rook and Whimster). Cancer 1955; 8:1047–1056.

Grinspan Bozza NO, Totaro II, Pocovi M, et al. Queratoacanthoma centrifugo de Miedzinski y Kozakiewicz. Med Cutan Ibero-Latin-America 1989; 17:234–238.

Grzybowski M. A case of peculiar generalized epithelial tumours of the skin. Br J Dermatol Syphil 1950; 62:310–313.

Guillot B, Fesneau H, Mourad G, et al. Kératoacanthomes multiples sous ciclosporine. Presse Med 1990; 19:1286.

Habel G, O'Regan B, Eissing A, et al. Intra-oral keratoacanthoma: an eruptive variant and review of the literature. Br Dental J 1991; 170:336–339.

Hashimoto Y, Matsuo S, Iizuka H. A flow cytometric study of the DNA content from paraffin-embedded samples of keratoacanthoma and squamous cell carcinoma. Nippon Hifuka Gakkai Zasshi 1991; 101:701–705.

Hackel H, Burg G, Lechner W, et al. Keratoacanthoma centrifugum marginatum. Hautarzt 1989; 40:763–766.

Haider S. Keratoacanthoma in a smallpox vaccination site. Br J Dermatol 1974; 90:689–690.

Hamada T, Fujimoto W, Okazaki F, et al. Lichen planus pemphigoides and multiple keratoacanthomas associated with colon adenocarcinoma. Br J Dermatol 2004; 151:252–254.

Habif TP. Extirpation of keratoacanthomas by blunt dissection. J Dermatol Surg Oncol 1980; 6:652–654.

Hellier FF, Rowell NR. Giant keratoacanthoma complicating dermatitis. Arch Dermatol 1962; 85:485–487.

Hendricks WM. Sudden appearance of multiple keratoacanthomas three weeks after thermal burns. Cutis 1991; 47: 410–412.

Henseler T, Christophers E, Honigsmann H, et al. Skin tumors in the European PUVA study. Eight-year follow-up of 1,643 patients treated with PUVA for psoriasis. J Am Acad Dermatol 1987; 16:108–116.

Herold WC, Nelson LM. Pseudoepitheliomatous reaction (pseudorecidive) following radiation therapy of epitheliomata. In: Hellerström S, Wikström K, Hellerstrom A-M, eds. The Eleventh International Congress of

Dermatology Stockholm 1957 Proceedings. :2Lund: Hakan Ohlssons Boktryckeri, 1959:426–432.

Herzberg AJ, Kerns BJ, Pollack SV, et al. DNA image cytometry of keratoacanthoma and squamous cell carcinoma. J Invest Dermatol 1991; 97:495–500.

Heslop JH. The histogenesis of experimental molluscum sebaceum. Br J Cancer 1958; 12:553–560.

Higuchi M, Tanikawa E, Nomura H, et al. Multiple keratoacanthomas with peculiar manifestations and course. J Am Acad Dermatol 1990; 23:389–392.

Hodak E, Jones RE, Ackerman AB, et al. Controversies in Dermatopathology. Solitary keratoacanthoma is a squamous-cell carcinoma: three examples with metastases; with responses by Grant-Kels JM, From L, Reed RJ, et al. Am J Dermatopathol 1993; 15:332–352.

Ho T, Horn T, Finzi E. Transforming growth factor a expression helps to distinguish keratoacanthomas from squamous cell carcinomas. Arch Dermatol 1991; 127:1167–1171.

Hoxtell EO, Mandel JS, Murray SS, et al. Incidence of skin carcinoma after renal transplantation. Arch Dermatol 1977; 113:436–438.

Hutchinson J. Morbid growths and tumours. 1. The "crateriform ulcer of the face," a form of acute epithelial cancer. Trans Pathol Soc London 1889; 40:275–281.

Hutchinson J. Demonstrations at the clinical museum. The crateriform ulcer — microscopic examination. Arch Surg 1896; 7:88–89.

Hutchinson J. A peculiar form of cancer of the skin. Illustrations of clinical surgery consisting of plates, photographs, woodcuts, diagrams, etc illustrating surgical diseases, symptoms and accidents also operative and other methods of treatment with descriptive letterpress. Philadelphia: P Blakiston & Son, 1888; 2:plate 92.

Inoshita T, Youngberg GA. Keratoacanthoma associated with cervical squamous cell carcinoma. Arch Dermatol 1984; 120:123–124.

Jablonska S, Schwartz RA. Giant condylomaacuminatum of Buschke and Lowenstein. In: Demis DJ, ed. Clinical Dermatology. 18th ed. Philadelphia: JB Lippincott, 1991:Unit 14–15:1–5.

Jackson IT, Alexander JO, Verheyden CN. Self-healing squamous cell epithelioma: a family affair. Br J Plast Surg 1983; 36:22–28.

Jackson IT. Diagnostic problem of keratoacanthoma. Lancet 1969; 1:490–492.

Jackson R, Williamson GS. Keratoacanthoma: incidence and problems in diagnosis and treatment. Can Med Assoc J 1961; 84:312–315.

Janecka IP, Wolff M, Crikelair GF, et al. Aggressive histologic features of keratoacanthoma. J Cutan Pathol 1978; 4:342–348.

Janniger CK, Kapila R, Schwartz RA, et al. Histoid lepromas of lepromatous leprosy. Inter J Dermatol 1990; 29:494–496.

Jaber PW, Cooper PH, Greer KE. Generalized eruptive keratoacanthoma of Grzybowski. J Am Acad Dermatol 1993; 29: 299–304.

Jolly HW Jr., Carpenter CL Jr. Multiple keratoacanthomas. A report of two cases. Arch Dermatol 1966; 93:348–353.

Jordan RCK, Kahn HJ, From L, et al. Immunohistochemical demonstration of actinically damaged elastic fibers in keratoacanthomas: an aid in diagnosis. J Cutan Pathol 1991; 18:81–86.

Job CK. Keratoacanthoma associated with leprosy. Indian J Pathol Bacteriol 1963; 6:160–162.

Jung-Grimm H. Pseudo-Rezidive nach Röntgenbestrahlung der Haut. Dermatol Wochenschr 1957; 135:210–215.

Karalas M, Homan S, Baba M, et al. Reactive multiple keratoacanthoma in a patient with chronic renal insufficiency. Br J Dermatol 2001; 145:846–847 (Karalos has Latin small letter "s" with ogoaek).

Kanitakis J, Hoyo E, Hermier C, et al. Nucleolar organizer region enumeration in keratoacanthomas and squamous cell carcinomas of the skin. Cancer 1992; 69:2937–2941.

Kannon G, Park HK. Utility of peanut agglutinin (PNA) in the diagnosis of squamous cell carcinoma and keratoacanthoma. Am J Dermatopathol 1990; 12:31–36.

Kerschmann RL, McCalmont TH, LeBoit PE. p53 oncoprotein expression and proliferation index in keratoacanthoma and squamous cell carcinoma. Arch Dermatol 1994; 130:181–186.

Kestel JL Jr., Blair DS. Keratoacanthoma treated with methotrexate. Arch Dermatol 1973; 108:723–724.

King DF, Barr RJ. Intraepithelial elastic fibers and intracytoplasmic glycogen: diagnostic aids in differentiating keratoacanthoma from squamous cell carcinoma. J Cutan Pathol 1980; 7:140–148.

Kingman J, Callen JP. Keratoacanthoma: a clinical study. Arch Dermatol 1984; 120:736–740.

Klein-Szanto AJP, Barr RJ, Reiners JJ, et al. Filaggrin distribution in keratoacanthomas and squamous cell carcinoma. Arch Pathol Lab Med 1984; 108:888–890.

Klein E, Helm F, Milgrom H, et al. Tumors of the skin-II: keratoacanthoraa: local effect of 5-fluorouracil. Skin 1962; 1:153–156.

Kopf AW, Bart RS. Development of more keratoacanthomas following skin testing with nitrogen mustard in a patient with the multiple keratoacanthoma syndrome. J Dermatol Surg Oncol 1979; 5:450–451.

Kopf AW, Bart RS. Giant keratoacanthoma. J Dermatol Surg Oncol 1978; 4:444–445.

Korenberg R, Penneys NS, Kowalczyk A, et al. Quantitation of S100 protein-positive cells in inflamed and. noninflammed keratoacanthoma and squamous cell carcinoma. J Cutan Pathol 1988; 15:104–108.

Koziorowska J, Dux K. Poszukiwanie etiologicznego czynnika w keratoacanthoma. Nowotwory 1959; 9:269–273.

Kuflik EG, Kuflik AS. Cryosurgery. In: Demis DJ, ed. Clinical Dermatology. 20th ed. Philadelphia: JB Lippincott, 1993:Unit 37–5:1–5.

Kvedar JC, Fewkes J, Baden HP. Immunologic detection of markers of keratinocyte differentiation. Its use in neoplastic and preneoplastic lesions of skin. Arch Pathol Lab Med 1986; 110:183–188.

Kwittken J. A histologic chronology of the clinical course of the keratocarcinoma (so-called keratoacanthoma). Mt. Sinai J Med 1975; 42:127–135.

Kwittken J. Dermatologic pseudobenignities. Mt Sinai J Med 1980; 47:34–37.

Lawrence N, Reed RJ. Actinic keratoacanthoma. Speculations on the nature of the lesion and the role of cellular immunity in its evolution. Am J Dermatopathol 1990; 12: 517–533.

Laaff H, Mittelviefhaus H, Wokalek H, et al. Eruptive Keratoakanthome Typ Grzybowski und Ektropium. Ein therapeuticsches Problem. Hautarzt 1992; 43:143–147.

Larson PO. Keratoacanthoma treated with Mohs' micrographic surgery (chemosurgery). A review of forty-three cases. J Am Acad Dermatol 1987; 16:1040–1044.

Levy EJ, Cahn MM, Shaffer B, et al. Keratoacanthoma. J Am Med Assoc 1954; 155:562–564.

LeBoit PE. Can we understand keratoacanthoma? Am J Dermatopathol 2002; 24:166–168.

Lejman K, Starzycki Z. Giant keratoacanthoma of the inner surface of the prepuce. Br J Venereol Dis 1977; 53:65–67.

Lever WF, Schaumburg-Lever G. Histopathology of the Skin. 7th. Philadelphia: JB Lippincott, 1990:560–563.

Lyell A, John Ferguson Smith (1888–1978). Am J Dermatopathol 1986; 8:525–528.

Markey AC, MacDonald DM. Identification of CD16/NKH-1 natural killer cells and their relevance to cutaneous tumour immunity. Br J Dermatol 1989; 121:563–570.

Maxwell TB, Lamb JH. Unusual reaction to application of podophyllum resin. AMA Arch Derm Syphilol 1953; 70: 510–511.

MacCormac H, Scarff RW. Molluscum sebaceum. Br J Dermatol Syph 1936; 48:624–627.

Marshall J, Pepler WJ. Mollusca pseudocarcinomatosa. Discussion of a case of the Ferguson Smith type of unilateral distribution. Br J Cancer 1954; 8:251–254.

Maddin WS, Wood WS. Multiple keratoacanthomas and squamous cell carcinomas occurring at psoriatic treatment sites. J Cutan Pathol 1979; 6:96–100.

Markey AC, Churchill LJ, MacDonald DM. Altered expression of major histocompatibility complex (MHC) antigens by epidermal tumours. J Cutan Pathol 1990; 17:65–71.

McGregor JM, Yu CC, Dublin EA, et al. Aberrant expression of p53 tumour-suppressor protein in non-melanoma skin cancer. Br J Dermatol 1992; 127:463–469.

McKee PH, Wilkinson JD, Black MM, et al. Carcinoma (epithelioma) cuniculatum: a clinico-pathological study of nineteen cases and review of the literature. Histopathol 1981; 5: 423–436.

McGlashan JA, Rees G, Bowdler DA. Solitary keratoacanthoma of the nasal vestibule. J Laryngol Otol 1991; 105:306–308.

Mehregan AH, Fabian L. Keratoacanthoma of nailbed: a report of two cases. Int J Dermatol 1973; 12:149–151.

Melendez ND, Smoller BR, Morgan M. VCAM (CD-106) and ICAM (CD-54) adhesion molecules distinguish keratoacanthomas from cutaneous squamous cell carcinomas. Mod Pathol 2003; 16:8–13.

Mehta VR. Keratoacanthoma with osteolysis (a case report with an isolated interdigital lesion). Indian J Dermatol Venereol Leprol 1980; 46:360–363.

Melton JL, Nelson BR, Stough DB, et al. Treatment of keratoacanthomas with intralesional methotrexate. J Am Acad Dermatol 1991; 25:1017–1023.

Miedziński F, Dratwiński Z, Brzozowski J, et al. Ein Beitrag zur nosologischen Stellung des Keratoakanthoma centrifugum. Hautarzt 1973; 24:120–123.

Miracco C, De Santi MM, Lio R, et al. Quantitatively evaluated ultrastructural findings can add to the differential diagnosis between keratoacanthoma and well differentiated squamous cell carcinoma. J Submicrosc Cytol Pathol 1992; 24:315–321.

Milewski B, Chorzelski T. Vergleichende histologische und histochemische Untersuchungen von Keratoakanthomen und höber differenzierten spinocellulären Epimeliomen. Hautarzt 1962; 13:7–12.

Miedziński F. Keratoacanthoma as a pathogenetic and clinicohistological problem, its 40th anniversary. Postepy Dermatol 1990; 7:61–70.

Miedziński F, Kozakiewicz J. Das Keratoakanthoma centrifugum—eine besondere Varietät des Keratoakanthoms. Hautarzt 1962; 13:348–352.

Michalowski R. Program tajnego nauczania dermatologii w klinice dermatologicznej w Warszawie podczas niemieckiej okupacji. Arch Hist Filoz Med 1988; 51:439–447.

Mittal RR, Popli R, Parsad D. Multiple keratoacanthoma in a female infant. Indian J Dermatol Venereol Leprol 1992; 58:227–228.

Molochkov VA, Ilyin II, Dolgushin II, et al. Histocompatibility antigens and solitary keratoacanthoma. Vopr Onkol 1989; 35: 286–288.

Morita H, Sagami S. Analysis of lymphocyte subpopulations using monoclonal antibodies in a case of keratoacanthomas. Acta Dermatol (Kyoto) 1985; 80:209–211.

Muir EG, Bell AJY, Barlow KA. Multiple primary carcinomata of the colon, duodenum, and larynx associated with kerato-acanthomata of the face. Br J Surg 1967; 54:191–195.

Musso L, Gordon H. Spontaneous resolution of a molluscum sebaceum. Proc Roy Soc Med 1950; 43:838–839; with abstract of discussion by Rook A, Whimster IW, Gordon H, et al.

Muller HK, Flannery GR. Epidermal antigens in experimental keratoacanthoma and squamous cell carcinoma. Cancer Res 1973; 33:2181–2186.

Mukunyadzi P, Sanderson RD, Fan CY, Smoller BR. The level of syndecan-1 expression is a distinguishing feature in behavior between keratoacanthoma and invasive cutaneous squamous cell carcinoma. Modern Pathol 2002; 15:45–49.

Nedwich JA. Evaluation of curettage and electrodesiccation in treatment of keratoacanthoma. Australas J Dermatol 1991; 32:137–141.

Nelson LM. Self-healing pseudocancers of the skin. Calif Med 1959; 90:49–54.

Neumann RA, Knobler RM. Argon laser treatment of small keratoacanthomas in difficult locations. Int J Dermatol 1990; 29:733–736.

Odom RB, Goette DK. Treatment of keratoacanthomas with intralesional fluorouracil. Arch Dermatol 1978; 114:1779–1783.

Odom RB. Keratoacanthoma. J Assoc Milit Dermatol 1980; 6(1):2–5.

Oettlè AG. Skin cancer in Africa. J Natl Cancer Inst Monogr 1963; 10:197–214.

Ogasawara Y, Kinoshita E, Ishida T, et al. A case of keratoacanthoma centrifugum marginatuim: response to oral etretinate. J Am Acad Dermatol 2003; 48:282–285.

Pattee SF, Silvis NG. Keratoacanthomas developing in sites of previous trauma: a report of two cases and review of the literature. J Am Acad Dermatol 2003; 48:S35–S38.

Patel MR, Desai SS. Subungual keratoacanthoma in the hand. J Hand Surg 1989; 14A:139–142.

Pavithran K. Multiple keratoacanthomas on the mons pubis and labia majora. Indian J Dermatol Venereol Leprol 1988; 54:262–263.

Pagani WA, Lorenzi G, Lorusso D. Surgical treatment for aggressive giant keratoacanthoma of the face. J Dermatol Surg Oncol 1986; 12:282–284.

Parker CM, Hanke CW. Large keratoacanthomas in difficult locations treated with intralesional 5-fluorouracil. J Am Acad Dermatol 1986; 14:770–777.

Pellicano R, Fabrizi G, Cerimele D. Multiple keratoacanthomas and junctional epidermolysis bullosa. A therapeutic conundrum. Arch Dermatol 1990; 126:305–306.

Peteiro MC, Caeiro JL, Toribio J. Keratoacanthoma centrifugum marginatum versus low-grade squamous cell carcinoma. Dermatologica (Basel) 1985; 170:221–224.

Philips P, Helm KF. Proliferating cell nuclear antigen distribution in keratoacanthoma and squamous cell carcinoma. J Cutan Pathol 1993; 20:424–428.

Pillsbury DM, Beerman H. Multiple keratoacanthoma. Am J Med Sci 1958; 236:614–623.

Piérard-Franchimont C, Piérard GE. Rates of epidermal carcinomas in the Mosan region of Belgium. Dermatologica (Basel) 1988; 177:76–81.

Popkin GL, Brodie SJ, Hyman AB, et al. A technique of biopsy recommended for keratoacanthomas. Arch Dermatol 1966; 94:191–193.

Ponti G, Losi L, Di Gregorio C, et al. Identification of Muir-Torre syndrome among patients with sebaceous tumors and keratoacanthomas: role of clinical features, microsatellite instability, and immunohistochemistry. Cancer 2005; 103:1018–1025.

Poleksic S. Keratoacanthoma and multiple carcinomas. Br J Dermatol 1974; 91:461–463.

Poth DO. Tumor-like keratoses: report of a case. AMA Arch Dermatol Syphilol 1939; 39:228–238.

Poleksic S, Yeung KY. Rapid development of keratoacanthoma and accelerated transformation into squamous cell carcinoma of the skin. A mutagenic effect of polychemotherapy in a patient with Hodgkin's disease. Cancer 1970; 41:12–16.

Prutkin L. An ultrastructure study of the experimental keratoacanthoma. J Invest Dermatol 1967; 48:326–336.

Puente Duany N. Squamous cell pseudoepithelioma (keratoacanthoma). A new clinical variety, gigantic, multiple, and localized. Arch Dermatol 1958; 78:703–709.

Randall MB, Geisinger KR, Kute TE, et al. DNA content and proliferative index in cutaneous squamous cell carcinoma and keratoacanthoma. Am J Clin Pathol 1990; 93:259–262.

Ramselaar CG, van der Meer JB. Non-immunological regression of dimethylbenz(A) anthracene-induced experimental keratoacanthomas in the rabbit. Dermatologica (Basel) 1979; 158:142–151.

Ramselaar CG. Spontaneous regression of keratoacanthoma. In: Proefschrift terverkrijging van de graad van Doctor in de Geneeskunde aan de Rijksuniversiteit te Utrecht, op gezag van de Rector Magnificus Prof. Dr. A. Verhoeff, volgens besluit van het College van Decanen in het openbaar te verdedigen op dinsdag 17 juni 1980 des namiddags te 2.45 uur. Doctoral Thesis. Amsterdam: Rodopi, 1980.

Ramselaar CG, van der Meer JB. The spontaneous regression of keratoacanthoma in man. Acta Derm Venereol (Stockh) 1976; 56:245–251.

Reiffers J, Laugier P, Hunziker N. Hyperplasies sébacées, kerato-acanthomes, épithéliomas du visage et cancer du côlon. Une nouvelle entité? Dermatologica (Basel) 1976; 153:23–33.

Reid BJ, Cheesbrough MJ. Multiple keratoacanthomata. A unique case and review of the current classification. Acta Derm Venereol (Stockh) 1978; 58:169–173.

Reid E, Grosshans E, Lazrak B, et al. Keratoacanthoma centrifugum marginatum. Ann Dermatol Venereol (Paris) 1979; 106:367–370.

Reymann F. Treatment of keratoacanthomas with curettage. Dermatologica (Basel) 1977; 155:90–96.

Requena L, Romero E, Sanchez M, et al. Aggressive keratoacanthoma of the eyelid: "malignant" keratoacanthoma or squamous cell carcinoma. J Dermatol Surg Oncol 1990; 16:564–568.

Rigdon RH. Histopathogenesis of "keratoacanthoma" induced with methylcholanthrene. AMA Arch Dermatol 1960; 81:381–387.

Rook A, Whimster I. Le kérato-acanthome. Arch Belg Dermatol Syphiligr 1950; 6:137–146.

Ro YS, Cooper PN, Lee JA, et al. p53 protein expression in benign and malignant skin tumours. Br J Dermatol 1993; 128:237–241.

Rook A, Champion RH. Keratoacanthoma. Nat Cancer Inst Monogr 1963; 10:257–273.

Rook A, Moffatt JL. Multiple self-healing epithelioma of Ferguson Smith type. Report of a case of unilateral distribution. Arch Dermatol 1956; 74:525–532.

Rossman RE, Freeman RG, Knox JM. Multiple keratoacanthomas. Arch Dermatol 1964; 89:374–381.

Rosen T. Keratoacanthoma arising within a linear epidermal nevus. J Dermatol Surg Oncol 1982; 8:878–880.

Rook A, Whimster I. Keratoacanthoma—a thirty year retrospect. Br J Dermatol 1979; 100:41–47.

Roth AM. Solitary keratoacanthoma of the conjunctiva. Am J Ophthalmol 1978; 85:647–650.

Sanders S, Busam KJ, Halpern AC, Nehal KS. Intralesional corticosteroid treatment of multiple eruptive keratoacanthomas:

case report and review of a controversial therapy. Dermatol Surg 2002; 28:954–958.

Santa Cruz DJ, Clausen K. Atypical sweat duct hyperplasia accompanying keratoacanthoma. Dermatologica (Basel) 1977; 154:156–160.

Sanchez Yus E, Requena L. Keratoacanthoma within a superficial spreading malignant melanoma in situ. J Cutan Pathol 1991; 18:228–292.

Santa Lucia P, Wilson BD, Allen HJ. Localization of endogenous beta-galactoside-binding lectin as a means to distinguish malignant from benign skin tissue. J Dermatol Surg Oncol 1991; 17:653–655.

Samochocki Z. Rogowiak kolczystokomórkowy (keratoacanthoma). Przegl Dermatol 1984; 71:177–180.

Schwartz RA. Skin Cancer Recognition and Management. New York: Springer Verlag, 1988:48–56.

Schwartz RA. Keratoacanthoma: a clinico-pathologic enigma. Dermatol Surg 2004; 30:245–252.

Schwartz RA, Tarlow MM, Lambert WC. Keratoacanthoma-like squamous cell carcinoma within a fibroepitheliomatous polyp. Dermatol Surg 2004; 30:332–333.

Schwartz RA, Flieger FN, Saied NK. The Torre syndrome with gastrointestinal polyposis. Arch Dermatol 1980; 116: 312–314.

Schwartz RA, Goldberg DJ, Mahmood F, et al. The Muir-Torre syndrome: a disease of sebaceous and colonic neoplasms. Dermatologica (Basel) 1989; 178:23–28.

Schwartz RA, Stoll HL Jr. Squamous cell carcinoma. In: Fitzpatrick TB, Eisen AZ, Wolff K, et al., eds. Dermatology in General Medicine. 4th ed. New York: McGraw-Hill, 1993:821–839.

Schwartz RA. Keratoacanthoma: an abortive squamous cell carcinoma that does not always have to fail. Giornale Italiano Dermatol Venereol 2003; 138:355–362.

Schwartz RA. The keratoacanthoma: a review. J Surg Oncol 1979; 12:305–317.

Schwartz RA. Keratoacanthoma. J Am Acad Dermatol 1994; 30:1–19.

Schwartz RA. Verrucous carcinoma. In: Demis DJ, ed. Clinical Dermatology. 18th ed. Philadelphia: JB Lippincott, 1991:Unit 21–22:1–8.

Schwartz RA, Klein E. Ultraviolet light-induced carcinogenesis. In: Holland JF, Frei E III, eds. Cancer Medicine. 2nd ed. Philadelphia: Lea & Febiger, 1982:109–119.

Schwartz RA. Multiple persistent keratoacanthomas. Oncology (Basel) 1979; 36:281–285.

Schaumburg-Lever G, Alroy J, Gavris V, et al. Cell-surface carbohydrates in proliferative epidermal lesions: distribution of A, B, and H blood group antigens in benign and malignant lesions. Am J Dermatopathol 1984; 6:583–589.

Schwartz RA, Burgess GH. Florid cutaneous papillomatosis. Arch Dermatol 1978; 114:1803–1806.

Schwartz RA, Blaszczyk M, Jablonska S. Generalized eruptive keratoacanthoma of Grzybowski: follow-up of the original description, and 50-year retrospect. Dermatology (Basel) 2002; 205:348–352.

Seidman JD, Berman JJ, Moore GW, et al. Multiparameter DNA flow cytometry of keratoacanthoma. Anal Quant Cytol Histol 1992; 14:113–119.

Shaw Dunn J, Ferguson Smith J. Self-healing primary squamous cell carcinoma of the skin. Br J Dermatol Syphil 1934; 46:519–523.

Shatkin BT, Hunter JG, Song IC. Familial subungual keratoacanthoma in association with ectodermal dysplasia. Plast Reconstr Surg 1993; 92:528–531.

Shimm DS, Duttenhaver JR, Doucette J, Wang CC. Radiation therapy of keratoacanthoma. Int J Radiat Oncol Biol Phys 1983; 9:759–761.

Shaw JC, Storrs FJ, Everts E. Multiple keratoacanthomas after megavoltage radiation therapy. J Am Acad Dermatol 1990; 23:1009–1011.

Shellito JE, Samet JM. Keratoacanthoma as a complication of arterial puncture for blood gases. Int J Dermatol 1982; 21:349.

Sina B, Adrian RM. Multiple keratoacanthomas possibly induced by psoralens and ultraviolet A photochemotherapy. J Am Acad Dermatol 1983; 9:686–688.

Silberberg I, Kopf AW, Baer RL. Recurrent keratoacanthoma of the lip. Arch Dermatol 1962; 86:92–101.

Smoller BR, Kwan TH, Said JW, et al. Keratoacanthoma and squamous cell carcinoma of the skin: immunohistochemical localization of involucrin and keratin proteins. J Am Acad Dermatol 1986; 14:226–234.

Snider BL, Benjamin DR. Eruptive keratoacanthoma with an internal malignant neoplasm. Arch Dermatol 1981; 117:788–790.

Sommerville J, Milne JA. Familial primary self-healing squamous epithelioma of the skin (Ferguson Smith type). Br J Dermatol Syphil 1950; 62:485–490.

Somlai B, Holló P. Die Anwendung von Interferon alpha (IFN α) in der Keratoakanthombehandlung. Hautarzt 2000; 51:173–175.

Spitler LE, Levin AS, Fudenberg HH. Transfer factor II: results of therapy. In: Bergsma D, Good RA, Finstad J, eds. Birth Defects: Original Article Series. Part I. Immunodeficiency in Man and Animals. Sunderland, Massachusetts: Sinauder Assoc, 1975; 11(1):449–456.

Sródka A. Akademickie nauczanie dermatologii i wencrologii w Warszawie w latach 1869–1939. Przegl Dermatol 1989; 76:188–193.

Sterry W, Steigleder GK, Pullmann H, et al. Eruptive keratoakanthome. Hautarzt 1981; 32:119–125.

Stewart WM, Lauret P, Hemet J, et al. Kerato-acanthomes multiples et carcinomes visceraux: syndrome de Torre. Ann Dermatol Venereol (Paris) 1977; 104:622–626.

Street ML, White JW Jr, Gibson LE. Multiple keratoacanthomas treated with oral retinoids. J Am Acad Dermatol 1990; 23:862–866.

Strumia R, Venturini D, Califano AL. Seasonality of presentation of keratoacanthoma. Int J Dermatol 1993; 32:691.

Stone OJ. Non-immunologic enhancement and regression of self-healing squamous cell carcinoma (keratoacanthoma)—ground substance and inflammation. Med Hypotheses 1988; 26:113–117.

Starzycki Z. Zastosowanie maści Efudix w leczeniu rogowiaka kolczystokomórkowego (keratoacanthoma). I. Kliniczna ocena wyników leczenia. Przegl Dermatol 1980; 67:470–474.

Starzycki Z. Zastosowanie maści Efudix w leczeniu rogowiaka kolczystokomórkowego (keratoacanthoma). II. Obserwacje histologiczne w przebiegu leczenia. Przegl Dermatol 1980; 67:475–479.

Stephenson TJ, Royds JA, Bleehen SS, Silcocks PB, Rees RC. 'Anti-metastatic' nm23 gene product expression in keratoacanthoma and squamous cell carcinoma. Dermatology (Basel) 1993; 187:95–99.

Stephenson TJ, Royds J, Silcocks PB, Bleehan SS. Mutant p53 oncogene expression in keratoacanthoma and squamous cell carcinoma. Br J Dermatol 1992; 127:566–570.

Stevanović DV. Pseudocarcinomatous hyperplasia. In: Pillsbury DM, Livingood CS, eds. Proceedings of the XII International Congress of Dermatology September 1962/ Washington D.C. Vol. 2. Amsterdam: Excerpta Medica Foundation, 1963:1577–1578.

Stevanović DV. Keratoacanthoma dyskeratoticum and segregans. Arch Dermatol 1965; 92:666–669.

Stevanović DV. Keratoacanthoma. Mucous membranes as the site of its localization. Dermatologica (Basel) 1960; 121:278–284.

Svirsky JA, Freedman PD, Lumerman H. Solitary intraoral keratoacanthoma. Oral Surg Oral Med Oral Pathol 1977; 43:116–122.

Takeda H, Kondo S. Differences between squamous cell carcinoma and keratoacanthoma in angiotensin type-1 receptor expression. Am J Pathol 2001; 158:1633–1637.

Tanigaki T, Endo H. A case of squamous cell carcinoma treated with intralesional injection of oil bleomycin. Dermatologica (Basel) 1985; 170:302–305.

Tham SN, Lee CT. Condyloma latum mimicking keratoacanthoma in patient with secondary syphilis. Genitourin Med 1987; 63:339–340.

Torre D, Lubritz RR, Kuflik EG. Practical Cutaneous Cryosurgery. Norwalk: Appleton & Lange, 1988:76.

Torre D. Multiple sebaceous tumors. Arch Dermatol 1968; 98: 549–551.

Trowell HE, Dyall-Smith ML, Dyall-Smith DJ. Human papillomavirus associated with keratoacanthomas in Australian patients. Arch Dermatol 1990; 126:1654.

Van De Staak WJ, Bergers AM. Intranuclear particles in keratoacanthoma: possible association with malignant degeneration. Dermatologica (Basel) 1979; 158:413–416.

Venkei T, Sugár J. Precancerous and cancerous varieties of keratoacanthoma. Acta Unio Int Contra Cancrum (Louvain) 1960; 16:1454–1457.

Vickers CF, Ghadially FN. Keratoacanthomata associated with psoriasis. Br J Dermatol 1961; 73:120–124.

Washington CV Jr., Mikhail GR. Eruptive keratoacanthoma en plaque in an immunosuppressed patient. J Dermatol Surg Oncol 1987; 13:1357–1360.

Weber G, Stetter H, Pliess G, Stickl H. Assoziiertes Vorkommen von eruptiven Keratoacanthomen, Tubencarcinom und Paramyeloblastenleukämic. Arch Klin Exp Dermatol 1970; 238:107–119.

Webb AJ, Ghadially FN. Massive or giant keratoacanthoma. J Pathol Bacteriol 1966; 91:505–509.

Whiting DA. Skin tumours in white South Africans. S Afr Med J 1978; 53:98–102; 131–133; 134–136; 162–176; 166–170.

Witten VH, Zak FG. Multiple, primary, self-healing prickle-cell epithelioma of the skin. Cancer 1952; 5:539–550.

Wilkinson SM, Tan CY, Smith AG. Keratoacanthoma arising within organoid naevi. Clin Exp Dermatol 1991; 16:58–60.

Wick MR, Manivel JC, Millns JL. Histopathologic considerations in the management of skin cancer. In: Schwartz RA, ed. Skin Cancer Recognition and Management. New York: Springer Verlag, 1988:246–275.

Yamagiwa K, Ichikawa K. Experimental study of the pathogenesis of carcinoma. J Cancer Res 1918; 3:1–29.

Yus ES, Simon P, Requena L, Ambrojo P, de Eusebio E. Solitary keratoacanthoma: a self-healing proliferation that frequently becomes malignant. Am J Dermatopathol 2000; 22:305–310.

Zalewska-Kubicka L, Mikulska D, Nowak A. The ultrastructure of squamous cell carcinoma and keratoacanthoma with morphological characterization of the mast cells. Dermatol Klin Zab (Wroclaw) 2001; 3(suppl 1):182.

40

Mohs Micrographic Surgery

Trephina Galloway and Sharon Thornton
Division of Dermatologic Surgery, Department of Dermatology, Cleveland Clinic Foundation,
Cleveland, Ohio, U.S.A.

John Louis Ratz
Center for Dermatology and Skin Cancer, Tampa, Florida, U.S.A.

Ronald G. Wheeland
University of Arizona College of Medicine, Tucson, Arizona, U.S.A.

Philip Bailin
Division of Dermatologic Surgery, Department of Dermatology, Cleveland Clinic Foundation,
Cleveland, Ohio, U.S.A.

HISTORY OF MOHS MICROGRAPHIC SURGERY

The concept of Mohs Micrographic surgery as we know it today had its beginnings in the early 1930s when Fredrick Mohs was a medical student/research assistant in the Department of Zoology at the University of Wisconsin. Mohs surgery arose from an initial chance discovery during experiments to account for the inhibition of implanted cancer in rats. During these experiments, Dr. Mohs found that injected irritants caused a dense leukocytic reaction in tissues surrounding the cancer, more than in the cancer itself. During these experiments, many irritants were injected. It was found that a 20% solution of zinc chloride, which caused tissue necrosis, also preserved the histologic architecture of the tissue when excised several days later. These discoveries lead Dr. Mohs to believe that the in situ tissue fixation technique might be useful in the excision and microscopic examination of cancers. Zinc chloride provided good in situ fixation preserving the microscopic features of the tissue without damaging subjacent normal tissue. It was safe to handle, had no systemic toxicity, and did not increase the tendency of cancers to metastasize.

In 1936, Dr. Mohs developed a paste vehicle for the zinc chloride that allowed accurate control of the depth of penetration. Dr. Mohs experimented with several formulations until he came up with a mixture of a matrix of fine granules of an inert substance with a high-specific gravity (stibnite) held together with a binder (Sanguinaria canadensis) to produce the correct consistency. The final paste formula contained 40 g stibnite, 10 g Sanguinaria canadensis, and 34.5 mL zinc chloride, to give a final concentration of 45% zinc chloride. The term "chemosurgery" was coined.

Development of the fresh tissue technique began in 1951 when R. Ray Allington, MD was training with Dr. Mohs. Dr. Allington demonstrated the technique of removing the bulk of the neoplasm with a scalpel or curet, achieving hemostasis, and then proceeding with the usual fixation–excision sequence. Dr. Mohs was excited about the reduction of time and discomfort using this technique, and in 1953 began making a movie for educational purposes using the technique. This film was of the removal of a pigmented basal cell carcinoma on the lower eyelid. The first level was removed with the fixed tissue technique. The margins were involved so as to expedite the filming; the next two layers were removed as fresh tissue. Maps were used to show the origin of the specimen, the edges were color coded, and the fresh tissue was fixed and histologically examined, the same as the fixed tissue. After this, most eyelid carcinomas were removed with the fresh tissue technique. However, interest in the fresh tissue technique did not pick up for many years.

In 1969, at the meeting of the American College of Chemosurgery, Dr. Mohs presented data on the use of fresh tissue technique for 66 basal cell carcinomas and for squamous cell carcinomas of the eyelid with 100% five-year cure rates. In 1970, at the meeting of the American Academy of Ophthalmology, Robins, Henkind, and Menn (two of them Mohs' trainees), again presented the results of the five-year 100% cure with the fresh tissue technique. A corroborating series was presented by Dr. Tromovitch in 1970 presenting 75 patients treated with fresh tissue technique and five-year follow-up. At this time, the fresh tissue technique became popular.

In 1967, the American College of Chemosurgery was formed. At that time it had only 23 attendees and preceded the annual meeting at the American Academy of Dermatology. From the 1950s to the 1970s, training in the technique was informal. Training occurred with Dr. Mohs in his chemosurgery clinic and with physicians who had trained with Dr. Mohs. Training lasted anywhere from days to months. In the 1980s, formal fellowships were initiated. In 1986, the American College of Chemosurgery officially changed its name to the American College of Mohs Micrographic Surgery and Cutaneous Oncology.

MOHS MICROGRAPHIC SURGERY TECHNIQUE

Mohs micrographic surgery is a technique first described by Dr Frederic Mohs and subsequently modified, which permits the complete removal of contiguously spreading skin cancers. When properly performed, this procedure allows for immediate and total microscopic evaluation of all surgical margins, and precise identification and localization of any residual tumor through the use of fresh frozen section. The location of residual tumor cells can be accurately identified on a detailed anatomic diagram or map, and the positive areas can be selectively removed. This serial or staged excision technique is repeated until no microscopic evidence of tumor remains, permitting all contiguous extensions of the tumor to be mapped and removed. This can be completed on an outpatient basis over several hours using local anesthesia. The resulting defect can be repaired immediately or allowed to heal by second intention.

Indications

Mohs micrographic surgery is the most effective form of treatment for cutaneous neoplasms that spread by contiguous growth. These include basal cell carcinoma, squamous cell carcinoma, sebaceous carcinoma, verrucous carcinoma, keratoacanthomas, squamous cell carcinoma in situ, and dermatofibrosarcoma protuberans. Other neoplasms that have been successfully treated with Mohs micrographic surgery include microcystic adnexal carcinoma, atypical fibroxanthoma, malignant fibrous histiocytoma, merkel cell carcinoma, extramammary Paget's disease, adenocystic carcinoma, lentigo maligna, desmoplastic trichilemmoma, granular cell tumor, mucinous carcinoma, leiomyosarcoma, and other eccrine carcinomas. Malignant melanoma has also been treated using the Mohs micrographic technique; however, its use is controversial. Although it is an effective form of therapy, it is not necessary to utilize Mohs micrographic surgery for the treatment of all these tumors. However, it is considered the treatment of choice for recurrent tumors, tumors greater than 2 cm in size, and tumors that occur in one of the known high-risk locations for recurrence. These areas include the H-zone of the face, ears, temple, and the mid-central portion of the face. Mohs surgery should be considered for the treatment of basal cell carcinoma that demonstrates aggressive clinical or histologic behavior such as the metatypical and morpheaform subtypes (Table 1).

Preoperative Evaluation

Ideally, a potential Mohs surgery patient would have an initial consultation prior to the day of surgery. However, many patients today make their first visit to the office on the day of surgery. Whether an initial consultation is performed in the office or through correspondence, a complete

history should be taken. The lesion should also be examined, measured, and photographed.

A history of previous treatment affects the prognosis of the tumor as well as the repair to be considered. Previous radiation exposure, intake of arsenic, or significant exposure to ultraviolet light should be noted to evaluate the potential for new tumors. The history should also include any previous medical conditions, including implantable devices such as pacemakers and deep brain stimulators, medications, dietary supplements, and medication allergies.

Patients on prescribed anticoagulants/antiplatelet drugs should continue these medications. No surgical complications have arisen from the continuance of blood thinners during Mohs Micrographic surgery. However, discontinuation of anticoagulants during Mohs surgery has been associated with the occurrence of thrombotic events and death.

Specific questions regarding dietary supplements should be included. Majority of the patients will not report the use of these supplements, many of which have anticoagulant properties alone or in combination with prescribed medications.

Patients with implantable devices require special consideration with the use of office-based electrosurgery. The use of battery-operated handheld heat devices, bipolar forceps or true electrocautery should be used during surgery to prevent interference with these devices.

Most cutaneous surgeries have a low incidence of infection and do not require antibiotic prophylaxis. Patients with an increased risk of infection who may require antibiotic prophylaxis include those with a history of prosthetic heart valve, history of endocarditis, mitral valve prolapse, valvular dysfunction, cardiac malformation, hypertrophic cardiomyopathy, orthopedic prosthesis, and CNS, peritoneal or ventriculoarterial shunts. The selection of an appropriate antibiotic should be evaluated on a case-by-case basis.

If the patient is required to take medications regularly for preexisting internal disease, he or she should take the usual dose on the day of surgery. Also, it is recommended that the patient eat a light breakfast during the morning of surgery.

Most patients are advised to come to the office with a family member or friend. Because the patient usually does not remain in the Mohs operating suite during tissue processing, it is often helpful to have someone present to lessen the

Table 1 Common Indications for Mohs Micrographic Surgery

Recurrent tumors
Size greater than 1 cm on face or greater than 2 cm on trunk/extremities
High-risk anatomic location (H-zone of face including ears, temples, and
   mid-central face)
Aggressive histologic subtype (morpheaform, infiltrating, metatypical)
Poorly defined borders
Locations requiring tissue-sparing (digits, genitals)
Immunosuppressed patients including patients with a history of organ
   transplant or radiation exposure
Incompletely excised tumors
Perineural invasion

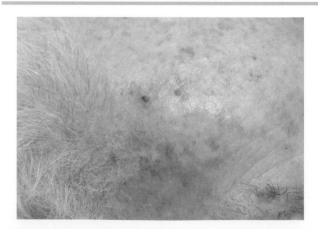

Figure 1 Preoperative clinical appearance of a primary squamous cell carcinoma of the scalp. (*See color insert.*)

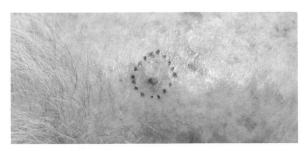

Figure 2 Apparent clinical extent of tumor is outlined with a surgical skin marker. (*See color insert.*)

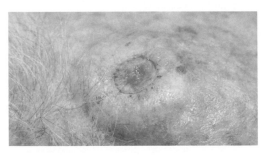

Figure 4 The margin is marked with several small incisions to orient the tissue. (*See color insert.*)

anxiety of waiting for the results of microscopic analysis. Additionally, if the lesion is located in the periorbital area, where a dressing may interfere with vision, a family member or friend can accompany the patient home.

Procedure

The extent of the tumor is first determined as accurately as possible (Fig. 1) and the apparent peripheral border is outlined with a surgical skin marker such as brilliant green or gentian violet (Fig. 2).

The outlined tumor is measured, and the size is recorded on an anatomic diagram from which the surgical map will be generated. The affected area is then prepped with surgical scrub such as Hibiclens or Betadine. Hibiclens should not be used around the eyes and ear canal because it has the potential to cause keratitis and ototoxicity. Local anesthesia, typically 1% lidocaine with epinephrine (1:100,000 or 1:200,000), is administered by intradermal injection. The operative field is covered with sterile towels or drapes.

If the tumor is large or particularly thick, debulking may be useful. This is accomplished by simple curettage or shave excision, with or without the use of electrodesiccation (Fig. 3). There is controversy surrounding the usefulness of curettage prior to taking the first Mohs layer. Curettage may be beneficial to determine the extent of primary tumors or to identify a biopsy site. There are studies suggesting that curettage is imprecise and is capable of removing normal and/or inflamed skin adjacent to a tumor beyond necessary margins.

The first micrographic specimen should include the entire clinically evident tumor plus a very small peripheral margin of normal-appearing tissue. Before the specimen is removed, the margin is marked with several small incisions or with inking such as methylene blue, a temporary tattoo to orient the removed tissue properly (Fig. 4). These marks are made in both the specimen and the adjacent normal tissue.

An incision is then made along the outlined margin with the scalpel angled in the traditional perpendicular position. Then the blade is beveled slightly inward and the incision is repeated along the margin. Subsequent cuts, each increasingly beveled inward, are made until the plane of the incision is horizontal. This is the plan of dissection along which the entire specimen is removed. This yields a thin disc of tissues. The tissue is held at only one edge with forceps to preserve the proper orientation of the specimen. Additionally, the elliptical technique allows for complete histologic margin control and tissue conservation. This technique involves planned elliptical incisions with 1 to 2-mm margins around the visible tumor. On the first layer, tissue is taken in a traditional fashion with a vertical incision through the epidermis and dermis down to superficial subcutaneous fat. The tissue is removed in depth, thus allowing for ease of repair. This technique should not be used in recurrent or sclerotic tumors, large tumors, or tumors in locations that are not amenable to a primary linear closure such as part of the nose, ear, and eye. Similarly, it should be avoided in areas where second intention healing of a partial-thickness wound would be preferred.

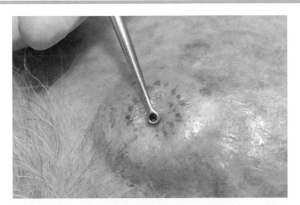

Figure 3 Curettage is performed to determine extent of tumor. (*See color insert.*)

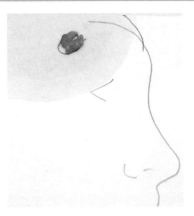

Figure 5 The specimen is placed on a card on which anatomic features are sketched to preserve orientation.

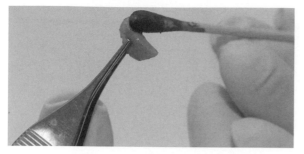

Figure 6 The cut edge of the specimen is color coded with special dyes to orient the sectioned tissue under the microscope.

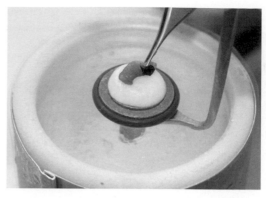

Figure 8 The specimen is turned over and placed horizontally on top of optimal cutting temperature medium so that the deepest margin now faces up. It is then frozen in liquid nitrogen.

Once the specimen has been removed, orientation must be verified. This is accomplished by aligning the specimen in its original position using the scored incisions made previously. The specimen is then placed with proper orientation on an anatomically marked transfer card (Fig. 5).

Although epinephrine will aid hemostasis, additional measures for limiting blood loss may be necessary. In most cases, this is achieved with standard electrosurgery, either as direct electrofulguration or as indirect electrocoagulation, with the aid of forceps or a hemostat. Larger transected blood vessels may require suture ligation. If the operative field is large and there is significant capillary bleeding from the skin edges, chemical cautery, bovine thrombin, or hemostatic gauze (Oxycel, Gelfoam) may be helpful. Between layers, a pressure dressing is applied. If immediate repair is anticipated, Gelfoam is placed in the wound as a temporary hemostatic aid. However, if the wound will be allowed to heal by second intention, oxidized cellulose cotton (Oxycel) can be used instead. An antibiotic ointment is applied topically followed by nonadherent gauze (Telfa). A simple bulk dressing is placed on the surface and, when appropriate, a pressure dressing is applied.

To ensure proper orientation of the specimen, an accurate schematic representation of the surgical defect is drawn on an anatomic diagram. The alignment is aided by the incisions or ink markings made for orientation, which are marked on the diagram. After the specimen has been removed, it is divided into smaller pieces that will fit on a microscope slide when processed. These subdivided pieces are indicated on the map. Relatively straight lateral epidermal margins must be obtained when dividing the specimen to facilitate histologic processing. Specimens with acutely curved epidermal margins are difficult to evaluate after processing because that edge is often deep in the frozen block.

After the specimen has been divided, each piece is lifted from the transfer card, and all margins not at the periphery are marked with colored dyes (Fig. 6). After being marked, the pieces are numbered consecutively, and the colored margins are recorded on the map. For diagrammatic purposes, a straight line on the map represents a red-colored margin, a dotted line on the map represents a blue one, and a jagged line on the map represents a black one. Each piece of the specimen is placed on a saline-moistened gauze pad in ordered sequence in a Petri dish so that the peripheral skin edge margin is pointed down. This routine simplifies handling by the technician (Fig. 7).

The technician begins the processing with piece number one and proceeds consecutively. Optimal cutting temperature (OCT) medium is placed on the cryostat chuck; the specimen is inverted and placed horizontally on the chuck so that the deepest margin now faces up. If the specimen is quick frozen in liquid nitrogen, the OCT partially

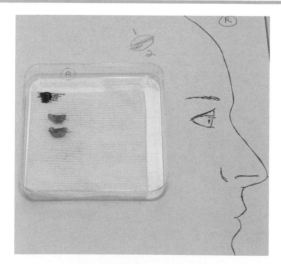

Figure 7 The specimens are placed on a saline-moistened gauze pad in order in a petri dish so that peripheral skin edge margin is pointed down. The orientation of the color-coding and tissue placement is marked on a map.

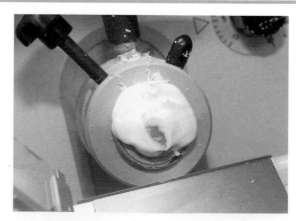

Figure 9 The chuck is mounted in the cryostat.

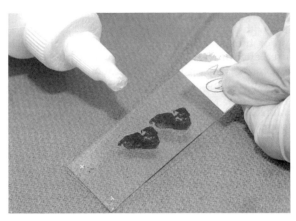

Figure 10 The sections are stained and a coverslip is applied to the slide.

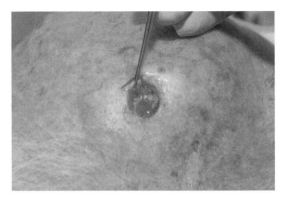

Figure 12 Residual tumor is removed in the next layer.

solidifies, and the specimen can be molded (Fig. 8). This may be done by using the flat portion of a Bard-Parker scalpel handle, a spatula, or similar instrument. After the instrument is warmed over an alcohol flame, it is used to compress the semirigid specimen into a flat plane. The peripheral skin margin is elevated until it is in the same plane as the rest of the specimen. Once this has been accomplished, the entire specimen is covered with OCT medium and frozen in liquid nitrogen.

The chuck with the attached specimen is then placed in the cryostat for storage until all specimens have been mounted. The specimens are stored in consecutive order to maintain proper identification. The tissue is the section (Fig. 9) at a thickness of 4 to 8 µm. The first sections processed represent the deepest and most lateral margins of that piece and are the most important. These sections are placed on a standard glass slide beginning at the end away from its frosted portion. Deeper sections into the block are actually close to the epidermal surface and are placed on the slide in sequence progressing toward the frosted end of the slide. Once all sections have been positioned on the slide, it is dried on a slide warmer and stained with hematoxylin and eosin (H and E).

After staining, a coverslip is applied (Fig. 10) and each slide is carefully examined microscopically. Residual tumor

can then be identified (Fig. 11) and its exact location determined because precise orientation is revealed by the colors on the dyed margins. If residual tumor is identified, the patient is returned to the operating room for removal of any areas with persistent tumor. Those areas positive for tumor are removed (Fig. 12) in a similar manner as in the first stage of the procedure. Each specimen encompasses the area of residual tumor and a small amount (1–2 mm) of surrounding clinically normal tissue. The mapping, marking, and processing of specimens from the second stage of the procedure are carried out exactly as in the initial stage.

If any areas still contain residual tumor, they are treated in a third stage. This process continues until there is no further evidence of tumor. Once a tumor-free plane has been reached, the final defect is measured and recorded. The resulting defect is evaluated to consider whether immediate repair should be undertaken or if the wound should be allowed to heal by second intention.

Special Stains

In Mohs micrographic surgery, frozen sections are typically stained with H and E. More recently, several adjunctive stains have been introduced. Rapid toluidine blue stains are useful in the detection of basal cell carcinoma with Mohs micrographic surgery. Rapid toluidine blue metachromatically stains the mucopolysaccharide stroma of basal cell carcinomas a pink or magenta color. This staining method also reduces traditional staining time with an automatic stainer from nine minutes for H and E to seven minutes, and with the addition of sodium borate, it can further reduce the time to less than 2.5 minutes.

Cytokeratin stains can be used to help delineate aggressive basal cell carcinoma. Cytokeratin stains are not specific for basal cell carcinoma. However, they will help to identify areas of tumor where only inflammation is detectable on traditional H and E sections. The widely available cytokeratin stain used is Ber-EP4.

The use of Mohs micrographic surgery for the treatment of lentigo maligna and invasive melanoma is very controversial. Many surgeons believe that atypical melanocytes cannot be visualized on frozen sections stained with H and E. Melanoma antigen recognized by T-cells (MART-1) and HMB-45 are two stains frequently used to aid in the visualization of atypical melanocytes.

HMB-45, a monoclonal antibody, stains immature melanosomes and not normal adult melanocytes and is thus helpful in the identification of melanoma. When positive, HMB-45 stains the cytoplasm of the melanocyte, pink.

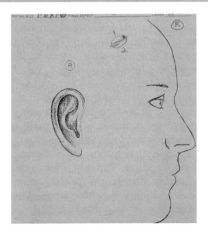

Figure 11 Residual tumor is identified microscopically and marked on the anatomic diagram.

41

Malignant Melanoma

Robert J. Friedman, Melanie Warycha, and Darrell S. Rigel
*Department of Dermatology, New York University School of Medicine,
New York, New York, U.S.A.*

INTRODUCTION

Malignant melanoma remains one of the most serious life-threatening cancers of the skin with over 55,100 new cases having been diagnosed in the United States in 2004. The incidence of melanoma has doubled over the last 25 years, with current reports stating that it is now the fifth and seventh most common cancer among men and women, respectively. Approximately one out of 64 Americans was estimated to have developed melanoma in 2004, with this number expected to rise in the future partially due to increased surveillance and a shift to intermittent sun exposure. The greatest increase in diagnosis has been in thin tumors, with the proportion of "in situ" melanomas having risen from less than 10% in the late 1970s to greater than 40% today. The fact that patients are now presenting at an earlier stage of tumor development may account for the disproportionate increase in incidence over mortality.

Sun and ultraviolet radiation exposure continue to be the major modifiable environmental risk factors for melanoma. Recent data suggest that cumulative exposure, in addition to intermittent or recreational exposure, is likely to impact melanoma risk, whether acquired as an adult or child. Elwood and Jopson found that sunburns at any time of life were associated with a two-fold risk of melanoma. An increased number of melanocytic nevi also confers an increased risk, with dysplastic nevi in particular having been established in the literature as independent risk factors for melanoma. Children with large congenital nevi are also at increased risk for melanoma primarily within the first decade of life. Of note, the majority of melanoma cases do arise de novo. In addition, a family history of melanoma, which is often defined as the presence of melanoma in two or more first-degree relatives, is of utmost importance. Despite the emphasis placed on family history, only between 6% to 14% of malignant melanomas are reported to occur in the context of a family history of melanoma. Two genes conferring susceptibility to melanoma have been identified within high-risk families, the CDKN2A tumor-suppressor gene and the CDK4 oncogene. Recently, loss of function MC1R mutations, which primarily account for the red hair phenotype, have been shown to function as low-penetrance melanoma-predisposition alleles with a high frequency in the population. Despite the genetic basis in a small number of melanoma cases, genetic testing for clinical care is still considered premature.

HISTOPATHOLOGY

Malignant melanoma is best defined as a malignant neoplasm comprised of atypical melanocytes that almost always begins within the epidermis (Figs. 1–7). A wholly intraepidermal (in situ) malignant melanoma is a biologically benign neoplasm that does not metastasize and thus is 100% curable if completely removed. Under the light microscope and with routine staining, they initially appear as a small proliferation of foci of melanocytes, increased in number and apparently cytologically normal at the dermoepidermal junction. As the tumor progresses, more nests of atypical melanocytes in addition to single atypical melanocytes develop, eventually spreading throughout the epidermis, including the cornified layer. This irregular proliferation of atypical melanocytes clinically manifests as an asymmetrical lesion with a jagged or notched border. It is at this point when the melanocytes are distributed in upper levels of the epidermis that the lesion is variably pigmented, with shades of dark brown or black. Once the lesion is 4 or 5mm in diameter, it may infiltrate into the dermis, entering what Clark described as the "vertical" growth phase. Once atypical melanocytes penetrate the dermis, the flat malignant melanoma becomes elevated. If the atypical melanocytes infiltrate into the dermis focally, a small papule or nodule may appear superimposed on the macule. Some melanomas never progress to this invasive phase but remain "in situ" for many years (e.g., melanomas on sun-damaged skin of head and neck, the so-called lentigo maligna), whereas others enter this phase early on (e.g., the so-called "nodular melanomas"). If not diagnosed and treated early in its evolution, melanocytes invade deeper structures such as the papillary and reticular dermis and subcutaneous fat. Once the neoplasm exceeds a certain size or volume, new blood vessels must form (neovascularization) to sustain a nutrient supply for continued growth. Metastases occur when the atypical melanocytes penetrate into local lymphatic and vascular channels. This event is directly proportional to both the thickness and volume of the neoplasm.

At times, the immune system may partially or, rarely, completely destroy the malignant melanoma manifesting itself clinically and histologically as focal or complete regression. Histologically, these changes are characterized by the finding of a thickened fibrotic papillary dermis with a few scattered lymphocytes and melanophages. Clinically, such areas are seen as focal zones of white or pink within (or at the site of) a malignant melanoma. The earliest histologic feature of regression is a dense band-like infiltrate of lymphocytes, often followed by broad zones of histiocytes laden with melanin (melanophages) resulting in the so-called melanosis.

(A)   **(B)**   **(C)**   **(D)**

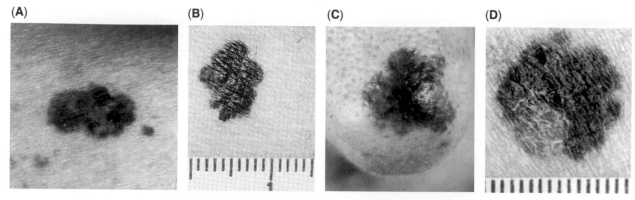

Figure 1 ABCDs of early malignant malanoma. **(A)** Asymmetry. **(B)** Border irregularity. **(C)** Color variegation. **(D)** Diameter greater than 6 mm.

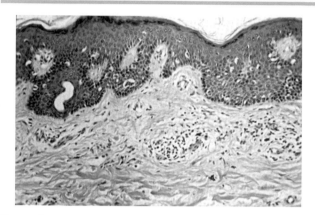

Figure 2 Malignant melanoma in situ evolving early, showing an increased number of cytologically normal-appearing melanocytes focally arranged, predominantly as single cells along the dermoepidermal junction and slightly above it.

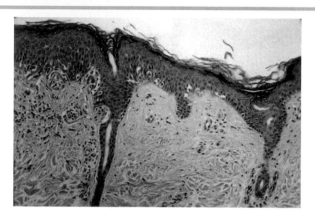

Figure 4 Malignant melanoma in situ showing an increased number of cytologically atypical melanocytes arranged both singly and in confluent nests within the epidermis and at somewhat higher levels of the epidermis.

CLINICAL FEATURES

In 1985, the "ABCD rule" (Fig. 8D) was established to draw attention to key clinical features (asymmetry, border irregularity, color variation, and diameter > 6 mm) of melanocytic lesions that warrant further evaluation. Since its implementation, it has served as an effective screening tool employed by both patients and physicians with the goal of early recognition of potentially curable cutaneous melanoma.

The clinical asymmetry ("A") of an early malignant melanoma is present when one-half of the lesion does not match the other half. Histologically, this is due to the asymmetrical proliferation of atypical melanocytes, both singly and in nests within the epidermis. Border irregularity ("B") describes edges that are either ragged, blotched, or blurred. Color variability ("C") refers to the presence of various shades of tan, brown, black, or at times, red, blue, or white within the same lesion. This could be seen secondary to

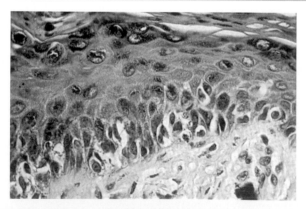

Figure 3 Malignant melanoma in situ: early changes show an increased number of cytologically atypical melanocytes arranged as single cells along the dermoepidermal junction and slightly above it.

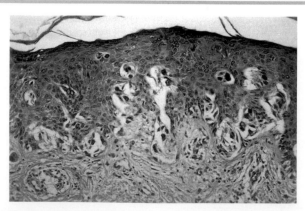

Figure 5 Malignant melanoma in situ showing an increased number of atypical melanocytes arranged both singly and in confluent nests throughout the epidermis

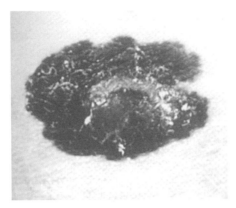

Figure 6 Malignant melanoma involving the epidermis and dermis.

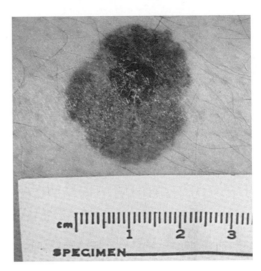

Figure 8 Malignant melanoma with small invasive component.

irregular amounts of melanin pigment within and at all levels of the epidermis. The peripheral growth or diameter ("D") of malignant melanoma provides the fourth letter of the mnemonic and has been established as any diameter greater than 6 mm. Recent reports documenting existence of invasive small diameter melanomas (those < 6 mm in diameter) has prompted discussion over the revision of this criterion. A review of the literature conducted at our institution, however, failed to identify sufficient evidence to support a lowering of the diameter criterion. Although it is difficult to estimate the frequency of invasive small-diameter melanomas as they are often considered benign and fail to undergo biopsy, we believe these lesions are uncommon among all known pigmented lesions of similar diameter. We thus concluded that lowering the diameter criterion of the ABCD framework would not increase sensitivity of melanoma diagnosis without seriously compromising specificity and generating millions of unnecessary skin biopsies.

In the same review, we also examined the evidence regarding expansion of the acronym to ABCDE, including a criterion for evolving ("E"). We defined "evolving lesions" as those noted to have changed with respect to size, shape, symptoms (e.g., itching and tenderness), surface (e.g., bleeding), or shades of color. The significance of lesion evolution as a precursor to malignant melanoma has been well documented, with one study by Cassileth et al. reporting changes in "size, elevation, and color" to be among the most frequent

cluster of symptoms reported by patients to have prompted medical evaluation. Furthermore, Thomas et al. concluded that lesion evolution (defined as horizontal enlargement) was the most specific criterion among the ABCD(E)s, with a specificity of 90%. Our review supported endorsement of the ("E") criterion, with the hope that future educational programs and literature will emphasize the importance of a changing lesion, a shift we believe will lead to diagnoses of melanoma at earlier stages of the disease.

In the past, primary cutaneous melanoma was divided into four major clinical–pathologic subtypes: (i) superficial spreading melanoma, (ii) nodular melanoma, (iii) acral lentiginous melanoma, and (iv) lentigo maligna melanoma. All of the clinicopathologic types of melanoma have been found to have a comparable prognosis for a given Breslow thickness. Superficial spreading is the most prevalent subtype of melanoma, accounting for about 70% of all cases, primarily in patients between 30 and 50 years of age. It commonly arises on the trunk in men and on the lower extremities of women. Nodular melanomas are the second most common subtype, occurring in 15% to 30% of patients. The most ominous feature of this subtype is its lack of a radial growth phase, allowing the melanoma to invade deeper layers of the dermis over weeks to months. Clinically, it presents as an elevated, dark brown to black papule or nodule, with ulceration and bleeding being common. Lentigo maligna melanoma accounts for 4% to 15% of melanoma cases, occurring most commonly on the head, neck, or arms of elderly, fair-skinned individuals. This form of melanoma is linked to cumulative, rather than intermittent, sun exposure. The so-called lentigo maligna, is the wholly "in situ" variant of this subtype and is usually present for over five to 20 years before the transformation into melanoma occurs. The lesion initially begins as an irregular tan-brown patch, which can grow to a large size and develop variably pigmented areas. Acral lentiginous melanoma is the least common subtype, however, it accounts for 29% to 72% of melanoma cases in dark-complexioned individuals. Clinically, it manifests as a brown to black irregular macule or papule on the palms, soles, or beneath the nail plate.

Currently, we view melanoma according to the unifying concept of Ackerman and Su. Melanoma, regardless of

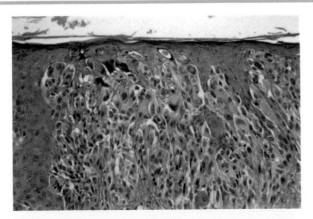

Figure 7 Malignant melanoma involving the epidermis and dermis.

their anatomic site of origin, arise, nearly all of the time, from a single, or small collection of transformed melanocyte(s) within the basilar epidermis. In time, these melanocytes proliferate first as single "typical appearing" melanocytes in a somewhat asymmetric array along the dermo-epidermal junction. Some melanocytes become "atypical appearing" having pleomorphic and hyperchromatic nuclei. With progression of the neoplastic process, these cells extend both peripherally along the dermo-epidermal junction and at higher levels of the epidermis. Some cells develop a nested pattern and these nests tend to vary in their sizes and shapes. Some tend toward confluence. Classic full-blown melanoma in situ consists of atypical melanoctyes arranged both singly and nests throughout the epidermis (in most cases). Classically, the melanocytic proliferation follows the ABCDE rule clinically. That is, the proliferation has a tendency to be asymmetric both along the dermo-epidermal junction, giving rise to a pigmented macule exhibiting clinically asymmetric and irregular borders. The initial proliferation of melanocytes along the dermo-epidermal junction and eventually as somewhat higher levels of the epidermis, gives rise to a pigmented macule having subtle nuances in tans, brown, and, where the pigment-laden melanocytes are present in the cornified layer, black. The varying sizes, shapes, and confluences of the nests of melanocytes also contribute to the variation in color. Once the melanoma proliferates such that it enters the subjacent dermis, variable elevation in the lesion occurs (Figs. 9–13). Inflammatory cell infiltrates, vascular dilatation and engorgement, fibrosis (regression), and deeper involvement of pigmented melanocytes and melanophages give the appearance of pink, red, white, and blue. In sum, the unifying concept of Ackerman and Su help explain the clinicopathologic features of both early melanoma in situ as well as more advanced disease without the confusion in terminology associated with the older classification schema.

There also exist other rare clinical and histologic variants of melanoma. Desmoplastic melanoma often presents as a nodule or plaque with up to 40% being amelanotic, thus delaying early diagnosis. Up to 40% have been reported to recur locally. Nevoid melanoma presents as either a verrucous or dome-shaped nodule that occurs most commonly on the trunk or limbs of young adults.

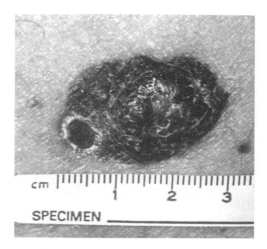

Figure 10 Malignant melanoma, ulcerated.

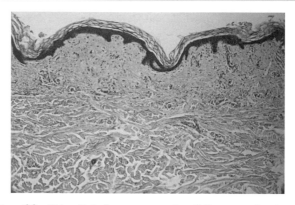

Figure 11 Histopathologic appearance of partially regressed melanoma shows a thickened fibrotic papillary dermis with a few scattered lymphocytes and melanophages.

The introduction of dermoscopy in 1989 allowed for a noninvasive approach to magnifying subsurface structures of the epidermis and papillary dermis. A consensus meeting held in Hamburg in 1989 identified the following six features as predictors of melanoma: irregular, prominent, and broad pigment network, black dots, radial streaming, irregular brown globules, gray-blue areas, and white scar-like areas. Since then, the presence of a pigment network

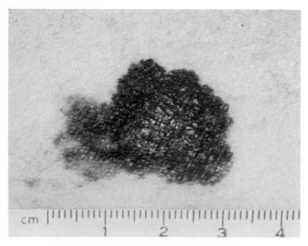

Figure 9 Plaquelike malignant melanoma.

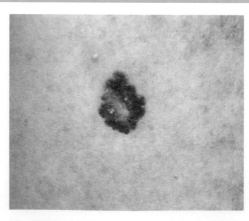

Figure 12 Malignant melanoma shows changes of partial regression.

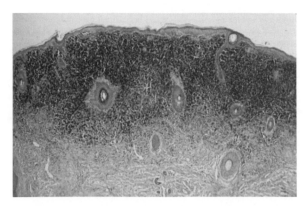

Figure 13 Histopathologic appearance of the early features of histologic regression shows a dense bandlike infiltrate of lymphocytes and melanophages.

with an abrupt margin, four or more colors, and a white veil have been shown to be the most specific predictors of melanoma. Multiple grading systems for predicting melanoma based upon dermoscopic features exist. The most widely accepted among them is the ABCD rule of dermatoscopy. This grading system allows for lesions to be scored on the bases of asymmetry in two axes, sharpness of margins, number of colors seen, and the presence of additional dermoscopic features. It has been shown that dermatologists trained in the use of dermoscopy can improve their diagnostic accuracy of melanoma from 65% to approximately 80% with the benefit of a dermoscope. With the introduction of digital imaging dermoscopes, these statistics are anticipated to improve dramatically.

PROGNOSIS

Malignant melanoma continues to be a fatal disease once widespread metastases develop, with mortality rates having steadily risen over the past three decades. In the United States, the age-adjusted melanoma mortality rate increased from 2.2/100,000 in white males in 1973 to 3.7/100,000 in white males in 1998. Despite increases in mortality rates, survival among melanoma patients has improved. The survival rate in Caucasians was approximately 60% between 1960 and 1963, however, it climbed to 89% from 1992 to 1997. Attempts to predict which patients have a better chance of surviving is dependent upon the identification of clinical and pathologic prognostic factors. It is with this knowledge that physicians may be better equipped at recognizing those patients with a greater risk of metastatic disease and thus poor survival.

The most important predictor of prognosis remains the Breslow thickness of the neoplasm. Breslow refined the concept of microinvasion using ocular micrometry to measure the precise thickness of the neoplasm in millimeters. The thickness of a malignant melanoma is measured vertically from the stratum granulosum to the deepest penetration of the neoplasm. This is in contrast to Clark et al. who described melanoma by its anatomic depth rather than its thickness. Clark's level has been shown to be less statistically significant than Breslow thickness as a prognostic variable. It has been proposed that Clark's level derives its prognostic capability through its secondary correlation with tumor thickness.

Another powerful predictor of patient survival is the status of regional lymph nodes. Dubois et al. found that the presence of one palpable lymph node predicted an approximately 50% five-year survival rate. Likewise, Buzaid et al. found that the five-year survival rate of patients with lymph node metastases decreased by approximately 30% to 50%. Sentinel lymph node status in particular has also been thoroughly studied in the literature in terms of its association with prognosis. Gershenwald found that patients with negative rather than positive sentinel nodes were 6.43 times more likely to survive. In a study by Vuylsteke et al., 55% of patients with a positive sentinel lymph node had a relapse, compared to only 14% in patients with a negative sentinel lymph node.

Melanoma ulceration has also proven to be a vital feature of primary melanoma that influences mortality rates. Ulceration primarily occurs in a subset of thick, nodular lesions and is a marker of the aggressive nature of the lesion. Balch et al. in 1980 found a decrease in survival associated with ulcerated (55%) compared with nonulcerated melanomas (80%) in Stage I melanoma patients. Furthermore, the same investigators evaluated five-year survival dates from 17,600 melanoma patients and found ulceration to be one of the most powerful predictors of survival.

Anatomic site appears to play a role in prognosis. With equivalent thickness, patients with malignant melanoma on the head and neck, trunk, hands, and feet have a poorer five-year survival than those with malignant melanomas on the remaining areas of the arms and legs (84% vs. 93%).

Age is also an important prognostic variable. Patients older than 50 years of age have worse five-year survivals (84%) than those who are younger (90%). Female patients have a better prognosis than males (90% five-year survival vs. 83% five-year survival).

The presence of local satellitosis has been found to be an important prognostic factor. Microscopic satellites are defined as deposits of tumor that are larger than 0.05 mm in diameter and are discontinuous from the main body of Stage IV or V melanoma. Both Day and Harrist have shown a decreased five-year survival rate with the presence of microsatellitosis, in addition to an increased frequency of occult regional lymph node metastasis.

In the presence of histologic evidence of a pre-existing melanocytic nevus, thickness for thickness, patients with those malignant melanomas arising in association with a pre-existing nevus had better five-year survivals than those not having an associated melanocytic nevus. In addition, mitotic rate has been shown to be an important marker of outcome, with higher rates of predictor of poor prognosis.

Tumor regression may also be associated with a worse prognosis, although these findings have been controversial. It may be reflective of a more aggressive lesion, having been correlated with metastasis. Clinically, it manifests as gray or whitish areas either within a melanoma or without obvious residual melanoma. Thin melanomas show regression more frequently than do thick melanomas. It is possible that these lesions are thin because they have undergone regression and the tumor depth has been underestimated.

Recently, new data on prognosis has been incorporated into a new melanoma staging system, which was developed by the American Joint Committee on Cancer in 2002. Modifications to the old staging system include: (i) incorporation of melanoma thickness and ulceration, but not level of invasion, into T classification, (ii) utilizing the number of metastatic nodes rather than their gross dimensions, in addition to distinguishing between microscopic versus macroscopic nodal metastases, to be used in the N

Table 1 The New American Joint Committee on Cancer TNM Melanoma Staging System

T classification	Thickness	Ulceration status
T1	≤1.0 mm	(a) Without ulceration and level II/III
		(b) With ulceration or level IV/V
T2	1.01–2.0 mm	(a) Without ulceration (b) With ulceration
T3	2.01–4.0 mm	(a) Without ulceration (b) With ulceration
T4	>4 mm	(a) Without ulceration (b) With ulceration
N classification	Number of metastatic nodes	Nodal metastatic mass
N1	One node	(a) Micrometastasis (b) Macrometastasis
N2	Two or three nodes	(a) Micrometastasis (b) Macrometastasis
		(c) In transit Metastasi(e)s/satellite(s) Without metastatic nodes
N3	Four or more metastatic nodes, or matted nodes, or in transit metastasi(e)s/satellite(s) with metastatic nodes	
M classification	Site	Serum lactate dehydrogenase
M1a	Distant skin, subcutaneous, or nodal metastases	Normal
M1b	Lung	Normal
M1c	All other visceral metastases Any distant metastasis	Normal Elevated

classification, (iii) specification of the site of distant metastases and the presence or absence of an elevated serum lactic dehydrogenase to be used in the M classification, (iv) upstaging of patients with Stage I, II, or III disease when ulceration is present, and (v) merging of satellite metastases and in transit metastases into a single staging entity grouped into Stage III disease (Table 1).

MANAGEMENT

The first step in the management of the patient with malignant melanoma is biopsy of the suspicious lesion. Clinical suspicion for malignant melanoma is guided by the clinical presentation ("ABCD" changes), along with history. In its early evolving stages, even the astute dermatologist often has difficulty making an unequivocal diagnosis. A properly obtained biopsy specimen and expert histologic interpretation are vital for the definitive diagnosis.

BIOPSY TECHNIQUE

The best way to biopsy a malignant melanoma is by total excision (Figs. 14–16). Exceptions to this include lesions that

are so large that their complete removal would result in a significant surgical procedure or those in difficult anatomic locations for which the deformity, if the lesion were benign, would be unacceptable. In such cases, an incisional biopsy is permissible. Many practitioners find that procedures such as punch biopsy, curette biopsy, and needle biopsy are not acceptable when the possibility of malignant melanoma is seriously entertained. It is important to emphasize that the histologic diagnosis of malignant melanoma requires the pathologist to assess breadth, circumscription, and depth of the lesion. Any biopsy technique that does not permit the assessment of the above features may lead to a misdiagnosis.

Excisional biopsy of most malignant melanomas is an office or outpatient procedure. The patient should be made aware of the fact that often the excisional biopsy of a malignant melanoma is only one part of the treatment. Generally, a margin of at least 2 mm around the clinically suspicious pigmented lesion is sufficient for an excisional biopsy. Local anesthesia is generally administered in a field block outside of the 2 mm margin. The incision should be directed such that the long axis of the ellipse is placed in the direction of the probable pathway of lymphatic drainage for that anatomic site. The incision should extend through the skin and into the subcutaneous adipose tissue but not to the level of the underlying fascia. The wound can be closed easily with

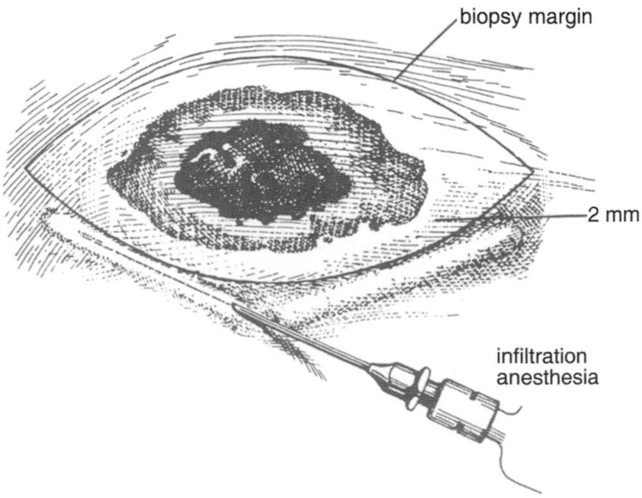

Figure 14 Biopsy in totos of a malignant melanoma. *Source*: Reproduced with permission from Roses DF, Harris MN, Ackerman AB. *Diagnosis and Management of cutaneous malignant melanoma*. Philadelphia, WB Saunders, 1983.

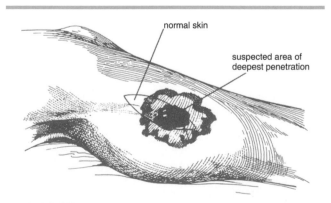

Figure 15 Biopsy in part for large malignant melanoma. *Source*: Reproduced with permission from Roses DF, Harris MN, Ackerman AB. *Diagnosis and Management of cutaneous malignant melanoma*. Philadelphia, WB Saunders, 1983.

(A)

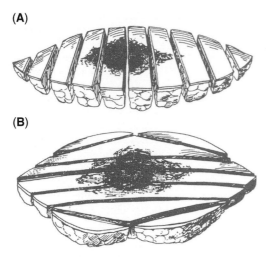

(B)

Figure 16 Laboratory preparation of a specimen of malignant melanoma. *Source*: From Roses DF, Harris MN, Ackerman AB. Diagnosis and Management of Cutaneous Malignant Melanoma. Philadelphia, WB Saunders, 1983.

simple, interrupted sutures. The specimen should be placed in 10% formalin solution for transport to the pathology laboratory. It is essential that an adequate clinical description of the lesion accompany the specimen, including the size of the lesion.

An incisional biopsy of a malignant melanoma should be done to include tissue that clinically contains the thickest portion of the lesion. The surgical technique is otherwise the same. The incisional specimen should include the thickest portion of the lesion and extend to include some of the surrounding normal skin. There appears to be evidence that a biopsy specimen obtained by incision into a malignant melanoma has a detrimental influence on the survival of patients.

HANDLING AND PROCESSING SPECIMENS SUSPECTED OF BEING MALIGNANT MELANOMA

Specimens submitted to be evaluated for malignant melanoma should be placed in neutral buffered 10% formalin solution in a bottle containing 20 times as much volume of fixative as specimen. "Grossing" of the specimen by the laboratory can be as important as the biopsy technique. The size of the excision, as well as the dimensions of the pigmented lesion, should be properly recorded as part of the gross description of the specimen. The specimen should be step-sectioned at 2 mm intervals. An alternative method is to section the specimen on the long axis of the specimen. This method may permit a better assessment of the breadth of the neoplasm.

In most instances, an accurate diagnosis can be obtained using routine hematoxylin and eosin staining. The diagnosis can also be confirmed by utilizing immunohistochemical analysis. Two of the most widely used antibodies in the detection of malignant melanoma include polyclonal S100 protein and monoclonal HMB-45. S100 exhibits significant crossreactivity with nonmelanocytic cell types, and thus its' utility is limited by low specificity. HMB-45 has advantages in specificity, functioning as a marker for "activated melanocytes." It has little utility in recognizing cases of desmoplastic melanoma however.

Newer monoclonal antibodies developed against melan-A and tyrosinase can serve as supplemental markers to the detection of melanocytes. Melan-A is a cytoplasmic protein expressed in mature melanocytes and has been reported to be positive in most primary and over 80% of metastatic melanoma. Tyrosinase, an enzyme that functions in melanin synthesis, has been shown to be effective in detecting micrometastasis in sentinel lymph nodes that were negative on histological examination.

In addition to employing immunohistochemistry as a means of identifying malignant melanoma, research efforts are turning towards cytogenetics to achieve a higher level of specificity. Initial studies of the use of reverse-transcriptase polymerase chain reaction to detect melanoma-specific messenger RNA in lymph nodes have been promising. This modality has been shown to exhibit greater sensitivity over routine histology or immunohistochemistry.

CLINICAL EVALUATION

A properly performed history and physical examination should include careful questioning concerning the pigmented lesion in question, sun exposure history, personal and family history of malignant melanoma or dysplastic nevi, as well as a history of other medical illnesses. The physical examination should be comprehensive. All patients, including those with malignant melanoma, should be completely undressed and the entire cutaneous and mucocutaneous surfaces examined. Examination of the site of the melanoma, including careful palpation for any subcutaneous satellite lesions, should be performed. A complete examination of the regional lymph nodes as well as examination for organomegaly should be done.

The routine evaluation of a patient with malignant melanoma at our institution also includes a complete blood count, urinalysis, chest X ray, electrocardiogram, serum chemistry screen, and when indicated, a computed tomographic scan of the chest and abdomen. This comprehensive assessment, however, has not been universally accepted among practitioners. In fact, there is evidence in the literature that routine imaging studies including chest X ray or blood work have limited value in the work-up of asymptomatic patients with melanoma less than 4 mm in thickness. Furthermore, the Melanoma Consensus Conference of 1992 concluded that staging work-up was not indicated in melanomas 1 mm or less in thickness. Thus, the extent to which a patient diagnosed with melanoma should be evaluated remains controversial.

Whenever possible, the principal treatment modality for primary cutaneous melanoma is surgery. Diagnosed early, well over 90% of primary melanomas can be cured with surgical excision alone. Local control of a primary melanoma requires wide excision of the tumor or biopsy site down to the deep fascia with a margin of normal-appearing skin. The optimal width of the primary tumor resection margins have been a subject of debate, but have tended to favor narrower margins. A prospective, randomized study conducted by the World Health Organization demonstrated that melanomas up to 2 mm in depth can safely be excised with a 1 cm margin with no adverse effects on patient survival. To date, there have been no specific randomized trials to determine the ideal margins to use in the treatment of tumors greater than 4 mm deep; however, retrospective data supports the use of 2 cm margins. Table 2 summarizes recommendations for surgical margins according to thickness of lesion.

Table 2 Recommended Surgical Margins

Breslow thickness	Surgical margin (cm)
In situ	0.5
< 2 mm	1
≥ 2 mm	2

Elective lymph node dissection in patients with cutaneous melanoma with no clinically detectable node metastasis has been long debated. Lymph node dissections were initially recommended as it was believed that lymph node involvement preceded more widespread metastatic disease. Elective lymph node dissection was applied to all patients, subjecting those without nodal disease (~80%) to the morbidity associated with this procedure without any therapeutic benefit. Then in 1992, Morton et al. proposed sentinel lymph node biopsy as a means to evaluate the primary draining lymph node for metastasis in a less invasive manner. He was able to show that the pathologic status of the sentinel node was an accurate assessment of whether or not metastases were present in that specific lymph node basin. Thus, this set the precedent that the histologic status of lymph nodes could serve as a prognostic factor. This technique has become the standard method for staging melanoma by determining the pathologic status of regional lymph nodes, in addition to stratifying which patients are candidates for adjuvant therapy. This procedure is conducted in patients with melanomas of intermediate or high-risk thickness (>1 mm), or in patients with lesions less than 1 mm thick that are at least Clark level IV or that are ulcerated. Sentinel lymph node mapping involves the intradermal injection of biologic blue dye and radiolabeled technetium sulfur colloid into the skin surrounding the primary melanoma. Selective identification of the sentinel lymph node is facilitated with lymphoscintigraphy once the agents have drained to the regional lymph node basin. A hand-held gamma probe approximates the position of the sentinel lymph node, which is then histologically examined by careful sectioning of the node as well as immunostaining with anti-S100, anti-MART-1, or anti-HMB-45 antibodies. Immediate complete lymph node dissection is undertaken if evidence of metastasis is noted on histopathologic examination. If no foci of metastasis are observed, then further excision of lymph nodes is not warranted.

Once the presence of metastases are documented in a patient with melanoma, there are not many effective options available for further management. Attempts to treat metastatic melanoma have been dismal, with response rates usually less than 40%. Chemotherapy is reserved for metastatic disease, however, its' efficacy is limited. Single and multiagent chemotherapy for metastatic melanoma has continued to be disappointing, with low complete response rates and no long-term survival benefit. Dacarbazine remains the single most active chemotherapeutic agent, with average response rates between 15% and 20%; however, response duration does not usually exceed five to six months. Ultimately, only 2% of all patients sustain a complete remission.

In addition to chemotherapy, there has been an impetus to explore various immunotherapies in the hopes of imparting a clinical impact. Multiple clinical trials exploring the effectiveness of interferon alpha (IFN-α) 2b . as an adjuvant therapy for melanoma have been undertaken, with two demonstrating a 5% to 10% improvement in overall survival. Based on the 1995 Eastern Cooperative Oncology Group (ECOG) trial E1684 which found a slight, but significant, advantage in terms of relapse-free survival and overall survival rates with the use of high-dose IFN-α2b, the U.S. Food and Drug Administration approved the use of IFN-α2b for stage IIB and III disease. Only high-dose IFN-α has had a significant impact upon survival, but it is associated with significant toxicity. Low-dose IFN-α has never been shown to impact overall survival in randomized controlled trials. Currently, clinical trials are underway to study the efficacy of intermediate IFN-α regimens. Despite the slight improvement in survival, the adjuvant use of interferon in the treatment of metastatic melanoma still remains controversial. The toxicities of IFN-α are too high for many physicians to prescribe it to patients with only intermediate risk of recurrence. Additional clinical trials are needed to elucidate the optimal dose regimen and selection of patients who will benefit the most from this treatment. Interleukin-2 has also been employed in the treatment of metastatic melanoma, leading to long-term remissions in an estimated 6% of patients. Lastly, vaccines are currently being investigated for therapeutic use in patients with extracutaneous melanoma in the hopes of enhancing or inducing an immune response against the neoplasm. Research has identified numerous antigens present on melanoma cells that could potentially function as targets for experimental vaccines, however, as of yet, none have been proven to provide significant benefits in terms of survival.

Due to the aggressive nature of melanoma, combined with its unresponsiveness to medical therapy, it is not surprising that the survival for patients with metastatic disease has not improved greatly since the 1970s. Only through patient education can melanoma be caught in its early stages when it is curable. The National Institutes of Health Consensus Conference on Early Melanoma, and the American Cancer Society recommend population-based screening. Patients should be familiar with the warning signs of melanoma, and those at risk for developing melanoma should be encouraged to undergo routine screening. Prevention of death from malignant melanoma is not only a possibility but should also be a reality and the goal of each and every physician managing diseases of the skin. Learn to recognize malignant melanoma when it is small, flat, and curable. Teach those around you to do the same.

"But what is the black spot, Captain?" I asked. "That's a summons, mate...."

Robert Louis Stevenson, *Treasure Island*

BIBLIOGRAPHY

Abbasi NR, Shaw HM, Rigel DS, et al. Early diagnosis of cutaneous melanoma: revisiting the ABCD criteria. JAMA 2004; 292(22): 2771–2776.

Ackerman AB, Su WPD. The histology of cutaneous melanoma. In: Kopf AW, Bart RS, Rodriguez-Sains RS, Ackerman AB, eds. Malignant Melanoma. New York: Masson Publishing Company, 1979:25.

Anderson C, Buzaid A, Legha S. Systemic treatment for advanced cutaneous melanoma. Oncology 1995; 9:1149–1154.

Balch CM, Wilkerson JA, Murad TM, et al. The prognostic significance of ulceration of cutaneous melanoma. Cancer 1980; 45:3012–3017.

Balch CM, Soong SJ, Gershenwald JE, et al. Prognostic factors analysis of 17,600 melanoma patients: validation of the American Joint Committee on Cancer melanoma staging system. J Clin Oncol 2001; 19(16):3622–3634.

Balch CM, Buzaid AC, Soong SJ, et al. Final version of the American Joint Committee on Cancer staging system for cutaneous melanoma. J Clin Oncol 2001; 19(16):3635–3648.

Balch C, Buzaid A, Soong S, et al. New TNM melanoma staging system: linking biology and natural history to clinical outcomes. Semin Surg Oncol 2003; 21:43–52.

Blessing K, McLaren KM, McLean A, Davidson P. Thin malignant melanomas (< 1.5 mm) with metastasis: a histological study and survival analysis. Histopathology 1990; 17:389–395.

Blessing K, Grant JJ, Sanders DS, et al. Small cell malignant melanoma: a variant of naevoid melanoma. Clinicopathological features and histological differential diagnosis. J Clin Pathol 2000; 53(8):591.

Blessing K, Sanders DS, Grant JJH. Comparison of immunohistochemical staining of the novel antibody melan-A with S100 protein and HMB 45 in malignant melanoma and melanoma variants. Histopathology 1998; 32:139–146.

Bostick PJ, Morton DL, Turner RR, et al. Prognostic significance of occult metastases detected by sentinel lymphadenectomy and reverse transcriptase-polymerase chain reaction in early-stage melanoma patients. J Clin Oncol 1999; 17(10):3238–3244.

Breslow A. Thickness, cross-sectional areas and depth of invasion in the prognosis of cutaneous melanoma. Ann Surg 1970; 172:902–908.

Brogelli L, Reali UM, Moretti S, Urso C. The prognostic significance of histologic regression in cutaneous melanoma. Melanoma Res 1992; 2:87–91.

Buzaid AC, Ross MI, Balch CM, et al. Critical analysis of the current American Joint Committee on Cancer staging system for cutaneous melanoma and proposal of a new staging system. J Clin Oncol 1997; 15(3):1039–1051.

Bulliard J-L, Cox B. Int J Epidemiol 2000; 29:416–423.

Cassileth BR, Lusk EJ, Guerry D, Clark WH Jr., Matozzo I, Frederick BE. "Catalyst" symptoms in malignant melanoma. J Gen Intern Med 1987; 2:1–4.

Chin L. The genetics of malignant melanoma: lessons from mouse and man. Nat Rev 2003; 3:559–570.

Cochran AJ, Wen DR, Morton DL. Management of the regional lymph nodes in patients with cutaneous malignant melanoma. World J Surg 1992; 16:214–221.

Day CL Jr, Sober AJ, Kopf AW, et al. A prognostic model for clinical stage I melanoma of the upper extremity. The importance of anatomical subsites in predicting recurrent disease. Ann Surg 1981; 193:436–440.

Desmond R, Soong S. Epidemiology of malignant melanoma. Surg Clin North Am 2003; 83.

Dubois RW, Swetter SM, Atkins M, et al. Developing indications for the use of sentinel node biopsy and adjuvant high dose interferon alfa-2b in melanoma. Arch Dermatol 2001; 137:1217–1224.

Elwood JM, Jopson J. Int J Cancer 1997; 73:198–203.

Gershenwald JE, Thompson W, Mansfield PF, et al. Multi-institutional melanoma lymphatic mapping experience: the prognostic value of sentinel lymph node status in 612 stage I or II melanoma patients. J Clin Oncol 1999; 17:976–983.

Gromet MA, Epstein WL, Blois MS. The regressing thin malignant melanoma: a distinctive lesion with metastatic potential. Cancer 1978; 42:2282–2292.

Harrist TJ, Rigel DS, Day CL, et al. "Microscopic satellites" are more highly associated with regional lymph node metastases than is primary melanoma thickness. Cancer 1984; 53(10):2183–2187.

Houghton AN, Legha S, Bajorin DF. In: Balch CM, Houghton AN, Milton GW, et al., eds. Cutaneous Melanoma. Philadelphia, PA: JB Lippincott, 1992:499.

Hussussian CJ, Struewing JP, Goldstein AM, et al. Nat Genet 1994; 8:15–21.

Jaroszewski DE, Pockaj BA, DiCaudo DJ, et al. Clinical behavior of desmoplastic melanoma. Am J Surg 2001; 182(6):590–595.

Jemal A, Murray T, Samuels A, Ghafoor A, Ward E, Thun MJ. Cancer statistics, 2004. CA Cancer J Clin 2004; 54(1):5–26.

Jemal A, Devesa SS, Fears TR, Hartge P. J Natl Cancer Inst 2000; 92:811–818.

Jungbluth AA, Busam KL, Gerald WL, et al. An anti-melan A monoclonal antibody for the detection of malignant melanoma in paraffin embedded tissues. Am J Surg Pathol 1998; 22:595–602.

Kamb A, Shattuck-Eidends D, Eleles R, et al. Analysis of the p16 gene (CDKN2) as a candidate for the chromosome 9p melanoma susceptibility locus. Nat Genet 1994; 8:23–26.

Kirkwood JM, Ibrahim JG, Sondak VK, et al. High- and low-dose interferon alfa-2b in high-risk melanoma: first analysis of Intergroup trial E1690/S9111/C9190. J Clin Oncol 2000; 18:2444–2458.

Koh HK. Cutaneous melanoma. N Eng J Med 1992; 325:171–182.

Kopf AW, Hellman LJ, Rogers GS, et al. Familial malignant melanoma. JAMA 1986; 256:1915–1919.

Legha SS, Ring S, Eton O, et al. Development of a biochemotherapy regimen with concurrent administration of cisplastin, vinblastine, dacarbazine, interferon alfa, and interleukin-2 for patients with metastatic melanoma. J Clin Oncol 1998; 16:1752–1759.

Martini L, Brandani P, Chiarugi C, et al. First recurrence analysis of 840 cutaneous melanomas: a proposal for follow-up schedule. Tumori 1994; 80:188–197.

Marks R. Recent Results Cancer Res 2002; 160:113–121.

Maize JC. Primary cutaneous malignant melanoma. J Am Acad Dermatol 1983; 8(6):857–863.

Mackie RM, Bray CA, Hole DJ, et al. for the Scottish Melanoma Group. Lancet 2002; 360:587–591.

Masback A, Olsson H, Westerdahl J, et al. Prognostic factors in invasive cutaneous malignant melanoma: a population-based study and review. Melanoma Res 2001; 11:435–445.

Magennis DP, Orchard GE. Malignant melanoma, death by image and ignorance, diagnosis by surgical excision and laboratory investigation. Br J Biomed Sci 1999; 56:134–144.

McCarthy WH, Shaw HM, Thompson JF, et al. Time and frequency of recurrence of cutaneous stage I malignant melanoma with guidelines for follow up study. Surg Gynecol Obstet 1988; 166:497–502.

Messina JL, Glass LF, Cruse CW, Berman C, Ku NK, Reintgen DS. Pathologic examination of the sentinel lymph node in malignant melanoma. Am J Surg Pathol 1999; 23:686–690.

Morton DL, Wen DR, Wong JH, et al. Technical details of intraoperative lymphatic mapping for early stage melanoma. Arch Surg 1992; 127:392–399.

Morton DL, Thompson JF, Essner R, et al. Validation of the accuracy of intraoperative lymphatic mapping and sentinel lymphadenectomy for early-stage melanoma: a multicenter trial. Multicenter Selective Lymphadenectomy Trial Group. Ann Surg 1999; 230:453–463.

National Cancer Institute, DCCPS, Surveillance Research Program, Cancer Statistics Branch. Surveillance, Epidemiology, and End Results (SEER) Program Public-Use Data (1973–1998). Bethesda, MD: National Cancer Institute. Released April 2001.

Nachbar F, Stolz W, Merkel T, et al. The ABCD rule of dermatoscopy: high prospective value in the diagnosis of doubtful melanocytic skin lesions. J Am Acad Dermatol 1994; 30:551–559.

Orchard GE. Comparison of immunohistochemical labeling of melanocyte differentiation antibodies melan-A, tyrosinase and HMB 45 with NKIC3 and S100 protein in the evaluation of benign naevi and malignant melanoma. Histochem J 2000; 32:475–481.

Orchard GE, Wilson JE. Immunocytochemistry in the diagnosis of malignant melanoma. Br J Biomed Sci 1994; 51:44–56.

Paladugu RR, Yonemoto RH. Biologic behavior of thin malignant melanomas with regressive changes. Arch Surg 1983; 118:41–44.

Prade M, Bognel C, Charpentier P, et al. Malignant melanoma of the skin: prognostic factors derived from a multifactorial analysis of 239 cases. Am J Dermatopathol 1982; 4: 411–412.

Rhodes AR, Weinstock MA, Fitzpatrick TB, Mihm MC Jr, Sober AJ. Risk factors for cutaneous melanoma: a practical method of recognizing predisposed individuals. JAMA 1987; 258:3145–3153.

Ries LAG, Eisner MP, Kosary CL, et al. SEER Cancer Statistics Review, 1973—1998. Vol. 2001. Bethesda, MD, U.S.: National Cancer Institute, 2001.

Salopek TG, Kopf AW, Stefanato CM, Vossaert K, Silverman M, Yadav S. Differentiation of atypical moles (dysplastic nevi) from early melanomas by dermoscopy. Dermatol Clin 2001; 19(2):337–345.

Schaffer J, Rigel D, Kopf A, Bolognia J. Cutaneous melanoma—past, present, and future. J Am Acad Dermatol 2004:51.

Schmoeckel C, Castro CE, Braun-Falco O. Nevoid malignant melanoma. Arch Dermatol Res 1985; 277:362.

Shivers S, Wang X, Li W, et al. Molecular staging of malignant melanoma: correlation with clinical outcome. JAMA 1998; 280:1410–1415.

Terhune MH, Swanson NA, Johnson TM. Use of chest radiography in the initial evaluation of patients with localized melanoma. Arch Dermatol 1998; 134:569–572.

Thomas L, Tranchand P, Berard F, Secchi T, Colin C, Moulin G. Semiological value of ABCDE criteria in the diagnosis of cutaneous pigmented tumors. Dermatology 1998; 197:11–17.

Veronesi U, Cascinelli N. Narrow excision (1 cm margins): a safe procedure for thin cutaneous melanoma. Arch Surg 1991; 126:438–441.

Veronesi U, Cascinelli N, Adams J, et al. Thin stage I primary cutaneous malignant melanoma: comparison of excision with margins of 1 or 3 cm. N Engl J Med 1988; 318:1159–1162.

Vuylsteke RJ, van Leeuwen PA, Statius MMG, Gietema HA, Kragt DR, Meijer S. Clinical outcome of stage I/II melanoma patients after selective sentinel lymph node dissection: long-term follow-up results. J Clin Oncol 2003; 21(6):1057–1065.

Weinstock MA, Sober AJ. The risk of progression of lentigo maligna to lentigo maligna melanoma. Br J Dermatol 1987; 116:303.

Zartman GM, Thomas MR, Robinson WA. Metastatic disease in patients with newly diagnosed malignant melanomas. J Surg Oncol 1987; 35:163–164.

Zuo L, Weger J, Yang Q, et al. Nat Genet 1996; 12:97–99.

42

Fibrohistiocytic Tumors

Jennifer Z. Cooper and Marc D. Brown
Department of Dermatology, University of Rochester Medical Center, Rochester, New York, U.S.A.

INTRODUCTION

Fibrohistiocytic tumors are a group of soft-tissue neoplasms composed of cells that resemble fibroblasts and/or histiocytes. Historically, fibrohistiocytic tumors were designated as such to imply their tissue origin from a pleuropotential tissue histiocyte that could assume fibroblastic properties. To date, the histogenesis of fibrohistiocytic tumors remains uncertain, although more recent immunohistochemical studies provide evidence that the fibroblast is the probable cell of origin. Despite efforts to reclassify these tumors to correlate with their distinct cell of origin, the term will be used to encompass the three tumors to be discussed in this chapter: dermatofibrosarcoma protuberans (DFSPs), atypical fibroxanthoma (AFX) and malignant fibrous histiocytoma (MFH).

Fibrohistiocytic tumors can be classified according to their malignant potential. For example, the benign fibrohistiocytic tumors are diverse. The most common tumor of this classification is the benign cutaneous fibrous histiocytoma. While there is debate in terminology, the benign fibrous histiocytoma includes the dermatofibroma, which is so commonly encountered in clinical practice. Fibrohistiocytic tumors of intermediate malignancy include DFSP, and now the angiomatoid fibrous histiocytoma. The angiomatoid fibrous histiocytoma was previously regarded as angiomatoid MFH. This tumor was reclassified by the World Health Organization due to its less aggressive behavior when compared to the other variants of MFH. Finally, the malignant fibrohistiocytic tumors include AFX and the various subtypes of MFH. Conventionally, AFX has been considered to follow a course more similar to the tumors of intermediate malignancy. However, due to its histologically identical nature to the pleomorphic MFH and reports of metastases, it may be better viewed as a cutaneous variant of the pleomorphic MFH. Table 1 outlines the fibrohistiocytic tumors based on malignant potential.

DERMATOFIBROSARCOMA PROTUBERANS

The DFSP is a spindle cell neoplasm, with a marked propensity for local recurrence but a low incidence of metastatic spread. The DFSP was initially described in 1924 as a "progressive and recurring dermatofibroma." Due to its histologic similarity to the benign fibrous histiocytoma, it has been classified in the fibrohistiocytic tumor subset despite debate regarding its true cell of origin. The DFSP presents as a nodular cutaneous tumor more commonly during early or mid-adult life. The DFSP is slightly more common in males than in females, and is more frequently seen on the trunk and proximal extremity. Typical anatomic areas of involvement include the thigh, groin, abdomen, back, and chest. About 15% of all DFSP tumors occur in a head and neck location. The initial DFSP lesion may be plaque-like and/or sclerotic, with a surrounding red to blue discoloration. Differential diagnosis includes a keloid, dermatofibroma, or even localized scleroderma or morphea. There is a slow but relentless growth over a period of several years, eventually giving rise to a more accelerated growth phase with the development of one or more nodules. Satellite lesions can appear around the original tumor. This gives the clinical "protuberant" appearance (Fig. 1). There is also a well-described atrophic variant (Fig. 2). Patients will tend to stay relatively asymptomatic. The tumor is firm to palpation, sometimes freely mobile, but at times fixed to underlying muscle fascia. The Bednar tumor is a pigmented variant of the DFSP, occurring primarily in blacks (Fig. 3). Melanin-containing cells cause this distinctive coloration. Electron microscopic studies suggest that the fibroblast is the cell from which a DFSP arises.

Histologically, the DFSP is characterized by a uniform storiform pattern of plump spindle fibroblasts. It may assume a classic cartwheel appearance. Mitotic activity is low, and nuclear pleomorphism is minimal. Occasional tumors may show myxoid areas, characterized by the interstitial accumulation of hyaluronic acid ground substance. Myxoid foci are more commonly seen in recurrent tumors. The DFSP tumor diffusely infiltrates the dermis and subcutis. It interdigitates the subcutaneous fat lobules, and spreads along connective tissue septa and between adnexal structures (Figs. 4 and 5). The tumor infiltrates outward and downward, sending off tentacle or finger-like projections from the central mass. It does spread well beyond obvious clinical margins. The tumor tends to follow the path of least resistance, including muscle fascia, nerves, vessels, and adnexal structures. Recurrent tumors are more likely to invade deeper structures such as skeletal muscle. Sarcomatous changes are sometimes seen in these tumors.

Due to the histologic similarity between DFSP and the benign fibrous histiocytoma, immunocytochemical analysis has been a helpful discovery in the analysis of these tumors. The use of CD34, a human progenitor cell antigen, and Factor XIIIa, a fibrin stabilizing factor, has

Table 1 Fibrohistiocytic Tumors

Benign
  Dermatofibroma
Intermediate malignancy
  Dermatofibrosarcoma protuberans
  Angiomatoid fibrous histiocytoma
Low to high-grade malignancy
  Malignant fibrous histiocytoma
  Atypical fibrous xanthoma

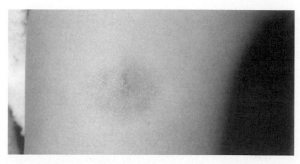

Figure 2 Subtle atrophic plaque on extremity consistent with atrophic variant of dermatofibrosarcoma protuberans. (*See color insert.*)

allowed better distinguishment between the two tumors. In general, DFSP stains positively for CD34, whereas the benign fibrous histiocytoma stains positively for Factor XIIIa. Other novel markers such as CD44, a membrane glycoprotein, and apolipoprotein D may have future applications as markers for DFSP.

DFSP is felt to arise on the nuclear level from atranslocation between chromosomes 17 and 22. Downstream this rearrangement results in continuous activation of the platelet-derived growth factor receptor beta protein tyrosine kinase by the collagen 1A1 promoter. This uncontrolled activation is felt to promote DFSP cell growth. Discovery of this important disregulation of pathways has led to the early development of targeted medical treatment for tumors such as the chemotherapeutic agent, Imantinib, both localized and metastatic, which exhibit this translocation.

Metastases are rare, occurring in only 1% to 4% of patients. It has been suggested that approximately 5% of DFSP tumors that show fibrosarcomatous change show a higher likelihood of recurrence and metastases. Although, it has been argued that with adequate and histologically clear resection margins, the recurrence rate of these tumors with sarcomatous change is no higher than the standard DFSP. The lung is the most common site of distant metastases, but they can also be seen in the brain, bone, and heart. Most cases of metastatic DFSP represent recurrent tumors (often multiple recurrences), with an interval of several years between initial diagnosis and the development of metastases. Unfortunately, the development of distant metastases is a poor prognostic sign, with most patients dying within two years.

Although the DFSP closely resembles the benign fibrous histiocytoma, it shows a marked tendency for locally aggressive growth, with local recurrence occurring in up to 50% of patients. The high recurrence is due to its extensive subcutaneous infiltration and initial inadequate surgical excisional margins. Most recurrences will be seen in the first two to three years, with 50% occurring within the first year. However, recurrences have been described as long as 20 years after surgical removal. Therefore, long-term follow-up is necessary. The recurrence rate correlates well with the surgical margin. Recurrence rates vary in the literature, but, in general, the larger the margin, the lower the recurrence rate. Gloster et al., and Parker and Zitelli analyzed data from patients cleared with Mohs surgery for DFSP. In a total of 38 patients, a 2.5 cm margin cleared the tumor in 100% of the patients. Recurrences remain highest for DFSP tumors of the head and neck (50–75%), reflecting the difficulty in achieving an adequate wide local excision. In a review of the literature, 15 studies with a total of 489 patients had recurrence rates varying from 0% to 60%. The potential subcutaneous spread of the tumor and standard bread loaf sectioning, which does not examine all margins probably accounts for the high rates of recurrence reported in various studies.

The primary treatment of DFSP is complete surgical excision. Current recommendations are for a wide local excision with a 1 to 3 cm margin down to and including the muscle fascia or periosteum. Due to the very low incidence

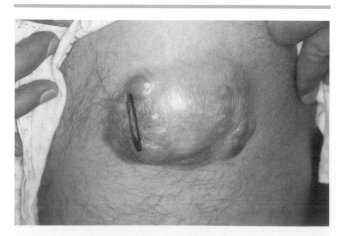

Figure 1 Dermatofibrosarcoma protuberans with classic protuberant appearance. Wedge biopsy to be performed. (*See color insert.*)

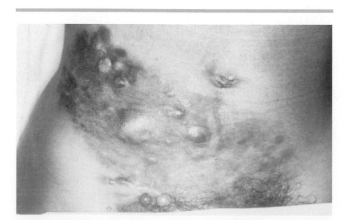

Figure 3 Pigmented dermatofibrosarcoma protuberans. (*See color insert.*)

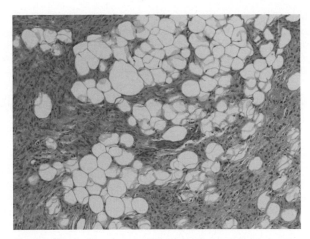

Figure 4 Microscopic image of DFSP (X20 H&E stain). (*See color insert.*)

of regional node involvement, elective lymph node dissection is not recommended.

Due to functional and cosmetic concerns, a wide excisional margin is not always feasible. To date, there have been multiple studies with significant follow-up data, confirming the utility of Mohs micrographic surgery (MMS) for tumor extirpation. The high cure rate of MMS is due to the ability of the procedure to carefully and meticulously track out the subclinical extensions of the DFSP tumor. The precise margin control of Mohs surgery (with simultaneous examination of the entire deep and/or peripheral margins) allows for complete tumor extirpation while preserving maximum normal tissue. Arbitrary margin guidelines thus become unnecessary. Multiple reports utilizing MMS for DFSP has shown an extremely low recurrence rate. A review of the literature in 1996 revealed a mean recurrence rate of 18% after wide local excision versus 0.6% with MMS. In a retrospective review of patients with more than five years follow-up, with an update of the literature in 2004, 136 patients had no recurrences or distant metastases in that time period. The suggestion of a multidisciplinary approach (MMS, wide local excision with circumferential and deep margin evaluation, or a combination of both) in the treatment of DFSP may lead to extremely high cure rates, even in the setting of a recurrent tumor.

ATYPICAL FIBROXANTHOMA

The AFX is probably best thought of as a superficial MFH or "MFH in situ." This tumor is histologically indistinguishable from pleomorphic form of MFH, but it does not invade deeper subcutaneous tissue, fascia, or muscle. Initially, the AFX was interpreted as a benign reactive lesion, but most dermatopathologists now view the AFX as a superficial or early form of the MFH.

Clinically, the AFX is typically seen on the actinically damaged skin of the elderly patient. It appears as an asymptomatic solitary nodule or nodular ulcer, most commonly on the nose, cheek, or ear (Fig. 4). Typically an AFX tumor is less than 2 cm in size; its clinical appearance is not distinctive and must be differentiated from a squamous cell carcinoma, basal cell carcinoma, or a necrotic pyogenic granuloma. As the tumor enlarges, it may erode, ulcerate, and bleed. Less commonly, the AFX tumor will present on the extremities and trunk of younger persons. These lesions are often larger, less well demarcated, and more nodular in appearance, with extension into the subcutaneous tissue.

The etiology of the AFX is uncertain, but ultraviolet exposure has to be a prime consideration given the common occurrence of this tumor on the actinically damaged face of elderly persons. p53 mutations have been noted in AFX tumors as well as AFX tumors, occurring in patients with xeroderma pigmentosum. Other actinic-related neoplasms are often associated with an AFX, including squamous cell carcinoma and melanoma (both locally aggressive and metastatic). In some cases, previous X-ray therapy has been proposed as an etiologic factor, although this is not consistently documented. The AFX is thought to be mesenchymal-derived neoplasm (like the MFH) rather than a spindled carcinoma. Electron microscopic studies have demonstrated fibroblastic and histiocytic-like cells and no features specifically suggesting epithelial differentiation.

Microscopic findings under low-power magnification show an expansile dermal nodule that often abuts the epidermis. Sometimes the tumor is separated from the epidermis by an area of uninvolved dermis or grenz zone. The AFX tumor can extend into the superficial subcutis, but by definition should not invade more deeply. Histologically, the AFX resembles a pleomorphic MFH. There is dense cellular infiltrate with pleomorphic hyperchromatic nuclei in an elongated irregular arrangement. A characteristic feature is that of large bizarre multinucleated cells arranged in a vague fascicular pattern. There can be marked nuclear atypia with many mitoses. Cells will vary from plump spindled cells to large rounded cells. A scattered inflammatory infiltrate can be seen sometimes. The histologic differential diagnosis of an AFX includes that of a spindle cell squamous cell carcinoma, melanoma, or metastatic cancer. Mucin and melanin stains are helpful, as are immunostains for cytokeratin and S-100 protein. The pleomorphic MFH differs from the AFX only by its deeper location in the subcutis or muscle, and its often larger size. Necrosis is also a prominent feature in the MFH, but is rarely seen in AFX. A clear cell variant has been described.

Because AFX is considered to be an early form of MFH, the distinction of the two is somewhat arbitrary; nonetheless, it is important to distinguish them because of their differing natural histories and recommended surgical treatment. It has been suggested that LN-2 (CD74) may

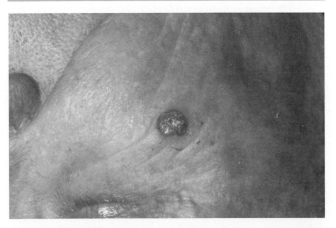

Figure 5 Atypical fibroxanthoma on sun-exposed areas of cheek and helical rim. Clinical differential diagnosis includes squamous cell carcinoma and basal cell carcinoma. (*See color insert.*)

aid in the distinguishment between the two tumors, with an MFH staining much more strongly that AFX. Deeper involvement, necrosis, and vascular or perineural invasion strongly suggest a diagnosis of MFH instead of AFX. An adequate biopsy is very important to distinguish AFX from MFH; if only a portion of the entire tumor is submitted for pathologic interpretation, it may be difficult to assess the true depth and nature of invasion.

The AFX has a very good prognosis. Due to its "in situ" dermal location, the risk of recurrence and/or metastatic disease is quite low. In one review, only 9 out of 140 patients developed a recurrence, and no metastatic lesions were found. There have been only 22 published cases of metastatic AFX since its first description in 1961. In rare instances, the AFX tumor can produce cutaneous metastatic disease, as well as regional lymph node and distant metastatic disease.

Recommended surgical treatment of an AFX should include complete excision and margin control. Due to the possible extension into superficial subcutaneous tissue, curettage and electrodessication or other superficial distinctive modalities are not recommended. Dissection should be carried well into the subcutaneous tissue or fascial plane in order to ensure a free deep margin. MMS can be utilized to treat AFX allowing for complete frozen section control. Brown and Swanson treated five patients with AFX. All tumors were less than 2 cm in size, none were recurrent, and all were excised easily with only one stage of Mohs surgery. Although a conservative excision may be a sufficient treatment for AFX, Mohs surgery does offer the advantage of tissue conservation in important facial areas as well as assurance of tumor-free margins at the time of surgery. If an AFX does recur in a deeper subcutaneous location, then it should be considered a MFH and treated accordingly. Due to the ambiguity in the distinguishment between AFX and pleomorphic MFH, most AFX tumors at this institution are treated with a combination of Mohs surgery with a 1 cm initial margin, with a deep margin sent for permanent sectioning.

MALIGNANT FIBROHISTIOCYTOMA

MFH is at present a diagnosis in evolution. It has been shown in several recent studies that tumors originally diagnosed as MFH are actually pleomorphic subtypes of other soft-tissue sarcomas. For the purposes of this chapter, the traditional subtypes of this tumor will be presented with the acknowledgment to the reader that the diagnosis of MFH may become obsolete in upcoming years.

The MFH has traditionally been considered the most common soft-tissue sarcoma of late adult life. MFH tumors can be classified as either superficial or deep. Superficial MFH tumors tend to be confined to the subcutaneous tissue, but may be attached to the fascia. Most MFH tumors presenting to the dermatologic surgeon will be of this superficial type, and overall will have a more favorable prognosis. However, the majority of MFH tumors are deeper lesions with approximately twice as many deeply situated tumors as superficial tumors. The deep MFH tumors can extend from subcutaneous tissue through fascia and into muscle. At times this tumor can be situated entirely within the muscle; this is especially true when MFH involves limb skeletal muscles.

Although there are several histologic subtypes of MFH, the clinical features are relatively similar. This neoplasm typically appears between the ages of 50 and 70.

The MFH tumor is extremely rare in patients under the age of 20. The tumor is slightly more common in males, and Caucasians are affected more frequently than Blacks or Orientals. Clinically, the MFH presents as a painless enlarging mass of several months duration. At times, growth of the tumor may be rapid. Accelerated growth has been observed during pregnancy. The tumor is usually solitary, can be multinodular, and may often be as large as 5 to 10 cm in size at the time of diagnosis. The more superficial of the MFH tumors are usually smaller at the time of diagnosis. The extremities are the most common sites of involvement, especially the thigh, buttocks, and limb skeletal muscles. The lower extremity is affected more commonly than the upper extremity. Any area of the body may be involved, and approximately 10% of the MFH tumors are on the head and neck region. Those MFH tumors located in the retroperitoneum are the largest because early diagnosis is difficult. If an MFH presents with evidence of metastatic disease, a primary source is usually readily diagnosable. This is in contrast to some other spindle squamous cell tumors, such as melanoma or spindle cell carcinomas, where there may be an unknown primary.

Most patients with MFH are asymptomatic. On occasion, there may be an associated fever and leukocytosis, which seems to resolve after the rumor is removed. Patients with retroperitoneal tumors may develop fatigue, weight loss, anorexia, and abdominal pain. The etiology of the MFH is unclear. There are sporadic reports suggesting that previous radiation exposure may be a predisposing factor, but this would explain only a minority of cases. Unlike AFX, sun exposure does not appear to be an important factor.

The MFH manifests a broad range of histologic appearances and is currently divided into four subtypes, which are not mutually exclusive (Table 2). However, to highlight the challenges of accuracy in making this diagnosis, Fletcher reviewed 159 cases of MFH and found only 100 would qualify as MFH by light microscopy standards and only 42 cases would qualify after rigorous immunohistochemistry and/or electron microscopy. More recently, Fletcher reviewed 100 tumors originally diagnosed as MFH. A specific line of differentiation was found in 84 of the tumors, and the tumors most commonly were identified to be high-grade myxofibrosarcoma and high-grade leiomyosarcoma. Tumors identified that showed myogenic differentiation had prognostic implications in a worse prognosis and shorter time to metastases.

The most common subtype is the *storiform-pleomorphic type*. This highly cellular tumor is composed of plump pleomorphic spindle cells, histiocytes, and frequent multinucleated giant cells. The morphologic pattern is highly variable with frequent transitions from storiform to pleomorphic areas. Mitotic figures are common and often atypical. Although the storiform-pleomorphic MFH may resemble a DFSP, there are distinctive histologic differences. The numerous atypical mitotic figures, less prominent storiform pattern, marked pleomorphism, and typical foamy giant cells seen with MFH are all key differential elements

Table 2 Malignant Fibrous Histiocytoma: Histologic Subtypes

Storiform-plemorphic

Myxoid

Giant cell

Inflammatory

Table 3 Malignant Fibrous Histiocytoma: Key Histologic Features

Focal storiform pattern
Marked plemorphism
Prominent atypical mitotic figures
Necrosis
Myxoid foci
Prominent foam cells and giant cells

Table 4 Prognostic Variables for Malignant Fibrous Histiocytoma

Good	Poor
Superficial	Deep
Intradermal	Skeletal muscle
Subcutis	Retroperitoneal
Small tumor size	Large tumor size
Distal extremity	Proximal extremity
Myxoid or angiomatoid variant	

(Table 3). The storiform-pleomorphic pattern would be the most common subtype presenting to the dermatologic surgeon. This shows the closest resemblance to its superficial counterpart, the AFX.

The *myxoid variant* of MFH is the next most frequent subtype, comprising approximately 25%. Histologically there is a prominent myxoid change of the stroma. Large areas appear hypocellular with widely spaced bizarre spindle-shaped cells in a myxoid matrix rich in acid mucopolysaccharides. For unclear reasons, the myxoid variant can be a slower-growing tumor and has a slightly better prognosis. The last two histologic subtypes are much less common. In the *inflammatory type*, there is diffuse neutrophilic infiltrate with numerous foam and xanthoma cells. The retroperitoneal MFH tumor is usually of the inflammatory type. The *giant cell* subtype shows osteoclastic-like giant cells. The histologic differential diagnosis of MFH includes pleomorphic variants of liposarcoma and rhabdomyosarcoma, pleomorphic carcinoma, histiocytic lymphoma, leiomyosarcoma, and epithelioid sarcoma, and as stated previously MFH may truly represent pleomorphic subtypes of these tumors. Prior to reclassification, there was an angiomatoid subtype, which has now been renamed as an angiomatoid fibrous histiocytoma due to its much better prognosis.

Although the MFH has a clinical appearance of being a circumscribed tumor, it often spreads for considerable distances along the fascial planes or between muscle fibers. Invasive behavior of the MFH accounts for its high rate of local recurrence, estimated to be 20% to 30% even after wide local excision for the storiform-pleomorphic subtype. Unfortunately, the metastatic rate is also in the range of 50% with a high associated mortality. The five-year survival is only about 65% to 70%. Metastatic disease occurs early (usually within two years of diagnosis) and most frequently affects the lung, liver, lymph nodes, and bone.

Prognosis appears to correlate best with the depth of the MFH tumor (not unlike other aggressive cutaneous tumors such as melanoma, squamous cell carcinoma, and Merkel cell cancers). For example, less than 10% of MFH tumors confined entirely to the subcutis without deeper fascial or muscle involvement will metastasize. The size of the tumor also correlates with the risk metastatic disease, but this may be a covariable with tumor depth. Anatomic location of the tumor also correlates with prognosis. Distally located MFH tumors have a better prognosis than proximally located tumors. Histologic features, including degree of anaplasia and the number of mitoses, appear to have little prognostic value. However, the histologic subtype of the myxoid variant appears to do slightly better. There is some evidence that tumors with a significant inflammatory response may have an improved prognosis, but the metastatic rate for the inflammatory subtype is still in the range of 30% to 35%. In a retrospective analysis of 109 patients with MFH (various subtypes), relapse-free five year survival was 39% and five year overall survival was 50%. However,

25% of patients underwent excision with margins less than 2 cm, but over half received adjuvant radiation. Table 4 outlines the prognostic variables for MFH.

Surgical excision is the mainstay of therapy for MFH. Because this tumor can spread a considerable distance beyond the gross tumor margins, aggressive wide and deep local excision or even possible amputation has been recommended. Recurrence rates are directly related to the adequacy of the surgical treatment and establishment of tumor-free margins. One of the major problems in dealing with this soft-tissue sarcoma is adequate local control of the primary tumor. MFH tumors with local recurrence do have a much worse prognosis, so complete excision of the primary tumor is important. Islands of tumor cells may extend well beyond what appears to be a well-encapsulated neoplasm. As with other aggressive cutaneous tumors, the MFH has a tendency to invade along fascial planes, muscle fibers, nerves, and blood vessels. Wide excisional margins of 3 to 5 cm may still result in recurrence rates of 30% to 40%, dependent somewhat on the previously described prognostic factors. Positive surgical resection margins will result in a local recurrence rate between 50% and 90%. Recurrence will usually recur within the first two years after surgery of the primary tumor. More radical surgical procedures such as complete muscle compartment excision or limb amputation will give higher cure rates, but with greater patient morbidity. Less radical surgery in conjunction with radiation and/or chemotherapy is becoming more popular for soft-tissue sarcomas. Even with adequate local control, metastatic disease will still occur. Only a minority of patients (less than 10%) will initially present with evidence of metastases. Because lymph node metastases are relatively infrequent, elective lymph node dissection of regional nodes is usually not recommended. Lymph node dissection should be reserved for those patients with clinically suspicious nodes and/or positive nodal biopsy.

For those more superficially located MFH tumors, MMS appears to be an excellent surgical modality. Although a more time-consuming and meticulous procedure, Mohs surgery is capable of tracing out the deepest and widest extensions of the MFH tumor as it spreads along anatomic planes. The MFH tumor is easily visualized with frozen section technology. Brown and Swanson, respectively, looked at 17 patients with a total of 20 MFH tumors who underwent MMS. Half of these patients already had local recurrence

Table 5 Malignant Fibrous Histiocytoma: Evaluation

Size and anatomic location
Fixation to deep structures
Lymph nodes
Chest X-ray
Malignant fibrous histiocytoma to asses depth and extent of local spread
Computed tomography of chest for high-risk patients
Consultation with radiation and medical oncology

Table 6   Treatment of Fibrohistiocytomas

Tumor	Excisional margins (cm)	Mohs surgery	Adjuvant radiation/chemo Rx
AFX	1	Tissue sparing for important cosmetic areas	No; XRT can be considered
MFH	35	Yes (except for deep skeletal and retroperitoneal tumors)	Yes, for high-risk tumors
DFSP	3	Yes	No; imantinib for metastases or unresectable tumors

Abbreviations: AFX, atypical fibroxauthoma; MFH, malignant fibrous histiocytoma; DFSP, dematofibrorarcoma protuberans; XRT, adjuvant radiotherapy.

of their MFH from a previous non-Mohs procedure. All patients were treated in an outpatient setting. Standard horizontal frozen sections were prepared in the usual manner after appropriate mapping and staining of the excised tissue. The locations of these tumors were widespread with the averages preoperative tumor size of 3 cm. The patients required an average of 2.5 stages and 16 tissue sections to achieve tumor-free margins. The average postoperative defect size was 4.8 cm. The average follow-up was approximately four years. There was local recurrence of only one tumor, and the patient subsequently underwent a second Mohs surgical procedure and remained tumor-free. One patient developed probable metastatic disease to the lungs, but an autopsy was not performed at the time of death. Thus, the overall success rate with Mohs surgery was excellent. These MFH tumors were primarily of the storiform-pleomorphic type with origin of the tumor in the dermis and subcutis. However, a number of these tumors did extend into the muscle. The more superficial location and relatively smaller size may have contributed to the higher success rate. Nonetheless, for select MFH tumors, Mohs surgery offered a precise surgical approach with careful tracking of the tumor and clear definition of tumor-free margins. There was also the value of tissue sparing, which becomes extremely important for the approximately 10% of MFH tumors located in the head and neck region. Local recurrence portends in this anatomic area portends a lower

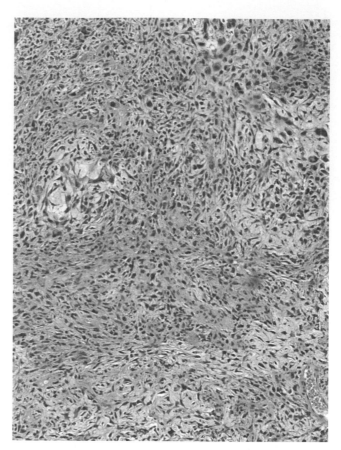

Figure 7   Cellular spindle cell lesion with marked nuclear pleomorphism (hematoxylin and eosin stain, x10).

five-year survival in patients with tumors of the head and neck over the extremity (in one study, 48% vs. 77%).

The preoperative evaluation of patients with MFH is outlined in Table 5,6. It is important to note the size of the tumor, its anatomic location, and possible fixation of the tumor to deeper structures such as muscle. Careful palpation of regional lymph nodes should be performed. Clinically suspicious nodes should be biopsied. Because the lungs are the most common site of metastatic disease, a chest X-ray should be performed for all MFH tumors. For the higher-risk, deep and large MFH tumors, a computed tomography (CT) of the chest should be undertaken. Evidence of metastatic disease may well alter the overall treatment plan. At times, resection of a solitary pulmonary metastasis can be performed, but only after a complete evaluation and staging of the metastatic disease. CT or magnetic resonance imaging scans can also be helpful to assess the depth and extent of local spread of these MFH tumors. With better classification strategies for these tumors previously labeled as MFH, better intervention for this aggressive subset of tumors may be on the horizon. Figure 6 outlines the treatment considerations for the fibrohistiocytic tumors.

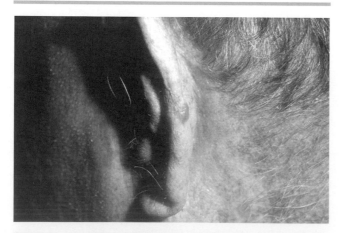

Figure 6   Atypical fibroxanthoma on sun-exposed areas of cheek and helical rim. Clinical differential diagnosis includes squamous cell carcinoma and basal cell carcinoma. (See color insert.)

BIBLIOGRAPHY

Alguacil-Garcia A, et al. Atypical fibroxanthoma of the skin: an ultrastructural study of two cases. Cancer 1977; 40(4): 1471–1480.

Barr RJ, Wuerker RB, Graham JH. Ultrastructure of atypical fibroxanthoma. Cancer 1977, 10(2).750–745.

Bertoni F, et al. Malignant fibrous histiocytoma of soft tissue. An analysis of 78 cases located and deeply seated in the extremities. Cancer 1985; 56(2):356–367.

Belal A et al. Malignant fibrous histiocytoma: a retrospective study of 109 cases. Am J Clin Oncol 2002; 25(1):16–22.

Beck HG, Lechner W, Wunsch PH. [Metastasizing soft tissue tumor of light damaged skin: atypical fibroxanthoma or malignant fibrous histiocytoma?] Z Hautkr 1985; 60(21):1702–1704, 1707–1710.

Bowne WB, et al. Dermatofibrosarcoma protuberans: a clinicopathologic analysis of patients treated and followed at a single institution. Cancer 2000; 88(12):2711–2720.

Brown MD, Swanson NA. Treatment of malignant fibrous histiocytoma and atypical fibrous xanthomas with micrographic surgery. J Dermatol Surg Oncol 1989; 15(12):1287–1292.

Calikoglu E et al. CD44 and hyaluronate in the differential diagnosis of dermatofibroma and dermatofibrosarcoma protuberans. J Cutan Pathol 2003; 30(3):185–189.

Cooper JZ et al. Metastasizing atypical fibroxanthoma (cutaneous malignant histiocytoma): report of five cases. Dermatol Surg 2005; 31(2):221–225; discussion 225.

Dahl I. Atypical fibroxanthoma of the skin. A clinico-pathological study of 57 cases. Acta Pathol Microbiol Scand [A] 1976; 84(2):183–197.

Darier J. FM. Dermatofibromas professifs et recidivants on fibrosarcomes de la peau. Ann Dermatol Venereol 1924; 5:545–562.

Dei Tos AP et al. Ultraviolet-induced p53 mutations in atypical fibroxanthoma. Am J Pathol 1994; 145(1):11–17.

Dilek FH et al. Atypical fibroxanthoma of the skin and the lower lip in xeroderma pigmentosum. Br J Dermatol 2000; 143(3):618–620.

Dupree WB, Langloss JM, Weiss SW. Pigmented dermatofibrosarcoma protuberans (Bednar tumor). A pathologic, ultrastructural, and immunohistochemical study. Am J Surg Pathol 1985; 9(9):630–639.

DuBay D et al. Low recurrence rate after surgery for dermatofibrosarcoma protuberans: a multidisciplinary approach from a single institution. Cancer 2004; 100(5):1008–1016.

Enzinger FM, Weiss WS. Soft Tissue Tumors. 4th. Philadelphia: Mosby, 2001.

Erlandson RA, Antonescu CR. The rise and fall of malignant fibrous histiocytoma. Ultrastruct Pathol 2004; 28(5–6):283–289.

Fletcher CD. Pleomorphic malignant fibrous histiocytoma: fact or fiction? A critical reappraisal based on 159 tumors diagnosed as pleomorphic sarcoma. Am J Surg Pathol 1992; 16(3):213–228.

Fletcher CD, et al. Dermatofibrosarcoma protuberans: a clinicopathological and immunohistochemical study with a review of the literature. Histopathology 1985; 9(9):921–938.

Fletcher CD et al. Clinicopathologic re-evaluation of 100 malignant fibrous histiocytomas: prognostic relevance of subclassification. J Clin Oncol 2001; 19(12):3045–3050.

Fletcher CD et al. Pigmented dermatofibrosarcoma protuberans (Bednar tumour): melanocytic colonization or neuroectodermal differentiation? A clinicopathological and immunohistochemical study. Histopathology 1988; 13(6):631–643.

Frierson HF, Cooper PH. Myxoid variant of dermatofibrosarcoma protuberans. Am J Surg Pathol 1983; 7(5):445–450.

Fretzin DF, Helwig EB. Atypical fibroxanthoma of the skin. A clinicopathologic study of 140 cases. Cancer 1973; 31(6):1541–1552.

Giuffrida TJ, Kligora CJ, Goldstein GD. Localized cutaneous metastases from an atypical fibroxanthoma. Dermatol Surg 2004; 30(12 Pt 2):1561–1564.

Gloster HM Jr., Harris KR, Roenigk RK. A comparison between Mohs micrographic surgery and wide surgical excision for the treatment of dermatofibrosarcoma protuberans. J Am Acad Dermatol 1996; 35(1):82–87.

Glavin FL, Cornwell ML. Atypical fibroxanthoma of the skin metastatic to a lung. Report of a case, features by conventional and electron microscopy, and a review of relevant literature. Am J Dermatopathol 1985; 7(1):57–63.

Goldblum JR, Tuthill RJ. CD34 and factor-XIIIa immunoreactivity in dermatofibrosarcoma protuberans and dermatofibroma. Am J Dermatopathol 1997; 19(2):147–153.

Grosso M, et al. Metastatic atypical fibroxanthoma of skin. Pathol Res Pract 1987; 182(3):443–447.

Helwig EB, May D. Atypical fibroxanthoma of the skin with metastasis. Cancer 1986; 57(2):368–376.

Hodl S. [Metastasizing atypical fibroxanthoma or malignant fibrous. Clinical and histological picture, nosology, nomenclature]. histiocytoma. Arch Dermatol Res 1982; 273(1–2):25–35.

Hudson AW, Winkelmann RK. Atypical fibroxanthoma of the skin: a reappraisal of 19 cases in which the original diagnosis was spindle-cell squamous carcinoma. Cancer 1972; 29(2):413–422.

Ivetzin DF, Helvig EB. Atypical fibrous xanthoma: a clinicopathologic study of 140 cases. Cancer 1973; 57:368.

Jacobs DS, Edwards WD, Ye RC. Metastatic atypical fibroxanthoma of skin. Cancer 1975; 35(2):457–463.

Kemp JD, et al. Metastasizing atypical fibroxanthoma. Coexistence with chronic lymphocytic leukemia. Arch Dermatol 1978; 114(10):1533–1535.

Kearney MM, Soule EH, Ivins JC. Malignant fibrous histiocytoma: a retrospective study of 167 cases. Cancer 1980; 45(1):167–178.

Kyriakos M, Kempson RL. Inflammatory fibrous histiocytoma. An aggressive and lethal lesion. Cancer 1976; 37(3):1584–1606.

Lautier R, Wolff HH, Jones RE. An immunohistochemical study of dermatofibrosarcoma protuberans supports its fibroblastic character and contradicts neuroectodermal or histiocytic components. Am J Dermatopathol 1990; 12(1):25–30.

Lazova R et al. LN-2 (CD74). A marker to distinguish atypical fibroxanthoma from malignant fibrous histiocytoma. Cancer 1997; 79(11):2115–2124.

Le Doussal V et al. Prognostic factors for patients with localized primary malignant fibrous histiocytoma: a multicenter study of 216 patients with multivariate analysis. Cancer 1996; 77(9):1823–1830.

McArthur G. Molecularly targeted treatment for dermatofibrosarcoma protuberans. Semin Oncol 2004; 31(2 Suppl 6):30–36.

Miller SJ, et al. Dermatofibrosarcoma protuberans clinical practice guidelines in oncology. JNCCN 2004; 2:74–78.

Parker TL, Zitelli JA. Surgical margins for excision of dermatofibrosarcoma protuberans. J Am Acad Dermatol 1995; 32(2 Pt 1):233–236.

Patterson JW, Konerding H, Kramer WM. "Clear cell" atypical fibroxanthoma. J Dermatol Surg Oncol 1987; 13(10):1109–1114.

Patterson JW, Jordan WP Jr. Atypical fibroxanthoma in a patient with xeroderma pigmentosum. Arch Dermatol 1987; 123(8):1066–1070.

Rutgers EJ, et al. Dermatofibrosarcoma protuberans: treatment and prognosis. Eur J Surg Oncol 1992; 18(3):241–248.

Sankar NM et al. Metastasis from atypical fibroxanthoma of skin. Med J Aust 1998; 168(8):418–419.

Sabesan T, et al. Malignant fibrous histiocytoma: Outcome of tumours in the head and neck compared with those in the trunk and extremities. Br J Oral Maxillofac Surg 2005.

Salo JC et al. Malignant fibrous histiocytoma of the extremity. Cancer 1999; 85(8):1765–1772.

Snow SN, et al. Dermatofibrosarcoma protuberans: a report on 29 patients treated by Mohs micrographic surgery with long-term follow-up and review of the literature. Cancer 2004; 101(1):28–38.

Taylor HB, Helwig EB. Dermatofibrosarcoma protuberans. A study of 115 cases. Cancer 1962; 15:717–725.

Weiss SW, Enzinger FM. Myxoid variant of malignant fibrous histiocytoma. Cancer 1977; 39(4):1672–1685.

West RB, et al. Apo D in soft tissue tumors: a novel marker for dermatofibrosarcoma protuberans. Am J Surg Pathol 2004; 28(8):1063–1069.

Weiss SW, Enzinger FM. Malignant fibrous histiocytoma: an analysis of 200 cases. Cancer 1978; 41(6):2250–2266.

Youssef N et al. Two unusual tumors in a patient with xeroderma pigmentosum: atypical fibroxanthoma and basosquamous carcinoma. J Cutan Pathol 1999; 26(9):4 30–435.

Zagars GK, Mullen JR, Pollack A. Malignant fibrous histiocytoma: outcome and prognostic factors following conservation surgery and radiotherapy. Int J Radiat Oncol Biol Phys 1996; 34(5):983–994.

43

Unusual Tumors

**Whitney A. High, James E. Fitzpatrick,
and Loren E. Golitz**

*Department of Dermatopathology, University of Colorado Health Sciences Center,
Denver, Colorado, U.S.A.*

INTRODUCTION

The tumors discussed within this chapter arise from epithelial cells differentiating toward adnexal structures, except for Merkel cell tumor, which is considered to be a primary neuroendocrine carcinoma of the skin. The derivation, classification, and nomenclature of the adnexal tumors are controversial, and important disagreements will be addressed. This chapter is organized into subunits based upon tumoral differentiation toward hair, sebaceous glands, apocrine glands, and eccrine glands, with the final section discussing Merkel cell carcinoma.

Management of most benign cutaneous tumors involves surgical excision, although important alternatives exist for some lesions. All the malignant tumors discussed are capable of metastasis, and their management is more controversial. Special emphasis will be placed upon the clinical and histologic diagnosis of the malignant tumors.

TUMORS OF FOLLICULAR DIFFERENTIATION

Trichofolliculoma

Trichofolliculoma is an uncommon benign hair follicle tumor, first described by Miescher in 1944. It is one of the few adnexal tumors with a distinct clinical appearance. The typical lesion is a solitary, firm, dome-shaped, skin-colored papule measuring 3 to 5 mm in diameter, with a dilated central pore. Trichofolliculomas are characteristically located upon the face or scalp (Fig. 1). Careful examination may often reveal a small wisp of fine white hairs emanating from the follicular orifice, referred to as a "wool-wisp" or "feather" hair.

Histologic examination reveals a central keratin-filled primary follicle, surrounded by multiple radiating secondary hair follicles. Epithelial strands may connect some of the secondary hair follicles. The primary follicle contains multiple vellus hairs, and the secondary follicles demonstrate variable degrees of follicular differentiation, ranging from immature basaloid islands to well-formed papillae with vellus hairs. The tumor is surrounded by a well-circumscribed fibrotic stroma. If mature sebaceous glands are

present, some authorities use the term "sebaceous trichofolliculoma." Furthermore, there is evidence to suggest that folliculosebaceous cystic hamartoma, a recently described entity, is in fact, a late stage of trichofolliculoma.

Within the gynecological literature, a small case series associated trichofolliculoma with severe vulvar intraepithelial neoplasia; however, the occurrence is likely coincidental, and no other significant associations have been reported. Surgical removal is curative. Exophytic lesions may be removed by shave biopsy, but the majority require punch or elliptical excision to extirpate the deeper component.

Fibrofolliculoma

Fibrofolliculomas are usually multiple, and may be associated with Birt–Hogg–Dube syndrome—an autosomal-dominant inherited disorder caused by defects in a novel protein, folliculin, and associated with kidney tumors and spontaneous pneumothorax. Solitary and incidental lesions may occur as well. The primary lesion is a 1 to 4 mm white or yellow-white, dome-shaped papule, with a central keratin plug demonstrated in some cases. Fibrofolliculomas are most often located upon the head and neck, but may also occur on the trunk and arms.

Histologic examination reveals a central keratin-filled follicle. Radiating from this follicle are thin strands of follicular epithelium that may anastomose with adjacent projections. Surrounding this abortive follicle is a well-demarcated mantle of fibrous tissue composed of collagen, elastin, and dermal mucin, which represents a proliferation of a rudimentary fibrous root sheath.

It had been thought that within Birt–Hogg–Dube syndrome, fibrofolliculomas occurred in association with trichodiscomas and acrochordons. More recently, however, it has been discovered that in all likelihood, the skin manifestations of this syndrome are all variations of the same lesion, namely fibrofolliculoma. Variations in histologic sectioning and clinical bias in tissue sampling (lesions resembling acrochordons are not typically sampled) account for differences in the histological appearance.

Fibrofolliculomas that are cosmetically unacceptable may be removed by punch or elliptical excision. Exophytic lesions may be removed by shave technique. When lesions are multiple, consideration of Birt–Hogg–Dube syndrome should be given, and a thorough history taken, particularly with respect to renal carcinoma within the family. Associated pulmonary findings necessitate a screening chest X ray, especially in younger family members, because of the

---

Many of the photos herein were obtained by one of the authors (James E. Fitzpatrick) during assignment to Fitzsimons Army Medical Center, Aurora, Colorado, U.S.A. The opinions or assertions contained herein are the views of the authors and are not to be considered as reflecting the views of the U.S. Department of the Army or the Department of Defense. This is a U.S. Government publication and is in the public domain.

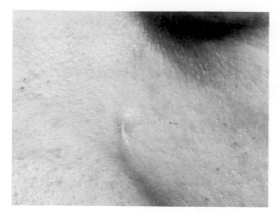

Figure 1   Trichofolliculoma: small, skin-colored papule with characteristic white feathery tuft composed of miniature hairs.

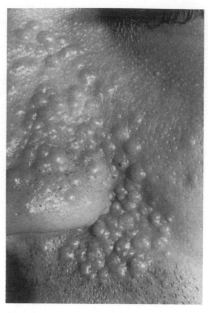

Figure 2   Multiple trichoepitheliomas: small papules and nodules in characteristic distribution. Small white areas representing foci of keratinization can be seen in several of the papules.

association with recurrent spontaneous pneumothorax, bullous emphysema, and lung cysts.

Trichoepithelioma

Trichoepitheliomas are poorly differentiated, benign follicular tumors that may be confused, both clinically and histologically, with basal cell carcinoma. Common variants include solitary conventional trichoepithelioma, multiple conventional trichoepitheliomas, and desmoplastic trichoepithelioma.

Solitary conventional trichoepithelioma occurs sporadically and is typically located on the midface, although it may occur elsewhere. The primary lesion is a firm, flesh-colored or slightly white papule usually measuring 2 to 10 mm. Multiple conventional trichoepitheliomas may be inherited in autosomal-dominant fashion and may be associated with other adnexal tumors, such as cylindromas or eccrine spiradenomas (Brooke–Spiegler syndrome). Multiple lesions are identical to the solitary form and are typically located on the nasolabial folds, nose, forehead, upper lips, and around the eyes (Fig. 2). Linear and dermatomal distributions have also been described. The clinical differential diagnosis includes tuberous sclerosis, basal cell nevus syndrome, multiple perifollicular fibromas, and multiple syringomas.

Histologic examination of conventional trichoepitheliomas reveals a proliferation of variably sized, basaloid islands of epithelium within the superficial dermis, forming a characteristic "lace-like" pattern. Unlike basal cell carcinoma, trichoepitheliomas are well demarcated and do not manifest an infiltrative growth pattern. Some epithelial islands may be solid, while others have central keratinizing centers yielding small cystic structures thought to be an abortive attempt at hair differentiation. Some lesions may demonstrate formation of primitive hair bulbs or distinct fibroblastic aggregations termed "papillary mesenchymal bodies," because they resemble normal follicular papillary mesenchyme. The surrounding stroma often demonstrates a fibroblastic response.

There exists evidence suggesting a qualitative immunohistological difference between basal cell carcinoma and trichoepithelioma when stained for *bcl-2*. Basal cell carcinoma is thought to stain homogenously with *bcl-2*, while trichoepithelioma demonstrates preferential staining at the periphery of the lobules. Immunohistochemical staining for p53 and Ki-67 (a proliferation marker) may also be discriminatory. In situations engendering confusion, such immunohistochemical studies may prove helpful.

Desmoplastic trichoepithelioma is a clinical and histologic variant that is typically solitary. The primary lesion is a firm, fleshy or white-yellow, often slightly annular papule measuring 3 to 8 mm. The most common location is the face, with almost one-half occurring on the cheek. The annular appearance is so characteristic that the diagnosis may be suspected clinically. Histologically, desmoplastic trichoepithelioma is characterized by the presence of narrow basaloid epithelial strands, horn cysts, and dense desmoplastic stroma. Some lesions demonstrate variable calcification and/or foreign body reaction. The relative absence of epidermal connections, invasive architecture, peripheral palisading of nuclei, and retraction artifact from the surrounding dermal stroma may assist in differentiation from morpheaform basal cell carcinoma.

Solitary conventional and desmoplastic trichoepitheliomas are managed by simple excision of the tumor. Multiple trichoepitheliomas represent a significant cosmetic problem. Being so numerous, they are not easily amenable to surgical removal. Methods that may restore normal facial contour include dermabrasion, multiple shave excisions, electrosurgery, or cryotherapy. Because these techniques do not usually remove the deeper aspects of the tumor, regrowth may occur over a period of years. Excellent results have been reported with carbon dioxide laser resurfacing procedures. There exists a single case report noting an approximate 80% clearing of multiple trichoepitheliomas using topical imiquimod and tretinoin over a three-year period. Other modalities, including irradiation, generally produce less satisfactory long-term results.

Pilomatricoma (Calcifying Epithelioma, Pilomatrixoma)

Pilomatricoma, also known as calcifying epithelioma of Malherbe, is a benign follicular tumor arising from the hair matrix. Lesions are typically single, but can be multiple. Multiple pilomatricomas may occur sporadically or may be inherited as an autosomal-dominant trait. Rare cases may be associated with myotonic dystrophy. Abnormalities in beta-catenin, a protein involved in developmental cascades, have been detected within pilomatricomas and also within some colon, hepatocellular, and other carcinomas.

Pilomatricomas typically arise in children and young adults, with 40% occurring before the age of 10 years. Three-quarters of all pilomatricomas occur on the head and neck. Most develop slowly, although a subset may demonstrate rapid growth. The primary lesion is a dermal or subcutaneous nodule, and the overlying skin is usually normal, although variants extruding granular calcified material have been described. The lesions may be skin colored, erythematous, or even violaceous. Calcification may yield a yellow or white discoloration near the surface (Fig. 3). When the skin is stretched, multiple facets of the tumor may be appreciated, producing the classic "tent sign." Clinically, the differential diagnosis includes epidermoid cyst, trichilemmal cyst, and other adnexal neoplasms.

Histologic examination of pilomatricomas demonstrates the tumor to be composed of two main cell types: a basophilic matrical cell typically located at the periphery, and a more eosinophilic "shadow cell" or "ghost cell" located centrally, which lacks nuclear staining, but instead demonstrates a faint unstained area at the site of the former nucleus. As the matrical element is proliferating, an increased numbers of mitotic figures may be present. The matrical cells may also demonstrate focal squamatization. Calcification, ossification, and foreign body reaction may also be observed.

Pilomatricoma is best managed by surgical excision, which is usually curative. Recurrence may follow incomplete removal. Tumors that recur should be excised because of the rare occurrence of pilomatrix carcinoma. Pilomatrical carcinoma, a rare entity, has the potential for metastasis and death, and wide local excision or complete micrographic removal is advocated.

Proliferating Trichilemmal Cyst (Pilar Tumor)

Most dermatopathologists believe proliferating trichilemmal cysts arise from the outer root sheath of the hair follicle, but at least nine terms have been used in the literature to describe this tumor. This neoplasm typically affects the scalp of elderly women. The primary lesion is a slow-growing, firm, subcutaneous nodule.

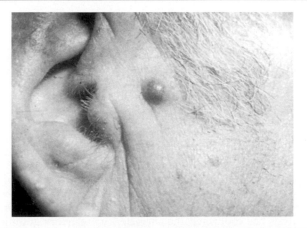

Figure 3 Pilomatricoma: violaceous nodule that was hard on palpation.

Histological examination reveals a large subcutaneous or dermal tumor that is well demarcated and composed of interlacing lobules of squamous epithelium. Abrupt trichilemmal keratinization is present in the center of at least some islands. Aggregates of squamous cells may extend focally into the surrounding dermis, but in general, the proliferation is mostly inwards. The tumor is particularly important because it can be confused histologically with squamous cell carcinoma. In the single largest study of proliferating trichilemmal cysts, conducted at the Armed Forces Institute of Pathology, it was determined that among 63 lesions, frank carcinomatous degeneration was revealed in 10, including a single lesion with lymph node metastases. These malignant variants of proliferating trichilemmal cyst have features in common with proliferating trichilemmal cyst, including abrupt keratinization and a hyperplastic squamous epithelium forming solid areas. In our opinion, the diagnosis of malignancy is determined by a high mitotic rate and the presence of atypical mitosis and severe nuclear pleomorphism, in association with demonstrable invasion of the adjacent tissues.

Proliferating trichilemmal cysts are best treated by surgical excision with clear surgical margins. Complete removal is of particular importance given the known recurrence of this lesion, the existence of a malignant variant, and confusion of the lesion with squamous cell carcinoma. Similarly, appropriate follow-up is essential. At least one such tumor has been inadvertently treated as a squamous cell carcinoma, using bleomycin and radiotherapy, and responded well to this regimen; however such treatment is not recommended.

SEBACEOUS GLAND TUMORS

Sebaceous Adenoma

Sebaceous adenoma is a benign adnexal tumor occurring most commonly as a solitary lesion on the face, scalp, or anterior trunk. Most patients report a history of slow growth, but rapid evolution may occur. The primary lesion is not distinctive clinically and is usually described as a tan/yellow, pink/red, or skin-colored papule of approximately 5 mm diameter. Larger lesions (up to 9 cm) have been described. Less commonly, the papules may be ulcerated or pedunculated.

Sebaceous adenomas are important; as they may be markers for Muir–Torre syndrome. Muir–Torre syndrome consists of the association of sebaceous neoplasms, possible keratoacanthomas, and colonic polyposis and carcinoma. In most cases, an autosomal-dominant pattern of inheritance has been implicated, although sporadic mutations exist. DNA mismatch repair enzymes have been implicated within the syndrome. In a large series of solitary sebaceous adenomas reviewed by the Armed Forces Institute of Pathology, 11 of 46 patients maintained a history of visceral malignancy. Although controlled studies are needed, preliminary evidence suggests that even solitary sebaceous adenomas may be markers for visceral malignancies.

Histologic examination reveals a well-demarcated tumor composed of sebaceous lobules connected to the overlying epidermis. The lobules are composed of two cell types: a germinative cell layer of basophilic cells arranged around the periphery and larger cells with variable sebaceous differentiation located centrally. Generally speaking, the sebaceous-appearing cells compose a greater fraction of the lesion. Tumors demonstrating incomplete differentiation, an increased numbers of mitotic figures, and limited sebaceous differentiation may be difficult to separate from basal cell carcinoma with sebaceous differentiation (sebaceous epithelioma) or sebaceous carcinoma.

Sebaceous adenomas are best managed by curettage or shave or elliptical excision. Cryosurgery may yield satisfactory cosmetic results. Short-term studies have demonstrated that multiple sebaceous adenomas, even those associated with Muir–Torre, will decrease in number and size following the administration of oral isotretinoin or oral isotretinoin with parenteral interferon-α. Because of the association with Muir–Torre syndrome, anecdotal reports have suggested that a thorough personal and family history of malignancy should be solicited from all patients with sebaceous adenoma, with a low threshold for age-appropriate or symptom-directed cancer screening.

Sebaceoma

Sebaceoma represents a benign sebaceous neoplasm, and its recognition has largely replaced the entities sebaceous epithelioma and basal cell with sebaceous differentiation. Like sebaceous adenoma, sebaceoma has been associated with Muir–Torre syndrome (see discussion above).

Clinically, sebaceoma presents as a yellow or yellow-orange papule or nodule in an adult. Almost all tumors have been located on the face or scalp. Lesions develop slowly and are sometimes multiple.

Histologically, sebaceomas are composed of circumscribed dermal aggregates of basaloid cells that demonstrate cystic spaces within the epitheloid islands. The cystic spaces frequently contain eosinophilic amorphous debris consistent with sebaceous holocrine secretion. Within the basaloid islands, there are differentiated sebaceous cells, either singly or in small clusters. The surrounding stroma is often sclerotic.

Sebaceomas are benign sebaceous tumors, and complete removal is not required unless cosmetic concerns exist. Of chief concern is possible histological confusion with basal carcinoma, leading to overly aggressive therapeutic intervention. Electrodessication and curettage, cryosurgery, shave removal, and elliptical excision are all curative. Because of the association with Muir–Torre syndrome, a complete history and evaluation are prudent.

Sebaceous Carcinoma

Sebaceous carcinoma is a cutaneous malignancy that can occur on the eyelid or other skin surface. Sebaceous carcinomas of the eyelid typically originate from the Meibomian glands, although they may also arise from the glands of Zeis. The tumor most often arises upon the upper eyelid and presents as a firm nodule (Fig. 4), Alternative presentations include papillomatous growths or as mimics of chronic inflammatory conditions such as chalazions, blepharoconjunctivitis, or keratoconjunctivitis. This particular subset of sebaceous carcinoma is quite important, as it is regarded as one of the most lethal tumors of the eye. Large reviews have reported high local recurrence rates (32%), frequent lymph node metastases (17%), and high mortality rates (6–25%).

Extraocular sebaceous carcinoma arising of the skin is less common. Such a lesion usually arises on the scalp or face (75%), trunk (15%), or extremities (10%). In the past, this tumor has been regarded as a locally invasive tumor that rarely metastasizes. Recent reports documenting metastatic disease suggest that this variant may be more aggressive than first appreciated.

Histologically, sebaceous carcinoma is distinguished by irregular lobules of cells with an invasive growth

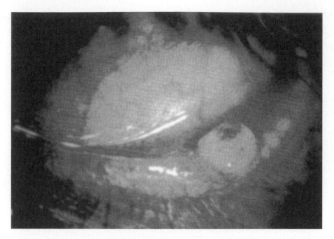

Figure 4 Ocular sebaceous carcinoma: tumor was cleared by Mohs micrographic surgery and referred back to ophthalmology for reconstruction.

pattern. The lobules are composed of variable numbers of basophilic germinative cells and larger cells, demonstrating sebaceous differentiation. The cells typically demonstrate increased numbers of atypical mitotic figures, pleomorphism, and hyperchromaticity; however, even occasional well-differentiated carcinomas may demonstrate aggressive clinical behavior. In some cases, the overlying epidermis may be ulcerated, or the tumor may demonstrate lymphovascular invasion or perineural extension. An important feature of the periocular variant is pagetoid spread across mucosa, leading to corneal involvement.

Treatment for primary lesions has traditionally included wide local excision with histological examination of margins using frozen and permanent sections, and possible corneal mapping, or even exenteration of the eye, where indicated. Mohs micrographic surgery is an alternative that may provide tissue conservation and lower recurrence rates. Radiation may be useful when surgery cannot be tolerated or is contraindicated. Metastatic sebaceous carcinoma is best managed by surgical excision of resectable lesions and radiation of nonresectable tumors.

APOCRINE GLAND TUMORS

Hidradenoma Papilliferum

Hidradenoma papilliferum is a benign apocrine gland tumor that occurs nearly exclusively in women, on the vulva or perineum, although occurrences in other sites such as eyelid, breast, or anus have been reported. The tumor is characteristically a solitary, dome-shaped nodule, 5 to 15 mm in size. Rarely, multiple lesions are present. The overlying epidermis is usually normal, although occasional lesions may demonstrate a red papular area if there is a large connection from the tumor to the overlying surface.

Histologic examination reveals a well-circumscribed dermal nodule not often connected to the overlying epidermis. The tumor is composed of intricate papillary structures lined by two distinct cell layers. The peripheral layer is composed of small or cuboidal cells, while the luminal cells are more columnar and demonstrate variable decapitation secretion. Characteristically, plasma cells are absent; although occasional plasma cells may be seen near the surface if a connection to the overlying epidermis is present. Ultrastructural analysis has confirmed the characteristic secretory granules and decapitation secretion of apocrine tissue.

Hidradenoma papilliferum is best treated with surgical excision.

Apocrine Hidrocystoma (Apocrine Cystadenoma, Apocrine Gland Cyst)

Apocrine hidrocystoma is a relatively common and benign cystic tumor that demonstrates ductal and glandular differentiation. This tumor typically affects older patients and is rare in children. Apocrine hidrocystoma is usually solitary, but multiple lesions may occur. The head and neck are the most common locations, with the majority of tumors being located around the eyes. Often a bluish hue is described. Periorbital lesions probably arise from the glands of Moll, which are modified apocrine glands. Apocrine hidrocystoma arising in other locations are less common. The primary lesion is a soft, translucent cyst varying in size from several millimeters to several centimeters. The lesions are typically skin colored, although less commonly they appear blue or brown (Fig. 5).

Histologic examination demonstrates the tumor to be composed of large, multiloculated cystic spaces. Superficial portions of the cyst are lined by ductal epithelium composed of two layers of cuboidal cells. At the deeper extents of tumor, the lining demonstrates a luminal layer composed of more columnar cells with eosinophilic cytoplasm and decapitation secretion. A peripheral layer of small cuboidal cells (myoepithelial cells) is often present, but may be difficult to appreciate. Areas with papillomatous hyperplasia projecting into the lumen may be present.

Incision and drainage provide temporary improvement, but to prevent recurrence the cyst lining must be destroyed or removed. Although the wall may be destroyed by electrodesiccation or thermal cauterization, better cosmetic results are usually obtained by surgical excision of the cyst. Treatment with an ablative carbon dioxide laser has been reported. Recently, chemical ablation of the cyst lining using tricarboxylic acid has been reported to be efficacious, cosmetically acceptable, and less time consuming than surgical removal.

Apocrine Adenoma (Tubular Apocrine Adenoma, Tubular Adenoma)

Apocrine adenoma is a rare tumor that typically occurs on the scalp, face, axillae, or anogenital area. This tumor may occur in association with an organoid nevus. The primary

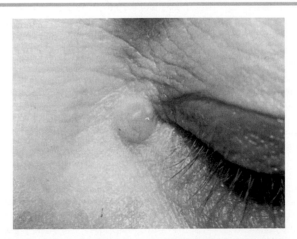

Figure 5 Apocrine cystadenoma: characteristic solitary translucent cyst near the eye.

lesion is a slow-growing, skin-colored papule or nodule in the dermis.

Histologic examination reveals a well-circumscribed tumor that may be focally connected to the overlying epidermis by stratified squamous epithelial conduits. The tumor itself is composed of small to medium-sized tubules or cystic spaces lined by cuboidal or columnar epithelium with papillary projections. The ratio of ductal to glandular areas is variable. The surrounding stroma may be fibrous, with a paucity of inflammatory cells. The lack of plasma cells distinguishes this lesion from syringocystadenoma papilliferum. Focal areas may demonstrate pleomorphism or perineural invasion, complicating differentiation from apocrine adenocarcinoma.

This tumor is best managed by surgical excision. Lesions that demonstrate pleomorphism or an abnormal growth pattern should be excised with clear surgical margins, as differentiation from apocrine adenocarcinoma may occasionally be difficult.

Apocrine Adenocarcinoma

Apocrine adenocarcinoma is a rare malignant neoplasm of the apocrine gland that most often arises in the axillae, but may occur in other apocrine-bearing areas such as the eyelid (Moll's glands), external auditory canal (ceruminous glands), and anterior chest. This tumor may also arise in organoid nevi. The primary lesion is not distinctive and is usually described as a nodular or multinodular, firm or cystic tumor measuring 1 to 8 cm. The tumor is erythematous to violaceous in color, with occasional ulceration.

Histologic examination reveals a dermal tumor with an invasive growth pattern. Marked variation in the appearance of the tumor may occur depending upon the degree of differentiation. The tumor is composed of irregular cystic spaces lined by cuboidal or columnar cells with varying degrees of cytologic atypia and abundant eosinophilic cytoplasm. The number of mitotic figures is variable, but may be as many as four per high-power field. Careful examination will reveal diagnostic areas of apocrine secretion into the lumina. Less differentiated areas may consist of solid sheets and cord-like infiltrations of cells. The surrounding stroma may demonstrate variable fibrosis. Apocrine gland carcinomas arising in the axilla of women may be difficult to differentiate from breast gland carcinomas.

This tumor is best managed by wide local excision with histologic examination of margins to ensure complete extirpation. Mohs micrographic surgery may be useful in areas where preservation of tissue and function is important. Metastasis occurs in up to 50% of cases, first to lymph nodes, but also to other organs. Death due to visceral metastases has been reported in up to 40% of cases. Reviews within the oncology literature note that although apocrine gland carcinoma responds poorly to chemotherapy, adjuvant radiotherapy may be used in advanced local or regional disease.

ECCRINE GLAND TUMORS

Eccrine Poroma

Eccrine poroma is a benign tumor arising from the intraepidermal portion of the eccrine sweat duct. The term "hidroacanthoma simplex" has been used to describe variants confined to the epidermis. This tumor is closely related to eccrine acrospiroma, and in some cases, both tumors may be present within the same histologic section. Some authorities even regard this as a variant of eccrine acrospiroma.

Clinically, eccrine poroma usually occurs as a solitary lesion, but linear variants and diffuse eccrine poromas have been reported in association with hidrotic ectodermal dysplasia. The tumors usually develop during adult life and are most commonly located on the plantar surface or lateral surface of the feet. The hands are less often involved. The primary lesion is a soft, skin-colored to red papule that may be pedunculated. The overlying epidermis is typically normal, but may be ulcerated if exposed to friction or pressure (Fig. 6).

Microscopic examination reveals a well-circumscribed tumor, typically connected to the epidermis. The tumor lobules are comprised of small, uniform basaloid cells that are clearly demarcated from the normal keratinocytes at the site of epidermal attachment. Palisading of nuclei at the periphery of the tumor is conspicuously absent. Focal accumulations of melanin or horn cyst formation may occur. Some cells may appear clear due to glycogen accumulation. Small eccrine ducts are often present within the lobules. The surrounding stroma is usually loosely aggregated with increased vascularity.

Pedunculated lesions may be effectively removed by a deep shave removal, while endophytic lesions require a deeper excision procedure to prevent recurrence.

Nodular Hidradenoma (Eccrine Acrospiroma, Solid and Cystic Hidradenoma, Clear Cell Hidradenoma)

Nodular hidradenoma is a benign eccrine gland tumor. Clinically, the lesion is usually solitary and typically occurs in adults. This tumor is a cyst or nodule that is skin colored or violaceous (Fig. 7). The overlying epidermis may be normal, thickened, or even verrucous. In sum, the clinical features are not distinctive. Although this tumor is generally regarded as benign, a malignant counterpart with aggressive clinical behavior has been described.

Microscopic examination reveals the tumor to be composed of multiple, well-circumscribed lobules. A demonstrated connection to the epidermis is variable. The superficial portion may be histologically identical to an eccrine poroma. The deeper lobules of the tumor are composed of varying proportion of small basaloid cells and larger clear cells rich in glycogen. In some areas, the cells may be fusiform. Most tumors demonstrate ductal structures varying from small, round ducts lined by cuboidal epi-

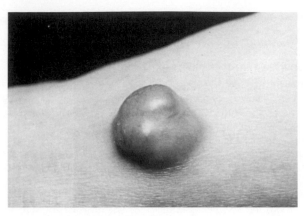

Figure 7 Eccrine acrospiroma: large, multilocular, cystic nodule of anterior shin. Histologic examination revealed the cystic hidradenoma variant of eccrine acrospiroma.

thelium to large cystic structures lined by flattened epithelium. The surrounding stroma varies from delicate to hyalinized.

Nodular hidradenomas are best managed by simple excision. Occasional lesions may be so large (up to 6 cm) that surgical flaps or grafts may be necessary to close the defect following removal.

Syringoma

Syringoma is a common, benign sweat gland tumor with differentiation toward the eccrine sweat duct. It more common in women than in men and usually appears after puberty. Syringomas may be familial, often inherited in autosomal-dominant fashion, or may be associated with Down's syndrome. These tumors are usually multiple and are characteristically located around the eyes, although scalp, genitalia, trunk, and extremities may also be involved. Linear or unilateral distributions have also been documented. The primary lesion is a small, 1 to 5 mm white or white-yellow papule that is firmer than the surrounding skin (Fig. 8). Rarely, syringomas may present as plaques several centimeters in diameter.

Histologically, syringomas are composed of small ductal structures in the upper dermis surrounded by a dense sclerotic stroma. The ducts are typically lined with two layers of flattened or cuboidal cells. Epithelial extensions may arise from the duct, producing a structure resembling a "tadpole" or "comma." The cells lining the duct have variable amounts of glycogen. In rare cases, this glycogen accumulation may be so significant that the term "clear cell syringoma" has been used. Clear cell variants have been reported in association with diabetes mellitus. Occasionally, structures resembling small epidermoid cysts may be seen, most often at the superficial extent of the tumor.

While single lesions may be excised with excellent cosmetic results, the large numbers of lesions present in many cases preclude the extensive use of this modality. Scissor excision using ophthalmologic spring-action scissors and secondary intention healing has been reported to produce excellent cosmetic results. Electrodesiccation has been advocated, but this may often result in incomplete destruction, recurrence, or unattractive scarring. Dermabrasion has been advocated by some, and it appears to work well in many locations, except for the thin skin just under the eye, which is a common location for syringomas. The carbon

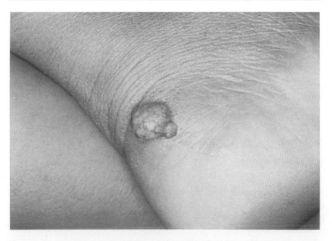

Figure 6 Eccrine poroma: large pedunculated nodule of heel with overlying erosion secondary to trauma. *Source*: Courtesy of Dr. Richard Gentry.

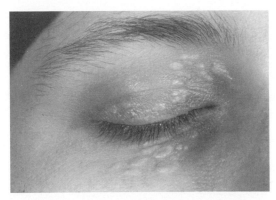

Figure 8 Multiple syringomas: multiple, small, firm papules in characteristic periocular location in a woman. *Source*: Courtesy of Dr. Richard Gentry.

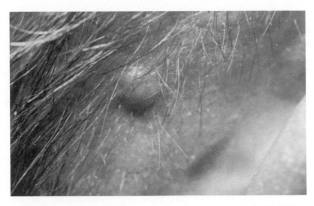

Figure 9 Eccrine spiradenoma: small violaceous papule behind the ear that was spontaneously painful.

dioxide laser has been reported to be an efficient and effective method for removing multiple small syringomas and usually produces favorable cosmetic outcomes. Appropriate precautions to avoid inadvertent eye injury should be undertaken when using this modality.

Eccrine Spiradenoma

Ecccrine spiradenoma is a benign sweat gland tumor regarded by many to be of eccrine in origin, although arguments have also been made for an apocrine origin. Lesions typically appear in adults, without sex predilection. The majority of lesions are asymptomatic, although a significant percentage is associated with pain or tenderness. Eccrine spiradenomas are usually solitary, although they may be rarely multiple or may be associated with cylindromas and trichoepitheliomas. The primary lesion is a 0.2 to 2.5 cm papule or nodule. The majority are skin colored or violaceous in appearance (Fig. 9). Malignant transformation is decidedly uncommon.

Histologic examination reveals one or more large, basophilic, well-circumscribed lobules without a connection to the overlying epidermis (blue balls in the dermis). The lobules are composed of two cell types with small, basaloid cells arranged at the periphery and larger clear cells located more centrally. Occasional ducts or hyaline droplets, similar to those seen in cylindromas, may be present. The associated stroma may be delicate or hyalinized. Occasional eccrine spiradenomas may occur in association with a nearby cylindroma, perhaps suggesting a common derivation or precursor cell.

Eccrine spiradenoma is best removed by surgical excision. Characteristically, the tumor shells out easily during excision.

Papillary Eccrine Adenoma

Papillary eccrine adenoma is a rare, benign sweat gland tumor usually located on the extremities of black patients. The primary lesion is a nodule measuring 0.5 to 3 cm. The overlying skin is normal, although occasional lesions may be verrucous. The color is usually red, brown, or gray.

The tumor is comprises a reasonably well-circumscribed dermal mass formed by ducts of varying sizes surrounded by a fibrous or sclerotic stroma. The ducts are lined by two cell layers, and in some areas may form complex intraluminal papillations. The cells are cytologically benign, and mitotic figures are rare or absent.

The treatment of papillary eccrine adenoma is surgical excision. Recognition of this variant of sweat gland tumors is important, as it has been often confused with eccrine adenocarcinoma, resulting in overly aggressive and disfiguring surgery.

Eccrine Carcinoma

Eccrine sweat gland carcinomas are an extremely rare class of malignant neoplasms that have been described by myriad of bewildering terms. The very rarity of this type of malignancy has led to multiple isolated case reports, as opposed to series, further confounding the subject. Some malignant sweat gland tumors are named in relation to their benign counterpart (eccrine porocarcinoma, malignant eccrine spiradenoma, hidradenocarcinoma, etc.), while others are classified by their histologic pattern (microcystic adnexal carcinoma, adenocystic carcinoma, mucinous carcinoma, ductal carcinoma, etc.). Eccrine porocarcinoma, adenocystic eccrine adenocarcinoma (mucinous adenocarcinoma), adenoid cystic carcinoma, ductal eccrine carcinoma, and microcystic adnexal carcinomas represent the best-understood and most widely accepted variants and will be discussed herein.

Eccrine carcinomas tend to affect older patients and typically have no distinguishing clinical characteristics. Radiation therapy has been identified as an important predisposing factor in some cases. Primary lesions are typically painless, slow-growing papules or nodules. The most characteristic locations are the head, neck, and extremities (Fig. 10).

Histologic examination of eccrine porocarcinoma reveals a tumor connected to the epidermis by cellular cords. As this tumor is thought to arise from the acrosyringium, it often presents intraepidermally. A benign eccrine poroma may be present. The dermal component is composed of an infiltrating pattern of tumor lobules that may demonstrate focal necrosis and calcification. Individual cells demonstrate cytologic atypia. Adenocystic carcinoma is composed of islands of atypical epithelial cells that may form ductal structures or demonstrate perineural extension. Such tumors may demonstrate focal mucin, or occasionally, the mucin may be so abundant that the term "mucinous carcinoma" is used. Adenoid cystic carcinoma is characterized by basaloid islands with a characteristic cribriform growth pattern. Eccrine ductal carcinomas are histologically similar to ductal carcinoma of the breast.

Microcystic adnexal carcinoma, a variant often encountered in the dermatological literature, demonstrates features of both follicular and sweat duct differentiation. While the tumor is composed of cytologically bland cells, an aggressive and infiltrative growth pattern is present, with aggregates extending to the deep dermis and beyond. Perineural extension is common. The superficial portions of the tumor often resemble a syringoma and may demonstrate small keratinous cysts, while the deeper extents demonstrate focal ductal differentiation. The surrounding stroma is typically fibrotic.

Optimal management has not been delineated for all forms of eccrine carcinoma. Microcystic adnexal carcinoma, mucinous carcinoma, and adenoid cystic carcinoma are low-grade sweat gland carcinomas that are locally invasive, but less commonly metastasize. Recurrence is common if these tumors are not completely excised, and Mohs micrographic surgery is an ideal modality.

Conversely, eccrine ductal carcinoma and eccrine porocarcinomas are locally aggressive, but may also frequently metastasize and cause death. Wide excision is the treatment of choice for these histologic variants (Figs. 11 and 12). Regional lymph node dissection has been recommended for the eccrine ductal carcinoma variant, but it is not of proven benefit. Radiation therapy for recurrent or metastatic disease does not appear to be effective. There are several reports of anti–estrogen-based therapy, including tamoxifen, successfully employed for metastatic eccrine carcinoma, but the role of such chemotherapeutic agents in this situation has not been determined conclusively.

SWEAT GLAND TUMORS OF MIXED OR UNCERTAIN HISTOGENESIS

Syringocystadenoma Papilliferum

Syringocystadenoma papilliferum is a benign tumor of the skin. The etiology of this tumor, with particular emphasis on eccrine or apocrine origin, is highly debated. One of the most recent immunohistochemical and ultrastructural studies found the tumor epithelium was composed of several cell types demonstrating various developmental stages, and concluded it was most likely a hamartomatous proliferation derived from pluripotent progenitor cells.

Clinically, these tumors most often present as congenital lesions of the scalp, but they may not be noticed until puberty, when they may suddenly enlarge. Approximately one-third of all such lesions are associated with an organoid

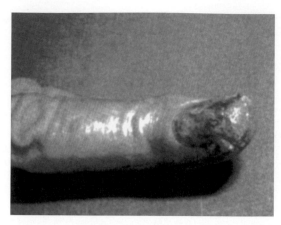

Figure 11 Eccrine porocarcinoma arising in an eccrine poroma: lesion was initially mistaken for a verruca vulgaris and treated with liquid nitrogen.

nevus (nevus sebaceus). In fact, in a recent series of 596 organoid nevi, syringocystadenoma papilliferum represented the most frequent associated tumor (occurring in 30 cases). Immature lesions tend to exist as smooth papules, while developed lesions may be papillomatous or verrucous. In some cases, the papules may be grouped, yielding large plaques, while in other cases they may be arranged in a linear or segmental fashion. The surface may demonstrate scale crust and/or dried blood; other lesions may demonstrate a clear or mucoid secretion.

Histologic examination at low power typically reveals a papillomatous appearance. The tumor itself is composed of ductal structures lined by twolayers of cells. The outer cell layer is more cuboidal, while the luminal layer appears more columnar. The ductal structures are contiguous with the overlying epidermis or, less commonly, can be seen originating from the infundibular portion of a hair follicle. The central collagenous stroma characteristically contains abundant plasma cells—a key histological feature.

Syringocystadenoma papilliferum is best managed by surgical excision, although cautery and electrodesiccation have been used successfully as well. Clearly, for syringocystadenoma occurring within an organoid nevus, the entire organoid nevus should be excised as well. A discussion of

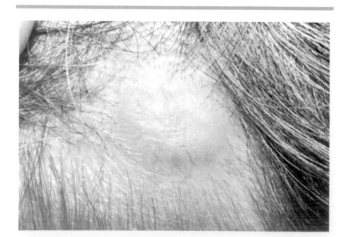

Figure 10 Eccrine carcinoma: slow-growing firm nodule of frontal scalp line. The patient had received radiation therapy for tinea capitis as a child.

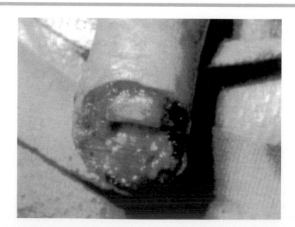

Figure 12 Eccrine porocarcinoma: distal amputation of tumor depicted in Figure 11. This was done in the dermatology clinic following Mohs micrographic surgery.

the merits and timing of prophylactic excision of organoid nevi is beyond the goals of the chapter.

Mixed Tumor of the Skin (Chondroid Syringoma)

Mixed tumor of the skin, or chondroid syringoma, is a benign sweat gland tumor that likely may be derived from either apocrine or eccrine origin. Over 30 years ago, it was first suggested that both apocrine and eccrine variants existed, but only recently has the contention reached broad acceptance. Apocrine-derived tumors are certainly more common that those of eccrine derivation. Mixed tumor of the skin demonstrates both histologic and ultrastructural similarities to mixed tumors of the salivary gland and breast.

Clinically, mixed tumor of the skin usually exists a slow-growing, solitary lesion of the head or neck in the middle-aged and elderly, although lesions of the trunk or extremities have been described. The lesion is a firm dermal or subcutaneous nodule with a normal overlying dermis (Fig. 13). Indeed, the clinical appearance is nondescript, and typically, the ultimate histological diagnosis is not suspected at the time of the clinical exam.

Histologic examination reveals a well-circumscribed dermal or subcutaneous nodule with both epithelial and stromal components. The epithelial component consists of nests of cuboidal or polygonal cells often arranged in a lace-like pattern with ductal structures. Ductile structures will often demonstrate apocrine decapitation secretion; however, those of eccrine origin will lack this finding. Eccrine variants also maintain smaller, nonbranching ducts resembling a syringoma. Keratinous cysts may be present in apocrine forms. In either type of lesion, the surrounding matrix is highly variable and may demonstrate sclerotic, myxoid, or chondroid elements.

This tumor is easily managed surgically because of its distinct tendency to shell out during removal. Recurrences are rare unless an alternate form of therapy, such as electro-desiccation, is utilized.

Cylindroma (Turban Tumor)

Cylindroma is a benign sweat gland tumor of uncertain origin. Immunohistochemical studies have, on occasion, demonstrated both eccrine and apocrine etiology. A recent study using IKH-4, a monoclonal antibody thought to be specific for eccrine epithelium, showed positive staining within cylindroma, reigniting the debate over the etiology of this tumor.

Cylindromas are most common on the head, particularly the forehead and scalp. The usual presentation is that of a solitary, firm, pink or violaceous nodule measuring from 0.2 to 6 cm (Fig. 14). Multiple cylindromas may occur sporadically or may be inherited in autosomal-dominant fashion with trichoepitheliomas (Brooke–Spiegler syndrome). In some cases, multiple cylindromas of the scalp may be so numerous and large that the descriptive label "turban tumor" is applied. There is a single report of a massive, but otherwise benign cylindroma resulting in erosion of the calvarium. Rarely, malignant transformation may occur.

Histologic examination reveals a poorly circumscribed dermal tumor that is only rarely connected to the overlying epidermis. The tumor is composed of numerous discrete, basaloid islands thatvaguely conform to adjacent islands, yielding a characteristic "jigsaw puzzle" pattern. The lobules are composed ofsmaller, basophilic cells at the

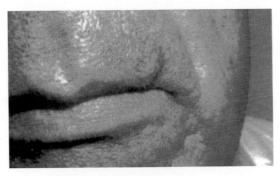

Figure 13 Mixed tumor of the skin: firm dermal nodule of left upper lip.

periphery of the lobule and larger, pale cells in the central portions. Many lobules demonstrate characteristic droplet-like accumulations of an eosinophilic, hyaline material, and some areas may demonstrate ductal structures lined by cuboidal epithelium. The individual lobules are ensheathed by a thick, periodic acid-Schiff–positive, diastase-resistant, hyalinized membrane.

Solitary cylindromas, or multiple lesions of limited extent, may be easily managed by simple excision. Recurrence is common if the entire tumor is not removed. For this reason, Mohs micrographic surgery has been advocated for cosmetically important areas or for cases with evidence of malignant transformation. Small cylindromas have also been successfully managed by electrocautery, cryotherapy, or even radiation therapy. Turban tumors may be so massive that simple excision with primary closure is not feasible. Rarely, such extensive cases have been managed by total excision of the scalp under general anesthesia, followed by split-thickness skin grafts. Dermabrasion may be palliative, but it is not curative.

MERKEL CELL CARCINOMA (TRABECULAR CELL TUMOR, TOKER TUMOR, PRIMARY NEUROENDOCRINE CARCINOMA OF THE SKIN)

Merkel cell carcinoma was originally thought to represent a poorly differentiated eccrine sweat gland carcinoma, but ultrastructural and histochemistry studies have convincingly identified it as a neuroendocrine tumor of the skin arising from the Merkel cell. This tumor typically affects older patients, and arises as a rapidly growing nodule on sun-exposed skin, although other sites such as the sacrum or buttocks are not uncommonly affected. Regional lymph node metastases may occur in up to 50% of all patients. The most recent and largest case series of 251 patients from Memorial Sloan-Kettering Cancer Center demonstrated an overall five-year survival of 64%.

Histologic examination reveals a dermal tumor composed of uniform, small, densely packed basophilic cells with scanty cytoplasm. Mitosis and apoptotic cells are numerous. Cells are arranged in both sheets and trabeculae in the dermis. Lymphatic invasion may be present. Epidermotropism may be observed on occasion. Merkel cell carcinoma typically stains positive with neuron-specific enolase, epithelial membrane antigen, chromogranin, C-kit (CD 117), and cytokeratin 20. Cytokeratin 20 staining often demonstrates a useful perinuclear dotting pattern. Because metastatic small cell lung cancer can yield nearly identical histological lesions, exclusion of this occurrence by negative

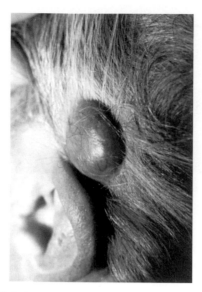

Figure 14 Cylindroma: large violaceous nodule of the scalp. The patient had similar lesions elsewhere on the scalp.

thyroid transcription factor-1 immunohistochemical staining is often useful.

Classically, wide local excision for Merkel cell carcinoma was advocated, although the optimal size of the surgical margin has not been convincingly established. Increasingly, Mohs micrographic surgery has been used, particularly when preservation of function ha been a prime concern. Sentinel lymph node positivity has been reported by some to be helpful in predicting the risk of recurrence or metastasis. The efficacy of regional lymphadenectomy has not been established, but it has been advocated on the basis of anecdotal cases. The tumor is radiosensitive, but the necessity of utility of adjuvant radiotherapy is controversial. In a retrospective analysis of 45 patients with stage 1 disease treated with Mohs surgery, 20 elected for postoperative radiation therapy while 25 did not. There did not appear to be any differences in recurrence, overall survival, relapse-free survival, or disease-free survival, but prospective matched studies are lacking.

Traditional chemotherapy has been recommended as adjunctive therapy for metastatic disease, but it does not appear to be curative. Advanced cases have been treated by primary excision followed by induction chemotherapy and radiotherapy. Recently, a trial using imatinib mesylate in metastatic or unresectable cases of Merkel cell carcinoma has been outlined and is hoped to exploit the C-kit (CD 117) positivity documented within this type of tumor.

BIBLIOGRAPHY

Allen PJ, Bowne WB, Jaques DP, et al. Merkel cell carcinoma: prognosis and treatment of patients from a single institution. J Clin Oncol 2005; 23:2300–2309.

Bickley LK, Goldberg DJ, lmaeda S, et al. Treatment of multiple apocrine hidrocystomas with the carbon dioxide (CO_2) laser. J Dermatol Surg Oncol 1989; 15:599–602.

Birt AR, Hogg GR, Dube WJ. Hereditary multiple fibrofolliculomas with trichodiscomas and acrochordons. Arch Dermatol 1977; 113:1674–1677.

Boyer JD, Zitelli JA, Brodland DG, et al. Local control of primary Merkel cell carcinoma: review of 45 cases treated

with Mohs micrographic surgery with and without adjuvant radiation. J Am Acad Dermatol 2002; 47:885–892.

Brooke JD, Fitzpatrick JE, Golitz LE. Papillary mesenchymal bodies: a histologic finding useful in differentiating trichoepitheliomas from basal cell carcinomas. J Am Acad Dermatol 1989; 21:523–528.

Brownstein MH, Shapiro L. Desmoplastic trichoepithelioma. Cancer 1977; 40:2979–2986.

Callahan EF, Appert DL, Roenigk RK, et al. Sebaceous carcinoma of the eyelid: a review of 14 cases. Dermatol Surg 2004; 30:1164–1168.

Chamberlain RS, Huber K, White JC, et al. Apocrine gland carcinoma of the axilla: review of the literature and recommendations for treatment. Am J Clin Oncol 1999; 22:131–135.

Chan EF. Pilomatricomas contain activating mutations in beta-catenin. J Am Acad Dermatol 2000; 43:701–702.

Chesser RS, Bertler DE, Fitzpatrick JE, et al. Primary cutaneous adenoid cystic carcinoma treated with Mohs micrographic surgery toluidine blue technique. J Dermatol Surg Oncol 1992; 18:175–176.

Crain RC, Helwig EB. Dermal cylindroma (dermal eccrine cylindroma). Am J Clin Pathol 1961; 35:504–515.

Cribier B, Scrivener Y, Grosshans E. Tumors arising in nevus sebaceus: a study of 596 cases. J Am Acad Dermatol 2000; 42:263–268.

Curry ML, Eng W, Lund K, et al. Muir-Torre syndrome: role of the dermatopathologist in diagnosis. Am J Dermatopathol 2004; 26:217–221.

Dailey RA, Saulny SM, Tower RN. Treatment of multiple apocrine hidrocystomas with trichloroacetic acid. Ophth Plast Reconstr Surg 2005; 21:148–150.

del Pozo J, Garcia-Silva J, Pena-Penabad C, et al. Multiple apocrine hidrocystomas: treatment with carbon dioxide laser vaporization. J Dermatol Treat 2001; 12:97–100.

Dixon RS, Mikhail GR, Slater HC. Sebaceous carcinoma of the eyelid. J Am Acad Dermatol 1980; 3:241–243.

Duhra P, Paul JC. Cryotherapy for multiple trichoepithelioma. J Dermatol Surg Oncol 1988; 14:1413–1415.

Feinmesser M, Halpern M, Kaganovsky E, et al. C-kit expression in primary and metastatic merkel cell carcinoma. Am J Dermatopathol 2004; 26:458–462.

Fenig E, Lurie H, Klein B, et al. The treatment of advanced Merkel cell carcinoma: a multimodality chemotherapy and radiation therapy treatment approach. J Dermatol Surg Oncol 1993; 19:860–864.

Fleischmann HE, Roth RJ, Wood C, et al. Microcystic adnexal carcinoma treated by microscopically controlled excision. J Dermatol Surg Oncol 1984; 10:873–875.

Forbis R, Helwig EB. Pilomatrixoma (calcifying epithelioma). Arch Dermatol 1961; 83:606–618.

Goldman B. Total excision of the scalp and portions of face; restoration by skin grafting: the surgical management of massive cylindroma of the scalp and face. Ann Surg 1951; 133:555–560.

Graefe T, Wollina U, Schulz H, et al. Muir-Torre syndrome—treatment with isotretinoin and interferon alpha-2a can prevent tumour development. Dermatology 2000; 200:331–333.

Gray HR, Helwig EB. Trichofolliculoma. Arch Dermatol 1962; 86:619–625.

Gray HR, Helwig ED. Epithelioma adenoides cysticum and solitary trichoepithelioma. Arch Dermatol 1963; 87:102–114.

Hanly AJ, Elgart GW, Jorda M, et al. Analysis of thyroid transcription factor-1 and cytokeratin 20 separates Merkel cell carcinoma from small cell carcinoma of lung. J Cutan Pathol 2000; 27:118–120.

Headington JT. Mixed tumors of skin: eccrine and apocrine types. Arch Dermatol 1961; 84:989–996.

Hirsch P, Helwig EB. Chrondroid syringoma. Arch Dermatol 1961; 84:835–847.

Janitz J, Wiedersberg H. Trichilemmal pilar tumors. Cancer 1980; 45:1594–1597.

Kersting DW, Helwig EB. Eccrine spiradenoma. Arch Dermatol 1956; 73:199–227.

Lo JS, Snow SN, Mohs FE. Cylindroma treated by Mohs micrographic surgery. J Dermatol Surg Oncol 1991; 17:871–874.

Lum CA, Binder SW. Proliferative characterization of basal-cell carcinoma and trichoepithelioma in small biopsy specimens. J Cutan Pathol 2004; 31:550–555.

Maloney ME. An easy method for removal of syringoma. J Dermatol Surg Oncol 1982; 8:973–975.

Mambo NC. Eccrine spiradenoma: clinical and pathologic study of 49 tumors. J Cutan Pathol 1983; 10:312–320.

Mammino JJ, Vidmar DA. Syringocystadenoma papilliferum. Int J Dermatol 1991; 30:763–766.

Miescher G. Trichofolliculoma. Dermatologica 1944; 89:193.

Mellette JR Jr., Amonette RA, Gardner JH, et al. Carcinoma of sebaceous glands on the head and neck. J Dermatol Surg Oncol 1981; 7:404–407.

Moehlenbeck FW. Pilomatrixoma (calcifying epithelioma). Arch Dermatol 1973; 10:532–534.

Nickerson ML, Warren MB, Toro JR, et al. Mutations in a novel gene lead to kidney tumors, lung wall defects, and benign tumors of the hair follicle in patients with the Birt-Hogg-Dube syndrome. Cancer Cell 2002; 2:157–164.

Okun MR, Finn F, Blumental G. Apocrine adenoma versus apocrine carcinoma. J Am Acad Dermatol 1980; 2:322–326.

Peterdy GA, Huettner PC, Rajaram V, Lind AC. Trichofolliculoma of the vulva associated with vulvar intraepithelial neoplasia: report of three cases and review of the literature. Int J Gynecol Pathol 2002; 21:224–230.

Pinkus H, Rogin JR, Goldman P. Eccrine poroma. Arch Dermatol 1956; 74:511–521.

Plewig G. Sebaceous trichfolliculoma. J Cutan Pathol 1980; 7:394–403.

Roenigk HH Jr. Dermabrasion for miscellaneous cutaneous lesions (exclusive of scarring from acne). J Dermatol Surg Oncol 1977; 3:322–328.

Roenigk RK, Goltz RW. Merkel cell carcinoma-a problem with microscopically controlled surgery. J Dermatol Surg Oncol 1986; 12:332–336.

Rulon DB, Helwig EB. Cutaneous sebaceous neoplasms. Cancer 1974; 33:82–102.

Rulon DB, Helwig EB. Papillary eccrine adenoma. Arch Dermatol 1977; 113:596–598.

Sable D, Snow SN. Pilomatrix carcinoma of the back treated by mohs micrographic surgery. Dermatol Surg 2004; 30:1174–1176.

Sau P, Graham JH, Helwig EB. Proliferating epithelial cysts. Clinicopathological analysis of 96 cases. J Cutan Pathol 1995; 22:394–406.

Schroder U, Dries V, Klussmann JP, et al. Successful adjuvant tamoxifen therapy for estrogen receptor-positive metastasizing sweat gland adenocarcinoma: need for a clinical trial? Ann Otol Rhinol Laryngol 2004; 113:242–244.

Schulz T, Hartschuh W. Folliculo-sebaceous cystic hamartoma is a trichofolliculoma at its very late stage. J Cutan Pathol 1998; 25:354–364.

Shaffelburg M, Miller R. Treatment of multiple trichoepithelioma with electrosurgery. Dermatol Surg 1992; 24:1154–1156.

Smith JD, Chemosky ME. Apocrine hidrocystoma (cystadenoma). Arch Dermatol 1974; 109:700–702.

Snow SN, Reizner GT: eccrine porocarcinoma of the face. J Am Acad Dermatol 1992; 27:306–311.

Troy JL, Ackerman AB. Sebaceoma: a distinctive benign neoplasm of adnexal epithelium differentiating toward sebaceous cells. Am J Dermatopathol 1984; 6:7–13.

Uede K, Yamamoto Y, Furukawa F. Brooke-Spiegler syndrome associated with cylindroma, trichoepithelioma, spiradenoma, and syringoma. J Dermatol 2004; 31:32–38.

Urquhart JL, Weston WL. Treatment of multiple trichoepitheliomas with topical imiquimod and tretinoin. Pediatr Dermatol 2005; 22:67–70.

Vincent A, Farley M, Chan E, et al. Birt-Hogg-Dube syndrome: a review of the literature and the differential diagnosis of firm facial papules. J Am Acad Dermatol 2003; 49:698–705.

Warkel RL, Helwig EB. Apocrine gland adenoma and adenocarcinoma of the axilla. Arch Dermatol 1978; 114:198–203.

Wheeland RG, Bailin PL, Kronberg E. Carbon dioxide (CO2) laser vaporization for the treatment of multiple trichoepithelioma. J Dermatol Surg Oncol 1984; 10:470–475.

Wheeland RG, Bailin PL, Reynolds OD, et al. Carbon dioxide (CO2) laser vaporization of multiple facial syringomas. J Dermatol Surg Oncol 1986; 12:225–228.

Wick MR, Goellner JR, Wolfe IT III, et al. Adnexal carcinomas of the skin. II. Extraocular sebaceous carcinomas. Cancer 1985; 56:1163–1172.

Woodworth H Jr., Dockerty MB, Wilson RB, et al. Papillary hidradenoma of the vulva: a clinicopathologic study of 69 cases. Am J Obstet Gynecol 1971; 110:501–508.

Wyld L, Bullen S, Browning FS. Transcranial erosion of a benign dermal cylindroma. Ann Plast Surg 1996; 36:194–196.

Yamamoto O, Doi Y, Hamada T, et al. An immunohistochemical and ultrastructural study of syringocystadenoma papilliferum. Br J Dermatol 2002; 147:936–945.

44

Keloids

Nathan Rosen
McGill University, Montreal, Quebec, Canada

Steven C. Bernstein
University of Montreal, Montreal, Quebec, Canada

Randall K. Roenigk
Mayo Clinic, Rochester, Minnesota, U.S.A.

HISTORY

The earliest recorded description of keloid scars is found in the Smith Papyrus dating back to approximately 3000 B.C. Reference is made to "the existence of swelling on his breast, large, spreading, and hard, touching them is like touching a ball of wrappings." The Yorubas, a tribe in West Nigeria, described many observations relating to the character and presentation of keloids as early as the 10th century A.D. The Yorubas practiced ritual facial markings and earlobe perforations. These acts were usually performed during the first week of life, as the Yorubas were aware that scarring during adolescence or adult life often became keloidal. They noted the tendency of the lesions to appear within the same family, but that not all family members were necessarily affected. Also, they described a time interval observed between a trauma and the appearance of a keloid. Finally, the Yorubas knew that once a lesion was present it had no remedy, except when "the Divine power is suitably appropriated to intervene in bringing about its resolution."

Jean Louis Alibert, a founder of the French School of Dermatology, is commonly credited with being the first to describe cicatricial tumors in the modern literature (1806) and to suggest the current name, keloid, in 1817. Retz in 1790 also described these tumors clinically, but he referred to them as "datre de graisse" or "fatty hernias." Initially, Alibert was convinced that these lesions were cancerous in origin and consequently chose the term "cancroids." When the noncancerous nature of these tumors became apparent, he modified the term to "cheloide," "chele" being derived from the Greek for crab's claw. This new term referred both to the clawlike extension of the lesions and to their tendency toward lateral growth.

Between 1825 and 1854, an artificial distinction was made between "true keloids" (spontaneously arising) and "false keloids" (arising secondary to trauma). In 1884, Addison described "true" keloids, which are now thought to be morphea or scleroderma.

It is now recognized that keloids are unique to humans. Keloid-like lesions have been reported in a few animals, but in all cases the excessive collagen that is deposited in animals is reabsorbed when the tissue insult ceases.

EPIDEMIOLOGY

The incidence of keloids in the general population varies with age, sex, race, anatomic location, and type of trauma. Additional confounding variables include difficulty in distinguishing keloids from hypertrophic scars and the broad time frame during which keloids form or reform. Accordingly, the reported incidence of keloids ranges from a high of 16% among adults in Zaire to a low of 0.09% in England. Keloids are more common among the darker-pigmented races. African-Americans form keloids more, often than Caucasians, with reported ratios ranging between 2 and 19:1. Arnold and Grauer found that in Hawaii, keloids are five times more common in Japanese and three times more common in Chinese than among Caucasians. There is also an increased incidence in people from East India, Aruba, and Polynesia. There are no known reports of keloids in Albinos.

Many theories have been espoused to explain the difference in keloid incidence between African-Americans and Caucasians. Bohrod suggested that it was based on the principle of long-term social and religious mores for scarification, which consequently determined genetic predisposition. Another theory implicates excessive secretion of melanocyte-stimulating hormone (MSH) and increased sensitivity of the melanocytes to this MSH in the pathogenesis of keloids, which may also account for the increased incidence in African-Americans.

Keloids are uncommon at the extremes of life. They may occur at any age but develop most commonly between the ages of 10 and 30. The median age of onset is equal in both sexes. The incidence of keloids is usually reported to be equal among males and females, although some studies do report a higher incidence among females. This is most likely considered attributable to the greater frequency of ear piercing and the greater cosmetic concern in the female population.

These are regional predilections as well. The most susceptible anatomic locations are the presternal area, anterior chest, back, shoulder, and posterior neck. Moderately susceptible are the ears, beard areas, and the rest of the neck. Mildly susceptible areas include the abdomen, forearms, and the rest of the face. Keloids are rarely seen on the scalp,

Table 1 Regional Susceptibility to Keloids

High risk	Mild risk
Presternal area	Abdomen
Anterior chest	Forearms
Superior back	Centrofacial area
Shoulder	Legs
Posterior neck	Negligible risk
Moderate risk	Scalp
Ear lobe	Eyelids
Beard	Genitalia
Anterior and lateral neck	Palms
Upper arms	Soles
	Mucous membranes

eyelids, genitalia, palms, soles, mucous membranes, tongue, and even the cornea (Table 1).

ETIOLOGY

Many factors are associated with keloid formations (Table 2). However, most lesions result from some form of trauma to a genetically susceptible individual. Keloids usually form within two weeks and up to one year following injury. Nevertheless, not all keloids result from trauma. Several authors have described spontaneous keloids. Notably, following trauma, sebaceous glands secrete sebum intradermally, which acts to elicit an autoimmune granulomatous response with progression to keloid formation. In support of this theory is the rarity of keloid scarring on areas lacking sebaceous glands such as the palms and soles. Other groups have suggested that it is the presence of an intralesional foreign body (e.g., ritual object, epidermal fragment, and suture material) that leads to keloid formation.

Infection has also been proposed as an etiologic agent in the initiation of keloids. Wound infection constitutes an adverse healing scenario and as such can lead to keloid formation. Over the years, many organisms have been incriminated as being "keloidogenic" (e.g., tuberculosis and syphilis), but there is currently no evidence to support this.

Endocrine factors have also been implicated in the cause of keloids. The ages of the most keloids correlate with the periods of physical (puberty) and pituitary growth. The pituitary has long been incriminated due to the observations that acromegalics are particularly susceptible to keloid formation. Additionally, keloid growth is increased during puberty and pregnancy, periods with augmented pituitary activity. The predisposition for keloid formation has been associated with abnormal function of the hypothalamus, thyroid, and parathyroid. It has been proposed that increased MSH may be the unifying feature of the endocrinologic disorders. The

Table 2 Etiological Factors in Keloid Formation

Trauma	Anatomic sites
Genetic susceptibility	Wound tension
Nonspecific skin injury	Sebum autoimmune mechanism
Dermatologic disease	Foreign body reaction
Follicular occlusion tetrad	Infection
Genodermatoses	Endocrine factors
Familial tendency	

Table 3 Clinical Features Distinguishing Keloids from Hypertrophic Scars

Keloid	Hypertrophic scar
Not limited to site of trauma	Limited to site of trauma
No spontaneous regression	Spontaneous regression
Onset 1 mo to 1 yr or longer	Onset <3 mo
High-risk anatomic areas	Anywhere
Familial tendency	Familial tendency
Associated symptoms	No associated symptoms
May be worsened by surgery	Improved with appropriate surgery

hypothesis is supported by the increased incidence of keloids in dark-skinned races and more deeply pigmented individuals; the anatomic site of predisposition being parts of the body with the greatest melanocyte distribution; the increased incidence during puberty and pregnancy, and even the response to intralesional steroid injections.

CLINICAL MANIFESTATIONS

Keloids are benign fibrous growths that result from the excessive dermal connective tissue that forms in response to trauma in predisposed individuals. Clinically, their appearance is highly variable, reflecting the variation in antecedent trauma. Their location and configuration, but not their size, appears predetermined by the site of skin trauma. Characteristically, keloids generally appear within one to two months of trauma, but onset may be delayed up to one year or more. Classically, keloids are said to grow beyond the margins of the original injury progressively invading the surrounding normal skin. In contrast, the hypertrophic scar, with which the keloid is often confused, is confined to the tissue damaged by the original injury. Additionally, keloids never spontaneously regress, whereas regression is frequently seen in hypertrophic scars within 12 to 18 months (see Table 3 for comparison of keloids and hypertrophic scars).

Keloids vary in size from small papules to large pendulous tumors. Shape may vary from evenly contoured, symmetric protrusions with regular margins to irregular claw-like projections from an unevenly twisted mass (Figs. 1–4). The physical characteristics of the keloid are somewhat dependent on anatomic location. Keloids on the anterior chest tend to be broad-based, raised, and may have irregular clawlike projections (Fig. 5). Earlobe keloids are clinically diverse (Figs. 6 and 7). Keloids range in consistency

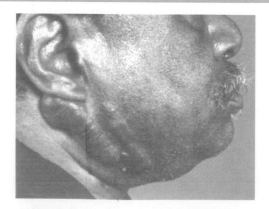

Figure 1 Keloids in pseudofolliculitis barbae.

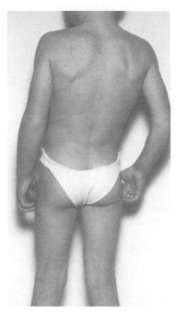

Figure 2   Keloids postvaricella.

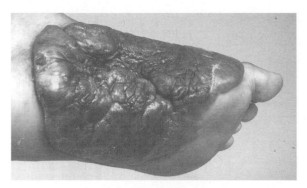

Figure 4   Unusual twisted mass on the dorsal and plantar foot.

from soft and doughy to rubbery to rock hard. The color is variable, ranging from mildly erythematous in new lesions to vivid purple in maturing lesions to hypo- or hyperpigmented in order lesions. The clinical course of keloids is also variable. Most keloids have a growth phase followed by a stable period of little or no growth. Often intense pruritus accompanies the growth phase. The epidermis commonly becomes thinned but only rarely ulcerates or drains necrotic material. Keloids rarely regress. Malignant transformation has been described, but such cases are rare and poorly documented. Patients consult physicians due to cosmetic concerns or symptomatology. Keloids following sternotomy or thoracotomy are notoriously painful (Figs. 8 and 9).

The clinical appearance is characteristic, and the differential diagnosis is limited. Aside from hypertrophic scar, lesions such as dermatofibrosarcoma protuberans, leiomyosarcoma, and other sarcomas may bear clinical resemblance. Infectious lesions such as lupus vulgaris and blastomycosis need to be eliminated by histopathology and culture. Sarcoidosis should be considered in the black population and superficial fascial fibromatoses in whites.

HISTOPATHOLOGY

Keloids are characterized histologically by the intradermal presence of highly compacted hyalinized collagen in nodular formations. The nodules gradually increase in size and ultimately show thick, highly compacted, and hyalinized bands of collagen lying in a concentric arrangement. The collagen fibers are thickened, glassy, pale staining, and faintly refractile. Individual fibrils are large and irregular. Blood vessels, the number of fibroblasts, and ground substance are all increased. Depending upon whether the nodules of collagen encroach upon the papillary dermis, the epidermis appears either flattened or normal.

Craig et al. reported that mast cells are present only in the dermis and never in the epidermis, as in normal skin. However, the mast cells are more diffusely distributed than the normal periadnexal location. The actual number of mast cells in keloids is increased due to the presence of a much thicker dermis.

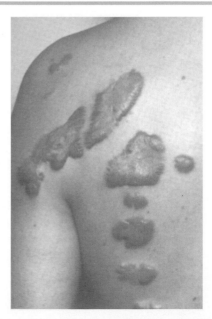

Figure 3   Broad-based posterior chest wall keloids.

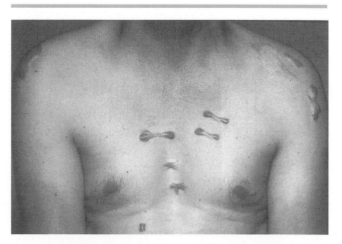

Figure 5   Typical dumbbell lesions of the anterior chest.

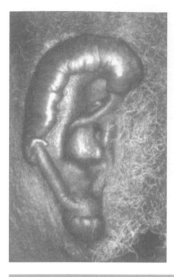

Figure 6 Unusual keloid of the helix and lobe of the ear. *Source*: Courtesy of Dr. John Ratz.

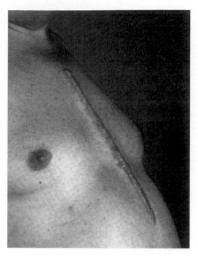

Figure 8 Postthoracotomy keloid.

According to Lever et al., hypertrophic scars and keloids are indistinguishable from one another on histologic exam. However, with time, the thick and hyalinized collagen bundles that compose the hypertrophic scar gradually become thinner and straighten out so that the collagen bundles assume an orientation parallel to the epidermal surface. In keloids, the nodular condensation of collagen persists indefinitely.

PATHOGENESIS

Keloid scars are a result of an aberrant form of wound healing in which factors necessary for regulation of normal healing and remodeling are defective (Table 4). These keloid tumors exhibit abnormal collagen metabolism and overabundance of extracellular matrix (ECM) components. Both the increased ECM and water account for the tissue bulk that forms a keloid.

Although the pathogenesis of keloids remains elusive, many advances have been made in uncovering the biochemical abnormalities that are found in keloid scars. The focus of this research has naturally centered on the fibroblast, which is the collagen and ECM-producing factory of the dermis, excessive collagen deposition being the histopathological hallmark of keloids. It has now been shown that "keloid fibroblasts" not only produce far increased

amounts of collagen, elastin, fibronectin, and proteoglycan, but also do that with reduced growth factor requirements as compared to the fibroblasts that are isolated from normal skin. TGF-β1 is the main trigger for fibroblast production of collagen and ECM, and levels of this cytokine, and its receptor on fibroblasts have been shown to be increased in keloids. Tamoxifen, which decreases levels of TGF-β, has been shown to decrease collagen synthesis of keloid fibroblasts. TGF-β may be released from endothelial cells of small capillaries, making vascular damage a possible initiating event to keloid formation. Daian et al. have shown that keloid fibroblasts also express increased numbers of insulin-like growth factor receptor (IGF-receptor), which when stimulated by IGF, leads to a synergistic effect with TGF-β–induced ECM protein production, likely via downstream signaling cross talk. They also propose that IGF may play a role in making these fibroblasts resistant to apoptosis, helping to explain why the collagen production by these fibroblasts continues on for years. Keloidal fibroblasts have also shown an increased growth response to platelet-derived growth factor. Phan et al. have demonstrated that

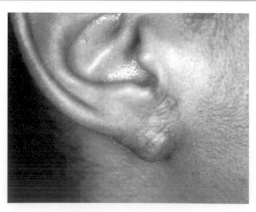

Figure 7 Earlobe keloid.

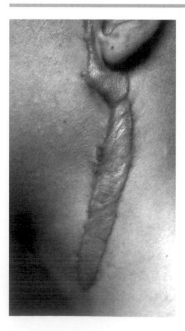

Figure 9 Postcarotidectomy keloid.

Table 4 Biochemistry of Keloids

Abnormal collagen synthesis
    Increased collagen synthesis
    Increased immature soluble collagen
    Increased type I and type III collagen
    Abnormal cross-linking between collagen molecules
    Increased proline hydroxylase
Abnormal collagen catabolism
    Increased concentration of collagen
    Defective collagenase
    Collagenase inhibitors
        α_1-antitrypsin
        α_2-macroglobulins
        Chondroitin-4-sulfate
    Increased collagenase
    Increased cellularity
    Increased concentration of DNA
    Increased fibroblast number
    Increased mastocyte number
Abnormal proteoglycans
    Increased total proteoglycans (water retention)
    Major increase in chondroitin-r-sulfate
    (Stimulates) fibroblast synthesis
Increased metabolic activity
    Increased glycolytic enzyme activity
    Increased glycoprotein synthesis
    Increased fibronectin deposition
Growth factors
    Transforming growth factor β
    Platelet-derived growth factor
    Insulin-like growth factor

the overlying keratinocytes are an important source of growth factors, acting in a paracrine manner to enhance collagen synthesis by the fibroblasts. The collagen that is produced by these "keloid fibroblasts" is predominantly type I and III, and the cross-links between individual fibers have been shown to be abnormal. This has been postulated to be due to a decrease in lysyl oxidase activity. This enzyme is copper dependant, and keloids have been shown to be copper deficient.

In addition to the increased production, collagen degradation has been shown to be defective in Keloids. Actual collagenase activity in keloids, hypertrophic scars, and mature scars is paradoxically greater than in normal skin. Keloids demonstrate as much as 14 times the collagenase activity and hypertrophic and mature scars four times as much. Nevertheless, this increased activity seemed to be overmatched by increased deposition, with a net result of excess scar formation. New data, demonstrating the presence of plasma proteins known as α-globulins has helped to explain why the increased collagenase activity seems to be ineffective in keloids. These proteins such as α1-antitrypsin and α2-microglobulin, have been shown to be serum proteinase inhibitors and thus inhibit degradation of connective tissue. The proteoglycan chondroitin-4-sulfate has been shown to be extremely abundant in keloidal tissue. This proteoglycan provides a stimulus to collagen production while coating the collagen fibers and inhibiting degradation by collagenase.

Keloids and hypertrophic scars are more cellular than normal dermis. This is reflected by an increased concentration of DNA. The collagen producing fibroblasts are increased in number and metabolic activity, and mast cells are also prominent, likely accounting for the pruritus often associated with these tumors.

TREATMENT

It is dogma in clinical medicine that the more treatment modalities described for any one malady, the more refractory it is to cure. Nowhere is this more evident than in the treatment of keloids. Kelly states that the cardinal rule of keloid therapy is prevention. He advises that nonessential cosmetic surgery be withheld from patients prone to keloid formation. However, he considers patients with only earlobe keloids and a negative family history not to be at increased risk.

It is clear that there is no ideal, uniformly effective treatment for all keloids. Therapy must be tailored to the unique characteristics of the individual keloid such as the location, size, depth, age of the patient, and the response to previous treatment. Also, the patient's goals and expectations must be considered. It is important to distinguish the keloid from the hypertrophic scar if appropriate treatment to be instituted. Hypertrophic scars may spontaneously regress and can be treated effectively surgically or with less invasive measures such as intralesional corticosteroid injections, pressure devices, topical retinoid therapy, or flashlamp dye laser. Many diverse treatment modalities have been described for keloids, but the search for a uniformly effective therapy has proved elusive. For any regimen to be deemed effective, there must be symptomatic and cosmetic improvement as well as normal function. Most importantly, a minimum two-year follow-up period is necessary to determine recurrence. Finally, one may have to accept the philosophy that treatments for keloids may last up to two years, but it is the nature of the disease that regular retreatment is required.

Surgery

Surgical excision of keloid tumors was described as early as 1844 by Druit. By 1903, DaCosta reported on the futility of surgical excision: "it is also useless to remove keloid by operation, as it will usually return and a study of the growth removed shows no reason for the inevitable return." Recent studies have shown that surgical excision alone has been associated with a 55% recurrence rate. Long-term follow-up studies have shown as many as 80% of keloids regrowing at two years and close to 100% over a lifetime. Although surgery alone is often ineffective, it remains the only method by which the larger, tumorous keloids can be effectively removed. This dilemma has led to the development of specialized surgical techniques to decrease wound tension and the implementation of adjuvant therapies such as intralesional corticosteroids, pressure devices, and radiation therapy.

Several surgical approaches are available. Very small lesions may be excised and closed primarily if the surrounding tissue is not under excessive tension. Such lesions must be removed atraumatically and closed precisely with a minimum amount of foreign material and without dead space or hematoma resulting. If a layered closure is necessary, sutures with low tissue reactivity such as polyglycolic acid should be chosen. Monofilament nylon may be used to close the epidermis, although monofilament polybutester sutures offer the advantage of greater elasticity and low tissue reactivity.

Larger lesions may be treated by excision and grafting or by various flap techniques to minimize tension. Unfortunately, excision followed by skin grafting has had a recurrence rate of 59%, and 50% develop a keloid at the donor site. One way to avoid this complication is to harvest the graft from the overlying epithelium of the keloid, thus creating no secondary wound. This technique is particularly useful for very large or flat pancake-like keloids. The surface epithelium is resected from the keloid using a scalpel or scissors, and the keloid is then resected or debulked. Finally, the harvested skin is sutured into the defect as a full-thickness skin graft. Excision of the keloid, while retaining a rim to which the graft is anchored, is thought to decrease recurrence. The scar rim serves as a splint and decreases the transmission of tensile forces to the rest of the graft. It is important to note that keloid remnants do not cause recurrence. Partial thickness skin grafts generally yield poor results, and the open donor site is at high risk for abnormal scar formation.

Skin flaps are useful for small- to medium-sized lesions or even larger pedunculated earlobe lesions. The skin overlying the keloid can be used to create a low-tension flap. A flap of epidermis may be gently folded down to create less skin tension than pulling surrounding skin over the defect. Additionally, the skin match is superior to that of a skin graft taken from another anatomic site. Earlobe keloids can also be managed by two other useful techniques. Dumbbell-shaped keloids can be completed excised using the core-excision technique whereby elliptical incisions are made at the base of the lesion on the anterior and posterior sides of the pinna and the scalpel pushed through the earlobe, dissecting the core of the keloid from normal tissue. Thus, most of the lower earlobe tissue is spared. Shave excision of posterior earlobe keloids has been advocated as a fast, efficient technique. Healing by second intention with accompanying wound pressure is often adequate for treatment of keloids on skin that is not readily visible.

For all surgical techniques in which suture closure is performed, adjuvant therapy is strongly recommended to diminish recurrence. Most clinicians suggest infiltration of 0.1 to 1.0 mL of 40 mg/mL triamcinolone acetonide into the operative bed after the placement of sutures. Some clinicians suggest injecting the base of the wound with 10 mg of triamcinolone before closing the wound. The quantity of steroid injected should be sufficient to infiltrate the entire lesion. Steroids are generally reinjected at the time of suture removal and then at monthly intervals for three to six months. Thereafter, the interval between treatments can be progressively increased to two, three and four months, and thereafter can be lengthened to a year. If there is any sign of recurrence such as pruritus of skin thickening, the patient should be encouraged to return as needed.

Carbon dioxide (CO_2) laser removal of keloids as opposed to "cold steel" surgery was originally reported to have a lower recurrence rate (Figs. 10 and 11). This method sterilizes tissue, seals blood vessels up to 0.5 mm as it cuts, and causes minimal necrosis to surrounding tissue. Unfortunately, once the initial enthusiasm subsided, there appeared to be no advantage if suture closure was subsequently performed. However, if the wound is left to heal by second intention and adjuvant therapy employed, the results are more encouraging. Intralesional triamcinolone acetonide at 40 mg/mL is injected after excision into the wound edges and then monthly for six months during healing. This time frame is arbitrary, and some clinicians have achieved better results by giving intralesional steroids at two-to-three-week intervals.

Surgical removal of keloid tissue is appropriate for some lesions if proper technique is observed and adjuvant therapy employed. Excision is the only technique that provides debulking of the keloidal mass. Patients must

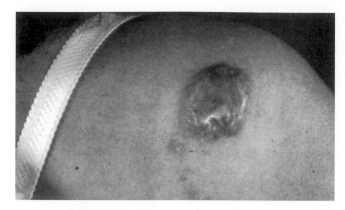

Figure 10 Keloid preoperative CO_2 laser.

understand the risk of recurrence and the consequent need for follow-up evaluation.

Pressure

Pressure therapy is useful both for therapy of established keloids and for prophylactic prevention. It is used for its proposed thinning effects. Bedridden patients resting on their sacrum of ischial tuberosities develop dermal thinning. In 1860, Herman Lawrence of Melbourne treated a keloid with multiple scarifications followed by compression for several months. After one year, only a thin scar remained. Rayer in 1894 was the first to use pressure alone in keloid treatment. Larsen in 1971 showed that nodules did not develop under pressure treatment. Kishcher et al. proposed in 1978 that pressure produced hypoxia, resulting in fibroblast degeneration and altering the ratio of collagen metabolism so that catabolism became dominant. Another group suggested that the decreased blood flow to the scar resulted in the reduced delivery of α_2-macroglobulin, an α-protein known to inhibit collagenase function. Asboe-Hansen reported that mast cells degranulate under edematous conditions and that their products encourage the formation of increased ground substance. Pressure, therefore, would decrease the availability of water and diminish the degranulation of mast cells.

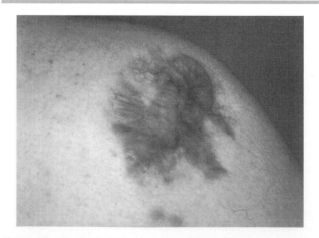

Figure 11 Six months post-CO_2 laser excision healing by second intention and two intralesional steroid treatments. Note recurrence.

Pressure therapy following surgical excision is an effective method to help prevent recurrence of earlobe keloids. Both spring-pressure earring devices and acrylic ear splints have been reported to be beneficial. Large clip-on earrings may be used with flurandrenolide tape for greater preventative effect. Pressure devices for other locations include elastic garments tightly fitted to involved anatomic sites. The pressure exerted should be at least 24 mmHg to exceed the inherent capillary pressure. It must be maintained day and night for a minimum of four to six months to one year or more. Daily discontinuances of pressure for hygiene should not exceed 30 minutes. Kelly suggests that a pressure gradient elastic garment should be worn at least 12 hour a day for four to six months after cutaneous trauma in patients at high risk for the development of keloids.

Radiation

Radiation therapy is used either alone or as an adjunct to surgical excision. In 1906, DeBeurman and Gougerot were the first to describe X-ray treatment for keloids. Homans, in 1940, recommended radiation after excision or pressure therapy. In 1961, Cosmon et al. found that radiation treatment given in the early postoperative period was most advantageous in the prevention of recurrence. No advantage has been shown for preoperative radiation therapy alone or in combination with postoperative therapy.

The rationale for radiotherapy involves the destruction of fibroblasts by ionizing radiation. These fibroblasts are not replaced by bloodborne cells from distant tissues. Through the destruction of a sufficient quantity of cells, a balance may be reached between collagen synthesis and degradation.

Inalsingh reported a series of 501 patients given either superficial radiation alone or radiation following excisional therapy. Patients received 400 rads monthly and five or fewer treatments. Good cosmetic results and relief of symptoms were reported in 26.5% of patients. Over a two-year follow-up, no adverse effects from radiation were observed. In 1989, Sallstrom et al. treated 124 patients with postoperative X-ray radiation begun within 24 hours of surgery. The treatment results were evaluated between 6 and 24 months after treatment. Good or excellent results were observed in 92% of the patients. Side effects included slight hyperpigmentation in 31% and telangiectasia in 15%. Other reported side effects include pruritus, paresthesias, and pain. More recently, Giux et al. have reported excellent results using high-dose-rate brachytherapy, with a 3.4% failure rate when combined with surgery, and 13.6% persistence rate when used alone. This study however followed a favorable group of patients with relatively small scars. The results of radiation alone are cosmetically inferior to surgery and radiation combined.

Many clinicians remain concerned about the possible carcinogenic effects of radiation therapy. In an effort to quantify this risk, Ragoowansi et al. reviewed the literature on radiotherapy for keloids, finding five cases of cancer in 6741 treatments. These include one case of thyroid cancer in a potential exit dose site eight years after treatment of a keloid on the chin; bilateral breast cancer developing 29 years following radiotherapy for chest wall keloids; a basal cell carcinoma 10 years postradiotherapy; a parathyroid adenoma 38 years after treatment of neck keloids; and finally, a case of fibrous mesothelioma of the pleura with ipsilateral breast carcinoma 23 years after external radiotherapy for a chest wall keloid. Four of these patients were between the ages of 10 and 36 years at the time of treatment. No age-matched controls were offered as comparison for cancer risk over the same time period. It appears that although radiation therapy appears to be an effective adjuvant therapy, it should be used with caution, and then only in elderly patients with significant symptoms or loss of function from their keloids.

Intralesional Therapy
Corticosteroids

A preferred initial approach to the treatment of keloids is the intralesional injection of steroids. Proper placement of the needle and medication within the lesion is important and often the reason this approach fails. Such injections may be used alone or in combination with other therapies such as surgery (as discussed above) or cryotherapy. Intralesional injections alone serve to diminish symptoms and soften and flatten the upraised scar. The patient must be informed that this treatment will not result in narrowing or disappearance of the scar. The response rate to intralesional steroid injections is variable. In 1970, Griffith et al. reported recurrence of only five of 56 treated keloids after four years of follow-up. However, Kiil in 1977 reported a 50% recurrence rate over five years.

Corticosteroids alter the balance between collagen synthesis and degradation. Collagen synthesis is diminished, and collagen breakdown is enhanced by decreasing levels of the known inhibitors α_2-macroglobulin and α_1-antitrypsin. It appears that early keloids are more responsive to treatment. This may be explained by the younger fibroblast's increased collagenase production in response to steroids.

Several preparations may be used for intralesional injection. Many clinicians routinely use triamcinolone acetonide (Kenalog) 40 mg/mL for initial treatment. However, others suggest starting with a 10 mg/mL dose and monitoring response. Lack of response after two or three injections would dictate the need to increase the concentration or switch to a triamcinolone diacetate (Aristocort 25 mg/mL) preparation. Another approach is to vary the concentrations of triamcinolone acetonide in different lesions or within different areas of the same lesion. Corticosteroids can also be diluted with equal parts of 2% lidocaine. The lidocaine is most useful in decreasing the pain of multiple injections as well as the pain immediately following treatment.

The steroid preparation may be delivered in a number of fashions. Usually, a needle and syringe delivery system is used. A Luer-Lok needle and syringe are necessary to prevent separation of the syringe from the needle while injecting. A small-gauge needle is used; ideally, a 30- or 27-gauge needle is recommended. Occasionally, clogging and near impossible injection result, necessitating the use of a 25-gauge needle, especially while using tyriamcinolone acetonide at 40 mg/mL. Other delivery systems include mechanical injectors such as the spring or CO_2-powered device. Mechanical injectors are said to cause less pain on injection, but most clinicians feel that steroid placement is less efficient and there is greater wastage. Dental syringes are preferred by some as they are said to facilitate injection.

Intralesional injections are directed at the center or bulk of the keloid mass. Care must be taken to inject only the keloid itself or the base of the keloid. Superficial infiltration beneath the epidermis or deep deposition within the adipose will increase the risk of side effects such as atrophy and hypopigmentation. Occasionally, injection will be extremely difficult due to the fibrotic nature of the tumor. A technique for facilitating injection involves creating a needle tract by inserting the needle into the keloid and injection while slowly withdrawing. Another effective method is to use light cryosurgery prior to injection. Cryosurgery induces tissue edema and provides the additional advantage of subsequent cellular and collagen disruption. The liquid nitrogen is applied only briefly to establish a skin frost. An alternative used by the author (RKR) is to inject local anesthesia, followed by a freeze–thaw cycle with liquid nitrogen for 1.5 minutes, which results in tissue necrosis plus the steroid effect. After 10 of 15 minutes, the lesion is injected. The technique also allows for better dispersal of the corticosteroid through the keloidal tissue and minimizes its deposition in the subcutaneous or surrounding tissue. Keloids become easier to inject with increasing treatment number. Treatment intervals are arbitrary, but most clinicians separate treatments by three to four weeks for maximal effect.

Intralesional steroid injections are not without potential risk. Hypopigmentation and atrophy are not uncommon side effects. Overenthusiastic use of steroids may result in telangiectases, necrosis, ulceration, and even cushingoid habitus. A rare complication results from the pooling of 40 mg/mL of triamcinolone acetonide in injected sites. This leads to the formation of subepidermal insoluble xanthomatous deposits, which must be removed for maximum cosmesis.

Other Steroids

In a comparative study of the effect of intralesional corticosteroids, intralesional 5-fluorouracil (5-FU), intralesional steroid plus 5-FU and 585-nm flashlamp-pumped pulsed dye laser treatments, Manuskiatti and Fitzpatrick showed that improvement in height, erythema, pliability, and histopathological changes, as well as patient self-assessment was similar between all of the above modalities, and significantly better than baseline and control segments. The study had a short follow-up period of 32 weeks, and the only persistent side effects were seen in the triamcinolone acetonide injection group, and these included hypopigmentation, telangiectasia, and skin atrophy.

5-FU has been shown to have an inhibitory effect on human fibroblast cell lines in culture, and inhibits myofibroblast proliferation and differentiation in Dupeytren fibroblasts in vitro. Two recent studies by Nanda et al. and Gupta et al., looking at the efficacy of intralesional 5-FU as a single modality therapy over a 12- to 24-week follow-up period showed similar results. More than half of the patients experienced more than 50% improvement in symptoms and flattening of the lesions. Neither of these trials was controlled, nor were their methods of assessment of improvement validated. The side effect profile was favorable, when compared with other injectable modalities, with patients experiencing pain on injection, injection site purpura, hyperpigmentation, and localized superficial tissue sloughing, none of which were permanent.

Another injectable agent that has been used in the adjuvant treatment of keloids is the calcium channel antagonist verapamil. Calcium channel blockers have been shown to inhibit synthesis/secretion of ECM molecules, including collagen, glycosaminoglycans, fibronectin, and additionally stimulates collagenase synthesis, all of which serves to reduce fibrous tissue production. In a controlled study comparing the effects of surgery and topical silicone combined with adjuvant intralesional verapamil hydrochloride versus surgery

and topical silicone alone, D'Andrea et al. found complete resolution of the keloids in 54% of the verapamil group versus no resolution in the control group at 18-month follow up.

Berman and Flores reported an 18.7% recurrence rate with adjuvant interferon (IFN)-α-2b injections versus 58.4% recurrence with IL triamcinolone versus 51.1% with excision alone. IFN-α and -γ are thought to reduce collagen types I and III messenger ribonucleic acid synthesis, with subsequent decreased protein production.

Bleomycin, which has been shown to induce both pulmonary and renal fibrosis, as well as scleroderma-like changes in cancer patients, has paradoxically been used to treat keloids. In an uncontrolled study by Espana et al., patients with keloids and hypertrophic scars were treated with bleomycin 1.5 IU/mL for one to five sessions separated by one to four months. After the lesions were anesthetized with mepivacaine, bleomycin was dripped onto the lesion, and the scar was subsequently pierced with a 25-gauge needle. All lesions showed subjective flattening, however, of the three patients who achieved complete flattening of their keloids, two showed nodular recurrences within 12 months.

Cryotherapy

Cryotherapy has already been discussed for use in conjunction with intralesional corticosteroids. Two recent studies have reported excellent results using cryotherapy alone. Zouboulis et al. in 1993 performed a prospective trial on 93 white patients including 32 months of average follow-up. They reported excellent response in 32%, good response in 29%, poor response in 29%, and no response in 10%. Treatment was administered using the contact method for one freeze–thaw cycle of 30 second per lesion. Treatment was repeated as needed every 20 to 30 days. Rusciani et al. treated 65 lesions with a hand-held liquid nitrogen spray unit. They reported complete flattening in 73% of the scars, most of which were less than two-years old. No recurrence was seen during follow-up of 17 to 42 months.

The major side effect associated with cryotherapy is hypopigmentation due to enhanced melanocyte sensitivity to such cold temperatures. When cryotherapy is combined with intralesional steroid injection, hypopigmentation is almost inevitable.

Silastic Gel Sheeting

A newer approach to the treatment of keloid scars is with silastic gel sheeting. However, these authors are skeptical, not having much success with our patients. This is a semiocclusive scar cover made of cross-linked polydimethylsiloxane polymer. Silicon gel was shown to be of value in the treatment of hypertrophic scars, especially following thermal injury. Quinn proposed that it is the low molecular weight of the silicone oil continuously released from gel sheeting that is responsible for the clinical effect. Mercer described 18 patients with 22 keloid scars treated for six months with silicone gel. He reported improvement in texture and color in greater than 80% and height in 68%.

Sawada and Sone compared a silicone cream containing 20% silicone oil covered with an occlusive dressing to the cream formulation alone. They reported remarkable improvement in the cream/occlusive dressing group (82%) and only mild improvement (22%) in the cream alone group. The authors consequently suggested that occlusion and hydration are the principal modes of action of both the silicone gel sheeting method and the silicone cream/occlusive dressing method. They recently went on to compare the efficacy of an occlusive dressing technique using cream that did not contain silicone with an application of Vaseline as a control. Greater scar improvement was noted in the cream-tested areas, and the authors once again emphasized the importance of hydration and occlusion.

A more recent study of silicone versus the nonsilicone Duoderm synthetic occlusive gel dressing using more objective means of comparing scar color and intracicatricial pressure showed that both modalities significantly reduce scar size, induration, and symptoms as compared with control. There was no significant difference between the two treatment groups.

It appears that sensitization to silicone oil does not occur, nor does it cause irritation. There is no evidence to date of silicone absorption.

Lasers

Laser surgery using the CO_2 laser has already been discussed. Disappointing results have consistently been reported with the argon laser. In the past, some authors have reported softening and flattening of lesions with the neodymium yttrium-garnet (Nd:YAG) laser. Abergel et al. reported initial success in two patients with three years of follow-up. They suggested that the mechanism of action was a specific bioinhibition of collagen production without altering the viability or replication of cells. Collagen production was selectively inhibited after treatment with the Nd:YAG laser. Sherman et al. in 1990 also reported improvement with the Nd:YAG laser in 20 patients with keloid scars. Long-term follow-up and larger population sampling are necessary to judge the ultimate utility of this treatment modality.

Like the CO_2 laser, which has already been discussed, keloid vaporization with the argon and Nd:Yag continuous wave lasers, have ultimately demonstrated no advantage over scalpel excision. These modalities have also produced significant side effects such as pain, atrophy, and dyspigmentation. Progress over the past decade, however, has raised new hope for laser in the treatment of hypertrophic scars and keloids.

Dierickx et al. reported the use of the flashlamp pulsed dye laser at 585 nm and 6.0 to 7.5 J/cm^2 fluence for the treatment of refractory hypertrophic scars. They reported that 47% of the patients had 100% improvement after one to three treatments. The authors had used the laser with the goal of improving scar color. An unexpected consequence was an improvement in the scar texture, with flattening and softening of the scar. Data suggest that patients with hypertrophic scars have an early increased microcirculatory perfusion. The authors suggest that selective photothermolysis of the increased vasculature by the flashlamp pulsed dye laser may reduce scar hypertrophy. The hypoxia induced by the laser treatment of the vessels has been proposed to alter the collagen metabolism, favoring catabolism by collagenase activity.

Unfortunately, the profound improvements in pliability, erythema, and bulk seem with the treatment of hypertrophic scars, do not seem to cross over to the treatment of keloid scars. In a recent study using remittance spectroscopy as an objective measurement of erythema, in order to assess the effect of the 585 nm flashlamp-pumped pulsed dye laser versus silicone gel sheeting for the treatment of keloids, no difference was found. Nevertheless, with the continued refinement of laser technology, the future holds promise.

Systemic Therapy

Many keloids are associated with significant symptoms such as pain and pruritus. These symptoms are frequently ascribed to histamine release. Additionally, there is some evidence that the elevated histamine content in keloid tissue may be responsible for the development of the lesion. Antihistamines have been reported to inhibit the growth of fibroblasts derived from human keloids in addition to alleviating pruritus.

Other oral medications have also been suggested to have antifibrotic effects. Systemic d-penicillamine has been used with some success in the treatment of keloids; it is a prototypical thiol that inhibits the synthesis of collagen cross-links. In vitro d-penicillamine chelates copper, which thereby reduces the activity of lysyl oxidase. Uncross-linked collagen is more susceptible to collagenase, and therefore conditions for collagen breakdown are more favorable.

Pentoxifylline, an analog of methyl xantine theobromine, causes a dose-dependent inhibition of collagen, fibronectin, and glycoaminoglycan production from keloid-derived fibroblasts. Colchicine and β-aminopropiontile (BAPN) fumarate are also effective antifibrotic agents. BAPN, like penicillamine, is a lysyl oxidase inhibitor, which interferes with collagen cross-linking Colchicine increases tissue collagenase degradation. These treatments are still largely experimental and require further study.

Topical Therapy

Topical retinoic acid is thought to have an inhibitory effect on DNA synthesis in fibroblasts. It has been reported to reduce growth and soften keloid scars. Delimpens reported 28 patients treated with 0.025% solution of retinoic acid daily for up to 22 months. Favorable results were achieved in 77% and consisted of decreased symptomatology, improved coloration, and decreased tumor bulk. Zinc, in the form of zinc oxide, has also been used topically. One study reported scars reduced to the level of the surrounding skin within six months. No further studies followed.

Based on its ability to increase the local concentration of IFNs at the site of application, Kaufman and Berman studied the use of adjuvant imiquimod cream in 12 patients, who applied the cream nightly for eight weeks following surgical excision and layered closure. None of the 10 completing the study had recurrence after 24 weeks of follow up. Most patients experience mild to marked irritation, occasionally requiring the suspension of applications for days to a week, before being able to resume therapy.

Cytokines

Two types of cytokine, IFN (α, β, and γ), and TGF-β have been investigated for their effects on collagen synthesis. The IFNs and especially IFN-γ have been shown to inhibit collagen synthesis, while TGF-β is a cytokine that enhances ECM production by a variety of cells in vitro and in vivo. Further study will likely exploit methods to inhibit the effect of TGF-β on collagen production.

ACNE KELOIDALIS

The first description of Acne keloidalis (AK) was by Kaposi in 1869, who termed the seemingly idiopathic chronic inflammation and excessive connective-tissue formation as "dermatitis papillaris capillitii." Contemporary authors most commonly refer to a disorder that typically affects the occipital scalp of young black men as AK nuchae (AKN), AK, acne keloid, and folliculitis keloidalis. Although the etiology is unknown, what is clear is that these lesions are neither keloids, nor variants of acne vulgaris. There has been one case report of familial AK in a father and his three sons (but not in his two daughters). In a Nigerian study, 15% of patients had a family history of AKN. Although overwhelmingly a problem of postpubertal black men, there have been reports of AKN occurring in black woman, and white men. The male to female ratio however, is approximately 20:1, and the disease accounts for 0.45% of all dermatoses in African-Americans.

Pathogenesis

Many theories on the pathogenesis of AKN have been put forward, yet none have been proven. Incriminated precipitating factors have included constant irritation from shirt collars, chronic low-grade folliculitis, and autoimmune processes. The notion that lesions of AKN are caused by ingrown tightly curled hair, analogous to the situation in pseudofolliculitis barbae has been disproved by Sperling et al. who argue, based on the histologic findings of early clinical lesions, that AKN is a form of primary inflammatory scarring alopecia against an as yet unidentified antigen. Previous studies have argued, largely based on histopathology that AKN represents a variant form of lichen simplex chronicus with fibrotic keloidal scarring, and that AKN is a transepithelial elimination disorder similar to perforating folliculitis. Drug-induced variants have been suggested, based on reports of scalp lesions in patients on cyclosporin and the anticonvulsants diphenylhydantoin and carbamazepine that resolved with discontinuation of the drug.

Clinical Pathogenesis

The primary lesions include small firm, smooth, often dome-shaped papules, and occasional pruritic pustules over the nape of the neck and the occiput of the scalp. In a minority of cases, lesions occur on the vertex and crown. Hair can be seen exiting the papules initially, however these are generally lost as the papules enlarge and coalesce into hairless, keloid-like plaques. The upper border of this band-like lesion over the occipital scalp is often fringed with tufted hair. Subcutaneous abscesses with draining sinuses may also be present in advanced lesions, and these often omit a malodorous discharge. Although AK may be asymptomatic, burning and itching are often reported, usually in association with pustules, which are often secondarily excoriated and traumatized. No comedones are present at any stage of AKN.

Histopathology

Sperling et al., in a study of the early clinical lesions of AK in 10 African-American patients, showed that the most consistent changes included a perifollicular chronic lymphoplasmacytic inflammation concentrated at the level of the isthmus and lower infundibulum, with disappearance of sebaceous glands associated with the inflamed follicles. Other findings included lamellar fibroplasia, thinning of the follicular epithelium at the level of the isthmus, and even total epithelial destruction with residual "naked" hair fragments. Noteworthy was the lack of evidence of bacteria, and only small numbers of Demodex organisms, and that even some clinically normal specimens showed significant abnormalities, including destruction of the individual follicles. More advanced lesions demonstrate a granulomatous foreign body reaction to broken hair fragments, producing tufted hairs, and dermal fibrosis resembling normal scar tissue.

Treatment

Although the pathogenetic theories are unproven, many authors continue to advocate avoidance of tight fitting clothing or hats that may cause mechanical irritation to the posterior hairline, and cutting the hairs in this area with a razor or clippers. For early and limited lesions, medical therapies have been met with a modicum of success. These therapeutic options include topical treatment with potent corticosteroids, retinoic acid gels, and when there are pustules, topical antibiotics. Intralesional steroids and cryotherapy may attenuate the process, but can also lead to postinflammatory hypopigmentation. The use of long-pulse diode laser therapy or long pulse Nd:YAG lasers have been used to eliminate the hair, which seems to be the focus of the inflammatory process.

Larger, more developed, late-stage lesions are traditionally dealt with surgically. Excision can be done with cold steel, electrosurgical excision using a cutting current, or CO_2 laser. The advantages of the latter two techniques being the improved hemostasis, however, thermal injury to the wound edges may theoretically increase the risk of dehiscence of a primary closure, and some authors argue that electrodissection may be associated with increased postoperative pain. There are no head-to-head, randomized, prospective trials to compare the efficacy of the various excision modalities. When excising the keloid tissue, it is imperative to cut to deep subcutaneous tissue or muscular fascia, as recurrence is more common if one does not achieve subfollicular destruction; if possible, optimal cosmetic result is achieved when a horizontal elliptical excision includes the posterior hairline. Excision may be followed by second intention healing, split-thickness skin grafting, primary closure, or staged excision with primary closure. Second intention healing generally results in contraction of the wound, resulting in a smaller and flatter scar than the original acne keloid. Unfortunately, the often large wound takes long to heel (usually 8–12 weeks), and requires diligent postoperative care, including twice daily dressing changes.

Split-thickness skin grafts eliminate the need for long-term postoperative wound care, however, they have shown to be of little cosmetic benefit, and leave a second wound at the donor site.

Primary closure has been maligned due to fact that the scars often stretch to as large an area as one produced by second intention healing, and has the added disadvantage of restricted movement if the patients head had to be bent back during suturing of the wound. In a recent study by Gloster, excision with primary closure or staged excision with primary closure achieved qualitative cosmetic result scores of 3.6/4 and 3.8/4 by the physician and patients, respectively. Side effects including recurrences of tiny pustules and papules occurred in 15 patients, and five patients developed hypertrophic scars within the incision site. No patients required analgesics stronger than acetaminophen.

BIBLIOGRAPHY

Abdalla Osman AA, Gumma KA, Satir AA. Highlights on the etiology of keloid. Int Surg 1978; 63(6):33–37.

Abergel RP, Pizzurro D, Meeker CA, et al. Biochemical composition of the connective tissue in keloids and analysis of collagen metabolism in keloid fibroblast cultures. J Invest Dermatol 1985; 84(5):384–390.

Abergel RP, Pizzuro RD, Meeker CA, et al. Biochemical composition of the connective tissue in keloids and analysis

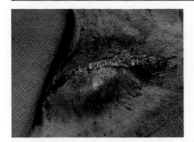

Fig. 11.5 Acute hematoma presenting 24 hours postoperatively at supraclavicular full thickness skin graft donor site. *(See p. 86)*

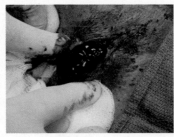

Fig. 11.6 Gelatin-like clots of a hematoma being expressed after removal of several staples. *(See p. 86)*

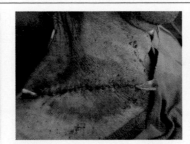

Fig. 11.7 A Penrose drain in place. *(See p. 86)*

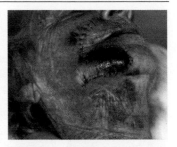

Fig. 11.8 Organized hematoma at postoperative day 7. *(See p. 87)*

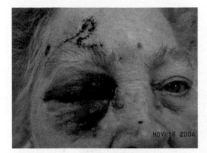

Fig. 11.9 Periorbital edema and ecchymoses the day after a procedure on the forehead. *(See p. 87)*

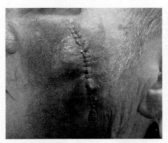

Fig. 11.10 Acute wound infection presenting several days postoperatively. The area is red, warm, swollen, and tender. *(See p. 89)*

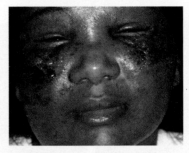

Fig. 11.11 Allergic contact dermatitis to topical antibiotic applied to periocular wounds. *(See p. 90)*

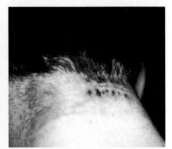

Fig. 11.12 Brightly erythematous suture reaction. *(See p. 90)*

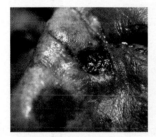

Fig. 11.13 Necrosis of distal portion of transposition flap. Note hyperpigmentation from full-thickness graft on distal nose. *(See p. 92)*

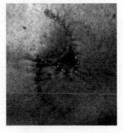

Fig. 11.14 Necrosis of a full-thickness skin graft in an area placed over exposed cartilage. *(See p. 92)*

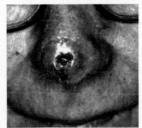

Fig. 11.15 Dehiscence at the site of necrosis. *(See p. 93)*

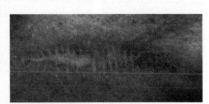

Fig. 11.18 "Railroad tracking" at suture sites and early scar spreading. *(See p. 95)*

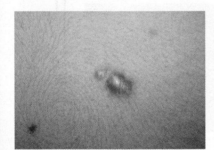

Fig. 11.19 Keloid formation at punch biopsy site. *(See p. 95)*

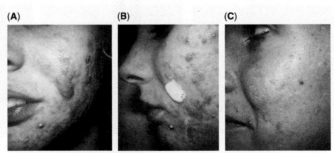

(A) **(B)** **(C)**

Fig. 20.3 **(A)** Acne cyst on left cheek prior to treatment. **(B)** Acne cyst immediately after treatment with cryosurgery. **(C)** Completely healed 10 months after treatment. *(See p. 176)*

(A) **(B)** **(C)**

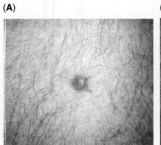
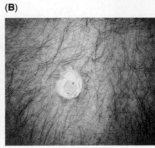
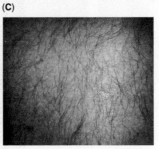

Fig. 20.4 **(A)** Dermatofibroma on left leg prior to treatment. **(B)** Cryosurgery to lesion. **(C)** Complete healing six months after treatment. *(See p. 177)*

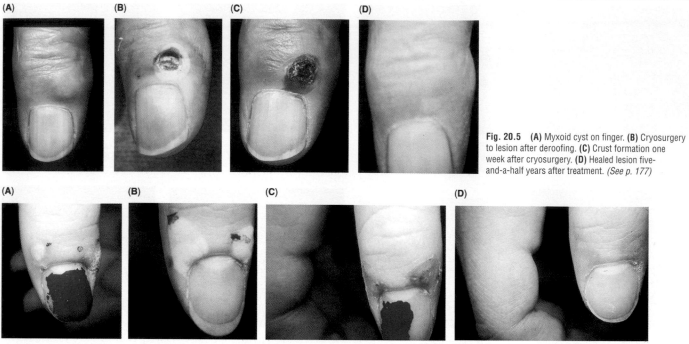

Fig. 20.5 **(A)** Myxoid cyst on finger. **(B)** Cryosurgery to lesion after deroofing. **(C)** Crust formation one week after cryosurgery. **(D)** Healed lesion five-and-a-half years after treatment. *(See p. 177)*

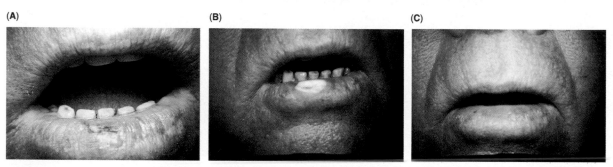

Fig. 20.9 **(A)** Periungual warts prior to treatment. **(B)** Cryosurgery to lesions. **(C)** Healing three weeks after treatment. **(D)** Excellent results four weeks after treatment. *(See p. 178)*

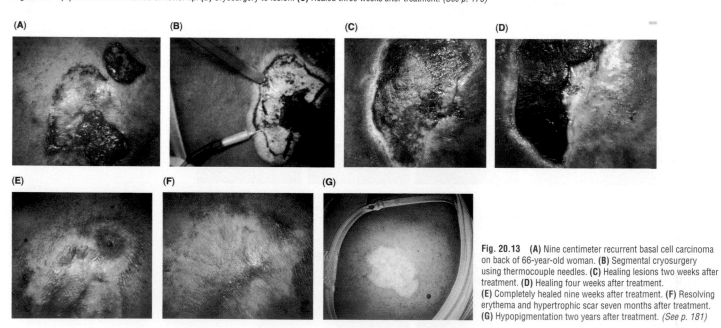

Fig. 20.11 **(A)** Small actinic cheilitis on lower lip. **(B)** Cryosurgery to lesion. **(C)** Healed three weeks after treatment. *(See p. 179)*

Fig. 20.13 **(A)** Nine centimeter recurrent basal cell carcinoma on back of 66-year-old woman. **(B)** Segmental cryosurgery using thermocouple needles. **(C)** Healing lesions two weeks after treatment. **(D)** Healing four weeks after treatment. **(E)** Completely healed nine weeks after treatment. **(F)** Resolving erythema and hypertrophic scar seven months after treatment. **(G)** Hypopigmentation two years after treatment. *(See p. 181)*

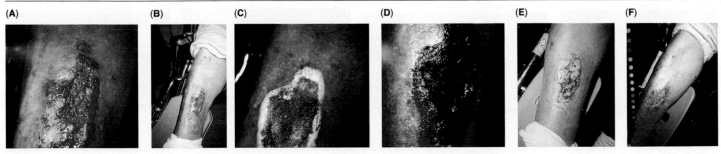

Fig. 20.14 **(A, B)** 11 cm ulcerative basal cell carcinoma on right lower leg in a 90-year-old man **(C)** Cryosurgery to entire tumor. **(D)** Sloughing and crusting one week after treatment. **(E)** Healing four weeks after treatment. **(F)** Completely healed three months after treatment. *(See p. 182)*

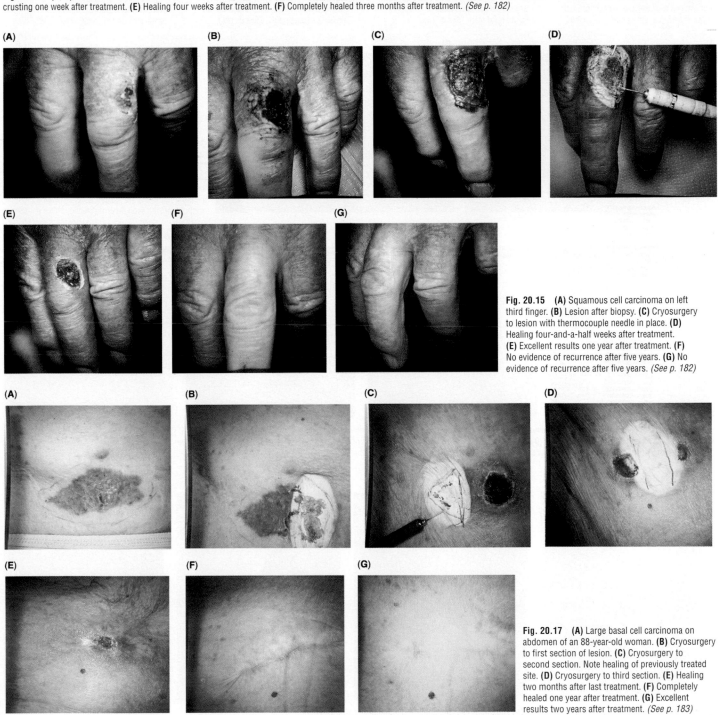

Fig. 20.15 **(A)** Squamous cell carcinoma on left third finger. **(B)** Lesion after biopsy. **(C)** Cryosurgery to lesion with thermocouple needle in place. **(D)** Healing four-and-a-half weeks after treatment. **(E)** Excellent results one year after treatment. **(F)** No evidence of recurrence after five years. **(G)** No evidence of recurrence after five years. *(See p. 182)*

Fig. 20.17 **(A)** Large basal cell carcinoma on abdomen of an 88-year-old woman. **(B)** Cryosurgery to first section of lesion. **(C)** Cryosurgery to second section. Note healing of previously treated site. **(D)** Cryosurgery to third section. **(E)** Healing two months after last treatment. **(F)** Completely healed one year after treatment. **(G)** Excellent results two years after treatment. *(See p. 183)*

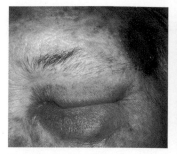

Fig. 20.22 Severe periorbital edema after treatment of a large basal cell carcinoma on the temple on a 67-year-old woman. *(See p. 185)*

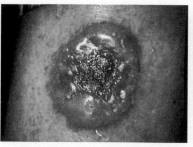

Fig. 20.23 Bulla formation after treatment of a large basal cell carcinoma on the thigh of a 75-year-old man. *(See p. 185)*

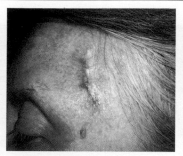

Fig. 20.24 Hypertrophic scar on forehead two months after treatment of a basal cell carcinoma. *(See p. 185)*

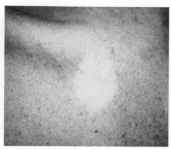

Fig. 20.25 Hypopigmentation 15 months after treatment of a basal cell carcinoma on the chest. *(See p. 185)*

(A)

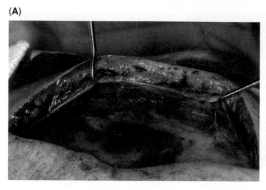

(B)

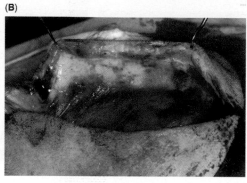

Fig. 21.2 Clinical photos demonstrating the layers of the scalp: **(A)** note the three top layers of the scalp (skin, subcutaneous tissue, and galea) are connected to one another. These three layers have been separated from the periosteum via the subgaleal space; **(B)** another photo of the forehead demonstrating the three top layers of the scalp separated from the periosteum via the subgaleal space. Note the frontalis muscle seen on cross-section. *(See p. 189)*

(A)

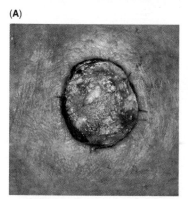

(B)

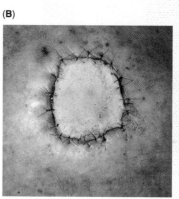

(C)

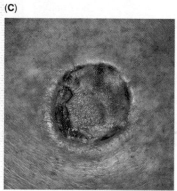

(D)

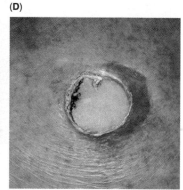

Fig. 21.4 Clinical photos demonstrating the adverse impact that a relative loss of the vascular network can have in defects extending to bone: **(A)** surgical defect extending to the periosteum; **(B)** skin graft placed at the surgical site; **(C)** signs of a failing graft with epidermal sloughing 13 days postoperatively; **(D)** completely failed skin graft with defect extending to bone three months after the original surgery. *(See p. 190)*

(A)

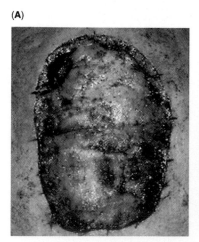

(B)

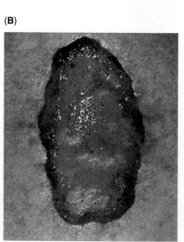

(C)

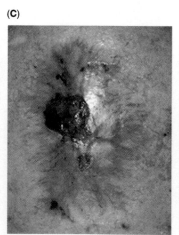

(D)

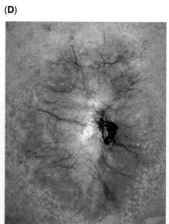

Fig. 21.7 Healing by second intention on the scalp: **(A)** squamous cell carcinoma; **(B)** immediately after resection; **(C)** two months after resection showing healthy granulation tissue; **(D)** one year after resection. *(See p. 192)*

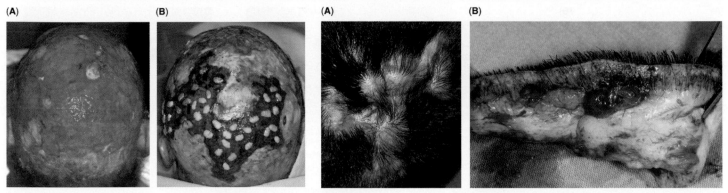

Fig. 21.8 **(A)** Ulcerative sarcoidosis involving the scalp. **(B)** Two sessions of split thickness pinch grafting four months after controlling the disease with immunosuppressive therapy. *(See p. 192)*

Fig. 21.9 **(A)** Keratosis follicularis spinulosa decalvans resulting in scarring alopecia. **(B)** Gross specimen after resection demonstrates hair, granulation tissue, and scar. *(See p. 192)*

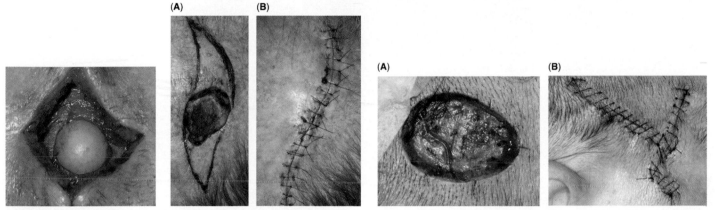

Fig. 21.10 Osteoma demonstrated intraoperatively. *(See p. 193)*

Fig. 21.11 Primary closure of a scalp defect: **(A)** defect after Mohs micrographic surgery; **(B)** primary S-plasty closure. *(See p. 193)*

Fig. 21.12 An A-to-T flap: **(A)** surgical defect after Mohs micrographic surgery; **(B)** A-to-T flap with a Burow's triangle inferiorly. *(See p. 193)*

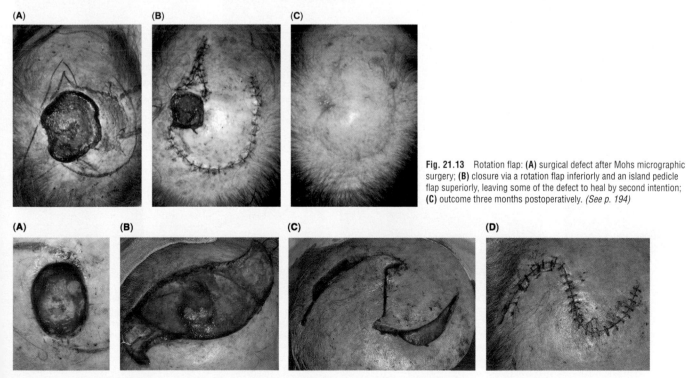

Fig. 21.13 Rotation flap: **(A)** surgical defect after Mohs micrographic surgery; **(B)** closure via a rotation flap inferiorly and an island pedicle flap superiorly, leaving some of the defect to heal by second intention; **(C)** outcome three months postoperatively. *(See p. 194)*

Fig. 21.14 Bilateral rotation flap on the scalp vertex: **(A)** surgical defect after Mohs micrographic surgery; **(B)** undermined flaps; **(C)** initial sutures holding the flaps in place; **(D)** outcome immediately after surgery. *(See p. 194)*

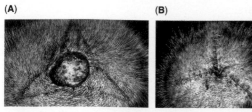

Fig. 21.15 Mercedes or tripolar advancement flap:
(A) surgical defect after Mohs micrographic surgery;
(B) immediate postoperative result. *(See p. 195)*

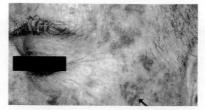

Fig. 36.1 Erythematous to yellow papules and plaques of actinic keratosis, with adjacent scale crust on the zygomatic area (*arrow*) of the cheek in a 60-year-old man with severe sun damage. *(See p. 330)*

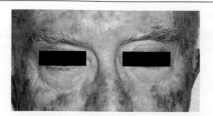

Fig. 36.2 Multiple erythematous plaques of actinic keratosis on the bridge of nose and cheek. *(See p. 330)*

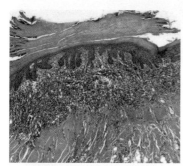

Fig. 36.4 Low-power view of an actinic keratosis, showing small buds and diffuse basal epidermal atypical keratinocytes. Note a dense upper dermal lymphocytic infiltrate and underlying severe solar elastosis of the dermal collagen (H&E, X100). *(See p. 331)*

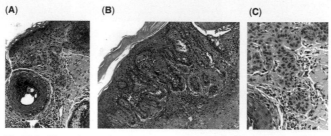

Fig. 36.7 Photomicrographs of invasive squamous cell carcinoma arising in actinic keratosis, displaying various depths of dermal invasion by carcinoma cells, branching down from the dermo–epidermal junction **(A and B)** (H&E, X60, X25). Higher magnification of **(A)** depicts dermal irregular strands of invasive tumor cells **(C)** (H&E, X125). *(See p. 332)*

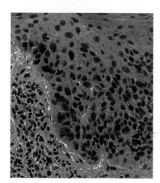

Fig. 36.11 A radiation keratosis on the skin of the chest at the site of a radiation port in a patient with esophageal carcinoma, displays disorderly, atypical keratinocytes, with pleomorphic and hyperchromatic nuclei involving the basal epidermis (H&E, X200). *(See p. 334)*

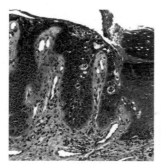

Fig. 36.13 Plaque-like lesion of Bowen's disease showing hyperkeratosis, and atypical keratinocytes replacing the entire thickness of the epidermis, absent normal keratinocytic maturation and marked nuclear atypia with abnormal mitoses (H&E, X250). *(See p. 335)*

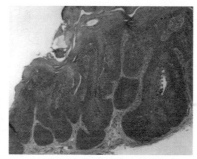

Fig. 36.15 Invasive adnexal carcinoma arising in Bowen's disease shows prominent basaloid and squamoid differentiation. Note marked nuclear anaplasia (H&E, X100). *(See p. 336)*

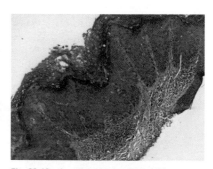

Fig. 36.16 A section of vulvar bowenoid papulosis, showing mild hyperkeratosis, acanthosis, and scattered dysplastic and dyskeratotic keratinocytes (H&E, X160). *(See p. 336)*

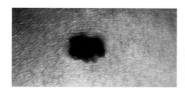

Fig. 36.20 An irregularly bordered, enlarging pigmented lesion of malignant melanoma in situ (precancerous melanosis) present on the arm of a 32-year-old-man. *(See p. 339)*

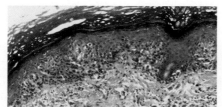

Fig. 36.21 A malignant melanoma in situ showing contiguous atypical melanocytic proliferation at the dermo–epidermal junction, with occasional intraepidermal pagetoid spread (H&E, X200). *(See p. 339)*

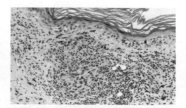

Fig. 36.22 Photomicrographs of a lentigo maligna melanoma illustrates extensive dermo–epidermal junction involvement by contiguous atypical melanocytes, with focal upper dermal invasion. Note spindle-shaped tumor cells (H&E, X250). *(See p. 339)*

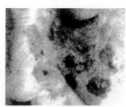

Fig. 36.23 A large, pigmented lesion of LM melanoma on the cheektemporal area of an 83-year-old fair-skinned individual. These tumors are characterized by a flat (macular) lesion with a prolonged radial growth phase, and developed invading tumor with pigmented nodule formation. *(See p. 340)*

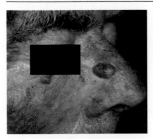

Fig. 37.1 Nodular basal cell carcinoma present on the nasal sidewall. Note the exophytic nature of the tumor with the characteristic pearly quality and overlying telangectasias. *(See p. 344)*

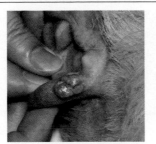

Fig. 37.2 Nodular basal cell carcinoma present on the superior helix of the ear. Sunexposed sites such as the face and ear are common locations for basal cell carcinoma. *(See p. 345)*

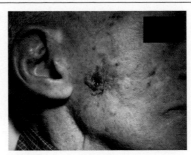

Fig. 37.3 Nodular pattern basal cell carcinoma of the face appearing decades after radiation therapy. Note extensive ulceration of the tumor. This patient has evidence of multiple prior surgical procedures for cutaneous malignancies. Patients treated with irradiation for benign dermatoses are prone to developing basal cell carcinoma in the treated areas. *(See p. 345)*

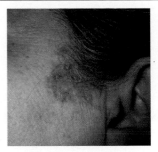

Fig. 37.4 Superficial pattern basal cell carcinoma on the cheek. Note its presentation as an erythematous, scaly patch, similar to that of benign processes such as psoriasis, seborrheic dermatitis, or of eczematous dermatitis such as atopic dermatitis or allergic contact dermatitis. *(See p. 345)*

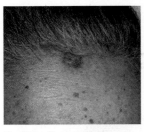

Fig. 37.5 Pigmented basal cell carcinoma on forehead. Note hyperpigmented nature, which might be confused with seborrheic keratosis, melanocytic nevus, or melanoma. *(See p. 345)*

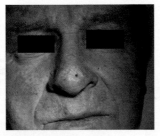

Fig. 37.6 Morpheaform pattern basal cell carcinoma present on lateral nasal tip. Note its scar-like indented appearance. These tumors can be easily overlooked because of their banal appearance. *(See p. 346)*

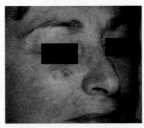

Fig. 37.7 Morpheaform pattern basal cell carcinoma in periorbital area. This tumor appears as an atrophic, indurated plaque. Minute telangectasias can be seen within the plaque. *(See p. 346)*

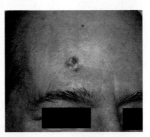

Fig. 37.9 Mixed pattern basal cell carcinoma located on forehead. Portions of this tumor are ulcerated and crusted; other areas resemble white scars. *(See p. 346)*

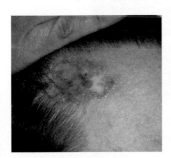

Fig. 37.10 Infiltrative pattern basal cell carcinoma located on upper forehead. The destructive nature is demonstrated by alopecia due to tumor invasion at hairline. *(See p. 347)*

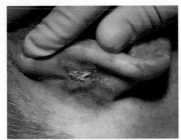

Fig. 37.11 Infiltrative pattern basal cell carcinoma of posterior ear. Note indistinct clinical margins and waxy appearance. *(See p. 347)*

(A) **(B)**

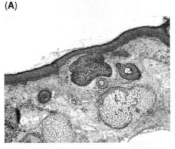

Fig. 37.12 **(A)** Low-power photomicrograph demonstrating the superficial subtype of basal cell carcinoma. A bud of basaloid cells connects to the epidermis. **(B)** High-power view of a separate section of the same tumor. Note the retraction artifact and peripheral palisading of cell nuclei. There is no intervening stroma in the tumor nodule. *(See p. 347)*

(A) **(B)**

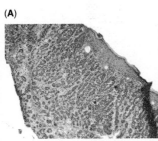

Fig. 37.13 **(A)** Low-power photomicrograph demonstrating micronodular subtype of basal cell carcinoma. Small islands of basaloid cells are present in the dermis. Note connection of tumor cells to the epidermis. **(B)** High-power photomicrograph of a micronodular subtype basal cell carcinoma shows characteristic peripheral palisading of tumor cell nuclei and retraction artifact. *(See p. 348)*

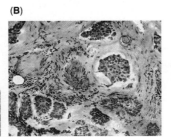

Fig. 37.14 Low-power photomicrograph demonstrating infiltrative subtype of basal cell carcinoma. Tumor islands with irregular borders are present in the dermis. *(See p. 348)*

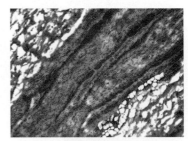

Fig. 37.15 High-power photomicrograph demonstrating intraneural involvement with basal cell carcinoma. Basal cell carcinoma tracking along nerves can travel far from the initial tumor presentation site and can be challenging to treat. *(See p. 348)*

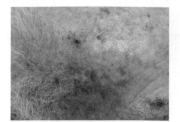

Fig. 40.1 Preoperative clinical appearance of a primary squamous cell carcinoma of scalp. *(See p. 386)*

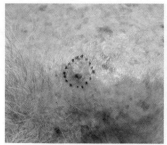

Fig. 40.2 Apparent clinical extent of tumor is outlined with a surgical skin marker. *(See p. 387)*

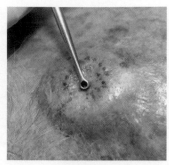

Fig. 40.3 Curettage is performed to determine extent of tumor. *(See p. 387)*

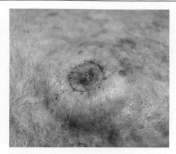

Fig. 40.4 The margin is marked with several small incisions to orient the tissue. *(See p. 387)*

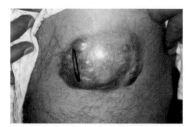

Fig. 42.1 Dermatofibrosarcoma protuberans with classic protuberant appearance. *(See p. 406)*

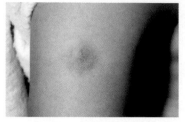

Fig. 42.2 Subtle atrophic plaque on extremity consistent with atrophic variant of dermatofibrosarcoma protuberans. *(See p. 406)*

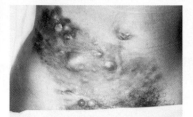

Fig. 42.3 Pigmented dermatofibrosarcoma protuberans. *(See p. 406)*

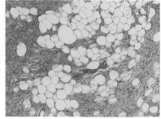

Fig. 42.4 Microscopic image of DFSP at X20, H&E stain. *(See p. 407)*

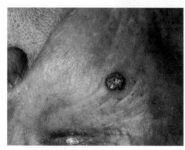

Fig. 42.5 Atypical fibroxanthoma on sun-exposed areas of cheek and helical rim. Clinical differential diagnosis includes squamous cell carcinoma and basal cell carcinoma. *(See p. 407)*

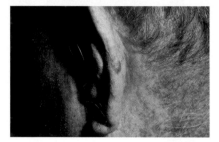

Fig. 42.6 Atypical fibroxanthoma on sun-exposed areas of cheek and helical rim. Clinical differential diagnosis includes squamous cell carcinoma and basal cell carcinoma. *(See p. 410)*

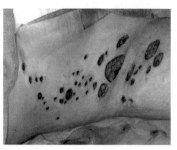

Fig. 45.7 Stage II hidradenitis suppurativa. Multiple foci of activity, independent from one another that was amenable to individual local surgical ablation. *(See p. 446)*

(A)

(B)

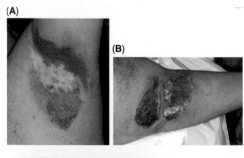

Fig. 45.8 Familial Benign Pemphigus involving the axilla. (A) Preoperative appearance. (B) Dermal wound immediately after CO2 laser vaporization. *(See p. 447)*

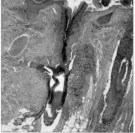

Transverse section: Lymphocytic Folliculitis

Fig. 46.3 Chronic cutaneous lupus erythematosus low-power vertical section with lymphocytic folliculitis and lichenoid infiltrate. *(See p. 452)*

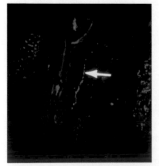

Fig. 46.4 Chronic cutaneous lupus erythematosus. Direct immunofluorescence "full house" immunoreactions linear deposition at follicular basement membrane. *(See p. 453)*

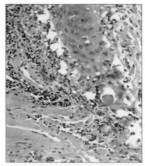

Fig. 46.6 Lichen planopilaris. Vertical sections. Lymphocytic folliculitis with civatte bodies. *(See p. 453)*

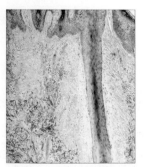

Fig. 46.7 Lichen planopilaris. Vertical section superficial wedge-shaped scar-perifollicular. *(See p. 454)*

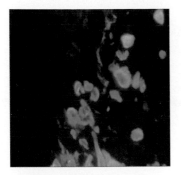

Fig. 46.8 Lichen planopilaris. Direct immunofluorescence, dermal clustered civatte bodies at basement membrane. *(See p. 454)*

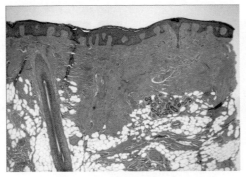

Fig. 46.14 Pseudopelade Brocq. Vertical section. Low power. End stage alopecia. *(See p. 456)*

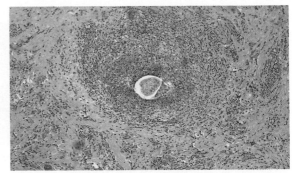

Fig. 46.16 Folliculitis decalvans. Transverse section mixed follicular and interfollicular inflammation and fibrosis. *(See p. 456)*

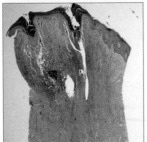
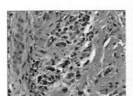

Fig. 46.18 Dissecting folliculitis. Vertical sections. Mixed follicular and interfollicular inflammation and fibrosis. *(See p. 457)*

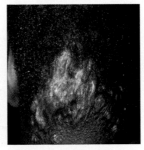

Fig. 46.20 Folliculitis keloidalis. Multiple shiny alopecic follicular papules and nodules. *(See p. 457)*

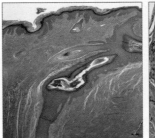
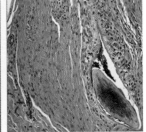

Fig. 46.21 Folliculitis keloidalis. Vertical sections. Chronic stage with follicular cysts and extensive perifollicular fibrosis. *(See p. 458)*

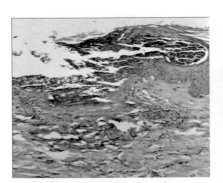

Fig. 46.23 Erosive pustular dermatosis. Vertical section. Superficial suppurative folliculitis. *(See p. 458)*

(A) **(B)**

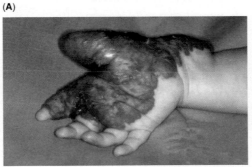
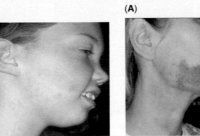

Fig. 66.1 Infant with hemangioma of hand. Before and after treatment with 577-nm flashlamp-pumped pulsed dye laser. *(See p. 673)*

(A) **(B)** **(C)**

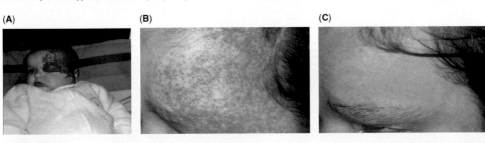

Fig. 66.3 **(A)** Infant with large facial hemangioma. **(B)** Several years later same infant as a child. Resolution of hemangioma with steroid use only. **(C)** Same child after treatment of residual hemangioma with 577-nm flashlamp-pumped pulsed dye laser. *(See p. 674)*

(A) **(B)**

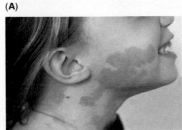
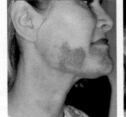

Fig. 66.4 Port-wine stain on child's face. Before and after treatment with 577-nm flashlamp-pumped pulsed dye laser. *(See p. 674)*

(A) **(B)**

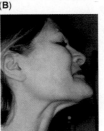

Fig. 66.5 Port-wine stain on face. Before and after treatment with 577-nm flashlamp-pumped pulsed dye laser. *(See p. 674)*

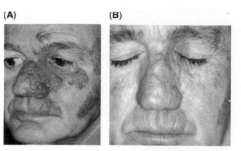

Fig. 66.6 Mature port-wine stain with bleb formation on face. Before and after treatment with 577-nm flashlamp-pumped pulsed dye laser showing reduction in texture changes and color. (See p. 674)

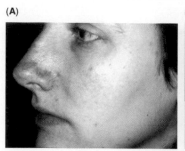
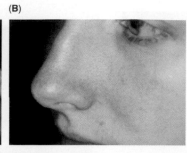

Fig. 66.7 Telengiectases on nasal ala. Before and after treatment with high-energy long-pulsed 532-nm Nd:YAG laser. (See p. 674)

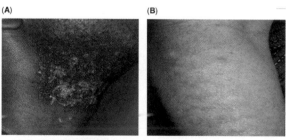

Fig. 66.8 Telengiectases in poikiloderma of civatte before and after treatment with 577-nm flashlamp-pumped pulsed dye laser. (See p. 675)

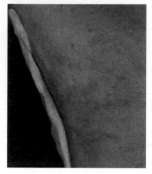
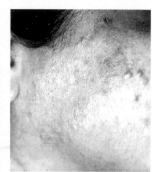

Fig. 67.4 Reactive erythema immediately following laser treatment. (See p. 686)

Fig. 67.5 Folliculitis following hair laser removal. (See p. 686)

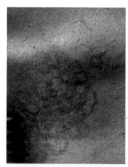
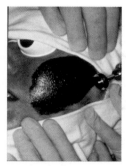
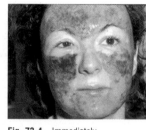

Fig. 67.6 Post-inflammatory hyperpigmentation with Fitzpatrick skin type VI after alexandrite laser treatment. (See p. 686)

Fig. 67.7 **(A)** Transient post-inflammatory hypopigmentation in dark-skinned patient following diode laser treatment for pseudofolliculitis barbae. **(B)** Post-inflammatory hypopigmentation occurring in tanned patient after alexandrite laser hair removal. (See p. 687)

Fig. 73.2. Dermabrasion operative site. Gentian violet to mark areas for dermabrasion, towels, and wire fraise on dermabrader. (See p. 752)

Fig. 73.4 Immediately postoperative after full-face dermabrasion. (See p. 753)

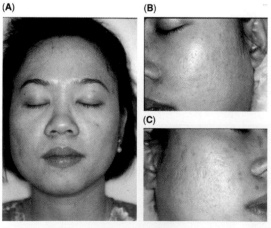

Fig. 73.6 **(A–C)** Preoperative pitted scars of moderate severity on entire face. (See p. 753)

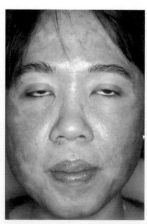

Fig. 73.7 Ten days postdermabrasion with edema and erythema. (See p. 753)

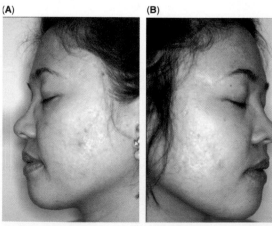

Fig. 73.8 **(A–B)** Six weeks after dermabrasion with return of normal colored skin and marked improvement in scars. (See p. 754)

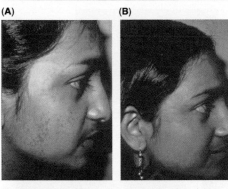
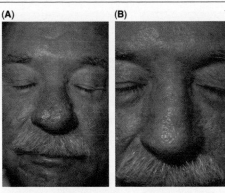
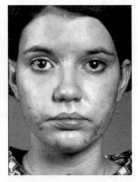

Fig. 73.9 Dark-skinned patient with facial epidermal nevus. Test spot dermabrasion in right temple, then entire cheek treated. Good repigmentation. *(See p. 754)*

Fig. 73.10 Rhinophyma before and after dermabrasion combined with CO_2 laser. *(See p. 754)*

Fig. 73.16 Complication—keloids on chin. *(See p. 759)*

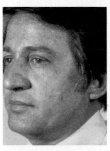
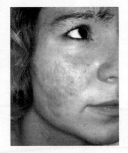
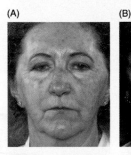
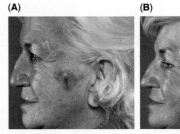

Fig. 73.17 Complication—hypopigmentation. *(See p. 759)*

Fig. 73.18 Complication—persistent erythema and telangiectasia. *(See p. 759)*

Fig. 74.3 (**A**) Prior to peel using 40%, 30%, 18% trichloroacetic acid w/v in different anatomic subunits. (**B**) Seven months postoperative. *(See p. 766)*

Fig. 74.4 (**A**) Note lentigo prior to 40% trichloroacetic acid w/v peel. (**B**) Five months postoperative. *(See p. 766)*

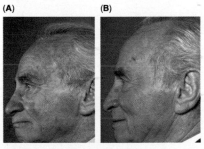
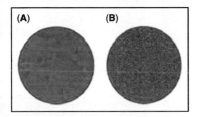
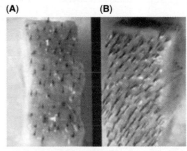

Fig. 74.5 (**A**) Solar elastosis, actinic keratoses, lentigines prior to 40% trichloroacetic acid w/v peel. (**B**) Six weeks postoperative. *(See p. 767)*

Fig. 75.A The impact of Finasteride on patients with male pattern baldness. Hair counts after five years demonstrated a 277-hair difference between the placebo (**A**) and patients maintained on 1mg Finasteride (**B**) for a five-year period. *(See p. 775)*

Fig. 75.B Donor density comparison between two individuals. (**A**) Donor hair with predominantly one and two hair follicular unit grafts of low density; (**B**) 2–4 hair follicular units with a high density of hairs per centimeter. *Source:* Courtesy of Bobby Limmer, M.D. *(See p. 777)*

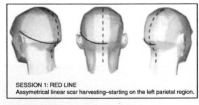
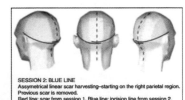
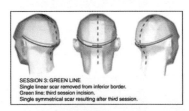

Fig. 75.C *(See p. 778)*

Fig. 75.D *(See p. 778)*

Fig. 75.E *(See p. 778)*

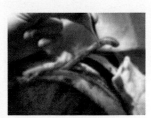
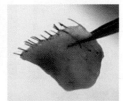
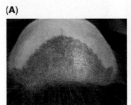
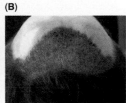

Fig. 75.F Donor Strip Removal: An 8-mm wide by 18-cm long area is removed. In cases of high density donor areas, this will consistently yield over 1500 grafts. *(See p. 778)*

Fig. 75.G Microscopic slivering (dissection): the process of producing follicular unit grafts initially involves cutting slivers of tissue approximately 2 mm in width from the donor strip. Slivering takes considerably skill and is best performed under a microscope. Further dissection of the slivering can be done under various magnification devices. *(See p. 778)*

Fig. 75.H (**A**) Before and (**B**) after placement of approximately 3000 follicular unit grafts. Perpendicular angle grafting. In Hair Transplantation. Procedures in Cosmetic Dermatology. Haber, Stough (eds), Elsevier, 2006. *Source:* Hassan V. *(See p. 779)*

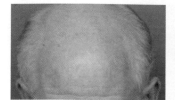

Fig. 75.I 65-year-old Caucasian male prior to transplantation. Patient has fine caliber red hair. *(See p. 779)*

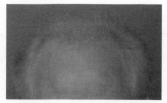

Fig. 75.J Patient in Fig. I shown after 2000 grafts; a mature recessed look can be achieved in one session. *Source*: Courtesy of Dow Stough, MD. *(See p. 779)*

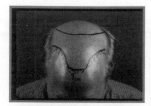

Fig. 75.K 53-year-old Caucasian male prior to transplantation. *(See p. 779)*

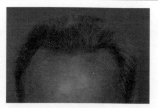

Fig. 75.L Patient in Fig. K after 3500 grafts achieved over three sessions. *(See p. 779)*

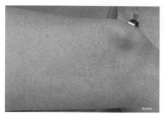
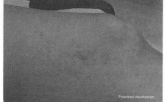

Fig. 76.5 Use of cross polarized lighting to increase visualization of telangiectasias. *(See p. 785)*

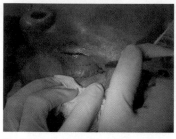

Fig. 79.11 The initial skin incision with the focused CO_2 laser. *(See p. 810)*

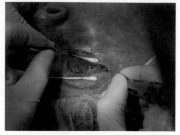

Fig. 79.12 Excising the skin/muscle flap with the focused CO_2 laser. *(See p. 810)*

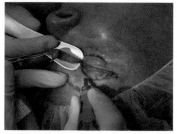

Fig. 79.13 A burnished bone plate is used as a backdrop for the laser near the medial canthus. *(See p. 811)*

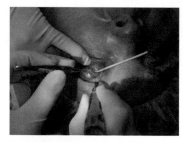

Fig. 79.14 Fragments of orbital fat are excised using defocused laser energy. *(See p. 811)*.

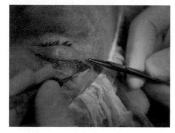

Fig. 79.15 Suture "bites" are taken 2 mm from the laser-incised wound edge. *(See p. 811)*

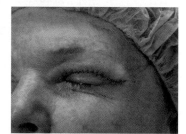

Fig. 79.16 Final sutures in place. *(See p. 811)*

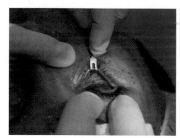

Fig. 79.17 The transconjunctival incision is made approximately 5mm from the lower lid margin and is directed toward the orbital rim. *(See p. 812)*

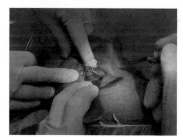

Fig. 79.18 The transconjunctival incision is deepened while gentle pressure is applied to the globe, causing the central orbital fat to extrude. *(See p. 812)*

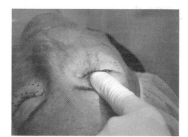

Fig. 79.19 Completeness of fat removal is assessed by applying gentle pressure to the globe and observing for bulging of fat pads. *(See p. 812)*

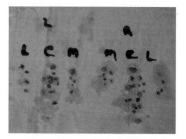

Fig. 79.20 The amount of excised fat from each fat pad (lateral, central, and medial) is assessed. *(See p. 812)*

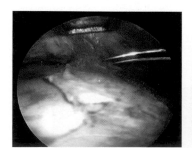

Fig. 79.23 Endoscopic view of lower zone of fixation. Scissors are used to release connective tissue. *(See p. 814)*

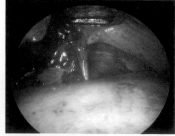

Fig. 79.24 Endoscopic view of supraorbital neurovascular bundle. Foreground is lower frontal bone. The periosteum (upper part of image) has been raised and incised just caudal to orbital rim. *(See p. 814)*

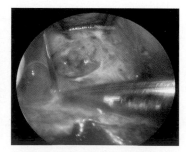

Fig. 79.25 Endoscopic view of lower temple dissection. Medial zygomaticotemporal vein (sentinel vein) is visible on the left side of the image. *(See p. 814)*

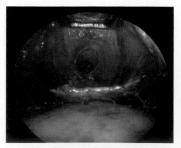

Fig. 79.26 Endoscopic view of glabella. Lower frontal bone is in the foreground. Left and right procerus muscles are visible below the steel dissector, separated by passage of a probe. To either side lay depressor supercilii muscles. Closer to foreground and obliquely oriented are corrugator supercilii muscles. *(See p. 815)*

of collagen metabolism in keloid fibroblast cultures. J invest Dermatol 1985; 84:284–290.

Acne Keloidalis

Adamson H. Dermatitis papillaris capillitii (Kaposi): acne keloid. Br J Dermatol. 1914; 26:69–83.

Addison T. On the keloid of Alibert and on true keloid. Med Chir Trans 1854; 37:27–47.

Alibert JL. Description des maladies de la peau observees a l <hopital Saint-Louis et exposition des meilleures methodes suivies pour leur traitement. Paris: Banois L'Aine et Fils, 1806; 113.

Alibert JL. Description des maladies de la peau observees a l <hopital Saint-Louis et exposition des meilleures methodes suivies pour leur traitement. Vol. 2. Bruxelles: Auguste Whalen, 1825:37.

Alibert JL. Quelques recherches sur la cheloide. Mem Soc Medicale d'Emulation 1817; 744.

Amar Inalsingh CH. An experience in treating 501 patients with keloids. Johns Hopkins Med J 1974; 134:284–290.

Apfelberg DB, Masr MR, Lash H. The use of epidermis over a keloid as an autograft after resection on the keloid. J Dermatol Surg 1976; 2(5):409–411.

Asboe-Hanson G. The mast cell in health and disease. Ann Dermatol Venereol 1973; 23:139.

Babu M, Diegelmann R, Oliver N. Fibronectin is overproduced by keloid fibroblasts during abnormal wound healing. Mol Cell Biol 1989; 9(4):1642–1650.

Bailly C, Dreze S, Asselineau D, et al. Retinoic acid inhibits the production of collagenase by human epidermal keratinocytes. J Invest Dermatol 1990; 94:47–51.

Berman B, Florcs F. Recurrence rates of excised keloids treated with post-operative triamcinolone acetonide injections or interferon alfa-2b injections. J Am Acad Dermatol 1997; 137:755–757.

Berman B, Villa A. Imiquimod 5% cream for keloid management. Dermatol Surg 2003; 29:1050–1051.

Breasted JH. The Edwin Smith surgical papyrus. In: Hieroglyphic Text Translation and Commentary. 1. Chicago: University of Chicago Press, 1930:403–406.

Brown LA Jr., Pierce HE. Keloids: scar revision. J Dermatol Surg Oncol 1986; 12(1):51–56.

Burkhart CG, Burkhart C. Acne keloidalis is lichen simplex chronicus with fibrotic keloidal scarring. J Am Acad Dermatol 1998; 39:661.

Califano J, Miller S, Frodel J. Treatment of occipital acne keloidalis by excision followed by secondary intention healing. Arch Facial Plast Surg 1999; 1:308–311.

Ceilley Rl, Babin RW. The combined use of cryosurgery and intralesional injection of suspension of fluorinated adrenocorticosteroids for reducing keloids and hypertrophic scars. J Dermatol Surg Oncol 1979; 5:54–56.

Chait LA, Kadwa MA. Hypertrophic scars and keloids. Cause and management–current concepts. S Afr J Surg 1988; 26(3):95–98.

Cohen IK, McCoy BS. Keloid: biology and treatment. In: Dineen P, Hildick-Smith G, eds. The Surgical Wound. Philidelphia: Lea & Febiger, 1981:123–131.

Combemale P, Cantaloube D. Traitement des cheloides. Ann Dermatol Venereol 1991; 118(9):665–673.

Cosman B, Crikelair GF, Ju DM, et al. The surgical treatment of keloids. Plast Reconstr Surg 1961; 27:335–358.

Craig RR, Schofield JD, Jackson DS. Collagen biosynthesis in normal and hypertrophic scars and keloid as a function of the duration of the scar. Br J Surg 1975; 62:741–744.

D'Souza P, Iyer VK, Ramam M. Familial acne keloidalis. Acta Derm Venereol 1998; 78(5):382.

Daly TJ, Weston WL. Retinoid effects on fibroblast proliferation and collagen synthesis in vitro and on fibrotic disease in vitro. J Am Acad Dermatol 1986; 15:900–902.

Datubo-Brown Department of Dermatology. Keloids: a review of literature. Br J Plast Surg 1990; 43(1):70–77.

De Cesare PE, Cheung DT, Perelman N, et al. Alteration of collagen composition and cross-linking in keloid tissues. Matrix 1990; 10(3):172–l78.

De Oliveira GV, Nunes TA, Magna LA, et al. Silicone versus nonsilicone gel dressings: a controlled trial. Dermatol Surg. 2001; 27:721–726.

Diegelmann RF, Cohen IK, McCoy BJ. Growth kinetics and collagen synthesis of normal scar and keloid fibroblasts in vitro. J Cell Physiol 1979; 98(2):341–346.

Dierickx C, Goldman MP, Fitzpatrick RE. Laser treatment of erythematous/hypertrophic and pigmented scars in 26 patients. Plast Reconstr Surg 1995; 95:84–92.

Dinehart SM, Herzberg AJ, Kerns BJ, Pollack SV. Acne keloidalis: a review. J Dermatol Surg Oncol 1989; 15(6):642–647.

Dinehart SM, Tanner L, Mallory SB, Herzberg AJ. Acne keloidalis in woman. Cutis 1989; 44:250–252.

Doyle-Lloyd DJ, White JA. Keloids. J La State Med Soc 1991; 143(12):9–12.

Edlich RF, Haines PC, Nichter LS, Silloway KA, Morgan RF. Pseudofolliculitis barbae with keloids. J Emerg Med 1986; 4(4):283–286.

English RS, Shenefelt PD. Keloids and hypertrophic scars. Dermatol Surg 1999; 25:631–638.

Espana A, Solano T, Quintanilla E. Bleomycin in the treatment of keloids and hypertrophic scars by multiple needle punctures. Dermatol Surg 2001; 27:23–27.

Fox H. Observations on skin diseases in the Negro. J cutan dis 1908; 28:67–79.

Friedman DW, Boyd CD, Mackenzie JW, et al. Regulation of collagen gene expression in keloids and hypertrophic scars. J Surg Res 1993; 55(2):214–222.

George AO, Akanji AO, Nduka EU, Olasode JB, Odusan O. Clinical, biochemical and morphologic features of acne keloidalis in a black population. Int J Dermatol 1993; 32(10):714–716.

Giux B, Henriquez I, Andres A, Finestres F, Tello Jl, Martinez A. Treatment of keloids by high-dose-rate brachytherapy: a seven-year study. Int J Radiat Oncol Biol Phys 2001; 50(1):167–172.

Gloster HM. Arch Dermatol 2000; 136:1376–1379.

Goethe DK, Berger TG. Acne keloidalis nuchae: a transepithelial elimination disorder. Int J Dermatol 1987; 26:442–424.

Griffith BH. Treatment of keloids with triamcinolone acetonide. Plast Reconstr Surg 1966; 30:202–208.

Gupta S, Kalra A. Efficacy and safety of intralesional 5-Fluorouracil in the treatment of keloids. Dermatol 2002; 204:13.

Inalsingh CH. An experience in treating five hundred and one patients with keloids. Johns Hopkins Med J 1974; 134:284–290.

Janssen Delimpens AM. The local treatment of hypertrophic scars and keloids with topical retinoic acid. Br J Dermatol 1980; 103:319.

Janssen de Limpens AM, Cormane RH. Keloids and hypertrophic scars–immunological aspects. Aesthetic Plast Surg 1982; 6(3):149–152.

Janssen de Limpens AM, Cormane RH. Studies on the immunologic aspects of keloids and hypertrophic scars. Arch Dermatol Res 1982; 274(3–4):259–266.

Jutley JK, Ng KY, Cunliffe WJ, Layton AM, Wood EJ. Analysis of collagen composition in acne keloids. Biochem Soc Trans 1993; 21(3):303S.

Kanthak FF, Cullen ML. Skin graft in the treatment of chronic furunculosis of the posterior surface of the neck (folliculitis keloidalis). South Med J 1951; 49:1154–1157.

Kaposi M. Ueber die sogennante Framboesia und mehrere andere arten von papiliaeren neubildungen der Haut. Arch Dermatol Syphilol 1869; 3:382–423.

Kaufman J, Berman B. Topical application of imiquimod 5% cream to excision sites is safe and effective in reducing keloid recurrences. J Am Acad Dermatol 2002; 47:S209–S211.

Keliey AP. Pseudofolliculitis barbae and acne keloidalis nuchae. Dermatol Clinic 2003; 21(4):645–653.

Kelly AP. Keloids. Dermatol Clin 1988; 6(3):413–424.

Ketchum LD, Cohen IK, Masters FW. Hypertrophic scars and keloids. A collective review. Plast Reconstr Surg 1974; 53(2):140–154.

Kiil J. Keloids treated with topical injections of triamcinolone acetonide (kenalog). Immediate and long-term results. Scand J Plast Reconstr Surg 1977; 11:169–172.

Kischer CW. The microvessels in hypertrophic scars, keloids, and related lesions: a review. J Submicroscopic Cytol Pathos 1992; 24(2):281–296.

Kischer CW, Shetlar MR, Chvapil M. Hypertrophic scars and keloids: a review and new concept concerning their origin. Scan Electron Microsc 1982:1699–1713.

Larson DL, Abston S, Evans EB, et al. Techniques for decreasing scar formation and contractures in the burned patient. J Trauma 1971; 11:807.

Layton AM, Yip J, Cunliffe WJ. A comparison of intralesional triamcinolone and cryosurgery in the treatment of acne keloids. Br J Dermatol 1994; 130(4):498–501.

Lever WF. Histopathology of the Skin. Philadelphia: JB Lippincott, 1990:668–669.

LowSQ, Moy RL. Scar wars strategies. Target collagen. J Dermatol Surg Oncol 1992; 18(11):981–986.

Luz Ramos M, Munoz-Perez MA, Pons A, Ortega M, Camacho F. Acne keloidalis nuchae and tufted hair folliculitis. Dermatology 1997; 194(1):71–73.

Manuskiatti W, Fitzpatrick RE. Treatment response of keloidal and hypertrophic sternotomy scars. Arch Dermatol 2002; 138:1149–1155.

Mercer NS. Silicone gel in the treatment of keloid scars. Br J Plast Surg 1989; 42(1):83–87.

Moulton-Levy P, Jackson CE, Levy HG, Fialkow PJ. Multiple cell origin of traumatically induced keloids. J Am Acad Dermatol 1984; 10(6):986–988.

Murray JC, Pollack SV, Pinnell SR. Keloids: a review. J Am Acad Dermatol 1981; 4(4):461–470.

Murray JC, Pollack SV, Pinnell SR. Keloids and hypertrophic scars. Clin Dermatol 1984; 2(3):121–133.

Murray JC. Scars and keloids. Dermatol Clin 1993; 11(4):697–708.

Nanda S, Reddy BSN. Intralesional 5–flourouracil as a treatment modality of keloids. Dermatol Surg 2004; 30:54–57.

Nemeth AJ. Keloids and hypertrophic scars. J Dermatol Surg Oncol 1993; 19(8):738–746.

Omo-Dare P. Yoruban contributions to the literature on keloids. J Natl Med Assoc 1973; 65:367–372.

Peltonin J, Hsiao LL, Jaakkoic S, et al. Activation of collagen gene expression in keloids: colocalization of type I and VI collagen and transforming growth factor-β_1, MRNA. J Invest Dermatol 1991; 97:240.

Placik OJ, Lewis VL Jr. Immunologic associations of keloids. Surg Gynecot Obstet 1992; 175(2):185–193.

Quinn KJ, Evans JH, Courtney JM, et al. Nonpressure treatment of hypertrophic scars. Burns 1988; 12:102.

Ragoowansi R, Cornes PGS, Al Glees MJP. Treatment of keloids by surgical excision and immediate postoperative single fraction radiotherapy. Plast Reconstr Surg 2003; 111(6):1853–1859.

Retz N. Des maladies de la peau et de celles de I'esprit. 3. Paris, Mequinon, 1790:155.

Rockwell WB, Cohen IK, Ehrlich HP. Keloids and hypertrophic scars: a comprehensive review. Plast Reconstr Surg 1989; 84(5):827–837.

Rusciani L, Rossi G, Bono R. Use of cryotherapy in the treatment of keloids. J Dermatol Surg Oncol 1993; 19:529–534.

Rudolph R. Wide spread scars, hypertrophic scars, and keloids. Clin Plast Surg 1987; 14(2):253–260.

Sallstrom KO, Larson O, Heden P, et al. Treatment of keloids with surgical excision and postoperative x-ray radiation. Scand J Plast Reconstr Surg Hand Surg 1989; 23(3):211–215.

Sawada Y, Sone K. Treatment of scars and keloids with a cream containing silicone oil. Br J Plast Surg 1990; 43(6):683–688.

Sawada Y, Sone K. Hydration and occlusion treatment for hypertrophic scars and keloids. Br J Ptast Sura 1992; 45(8):599–603.

Sahl WJ Jr., Clever H. Cutaneous scars. Part I. Int J Dermatol 1994; 33(1):681–691.

Seimanowitz VJ, Stiller MJ. Rubinstein-Taybi syndrome. Cutaneous manifestations and colossal keloids. Arch Dermatol 1981; 117(8):504–506.

Sherman R, Rosenfeld H. Experience with the Nd:YAG laser in the treatment of keloid scars. Ann Plast Surg 1988; 21:231–235.

Sherman R, Rosenfeld H. Differential oxygen sensitivities in G6PDH activities of cultured keloid and normal skin dermis single cells. J Dermatol 1991; 19(10):572–579.

Sperling Col LC, Homoky C, Pratt LTC L, Sau P. Acne keloidalis is a form of primary scarring alopecia. Arch Dermatol 2000; 136:479–484.

Topol BM, Lewis VL Jr., Benveniste K. The use of antihistamine to retard the growth of fibroblasts derived from human skin, scar, and keloid. Plast Reconstr Surg 1981; 68(2):227–232.

Zouboulis C, Blume V, et al. Outcomes of cryosurgery in keloids and hypertrophic scars. Arch Dermatol 1993; 129:1146–1151.

Zubert TJ, DeWitt DE. Earlobe keloids. Am Fam Phys 1994; 49(8):1835–1841.

45

Vault Disorders

Daniel C. Dapprich and P. Kim Phillips
Mayo Clinic, Rochester, Minnesota, U.S.A.

Harry J. Hurley
West Chester, Pennsylvania, U.S.A.

INTRODUCTION

Several axillary dermatoses for which medical or dermatologic treatment may be unsuccessful respond favorably to surgical management. They include axillary hyperhidrosis, apocrine bromhidrosis, hidradenitis suppurativa, and familial benign pemphigus (Hailey-Hailey disease). The essential pathogenetic and clinical features will be discussed here, followed by a description of the surgical therapy and its rationale.

AXILLARY HYPERHIDROSIS

About 3% of the U.S. population is afflicted with hyperhidrosis of some form, and about half of these people have axillary hyperhidrosis. The condition results from hyperactivity of the eccrine glands of the axillae. Because 60% to 80% of patients with this condition report a family history, an autosomal dominant mode of inheritance is suggested. Hyperhidrosis results from increased sudomotor impulses from the cerebral cortex that are generated almost exclusively during waking hours by mental, emotional, and sensory stimuli. The disappearance of such stimuli during sleep coincides with virtual cessation of the excessive sweating at such times. Moreover, anatomic, histologic, histochemical, electron microscopic, and physiologic studies fail to reveal any abnormalities of the hyperactive glands that would explain their increased secretory activity. The glands cannot be distinguished from axillary eccrine sweat glands of the normohidrotic individual. Axillary hyperhidrosis knows no geographic, racial, or gender-related bounds.

The onset of axillary hyperhidrosis is typically post-pubertal, usually occurring between the ages of 14 and 17. Axillary eccrine sweating normally begins just before or at puberty. This contrasts with eccrine sweating on most other skin surfaces, including the palms and soles, where sweating starts shortly after birth. Eccrine sweat is typically clear or watery (Fig. 1) and not turbid, opalescent, or occasionally colored as is apocrine sweat. Moreover, careful visualization defines the points of origin of individual droplets as nonfollicular, consistent with their eccrine origin.

Axillary hyperhidrosis is defined as sweating in an axilla exceeding 125 mg per five minutes measured gravimetrically. Not all patients with a rate of sweating this high complain of clinical wetness, because some simply tolerate the problem. Women are more likely to find this sweating distressing, and some with rates below 125 mg per five minutes seek professional help for the problem. The concurrence of axillary and volar (palmoplantar) hyperhidrosis is common, although each may exist separately.

The quantities of sweat in axillary hyperhidrosis can be dramatically excessive. In most patients, clothing is stained with the moisture after 15 to 30 minutes of active sweating due to emotional or mental excitation. As much as 2000 mg can be produced in a single axilla within five minutes. No mere cosmetic problem, it can alter a patient's life so that work is impaired or modified markedly, and social activities become difficult or are simply avoided. In fact, one third of those with axillary hyperhidrosis report at least frequent interference with daily activities. This problem can be costly, because clothes must be dry cleaned more frequently or discarded because of the stains.

Because it is an eccrine disorder, axillary hyperhidrosis does not normally coexist with axillary bromhidrosis. Excessive amounts of eccrine sweat wash away odor-producing apocrine sweat, preventing its accumulation on the axillary skin and hair. It is virtually axiomatic that patients complaining of axillary odor do not have axillary hyperhidrosis. Patients with axillary odor rarely have gravimetric sweating rates above 50 mg per five minutes, and their sweating patterns are distinctively different.

Seasonal variation in axillary sweating rates is not marked, although, in general, eccrine glands are conditioned by heat. They secrete earlier and at higher rates under hot ambient conditions. Patients with axillary hyperhidrosis notice little or no difference in sweating rates in winter and summer; however, many are less bothered in the summer when open or lighter-weight apparel permits more evaporative loss of sweat. Clearly this sweating is not induced by ambient or metabolic heat.

It should be emphasized that not only is the axillary sweating diurnal, beginning on awakening (coincident with the onset of mental activity), but is also generally continuous, varying only moderately through the day. If a particularly intense emotional stimulation is experienced, however, sweating rates sharply increase and then recede as the stimulation subsides. During sleep, sweating decreases dramatically or ceases completely.

Commercial antiperspirants are ineffective in these patients, with the exception of 12.5% aluminum chloride hexahydrate in anhydrous ethanol, applied under occlusion during sleep. Moreover, there is usually little or no relief from ataractic or anticholinergic medications.

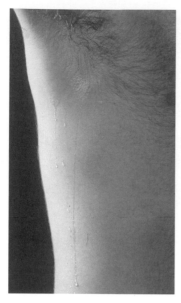

Figure 1 Axillary hyperhidrosis. Clear, watery sweat droplets extending onto the flank.

most active, the droplets become confluent, and puddles of bluish sweat are noted at sites with high rates of sweating.

Studies of axillary sweating patterns in patients with hyperhidrosis as well as normal controls reveal that eccrine sweating is not diffuse and even across the axilla. Also, it is not necessarily most active in the center or dome of the vault. There is considerable variation from person to person to the point of being individually unique, much like a fingerprint. Furthermore, the pattern is consistently reproducible, varying only in degree with the intensity of stimulation. These constant, individual sweating patterns reflect the regular responsiveness of identifiable groups of glands to emotional, mental, or sensory stimuli. This forms the rationale for the Hurley-Shelley axillary resection technique and others to be discussed later that require preliminary mapping of the axillary sweating patterns. It should be noted that thermally-induced sweating patterns differ from those of emotional induction in that the former involve more marginal glands, that is, those of thoracic or brachial areas outside the axilla.

In most hyperhidrotic patients, one, two, or occasionally three, loci of high rates of sweating can be defined in the axilla. The areas may vary in size, shape, and location, measuring from 2 to 6 cm in diameter. Smaller satellite loci of sweating may also be noted. The largest locus is most often in the center or dome of the axilla but may also be found at either end of the axilla. In exceptional cases, a diffuse pattern of sweating over the entire axilla can be seen, but even in such patients, pooling of sweat on the blue-black background will delineate one or two areas that are the most active. Axillary sweating patterns are different qualitatively and quantitatively on opposite sides. While the right axilla usually exceeds the left in sweat secretion, this asymmetry is not based on right- or left-handedness. The cortical center for sweating is not necessarily in the dominant cerebral hemisphere. The difference quantitatively in sweating between opposing axillae is usually small but may be extreme at times.

Patterns of sweating in axillary hyperhidrosis do not follow the distribution of apocrine glands in the axilla.

Sweating Patterns

When one examines patients with axillary hyperhidrosis, axillary sweating patterns can be evaluated by one of several colorimetric techniques to visualize eccrine sweat. The method used most commonly is the Minor technique, involving iodine and starch (Fig. 2). This provides a topographic, semiquantitative determination of the axillary sweating response. It permits an estimate of the sweating rate and a delineation of the glandular loci from which the sweat derives with a 7.5% povidone-iodine scrub solution and allowed to dry. Cornstarch powder is dusted over the painted areas. Sweat droplets appear at ductal orifices and solubilize the iodine, which reacts with the starch to produce a blue–black color at each sweat pore. Where sweating is

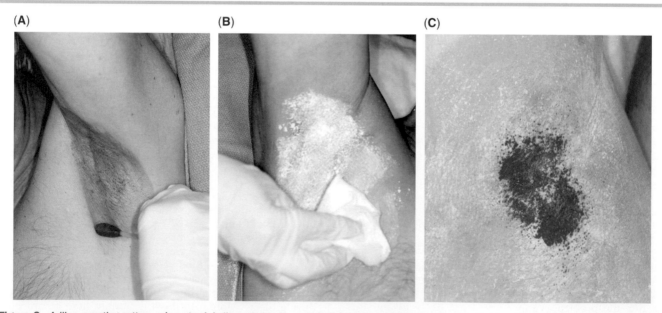

Figure 2 Axillary sweating pattern: minor starch-iodine colorimetric technique for demonstration of active sweating loci. **(A)** The axilla is painted with iodine and allowed to dry. **(B)** Starch is then applied. **(C)** Note demarcation of loci of most active sweating.

Apocrine glands are characteristically most dense in the center of the axilla and are smaller and less numerous peripherally. This distribution is evidence against proposals identifying apocrine glands as the source of excessive secretion in axillary hyperhidrosis.

Medical Treatment

Some patients can accept greater sweating activity more readily than others. Only 38% of those with hyperhidrosis discuss their sweating with a health care professional. It is regrettable that so many patients with axillary hyperhidrosis do not consult dermatologists or other physicians for treatment. They live with the problem, convinced that the failure of modern commercial antiperspirants leaves them without any other recourse. Even many physicians outside the field of dermatology do not realize that successful treatment is available.

Patients with axillary hyperhidrosis deserve a trial with one of several medical approaches before surgical management is recommended. The least invasive and least costly method is the topical application of aluminum chloride under occlusion at bedtime. Several such products are available. Certain Dry® (12%) is available over-the-counter, whereas Drysol® (20%) and Xerac AC® (6.25%) are prescription medications.

Some patients find these formulations irritating. Decreasing the pH with topical triethanolamine 50% in ethanol applied after the aluminum chloride has been shown to decrease irritation. Although this did decrease objective measurements of the effectiveness of the treatment in the study, there was no subjective difference in effectiveness. If aluminum chloride is effective in a patient, it can be used indefinitely because there is little risk of allergic sensitization or toxicity.

The use of botulinum toxin type A to treat axillary hyperhidrosis has revolutionized the medical therapy of this disorder. The toxin was first used clinically for ophthalmologic diseases starting in the early 1980s. Its use was soon expanded to the treatment of dystonias of the limbs, torticollis, leg spasm, cerebral palsy, and various motility disorders. Before its widespread use in dermatology, it was also found to be beneficial for spasms in various gastrointestinal and urinary sphincters, spasmodic dysphonia, and other muscle spasm disorders. Its first application for sweating was in the treatment of the gustatory hyperhidrosis of Frey's syndrome in 1994. In addition to blepharospasm, strabismus, cervical dystonia, and moderate to severe glabellar lines, it is currently Food and Drug Administration (FDA)-approved for severe cases of primary axillary hyperhidrosis that are inadequately managed by topical agents. Botox®, Botox Cosmetic®, and Dysport® are the brands of botulinum toxin type A that are currently commercially available. The first two are available in the United States, whereas the third is not. Dysport is significantly less potent than Botox. These toxins work by blocking the release of acetylcholine by sympathetic fibers innervating sweat glands.

The procedure is straightforward. If medically acceptable, aspirin and other nonsteroidal antiinflammatory drugs should be temporarily discontinued in advance of treatment one week and one day, respectively. This theoretically minimizes loss of the toxin via bleeding from the injection sites. Although injection of the palms and soles is often limited by pain, local anesthesia is generally unnecessary in the axillae. Topical anesthetics may be used after the sweat pattern has been mapped with the starch-iodine test. Injections should obviously be focused on the sites highlighted by this test.

Ideal dilution, dosage, and injection pattern are not known. The Botox® product information recommends the following for axillary hyperhidrosis:

- Dilute 100 units with 4 mL of preservative-free saline
- Use a 30-gauge needle
- Inject intradermally to a depth of 2 mm, at a 45° angle with the bevel up
- 0.1 to 0.2 mL aliquots to multiple sites (10–15) in each axilla
- Evenly distributed (1–2 cm apart)
- Total of 50 units per axilla

These recommendations are reasonable and there is no strong evidence to sway from them. Previous studies using Botox for axillary hyperhidrosis have reported dilutions of 1 to 5 mL per 100 units, dosages of 20 to 200 units per axilla, spacing of 1 to 3 cm, and 7- to 15-injection sites per axilla. Patients should be seen back after two weeks for touch-up of any areas that may have been missed by the initial treatment. The duration of effect for axillary hyperhidrosis is somewhat longer than that for palmar hyperhidrosis. The reported range is 4 to 10 months.

One author has suggested that reconstitution with bacteriostatic normal saline has the advantage of retaining potency for a week or more. The product information recommends reconstitution with preservative-free saline and storage for no more than four hours at 2°C to 4°C. Reconstitution with bacteriostatic saline may also have the benefit of decreased pain with injection.

Although multiple theoretical risks exist in the treatment of axillary hyperhidrosis with botulinum toxin, their occurrence is extremely rare. Those listed on the package insert include: anxiety, back or neck pain, fever, flu syndrome, headache, infection, injection site hemorrhage, pharyngitis, pruritus, and nonaxillary sweating. A literature search revealed no reported cases of compensatory hyperhidrosis after treatment of axillary hyperhidrosis with this modality. Botulinum toxin should be used with caution in those less than 18 years of age because it has not been tested for this indication in such people. Because its effects in pregnancy and breastfeeding are not known, use in these settings is to be avoided. Neither should it be used in patients with neuromuscular diseases such as myasthenia gravis or Eaton-Lambert syndrome. Epinephrine should be available should an anaphylactic reaction occur.

Evidence is beginning to accumulate for the use of botulinum toxin type B (Myobloc®) for axillary hyperhidrosis as well, though it is FDA approved only for cervical dystonia. It may be considered in doses of 2000 units per axilla when a patient has developed antibodies against botulinum toxin type A. Injections tend to be somewhat more painful, and there are often anticholinergic side effects. Its onset of action may be slightly sooner than that of type A.

It is generally not advisable to administer systemic medications, such as anticholinergics or calcium channel blockers, for long periods of time. Some of these drugs, especially the anticholinergics, suppress sweating only at dosages that produce unpleasant side effects. A possible special use of systemic anticholinergics is in the initial phases of use of the topical aluminum chloride technique cited above, when two to three days' dosage of glycopyrrolate or its equivalent inhibits axillary sweating enough to prevent the aluminum chloride from being washed away from the sweat pores. Glycopyrrolate (1 mg) given 45 to 60 minutes before applying the aluminum chloride works well in this regard. While propoxyphene is reportedly suppressive in some patients with spinal sweating and clonidine is helpful in some patients with gustatory hyperhidrosis, neither drug has been evaluated in axillary hyperhidrosis and should not be used on a long-term basis.

Topical anticholinergics suppress axillary sweating in some normohidrotic individuals but are not similarly suppressive in hyperhidrotic patients. They also carry the risk of side effects, especially in patients with undiagnosed glaucoma or prostatic hypertrophy. Topical anesthetics have also been used to inhibit axillary eccrine sweating but are not as effective as aluminum chloride. Tap water iontophoresis, biofeedback, and behavioral therapy should also be considered as alternatives to surgical treatment.

Surgical Treatment

Until the early 1960s, axillary hyperhidrosis was managed surgically by thoracic sympathectomy. While this is effective for volar hyperhidrosis, it is not routinely helpful for axillary hyperhidrosis, usually because the fifth thoracic autonomic ganglion is not included or because anatomic variations preclude complete denervation of the axillary skin.

Side effects such as Horner's syndrome and a distressing compensatory hyperhidrosis (thermal, emotional, and/or gustatory) of other areas, notably the trunk, may occur after sympathectomy.

Therefore, sympathectomy is not routinely recommended for axillary hyperhidrosis. Only in patients with combined palmar and axillary hyperhidrosis is it now indicated. An upper thoracic sympathectomy, which removes the second and third thoracic ganglia, controls the palmar hyperhidrosis of these patients, and local (axillary) ablative surgery is recommended for their axillary hyperhidrosis.

Local Axillary Surgical Treatment

Women who undergo radical mastectomy with extensive axillary dissection to remove lymph nodes and breast tissue in the axillary tail of Spence detect appreciable reduction or cessation of axillary sweating on that side. The effect is permanent and obviates the need for antiperspirants. While this effect has been known for years, these observations did not stimulate the development of local surgical techniques to control axillary hyperhidrosis until the early 1960s, when Skoog and Thyresson, and Hurley and Shelley independently described the first two procedures for this condition.

The Skoog-Thyresson technique does not involve mapping of sweat patterns. The goal is to inactivate all glands across an axilla. Carefully placed incisions permit reflection of skin flaps for dissection of the sweat gland layer over the entire axilla. This results in marked reduction in sweating. Residual sweating can be eradicated by smaller localized procedures.

The Hurley-Shelley operation is based on identification of the most active sweating loci by mapping out sweating patterns, as described above. Surgery is tailored to fit the sweating pattern. Because the pattern of axillary sweating is constant and reproducible in a given axilla, this tissue can be selectively ablated.

Most patients can be treated satisfactorily with the Hurley-Shelley procedure. Those with extreme hyperhidrosis and axillary sweating rates greater than 2000 mg per five minutes with diffuse sweating over the entire axilla may require the Skoog-Thyresson operation or total excision of the axilla, as in the Bretteville-Jensen procedure. Many modifications of these procedures have been described

Table 1 Surgical Treatment of Axillary Hyperhidrosis

Selective glandular removal based on sweating patterns
Hurley–Shelley procedure
Eldh–Fogdestam operation (M or W excision)
Broad glandular removal across axilla: no preliminary sweating patterns
Skoog–Thyresson technique
Bretteville-Jensen (Z-plasty)
Total excision of axilla
Subcutaneous tissue shavers
Curettage removal through skin incisions
Cryosurgical ablation
Liposuction with or without curettage

(Table 1). Cryosurgical removal of axillary sweat glands through a small incision has also been utilized. Some have advocated the use of subcutaneous tissue shavers, liposuction, or curettage removal of sweat glands through skin incisions, but the efficacy of these methods has been questioned.

In the Hurley-Shelley operation, the patient is informed that there should be 70% to 90% reduction in sweating following surgery. Details of the procedure, the postoperative period, and possible complications are discussed. The medical history should include questions about platelet disorders and other causes of bleeding tendencies, including use of anticoagulants, aspirin, and nonsteroidal antiinflammatory medications. Other pertinent information such as keloid formation and reactions to medications (specifically antibiotics) should be ascertained. An informed consent form should be signed and witnessed.

Examination of the patient preoperatively should include both gravimetric measurement of the axillary sweating using tared gauze pads (5 minute collection), and axillary sweating patterns using the starch-iodine method. The pattern should be drawn or photographed during the initial examinations and compared with a second pattern prepared just prior to the operation, when the patient should be anxious. This ensures adequate emotional stimulation and a marked sweating response. Mental stimulation such as doing arithmetic may also be used to stimulate axillary sweating. The areas of greatest sweating are marked with a sterile dye.

Preoperative preparation includes shaving the axillary hair and two cleansings of the axillary skin, 6 to 12 hours apart, with a germicidal soap or detergent. Sedatives and anticholinergics are avoided until after the sweat patterns are obtained immediately before the operation because these drugs alter the sweat rate significantly. Local anesthesia is obtained using lidocaine with epinephrine infiltrated superficially into or just below the dermis along the marked excision lines. If necessary, sedation may be administered after the sweat patterns have been established.

The operation is performed with the patient in the supine position and the axilla exposed with the arm extended and flexed at the elbow and the hand placed under the head. This is also the position used to obtain the preoperative sweat patterns. Be aware of possible brachial plexus injury, particularly when general anesthesia or deep sedation is used and when both axillae are operated on simultaneously.

The Hurley-Shelley procedure involves a fusiform excision, transversely oriented, to remove the center of each sweating locus based on the starch-iodine test. This is followed by undermining on each side of each excision to reflect lateral flaps and permit resection of sweat glands on the undersurface of the dermis to the limits of each locus of sweating. The primary excision usually measures 5 to 6 cm in length and 1.5 to 2.5 cm in width at its midpoint (Fig. 3A). Depending on the size and shape of the sweating loci, the excisions may occasionally be directed obliquely across the axilla. Transverse orientation is preferred, however, to minimize longitudinal contracture of the scar that could inhibit abduction of the limb. Undermining laterally is done just below the dermis for 2 to 4 cm on each side, depending on the sweating pattern.

In the subdermal glandular resection, the skin is reflected over the fingertip so that sweat gland lobules can be carefully resected with fine-curved scissors (Fig. 3B). While the eccrine glands are not grossly visible, apocrine gland lobules are, and these lobules must be visualized and resected. Because the eccrine glands are closely intermixed with or adjacent to the apocrine glands, this resection ensures removal of most of the eccrine glands. Trimming the undersurface too closely should be avoided so that as many hair follicles as possible are preserved. This contrasts with some techniques that stress close stripping of the dermal undersurface with a safety razor. Although hair follicle removal, especially in female patients, may be desirable, we are of the opinion that damage to hair follicles should be minimized to avoid damage to the deep dermal plexus, which may compromise flap survival.

Additional minor areas of sweating are treated with excisions that vary in size based on the sweating pattern, with proportionately less undermining and subdermal glandular resection. When more than one area is ablated, undermining should not overlap. This leaves some skin between the wounds not traumatized to ensure adequate blood supply for wound healing in the axilla.

Hemostasis is essential and must be established before closure. Electrocoagulation or suture ligature will control major sources of bleeding. Moderate pressure may be applied for 5 to 10 minutes to arrest small vessel bleeding. Drains (1/4–3/8 in. wide) are placed if there is uncertainty about hemostasis, but these are usually unnecessary. Deep sutures to obliterate dead space may decrease the risks of developing a seroma or hematoma, which could lead to infection. These should be followed by buried vertical mattress sutures. Finally, skin edges should be precisely approximated with skin sutures (Fig. 3C).

Pressure dressings are applied directly over each wound, with the pressure directed upward toward the apex of the axilla. A gauze dressing may also be tied in place with retention sutures. Patients are advised to keep their arms at their sides for 48 hours postoperatively. The skin sutures are removed in 10 to 14 days. Normal activity can be resumed two to three days postoperatively except for work or exercise that involves raising the arms above the head. Although avoidance of early abduction of the arms decreases the risk for wound dehiscence and scar widening, being too strict in this regard may lead to a frozen shoulder. A reasonable compromise would be gentle stretching several times a day, with gradual resumption of normal activities at about three weeks.

A side effect of this procedure is increased axillary odor, usually noticed within two days of the operation. The reduction in eccrine sweating permits retention of odorogenic apocrine sweat that was previously washed away by the excessive perspiration. Deodorants may be used as soon as the wounds are healed. Topical gentamicin can be used while sutures are in place for a deodorant effect.

The Hurley-Shelley operation results in sweat reduction of approximately 70% to 90%. The removal of skin and contained sweat glands by excision alone significantly reduces eccrine sweating. The additional reduction resulting from resection of glands from the dermal undersurface of

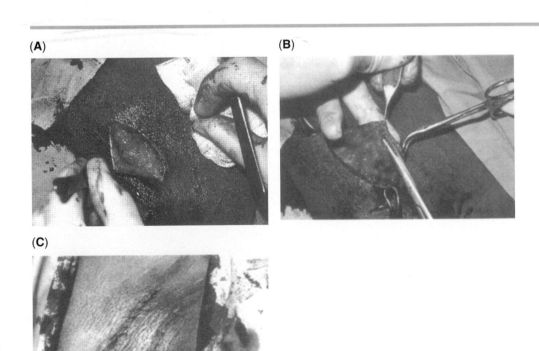

(A) **(B)**

(C)

Figure 3 Hurley–Shelley operation for axillary hyperhidrosis. **(A)** Elliptical excision of primary sweating locus. **(B)** Subdermal resection of sweat gland lobules on undersurface of flaps on each side of sweating locus. **(C)** Sutured wounds (with drain in one wound) at completion of operation.

the flaps usually brings the sweating rate down to acceptably low levels. Thus a preoperative sweating rate of 500 mg per five minutes is normally decreased to 100 mg per five minutes or lower. Diminished sweating is also evident in postoperative sweating patterns (Fig. 4). Occasionally, patients may require a second operation. Sweating patterns will reveal residual active loci of sweating, and they can be readily ablated using the same basic surgical approach on a smaller scale. It is not necessary to perform surgery beyond a second minor procedure.

Results from the operation are permanent. Examination 6 to 24 months later has shown no change from the postoperative sweating patterns. Results are best assessed at six to eight weeks postoperatively, when edema and inflammation have subsided.

Scars resulting from this operation are characteristically soft and pliable and do not inhibit mobility of the arms. Keloids may occur but are rare in the axilla, and they have not developed in our series of patients. Infection or hematoma is uncommon, as for most dermatologic surgery, if care is given to operative details. One problem that occurs occasionally, one to two weeks after the operation, is a retrograde lymphangitis of a major brachial lymphatic vessel. A cordlike thickening is noted extending from the lower, brachial pole of the axilla down the arm. It may feel like a tendon or vein to the patient. This resolves without treatment in about three weeks and results in no permanent sequelae. Compensatory hyperhidrosis at another location, a common complication of sympathectomy, does not occur after this procedure.

A completely dry axilla is not expected and is probably undesirable because of fictional irritation that might occur with normal movement of the arms. The objective is a reduction of sweating to levels compatible with work and social activities without appreciable wetting of undergarments. Topical antiperspirants may still be necessary in some patients and are useful also for their deodorant effect.

APOCRINE BROMHIDROSIS

Bromhidrosis, also known as bromidrosis, osmidrosis, or ozochrotia, means excessive or abnormal body odor and includes both apocrine and eccrine varieties (Table 2). Apocrine bromhidrosis is far more common and is the only form for which local surgery may be indicated.

Epidemiology, Causes, and Clinical Features

Apocrine bromhidrosis occurs only in the axilla because it is the only site where there is a large number of actively functioning apocrine glands. Like all apocrine disorders, apocrine bromhidrosis does not occur until puberty or

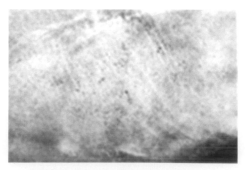

Figure 4 Postoperative sweating patterns.

Table 2 Types of Bromhidrosis

Apocrine
Axillary
Eccrine
Keratinogenic
Plantar
Intertriginous
Metabolic
Heritable aminoacidurias
Phenylketonuria
Maple syrup urine disease
Oasthouse syndrome
Methionine malabsorption syndrome
Hypermethionemia
Isovaleric academia
n-Butyric/*n*-hexanoic academia
Trimethylaminuria
Exogenous
Foods
Drugs
Chemicals

Source: Reprinted with permission from Hurley (1987).

thereafter, when the apocrine glands begin secretion. Blacks have the largest and most active apocrine glands, while eastern Asians have the least active; these races represent the extremes in frequency of apocrine bromhidrosis.

Some apocrine odor is expected in all individuals with axillary apocrine glandular function. When the odor is excessive or qualitatively distinctive, the diagnosis of bromhidrosis can be made. Apocrine sweat is probably the only cutaneous secretion or breakdown product whose degradation yields the classic acrid axillary odor, though certain androgenic steroidal compounds with odors similar to natural axillary odor may also be important. While apocrine sweat is odorless and sterile when it first appears on the skin surface, bacterial action on it produces odorogens such as short-chain fatty acids and ammonia. Aerobic diphtheroids generate the most common odor, while micrococci produce a different, less offensive smell. Unusual odors reflect individual variation in the composition of apocrine sweat. Thus, odors described as rancid, musty, pungent, fecal, sour, and sweet may be encountered. Factors that intensify axillary odor and apocrine bromhidrosis are poor bathing habits and the presence of axillary hair on which apocrine sweat can be retained. Concurrent axillary eccrine hyperhidrosis usually prevents significant apocrine bromhidrosis, because excessive quantities of eccrine sweat wash away odorogenic apocrine sweat.

The diagnosis of apocrine bromhidrosis is made clinically. It is essential to confirm its presence; bromhidrosiphobia, which may be indicative of impending schizophrenia, should be excluded. Moreover, temporal lobe tumors may produce olfactory hallucinations. A neurologic examination is indicated in patients who complain of body odor but have none discernible by the examiner. A thorough intranasal exam should also be performed because nasal foreign bodies can cause one to have an illusion of having bromhidrosis.

Treatment

In most patients, apocrine bromhidrosis is satisfactorily managed by nonsurgical methods to remove excessive apocrine sweat from the axilla or reduce axillary microflora. Thorough cleansing with an antibacterial soap, shaving of axillary hair, and application of a topical antibacterial agent may help. Commercial aluminum, zirconium, or zinc formulations and topical antibiotics such as neomycin, gentamicin, and clindamycin are effective deodorants. Because neomycin is a relatively common cause of allergic contact dermatitis, it should not be a first choice. Absorption of odorogens with ion-exchange resins or powders or masking the odor with perfumes is less helpful. Systemic antibiotics generally do not suppress axillary odor.

The most effective topical deodorant is aluminum chloride as described for the management of axillary hyperhidrosis. Its eccrine antiperspirant action is also helpful, but in apocrine bromhidrosis, aluminum chloride is acting as an antibacterial. A weaker concentration (Xerac AC®, 6.25% or Certain Dry®, 12%) may be tried first, but the stronger concentration (Drysol®, 20%) is often necessary for more severe forms of apocrine bromhidrosis. There are a limited number of anecdotal reports of successful use of botulinum toxin type of help in this condition.

Surgical treatment of apocrine bromhidrosis is rarely necessary. When it is required, however, either of the two techniques described for axillary hyperhidrosis (the Skoog-Thyresson operation or the Hurley-Shelley operation and their variants) may be used. Rather than outline patterns of high-eccrine activity, an effort is made to remove as many apocrine sweat glands as possible through a fusiform excision in the center of the axilla and subdermal resection of glands. Smaller procedures may be done at the thoracic and brachial poles of the axilla to remove additional apocrine glands. Because the largest and most active apocrine glands are located in the center or dome of the axilla and glandular density, size, and activity decrease toward the axillary poles and the periphery, this surgery markedly decreases the amount of apocrine sweating and thus controls bromhidrosis. Other less invasive options include, in decreasing order of effectiveness: subdermal shaving (92–97%), ultrasound-assisted liposuction (95%), ultrasonic aspiration (86–92%), tumescent liposuction with curettage (53–80%), frequency-doubled Q-switched Nd:YAG laser (80%), carbon dioxide laser (78%), and simple tumescent liposuction (10–81%).

HIDRADENITIS SUPPURATIVA

Hidradenitis suppurativa is a distinctive inflammatory disorder of the apocrine gland-bearing skin. Inflammatory and pustular in its earliest stages, it is chronic and cicatrizing in its late, recurrent forms. It is a painful, at times disabling, disease causing high morbidity. Moreover, it is misdiagnosed and mismanaged commonly and may involve several different medical specialists including the dermatologist, plastic surgeon, general surgeon, gynecologist, urologist, proctologist, and family practitioner. Hidradenitis suppurativa is a disease clearly made more troublesome and recalcitrant by delaying definitive surgical treatment when it is indicated. Although hidradenitis suppurativa was described and erroneously attributed to a disturbance of the apocrine glands in the early 19th century, clinical study of the disease did not take place until almost 100 years later.

Epidemiology

The prevalence of hidradenitis suppurativa has never been precisely established. It is not a common disorder, but it is by no means rare and is undoubtedly underdiagnosed. Axillary, mammary, and inguinal hidradenitis suppurativa is more common in women, but perianal disease occurs more frequently in men. Blacks and whites are both affected, while Asians do not appear to develop it as often.

Pathogenesis

Hidradenitis suppurativa was originally considered a disease of apocrine glands because of its distribution and the frequent histopathologic finding of inflammation and rupture of apocrine glands and ducts. However, this does not explain the reasons as to why many specimens lack apocrine involvement and why lesions typical of hidradenitis suppurativa may be found in skin devoid of apocrine glands. Additional microscopic analysis indicates that small cystic changes commonly arising from follicles are the most important early lesions in hidradenitis. Such cysts form and eventually become inflamed, probably secondary to a folliculitis, which is commonly induced by frictional trauma, If apocrine glands are present and are in the vicinity of the cystic lesions, they can be involved secondarily in the inflammatory process. Spread of infection and inflammation to adjacent tissue and glands results in an expanding abscess and, eventually, fibrosis and sinus tract formation. With recurrent, chronic disease, there is increased scarring and sinus tract formation, and this is often accompanied by persistent low-grade inflammation, with or without drainage. Clinical flares are marked by acute inflammation, infection, and suppurative drainage. It is difficult to distinguish end-stage hidradenitis suppurativa from other cicatrizing, sinus tract-producing diseases, including acne.

Thus, based on current information, hidradenitis suppurativa is best regarded as a follicular disorder with cyst formation, and not a primary alteration of the apocrine glands. A number of pathogenetic factors have been considered in the development or recrudescence of the disease and are worthy of discussion.

Local Frictional Trauma

A common, indeed the usual, incitant in hidradenitis suppurativa is local frictional trauma that is produced by the rubbing of apposing or redundant skin folds or tight-fitting clothing, such as brassieres or panty hose, or athletic equipment. The local edema and inflammation produced may result in ductal or follicular occlusion, cystic change and rupture, and abscess formation typical of the disease. Epithelial encapsulation results in large cyst formation and eventually inflammation and rupture as the process repeats itself. If apocrine glands are present, they may become involved but can be spared. It is likely that a preliminary pustular folliculitis represents the primary lesion in the pathogenesis of hidradenitis with cysts, sinus tracts, and scarring sequential developments. Yu and Cook have identified these changes histologically, emphasizing that apocrine involvement is not essential in the genesis of hidradenitis suppurativa.

Folliculitis

Subtle or obvious bacterial folliculitis can be found in almost all areas of hidradenitis suppurativa (Fig. 5) at some time. The importance of folliculitis in pathogenesis has been stressed above. It is important to realize that most such folliculitis lesions usually regress without incident, but some persist and extend more deeply to result in the classical alterations of hidradenitis suppurativa.

Specific Bacteria

Data from cultures of axillary hidradenitis suppurativa show polymicrobial infections with a predominance of anaerobes. Common anaerobes isolated include

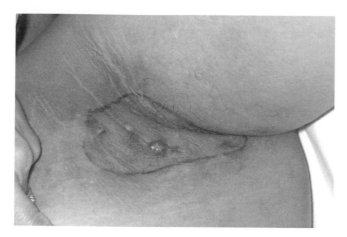

Figure 5 Hidradenitis suppurativa folliculitis in the axilla.

Peptostreptococcus, *Prevotella*, micro-aerophilic *Streptococci*, *Fusobacterium*, and *Bacteroides*. Frequently identified aerobic bacteria include *Staphylococcus aureus*, *Streptococcus pyogenes*, and Pseudomonas aeruginosa. Another study showed frequent *S. aureus*, coagulase-negative staphylococci, *Peptostreptococcus* species and *Propionibacterium* acnes.

The significance of this information is unclear. The bacteria may be essential to ductal occlusion or simply part of concomitant bacterial folliculitis. Certainly bacteria produce most of the inflammation once the disease process has begun, as well as in its late stages. To state that hidradenitis suppurativa is caused by any bacterial species and, thus, suggest that antibacterial therapy is curative is not justified by our experience to date.

Associated Acne

Contrary to popular belief, acne is not a sine qua non of hidradenitis suppurativa. Over half of these patients, especially women and those with axillary involvement alone, have no acne, whether active or quiescent. Only a small percentage of patients, usually those with chronic multiple site disease, have had an active pilonidal sinus or cicatrizing folliculitis of the scalp.

Associated Systemic Disease

These patients are usually healthy. No systemic disease has been associated with hidradenitis suppurativa. While obesity is common in patients with hidradenitis suppurativa, it is not found universally. Diabetes mellitus is not seen more frequently in patients with hidradenitis suppurativa, but impaired glucose tolerance has been noted.

Hormonal Factors

Pubertal or postpubertal onset of hidradenitis suppurativa and premenstrual exacerbations indicate an endocrine influence that is as yet unidentified. Pregnancy may result in amelioration of hidradenitis suppurativa, but much less regularly than it does Fox-Fordyce disease. There tends to be some relief after menopause. Although previous studies suggested androgen excess in these patients, more recent studies showed no such association when subjects and controls were matched for body weight.

Genetic Predisposition

Survey-based studies have shown that 27% to 38% of patients have a family history of the disorder, suggesting a genetic predisposition. Human leukocyte antigen (HLA) frequencies do not differ from those in the normal population.

Defective Immune Response

Patients' neutrophils have normal intracellular elastase activity, total elastase, release of elastase, total content and membrane expression of the receptors. The generation of free oxygen radicals, after stimulation with the protein kinase C activator phorbol myristate acetate, is significantly higher compared to that in normal subjects. There is no difference after Fc-receptor–mediated stimulation. Dysfunctional neutrophils might be involved in the pathogenesis of hidradenitis suppurativa, but these data are based on only 15 patients and 15 controls.

Local Eccrine Sweating

In patients with hidradenitis suppurativa, increased eccrine sweating in affected skin tends to aggravate existing lesions and precipitate the development of new ones. Patients with axillary hyperhidrosis show no increased incidence of hidradenitis suppurativa; so increased eccrine sweating alone is not enough to induce hidradenitis suppurativa.

Antiperspirant Deodorant Formulations and Depilatories

Antiperspirants and deodorants containing aluminum or zirconium salts do not promote or aggravate hidradenitis suppurativa, with the possible exception of those in a stick or ointment base. The use of an aluminum chloride may be helpful. No special pathogenic significance can be attached to depilatories, and very few patients give a history of their antecedent use in affected areas.

Smoking

A case-control study showed 89% of patients were current smokers, whereas only 46% of control patients were ($p < 0.001$). Though no causal relationship can be assumed, smoking cessation should be a part of the treatment plan for all patients who smoke.

Drugs

Lithium has been reported to induce hidradenitis suppurativa.

Clinical Course

Hidradenitis suppurativa develops after puberty, usually in the second or third decade. Classically, early lesions are solitary, painful, erythematous abscesses in an area rich in apocrine glands. Often described as blind boils or inflamed pilar cysts, they ultimately rupture, draining purulent material. Healing with fibrosis results and is usually followed by recurrences in or near the original site. Sinus tracts eventually form with dense bridges of scar tissue (Fig. 6). The majority of patients with hidradenitis suppurativa have small follicular lesions in the affected areas. Some are clearly pustular, others simply erythematous and macular. Cysts and comedones are noted in chronic hidradenitis suppurativa, but they are absent in early disease. Of note, comedones are absent in furunculosis, a major differential diagnosis.

The axillae are involved most commonly in hidradenitis suppurativa, though involvement of more than one site, including the inguinal, perianal, and breast skin, is not uncommon. However, with extensive hidradenitis across an axilla, diminished apocrine sweating and reduction in the usual axillary odor are noted. Regional adenopathy is usually insignificant or absent. During the acute phase with abscess formation, there may be mild constitutional symptoms.

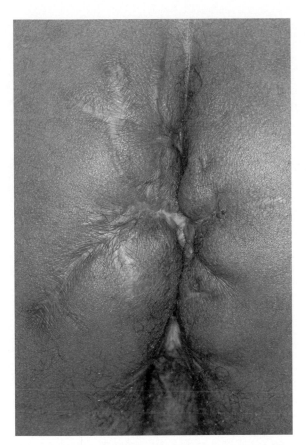

Figure 6 Recurrent hidradenitis suppurativa, with dense scarring and sinus tracts.

Untreated hidradenitis suppurativa is typically an unrelenting, progressive disease. In the affected sites there are periodic abscess and sinus tract formation, marked scarring, interference with local lymphatic drainage, and decreased mobility of the affected limb. In the anal and inguinal regions, fistulous tracts may involve the rectum, urethra, and vagina. Anemia, interstitial keratitis, inflammatory arthritis, and secondary amyloidosis are also possible with severe disease. Occasionally the process may burn out but usually not before there is extensive fibrosis and tissue destruction. Squamous cell carcinoma may develop in chronic lesions, especially those with ulceration.

Less than half of the patients with hidradenitis suppurativa also have acne of the face or trunk, while a smaller number have cicatrizing folliculitis of the scalp and a pilonidal sinus.

Histopathologic Findings and Laboratory Studies

Microscopic study of early lesions may reveal keratinous obstruction of the distal apocrine duct with dilation and rupture of the subjacent apocrine tubule. Neutrophils are present within the tubule before its rupture and afterwards in the surrounding dermis. Gram stain reveals bacteria within the neutrophils and extracellularly. A chronic lymphocytic infiltrate (mostly T-cells with a decreased helper to suppressor ratio), granulation tissue, fibrosis, sinus tract formation, pseudoepitheliomatous hyperplasia, and obliteration of glandular elements occur as the disease progresses. While the early lesions of hidradenitis suppurativa are diagnostic,

later the disease cannot be distinguished from severe acne or other disorders that cause chronic sinus tract formation.

A study of multiple specimens showed various combinations of poral occlusion, folliculitis, sinus tracts, epithelial cyst, abscess, apocrinitis, diffuse dermal inflammation, and pyogenic granuloma and scarring. Secondary involvement of eccrine glands was actually seen more commonly (25%) than was that of apocrine glands (12%). The authors of this study concluded that hidradenitis suppurativa is primarily follicular in nature.

Blood counts, blood chemistry tests, cell-mediated and immediate immune responsiveness, T- and B-cell levels, and routine endocrine assays are usually normal. Reports of abnormal hypothalamic-pituitary and T-cell response suggest the need for special study along these lines. Smears and cultures may be helpful as mentioned above.

Treatment

Medical Therapy and General Measures

Systemic antibiotics and topical therapy are ineffective once hidradenitis suppurativa shows evidence of progression or recurrence. Early solitary lesions may be treated by simple nonsurgical measures, but surgery is imperative once reactivation or chronic hidradenitis suppurativa is recognized.

In the axilla, it is convenient to approach treatment in a staged fashion (Table 3). Stage I, the initial manifestation of hidradenitis suppurativa, may be treated nonsurgically as follows. Intralesional triamcinolone (acetonide or diacetate suspension) is injected into the abscess. Distention of the inflamed abscess or tract with 5 to 10 mg triamcinolone suspension, diluted with saline, often results in involution within 12 to 24 hours. Incision and drainage of the abscess prior to the injection are avoided unless rupture is imminent.

Minocycline 100 mg twice daily should be given for a week or longer until the abscesses involute and should be maintained at 100 mg daily until all signs of inflammation are gone. This usually requires at least two weeks of antibiotic therapy but must be extended if necessary. Cephalosporins in the usual dosage for soft tissue infections are also effective. Drainage should be cultured and antibiotic sensitivities determined. Patients with slowly responsive or recalcitrant cases should be given antibiotics based on these findings. Some authors have pointed out that the average duration of individual lesions is six to nine days (with or without treatment) and that it is impossible to know whether the improvement is due to the antibiotics or to the natural course of the lesions.

High-dosage corticosteroids (prednisone 60–80 mg daily) have been advocated to reduce inflammation in recurrent, extensive hidradenitis suppurativa. This is only adjunctive therapy to hasten involution of the acute changes. Other treatment, particularly surgery, must be undertaken.

Table 3 Clinical Staging in Hidradenitis Suppurativa

Stage I
    Abscess formation, single or multiple, without sinus tracts and cicatrization

Stage II
    Recurrent abscesses with tract formation and cicatrization
    Single or multiple, widely separated lesions

Stage III
    Diffuse of near diffuse involvement, or multiple interconnected tracts and abscesses across entire area

Isotretinoin in dosages of 0.5 to 1.17 mg/kg/day has been used in courses of four to six months. Benefits have been minimal. Out of the approximately 107 patients studied to date, 22% have experienced clearing, and 21% have had marked improvement. However, many relapses occurred even with relatively short follow-up. Therefore, it appears far less useful for hidradenitis suppurativa than for cystic acne. There are a few anecdotal reports of successful treatment with finasteride and antiandrogens.

Daily, gentle cleansing should be done with a germicidal soap. Warm compresses with saline or Burow's solution (1:40) are helpful during the acute stages. Topical antibiotics, such as clindamycin lotion, may be applied but are not very effective. They may be helpful for prophylaxis after surgical or adjunctive therapy.

Avoidance of tight-fitting garments that cause frictional trauma, such as T-shirts, snug-fitting blouses or shirts, or straps from athletic equipment, is essential. Skintight blue jeans are a problem, particularly in the groin.

If a Stage I lesion heals after conservative management with no recurrence, further therapy is not required. Gentle cleansing and avoidance of tight-fitting clothing should be maintained. There is no restriction on the use of antiperspirants. Aluminum chloride may be used. It has a strong, local antibacterial and deodorant effect as well as an antiperspirant action. This provides prophylaxis against regional folliculitis and hidradenitis suppurativa.

At the first sign of recurrent hidradenitis suppurativa, surgical intervention is warranted. For unresponsive or recurrent diseases of Stage I to II, the following surgical approach is recommended.

Exteriorization

This technique is designed to destroy completely the hidradenitis tract and abscess. Healing is by second intention, obliterating the defect with fibrosis. The scar may be depressed or irregular but is surprisingly smooth and insignificant in most instances. It has been called marsupialization by some observers, which is an inappropriate designation, because formation of a pouch is certainly to be avoided.

Preoperative preparation is routine, and local anesthesia is administered using lidocaine with epinephrine. Complete anesthesia may be difficult to obtain in larger fibrotic areas; therefore, supplemental analgesia, sedation, or general anesthesia, is sometimes necessary.

Where there is an opening in the tract, a soft probe can be inserted to guide the incision. Secondary tracts that emanate from the primary one should be probed as well. If tract openings are not detectable, an incision is made over the abscess, and it is drained. The roof of the abscess or tract is then excised, exposing the interior of the lesion. In Stage I lesions with little or no fibrosis or tract formation, palpation and visualization will reveal whether all the indurated disease tissue has been removed. Curettage is performed along the base of the entire lesion to remove granulation tissue and debris even from the smaller fibrotic pockets. Electrocoagulation of the sides and base of the wound is done both for hemostasis and to destroy residual necrotic epithelial and fibrotic tissue. In some instances, when the base of the wound is clean and free of deeply placed tracts, electrocoagulation is kept to a minimum (Fig. 7). The wound may be quite large and irregularly shaped. Upon completion of surgery, there is often an appreciable reduction or absence of pain.

Postoperative care includes cleansing two to three times daily with soap and water or saline solution. Petrolatum

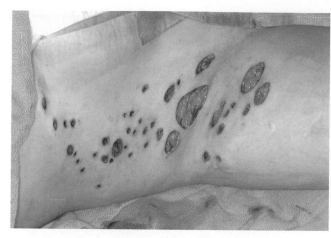

Figure 7   Stage II hidradenitis suppurativa. Multiple foci of activity, independent from one another that was amenable to individual local surgical ablation. (*See color insert.*)

ointment is then applied under a non-stick dressing such as sterile petroleum jelly-impregnated gauze.

Exteriorization can be used on the axillary, inguinal, inframammary, suprapubic, and trunk skin, including the buttock. It is generally not used in the perianal region. While it should be applicable to that site as well, injury to the anal sphincter, either directly or by postoperative wound contraction, must be avoided. The scars produced are usually quite acceptable and become soft and increasingly pliable with time.

Excision and Primary Closure

A sinus tract or fibrotic area may be sharply defined and limited in size, without irregular or poorly outlined tract extensions. In such instances, surgical excision of the entire area with primary closure may be used. If no residual disease has been missed, it produces a good result with minimal scarring. If there is any doubt about the complete removal of the lesion, however, these areas are best left to heal by second intention. Generally, excision and closure is more likely to be complicated by recurrent disease than is exteriorization, and the former is only recommended for selected patients.

Total Excision

Eradication of Stage III hidradenitis suppurativa usually requires total excision of the diseased region with closure utilizing flaps or grafts. In certain situations, such as involvement of the genital and perianal areas, closure or resurfacing may be best avoided, with healing by second intention aided by specialized dressings such as Silastic® foam. In the axilla, total excision followed by transverse primary closure has been successful. Limited upward extension of the arm on the operated side is anticipated and at times is unacceptable. The use of flaps, including Z-plasty, balloon tissue expansion with flaps, and grafting techniques such as mesh, split-thickness, and full-thickness grafts, are discussed elsewhere in this book. All these techniques may be useful in closing the remaining wound after removal of all the diseased tissue. There is also reported benefit from negative pressure dressings with split thickness skin grafts.

While results from total excision are very good and the disease is usually arrested, freedom from recurrence cannot be ensured. In a study of the efficacy of surgery, there was 100% recurrence after drainage, 42.8% after limited excision, and 27% after radical excision. The recurrences occurred at a median of 3, 11, and 20 months, respectively. Proper skin care, avoidance of frictional trauma, and smoking cessation may help to minimize the risk of recurrence.

Other Modalities

Cryosurgery with liquid nitrogen for treatment of Stage I lesions is an acceptable option and may result in minimal scarring. Despite significant pain during and after treatment, frequent infection, ulceration, and prolonged healing time (25 days on average), 70% of patients prefer this treatment to oral antibiotics. One freeze–thaw cycle should be used until a temperature probe reads 20°C.

Carbon dioxide laser therapy is another option. In a study of 34 patients with Hurley Stage II disease, only four had recurrences in the treated areas, and 31 thought the treatment improved their condition. The average follow-up was 35 months. Patients generally had moderately severe postoperative pain. The procedure these authors describe involves locally anesthetizing the areas to be treated and using the scanner-assisted carbon dioxide laser to repeatedly vaporize tissue downward until fresh yellow adipose tissue is reached, and outward to clinically-normal skin. The settings used were 20 to 30 W, a spot size of 3 to 6 mm, and a focal length setting of 12.5 or 18 cm. Care must be taken in the axillary region not to damage, major vessels and the nerve plexus. Ideally, carbon dioxide laser offers a bloodless field, but it may be necessary to use electrocoagulation or ligation for hemostasis involving vessels larger than 0.5 to 1 mm in diameter. After the procedure, the wound should be covered with petrolatum and a dressing applied. Healing is by second intention.

Liposuction may also be helpful in certain obese patients in an effort to minimize the local frictional trauma produced by apposing skin surfaces or folds, especially in hidradenitis involving the upper medial thigh or lower abdominal fold. Although there are no reports of its efficacy, in principle it is worthy of consideration in the appropriate patient.

Radiation

The use of radiation for hidradenitis suppurativa has essentially been abandoned. Popular in the 1930s and 1940s, it has been supplanted by the treatments described above.

Conclusions

The management of hidradenitis suppurativa has improved but is far from perfect. Surgical eradication of lesions is necessary in all but the earliest forms of the disease. Clinical staging is useful to define and quantify appropriate treatment and response. Dermatologic care must be continued to avoid recurrences. The best chance for cure is by proper treatment of Stage I or early Stage II hidradenitis suppurativa. The need for early diagnosis and proper treatment cannot be overemphasized. Despite the best available treatment, hidradenitis suppurativa recurs in some patients.

FAMILIAL BENIGN PEMPHIGUS

Familial benign pemphigus or "Hailey-Hailey disease" was described by the Hailey brothers in 1939. It is an uncommon genodermatosis of autosomal dominant inheritance, though nearly one-third of cases are sporadic. It is due to a defect in the ATP2C1 gene, which encodes an ATP-driven calcium pump. This disrupts the regulation of cytosolic calcium concentrations, which leads to acantholysis and the eruption seen clinically. The histologic hallmark of familial benign pemphigus is acantholysis. Initially, suprabasal clefting occurs. As time passes, the clefts expand into vesicles and bullae, and the epidermis is said to take on the appearance of a dilapidated brick wall due to partial acantholysis among large groups of cells. Direct immunofluorescence shows no consistent staining pattern.

Clinical Features

Familial benign pemphigus usually appears in late adolescence or early adult years. The eruption is characterized by clustered vesicles and bullae, which rapidly evolve into crusted erosions. The most common areas of involvement are the axillae, inframammary creases, groin folds, lateral neck, and anywhere there are apposing skin surfaces. Extension to portions of the trunk, especially the upper back and

(A)

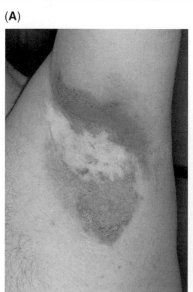

(B)

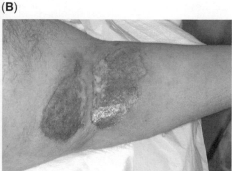

Figure 8 Familial Benign Pemphigus involving the axilla. **(A)** Preoperative appearance. **(B)** Dermal wound immediately after CO_2 laser vaporization. (*See color insert.*)

suprapubic area, may also occur. In the anogenital area, verrucous papules must be distinguished histopathologically from viral verrucae. Mucosal lesions (mouth, larynx, esophagus, and vagina) occur rarely. Otherwise, involvement of other organ systems has not been seen, and patients' general health is unaffected. Pruritus and burning pain are common, as is malodor. Large erosive areas become fissured with time. Asymptomatic longitudinal white bands in the fingernails were seen in a majority of patients in one study (38 out of 50). Unusual chronic variants may be hyperkeratotic, verrucous, neurodermatitic, and papular.

Sweat, heat, various forms of local trauma including friction from clothing or apposing skin folds, including patch testing for contact allergy, bacterial, candidal, and herpes simplex infections, are important in precipitating or aggravating the disease. Ultraviolet light induces acantholysis and can be used to diagnose the disease when it is in remission. It follows that the disease tends to be worse in the summer months.

Remissions and exacerbations are the rule. Disease-free periods last from months to years; however, the disease tends to persist well into the later years of life. During its active phase, familial benign pemphigus makes normal occupational and social activities difficult and causes considerable discomfort.

Diagnosis

The clinical features are usually characteristic, as are histologic findings. There are no other laboratory abnormalities of importance. The clinical differential diagnosis includes impetigo, pemphigus vulgaris, pemphigus foliaceus, pemphigus vegetans, keratosis follicularis (Darier's disease), and subcorneal pustular dermatosis. Histologically, it can be distinguished from Grover's disease by the focal nature of the acantholysis in the latter. Pemphigus vulgaris is also in the histological differential. Compared with Hailey-Hailey, it shows predominantly suprabasal acantholysis without the dilapidated brick wall appearance, and direct immunofluorescence shows characteristic intercellular space staining.

Treatment

Nonsurgical

Systemic antibiotics are predictably effective therapy. Tetracycline, in daily dosages of 1 to 2 g initially and tapered to 250 to 500 mg for maintenance, is helpful during the first attack and early recurrences of the disease. Minocycline, erythromycin, and penicillin are also effective. Topical antibiotics such as clindamycin and erythromycin, in lotion or cream bases, are helpful less regularly, as are topical corticosteroids. The local application of cyclosporine or tacrolimus has also been advocated. Systemic corticosteroids will suppress the disease if given in adequate doses but are not recommended for long-term use. Resistant cases may respond to dapsone 100 to 200 mg daily until clearing and then a maintenance dosage of 50 to 100 mg per day. Radiotherapy for this condition is controversial and is probably only of short-term benefit. One case that was recently reported was successfully treated with photodynamic therapy with 5-aminolevulinic acid. Several case reports have documented successful treatment with botulinum toxin type A. Presumably the beneficial effect is a result of the hypohidrosis that the toxin brings about. The procedure is outlined above under axillary hyperhidrosis. As with most uncommon dermatoses, there is a dearth of evidence on which to base treatment decisions.

Surgical

When familial benign pemphigus is persistent locally in one area, and especially if it is resistant to other forms of treatment, surgical management should be considered. Dermabrasion is reportedly beneficial, as is carbon dioxide (Fig. 8) and erbium:YAG laser vaporization of lesions. Excision of the affected area with skin grafting may also be helpful. Split-thickness grafts, usually of the thick type, are used to cover the defect, although mesh grafts could be used in certain situations. Any affected area is amenable to this approach, and it has been used in the axillae, groin, scrotum, perineum, and perianal sites. Donor skin for the grafts is taken from normal, uninvolved sites such as the thigh. Generally there is no recurrence of the disease, although occasionally this has been observed within the grafted skin.

BIBLIOGRAPHY

Adams DR, Gordon KB, Devenyi AG, Ioffreda MD. Severe hidradenitis suppurativa treated with infliximab infusion. Arch Dermatol 2003; 139(12):1540–1542.

Ashby EC, Williams JL. Cryosurgery for axillary hyperhidrosis. Br Med J 1976; 2(6045):1173–1174.

Baumann LS, Halem ML. Botulinum toxin-B and the management of hyperhidrosis. Clin Dermatol 2004; 22(1):60–65.

Boer J, van Gemert MJ. Long-term results of isotretinoin in the treatment of 68 patients with hidradenitis suppurativa. J Am Acad Dermatol 1999; 40(1):73–76.

Bong JL, Shalders K, Saihan E. Treatment of persistent painful nodules of hidradenitis suppurativa with cryotherapy. Clin Exp Dermatol 2003; 28(3):241–244.

Bovell DL, Clunes MT, Elder HY, Milsom J, Jenkinson DM. Ultrastructure of the hyperhidrotic eccrine sweat gland. Br J Dermatol 2001; 145(2):298–301.

Bretteville-Jensen G, Mossing N, Albrechtsen R. Surgical treatment of axillary hyperhidrosis in 123 patients. Acta Derm Venereol 1975; 55(1):73–77.

Brook I, Frazier EH. Aerobic and anaerobic microbiology of axillary hidradenitis suppurativa. J Med Microbiol 1999; 48(1):103–105.

Burge SM. Hailey-Hailey disease: the clinical features, response to treatment and prognosis. Br J Dermatol 1992; 126(3):275–282.

Bushara KO, Park DM, Jones JC, Schutta HS. Botulinum toxin— a possible new treatment for axillary hyperhidrosis. Clin Exp Dermatol 1996; 21(4):276–278.

Conway H, Stark RB, Climo S, Weeter JC, Garcia FA. The surgical treatment of chronic hidradenitis suppurativa. Surg Gynecol Obstet 1952; 95(4):455–464.

Crotty CP, Scheen SR III, Masson JK, Winkelmann RK. Surgical treatment of familial benign chronic pemphigus. Arch Dermatol 1981; 117(9):540–542.

Dobson-Stone C, Fairclough R, Dunne E, et al. Hailey-Hailey disease: molecular and clinical characterization of novel mutations in the ATP2C1 gene. J Invest Dermatol 2002; 118(2):338–343.

Dressler D, Adib Saberi F, Benecke R. Botulinum toxin type B for treatment of axillar hyperhidrosis. J Neurol 2002; 249(12):1729–1732.

Dvorak VC, Root RK, MacGregor RR. Host-defense mechanisms in hidradenitis suppurativa. Arch Dermatol 1977; 113(4):450–453.

Eldh J, Fogdestam I. Surgical treatment of hyperhidrosis axillae. Scand J Plast Reconstr Surg 1976; 10(3):227–229.

Elwood ET, Bolitho DG. Negative-pressure dressings in the treatment of hidradenitis suppurativa. Ann Plast Surg 2001; 46(1):49–51.

Fitzsimmons JS, Guilbert PR, Fitzsimmons EM. Evidence of genetic factors in hidradenitis suppurativa. Br J Dermatol 1985; 113(1):1–8.

Glent-Madsen L, Dahl JC. Axillary hyperhidrosis. Local treatment with aluminium-chloride hexahydrate 25% in absolute ethanol with and without supplementary treatment with triethanolamine. Acta DermVenereol 1988; 68(1):87–89.

Glogau RG. Treatment of hyperhidrosis with botulinum toxin. Dermatol Clin 2004; 22(2):177–185.

Harrison BJ, Kumar S, Read GF, Edwards CA, Scanlon MF, Hughes LE. Hidradenitis suppurativa: evidence for an endocrine abnormality. Br J Surg 1985; 72(12):1002–1004.

Hecht MJ, Birklein F, Winterholler M. Successful treatment of axillary hyperhidrosis with very low doses of botulinum toxin B: a pilot study. Arch Dermatol Res 2004; 295(8–9): 318–319.

Highet AS, Warren RE, Staughton RC, Roberts SO. Streptococcus milleri causing treatable infection in perineal hidradenitis suppurativa. Br J Dermatol 1980; 103(4):375–382.

Hurley HJ. Local surgical treatment of axillary hyperhidrosis. In: Epstein E, Epstein E Jr., eds. Skin Surgery. 6th ed. Philadelphia: WB Saunders, 1987:598–606.

Hurley HJ, Shelley WB. A simple surgical approach to the management of axillary hyperhidrosis. JAMA 1963; 186:109–112.

Hurley HJ, Shelley WB. Axillary hyperhidrosis. Clinical features, and local surgical management. Br J Dermatol 1966; 78:127–141.

Hynes PJ, Earley MJ, Lawlor D. Split-thickness skin grafts and negative-pressure dressings in the treatment of axillary hidradenitis suppurativa. Br J Plast Surg 2002; 55(6):507–509.

Inaba M, Anthony J, Ezaki T. Radical operation to stop axillary odor and hyperhidrosis. Plast Reconstr Surg 1978; 62(3):355–360.

James WD, Schoomaker EB, Rodman OG. Emotional eccrine sweating. A heritable disorder. Arch Dermatol 1987; 123(7):925–929.

Jemec B. Abrasio axillae in hyperhidrosis. Scand J Plast Reconstr Surg 1975; 9(1):44–46.

Jemec GB, Hansen U. Histology of hidradenitis suppurativa. J Am Acad Dermatol 1996; 34(6):994–999.

Jitsukawa K, Ring J, Weyer U, Kimmig W, Radloff H. Topical cyclosporine in chronic benign familial pemphigus (Hailey-Hailey disease). J Am Acad Dermatol 1992; 27(4):625–626.

Juhlin L, Rollman O. Vascular effects of a local anesthetic mixture in atopic dermatitis. Acta Derm Venereol 1984; 64(5):439–440.

Kang NG, Yoon TJ, Kim TH. Botulinum toxin type A as an effective adjuvant therapy for Hailey-Hailey disease. Dermatol Surg 2002; 28(6):543.

Kartamaa M, Reitamo S. Familial benign chronic pemphigus (Hailey-Hailey disease). Treatment with carbon dioxide laser vaporization. Arch Dermatol 1992; 128(5):646–648.

Kaufmann H, Saadia D, Polin C, Hague S, Singleton A, Singleton A. Primary hyperhidrosis—evidence for autosomal dominant inheritance. Clin Auton Res 2003; 13(2):96–98.

Kenkel JM. Ultrasound-assisted lipoplasty treatment for axillary bromidrosis: clinical experience of 375 cases. Plast Reconstr Surg 2004; 113(6):1897–1898.

Kirtschig G, Gieler U, Happle R. Treatment of Hailey-Hailey disease by dermabrasion. J Am Acad Dermatol 1993; 28(5 Pt 1):784–786.

Konig A, Lehmann C, Rompel R, Happle R. Cigarette smoking as a triggering factor of hidradenitis suppurativa. Dermatology 1999; 198(3):261–264.

Konrad H, Karamfilov T, Wollina U. Intracutaneous botulinum toxin A versus ablative therapy of Hailey-Hailey disease—a case report. J Cosmet Laser Ther 2001; 3(4):181–184.

Kunachak S, Wongwaisayawan S, Leelaudomlipi P. Noninvasive treatment of bromidrosis by frequency-doubled Q-switched Nd:YAG laser. Aesthetic Plast Surg 2000; 24(3): 198–201.

Langenberg A, Berger TG, Cardelli M, Rodman OG, Estes S, Barron DR. Genital benign chronic pemphigus (Hailey-Hailey disease) presenting as condylomas. J Am Acad Dermatol 1992; 26(6):951–955.

Lapiere JC, Hirsh A, Gordon KB, Cook B, Montalvo A. Botulinum toxin type A for the treatment of axillary Hailey-Hailey disease. Dermatol Surg 2000; 26(4):371–374.

Lapins J, Asman B, Gustafsson A, Bergstrom K, Emtestam L. Neutrophil-related host response in hidradenitis suppurativa: a pilot study in patients with inactive disease. Acta Derm Venereol 2001; 81(2):96–99.

Lapins J, Jarstrand C, Emtestam L. Coagulase-negative staphylococci are the most common bacteria found in cultures from the deep portions of hidradenitis suppurativa lesions, as obtained by carbon dioxide laser surgery. Br J Dermatol 1999; 140(1):90–95.

Lapins J, Sartorius K, Emtestam L. Scanner-assisted carbon dioxide laser surgery: a retrospective follow-up study of patients with hidradenitis suppurativa. J Am Acad Dermatol 2002; 47(2):280–285.

Leach RD, Eykyn SJ, Phillips I, Corrin B, Taylor EA. Anaerobic axillary abscess. Br Med J 1979; 2(6181):5–7.

Lebwohl B, Sapadin AN. Infliximab for the treatment of hidradenitis suppurativa. J Am Acad Dermatol 2003; 49(Suppl 5):S275–S276.

Levit F. Simple device for treatment of hyperhidrosis by iontophoresis. Arch Dermatol 1968; 98(5):505–507.

Mantell AM. Dilution, storage, and electromyographic guidance in the use of botulinum toxins. Dermatol Clin 2004; 22(2):135–136.

Menz P, Jackson IT, Connolly S. Surgical control of Hailey-Hailey disease. Br J Plast Surg 1987; 40(6):557–561.

Morgan WP, Harding KG, Hughes LE. A comparison of skin grafting and healing by granulation, following axillary excision for hidradenitis suppurativa. Ann R Coll Surg Engl 1983; 65(4):235–236.

O'Loughlin S, Woods R, Kirke PN, Shanahan F, Byrne A, Drury MI. Hidradenitis suppurativa. Glucose tolerance, clinical, microbiologic, and immunologic features and HLA frequencies in 27 patients. Arch Dermatol 1988; 124(7):1043–1046.

Paletta FX. Hidradenitis suppurativa: pathologic study and use of skin flaps. Plast Reconstr Surg 1963; 31:307–315.

Park YJ, Shin MS. What is the best method for treating osmidrosis? Ann Plast Surg 2001; 47(3):303–309.

Peppiatt T, Keefe M, White JE. Hailey-Hailey disease—exacerbation by herpes simplex virus and patch tests. Clin Exp Dermatol 1992; 17(3):201–202.

Pollock WJ, Virnelli FR, Ryan RF. Axillary hidradenitis suppurativa. A simple and effective surgical technique. Plast Reconstr Surg 1972; 49(1):22–27.

Product Information: Botox®, botulinum toxin type A. Allergan, Irvine, CA, (PI revised 07/2004).

Ramasastry SS, Conklin WT, Granick MS, Futrell JW. Surgical management of massive perianal hidradenitis suppurativa. Ann Plast Surg 1985; 15(3):218–223.

Ritz JP, Runkel N, Haier J, Buhr HJ. Extent of surgery and recurrence rate of hidradenitis suppurativa. Int J Colorectal Dis 1998; 13(4):164–168.

Roos DE, Reid CM. Benign familial pemphigus: little benefit from superficial radiotherapy. Australas J Dermatol 2002; 43(4):305–308.

Rosner IA, Richter DE, Huettner TL, Kuffner GH, Wisnieski JJ, Burg CG. Spondyloarthropathy associated with hidradenitis suppurative and acne conglobata. Ann Intern Med 1982; 97(4):520–525.

Scott AB. Development of botulinum toxin therapy. Dermatol Clin 2004; 22(2):131–133.

Shelley WB, Cahn MM. The pathogenesis of hidradenitis suppurativa in man; experimental and histologic observations. AMA Arch Dermatol 1955; 72(6):562–565.

Skoog T, Thyresson N. Hyperhidrosis of the axillae. A method of surgical treatment. Acta Chir Scand 1962; 124:531–538.

Strutton DR, Kowalski JW, Glaser DA, Stang PE. US prevalence of hyperhidrosis and impact on individuals with axillary hyperhidrosis: results from a national survey. J Am Acad Dermatol 2004; 51(2):241–248.

Sullivan TP, Welsh E, Kerdel FA, Burdick AE, Kirsner RS. Infliximab for hidradenitis suppurativa. Br J Dermatol 2003; 149(5):1046–1049.

Tashjian EA, Richter KJ. The value of propoxyphene hydrochloride (Darvon) for the treatment of hyperhidrosis in the spinal cord injured patient: an anecdotal experience and case reports. Paraplegia 1985; 23(6):349–353.

Torch EM. Remission of facial and scalp hyperhidrosis with clonidine hydrochloride and topical aluminum chloride. South Med J 2000; 93(1):68–69.

Tung TC, Wei FC. Excision of subcutaneous tissue for the treatment of axillary osmidrosis. Br J Plast Surg 1997; 50(1):61–66.

von der Werth JM, Williams HC. The natural history of hidradenitis suppurativa. J Eur Acad Dermatol Venereol 2000; 14(5):389–392.

Yamauchi PS, Lowe NJ. Botulinum toxin types A and B: comparison of efficacy, duration, and dose-ranging studies for the treatment of facial rhytides and hyperhidrosis. Clin Dermatol 2004; 22(1):34–39.

Yu CC, Cook MG. Hidradenitis suppurativa: a disease of follicular epithelium, rather than apocrine glands. Br J Dermatol 1990; 122(6):763–769.

46

Cicatricial Alopecia Diagnosis and Therapeutic Options

Wilma F. Bergfeld
*Department of Dermatology and Pathology, Cleveland Clinic Foundation,
Cleveland, Ohio, U.S.A.*

Dirk M. Elston
Department of Dermatology, Geisinger Medical Center, Danville, Pennsylvania, U.S.A.

INTRODUCTION

Cicatricial alopecia (permanent alopecia) is the result of primary inflammatory attack on the infundibular portion of the hair follicle/sebaceous gland with ultimate destruction of the follicular bulge area, pilosebaceous unit, and eccrine ducts that results in "follicular drop out." A secondary growth site, the anagen dermal papillae is intimately in contact with the external root sheath, both of which are involved in follicular regeneration. Destruction of the secondary regeneration site will also result in partial cicatricial alopecia.

Encompassed in the diagnosis of cicatricial alopecia are a group of heterogeneous disorders that are characterized by an end stage cicatricial alopecia. The diagnosis of a specific cicatricial alopecia is dependent on the clinical presentation and the histological features with clinicopathologic correlations. It is important to recognize that within each disorder there is a spectrum of activity from the acute to the chronic, which frequently complicates the ability to make an accurate diagnosis.

In 2001, "Working Classification of Primary Cicatricial Alopecia" was proposed by a Consensus Report from the American Hair Research Society (Table 1). The consensus report suggested that at least one 4 mm biopsy, which includes the subcutaneous tissue be obtained from the active border of the alopecic patch/plaque. It is recommended that horizontal sections be done so that all the follicles can be examined simultaneously. If possible, an additional biopsy for vertical sections is also recommended. To determine the presence of reparative fibrosis, an elastic stain is recommended, and for mucin deposition a PAS and Colloidal iron with hyaluronidase. Additional biopsies from less involved or normal sites are considered helpful and additive but not necessary. Direct immunofluorescence (DIF) is also helpful in confirmation of the diagnosis of discoid lupus erythematosus and lichen planopilaris (LPP).

CLINICAL AND HISTOLOGICAL PRESENTATION OF PRIMARY CICATRICIAL ALOPECIA
Lymphocytic Infundibular Folliculitis—Lymphocyte Predominant
Lupus Erthematosus
Acute and Subacute

The acute and subacute Lupus Erthematosus (LE) presents as scalp erythema with or without a fine white scale.

Frequently a telogen effluvium is the presenting sign. Scalp tenderness or pain is common. Erythema and scalp skin atrophy may also be present with diminished scalp hair density. This stage is difficult clinically to distinguish from other early inflammatory alopecias such as seborrheic dermatitis, LPP, and central centrifugal cicatricial alopecia. The more inflammatory plaques have an adherent white scale and are hairless. The cutaneous lesions frequently occur on sun-exposed areas and may be associated with the localized or diffuse scalp involvement (Fig. 1).

Chronic cutaneous lupus erythematosus (DLE) occurs more frequently in females than males with a higher prevalence in adults than children. Clinical features include keratotic follicular plugs, papules, telangiectasia, skin atrophy and variable mottled pigmentation and macules or patches of complete alopecia. The involved areas may be tender or pruritic (Fig. 2).

Histology

The histological features are those common to those of acute, subacute, chronic and subcutaneous lupus erythematosus. The acute and subacute findings are superficial and involve primarily the epidermis with interface changes of basilar vacuolar degeneration, necrotic keratinocytes, and a scant perivascular predominately lymphocytic infiltrate. Subepidermal bulla may be present in the acute LE. In chronic LE, there is basilar vacuolar degeneration of the epidermis and follicles, necrotic keratinocytes, thickened basement membrane (BMZ), a lymphoid interface infiltrates and a patchy lymphocytic perivascular and periadnexal infiltrate. In the chronic stage, dermal mucinosis (colloidal iron positive and digests with hyalurondase), may be extensive. Early, hyalinization of the follicular fibrous tracts (stellae) occurs and only late is there follicular scarring "tree trunk-like" hyalinization (Fig. 3). In chronic LE and lupus profundus there is a diffuse and angiocentric lymphocytic panniculitis with or without the classic epidermal changes.

DIF can be supportive of the LE diagnosis. The classical findings are a continuous IgG, IgM, C3 or "full house" (all immunoreactins; IgG, IgM, IgA, C3, Clq) and a shaggy deposition of fibrin at the BMZ (Fig. 4).

Medical Treatment of Cutaneous Lupus Erthematosus

Aggressive therapy for the acute inflammatory disease is necessary to prevent destruction of the folliculosebaceous

Table 1 Modified Proposed Working Classification of Primary Cicatricial Alopecia (Based on Histology)[a]

Lymphocytic folliculitis
    Chronic lupus erythematosus
    Lichen planus and variants
        Classic lichen planopilaris
        Frontal fibrosing alopecia
        Graham-Little syndrome
    Classic pseudopelade (Brocqo)
    Central centrifugal cicatricial alopecia
    Alopecia mucinosis
    Keratosis follicularis spinulosa decalvans
Neutrophilic folliculitis
    Folliculitis decalvans
    Dissecting folliculitis/cellulites (perifolliculitis abscedens et suffodiens)
    Central centrifugal cicatricial alopecia
Mixed suppurative folliculitis
    Folliculitis (acne) keloidalis
    Folliculitis (acne) necrotica
    Erosive pustular dermatosis
Nonspecific (histological changes)
    End stage permanent alopecia

[a]Combination medical and surgical therapies are need for the treatment primary and secondary cicatricial alopecia.
Source: From Olsen, Bergfeld, Cotsarelis, et al. (2003).

units and the follicular bulge area. Corticosteroids are the mainstay of therapy. Both class I and II topical corticosteroids may be effective. Intralesional steroids have also proved helpful in doses ranging from 2.5 to 10 mg/cc, in minute amounts into the dermis of the involved sites. Alternate therapies have included antimalarials, retinoids, dapsone, and thalidomide. In chronic LE, sulfasalazine, mycophenolate mofetil, and methotrexate have had some efficacy. Other infrequent therapies have included intralesional and systemic interferon, anti-CD4 antibodies and topical tazarotene. Regrowth has been assisted by the use of topical minoxidil when the inflammation is reduced. More recent reports suggest that topical tacrolimus and pimecrolimus are helpful.

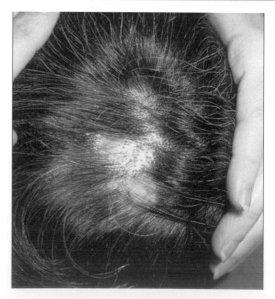

Figure 1 Chronic cutaneous lupus erythematosus. Seborrheic dermatitis like changes of mild erythema and keratotic follicular papules.

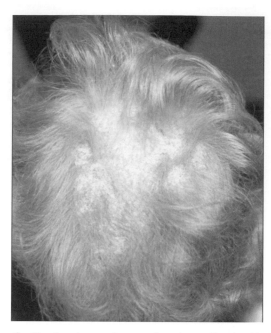

Figure 2 Chronic cutaneous lupus erythematosus. Chronic with discoid plaques and mottled pigmentation.

Lichen Planus and Variants

LPP was first described as a clinical syndrome of lichen planus (LP) associated with cicatricial alopecia. LPP is most prevalent in women and represents at least one-third of all the cicatricial alopecias. Fifty percent of those with LPP lack other cutaneous signs of LP. In the absence of cutaneous, mucosal and nail changes of LP, the diagnosis may be challenging.

    LPP presents clinically with perifollicular erythema and keratotic follicular papules that are observed primarily at the advancing margin. The central area is a hairless macule or patch with indistinct follicular keratin plugs, which is similar to acute and late/chronic LE. The most common sites of involvement include the frontal-central scalp and crown with slowly progressive peripheral centrifugal spread (Fig. 5). Linear progression on the scalp and beard is recognized. Tuffed folliculitis is common.

    The etiology of LP/LPP is unknown but they are considered to be an immunological disorder. ANA and

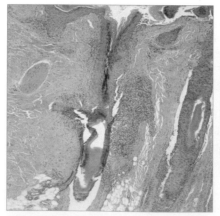
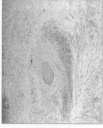

Transverse section:
Lymphocytic Folliculitis

Figure 3 Chronic cutaneous lupus erythematosus low power vertical section with lymphocytic folliculitis and lichenoid infiltrate. (*See color insert*.)

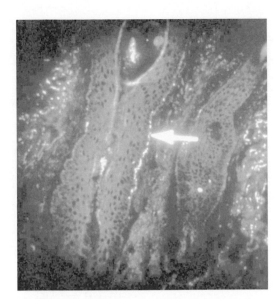

Figure 4 Chronic cutaneous lupus erythematosus. Direct immunofluorescence "full house" immunoreactions linear deposition at follicular basement membrane. (*See color insert.*)

microsomal antibodies can be seen in some patients. On occasions a drug induced LPP has been suspected.

The other variants of LPP include Graham-Little syndrome and keratosis follicularis spinulosa decalvans.

Histology

The epidermal changes classic of LP may be observed. There is an interface-lichenoid lymphocytic infiltrate with basalar vacuolar degeneration, Civatte bodies (globular cytoid bodies layer with immunoreactins), which involves the infundibular follicular epithelium and less frequently the epidermis (Fig. 6). When the epidermis is involved, the characteristic findings of LP are observed. They include irregular epidermal hyperplasia with saw tooth rete ridges with superficial hypergranulosis.

Late in LPP, a superficial wedge-shaped scar is seen, which can be defined by elastic stain. This scar represents the infundibular area and the superficial portion of the -follicular fibrous tract (stellae). PAS stain can help to identify the early BMZ changes. LE can be differentiated from LPP/LP by the presence of a thickened BMZ, large aggregates of lymphocytes and dermal mucin. The late changes of LE and LPP are similar. In both, there are decreased numbers of folliculosebaceous units, superficial perifollicular angiofibroplasia (scar), and occasional hair fiber granulomas (Fig. 7).

DIF studies demonstrate numerous superficial Civatte bodies that have a "full house" of immunoreactins: IgG, IgA, IgM, and C3. These bodies are observed adjacent to the involved epidermis and follicle. Shaggy linear fibrin at the BMZ is also noted, which is similar to LE (Fig. 8).

Frontal Fibrosing Alopecia

Frontal fibrosing alopecia (FFA) is a recently described variant of LPP. It affects older women with a mean age 67. It presents as a band-like frontal-temporal cicatricial alopecia that progress to involve the parietal scalp. The band of alopecia has fine follicular keratotic papules and mild perifollicular erythema. The older lesions leave the skin smooth and hairless with complete alopecia similar to the late findings of LE and LPP. To date, there have been no reported cases of FFA (LPP) associated with cutaneous LP (Fig. 9).

Histology

The histological features are similar to LPP.

Medical Treatment of Lichen Planopilaris

Like LE, corticosteroids are the mainstay of therapy. Retinoids and cyclosporine have proven helpful. Historically, grisofulvin has been proven a benefit especially if the patient has had tinea pedis, corporis, or onychomycosis. More recent reports suggest that topical tacrolimus and pimecrolimus are helpful.

Central Centrifugal Cicatricial Alopecia

Central centrifugal cicatricial alopecia (CCCA) is the new terminology, which has replaced follicular degeneration syndrome, hot comb alopecia, and central elliptical

(A) **(B)**

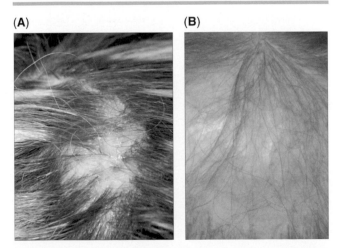

Figure 5 Lichen planopilaris. Large area of alopecia with peripheral erythema and keratotic follicular papules: (**A**) early and (**B**) late.

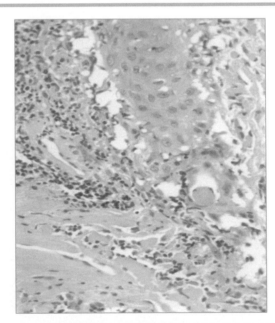

Figure 6 Lichen planopilaris. Vertical sections: Lymphocytic folliculitis with civatte bodies. (*See color insert.*)

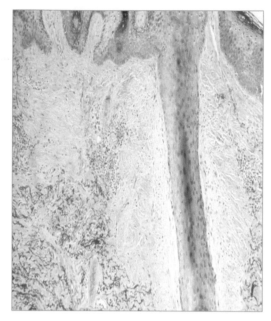

Figure 7 Lichen planopilaris. Vertical section; superficial wedge-shaped scarperifollicular. (*See color insert.*)

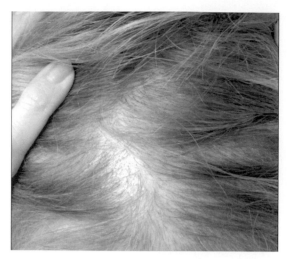

Figure 9 Frontal fibrosing alopecia. Mild erythema and subtle keratotic follicular papules (variant of lichen planopilaris).

pseudopelade. It is primarily seen in African–American women but it has been observed in African–American men, Indians from the Indian subcontinent and Caucasians. It commonly presents as central scalp alopecia (parietal and crown) with subtle progressive alopecia, which can be initially mistaken for female pattern hair loss (Fig. 10). On history and clinical examination, inflammatory papules, pustules, nodules and inflammatory keratotic follicular papules can be observed. A progressive alopecia evolves with late findings of severe central cicatricial alopecia with a peripheral localized or diffuse Hippocratic wreath of hair (Fig. 11). Because of its varied clinical presentation it is not surprising on biopsy to see changes of LPP and suppurative folliculitis, such as, observed in folliculitis decalvans (FD)/ dissecting folliculitis (DF).

Histology

The consistent histological findings of CCCA include complete loss of the folliculosebaceous unit and diminished adnexal structures, with widened hyalinization follicular fibrosis tracts (tree trunk-like) with preservation of the dermal elastin. Premature disintegration of the inner root sheath is characteristic but may not be a specific finding. The late findings reveal hyalinized "tree trunk" fibrosis tracts and interfollicular fibrosis with hair granulomas.

Medical Treatment of Central Centrifugal Cicatricial Alopecia

The treatment of CCCA is unsatisfactory and employs the common therapies used in the lymphocytic and suppurative folliculitis cicatricial alopecic disorders. In the inflammatory stage, antibiotic therapies can be helpful in reducing the inflammation and progression. Discontinuation of the common

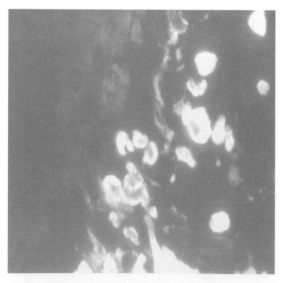

Figure 8 Lichen planopilaris. Direct immunofluorescence dermal clustered civatte bodies at basement membrane. (*See color insert.*)

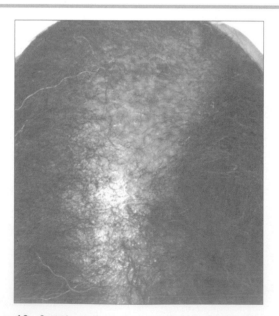

Figure 10 Central centrifugal cicatricial alopecia. Central alopeica with keratotic follicular papules.

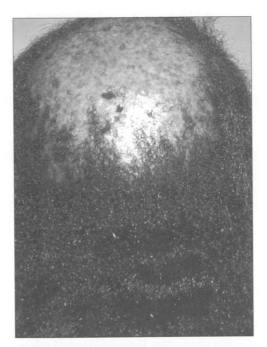

Figure 11 Central centrifugal cicatricial alopecia. Severe central thinning with Hippocratic wreath of hair.

African–American hair styling techniques, procedures, and chemicals appears essential in preventing progression. The use of topical minoxidil can be helpful in restoring hair growth in the early stages after the inflammation is reduced which also, is similar to the other inflammatory cicatricial alopecic disorders.

Pseudopelade of Brocq

The classic description of pseudopelade of Brocq (PPB) is the persistence of small, discrete, smooth, and flesh colored or white noninflammatory macules without follicular plugging or keratotic follicular papules. Over time the macules coalesce into larger patches "foot prints in the snow" (Fig. 12). PPB affects mainly adult women but has been reported in children (71–74). The natural course is a slowly progressive cicatricial permanent alopecia (Fig. 13).

Histology

PPB represents end stage alopecia with loss of the folliculosebaceous units and diminished adnexa. The follicular tracts are hyalinized and have widened "tree trunk-like" similar appearance to the findings in CCCA. Inflammation is absent or sparse. If inflammation is present, it is a chronic lymphocytic infundibular folliculitis. On DIF, there are occasional Civatte bodies with mixed immunoreactins similar to LPP (Fig. 14).

Medical Treatment of Pseudopelade of Brocq

Effective therapies are not available. PPB responds poorly to the mainstay therapies: corticosteroids and antimalarials. Clinically and histologically PPB is end stage alopecia.

NEUTROPHILIC FOLLICULITIS—NEUTROPHILS PREDOMINATE (SUPPURATIVE FOLLICULITIS)

Folliculitis Decalvans and Variants

This heterogeneous group of inflammatory scalp cicatricial alopecias begins as a suppurative folliculitis, which prog-

resses to cicatricial alopecia. This group includes FD, DF, FK, and pustular erosive dermatosis of the scalp. These disorders are more common in African Americans, affecting males greater than the females. The clinical presentation is that of inflammatory papules, pustules, nodules and large soft boggy nodules, which are associated with tenderness and pain. These lesions slowly extend and coalesce to larger hairless boggy or firm nodule and in the late stage results in large scarred patches and plaques. Cultures from the superficial crusts and or the acute boggy nodules reveal predominately *Staphylococcus aureus*. Other reported organisms include gram negative bacilli and other gram positive cocci. Antibiotic therapy is only temporally helpful.

Folliculitis Decalvans

The clinical presentation of FD is usually as inflammatory papules, pustules, and keratotic follicular papules, which may progress to tender inflammatory nodules and eventually cicatricial permanent alopecia (Fig. 15). Scalp tenderness and pain is common. This disorder may be associated with the cutaneous signs of follicular occlusive diseases, i.e., hidradenitis suppurativa and lupoid sycosis.

Histology

The early changes consist of ectatic follicles with keratin plugs and neutrophilic infundibular folliculitis with rupture. Later findings include the involvement 4of numerous infundibular follicles with rupture and interfollicular neutrophilic infiltrate (dermal abscesses) with coalescence of inflammation to involve the entire dermis and the deep follicle.

Later, there is a mixed acute infiltrate with neutrophils and eosinophils and chronic inflammatory infiltrate with a lymphoplasmic infiltrate. Hair fiber granulomas embedded in scar are common. The result is scarring with loss of elastin and extensive follicular and interfollicular full-thickness scarring. The result is a permanent cicatricial alopecia (Fig. 16).

Dissecting Folliculitis

The severe variant of FD is DF. In this disorder, the early presentation is similar to FD but it progresses to an expansive network of large coalescing erythematous tender nodules with sinus tracts. The end result is an extensive severe permanent cicatricial alopecia (Fig. 17).

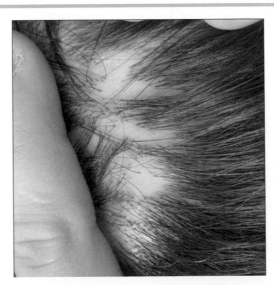

Figure 12 Pseudopelade of Brocq. "Finger print" alopecia macules.

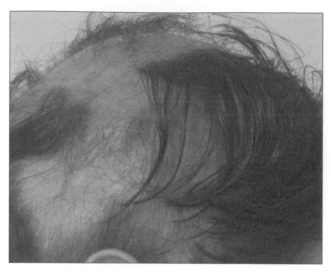

Figure 13   Pseudopelade of Brocq. Alopecia patches coalesce and result progressive alopecia.

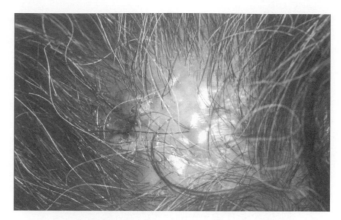

Figure 15   Folliculitis decalvans. Alopecic shiny follicular papules and plaques.

Histology

The histological changes are similar to FD with the exception of the increased severity and sinus tract development. Extensive full thickness dermal fibrosis is the final event and presents as both follicular and interfollicular fibrosis. Elastic stain reveals loss of elastin through out the dermis, reparative fibrosis (Fig. 18).

Tufted Folliculitis

Tufted folliculitis clinically presents as tufts of hair within a keratotic follicular papule or denovo within an alopecic patch. The tuff is composed of numerous hairs exiting from a single follicle. This change is considered a late clinical feature of an inflammatory cicatricial alopecia (Fig. 19). Tufted folliculitis has been reported to occur in LE, LP and variants, FD and variants, pemphigus vulgaris, and infectious folliculitis.

Histology

The histology varies and is dependent on the primary disorder. However, common to all is the presence of compounded hair follicles within keratotic follicular plugs.

MIXED INFLAMMATORY INFILTRATE (ACUTE AND CHRONIC FOLLICULITIS WITH INTERFOLLICULAR FIBROSIS)

Folliculitis Decalvans and Variants—Late Features

See folliculitis decalvans.

Folliculitis Keloidalis and Variants

FK or acne keloidalis presents shiny follicular papules that involve primary the nape of neck in African–American males. Similar lesions can be seen in the beard, central scalp, and crown. Initially, hair protrudes from the papules. These papules progress to shiny firm hairless irregular plaques (Fig. 20).

Histology

The early histological changes are similar to FD and include abscesses and sinus tract formation. Unique to this disorder is the extensive hypertrophic perifollicular fibrosis and follicular cysts. The result is a permanent cicatricial alopecia with loss of the folliculosebaceous units and adnexal structures. Hair fiber granulomas are common (Fig. 21).

Folliculitis Necrotica Varioliforme

Folliculitis necrotica or acne necrotica presents in adults. It is seen more frequently in males than females. It presents as a pruritic or painful infundibular folliculitis with keratotic

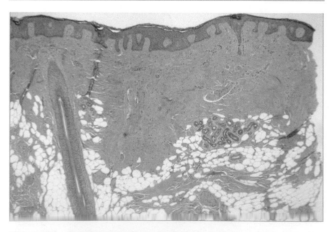

Figure 14   Pseudopelade Brocq (vertical section; low power). End stage alopecia. (See color insert.)

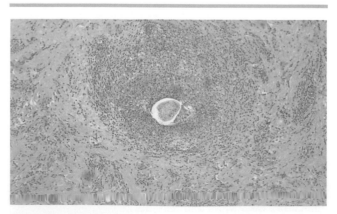

Figure 16   Folliculitis decalvans. Transverse section mixed follicular and interfollicular inflammation and fibrosis. (See color insert.)

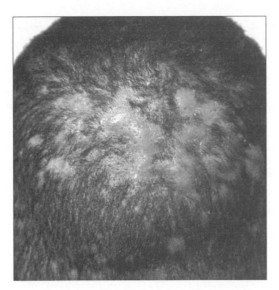

Figure 17 Dissecting folliculitis. Large tender alopecic coalescing nodules

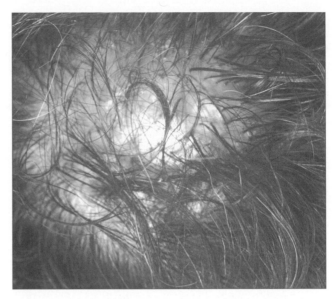

Figure 19 Tufted folliculitis. Grouped hairs exiting one follicle in an alopecic patch.

follicular papules or papulopustules that develop central umbilication with an adherent yellow crust. The common site of involvement is the frontal and parietal scalp but other sites such as face, neck, and chest have been reported. There are usually 5 to 20 necrotic pustules, which evolve to irregular varioliforme scars.

Histology

The common finding is a suppurative necrotic infundibular folliculitis. Initially it is a lymphocytic folliculitis, which evolves to a suppurative necrotic infundibular folliculitis. A permanent alopecia is uncommon, especially if the inflammation remains in the superficial portion of the follicle and/or involves only a few follicles.

Erosive Pustular Dermatosis of the Scalp

Erosive pustular dermatosis is a rare and unusual scalp folliculitis, which can result in a permanent cicatricial alopecia. It most commonly affects Caucasian adult women but has been reported in African Americans. The clinical presentation is diffuse superficial pustules with yellow crusts. Cultures have grown diphtheroids and *Staphylococcus epidermidis*. Immunological studies suggest a defect in immunologic host response to *Staphylococcus aureus* (Fig. 22).

Histology

The histological changes are similar to FD but a more extensive neutrophilic infundibular folliculitis with associated lymphoplasmocytic folliculitis and interfollicular acute and chronic inflammatory infiltrate with extensive dermal reparative fibrosis with loss of elastin (Fig. 23).

Medical Treatment of the Acute and Chronic Folliculitis Cicatricial

The identification of infectious organisms and specific prolonged antibiotic therapy can be suppressive and *Staphylococcus aureus* control will temporarily slow the progression of these disorders.

Because *Staphylococcus aureus* is the most common identified organism prolonged antibiotic therapy includes erythromycin, cephalosporins, trimethoprim/sulfamethoxozole, clindamycin, or a fluoroquinalone with or without

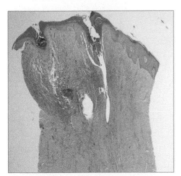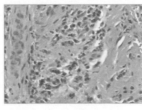

Figure 18 Dissecting folliculitis (vertical sections). Mixed follicular and interfollicular inflammation and fibrosis. (*See color insert*.)

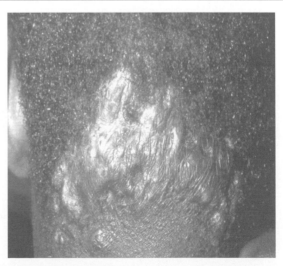

Figure 20 Folliculitis keloidalis. Multiple shiny alopecic follicular papules and nodules. (*See color insert*.)

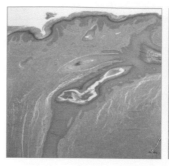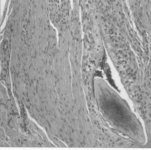

Figure 21 Folliculitis keloidalis (vertical sections). Chronic stage with follicular cysts and extensive perifollicular fibrosis. (*See color insert.*)

rifampin and fusidic acid. The combination of incision and drainage, corticosteroids, antibiotics, and retinoids is recommended for inflammatory nodules, cysts, and sinus tracts. On occasion, single therapies of high dose zinc or oral retinoids can be beneficial.

In FK, the prevention of the inflammatory papule results in decreased hypertrophic scarring. When scarring is present, topical high potency class I and II corticosteroids and intralesional corticosteroids, 5 to 10 mg/cc, with minute volume injections of less than 0.05 cc., will flatten the papules. In all these disorders, recurrence is common especially when therapies are reduced or discontinued.

Nonspecific (End Stage Cicatricial Alopecia)
This category represents the end stage of the inflammatory and noninflammatory (PPB) alopecic disorders with the resultant permanent cicatricial alopecia. The clinical presentation is flesh-colored alopecic macules and patches primarily involving the central scalp with centrifugal progression (Fig. 24).

Histology
The histological features are a complete or almost complete loss of the folliculosebaceous units with either dermal

hyalinization of the fibrosis tracts or the "full" dermis and loss of or reduced adnexal structures. Superficial wedge scars devoid of elastin can be seen. Inflammation is usually sparse to absent. The specimen rarely has histological features of the initial process. If the fibrosis is reparative and involves the follicular fibrosis tract and interfollicular areas, than folliculitis declavans and variants (neutrophilic and mixed inflammatory alopecic disorders) should be suspected. If the fibrous tracts are hyalinized and widened "tree trunk-like," then the primary differential includes CCCA, LE, and PPB. The superficial wedge scars are more common in LPP but can also be seen in DLE.

Secondary Cicatricial Alopecia
There are many causes of (secondary) cicatricial alopecia, which should be excluded when evaluating primary cicatricial alopecia. These include infections, dermatoses, familial alopecia, physical and chemical follicular insult, drugs, autoimmune disease, neoplastic disorders and developmental and hereditary disorders, and miscellaneous disorders (Table 2).

Surgical Treatment of Cicatricial Alopecia
The surgical treatment of cicatricial alopecia can be life altering for these patients. Surgical treatment is most effective for end stage disease when the inflammatory process is controlled. It is potentially hazardous to embark on a surgical correction in patients with active disease. Even in patients with apparent inactive disease, the disease can flare and progress after the surgical procedure. Therefore, the treatment recommendation is to confirm the diagnosis and employ adequate medical management prior to surgical correction (Table 3).

Erosive pustular dermatosis of the scalp can be a secondary phenomenon, which follows hair transplantation grafting or scalp reduction procedures. Unless the surgeon recognizes this disorder as both a primary and secondary phenomena and distinguishes it from a simple staphylococcal surgical wound infection, it can lead to a progressive cicatricial alopecia with unsatisfactory surgical results. The therapy would include diagnosis, antistaphylococcal

Figure 22 Erosive pustular dermatosis. Erythema, crusting and alopecia.

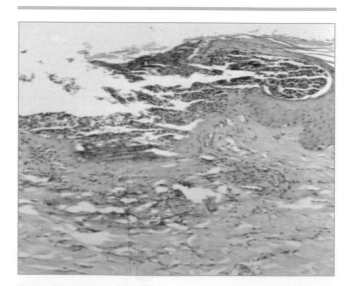

Figure 23 Erosive pustular dermatosis (vertical section). Superficial suppurative folliculitis. (*See color insert.*)

antibiotic therapy, topical potent corticosteroids and oral antineutrophil agents.

Although men currently comprise the majority (90%) of patients who have surgical hair restoration, excellent results are seen in women who have a variety of scalp disorders. Women, with cicatricial alopecia represent an important subgroup seeking hair restoration. These women are more complex than, those with Female Patterned Hair Loss and require special consideration of the surgical options and continued medical management.

In the African–American women with CCCA, physical trauma from traction, chemical procedures, and hair care play important roles in the initiation of their disorder and will need to be addressed along the surgical options. Recommendation on hair care and styling may be needed, and the surgeon should be prepared to advise these patients.

Surgical Options

The surgical options for hair restoration include follicular grafting, scalp reduction, flat rotations, tissue expansion, or some combination of these. Although grafting techniques are most widely use in the setting of common familial pattern alopecia, it can benefit the patients with cicatricial alopecia. Each technique has both advantages and disadvantages. For example, scalp reduction and rotation flaps are well suited for large localized areas of cicatricial alopecia. They are able to provide hair density unmatched by grafting techniques. However, they carry the risk of large surgical scars if unsuccessful.

Localized primary excision with closure is satisfactory for cicatricial areas one centimeter or less. Tissue expansion is often used for the larger areas of alopecia but again may be complicated by the enlargement of scar similar to the rotation grafts. The combination of single or staged tissue expansion and rotation flap was reported as the most suitable technique in children. Staged scalp reduction is also effective for large areas of cicatricial alopecia.

In individuals with numerous small alopecic macules or patches, hair transplantation may be preferred.

Hair Transplantation

Improvements of hair transplantation that involve follicular unit transplantation have vastly improved the cosmetic appearance. Follicular unit transplantation duplicates the naturally occurring hair patterns and minimizes trauma to the follicles.

Follicular units are obtained by strip harvesting and stereomicroscopic dissection. Follicular unit extraction with very small punch excisions may be a suitable alternative. The uses of micro–minigrafts containing one to four follicular units have used to treat secondary cicatricial in burns, surgical scars, and congenital cicatricial alopecia. If an individual has had hair transplantation by the older methods with resultant "corn row plugs," these can be improved with the added micro–minigrafts.

Follicular stem cell implantation has the potential to overcome the limitations of the donor supply. The in vivo immunodeficient mouse studies show that human vellus hair follicles from balding areas grow as well or better than terminal follicles from the same individuals. These studies suggest that follicular cells remain capable of regenerating a terminal follicle even after miniaturization of the follicular

Table 2 Secondary Cicatricial Alopecia[a]

Infections	Neoplasia
Bacterial	Malignant
Fungal	Primary
Viral	Metastatic
Dermatoses	Atypical lymphoproliferative
Psoriasis	disorders
Pityriasis amiantacea	Hamartoma
Seborrheic dermatitis	Syringoma
Lichen simplex chronica	Generalized follicular
Familial patterned hair loss/	hamartoma
senescent alopecia	Organoid nevus
Bullous disorders	Granulomatous
Cicatricial bullous pemphoid	Sarcoid
Epidermolysis injury	Necrobiosis lipoidica
Epidermolysis bullosa	Granuloma annulare
Physical and chemical causes	Crohn's disease
Ischemia/pressure	Development/hereditary disorders
Thermal injury	Fibrodysplasia
Corrosive/toxic injury	Darier's disease
Traction/trichotillomania	Ichthyosis
Chemical/physical-trichodystrophy	Congenital ichthyosiform
Radiation	erythroderma
Drugs	Lamellar ichthyosis
Autoimmune disorders	Keratitis–ichthyosis–deafness
Graft vs. host disease	syndrome
Scleroderma	Conradi-Hunermann
En coup de sabre	chondrodysplasia punctata
Lichen sclerosis	Incontentia pigmenti
	Aplasia cutis congenita
	Miscellaneous
	Lipedematous alopecia
	Porokeratosis
	POEMS syndrome

[a]Combination medical and surgical therapies are need for the treatment primary and secondary cicatricial alopecia.
Source: Bergfeld, Elston (2003).

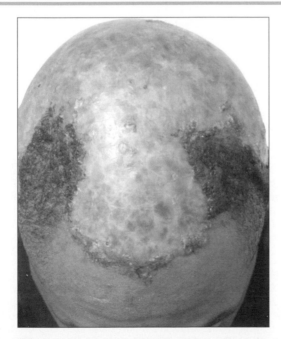

Figure 24 End stage alopecia. Extensive alopecic patches with peripheral crusting shiny papules and keratotic follicular papules.

unit. It also suggests that the scalp environment is a critical determinant for hair growth.

Flaps

Older techniques included temperoparieto-occipital (Juri) flaps and temperoparietal flaps that resulted in straight abrupt hair lines, posterior hair direction, inappropriate hair density, and blunted temperofrontal angles. Despite these limitations, the Juri flap repair with scalp reduction still has proved helpful for the treatment of large areas of scarring alopecia.

The temperoparietal fascial flap is richly vascularized and may be transferred as either a pedicle or free graft. These grafts have proved useful reconstruction of large scalp defects that are unsuitable for other techniques. Careful patient selection is recommended.

Modified bilobed flaps have been used successfully in scalp defects as large as 2 to 17 cm in length and 0.5 to 2 cm in width. Dispersion of flap tension reduces the expansion of the scar. Flaps used to repair alopecia can be random pattern using any part of the scalp. Scalp reduction combined with small random flaps can reduce the linear scars.

Most cases of stable, inactive, end stage cicatricial alopecia can be approached with a combination of scalp reduction, flaps, and follicular unit grafting.

Scarring alopecia of the vertex that involves the hair cowlick is especially difficult to camouflage. The use of multiple small scalp flaps can be helpful. Any residual scar can be treated with micro and minigrafts.

Minimizing Linear Surgical Scars

As mentioned above, the use of small random flaps can reduce the appearance of linear scars. Micro–mini hair grafts can be used to correct and camouflage the resultant scars. The use of double relaxation galea suturing reduces the skin tension, reduces scarring and preserves the follicular units.

Tissue Expansion

Tissue expansion has created new opportunities for scalp flaps and has allowed reconstruction of extensive alopecia. This technique has been used successfully but has a significant complication rate of 5% to 15%. The major complication is the erosion of the outer table of the skull. For this reason, this technique is reserved for the skilled surgeon.

Aplasia Cutis Congenita (Secondary Cicatricial Alopecia)

Successful treatment of aplasia cutis has been reported with staged excision, flaps, and tissue expansion. Prior to surgery, imaging studies are recommended to identify underlying bony defects. The literature reveals that conservative therapy has also produced good results.

Table 3 Surgical Options of Cicatricial Alopecia[a]

Scalp reduction
Primary excision (primary closure or heal by secondary intention)—scalp reduction
Staged excision
Hair transplantation-stem cells, follicular units (micro, mini, or punch grafts)
Flaps (pedicle or free, bilobed, Juri, or multiple mini flaps)
Tissue expansion
Combinations (primary or staged)

[a]Combination medical and surgical therapies are need for the treatment primary and secondary cicatricial alopecia.

Folliculitis Keloidalis Nuchae

Successful surgical treatment has been primary single and serial staged excision and closure. Other reports indicated the primary excision and healing by secondary intention had excellent results. Isolated cases have needed a combination of surgery procedures, i.e., tissue expansion.

Combination Medical and Surgical Management: Optimizing the Outcome

In the common familial pattern hair loss (androgenetic alopecia), the combined medical and surgical treatment has improved the outcome and cosmesis. These therapies have included topical minoxidil and oral finasteride (males only). The use or continuation of topical minoxidil has proven to reduce hair loss that follows hair transplantation and to reduce temporal hair loss seen following rhytidectomy.

The effective treatment of patient with cicatricial alopecia requires effective medical treatment and management with the primary goal to control the inflammation, which damages the folliculosebaceous units as well as careful surgical planning with selection of the optimal surgical technique(s). Optimal surgical management may require combined primary excision, staged excision, flaps, tissue expansion, and hair transplantation with additional surgeries to achieve the desired cosmetic camouflage and benefit.

Patients with cicatricial alopecia are a challenge in diagnosis, medical treatment, and management, and require dual management of their disorders by both the medical and surgical dermatologists.

BIBLIOGRAPHY

Annessi G, Lombardo G, Gobello T, Puddu P. A clinicopathologic study of scarring alopecia due to lichen planus. Am J Dermatopathol 1999; 21:324–331.

Avram Mr, Cole JP, Gandelman M, et al. Roundtable Consensus Meeting of the 9th Annual Meeting of The International Society of Hair Restoration Surgery. The potential role of minoxidil in the hair transplanting setting. Dermatol Surg 2002; 28(10):894–900.

Bang RL, Ghoneim IE, Gang RK, Al Najjadah I. Treatment dilemma: conservative versus surgery in cutis aplasia congenita. Eur J Pediatr Surg 2003; 13(2):125–129.

Bergfeld WF, Elston DM. Cicatricial alopecia. In: Elise Olsen, ed. Disorders of Hair Growth; Diagnosis and Treatment. McGraw-Hill Companies Inc., 2003:363–398.

Bilkay U, Karem H, Ozek C, Erdem O, Solngur E. Alopecia treatment with scalp expansion: some surgical fine points and a simple modification to improve results. J Craniofac Surg 2004; 15(50):758–765.

Bouhanna P. Androgenetic alopecia: combining medical and surgical treatments. Dermatol Surg 2003; 29(11):1130–1134.

Brandy DA. Corrective hair restoration techniques for the aesthetic problems of temperoparietal flaps. Dermatol Surg 2003; 29(3):230–234.

Burm JS, Oh SJ. Prevention and treatment of wide scar and alopecia in the scalp: wedge excision and double relaxation suture. Plast Reconstr Surg 1999; 103(4):l143–1149.

Callender VD, McMichael AJ, Cohen GF. Medical and surgical therapies for alopecias in black women. Dermatol Ther 2004; 17:162–176.

Cooley J. Follicular cell implantation: an update on "hair follicle cloning.". Surg Clin North Am 2004; 12(2):2119–2124.

Dawber RPR, Ebling FJG, Woynarowska FT. Disorder of hair. In: Champion RH, Burton JL, Ebling FJG, eds. Text Book of

Dermatology. 5th ed. Oxford: Blackwell Scientific Publications, 1992:2533.

De la Rosa Carrillo D, Christensen OB. Treatment of chronic discoid lupus erythematosus with topical tacrolimus. Acta Derm Venereol 2004; 84(3):233–234.

Duteille F, Le Fourn B, Hepner Lavergne D, Pannier M. The limitation of primary excision of cicatricial alopecia: a report of 63 patients. Ann Plast Surg 2000; 45:145–149.

El Kabbajn, Derurec O, Guillot B. Erosive pustulosis of the scalp: 3 cases. Ann Dermatol Venereol 2005; 132(5):4577.

Elston DM, McCollugh ML, Warschaw KE, Bergfeld WF. Elastic tissue in scars and alopecia. J Cutan Pathol 2000; 27:147–152.

Epstein JS. Follicular unit hair grafting: state of the art surgical technique. Arch Facial Plast Surg 2003; 5(5):439–444.

Epstein JS. The treatment of female patterned hair loss and other application of surgical hair restoration in women. Facial Plast Surg Clin North Am 2004; 12(2):241–247.

Eremia S, Umar SH, Li CY. Prevention of temporal alopecia following rhytidectomy: the prophylactic use of minoxidil. A study of 60 patients. Dermatol Surg 2002; 28(1):66–74.

Eren S, Hess J, Larkikn GC. Total scalp replantation based on one artery and one vein. Microsurgery 1993; 14(4):266–271.

Felman G. Post-thermal burn alopecia and its treatment using extensive horizontal scalp reduction in combination with a Juri flap. Plast Reconstr Surg 1994; 93(6):1268–1273.

Frechet P. A new method for correction of the vertical scar observed following scalp reduction for extensive alopecia. J Dermatol Surg Oncol 1990; 16(7):640–644.

Geertz G, Kind R, Lehmann P. Cicatricial alopecia. In: Orfanos CE, Happle R, eds. Hair and Hair Diseases. Berlin: Springer-Verlag, 1990:611–639.

Glenn MJ, Bennett RG, Kelly AP. Acne keloidalis nuchae: treatment with excision and second-intention healing. J Am Acad Dermatol 1995; 33(2 pt l):243–246.

Gloster HM Jr. The surgical management of extensive cases of acne keloidalis nuchae. Arch Dermatol 2000; 136(11):1376–1379.

Gurlek A, Alaybeyoglu N, Demir CY, Aydogan H, Bilen BT, Ozturk A. Aesthetic reconstruction of large scalp; defects by sequential tissue expansion with interval. Aesthetic Plast Surg. 2004; 28(4):245–250.

Harris JA. Follicular unit transplantation: dissecting and planting techniques. Facial Plast Surg Clin North Am 2004; 12(2):225–232.

Headington JT. Cicatricial alopecia. Dermatol Clin 1996; 14: 773–782.

Iida N, Ohsumi N, Tonegqwa M, Tsutsumi Y. Reconstruction of scalp defects using simple designed bilobed flap. Aesthetic Plast Surg 2000; 24(2):137–140.

Inaba Y, Inaba M. Prevention and treatment of linear scar formation in the scalp: basic principles of the mechanism of scar formation. Aesthetic Plast Surg 1995; 19(4):369–378.

Jordan RE. Subtle clues to diagnosis by immunopathology: scarring alopecia. Am J Dermatopathol 1980; 2:157–159.

Kolasinski J, Kolenda M. Algorithm of hair restoration surgery in children. Plast Reconstr Surg 2003; 112(2):412–422.

Krajcik RA, Vogelman JH, Malloy VL, Orentreich N. Transplants from balding and hairy Androgenetic alopecia scalp regrow hair comparably well on immunodeficient mice. J Am Acad Dermatol 2003; 48(5):752–759.

Lam SM, Hempstead BR, Williams EF. A philosophy and strategy for surgical hair restoration: a 10 year experience. Dermatol Surg 2002; 28(11):1035–1042.

Lampropoulos CE, Sangle S, Harrison P, Huges GR, D'Cruz DP. Topical tacrolimus therapy of resistant cutaneous lesions in lupus erythematosus: a possible alternative. Rheumatology (Oxford) 2004; 43(11):1383–1385.

Lubojevic S, Pasic A, Lipozencic J, Skerlev M. Perifolliculitis capitis abscedens et suffodiens. J Eur Acad Dermatol 2005; 19(6):719–721.

Martin FJ, Herrera A, Rios JJ, Moreno JC, Camacho F. Erosive pustular dermatosis of the scalp after skin grafting. Dermatol Surg 2001; 27(8):766–767.

Martinick JH. The latest developments in surgical hair restoration. Facial Plast Surg Clin North Am 2004; 12(2):249–252.

Mirmirani P, Willey A, Headington JT, Stenn K, McCalmont TH, Price VH. Primary cicatricial alopecia: histopathologic findings do not distinguish clinical variants. J Am Acad Dermatol 2005:637–643.

Mobini N, Tam S, Kamino H. Possible role of the bulge region in the pathogenesis of inflammatory scarring alopecia. J Cutan Pathol 2005; 32(10):675–679.

Mossard S, Shiell RC. Frontal fibrosing alopecia developing after hair transplantation for Androgenetic alopecia. Int J Dermatol 2005; 44(4):321–323.

Nnoruka NE. Hair loss: is there a relationship with hair care practices in Nigeria? Dermatol 2005; 44(31):13–17.

Olsen E, Bergfeld WF, Cotsarelis G, et al. Summary of North American Hair Research Society (NAHRS) sponsored workshop on Cicatricial alopecia, Duke University Medical Center February 10 and 11, 2001. J Am Acad Dermatol 2003; 48:454–457.

Pertonic-Rosic V, Krunic A, Mijuskovic M, Vesic S. Tufted hair folliculitis. A pattern of scarring alopecia? J Am Acad Dermatol 1999; 41:112–114.

Pestalardo CM, Cordero A Jr., Ansorena JM, Bestu M, Martinho A. Acne keloidalis nuchae. Tissue expansion treatment. Dermatol Surg 1995; 21(8):723–724.

Pinkus H. Differential patterns of elastic fibers in scarring and nonscarring alopecias. J Cutan Pathol 1978; 5:93–104.

Powell JJ, Dawber RP, Gattrer K. Folliculitis decalvans including tufted folliculitis. Clinical, histologic and therapeutic findings. Br J Dermatol 1999; 140:328–333.

Price VH, Roberts JL, Hordinsky M, et al. Lack of efficacy of finasteride in postmenopausal women with Androgenetic alopecia. J Am Acad Dermatol 2000; 43(5 pt 1):768–776.

Rassman WR, Bernstein RM, McClellan R, Jones R, Worton E, Uyttendaele H. Follicular unit extraction: minimally invasive surgery for hair transplantation. Dermatol Surg 2002; 28(8):720–728.

Rhee ST, Colville C, Buchman SR, Muraszko K. Complete osseous regeneration of a large skull defect in a patient with Cutis Aplasia. A conservative approach. J Craniofac Surg 2002; 13(4):497–500.

Roberts JL, DeVillez RL. Infectious, physical and inflammatory causes of hair and scalp; abnormalities. In: Elise Olsen, ed. Disorders of Hair Growth; Diagnosis and Treatment : McGraw-Hill Companies Inc., 2003:87–122.

Roenigk RK, Wheeland RG. Tissue expansion in cicatricial alopecia. Arch Dermatol 1987; 123(5):641–646.

Schultz BC, Roenigk HH Jr. Scalp reduction for alopecia. J Dermatol Surg Onco 1979; 5(10):808–811.

Seyhan A, Yoleri L, Barutcu A. Immediate hair transplantation into a newly closed wound to conceal the final scar on the hair bearing skin. Plast Reconstr Surg 2000; 105(5):1866–1870.

Silfen R, Hudson Da, Soldin MG, Skoll PJ. Tissue expansion for frontal hairline restoration in severe alopecia in a child. Burns 200; 26(3):294–297.

Sperling LC, Solomon AR. A new look at scarring alopecia. Arch Dermatol 2000; 136:235–242.

Stenn KS, Sundberg JP. Hair follicle biology, the sebaceous gland and scarring alopecias. Arch Dermatol 1999; 135:973–974.

Tan E, Shapiro J. Update on primary Cicatricial alopecia. J Am Acad Dermatol 2005; 53(l):l–37,38–40.

Trachsler S, Treub RM. Value of direct immunofluorescence for differential diagnosis of cicatricial alopecia. Dermatology 2005; 211(2):98–102.

Unger WP. Surgical approach to hair loss. In: Elise Olsen, ed. Disorders of Hair Growth; Diagnosis and Treatment. McGraw-Hill Companies Inc., 2003:453–480.

Valenzuela R, Bergfeld WF, Deodhar SD. Lupus erythematosus. Immunohistopathology. In: Interpretations of Immunofluroescent Patterns in Skin Diseases. Chicago: Am Society of Clinical Pathologists Press, 1984:66–79.

Viglizzo G, Verrini A, Rongioletti F. Familial Lassuerur-Graham-Little-Piccardi syndrome. Dermatology 2004; 208(2):142–144.

Vogel JE. Correcting problems in hair restoration surgery: an update. Facial Plast Surg Clin North Am 2004; 12(2):263–278.

Whiting DA. Cicatricial alopecia: clinico-pathologic findings and treatment. Clin Dermatol 2001; 19:211–225.

Wilson CLL, George SM, Dean D, et al. Scarring alopecia in discoid lupus crythematosus. Br J Dermatol 1992; 126:307–314.

Yotsuyanagi I, Watanabe Y, Yamashita K, Urushidate S, Yokoi K, Sawada Y. New treatment of a visible linear scar in the scalp: multiple hair bearing flap technique. Br J Plast Surg 2002; 55(4):324–329.

47

Evaluation and Management of Leg Ulcers

Gregory J. Wilmoth and Thom W. Rooke
Mayo Clinic, Rochester, Minnesota, U.S.A.

INTRODUCTION

Lower extremity ulcers are a common and troublesome problem affecting up to 1% of the adult population. They occur more frequently in the elderly, and their prevalence is likely to increase with the changing demographics of an older population. While the differential diagnosis of leg ulcerations is broad (Table 1), the majority are caused by venous insufficiency, arterial insufficiency, or neuropathy (in patients with diabetes mellitus). Fortunately, with a careful history, good physical examination, and select laboratory evaluations, a prompt diagnosis can usually be reached. Ulcers that elude initial investigations, are of unusual location or morphology, or are unresponsive to treatment may need further evaluations (Table 2), such as biopsy and culture.

DIAGNOSIS

History

Directed questions can be extremely helpful in establishing the cause of a leg ulcer.

1. *How did the ulcer develop*? Injury, infection, cold, or thrombophlebitis can be factors precipitating ulcerations. Neuropathic ulcers are often unnoticed.
2. *Did it develop rapidly or slowly*? Rapidly developing ulcers suggest venous insufficiency, acute thrombosis, embolic causes, or pyoderma gangrenosum. Slowly developing ulcers may reflect chronic arterial insufficiency or malignancy.
3. *How painful is the ulcer*? Ulcers from arterial insufficiency, livedoid vasculitis, sickle cell anemia, and cutaneous polyarteritis nodosa are typically very painful. Pain is not a prominent feature of venous ulcers. Neuropathic ulcers are often painless; however, there may be associated paresthesias or burning pain generalized to the leg. These neuropathic pains can also be seen in systemic vasculitis or cutaneous polyarteritis nodosa.
4. *Are there exacerbating or relieving factors*? Pain from arterial ulcers worsens with elevation or exercise and may be relieved with dependency and rest. The discomfort of venous ulcers may improve with elevation.
5. *Are there predisposing factors*? Is there a history of claudication (arterial) or edema and blood clots (venous)?
6. *What is current treatment*? Topical agents may impair healing or promote contact dermatitis. Compression therapy in a patient with arterial insufficiency may lead to new ischemic ulcerations.
7. *What are current medications*? Systemic corticosteroids, methotrexate, and immunosuppressive or chemotherapeutic agents can inhibit wound healing. Coumadin and hydroxyurea can cause ulcers. There may be a drug-induced vasculitis or lupus erythematosus.
8. *What is past medical history*? Systemic diseases contributing to ulcers can be identified. These include diabetes mellitus, rheumatoid arthritis, systemic lupus erythematosus, hematologic disorders, thrombosis or pregnancy loss (suggesting antiphospholipid antibodies), inflammatory bowel disease (suggesting pyoderma gangrenosum), and ischemic heart disease or stroke (suggesting atherosclerosis).
9. *How is general health*? Weight loss and fever may signal infection or malignancy. Smoking can impair wound healing and is an important aggravating factor in atherosclerosis and thromboangiitis obliterans.
10. *What is social history*? Does the patient have proper housing and nutrition? Is there anyone available to help with wound care?
11. *What is family history*? Are there inherited diseases present such as diabetes mellitus, hemoglobinopathies, connective tissue diseases, or atherosclerosis?

Physical Examination

The physical examination can help differentiate causes of leg ulcers. Questions to ask include the following.

1. *What is the location*? Venous ulcers tend to develop on the distal third of the leg. They may occur anywhere at this level, but commonly the medial malleolar area is involved. Ischemic ulcers affect the toes and distal foot. Embolic processes usually involve the toes. Neuropathic ulcers predominate under pressure points on the sole of the foot or at sites of trauma from shoes.
2. *What is the appearance*? Venous ulcers tend to be shallow and exudative, with ample granulation tissue. Arterial ulcers are usually dry and deep, with necrotic tissue or eschar at the base. Vasculitic ulcers are commonly well demarcated with necrotic base, giving a "punched-out" appearance, or they may have irregular serpiginous borders. Pyoderma gangrenosum has an exudative necrotic center to the ulcer with a ragged undermined violaceous border bounded by a halo of erythema. Ulcers of livedoid vasculitis tend to be shallow and sharply demarcated with linear and angled configurations.
3. *Are the foot and leg pulses present, adequate, and symmetrical*? Pulse changes or asymmetry indicate large vessel arterial occlusive disease.

Table 1 Classification of Leg Ulcers

I. Vascular diseases	*V. Hematologic diseases (contd.)*
A. Venous	E. Coagulation defects
B. Arterial	Protein S and C deficiencies
Atherosclerosis obliterans	Antithrombin III deficiency
Thromboangiitis obliterans	Antiphospholipid antibody
Arteriovenous malformations	syndromes
Cholesterol embolism	
Hypertension	*VI. Drugs*
C. Lymphatics	Ergotism
Lymphedema	Methotrexate
Halogens	Illicit drugs (injected)
	Vasopressors
II. Vasculitis	Hydroxyurea
A. Small vessel	Coumadin
Hypersensitivity vasculitis	
Drugs	*VII. Trauma*
Cryoglobulinemia	Pressure
Infection	Cold injury (frostbite, pernio)
Henoch-Schönlein purpura	Radiation
Malignancy	Burns (chemical, thermal)
Autoimmune associated	Factitial
Rheumatoid arthritis	
Lupus erythematosus	*VIII. Neoplastic*
Scleroderma	Squamous cell carcinoma
Sjogrens syndrome	Basal cell carcinoma
Behcets disease	Melanoma
Livedoid vasculitis	Sarcoma (Kaposi's)
B. Medium and large vessel	Lymphoma
Polyarteritis nodosa	Cutaneous T-cell lymphoma
Cutaneous polyarteritis nodosa	
Wegener's granulomatosis	*IX. Infection*
Churg-Strauss granulomatosis	A. Bacterial
Giant cell arteritis	Furuncle
	Ecthyma gangrenosum
III. Neuropathic	Septic emboli
Diabetes	Anthrax
Tabes dorsalis	Diphtheria
Poliomyelitis	Gas gangrene
Leprosy	Necrotizing fascitis
Traumatic and toxic neuropathies	Tuberculosis (lupus vulgaris)
Inherited sensory deficiency	Leprosy
Synergistic anaerobic infections	Atypical mycobacteria
	B. Fungal
IV. Metabolic	Blastomycosis
Diabetes	Coccidiomycosis
Gout	Histoplasmosis
Prolidase deficiency	Sporotrichosis
Vitamin C deficiency	Majocchi's granuloma (dermatophyte)
Syphilis	C. Actinomycosis (Madura foot)
	D. Leishmania
V. Hematologic diseases	E. Infestations and bites
A. Red blood cell disorders	
Sickle cell anemia	*X. Dermatosis*
Thalassemia	Pyoderma gangrenosum
Polycythemia rubra vera	Necrobiosis lipoidica diabeticorum
B. Leukemia	Lichen planus
C. Thrombocythemia	Sarcoidosis
D. Dysproteinemias	Necrobiotic xanthogranuloma
Cryoglobulinemia	Papulonecrotic tuberculid
Cryofibrinogenemia	
Macroglobulinemia	*XI. Panniculitis*
	Pancreatic fat necrosis
	Lupus panniculitis
	α_1-Antitrypsin deficiency

Table 2 Laboratory Tests

I. Routine	*III. Skin biopsy*
Complete blood count	Routine histopathology
Differential blood count	Immunohistochemical stains
Peripheral smear	Cultures
Urinalysis	Bacterial
Serum chemistry group	Fungal
Bacterial culture	Mycobacterial
Syphilis serology	Molecular genetic analysis
	lymphomatous infiltrates
II. Special laboratory tests	
Antinuclear antibodies	*IV. Vascular*
Lupus antibodies (ENA, anti-DNA)	A. Arterial
Total complement, C3, C4	Ankle brachial pressure ratio
Rheumatoid factor	Segmental pressures
Antineutrophilic cytoplasmic	Cutaneous temperature
antibodies	Doppler waveforms
Sickle cell preparation	Pulse volume recordings
Hemoglobin electrophoresis	Duplex ultrasound
Serum protein electrophoresis	B. Venous
Immunoelectrophoresis	Volume plethysmography
Cryoglobulins	Photoplethysmography
Routine and special coagulation	Doppler directional analysis
Chest radiograph	Duplex ultrasound
Limb radiographs	C. Cutaneous flow correlates
CT and MRI for malignancy detection	Laser Doppler flowometry
Colonoscopy (ulcerative colitis)	Transcutaneous oxygen tension
Vitamins C and A, iron, zinc	D. Angiography

Abbreviations: CT, computed tomography; MRI, magnetic resonance imaging.

erythematosus, livedoid vasculitis, cutaneous polyarteritis nodosa, cholesterol emboli, or antiphospholipid disease. The scarring of atrophie blanche is seen in livedoid vasculitis and venous disease. Is there infection with signs of lymphangitis or cellulitis? Subcutaneous nodules suggest panniculitis or cutaneous polyarteritis nodosa. An elevated "heaped-up" border suggests squamous cell carcinoma.

5. *Are there associated signs?* Arthritis may indicate rheumatoid disease or systemic lupus. Are there signs of scleroderma? Are there sensory losses or other signs of neuropathy such as altered gate? Are there heart or lung findings indicating endocarditis, tuberculosis, or systemic fungal disease? Does the patient's general appearance suggest malnutrition or malignancy?

LABORATORY STUDIES

Routine laboratory screening is helpful for any ulceration of the leg and includes complete blood count, serum chemistries, urinalysis, and syphilis serology. Testing may demonstrate evidence of hematologic disorders, infection, diabetes mellitus, nutritional deficiency, and systemic diseases such as vasculitis or systemic lupus erythematosus. Local radiographs are useful to rule out osteomyelitis.

Swab cultures of the wound should be obtained even without evidence of infection because they may reveal occult fungal or mycobacterial disease, identify Candida yeast overgrowth that can slow wound healing, and guide empiric antibiotic coverage pending definitive culture and sensitivity if infection should occur.

Any ulceration that is not felt to be from venous, arterial, or neuropathic causes should probably have a biopsy. Biopsy is essential in the diagnosis of malignancy, vasculitis, infection, panniculitis, and small-vessel occlusive

4. *What is the appearance of the surrounding skin?* Is there evidence of venous insufficiency with edema, varicosities, and hemosiderin pigmentation? Is there pallor or reactive dependent hyperemia from ischemic disease? Evidence of livedo reticularis suggests systemic lupus

diseases such as those associated with antiphospholipid syndromes or cryoglobulinemia. Tissue should be taken from skin at the ulcer edge, not the healing tissue or necrotic debris of the base. Ideally, it should be deep enough to contain ample pannicular tissue. The wound should be closed unless obvious necrosis and infection are encountered. Tissue should be submitted for bacterial, fungal, and mycobacterial culture. Of note, several ulcer-causing atypical mycobacteria have temperature requirements in culture of 30°C to 33°C instead of the routine 37°C. The laboratory should therefore be notified so that they may set up appropriate cultures. It is also wise to freeze a portion in liquid nitrogen and set it aside in the event that special immunohistochemical stains or molecular genetic studies are required. Specialized testing can be useful and should be directed by clinical suspicion. Helpful tests are summarized in Table 2.

NONINVASIVE VASCULAR STUDIES

Differentiation between venous and arterial ulcers is important in planning appropriate therapy and avoiding iatrogenic complications. A useful office procedure to evaluate arterial insufficiency is the ankle-to-brachial systolic blood pressure ratio, or ankle-brachial index (ABI). With the patient in supine position, a blood pressure cuff is placed over the calf while arterial flow is monitored over the dorsalis pedis or posterior tibial arteries with a handheld Doppler instrument. The cuff is inflated until no flow is detected, then the cuff is slowly released until the pressure at which return of flow occurs is identified. This is the systolic blood pressure. A similar reading is obtained over the brachial artery. Normally the ankle systolic pressure is equal to or greater than the brachial systolic pressure. Thus a normal ABI is between 0.8 and 1.1, but may be greater on occasion. An ABI of less than 0.8 indicates significant arterial obstructive disease. It is important to note that leg systolic pressure can be falsely elevated in patients with noncompressible arteries caused by medial calcification or severe atherosclerosis. Thus, in diabetic patients, a normal ABI may overlook significant ischemic disease. Other noninvasive techniques can be used to identify arterial insufficiency in diabetic patients.

If arterial insufficiency alone, arterial and venous insufficiency combined, or diabetes mellitus is identified, then the noninvasive vascular laboratory can be extremely helpful in reaching a diagnosis. The laboratory can determine if underlying arterial or venous disease is complicating other causes of ulcers. Localization of disease to certain segments or locations can be helpful. Vasculitis and thromboangitis obliterans typically involve more peripherally located vessels than atherosclerosis. Venous studies are useful in detecting thrombosis, obstruction, or incompetent valves. Disease can be localized to the superficial system, the perforators, or the deep system. These distinctions have prognostic and therapeutic implications regarding surgical options and anticoagulation. Techniques such as transcutaneous partial pressures of oxygen ($TcPO_2$) may be able to yield prognostic and therapeutic information. Several reports have associated threshold $TcPO_2$ levels (20–40 mmHg) below which healing is severely impaired.

SPECIFIC CLINICAL TYPES
Venous Insufficiency Ulcers

The primary pathologic event leading to venous ulceration is failure of the calf muscle pump, which is responsible for venous return against gravity. The venous systems of the leg consist of the superficial system (short and long saphenous veins with their tributaries), the perforating veins, which connect the superficial to the deep system, and the deep veins within the musculature. One-way valves, which are present throughout the system, direct flow from the superficial to deep system via the perforators, then cephalad to the pelvic veins. The calf muscle group is invested in a tough fibrous fascia, preventing distension and providing support. During ambulation and muscle contraction, pressure increases in the deep venous system, forcing blood cephalad. Backflow and high pressures in the superficial system are prevented by valves in the perforators. During muscle relaxation, the cephalad blood is held in check by valves, deep venous pressure falls, and filling of the deep veins occurs from the muscular tributaries and the superficial system. The siphoning effect of the pump is extremely effective in draining the superficial system and skin, maintaining a low superficial venous pressure during exercise.

Obstruction or valve incompetence in the deep system and perforators prevents the fall in pressure normally seen with ambulation and exposes the venous system to hydrostatic pressures. This persistent venous hypertension leads to chronic venous changes and ulcerations. Previous deep thrombosis with valve damage, primary valve incompetence, obstruction, or pump failure secondary to neuropathies, arthropathies, or inflammatory diseases all may find a common endpoint leading to persistent venous hypertension.

Several theories exist on how venous hypertension leads to ulcerations. One idea is that venous hypertension is transmitted to the capillary system leading to microvascular distension, fluid migration, and widened endothelial pores. This allows leakage of macromolecules and fibrin into the interstitial space, where the fibrin forms pericapillary cuffs. The fibrin cuffs then become a barrier to oxygen and metabolites, leading to ulceration. Fibrin deposition has not been well documented in other causes of leg ulcers. Of interest, defects in fibrinolysis and decreased protein C levels have been documented in some patients with venous disease. Another theory proposes that leukocytes are attracted to pressure-altered endothelial cells and trigger the release of inflammatory mediators, leading to subsequent capillary damage, increased permeability, and fibrin accumulation. Again, diffusion barriers are created. A recently formulated hypothesis unrelated to barrier effects is the "trap" hypothesis, in which macromolecules and fibrin leak into the dermis because of pressure or inflammation. They then bind up essential growth factors, rendering them unavailable for routine tissue homeostasis and repair. Venous ulcers can be located anywhere on the distal third of the leg (Fig. 1). They are relatively shallow with granulation tissue and exudation. Pain is not a prominent symptom. The pulses are typically intact. Pigment changes are common with "cayenne pepper" purpura and hemosiderin deposition leading to a red–brown color. Edema is often a prominent sign but may be absent. Varices are commonly present. In long-standing cases, the dermis and panniculus become fibrotic and woody hard, a change known as lipodermatosclerosis. In severe cases, the fibrotic area on the distal third of the leg excludes edema, which persist cephalad, giving the leg an inverted "champagne bottle" appearance. Repeated episodes of cellulitis may damage lymphatics, producing a component of lymphedema.

Often, there is an associated dermatitis with erythema, scaling, pruritus, and excoriation. This may be a direct

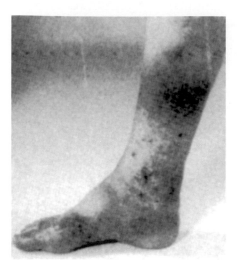

Figure 1   Venous ulcer.

consequence of venous disease or secondary to contact allergy. Common sensitizers include adhesives, neomycin, bacitracin, balsam of Peru, lanolins, benzocaine, parabens, and ethylenediamine.

The diagnosis of venous ulceration is usually made based on clinical impression supported by noninvasive vascular labs.

Ischemic Ulcers

Leg ulcers caused by arterial insufficiency may be associated with ischemic heart disease, cerebrovascular disease, diabetes mellitus, and hypertension. Atherosclerosis is the leading cause, usually occurring in patients who are 45 years of age or greater. In younger patients who smoke, thromboangiitis obliterans should be considered.

Ischemic ulcerations are usually painful and exhibit increased pain with elevation and exercise, while pain is relived with dependency and rest. Rest pain is a sign of more severe disease. These ulcerations usually appear sharply demarcated and occasionally punched out (Fig. 2). They are dry with a necrotic base and poor granulation response. Typically, they occur on distal points such as the toes or the distal foot and at sites of pressure or trauma such as bony prominences. The peripheral pulses are usually diminished, asymmetric, or absent. They are rarely normal. Capillary refill time is prolonged. Elevation of the leg leads to pallor, and subsequent leg lowering leads to a reactive hyperemia and erythema. Upon lowering, there will also be a delay

in venous filling beyond 15 to 20 seconds. This is valid only in the absence of venous incompetence, because if present, it would lead to erroneously normal findings.

The diagnosis can be confirmed with noninvasive vascular testing, and subsequent referral should be made to a vascular specialist to plan medical, interventional, or surgical management.

Neuropathic Ulcers

Sensory neuropathic ulcers arise from frequent trauma or persistent pressure leading to tissue ischemia, necrosis, and ulceration. Concurrent autonomic neuropathy may lead to the absence of vasodilator reflexes, which can contribute to ischemia. Traumatic tissue damage of this magnitude would not be tolerated in a sensate limb because of the pain. Diabetes mellitus is the most common cause, but neuropathic ulcers may be seen in leprosy, tabes dorsalis, traumatic neuropathy, or in children with inherited sensory neuropathies.

Neuropathic ulcers are usually located over points of pressure, especially on the plantar foot surfaces under the metatarsal heads or heel (Fig. 3). Footwear may also cause enough trauma for ulceration. Motor neuropathies may lead to altered weight bearing and gate, creating preferred areas of trauma. The ulcers are usually painless, with a necrotic or purulent base, and are surrounded by a rim of thick callus. Often, the extent of the ulcer is not appreciated upon surface inspection. Deep ulcers with extension to tendon or bone are common. Many of the ulcers will show signs of infection with surrounding erythema, cellulitis, or purulent drainage. Wounds that appear trivial at first inspection can rapidly expand and necrose secondary to infection. Baseline immune deficiencies in diabetes mellitus combined with ischemia and neglect often lead to gangrene and amputation.

Radiographic evaluation is required to evaluate osteomyelitis. Special studies such as plain films of the involved bones, nuclear medicine scans, computed tomography, and magnetic resonance imaging may help in distinguishing osteomyelitis from noninfected osteopathy in a diabetic foot.

Noninvasive vascular studies can identify underlying ischemia and diagnose major vessel obstructive disease that can benefit from revascularization procedures. In contrast, a subset of patients will not have ischemia, but only pure neuropathic ulcerations, and may heal with conservative measures.

Simple neurologic evaluation with soft touch and vibration testing will reveal sensory neuropathy. Special nylon filaments of a uniform diameter are available to aide clinical evaluation. Inability to sense 10 g of pressure (normal sensation senses 1–2 g) indicates a high risk of ulceration.

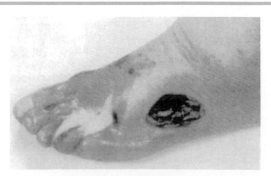

Figure 2   Ischemic ulcer.

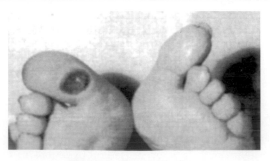

Figure 3   Neuropathic ulcer.

Autoimmune and Vasculitic Ulcerations

The incidence of leg ulcers attributed to autoimmune and vasculitic causes is around 7%. Many, but not all, of these ulcers will reveal vasculitis upon biopsy of skin at the lesion's edge. A finding of vasculitis directly under the ulcer base is nonspecific and can be seen with any ulceration. Excisional biopsy of suspected lesions, including panniculus, is important because it provides enough tissue that the pathologic architecture is preserved, it increases sampling of the process, and it provides information on the location and type of vessel involved in the process. Findings of vasculitis on biopsy may reflect a primary vasculitic syndrome or a vasculitis associated with infection, drug, autoimmune disease, or neoplasm. If vasculitis is noted on biopsy, then historical, physical, and laboratory evidence of other organ system involvement should be sought with attention to vasculitic syndromes and associated causes. Lower extremity pulses are usually intact if autoimmune disease or vasculitis is the only cause of the ulceration.

Leg ulcers may affect up to 10% of patients with rheumatoid arthritis. The etiology is multifactorial. Necrotizing vasculitis is seen in the majority of biopsies; however, other factors may contribute to poor healing and ulceration. These factors include corticosteroid therapy (which leads to thin, fragile, poorly healing skin), peripheral neuropathies (causing neuropathic ulcerations), arid venous insufficiency due to poor calf muscle pump function (resulting from neuropathy, deformity, and immobility). Rheumatoid ulcerations may have multiple appearances related to the underlying causes: ulcerative infarction and necrosis, deep punched-out dry ulcers of the feet, or shallow geographic exudative ulcers of the legs (Fig. 4).

Systemic lupus erythematosus can cause leg ulcerations, which are usually due to vascular occlusion associated with vasculitis or thrombosis. Patients with the lupus anticoagulant and antiphospholipid antibodies are at a greater risk of ulceration, and the ulcers are usually of the thrombotic

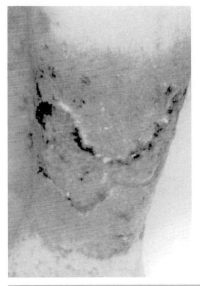

Figure 5 Lupus erythematosus ulcer.

occlusive nature. Vasculitic ulcers are usually seen in patients with active systemic disease (Fig. 5). Livedo reticularis, periungual erythema, a malar rash, oral ulcerations, and photosensitivity may be important differential clues. Systemic disease is often found with testing. Antiphospholipid antibodies may be seen primarily without evidence of systemic lupus erythematosus. These patients have a similar risk of ulceration. Ulcers related to antiphospholipids usually have a similar appearance to the ulceration of livedoid vasculitis.

Scleroderma may ulcerate, particularly long-standing severely involved lower limbs. Smaller ulcerations are common on the tips of involved digits. The etiology is multifactorial relating to functional (vasospasm) and structural (intimal proliferation and occlusion) vascular abnormalities supplying sclerotic and easily traumatized skin.

Livedoid vasculitis is a chronic relapsing segmental hyalinizing occlusive process of the dermal vessels accompanied by lymphocytic perivascular inflammation. Clinically, the ulcers are small, extremely painful, and have stellate or linear configurations associated with livedo reticularis of the involved limb. The ulcers often heal with

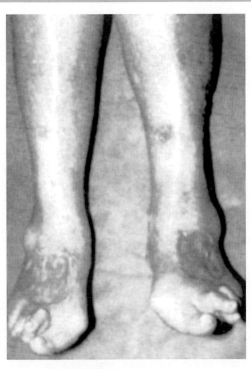

Figure 4 Rheumatoid vasculitis ulcer.

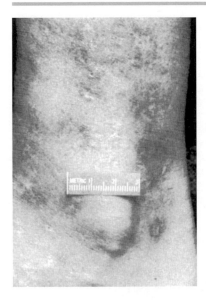

Figure 6 Livedoid vasculitis ulcers and atrophie blanche scarring.

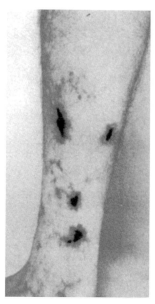

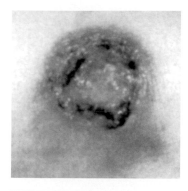

Figure 8 Pyoderma gangrenosum.

Figure 7 Polyarteritis nodosa ulcers.

the white scars of atrophie blanche (Fig. 6). The process is often idiopathic but has been associated with autoimmune disease such as systemic lupus erythematosus or antiphospholipid antibodies.

Necrotizing venulitis or leukocytoclastic vasculitis causes palpable purpuric lesions, vesicles, pustules, or necrotic papules. Occasionally, these lesions will progress to ulcerations. This vasculitis is usually a reactive process, but in the proper clinical setting may be a primary finding, as occurs, for example, in Henoch-Schönlein purpura. Inciting events include infection, autoimmune disease, drug reactions, cryoglobulinemia, malignancy, or systemic vasculitis.

Cutaneous polyarteritis nodosa and systemic polyarteritis nodosa can both cause leg ulcerations. In the cutaneous group, findings are limited to the skin and tend to have a chronic, recurrent course. Both diseases present with punched-out painful ulcerations on the legs associated with tender, erythematous, deep dermal, and subcutaneous nodules (Fig. 7). Often, there is a "star-burst" or linear irregular "lightning bolt" livedo pattern radiating from the ulcerated areas. Biopsy of a nodule (including panniculus) will often reveal necrotizing vasculitis of a small- to medium-sized artery at the dermal-pannicular junction.

Leg ulcer biopsies revealing vasculitis can be seen in Wegener's granulomatosis or Churg-Strauss vasculitis. Other common findings include erythematous papules and nodules. Systemic associations are necessary for diagnosis. In Wegener's granulomatosis, a necrotizing granulomatous vasculitis is noted in the upper respiratory tract and lung. Glomerulonephritis is seen in the kidney, and antineutrophil cytoplasmic antibodies are detected in the plasma. In Churg-Strauss granulomatosis, patients have a history of asthma, peripheral blood and tissue eosinophil, necrotizing granulomatous vasculitis (affecting the lung and other organs), and extravascular granulomas in the lung and the skin.

Miscellaneous Causes

Pyoderma gangrenosum is a well-recognized clinical entity. The lesions commonly begin as a purple nodule or pustule that rapidly spreads to produce necrosis and ulceration (Fig. 8). The border is characteristically undermined with a violaceous color and a surrounding erythematous halo. Central healing often leads to cribriform scarring. The lesions frequently begin at sites of minor trauma or after skin incision, ulcerating to a larger size than initially damaged. This process is known as pathergy. The most common systemic associations are inflammatory bowel disease and the presence of a monoclonal gammopathy. Biopsies are not specific and reveal neutrophilic central inflammation surrounded by intense perivascular lymphocytic inflammation at the periphery. The diagnosis is based on characteristic clinical findings and the exclusion of other causes by history, examination, vascular evaluation, biopsy, and cultures. Case reports exist where necrotizing fascitis has been mistaken for pyoderma gangrenosum, resulting in inappropriate steroid treatment with severe consequences.

Necrobiosis lipoidica diabeticorum may ulcerate. Diagnosis is established by the characteristic yellow-brown, atrophic, telangiectatic plaques on the pretibial leg in a patient who often has diabetes mellitus. Biopsy reveals palisading necrobiotic granulomas in the dermis.

Hematologic causes are an important consideration. The ulcers typically involve the ankle area and are often painful, shallow, and small. Upon biopsy, the majority of these processes reveal thrombotic occlusive phenomena. Red blood cell disorders such as sickle cell anemia, thalassemia, and polycythemia vera are common causes. Other disorders such as thrombocytosis and dysproteinemias (cryoglobulins, cryofibrinogenemia) may produce thrombotic or vasculitic ulcers. Fibrinolytic defects are a recently recognized cause of ulcers; they include protein C and S deficiencies and antithrombin III deficiency.

Emboli from atheroma, aneurysms, or endocarditis usually cause ulcerations in the distal extremities and the digits. There may be a preceding history of intravascular manipulations such as angiography. Initiation of coumadin therapy can sometimes cause showers of emboli from atheromatous plaques.

Infection is an important cause of leg ulcers, particularly in the immunocompromised patient. Causes that should be considered include deep fungal infections, tuberculosis, atypical mycobacteria, leprosy, syphilis, actinomycosis, septic emboli, and synergistic bacterial infections such as necrotizing fasciitis. Appropriate tissue must be submitted for culture and the biopsy examined with special stains.

Malignancy should be excluded with biopsy. Common malignant causes include squamous cell carcinoma (particularly in old burn scars and indolent ulcers of any cause), basal cell carcinoma, Kaposi's sarcoma, classic

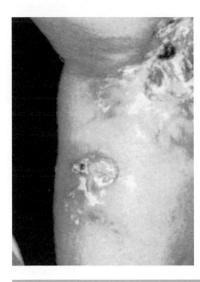

Figure 9 Angiocentric T-cell lymphoma ulcer.

cutaneous T-cell lymphoma (mycosis fungoides), and peripheral T-cell lymphomas (Fig. 9).

Several drugs may contribute to leg ulceration, including hydroxyurea, methotrexate, halogen ingestion, coumadin, infiltrated vasopressors, and intravenous or subcutaneous illicit drugs, particularly amphetamines.

Factitial ulcers are not a rare problem, and diagnosis can be difficult. The location, pattern, size, and shape of the ulcers can provide clues (Fig. 10). History of "physician shopping" or an indifferent attitude and obvious secondary gain may also help in diagnosis.

Panniculitis can ulcerate. The most likely causes of ulcerating panniculitis include pancreatic fat necrosis, α_1-antitrypsin deficiency, and lupus.

GENERAL TREATMENT MEASURES

Impairments to wound healing should be recognized and corrected. Nutritional deficiencies of protein, vitamin C, magnesium, iron, and zinc are important considerations. Glucocorticoids and cytotoxic agents will impair healing, although in autoimmune or malignant ulcers these agents can also promote healing.

If any evidence of active infection such as cellulitis, lymphangitis, leukocytosis, fever, or persistent drainage is encountered, then treatment with systemic antibiotics is

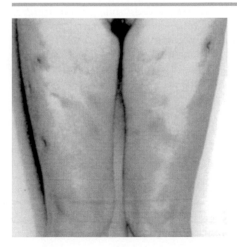

Figure 10 Factitial ulcers.

essential. This should be based upon culture and sensitivities. Empiric coverage of common skin organisms such as *Staphylococcus* and *Streptococcus* species should be started pending culture data. If deep or necrotic wounds are present, empiric coverage for anaerobic species should also be provided. *Candida* overgrowth under occlusive dressings or in topically treated wounds can be a cause of delayed wound healing. If cultures indicate *Candida* in high numbers, the addition of several days of topical antifungal therapy can be extremely helpful.

Treatment of dermatitis from venous disease or contact allergy will speed healing and decrease portals of entry for infection. A few days of topical steroids and nonirritating wet dressings (saline, water, or mild antiseptics such as aluminum subacetate or dilute acetic acid) will provide rapid control. The steroids may then be discontinued and the liberal use of lubricating creams begun as a protective measure.

Wound Care

Standard wound care consists of infection control, removal of necrotic debris (a sanctuary and media for bacteria and fungi), and provision of a moist wound environment promoting granulation tissue and epithelialization.

Mild antiseptic wet dressings are a historic and effective method of microbial control and gentle debridement. Wetting agents include aluminum subacetate and acetic acid. Povidone iodine inhibits wound healing in concentrations above 0.001% solution, as does Dakin's sodium hypochlorite solution above 0.005% solution and hexachlorophene at any concentration. Because of inhibition of wound healing, these last three should probably be avoided. All five of these compounds have shown in vitro fibroblast toxicity; therefore it seems prudent to use normal saline once debridement has been accomplished.

Wet-to-dry dressing changes can be very effective in debridement of necrotic wounds. The original moist wound surface dries as the wetting agent evaporates, binding wound exudate and debris to the gauze dressing material. When the dressing is removed, the necrotic debris is mechanically pulled away. Unfortunately, it may also pull away new epithelium and granulation tissue, so it should be stopped once debridement has been achieved. Newer occlusive dressings have the capacity to provide painless debridement by holding autolytic wound exudates against the ulcer bed. This process may lead to an erroneously perceived worsening and increase in size when actually it reflects loss of necrotic tissue.

Surgical debridement may be necessary for thick eschars, infectious ulcers, and deep ulcers extending to tendon and bone. Caution must be used to limit the debridement to devitalized tissues only, particularly in ischemic and neurotrophic ulcers. For superficial ulcers, topical 2% lidocaine gel followed by sharp curettage may be sufficient debridement.

Once granulation tissue is forming and the wound is clean, maintenance of a moist nontraumatic environment is desired for the fragile new tissues. This can be done with continuous wet dressings of saline or water, being careful not to macerate or overly dry the wound through evaporative losses. Gauze- and bandage-covered bland ointments and creams can be effective, including erythromycin ointment, silver sulfadiazine cream, or petrolatum-impregnated gauze. Harsh antiseptics and sensitizing chemicals are to be avoided. Care should be taken to remove cream buildup with occasional wet dressings or soaks. Occlusive dressings are helpful at this stage of healing as well.

Wound Dressings

There are a variety of new dressing materials available (see the chapter on wound dressings). In general, these dressings provide painless debridement, stimulate granulation tissue, encourage epithelialization, reduce wound pain, provide protection, and decrease dressing change needs. Initial concerns that increased bacterial counts in the trapped wound fluid would lead to greater incidence of infection have proved unfounded. Indeed, wounds treated with these dressings have a decreased infection rate. Infected draining wounds should not be occluded. Disadvantages are expense, availability, adhesives that rip away new epithelium if dressings are changed too frequently, malodorous leakage of wound fluid, and induction of an exudative wound phase in a previously dry wound. For chronic wounds, several types of occlusive dressings seem to have an advantage. The hydrocolloids are useful in all stages of wound healing because they have some ability to debride, absorb exudate, provide protection, and maintain moisture. These dressings are self-adhesive and may be used under compression therapy. Hydrogels will absorb and allow the passage of exudate to overlying gauze while maintaining a moist wound environment. They must be held in place with bandages. For exudative wounds the alginates have the unique ability to absorb abundant exudate into a gel-like matrix. These dressings promote exudative wounds into dry wounds, so it is recommended that a moisture-maintaining regime be used once the exudation ceases.

Skin Grafting

Any ulcer that is clean and granulating may benefit from skin grafting. Well-granulating but poorly epithelialized ulcers from venous insufficiency or previous occlusion therapy may show particular benefit. Often, the graft will stimulate epithelial healing even at sites not covered by the graft. This may relate to growth factor release or production of matrix materials for epithelial migration.

Given the compromised healing in chronic wounds, the most successful grafting methods have been pinch grafts and split-thickness skin grafts. Both of these grafts have fewer metabolic requirements than full-thickness grafts. Advantages of pinch grafts include the fact that they can be harvested in the office and will allow passage of wound exudate. Split-thickness grafts generally cover greater areas, leave better-appearing donor and recipient sites, and may heal faster. Fenestrations should be provided to allow passage of exudate. Meshing of split-thickness grafts offers wider coverage from a given size donor site and allows passage of exudate. Routine procedures for these grafting techniques should be followed (described elsewhere in this text). For small areas, all may be done in the office under local anesthesia.

Any large ulcer or ulcer with exposed bone and poorly vascularized deep structures, such as tendon, should have full-thickness skin and soft tissue coverage via flaps or free microvascular reconstructed flaps.

Systemic Agents

Systemic agents are sometimes used as primary or supportive treatment in leg ulcer management. Platelet-inhibiting drugs such as aspirin and dipyridamole have proven beneficial adjuncts to routine wound care. Processes where they are used include livedoid vasculitis, necrobiosis lipoidica diabeticorum, atheromatous and cholesterol emboli, and antiphospholipid antibody disease. Anticoagulation with heparin and coumadin has been useful in patients with livedoid vasculitis, coagulopathies, and antiphospholipid antibody disease.

Fibrinolytic agents such as phenformin and the anabolic steroid stanazolol are used to treat antiphospholipid antibody disease, livedoid vasculitis, and cryofibrinogenemia. Controversy remains whether stanazolol provides benefit in venous ulcerations. Low-dose tissue plasminogen activator has been successful in healing ulcerations of livedoid vasculitis and antiphospholipid antibody disease.

Ketanserin, a serotonergic blocker, has direct vasodilating effects and indirect effects via blocking serotonin-mediated platelet degranulation and the inflammatory and vasoconstricting sequelae. This also inhibits the serotonin-driven platelet degranulation-amplification loop. It has shown benefit in treating ischemic ulcers, venous ulcers, livedoid vasculitis and systemic scleroderma.

Pentoxifylline produces hemorrheologic effects by increasing red blood cell deformity, thereby allowing easier passage through the microvasculature and preventing sludging. Recent support on fibrinolytic effects, platelet aggregation effects, and changes in prostacyclin synthesis have been published. Studies support its use in a wide variety of ulcerations including ischemic ulcers, venous ulcers, necrobiosis lipoidica diabeticorum, sickle cell anemia, and thalassemia.

Corticosteroids and immunosuppressive agents are the mainstay of treatment for vasculitis, pyoderma gangrenosum, and autoimmune diseases. Antibiotics, antifungals, and antimycobacterials are essential in the treatment of infectious ulcerations.

TREATMENT OF SPECIFIC ULCERATIONS
Venous Ulcers

Specific measures to reduce ambulatory venous hypertension are essential in the treatment of venous ulcers. While hospitalization (for bed rest and wound care) has been a standard and effective treatment for venous and other ulcers, cost-control measures are quickly making this impossible. Benefits from an outpatient approach to ulcer management include less deconditioning and lower risks of falls, decreased risk of deep venous thrombosis, and patients who can remain active and at work.

One method to decrease venous hypertension is by using support hose that provide 30 to 40 mmHg of pressure. They should be put on first thing in morning and worn until retiring for the night, and in most cases they need to be worn indefinitely. Hose will lose elasticity over time and should be replaced on a regular basis. Routine wound care can usually be done with dressings underneath the stockings. Ischemic disease should always be sought and ruled out, because with any compression therapy, ischemia can be exacerbated.

Several problems make the use of compression hose difficult; for example, exudative wounds require frequent dressing changes, resolution of initial edema causes poor stocking fit, and mobility limitations make it hard to treat the disabled and elderly. One method that addresses some of these problems is the Unna boot. This impregnated bandage consists of a mixture of zinc oxide, calamine lotion, and glycerin. It is used to wrap the extremity from forefoot to knee, creating a semirigid cast that provides compression, occlusion, and protection. During the initial treatment of exudative or edematous wounds, the dressing must be changed every two to four days. After the edema and exudation resolve, the dressing can be changed every 7 to 10 days. Experience in application is required to provide adequate compression without inducing ischemia or creating pressure points. The Unna boot is particularly suited to disabled and noncompliant patients because the only requirements on the wearer are to come for office visits and keep the boot dry. Once the ulcer is healed, use of Unna boots or compression hose may continue. Continued boot use can provide prophylactic compression for patients unwilling or unable to use support hose. Problems with continued boot use include maceration and sensitization to the boot compounds. Intermittent pneumatic compression devices are helpful for rapidly reducing edema in a day or two, allowing support hose or Unna boots to be fit.

Elastic wraps are another compression method for treating venous ulcers, especially when they are exudative wounds, alternative limb shapes, changing states of limb edema, or in disabled patients. By nature they adapt to changing limb size and shape and are easily applied by health care providers. Some patients may also find them easier to use. They are inexpensive and can easily be replaced when soiled or when elasticity is lost. While wrapping a limb requires some degree of skill, it can usually be learned without difficulty. The wrap is started at the malleolar area for the first turn, then down over the ankle and forefoot. It is then reversed back up over the ankle to the knee. Wrapping direction should be from medial to lateral on the way up the leg. The overlap should be one-half to one-third of the width. Because the elastic recoil can be quite significant, care should be used not to wrap the limb too tightly. Underlying gauze pads can be used to absorb exudate and supply additional pressure over concave areas such as ulcers and the perimalleolar areas. Once healing occurs, the wraps may be continued or compression hose may be used.

The role of venous surgery in healing and preventing leg ulceration remains controversial. Procedure choices include sclerotherapy of superficial system and perforators, superficial system ligation, stripping with perforator ligation, bypass techniques, and deep venous valve reconstruction or brachial vein segment transplants. Proper patient selection appears to be important to outcome. In general, if deep venous system disease is present (as it is in the majority of the cases), then neither superficial nor perforator surgery is likely to help healing or prevent recurrence. Deep venous procedures combined with superficial procedures may play a role, but this remains to be proven conclusively. Isolated superficial system disease and ulceration will likely respond to surgical therapy, although this is a small portion of venous ulcer patients.

Arterial Disease

Simple measures can be done to benefit patients with ischemic ulcers. Smoking should be prohibited. Diabetes mellitus and hypertension should be controlled. The limbs should be protected from trauma (going barefoot, ill-fitting shoes) and protected from direct heat and cold environments. Surgical debridement should be undertaken cautiously. In general, despite theoretical advantages, vasodilator drugs such as calcium channel blockers have not been beneficial in ischemic ulcers. This may be due to a "shunting" effect into the muscle vasculature, resulting

from the muscle's ability to increase blood flow beyond that of damaged skin. Invasive interventions that are beneficial in selected patients include angioplasty, atherectomy, reconstruction, and bypass procedures.

Neuropathic Ulcerations

Prevention of trauma to the healing ulcer or surrounding tissues is the main therapeutic goal. Patients should inspect their feet daily for any evidence of trauma, fissuring, persistent erythema, or nonhealing wounds, no matter how minor. A similar examination should be done at each physician visit. Before dressing, shoes should be inspected by the patient to avoid walking on unnoticed foreign objects. Inspection may also reveal pressure points on the shoes. The shoes should fit, support, and distribute weight well. Consultation with orthopedics and podiatry can be extremely helpful in providing orthotics and special shoes for these patients. Tinea pedis should be sought and treated to decrease portals of entry for infection. Extreme care should be undertaken during nail trimming and corn or callus management. In many patients, this is best done by a physician or podiatrist. Patients must not go barefoot, wear pressure-inducing sandals or thongs, or apply heat or hot water to the feet. Bath water should always be tested before stepping into the tub. Patients should quit smoking and control their diabetes and hypertension.

Once ulceration develops, the severity of tissue destruction may not be apparent. It is important to inspect the wound for undermined areas that might extend to deep structures. Adequate debridement is important and should be done by a physician experienced in these wounds. Relief of pressure over the ulcer and nonweight bearing are essential until full healing has occurred. If this cannot be done adequately with crutches or a wheelchair, then total contact casting is recommended so that the patient can ambulate without placing pressure on the ulcer. Frequent inspections of the ulcer are needed to avoid overlooking complications.

Evaluation of infection is essential, and studies to rule out underlying osteomyelitis must be done. Treatment of ulcer-associated infection may require intravenous antibiotics, and six to eight weeks of antibiotics may be needed to eradicate osteomyelitis. Necrotic tissue, including bone, should be debrided. Antibiotic therapy should be guided by culture and sensitivity. Once healing occurs, preventive measures remain essential to prevent recurrence.

Autoimmune and Vasculitic Ulcers

Identification of the cause is the most important aspect in proper treatment of these ulcers. Once a diagnosis is reached, treatment of specific autoimmune or vasculitic disorders is the goal. General wound care measures are important. The main therapeutic agents for the vasculitic syndromes are systemic corticosteroids. Dosing depends upon the specific syndrome and response to therapy. Other useful agents include azathioprine and cyclophosphamide. The ulcers will often heal when the vasculitic syndrome is treated. In other cases, once the underlying process is controlled, the immunosuppressive medications may need tapering to a minimal beneficial level, so that wound healing may progress.

The treatment for autoimmune diseases is specific according to the disease process and ulcer cause. Vasculitic ulcers associated with rheumatoid arthritis usually require systemic corticosteroids. If associated with systemic vasculitis as well, cyclophosphamide or chlorambucil has been used. Vasculitis limited to the skin may respond to methotrexate or dapsone. Nonvasculitic rheumatoid leg ulcers may benefit from routine agents used in rheumatoid arthritis, including hydroxychloroquine, methotrexate, azathioprine, and penicillamine.

Systemic lupus erythematosus ulcerations are treated according to the cause. In cases revealing vasculitis, corticosteroids and immunosuppressants are used. If they are thrombotic in nature (usually associated with antiphospholipid antibodies), they are treated with antiplatelet agents, fibrinolytics, and anticoagulants (as in livedoid vasculitis).

Livedoid vasculitis has been treated successfully as a thrombotic occlusive disease without the need for immunosuppression. Methods that have been used include anticoagulation with heparin and coumadin, aspirin, low-dose tissue plasminogen activator, pentoxifylline, nicotinic acid, phenformin, and ketanserin.

Necrotizing venulitis (hypersensitivity vasculitis) is treated by removal of inciting agents and treatment of any stimulating disease processes. In idiopathic cases, dapsone and colchicine have been used.

Scleroderma ulcers have been treated with vasodilating agents such as nifedipine, nitrates, prazosin, hydralazine, and methyldopa. Other approaches have used antiplatelet therapy with aspirin, dipyridamole, and ketanserin. Pentoxifylline and immunosuppressives have also been reported as beneficial.

Miscellaneous Conditions

Pyoderma gangrenosum is generally treated with corticosteroids. For small superficial lesions, intralesional triamcinolone may be effective. For larger and multiple lesions, systemic prednisone is required. In refractory cases other agents are used, including rifampin, minocycline, dapsone, azathioprine, cyclosporin, and cyclophosphamide. Standard wound care measures support systemic therapy.

Necrobiosis lipoidica diabeticorum may respond to aspirin, dipyridamole, and pentoxifylline when combined with wound care.

Hemoglobinopathy-associated ulcers often respond to transfusion therapy, antiplatelet therapies, and pentoxifylline. Coagulation disorders and dysproteinemias may respond to antiplatelet therapies, anticoagulation, or fibrinolytics. Thrombocythemia-related ulcers often respond to therapy directed at lowering the platelet count.

Malignant lesions are treated according to type, location, extent, size, and distribution. Methods include local excision, Mohs micrographic surgery, amputation, radiation therapy, and systemic chemotherapy.

FUTURE DIRECTIONS IN LEG ULCER TREATMENT
Cultured Epidermal Grafting

Keratinocytes can now be propagated in tissue culture to produce sheets of cells. If grown on a collagen matrix, these sheets resemble normal epidermis. This allows coverage of large defects with minimal donor skin and has been used successfully in patients with widespread severe burns. These grafts are now being tested on chronic wounds including leg ulcers. Autografts are created from a sample of the patient's own skin. These grafts have been used on leg ulcers to speed healing of large or refractory ulcers. The main disadvantages are the patient-specific costs of individual preparation, time waiting for cultures to grow, and increased risks of fungal and bacterial contamination of the tissue culture due to harvesting from patients with colonized wounds.

Allografts provide improved efficiency through economies of time and scale, which has led to experiments using allograft keratinocyte cultures from unrelated donor. Neonatal foreskin cultures may have added benefits through increased response to growth factors and more rapid wound coverage. Allografts may also be frozen, allowing long-term storage and banking benefits as well as easing transportation pressures. Allografts have also been shown to speed healing in chronic leg ulcerations from a variety of causes. While originally thought to be immune tolerant (because no detectable signs of rejection were originally noted), this theory has been disproven using chromosomal analysis of wound-covering keratinocytes. It appears that the allografts serve as temporary dressings that stimulate wound healing and growth of host keratinocytes. No donor keratinocytes are noted in the wound after about day 14. One hypothesis to explain these findings is that the allograft provides growth factors or manufactures matrix protein structures that stimulate wound healing.

Growth Factors

The basic science literature on wound healing and growth factors has expanded exponentially over the last several years. Clinical applications of growth factor research are now being tested in a variety of settings. The most successful approach reported thus far utilizes an extract of autologous platelets isolated by apheresis. The platelets are then stimulated to release their storage granules, producing a variety of peptide growth factors including platelet-derived growth factor, transforming growth factors alpha and beta, and epidermal growth factor. This growth factor-rich extract is then applied to the wound surface, where it can speed healing of refractory leg ulcers from a variety of causes. This platelet-derived wound healing extract can also be prepared from donor platelets. Trials of individual and combined growth factor treatment in chronic wounds are currently underway.

Electrical Stimulation

Numerous human and animal studies have demonstrated that direct galvanic electrical stimulation can dramatically improve healing of skin wounds. The majority of the clinical studies have been in the treatment of pressure ulcers in bedridden patients or in patients with diabetic neuropathy. Even when compared to routine therapies, electrical stimulation showed improved healing. Several theoretical benefits exist which are supported by experimental data. They include attraction of macrophages, stimulation of fibroblast activity, induction of keratinocyte migration, bacteriostasis, improving edema, liquefaction of necrotic debris, expression of growth factor receptors, and stimulation of neurite growth and associated trophic factors. Devices manufactured for other uses are available, but none have Federal Drug Administration approval for use in wound healing.

Topical Hyperbaric Oxygen Therapy

Total body hyperbaric oxygen chambers have proven useful in the healing of chronic wounds. The main disadvantage has been oxygen toxicity affecting multiple organs. A simple method of local topical hyperbaric oxygen therapy has been described using routinely available oxygen delivery systems and disposable polyethylene bags. It has been used with success in the treatment of chronic wounds including leg ulcers secondary to venous disease, arterial disease, diabetes mellitus, vasculitis, and pyoderma gangrenosum.

BIBLIOGRAPHY

Alegre VA, Gastineau DA, Winkelmann RK. Skin lesions associated with circulating lupus anticoagulant. Br J Dermatol 1989; 120:419–429.

Angelides NS, Angastiniotis C, Pavlides N. Effect of pentoxifylline on treatment of lower limb ulcers in patients with thalassemia major. Angiology 1992; 43:549–554.

Bard JW, Winkelmann RK. Livedoid vasculitis: segmental hyalinizing vasculitis of the dermis. Arch Dermatol 1967; 96:489–499.

Bernstein EF. Vascular Diagnosis. 4th ed. St. Louis: Mosby, 1993.

Bennett NT, Schultz GS. Growth factors and wound healing: Part II. Role in normal and chronic wound healing. Am J Surg 1993; 166:74–81.

Beck SL, DeGuzman L, Lee WP, et al. One systemic administration of transforming growth factor-β1 reverses age- or glucocorticoid-impaired wound healing. J Clin Invest 1993; 92:2841–2849.

Bishop JB, Phillips LD, Musto TA, et al. A perspective randomized evaluator-blinded trial of 2 potential wound healing agents for the treatment of venous stasis ulcers. J Vasc Surg 1992; 16:251–257.

Blair SD, Wright DD, Blackhouse CM, et al. Sustained compression and healing of chronic venous ulcers. Br Med J 1988; 297:1159–1161.

Bockers M, Benes P, Bork K. Persistent skin ulcers, mutilations, and acro-osteolysis in hereditary sensory and autonomic neuropathy with phospholipid excretion. J Am Acad Dermatol 1989; 21:736–739.

Brown CD, Zitelli JA. A review of topical agents for wounds and methods of wounding: guidelines for wound management. J Dermatol Surg Oncol 1993; 19:732–737.

Brennan SS, Leper DJ. The effect of antiseptics on the healing wound: a study using the rabbit ear chamber. Br J Surg 1985; 72:780–782.

Brain A, Purkis P, Coates P, et al. Survival of cultured allogeneic keratinocytes transplanted to deep dermal bed assessed with probes specific for Y chromosome. Br Med J 1989; 298:917–919.

Brown GL, Naney LB, Griffin J, et al. Enhancement of healing by topical treatment with epidermal growth factor. N Engl J Med 1989; 321:76–79.

Burnand KG, Clemenson G, Morland M, et al. Venous lipodermatosclerosis: treatment by fibrinolytic enhancement and elastic compression. Br Med J 1980; 280:7–11.

Burnand KG, Whimster I, Naidoo A, et al. Pericapillary fibrin disposition in the ulcer-bearing skin of the lower limb: the cause of lipodermatosis sclerosis in venous ulceration. Br Med J 1982; 285:1071–1072.

Carley PJ, Wainapel SF. Electrotherapy for acceleration of wound healing: low intensity direct current. Arch Phys Med Rehabil 1985; 66:443–446.

Callen JP, Spencer LV, Bhatnagar Burruss J, Holtman J. Azathioprine. An effective corticosteroid sparing therapy for patients with recalcitrant cutaneous lupus erythematosus or with recalcitrant cutaneous leuko-cytoclastic vasculitis. Arch Dermatol 1991; 127:515–522.

Callen JP. Pyoderma gangrenosum and related disorders. Adv Dermatol 1989; 4:51–70.

Callen JP, Case JD, Sager D. Chlorambucil—an effective corticosteroid sparing therapy for pyoderma gangrenosum. J Am Acad Dermatol 1989; 21:514–519.

Cawley M. Vasculitis and ulceration in rheumatic diseases of the foot. Clin Rheumatol 1987; 1:315–333.

Chen WYJ, Lydon MJ. Identification of growth factor activities of wound fluid collected under hydrocolloid dressings. J Invest Dermatol 1990; 94:513.

Christensen JH, Freundlich M, Jacobsen BA, et al. Clinical relevance of pedal pulse palpation in patients suspected of peripheral arterial insufficiency. J Int Med 1989; 226:95–99.

Cikrit DF, Nichols WK, Silver D. Surgical management of refractory venous stasis ulceration. J Vasc Surg 1988; 7:473–477.

Comp PC, Esman CT. Recurrent venous thromboembolism in patients with partial deficiency of protein S. N Engl J Med 1984; 311:1526–1528.

Colgan MP, Dormandy JA, Jones PW, et al. Oxpentifylline treatment of venous ulcers of the leg. Br Med J 1990; 300:972–975.

Davis SC, Ovington LG. Electrical stimulation and ultrasound in wound healing. Derm Clin 1993; 11:775–782.

De Luca M, Albanese E, Cancedda R, et al. Treatment of leg ulcers with cryopreserved allogeneic cultured epithelium. Arch Dermatol 1992; 128:633–638.

Diaz-Perez JL, Winkelmann RK. Cutaneous periarteritis nodosa. Arch Dermatol 1974; 110:407–414.

Duncan HJ, Faris IB. Martorell's hypertensive ischemic leg ulcers are secondary to an increase in the local vascular resistance. J Vasc Surg 1985; 2:581–584.

Eaglstein WH. Occlusive dressings. J Dermatol Surg Oncol 1993; 19:716–722.

Ely H, Bard JW. Therapy of livedo vasculitis with pentoxifylline. Cutis 1988; 42:448–453.

Falanga V, Eaglstein WH. The "trap" hypothesis of venous ulceration. Lancet 1993; 341:1006–1008.

Falanga V, Kirsner RS, Eaglstein WH, et al. Stanozolol in the treatment of leg ulcers due to cryofibrinogenemia. Lancet 1991; 338:347–348.

Falanga V. Venous ulceration. J Dermatol Surg Oncol 1993; 19:764–771.

Falanga V. Growth factors in wound healing. J Dermatol Surg Oncol 1993; 19:711–715.

Falanga V, ed. Wound healing. J Dermatol Surg Oncol 1993; 19:677–812.

Falanga V, Moosa HH, Nemeth AJ, et al. Dermal pericapillary fibrin in venous disease and venous ulceration. Arch Dermatol 1987; 123:620–623.

Falanga V, Bontempo FA, Eaglstein WH. Protein C and protein S plasma levels in patients with lipodermatosclerosis and venous ulceration. Arch Dermatol 1990; 126:1195–1197.

Falanga V. Growth factors in chronic wounds: the need to understand the microenvironment. J Dermatol 1992; 19:667–672.

Fellner MJ, Ledesma GN. Leg ulcers secondary to drug reactions. Clin Dermatol 1990; 8:144–149.

Flynn MD, Tooke JE. Microcirculation in the diabetic foot. Vasc Med Rev 1990; 1:121–138.

Friedman SA. The diagnosis and medical management of vascular ulcers. Clin Dermatol 1990; 8:30–39.

Fredenberg MF, Malkinson FD. Sulphonamide on therapy in the treatment of leukocytoclastic vasculitis. J Am Acad Dermatol 1987; 17:355–359.

Gaylarde PM, Dodd HJ, Sarkany I. Venous leg ulcers and arthropathy. Br J Rheum 1990; 29:142–144.

Galinberti RL, Flores V, Gonzalez Ramos MC, et al. Cutaneous ulcers due to *Candida albicans* in an immunocompromised patient: response to therapy with itraconazole. Clin Exp Dermatol 1989; 14:295–297.

Gentzkow GD. Electrical stimulation to heal dermal wounds. J Dermatol Surg Oncol 1993; 19:753–758.

Geronemus RG, Mertz PM, Eaglstein W. Wound healing: the effects of topical antimicrobial agents. Arch Dermatol 1979; 115:1311–1314.

Geller JD, Peters MS, Su WPD. Cutaneous mucormycosis resembling superficial granulomatous pyoderma in an immunocompetent host. J Am Acad Dermatol 1993; 29:462–465.

Gilchrist T, Martin AM. Wound treatment with Sorbsan: an alginate fiber dressing. Biomaterials 1983; 4:317–320.

Gilliam JN, Herndon JH, Prystowski SD. Fibrinolytic therapy for vasculitis of atrophie blanche. Arch Dermatol 1974; 109:664–667.

Goslen JB. Autoimmune ulceration of the leg. Clin Dermatol 1990; 8:92–117.

Goodfield MJD. A relative thrombocytosis and elevated mean platelet volume are features of gravitational disease. Br J Dermatol 1986; 115:521–528.

Grattan CEH, Burton JL. Antiphospholipid syndrome and cutaneous vasoocclusive disorders. Semin Dermatol 1991; 10:152–159.

Gupta A, Ellis C, Nickoloff B, et al. Oral cyclosporine in the treatment of inflammatory and noninflammatory dermatoses. Arch Dermatol 1990; 126:339–350.

Harahap M, ed. Leg ulcers. Clin Dermatol 1990; 8:1–175.

Hansson C, Jekler J, Swanbeck G. *Candida albicans* infections in leg ulcers and surrounding skin after the use of ointment impregnated stockings. Acta Dermato-Vener 1985; 65:424–427.

Harahap M. Leg ulcers caused by bacterial infections. Clin Dermatol 1990; 8:49–64.

Harris IR, Bottomley W, Wood EJ, Cunliffe WJ. Use of autografts for the treatment of leg ulcers in elderly patients. Clin Exp Dermatol 1993; 18:417–420.

Heng MCY, Song MK, Heng MK. Healing of necrobiotic ulcers with antiplatelet therapy: correlation with plasma thromboxane levels. Int J Dermatol 1989; 28:195–197.

Helm KF, Su WPD, Muller SA, Kurtin PJ. Malignant lymphoma and leukemia with prominent ulceration: clinicopathologic correlation of 33 cases. J Am Acad Dermatol 1992; 27:553–559.

Herrick SE, Sloan P, McGurk M, et al. Sequential changes in histologic pattern and extracellular matrix deposition during the healing of chronic venous ulcers. Am J Pathol 1992; 141:1085–1095.

Hefton JM, Caldwell D, Biozes DG, et al. Grafting of skin ulcers with cultured autologous epidermal cells. J Am Acad Dermatol 1986; 14:399–405.

Heng MCY. Topical hyperbaric therapy for problem skin wounds. J Dermatol Surg Oncol 1993; 19:784–793.

Hopkins NFG, Spinks TJ, Rodes CG, et al. Positron emission tomography in venous ulceration and lipodermatosclerosis: study of regional tissue function. Br Med J 1983; 286:333–336.

Huntley AC. The cutaneous manifestations of diabetes mellitus. J Am Acad Dermatol 1982; 6:427–455.

Hutchinson JJ. Prevalence of wound infection under occlusive dressings, a collective survey of reported research. Wounds 1990; 1:123–133.

Janssen PAJ, Janssen H, Cauwenbergh G, et al. Use of topical ketanserin in the treatment of skin ulcers: a double-blind study. J Am Acad Dermatol 1989; 21:85–90.

Jarrett F. Leg ulcers of vascular etiology. Clin Dermatol 1990; 8:40–48.

Jemic GBE, Konradsen L. Pyoderma gangrenosum complicated by a necrotizing fasciitis. Cutis 1994; 53:139–141.

Johnson RB, Lazarus GS. Pulse therapy: therapeutic efficacy in the treatment of pyoderma gangrenosum. Arch Dermatol 1982; 118:76–84.

Joyce JW. Thromboangiitis obliterans (Buerger's disease). In: Young JR, Graor RA, Olin JW, Bartholomew JR, eds. Peripheral Vascular Diseases. St. Louis: Mosby, 1991:331–337.

Katz MH, Alvarez AH, Eaglstein WH, et al. Human wound fluid from acute wound stimulates cellular proliferation. J Invest Dermatol 1990; 94:541A.

Kerdel FA. Inflammatory ulcers. J Dermatol Surg Oncol 1993; 19:772–778.

Kirsner RS, Pardes JB, Eaglstein WH, et al. The clinical spectrum of lipodermatosclerosis. J Am Acad Dermatol 1993; 28:623–627.

Kirsner RS, Falanga V. Techniques of split-thickness skin grafting for lower extremity ulcerations. J Dermatol Surg Oncol 1993; 19:779–783.

Klein KL, Pittekow MR. Tissue plasminogen activator for treatment of livedoid vasculitis. Mayo Clin Proc 1992; 67:923–933.

Knighton DF, Ciresi K, Fiegel VD, et al. Stimulation of repair in chronic nonhealing cutaneous ulcers using platelet-derived wound-healing formula. Surg Gynecol Obstet 1990; 170:56–60.

Koshy M, Entsuah R, Koranda A, et al. Leg ulcers in patients with sickle cell disease. Blood 1989; 74:1403–1408.

Krajewski LP, Olin JW. Atherosclerosis of the aorta and lower extremity arteries. In: Young JR, Graor RA, Olin JW, Bartholomew JR, eds. Peripheral Vascular Diseases. St. Louis: Mosby, 1991:179–200.

Layton AM, Ibbotson SH, Davies JA, et al. Randomized trial of oral aspirin for chronic venous leg ulcers. Lancet 1994; 344:164–165.

Lawley TJ, Kubota Y. Vasculitis. Dermatol Clin 1990; 8:681–687.

Leoni A, Cetta G, Tenni R, et al. Prolidase deficiency in two siblings with chronic leg ulcerations. Clinical, biochemical, and morphologic aspects. Arch Dermatol 1987; 123:493–499.

Levin ME. Diabetic foot lesions. In: Young JR, Graor RA, Olin JW, Bartholomew JR, eds. Peripheral Vascular Diseases. St. Louis: Mosby, 1991:pp. 669–711.

Logerfo FW, Coffman JD. Vascular and micro vascular diseases of the foot in diabetes: implications for foot care. N Engl J Med 1984; 311:1615–1619.

Luetolf O, Bull RH, Bates DO, et al. Capillary under perfusion in chronic venous insufficiency: a cause for leg ulceration? \questBrJDermatol1993; 128 : 249–254.

Lundeberg TC, Eriksson SV, Malm M. Electrical nerve stimulation improves healing of diabetic ulcers. Ann Plast Surg 1992; 29:328–331.

Lydon MJ, Hutchinson JJ, Rippon M, et al. Dissolution of wound coagulum and promotion of granulation tissue under DuoDerm. Wounds 1990; 1:95–106.

Mani R, Gorman FW, White JE. Transcutaneous measurement of oxygen tension at edges of leg ulcers: preliminary communication. J R Soc Med 1986; 79:650–654.

McGoey JW. Metabolic causes of leg ulcers. Clin Dermatol 1990; 8:86–91.

Mertz PM, Eaglstein WH. The effect of semiocclusive dressing on the microbial population in superficial wounds. Arch Surg 1984; 119:287–289.

Mertz PM, Ovington LG. Wound healing microbiology. Derm Clin 1993; 11:739–748.

Miller OF. Essentials of pressure ulcer treatment: the diabetic experience. J Dermatol Surg Oncol 1993; 19:759–763.

Milligan A, Graham-Brown RA, Burns DA, et al. Prolidase deficiency: a case report and literature review. Br J Dermatol 1989; 121:405–409.

Nemeth AJ, ed. Wound healing. Dermatol Clin 1993; 11:629–809.

Nemeth AJ, Falanga V, Alstadt SP, Eaglstein WH. Ulcerated edematous limbs: effect of edema removal on transcutaneous oxygen measurements. J Am Acad Dermatol 1989; 20:191–197.

O'Donnell TF. Chronic venous insufficiency and varicose veins. In: Young JR, Graor RA, Olin JW, Bartholomew JR, eds. Peripheral Vascular Diseases. St. Louis: Mosby, 1991:443–480.

O'Donnell TF, MacKay WC, Shepherd AD, et al. Clinical, hemodynamic, and anatomic follow-up of direct venous reconstruction. Arch Surg 1987; 122:474–482.

Parish LC, Witkowski JA. Leg ulcers due to miscellaneous causes. Clin Dermatol 1990; 8:150–156.

Petry M. Antiphospholipid antibodies: lupus anticoagulant and anticardiolipin antibody. Curr Probl Dermatol 1992; 4:171–201.

Peters MS, Su WPD. Panniculitis. Dermatol Clin 1992; 10:37–57.

Phillips TJ, Bhawan J, Leigh IM, et al. Cultured epidermal allografts: a study of differentiation and allograft survival. J Am Acad Dermatol 1990; 23:189–198.

Phillips TJ, Dover JS, eds. Leg ulcers. J Am Acad Dermatol 1991; 25:965–987.

Phillips TJ. Cultured skin grafts: past, present, and future. Arch Dermatol 1988; 124:1035–1038.

Phillips TJ. Biologic skin substitutes. J Dermatol Surg Oncol 1993; 19:794–800.

Phillips TJ, Dover JS. Leg ulcers. J Am Acad Dermatol 1991; 25:965–987.

Phillips TJ, Kehinde O, Green H, et al. Treatment of skin ulcers with cultured epidermal allografts. J Am Acad Dermatol 1989; 21:191–199.

Pittelkow MR. Growth factors in cutaneous biology and disease. Adv Dermatol 1991; 7:55–81.

Piette WW. Hematologic associations of leg ulcers. Clin Dermatol 1990; 8:66–85.

Roenigk HH, Young JR. Leg ulcers. In: Young JR, Graor RA, Olin JW, Bartholomew JR, eds. Peripheral Vascular Diseases. St. Louis: Mosby, 1991:605–638.

Roenigk HH, Young JR. Leg ulcers. In: Young JR, Graor RA, Olin JW, Bartholomew JR, eds. Peripheral Vascular Diseases. St. Louis: Mosby, 1991:605–638.

Rothe M, Falanga V. Growth factors: their biology and promise in dermatologic diseases and tissue repair. Arch Dermatol 1989; 125:1390–1398.

Rustin MAJ, Bunker CB, Dowd PM. Chronic leg ulceration with livedoid vasculitis, and response to oral ketanserin. Br J Dermatol 1989; 120:101–105.

Sarkany I, Dodd HJ, Gaylarde PM. Surgical correction of venous incompetence restores normal skin blood flow and abolishes skin hypoxia during exercise. Arch Dermatol 1989; 125:223–226.

Sawada K, Segal AM, Malchesky PS, et al. Rapid improvement in patient with leukocytoclastic vasculitis with secondary mixed cryoglobulinemia treatment with cryofiltration. J Rheumatol 1991; 18:91–94.

Samlaska CP, Winfield EA. Pentoxifylline. J Am Acad Dermatol 1994; 30:603–621.

Schabauer AMA, Rooke TW. Cutaneous laser doppler flowmetry: applications and findings. Mayo Clin Proc 1994; 69:564–574.

Sehgal VN. Leg ulcers caused by deep mycotic infection. Clin Dermatol 1990; 8:157–165.

Sedgwick-O'Donnell SK, Kaplan RP. Primary and secondary skin cancers affecting the lower extremities: tumorous leg ulcers. Clin Dermatol 1990; 8:118–143.

Sehgal VN. Leg ulcers caused by yaws and endemic syphilis. Clin Dermatol 1990; 8:166–175.

Sporn MB, Roberts AB. A major advance in the use of growth factors to enhance wound healing (editorial). J Clin Invest 1993; 92:2565–2566.

Steed DL, Goslen JB, Holloway GA, et al. Randomized prospective double-blind trial in healing chronic diabetic foot ulcers. Diabetes Care 1992; 15:1598–1604.

Telfer NR, Moi RL. Drug and nutrient aspects of wound healing. Derm Clin 1993; 11:729–738.

Teepe RGC, Roseeuw DI, Hermans J, et al. Randomized trial comparing cryopreserved cultured epidermal allografts with hydrocolloid dressings in healing chronic venous ulcers. J Am Acad Dermatol 1993; 29:982–988.

Tuffanelli DL, Winkelmann RK. Systemic scleroderma: a clinical study of 727 cases. Arch Dermatol 1961; 84:359–371.

Wallace DJ, Dubois EL. Dubois-Lupus Erythematosus. 3rd ed. Philadelphia: Lea & Febiger, 1987.

Weiss DS, Kirsner R, Eaglstein WH. Electrical stimulation in wound healing. Arch Dermatol 1990; 126:222–225.

White RR, Lynch DJ, Verheyden CN, et al. Management of wounds in the diabetic foot. Surg Clin North Am 1984; 64:735–42.

Winter GD. Formation of scab and the rate of epithelialization of superficial wounds in the skin of the young domestic pig. Nature 1962; 193:293–294.

Wolfe JHN, Morland M, Browse NL. The fibrinolytic activity of varicose veins. Br J Surg 1979; 66:185–187.

Yamamoto M, Danno K, Shio H, Imanura S. Antithrombotic treatment in livedoid vasculitis. J Am Acad Dermatol 1988; 18:57–62.

48

Cure Rates for Cancer of the Skin: Basal Cell Carcinoma, Squamous Cell Carcinoma, Melanoma, and Soft Tissue Sarcoma

Clark C. Otley
Mayo Clinic, Rochester, Minnesota, U.S.A.

Katherine K. Lim
Mayo Clinic, Scottsdale, Arizona, U.S.A.

Randall K. Roenigk
Mayo Clinic, Rochester, Minnesota, U.S.A.

GENERAL CONSIDERATIONS

The goal of this chapter is to present an overview of the cure rates for local, regional, and distant metastatic involvement with malignant cutaneous neoplasms. Because the neoplasms discussed range from locally invasive basal cell carcinomas (BCCs) to highly lethal soft-tissue sarcomas, discussion will focus on either recurrence rates or survival rates, as indicated by the biologic tendencies of specific neoplasms. The quality of the literature with regard to consistency and depth is less than optimal in many areas, and attempts will be made to highlight controversial points. Finally, it is important to realize that the majority of therapies have not been subjected to head to head comparison, and the inevitable selection bias between study populations has a major impact on the cure rates cited. Therefore, direct comparisons of cure rates for different modalities should be viewed in the context of these inherent biases.

BASAL CELL CARCINOMA

BCC is a low-grade epithelial neoplasm, which grows in a contiguous manner with rare metastasis, making local control the primary therapeutic objective. Because of the locally invasive nature of BCC, cure rates are generally presented in terms of absence of local recurrence, rather than survival. Because BCC can recur five years or longer after treatment, the cure rates cited in this chapter are derived from those studies with follow-up of five years or greater. Cure rates will also be analyzed according to a variety of clinical and histologic variables, including location, size, histologic subtype, and patient characteristics. Discussion will focus on cure rates for primary BCC, with additional discussion of recurrent BCC.

Cure Rates: Summary for Primary BCC

Rowe et al. systematically reviewed the literature between 1947 and 1987 regarding recurrence rates after treatment of BCC. Recurrence rates based on studies with five-year follow-up were generally two to 3.5 times higher than in studies with less than five-year follow-up, emphasizing the inadequacy of studies with less than five-year follow-up. In fact, 18% of recurrences occurred between the fifth and 10th year after treatment. The authors conclude that recurrence rates should be standardized using five-year life-table analysis as outlined by Cutler, which compensates for patients lost to follow-up. The overall five-year cure rates according to Rowe's review divided by treatment modality is presented in Figure 1.

Thissen et al. systematically reviewed the studies between 1970 and 1997 that prospectively examined recurrence rates for at least 50 patients with primary BCCs observed for at least five years after treatment. Only 18 of the 298 studies found were large prospective studies of primary BCC with a follow-up of greater than five years. Due to different statistical methods for calculation of results, the authors were unable to determine overall mean recurrence rates. The strict recurrence rates (absolute number of patients with recurrence divided by number of patients) by modality are as follows: Mohs micrographic surgery, 1.1% cryosurgery, 4.3% immunotherapy (5-fluorouracil ointment), 21.4%. The cumulative five-year recurrence rates for the following treatment modalities are as follows: surgical excision, 5.3% curettage and electrodessication, 13.2% radiotherapy, 7.4%.

For curettage and electrodesiccation (C&E), overall recurrence rates as reported by Rowe et al. (7.7%) and Thissen et al. (13.2%) are relatively higher than that reported by Silverman et al. In Silverman et al.'s review of 2314 primary BCCs treated by C&E between 1955 and 1982, the overall five-year recurrence rate for low-risk sites (neck, trunk, extremities) was 3.3% as determined by the life-table method. According to this study, anatomic location and the size of the tumor are key determinants of recurrence.

For treatment of BCC with surgical excision, the relatively higher rate of recurrence of 10.1% reported by Rowe et al. as compared to the 5.3% cumulative five-year recurrence rate by Thissen et al. may be partially explained by a bias toward referral of more complicated tumors for excision as opposed to other non-Mohs modalities. Similarly, in Silverman's review of 588 primary BCCs treated with surgical excision between 1955 and 1982, the cumulative five-year recurrence rate was 4.8%. Statistically significant risk factors for recurrence included location on the head; the five-year recurrence rate for BCC on the head was 6.6% in contrast to 0.7% at all other sites. With regard

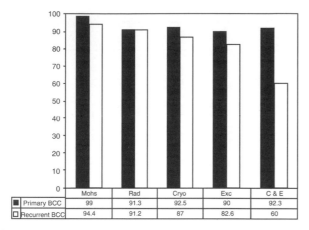

Figure 1 Five-year cure rates (in percentages) for primary and recurrent basal cell carcinoma by treatment modality: Mohs micrographic surgery (Mohs), radiation therapy (Rad); cryosurgery (Cryo), surgical excision (Exc) and curettage and electrodessication (C&E). *Source*: From Rowe, Carroll, Day (1989).

to the impact of surgical margins on recurrence rates for BCCs, Wolf and Zitelli's study demonstrated an inverse correlation between width of margins and rate of recurrence with BCC. A surgical margin of 4 mm resulted in the eradication of 98% of tumors less than 2 cm, whereas margins of 3 and 2 mm resulted in eradication of only 85% and 75% of tumors, respectively.

In regards to cryosurgery of BCC, the 7.5% recurrence rate cited by Rowe et al. was based on one retrospective study of 164 eyelid tumors by Fraunfelder et al. The 4.3% recurrence rate cited by Thissen et al. was based on four prospective studies, three involving tumors on the eyelid and one involving tumors >10 mm on the nose; however, 38% of the patients were lost to follow-up. In a retrospective review by Kuflik of 4406 new and recurrent BCC, squamous cell carcinoma (SCC), basosquamous carcinomas treated with cryotherapy between 1971 and 2001, the overall three-year cure rate was 98.6%; five-year cure rate in 415 BCCs treated between 1990 and 1996 was 99%. In an evidence-based review by Kokoszka and Scheinfeld of studies published between 1966 and 2001 revealed 13 noncontrolled prospective studies and four randomized clinical trials comparing cryosurgery to other treatment modalities. In the 13 noncontrolled studies, recurrence rates ranged from 0% to 8.2%, based mostly on clinical rather than histologic evaluation. Most studies included tumors less than 2 cm in size and those with superficial or nodular subtypes and follow-up times varied. A randomized, nonblinded clinical trial of 88 patients by Wang et al. revealed that the frequency of histologic recurrence of BCC after treatment with aminolevulinic acid photodynamic therapy (PDT) (25%) or cryosurgery (15%) was not statistically different. In a prospective randomized trial by Hall et al., histological recurrence rates were higher after treatment with cryosurgery (39%) versus radiotherapy (2%) group at one year. The combination of curettage and cryosurgery is associated with an excellent cure rate of 98% according to Nordin's study of 50 patients with non-morpheaform BCCs followed for at least five years. Cryosurgery is an effective therapeutic modality for the management of BCCs in a variety of

clinical settings, but does not permit histologic verification of tumor eradication.

Radiation therapy of BCC has a five-year recurrence rate of 7.4% based on the study by Silverman et al. in which 862 primary BCCs were treated with radiation between 1955 and 1982. Increased diameter of tumor correlated with increased recurrence, with 4.4% of BCCs 9 mm or less on the head recurring over five years in contrast to 9.5% of tumors 10 mm or greater. Cosmetic outcome was felt to diminish with time. A randomized study by Avril et al. showed statistically significant higher recurrence with radiotherapy as compared to surgical excision with frozen section examination.

Mohs micrographic surgery is associated with impressive cure rates of approximately 99% as reported by Rowe et al. and Miller et al. More recent European retrospective studies by Boztepe et al. and Smeets et al. show slightly higher recurrence rates of 3.3% and 3.2%, respectively. Treatment failures with Mohs micrographic surgery, which theoretically should have a 100% cure rate, have been traced to technical or interpretive difficulties or rare instances of discontiguous growth in studies by Hruza et al. and Madsen et al.

Clearly, the highest cure rate is obtained by Mohs micrographic surgery, which relies on immediate and complete histologic confirmation of tumor-free margins and the additional advantage of significant tissue conservation. It is the treatment of choice for many recurrent or large BCCs as well as those arising in high-risk sites, with ill-defined margins or with aggressive histologic subtype. However, for well-defined tumors with favorable histology in low-risk areas, the cost:benefit ratio may favor other modalities when applied to a large population.

Cure Rates: Summary for Recurrent BCC

Recurrent tumors are often embedded in a cicatricial stroma and have prolonged opportunity to infiltrate into deeper levels of dermis and subcutaneous tissue. It is intuitively obvious that recurrent tumors would be associated with higher rates of recurrence regardless of retreatment modality, a notion supported by the literature. Recurrent BCC treated with non-Mohs modalities is associated with an average 19.9% five-year recurrence rate, while the precision offered by Mohs micrographic surgery reduces this rate to 5.6%. By modality, five-year recurrence rates for recurrent BCC are 17.4% for surgical excision, 40.0% for curettage and electrodesiccation, 13% for cryotherapy, and 9.8% for radiation therapy, as demonstrated in Figure 1. Given the high rates of local recurrence when non-Mohs modalities are applied to recurrent BCCs, caution should be used when considering such therapy.

Cure Rates: Anatomic Location

An analysis by Roenigk et al. utilized odds ratios to demonstrate the increased risk of recurrence of BCC at certain anatomic units, such as the nose, ears, and periorbital region. Odd ratios of greater than 1.00 connote higher risk of recurrence for a particular site, and values less than 1.00 indicate a lower risk. BCCs of the nose are associated with a high risk of 2.38, while other sites such as the ears (1.43), periorbital region (1.17), and remaining face (1.04) have slight-to-moderate increased risk.

Managed by non-Mohs techniques, nasal BCCs have a 24% recurrence rate, compared with recurrence rates of 0.9%

to 2.6% for a combination of primary and recurrent BCCs treated with Mohs micrographic surgery in studies by Robins et al. and Mohs. Recurrence rates for primary BCCs of the periorbital area, inner canthus, retroauricular area, and scalp managed by Mohs micrographic surgery were 1.9%, 4.7%, 14%, and 1.3%, respectively, in the study by Robins et al. Recurrent BCCs of the periorbital area and inner canthus managed by Mohs micrographic surgery have 6.4% and 9.5% recurrence rates, respectively. Because of a higher propensity for perichondral spread, BCCs and SCCs of the ear have a 6.8% recurrence rate in the study by Robins et al.

Cure Rates: Histologic Subtype

BCCs with histologic evidence of infiltration, sclerosis, or multifocality are associated with increased rates of recurrence, estimated at 12% to 30%. In a histopathologic study of 156 BCCs by Sloane, infiltrative and multifocal types had recurrence rates of 20% to 30% as compared to 6% to 12% for nodular BCCs with or without infiltrative marginal features. A review of 51 recurrent BCCs by Lang and Maize revealed that 65% were characterized by poor palisading and a micronodular or infiltrative growth pattern. A multivariate analysis of prognostic histologic features for recurrent BCCs revealed that infiltrative, multicentric, or morpheaform growth patterns within 0.38 mm of the surgical margin were predictive of 82% probability of recurrence. Salasche et al. found that morpheaform BCCs had, on an average, 7.2 mm of subclinical extension beyond clinical borders. Roenigk et al. found statistically significant odds ratios for recurrence with multicentric and morpheaform BCCs of 5.80 and 3.62, respectively. The effect of histologic subtypes on recurrence rates makes pretherapy biopsy and knowledge of the prognostic significance of histologic features essential. BCCs evidencing aggressive histologic subtypes may best be managed with Mohs micrographic surgery.

Cure Rates for Alternative Therapeutic Modalities

A variety of nonsurgical, innovative modalities have been utilized in the treatment of BCCs. There are no studies in the literature citing recurrence rates for patients observed for over five years.

Brenner et al. demonstrated that twice-daily 0.05% tretinoin was ineffective in treating arsenic-induced BCCs. Treatment of BCC with isotretinoin and etretinate results in complete and partial remission rates of less than 20% and 70%, respectively, far inferior to conventional therapies.

Four randomized controlled trials of treatment of BCC with intralesional interferon are reported in the literature. Cornell et al. treated 172 patients with noduloulcerative or superficial BCCs with intralesional interferon alpha-2b (1.5 million IU three times weekly for three weeks) or placebo. Eighty-six percent of interferon-treated BCCs and 29% of placebo-treated BCCs were histologically negative after 16 to 20 weeks; after one year, 81% of the treatment group and 20% of the placebo group remained tumor free. Alpsoy et al. found 66.6% complete response after treatment with interferon alpha-2a as well as 66.6% complete response with interferon alpha-2b; combination of both did not significantly increase complete response (73.3%). Inferior cure rates, high cost, and need for repeated administration are distinct disadvantages.

Imiquimod is a promising new treatment modality. Seven randomized controlled trials have been reported, of which three addressed efficacy. The three trials by Beutner et al., Geisse et al., and Robinson et al. used similar regimens and confirmed reduction of early treatment failure of 5% imiquimod cream in treating superficial and nodular BCCs versus vehicle. Pooled data show that 120 of 168 (80%) patients treated with topical imiquimod versus 10 of 67 (15%) tumors treated with vehicle had clinical cure. Further longer-term studies are needed to address five-year cure rates.

PDT is a promising therapeutic modality in which a systemic or topical photosensitizer is preferentially absorbed by neoplastic cells with resultant selective killing of tumor cells after exposure to photons. Wilson et al. treated 37 patients with 151 tumors with intravenous Photofrin II and visible light with complete response in 88% of lesions but with an 18% recurrence rate. Retreatment of the recurrent BCCs resulted in 100% complete response, but with an eventual 26% recurrence rate. Introduction of 5-aminolevulinic acid (ALA), a potent topical photosensitizer, allows treatment without significant phototoxicity. In a review by Marmur et al. of all clinical trials of laser and PDT from the mid-1960s to the present, 10 clinical trials examining treatment of BCC with topical ALA-PDT were identified. There were varied treatment regimens, laser or light sources, study end points, and histologic subtypes, although most were superficial or nodular BCCs. The clearance rates ranged from 66% to 100% with mean duration of follow-up between 12 and 36 months. In a randomized controlled trial by Wang et al. for treatment of superficial and nodular BCCs, histologically verified recurrence rates at a year were comparable in the PDT group (25%) and cryotherapy group (15%). Rhodes et al. reported a multicenter randomized trial comparing topical methyl aminolevulinate-PDT with surgery in nodular BCC and found that complete response rates were similar at three months: 91% for PDT and 98% for surgery; however, at 24 months, there were five recurrences in the PDT group and only one in the surgery group. Studies with longer-term follow-up over five years are needed.

Another alternative modality, intralesional 5-fluorouracil implants, has been associated with 25% to 50% cure rates depending on the dosage. There are two randomized controlled trials of fluorouracil, one of which was an open-label randomized study by Miller et al. of 122 patients with six different treatment regimens and average early histologic treatment failure of 9%.

Locally advanced BCCs unsuitable for salvage therapy with either surgery or radiation therapy have been treated with cisplatin-based chemotherapy, with a durable (>5 years) complete response rate of 14% according to a study by Guthrie et al. Neoadjuvant, cisplatin-based chemotherapy has also been utilized with 12% complete and 62% partial response rates to shrink locally advanced BCCs in order to make definitive surgical resection or radiation therapy technically feasible. Systemic chemotherapy is best viewed as primarily a palliative modality in the management of advanced BCC.

Survival Rates for Metastatic BCC

Although very uncommon, metastasis from large, neglected, or highly aggressive BCC does occur. As reviewed by von Domarus and Stevens, 50% of patients with metastatic BCC are deceased within eight months after metastasis. Patients with isolated lymph node metastases survive for an average of 3.6 years, whereas prognosis after distant, visceral metastasis is extremely poor. Once distant spread occurs, response to chemotherapy with methotrexate, 5-fluorouracil, bleomycin, and cisplatin is marginal and survival rarely exceeds 1.5 years.

SQUAMOUS CELL CARCINOMA

SCC is the second most common skin cancer in the United States. The majority of SCCs are small, low-risk tumors associated with high cure rates with standard treatment modalities. Unlike BCC, SCC is associated with a measurable risk of nodal and disseminated metastasis and even death. Therefore, discussion will include cure rates not only for local SCC but also for regional and distant metastasis. Factors significant in the selection of treatment modality include tumor size, location, and histologic differentiation as well as patient characteristics.

Local Cure Rates of Cutaneous SCC

Local Cure Rates for Conventional Modalities

Conventional modalities for the treatment of primary cutaneous SCC include surgical excision, radiation therapy, curettage and electrodesiccation, cryosurgery, and Mohs microscopic surgery. In a systematic review of the literature between 1947 and 1987 on recurrence rates for SCC of the lip, ear, and skin, Rowe et al. found that Mohs microscopic surgery provided the highest cure rates for primary tumors in all locations. As shown in Figure 2, management of SCC of skin other than lip or ear by Mohs micrographic surgery affords a five-year local cure rate of 96.9% versus 92.1% for non-Mohs modalities. Similarly, primary SCC of the lip and ear had higher local cure rates with Mohs micrographic surgery than non-Mohs modalities as seen in Figure 3. With regard to local cure rates of specific non-Mohs modalities, Rowe et al. cite five-year cure rates of 90.0%, 91.9%, 96.3%, and 96.8% for primary SCC treated with radiation therapy, surgical excision, C&E, and cryosurgery, respectively (Fig. 2). It is important to note, however, that the majority of tumors treated by C&E and cryosurgery were smaller than 1 cm and that the follow-up for cryosurgery was less then five years. An earlier study of cryosurgery of SCC less then 2 cm by Kuflik et al. reported a five-year local cure rate of 96.1%. In a later study, Kuflik did not note any recurrences in a retrospective review of 132 SCCs treated with cryosurgery between 1990 and 1996. As noted in the introduction, the presence of selection bias between studies of different treatment modalities is inevitable, rendering direct comparison of cure rates imprecise. In general, high-risk tumors are more frequently managed by Mohs

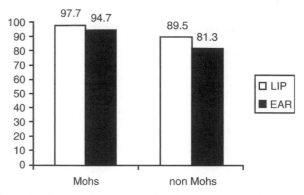

Figure 3 Cure rates by percentage for primary squamous cell carcinoma by anatomic site and treatment modality. *Source*: From Rowe, Carroll, Day (1992).

micrographic surgery then by non-Mohs modalities, resulting in lower cure rates for Mohs micrographic surgery than might occur with a random selection of tumors.

Recurrent SCC is associated with an increased risk of recurrence and metastasis regardless of treatment modality. As with primary SCC, Mohs micrographic surgery is associated with superior five-year local cure rates of 90% to 93.3% in studies by Rowe et al. and Dzubow et al. as shown in Figure 4. Recurrence rates were higher with tumors on the lower extremities, in male patients younger then 60 years of age, and in male patients requiring five or more Mohs stages. A study of Mohs micrographic surgery for recurrent SCC by Hruza with four-year follow-up had a 98.6% local cure rate. Surgical excision was associated with recurrence rates of 23.3% for recurrent SCC in the study by Rowe et al.

Clinical Predictors of Local Recurrence and Metastasis

Because SCC has a definite potential for metastasis and death, factors predictive of increased risk of dissemination have been extensively investigated. Clinical features predictive of increased metastatic risk include size greater than 2 cm, history of recurrence, high-risk location (ear, lip), rapid growth, association with a pre-existing scarring process (burn, ulcer, scar), and immunosuppression of the patient. Figure 5 presents the prognostic significance of various factors in local recurrence and metastasis of SCC based on

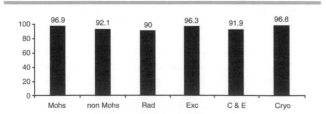

Figure 2 Cure rates by percentage for primary squamous cell carcinoma by treatment modality: Mohs micrographic surgery (Mohs), non-Mohs modalities (non-Mohs), radiation therapy (Rad), surgical excision (Exc), curettage and electrodessication (C&E), cryotherapy (Cryo). *Source*: From Rowe, Carroll, Day (1992).

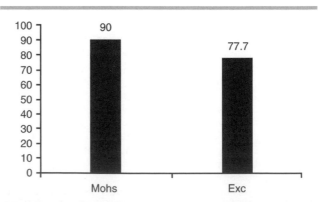

Figure 4 Cure rates by percentage for locally recurrent squamous cell carcinoma by treatment modality: Mohs micrographic surgery (Mohs) versus surgical excision (Exc). *Source*: From Rowe, Carroll, Day (1992).

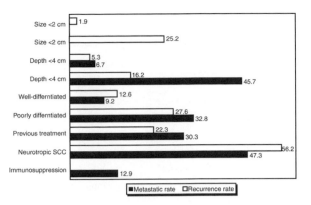

Figure 5 Influence of prognostic variables on recurrence and metastatic rates as percentage of cases. *Source*: From Rowe, Carroll, Day (1992).

more than 30 studies summarized by Rowe et al. For SCCs greater than 2 cm, the local recurrence rates are more than double and metastatic rates triple those of SCCs less than 2 cm. A study of Breuninger et al. found rates of metastasis of 1.4%, 9.2%, and 14.3% for 500 primary cutaneous SCCs of less than 2, 2 to 5, and greater than 5 cm, respectively. Five-year local cure rates after Mohs micrographic surgery are 98.1% for tumors less than 2 cm versus 74.8% for SCCs greater than 2 cm.

As mentioned before, recurrent SCCs have high local recurrence rates of 23.3% and metastatic rates of 30.3% with excision and a 10% local recurrence rate with Mohs micrographic surgery according to Rowe et al. Recurrent SCCs of the lip and ear are associated with high metastatic rates of 31.5% and 45%, respectively, according to Salasche et al. SCCs arising in association with a chronic ulcer or sinus tract have an 18% to 30% metastatic rate, while those arising in radiation dermatitis or scar have 20% to 26% and 26.2% to 37.9% metastatic rates, respectively. A report of SCCs in immunosuppressed patients noted a 12.9% metastatic rate.

SCCs in particular anatomic locations, especially ear and lip, have an increased risk of recurrence and distance metastasis. According to Rowe et al., SCC of the lip has local recurrence and metastatic rates of 10.5% and 13.7%, respectively, compared to 7.9% and 5.2%, respectively, for tumors at other sites. The relatively high recurrence rates may be related to horizontal spread of SCC on the mucosa not adequately treated by wedge excision, as suggested by Mehregan and Roenigk. SCC of the ear has more than double the rate of local recurrence and metastasis at 18.7% and 11%, respectively, compared with other sites. Mohs et al. reported a five-year local cure rate of 92.3% for SCC of the ear managed by Mohs micrographic surgery. Experience at the Mayo Clinic as studied by Holmkvist and Roenigk revealed a 92% cure rate with a mean follow-up at five years for auricular SCCs in 50 patients.

Mohs and Zitelli reported a five-year local cure rate of 98.8% for SCC of the scalp treated by Mohs micrographic surgery. However, because of unpredictable peripheral tumor extension with SCC on the scalp, modalities lacking in histologic confirmation of tumor-free margins suffer from inferior cure rates, with a 66% five-year local cure rate for radiation therapy. In a review of SCC of the trunk and limbs, Joseph et al. reported a 4.9% metastatic rate, a 3.4% overall mortality rate, and a 70.6% mortality rate among patients

with metastatic disease. Risk factors associated with metastasis include delayed presentation, large neglected tumors, misdiagnosis, and recurrence.

Histologic Predictors of Local Recurrence and Metastasis

Histologic features correlating with worse prognosis include depth greater than 4 mm, poor histologic differentiation, and neurotropism. Several studies have suggested that risk of recurrence and metastasis increases with invasion of SCC into or through the reticular dermis (Clark level IV/V). Rowe et al. found that SCCs less than 4 mm in depth have rates of local recurrence and metastasis of 5.3% and 6.7%, respectively, whereas tumors 4 mm or greater carry rates of 17.2% and 45.7%, respectively. Seemingly more reasonable estimates were derived from a study by Breuninger in which 0%, 4.5%, and 15% rates of metastasis were found with SCCs less than 2, 2 to 6, and greater than 6 mm in depth, respectively.

Poorly differentiated (Broders grades 3 and 4) SCCs are twice as likely to recur locally (28.6% vs. 13.6%) and three times more likely to metastasize (32.8% vs. 9.2%) than well-differentiated SCCs according to Rowe et al. Mohs micrographic surgery offers significant advantages when managing both well and poorly differentiated SCCs. Well-differentiated SCCs treated with non-Mohs modalities or Mohs micrographic surgery have local cure rates of 81.0% and 97.0%, respectively, while poorly differentiated SCCs have local cure rates of 46.4% and 67.4%, respectively.

The presence of tumor within the perineural space, known as neurotropism, has been associated with a poor prognosis in several studies. SCCs with histologic evidence of perineural invasion managed with excision have local recurrence and metastasis rates of 47.2% and 47.3%, respectively, according to Rowe et al. Mohs micrographic surgery offers improved outcome for neurotropic SCC compared with local recurrence and metastatic rates of 0% and 8.3%, respectively. Lawrence and Cottel reported a survival probability of 88.7% for SCC with perineural invasion managed with Mohs micrographic surgery. Adjuvant radiation therapy has been employed in the management of neurotropic SCCs with 100% and 50% local cure rates for primary and recurrent tumors, respectively, as reported by Barrett et al.

A retrospective analysis by Cherpelis et al. comparing characteristics of patients with metastatic SCC and those with nonmetastatic SCC showed that size, Clark's level, degree of differentiation, the presence of small tumor nests, infiltrative tumor strands, single-cell infiltration, perineural invasion, acantholysis, and recurrence all correlated strongly with metastasis, whereas location, ulceration, inflammation, and Breslow depth did not. On the other hand, Griffiths et al. found that the tumor diameter and tumor thickness were significant for metastatic disease, whereas there were no significant differences with regard to deep resection margin clearance, lateral epidermal resection margin clearance, lymphocyte response, or degree of tumor differentiation. Retrospective analysis and small numbers of patients may contribute to differences in statistical analysis, and thus large prospective studies are most ideal in determining significant factors.

Local Cure Rates with Alternative Modalities

PDT has been investigated as an alternative therapeutic modality and there are six published clinical trials utilizing ALA. Cairnduff et al. conducted a phase I trial of PDT with 20% topical ALA (ALA-PDT) irradiated with 630 nm light from copper vapor/dye laser in the treatment of Bowen's disease; there was a 97% complete response rate at two months, falling to 89% at a median of 18 months follow-up. On the other hand, Fink-Puches et al. retrospectively reviewed the effects of ALA-PDT plus UVA or differing wavelengths of visible light on superficial SCC and found that the disease-free rate was only 8% at 36 months. Morton et al. conducted three clinical studies on the use of ALA-PDT in Bowen's disease with the following conclusions: PDT using a nonlaser light source at 630 nm appeared to be as effective as cryotherapy, ALA-PDT utilizing red (630 nm) versus green (540 nm) light had superior results (88% vs. 48%, respectively); ALA-PDT for treatment of large and multiple lesions resulted in clearance rates of 79% and 89% and could be considered for these indications. Varma et al. utilized a different light source, an incoherent lamp with diameter of 15 cm and found a clearance rate of 69% at 12 months. ALA-PDT can be considered a therapeutic option in select cases of SCC in situ and superficial SCCs in the appropriate clinical setting, but response rates will understandably vary due to differences in lesion size and light sources.

Interferon has been utilized in the treatment of cutaneous SCC as well as BCC. Edwards et al. treated 36 SCCs ranging from 0.5 to 2.0 cm with 1.5 million units of intralesional interferon alpha-2a three times weekly for 3 weeks with an 88.2% complete response, histologically confirmed. Combination subcutaneous interferon alpha-2a with oral isotretinoin has been utilized in a study by Lippman et al. in 28 patients with inoperable SCC, with 25% complete remission and 43% partial remission. The use of topical imiquimod has been shown to be effective for SCC in situ or Bowen's disease in several case reports, but further clinical trials are needed to establish long-term cure rates. As with BCC, treatment of SCC with isotretinoin or etretinate alone has been disappointing, with three of 13 patients experiencing complete remission in one study.

As with BCC, cisplatin-based chemotherapy has resulted in 40% complete response rates in patients with locally advanced SCC unsuitable for salvage therapy with either surgery or radiation according to a study by Guthrie et al. When used neoadjuvantly to shrink SCCs to allow for easier surgical or radiation therapy, cisplatin-based chemotherapy has resulted in 25% complete and 25% to 50% partial response rates in the studies of Guthrie et al. and Sadek et al. Systemic chemotherapy may have a palliative or neoadjuvant role in the management of advanced SCC.

Survival Rates: Regional Lymph Node Metastasis

Salasche et al. estimated that 2% to 6% of actinically derived SCCs would metastasize to regional lymph nodes, contrary to earlier estimates of 0.5%. Once histologically confirmed lymph nodes metastases are present, therapeutic options include lymphadenectomy, radiation therapy, or combination therapy. Overall, survival rates after lymph node metastasis are poor, with 34.4% of patients alive after five years. Therapeutic lymphadenectomy results in five-year survival rates of 26.8% and 47.5% for SCC of the ear, and lip, respectively, according to Rowe et al. Radiation therapy is associated with five-year survival rates of 28.6% and 26.5% for ear and lip SCCs metastatic to regional nodes, respectively. Combination therapy with lymphadenectomy and radiation therapy results in improved five-year survival rates of 45.5% and 58.6% for ear and lip SCCs with nodal metastases, respectively, as shown in Figure 6. To date, systemic chemotherapy has not been shown to improve survival

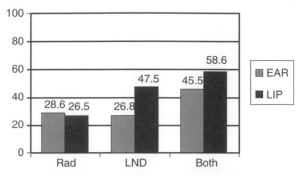

Figure 6 Cure rates by percentage for squamous cell carcinoma with clinical lymph nodes by anatomic location and treatment—postoperative radiation (Rad), lymph node dissection (LND) or both. *Source*: From Rowe, Carroll, Day (1992).

significantly beyond that achieved with surgery and radiation in patients with metastatic nodal involvement of the neck.

Since the prognosis is poor, before clinically detectable nodal metastasis develop, some advocate the use of sentinel lymph node biopsy in patients with high-risk SCC. Sentinel lymphadenectomy has been shown to be technically feasible for cutaneous SCC, even in conjunction with Mohs micrographic surgery. Sentinel lymph node biopsy has not yet been proven to influence survival.

Survival Rates: Distant Metastasis

Fifteen percent to 20% of metastatic SCC will bypass the regional lymph nodes and directly affect other organs according to Salasche et al. Additionally, patients with regional nodal metastases in whom the SCC is not cured by therapeutic lymphadenectomy may develop distant metastases. Once extranodal SCC is present, prognosis is grim. However, unlike melanoma, there are few data regarding survival rates once SCC is distantly disseminated.

SURVIVAL RATES FOR MELANOMA

Unlike BCC, in which cure rates are defined in terms of local recurrence, cure with a potentially lethal melanoma is best defined by prolonged disease-free survival. Sophisticated prognostic models based on well-defined clinical and histologic variables have been developed for melanoma. Thus, discussion of cure rates for melanoma centers on the predictive value of various prognostic factors for survival. The utility of carefully defining prognostic factors in melanoma relates to the potential to target aggressive surgical or systemic, adjuvant or neoadjuvant therapy to those patients at highest risk of metastasis. The most recent updated American Joint Committee on Cancer (AJCC) staging system was issued in 2002 (Tables 1 and 2). Table 3 outlines specific one-, two-, five-, and 10-year survival rates for each stage of melanoma. These data are highly specific and can be relied on for accurate prognostic information for melanoma. Figures 7–9 demonstrate the survival curves for stage I to IV melanoma. Survival rates in these tables are calculated with the exclusion of level I, in situ melanoma, which are considered to have no metastatic potential.

Historical Considerations

Advances in the early diagnosis of melanoma, independent of changes in therapeutic modalities, have had a major

Table 1 Melanoma TNM Classification

T classification	Thickness	Ulceration status
T1	1.0 mm	(a) Without ulceration and level II/III
		(b) With ulceration or level IV/V
T2	1.01–2.0 mm	(a) Without ulceration
		(b) With ulceration
T3	2.01–4.0 mm	(a) Without ulceration
		(b) With ulceration
T4	>4.0 mm	(a) Without ulceration
		(b) With ulceration
N classification	No. of metastatic nodes	Nodal metastatic mass
N1	1 node	(a) Micrometastasis
		(b) Macrometastasis
N2	2–3 nodes	(a) Micrometastasis
		(b) Macrometastasis
		(c) Macrometastasis
N3	4 or more metastatic nodes, or matted nodes, or in transit met(s)/satellite(s) with metastatic node(s)	
M classification	Site	Serum lactate dehydrogenase
M1a	Distant skin, subcutaneous, or nodal mets	Normal
M1b	Lung metastases	Normal
M1c	All other visceral metastases	Normal
	Any distant metastasis	Elevated

Micrometastases are diagnosed after sentinel or elective lymphadenectomy. Macrometastases are defined as clinically detectable nodal metastases confirmed by therapeutic lymphadenectomy or when nodal metastasis exhibits gross extracapsular extension.
Source: From Balch, Buzaid, Soong (2001).

impact on the cure rate for melanoma over the past few decades. As awareness of melanoma increases between both the public and the medical professionals, there has been a trend toward clinical presentation with lower stage, less ulceration, and decreased thickness and level as outlined by Little et al. As a result of earlier diagnosis, cumulative five-year survival rates for stage I and II malignant melanoma exclusive of in situ disease improved from 78% to 86% between 1970 and 1980 in a series from the Sydney Melanoma Unit, likely independent of any therapeutic innovations. For this reason, comparison of new survival data with historical controls not stratified by other variables is inappropriate.

Breslow Thickness

In the absence of pathologic data from lymph node dissection, the most reliable predictor of survival in melanoma is the measured histologic thickness of the tumor from the top of the granular cell layer to the deepest malignant cell, known as the Breslow thickness. As shown in Table 3, increased thickness correlates with worsening prognosis. Five-year survival data for stage I and II (localized) melanoma stratified by thickness are presented in Table 3. It is important to note that of patients with melanomas 4 mm thick or greater approximately 30% survive long term. Predictions of inevitable metastasis in patients with thick melanomas should thus be avoided. When compared with other non-nodal prognostic factors in melanoma, Breslow thickness is the most sensitive, with most other factors deriving significance from their secondary relation to thickness.

Clark's Level

As melanoma cells penetrate to deeper levels in the skin, known as Clark's levels, survival decreases according to univariate analysis. However, when level is compared to thickness as a prognostic indicator, Breslow thickness is a more accurate predictor of metastasis and survival as demonstrated in the studies of Balch et al. and Day et al.,

among others. Thus, a 0.6 mm, level IV tumor extending into the midreticular dermis is associated with a favorable prognosis, while a 4 mm level IV melanoma carries a poor prognosis. In the majority of cases, increased thickness correlates with deeper levels, resulting in fair correlation between the two prognostic indicators. However, when thickness and level are discordant, prognosis is more accurately predicted by measurement of thickness. The prognostic significance of Clark's level may be greater for melanomas arising from regions with thin skin, such as eyelid or ear. The new AJCC staging system for melanoma upstages patients with melanoma greater than or equal to 1 mm thick with level IV and V to the same extent as ulceration upstages to a worse prognosis.

Additional Histologic Factors

Ulceration has been shown to be an additional adverse prognostic feature, independent of Breslow thickness. For this reason, the presence of histologic ulceration upstages patients in the new AJCC staging system. Nodular and acral lentiginous melanomas tend to be thicker at presentation and are thus associated with a worse prognosis. However, when a tumor thickness is controlled for, nodular and superficial spreading melanomas have similar 10-year survival rates. Lentigo maligna melanoma may be associated with a slightly better 10-year survival rate and acral lentiginous melanoma with a slightly worse survival rate than either superficial spreading or nodular melanoma, even after controlling for thickness according to McGovern et al.

Gender and Anatomic Location

Although melanoma in women is associated with a more favorable prognosis than in men, the survival difference is due to the decreased thickness of melanoma at presentation in women. Melanoma of the scalp is associated with a worse prognosis than other sites on the head.

Table 2 Stage Groupings for Cutaneous Melanoma

Clinical staging				Pathologic staging		
	T	N	M	T	N	M
0	Tis	N0	M0	Tis	N0	M0
IA	T1a	N0	M0	T1a	N0	M0
IB	T1b	N0	M0	T1b	N0	M0
	T2a	N0	M0	T2a	N0	M0
IIA	T2b	N0	M0	T2b	N0	M0
	T3a	N0	M0	T3a	N0	M0
IIB	T3b	N0	M0	T3b	N0	M0
	T4a	N0	M0	T4a	N0	M0
IIC	T4b	N0	M0	T4b	N0	M0
III	Any T	N1	M0			
		N2				
		N3				
IIIA				T1-4a	N1a	M0
				T1-4a	N2a	M0
IIIB				T1-4b	N1a	M0
				T1-4b	N2a	M0
				T1-4a	N1b	M0
				T1-4a	N2b	M0
				T1-4a/b	N2c	M0
IIIC				T1-4b	N1b	M0
				T1-4b	N2b	M0
				Any T	N3	M0
IV	Any T	Any N	Any M1	Any T	Any N	Any M1

Clinical staging includes microstaging of the primary melanoma and clinical/radiologic evaluation for metastases. By convention, it should be used after complete excision of the primary melanoma with clinical assessment for regional and distant metastases. Pathologic staging includes microstaging of the primary melanoma and pathologic information about the regional lymph nodes after partial or complete lymphadenectomy. Pathologic stage 0 or stage 1A patients are the exception; they do not require pathologic evaluation of their lymph nodes. There are no stages in subgroups for clinical staging.
Source: From Balch, Buzaid, Soong (2001).

Sentinel Lymph Node Status

With the advent of sentinel lymph node biopsy in the management of melanoma, Breslow thickness has been supplanted as the most accurate prognostic factor. Given the value of prognostic information for triaging patients to clinical trials in melanoma, many centers are offering sentinel lymph node biopsy for melanoma with a Breslow thickness of 1 mm or greater, or for tumors less than 1 mm, but with histologic ulceration or Clark's level IV or V penetration. The prognosis for patients with a negative sentinel lymph node is much more favorable than that with a sentinel node affected by melanoma, as shown in Figure 10. Therefore, patients with positive sentinel lymph nodes usually undergo completion lymphadenectomy and consideration of adjuvant interferon or protocol therapy.

Lymph Node Metastases

Approximately 21% of patients with stage I or II melanoma (localized) eventually develop local recurrence or metastases. For patients with occult metastatic nodal melanoma detected by elective lymph node dissection, the 10-year survival rate is 48%. The five-year survival rate for all stage III (nodal metastases) patients is approximately 27% to 42%, with 15-year survival rates of 20% to 25%. Prognosis worsens with an increase in the number of involved nodes and a primary melanoma with axial location and ulceration.

Distant Metastases

Once distant metastases are present, median survival is six months, with one-year survival rates of 8% in the study by Balch et al. Patients with a greater number of metastatic sites, shorter duration of remission after primary treatment, and metastases to visceral organs tend to have significantly

Table 3 Survival Rates for Melanoma TNM and Staging Categories

Pathologic stage	TNM	Thickness (mm)	Ulceration	No. of nodes	Nodal size	Distant metastasis	No. of patients	Survival ± SE			
								1 Yr	2 Yr	5 Yr	10 Yr
IA	T1a	1	No	0	–	–	4,510	99.7 ± 0.1	99.0 ± 0.2	95.3 ± 0.4	87.9 ± 1.0
IB	T1b	1	Yes or level IV, V	0	–	–	1,380	99.8 ± 0.1	98.7 ± 0.3	90.9 ± 1.0	83.1 ± 1.5
	T2a	1.01–2.0	No	0	–	–	3,285	99.5 ± 0.1	97.3 ± 0.3	89.0 ± 0.7	79.2 ± 1.1
IIA	T2b	1.01–2.0	Yes	0	–	–	958	98.2 ± 0.5	92.9 ± 0.9	77.4 ± 1.7	64.4 ± 2.2
	T3a	2.01–4.0	No	0	–	–	1,717	98.7 ± 0.3	94.3 ± 0.6	78.7 ± 1.2	63.8 ± 1.7
IIB	T3b	2.01–4.0	Yes	0	–	–	1,523	95.1 ± 0.6	84.8 ± 1.0	63.0 ± 1.5	50.8 ± 1.7
	T4a	>4.0	No	0	–	–	563	94.8 ± 1.0	88.6 ± 1.5	67.4 ± 2.4	53.9 ± 3.3
IIC	T4b	>4.0	Yes	0	–	–	978	89.9 ± 1.0	70.7 ± 1.6	45.1 ± 1.9	32.3 ± 2.1
IIIA	N1a	Any	No	1	Micro	–	252	95.9 ± 1.3	88.0 ± 2.3	69.5 ± 3.7	63.0 ± 4.4
	N2a	Any	No	2–3	Micro	–	130	93.0 ± 2.4	82.7 ± 3.8	63.3 ± 5.6	56.9 ± 6.8
IIIB	N1a	Any	Yes	1	Micro	–	217	93.3 ± 1.8	75.0 ± 3.2	52.8 ± 4.1	37.8 ± 4.8
	N2a	Any	Yes	2–3	Micro	–	111	92.0 ± 2.7	81.0 ± 4.1	49.6 ± 5.7	35.9 ± 7.2
	N1b	Any	No	1	Macro	–	122	88.5 ± 2.9	78.5 ± 3.7	59.0 ± 4.8	47.7 ± 5.8
	N2b	Any	No	2–3	Macro	–	93	76.8 ± 4.4	65.6 ± 5.0	46.3 ± 5.5	39.2 ± 5.8
IIIC	N1b	Any	Yes	1	Macro	–	98	77.9 ± 4.3	54.2 ± 5.2	29.0 ± 5.1	24.4 ± 5.3
	N2b	Any	Yes	2–3	Macro	–	109	74.3 ± 4.3	44.1 ± 4.9	24.0 ± 4.4	15.0 ± 3.9
	N3	Any	Any	4	Micro/Macro	–	396	71.0 ± 2.4	49.8 ± 2.7	26.7 ± 2.5	18.4 ± 2.5
IV	M1a	Any	Any	Any	Any	Skin, SQ	179	59.3 ± 3.7	36.7 ± 3.6	18.8 ± 3.0	15.7 ± 2.9
	M1b	Any	Any	Any	Any	Lung	186	57.0 ± 3.7	23.1 ± 3.2	6.7 ± 2.0	2.5 ± 1.5
	M1c	Any	Any	Any	Any	Other visceral	793	40.0 ± 1.6	23.6 ± 1.3	9.3 ± 1.1	6.0 ± 0.9
Total							17,600				

Abbreviation: TNM, tumor node metastasis.

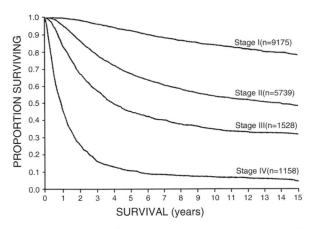

Figure 7 Survival curves for stage I–IV melanoma. *Source*: From Balch, Buzaid, Soong (2001).

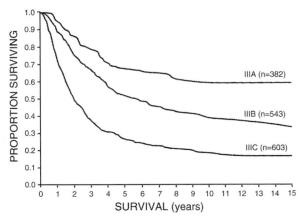

Figure 9 Survival curves for stage III melanoma. *Source*: From Balch, Buzaid, Soong (2001).

worse prognoses. Occasionally, patients with metastatic melanoma survive more than five years. Also intriguing is the fact that 2% to 3% of patients with melanoma will develop recurrences 10 years or more after treatment of their primary tumor, with rare relapses more than 30 years after initial diagnosis.

Surgical Margin

Many studies support the concept that the width of surgical margin has no effect on survival in cutaneous melanoma. Two prospective, randomized, controlled trials on patients with thin-to-intermediate thickness (<4 mm) melanomas by Veronesi et al. and Balch et al. recently demonstrated no statistically significant difference in survival rates between those receiving narrow (1–2 cm) versus wide (3–4 cm) margins. Based on these studies, recommended resection margins have decreased to 1 cm for thin melanomas (<1 mm), 1 to 2 cm for melanomas 1 to 2 mm thick, and 2 cm for melanomas 2 to 4 mm thick. Thick (>4 mm) melanomas may be managed with 2 or 3 cm surgical margins. Several studies, including Veronesi's, have demonstrated that narrow surgical margins may be associated with

increased local recurrence rates. The discordance between the negative effect of narrow surgical margins on local recurrence but not on survival challenges the concept that melanoma spreads via localized lymphatics prior to nodal or hematogenous dissemination.

Mohs Micrographic Surgery

Mohs micrographic surgery ideally offers the possibility of decreased surgical margins without increased risk of local recurrence, distant metastasis, or death. Although not universally accepted, the use of Mohs micrographic surgery for the removal of cutaneous melanoma is supported by clinical experience as outlined by Zitelli. According to most complete records, survival and local recurrence rates obtained with Mohs micrographic surgery are comparable to those of standard wide excision. Of 20 patients with invasive melanoma, Zitelli reported a 95% five-year survival, comparable to that expected from life-table analysis from other studies involving standard excisions. Mohs micrographic surgery for melanoma can be regarded as an extension of the general trend towards narrower margins for melanoma with the additional security of immediate and complete histologic verification of tumor-free margins. Prospective, randomized comparison with standard excision

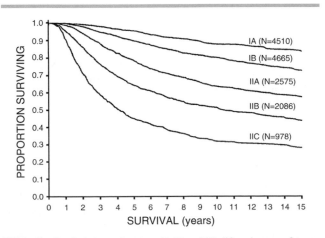

Figure 8 Survival curves for stage IA–IB and IIA–IIC melanoma. *Source*: From Balch, Buzaid, Soong (2001).

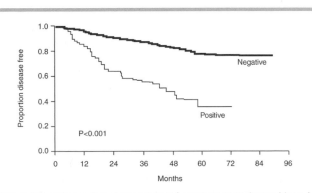

Figure 10 Disease-free survival curves for melanoma patients with positive and negative sentinel lymph node biopsy. *Source*: From Gershenwald et al. (1999).

would clarify the role of Mohs micrographic surgery in the management of melanoma.

Lymph Node Dissection

Results of studies regarding the impact of elective lymph node dissection in clinical stages I–II melanoma are conflicting, with some studies demonstrating improved survival while others reveal no impact on ultimate outcome. Four randomized, controlled, prospective trials of elective lymph node dissection for high-risk melanoma failed to reveal any efficacy in prolonging overall survival. The first two trials, the Mayo Clinic trial and the first WHO trial, relied on anatomic maps to select the dissected nodal basin. The latter portion of the second WHO trial and the Balch study employed preoperative lymphoscintigraphy to identify the at-risk nodal basin. The only therapeutic efficacy from elective lymph node dissection identified in four studies was from subgroup analysis of Balch's trial, where a potential benefit was identified for a subset of patients less than 60 years old, with nonulcerated, 1- to 2-mm-thick melanomas. The subgroup analysis in this study has been criticized as excessive. For patients with metastatic melanoma localized to regional lymph nodes, therapeutic nodal dissection has been associated with a 20% 10-year survival rate. Thus, therapeutic lymph node resection can result in long-term survival in patients with metastatic melanoma of the lymph nodes.

Treatment of Disseminated Metastatic Disease

At the present time, no nonsurgical modality has been shown in randomized, blinded trials to consistently and significantly improve survival in patients with metastatic melanoma. As shown in the study by Wong et al., 5% to 20% of patients with solitary visceral metastasis amenable to resection will survive more than five years. However, chemotherapy, radiotherapy, and biologic therapies have shown poor efficacy with regard to curative intent in metastatic melanoma and are best regarded as palliative. Chemotherapy with dacarbazine (DTIC) or paclitaxel (Taxol) is associated with objective response rates of 20%, while combination of DTIC, carmustine, cisplastin, and tamoxifen has been associated with response rates of 46%. Neither regimen has demonstrated the ability to improve survival rates. Autologous bone marrow transplantation after high-dose combination chemotherapy has been attempted, with overall response rates of 65%. For patients with extremity-based in-transit metastases, isolated limb perfusion with combination melphalan, tumor necrosis factor, and interferon-alpha has been associated with a 90% response rate and is currently being evaluated in controlled trials. None of the above regimens has been shown to improve disease-free or overall survival significantly and consistently. Ongoing investigations of isolated limb perfusion, adjuvant radiotherapy, megestrol acetate, and levamisole will hopefully identify treatments with more significant impact on metastatic melanoma than current regimens.

Biologic therapy with interferon-alpha in patients with metastatic melanoma is associated with a 15% objective response rate The efficacy of this therapy is hotly debated, with only one of four trials showing prolongation of overall survival. High-dose interleukin-2 has been associated with occasional long-term remissions in an uncontrolled trial in patients with metastatic melanoma. Such promising results must be viewed with caution, however, until interleukin-2 can be evaluated in a controlled trial. Trials of adjuvant interferon-alpha and vaccines in high-risk stage II patients are ongoing.

SOFT TISSUE SARCOMA

With only 5700 new cases reported in 1990, soft tissue sarcomas are relatively uncommon, and extensive prognostic data on specific sarcoma histologic types is not readily available. Because histologic type is not the most sensitive prognostic factor for soft tissue sarcomas, the majority of prognostic date regarding cure rates and survival are derived from grading and staging systems based on collective series of all types of soft tissue sarcomas. In many systems, the histologic characteristics of specific tumors are integrated into the overall grade of the tumor. Analogous to melanoma, "cure" rates for high-grade soft tissue sarcomas are more appropriately defined in terms of long-term survival, given the potentially lethal nature of these neoplasms. Conversely, for low-grade sarcomas local recurrence is a more relevant concept, given their indolent, locally invasive nature. As with melanoma, current therapy of soft tissue sarcomas centers on surgical resection, with adjuvant modalities essential but inadequately curative themselves. Most available data are based on the 2002 AJCC staging system (Table 4), which will be referred to in this section. Table 5 outlines the most common soft tissue sarcomas.

Survival Rates

Grade and Histologic Type

Grading systems attempt to objectify the degree on malignancy of a particular tumor. The grade of a soft tissue sarcoma is the most reliable predictor of survival. A variety of grading systems for soft tissue sarcomas have been proposed based on factors including cellularity, cellular pleomorphism, growth pattern, tumor necrosis, specific tumor type, vascular invasion, and mitotic rate. Of these prognostic factors, mitotic rate, vascular invasion and necrosis are the most reliable. Depth of tumor penetration has also been shown to predict decreased survival. As pathologists are concordant on histologic type, mitotic rate, and tumor necrosis in only 61%, 73%, and 81% of cases, respectively, examination by a pathologist experienced with soft tissue sarcomas is paramount for prognostic and therapeutic information.

In general, increasing grade correlates with decreased survival. There are notable exceptions as in malignant granular cell tumors, which display only moderate pleomorphism and little mitotic activity yet behave aggressively. Intermediate- and high-grade sarcomas are associated with a poor prognosis in general, with 50% of patients dying within five year according to Myhre Jensen et al. Table 6 outlines the differences in trends toward decreased survival in various grading systems. Figure 11 demonstrates typical corrected survival curves for grade 1, 2, and 3 sarcomas based on the grading system of Myhre Jensen et al. As can be seen in the curves, death from soft-tissue sarcomas can occur as much as 10 years after initial presentation, although 80% of local or distant recurrences occur within five year.

Five-year survival rates for specific histologic types of intermediate- and high-grade sarcomas are compiled in Table 7. As many of these sarcomas arise in the deep soft tissues and retroperitoneum, dermatologic surgeons have infrequent exposure to many of these tumors. A notable exception is cutaneous leiomyosarcoma, which rarely metastasizes, in contrast to the highly aggressive deep leiomyosarcoma, as shown by Fields and Helwig

Table 4 2002 American Joint Committee on Cancer Staging System for Soft Tissue Sarcomas

TNM categorization				
Primary tumor (T)				
TX	Primary tumor cannot be assessed			
T0	No evidence of primary tumor			
TI	Tumor 5 cm or less in greatest diameter			
	T1a—superficial tumor			
	T1b—deep tumor			
T2	Tumor more than 5 cm in greatest diameter			
	T2a—superficial tumor			
	T2b—deep tumor			
Regional lymph nodes (N)				
NX	Regional lymph nodes cannot be assessed			
N0	No regional lymph node metastasis			
NI	Regional lymph node metastasis			
Distant metastasis (M)				
MX	Distant metastasis cannot be assessed			
M0	No distant metastasis			
MI	Distant metastasis			
Stage groupings				
Stage I	TIa, Ib, 2a, 2b	N0	M0	Low grade
Stage II	TIa, Ib, 2a	N0	M0	High grade
Stage III	T2b	N0	M0	High grade
Stage IV	Any T	N0/1	M0/1	Low or high grade

Source: American Joint Committee on Cancer (2002).

Leiomyosarcomas localized to the dermis are associated with a 32% local recurrence rate after standard excision and have been successfully managed with Mohs micrographic surgery, as reported by Davidson et al.

Low-grade or locally invasive soft tissue sarcomas rarely metastasize but frequently recur, which makes complete surgical resection imperative. Dermatologic surgeons have made significant contributions to the therapeutic options available for these tumors. Table 8 outlines recurrence rates for low-grade, locally invasive soft tissue sarcomas.

Tumor Size, Depth, and Anatomic Location

Although tumor grade is the most important prognostic indicator in soft tissue sarcomas, the size of the primary tumor is the clinical variable most predictive of disease-free survival. Tumor size and duration of survival are inversely related, as shown in Table 9. Although soft tissue sarcomas arising in the subcutaneous tissue are associated with a better prognosis than deeper sarcomas, the difference is attributable to the smaller size of subcutaneous tumors when subjected to multivariate analysis, according to the a study by Peabody et al.

Due to compromise of surgical margins at locations adjacent to vital structures, the risks of local recurrence and death are increased in sarcomas on the head and neck. According to the large study by Gustafson, the increased rate of local recurrence and decreased survival associated with proximal as opposed to distal sarcomas is secondary to the larger size of proximal tumors when analyzed by multivariate analysis. Treatment of distal extremity sarcomas with radical excision or amputation results in local control rates near 100% according to Owens et al. Sarcomas arising in the abdomen, retroperitoneum, and body wall are all associated with worse prognosis than extremity sarcomas, largely due to advanced local and distant disease by the time of presentation.

Extent of Surgery and Local Recurrence

Soft tissue sarcomas grow in an expansile and microscopically infiltrative manner, which results in a 60% to 80% local recurrence rate if excisions are performed at the periphery of the pseudocapsule. En bloc wide excisions, which encompass a 1 to 3 cm margin of clinically normal tissue around the entire periphery of the tumor but remain within the muscular compartment of origin, result in an overall 30% recurrence rate. Wide excision alone is considered adequate therapy for small, superficial, or low-grade sarcomas, as supported by the study of Rydholm et al. Wide excision or lesser procedures can be utilized for higher grade sarcomas only with the addition of adjuvant radiation or chemotherapy, as demonstrated by Rosenberg et al. Radical excision involves extirpation of the entire compartment from which the sarcoma arose, either by radical muscle compartment excision or by radical amputation. Eighty percent of patients treated with radical excision or amputation

Table 5 Common Soft Tissue Sarcomas

Malignant fibrous histiocytoma (25.1%)[a]
Liposarcoma (11.6%)
Rhabdomyosarcoma (9.7%)
Leiomyosarcoma (9.1%)
Synovial sarcoma (6.5%)
Malignant schwannoma (5.9%)
Fibrosarcoma (5.2%)

[a]Percent of total soft-tissue sarcomas.

Table 6 Five-Year Survival Rates for Grade 1–3 Soft Tissue Sarcomas

Grading system	Grade 1	Grade 2	Grade 3	Grade 4
Markhede	100	100	68	47
Myhre Jensen	97	67	38	
Costa	100	73	46	

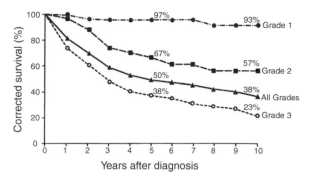

Figure 11 Survival rates by grade for soft tissue sarcomas. *Source*: From Myhre Jensen, et al. (1983).

achieve local control; of the 20% with local recurrences, 69% will be alive for three years after re-excision.

Stage

Staging systems attempt to define the extent to tumor involvement at presentation. The AJCC staging system for soft tissue sarcomas is based on the Tumor, Node, Metastasis (TNM) staging system, with the addition of histologic grade as an additional feature (GTNM) (Table 4). Survival decreases with increased stage at presentation, as shown in Figure 12.

Lymph Node Metastases

Whereas lymph node metastasis commonly occurs in metastatic melanoma and SCC, regional lymph nodes are involved in < 4% of patients at presentation and only 5% overall with soft tissue sarcomas. Because of this, elective lymph node dissection is not recommended. The histologic type rather than grade of the tumor is the most important factor predicting lymph node metastasis. Nodal metastasis carries the same prognosis as distant metastasis, uniformly poor, with a 2% to 3% 10-year survival rate. Radical lymphadenectomy for sarcoma metastatic to lymph nodes alone can

be curative, with five-year survival rates of 34% to 46%, as reported by Fong et al.

Distant Metastases

At presentation, 10% to 23% of patients with soft-tissue sarcomas will have distant metastases, most commonly to the lung, liver, bone, and central nervous system, according to Lawrence et al. Metastatic soft tissue sarcomas are associated with a dismal prognosis, with 10-year survival rates of 2% to 3%. A report by Verazin et al. documented a 21% overall five-year survival and an 11% disease-free survival after complete resection of lung metastases from soft tissue sarcomas of various types. Whereas isolated distant metastases can be surgically resected, chemotherapy would be appropriate palliative therapy for disseminated metastases. Novel therapeutic modalities such as cytokines and monoclonal antibodies have not shown efficacy in metastatic sarcoma.

Adjuvant Radiation Therapy

Radical excision and amputation can be associated with considerable functional morbidity, which has stimulated therapeutic approaches based on less radical surgical therapy. Other than small, superficial, and low-grade sarcomas, most surgically excised sarcomas are treated with adjuvant radiation therapy to optimize cure rates, as reviewed by Suit et al. Radiation can be administered pre- or postoperatively, either externally or via implanted brachytherapy. Radiation therapy alone, as discussed by Tepper and Suit, is associated with a 28% five-year survival, inadequate for monotherapy when compared with adequate surgical resection. When used in conjunction with surgical excision, control rates are superior to either approach alone, with decreased surgical morbidity.

Adjuvant Chemotherapy

Intermediate- and high-grade sarcomas are associated with a 50% five-year survival rate despite aggressive local therapy. The high propensity of sarcomas toward early microscopic metastasis has prompted trials of adjuvant systemic chemotherapy in an attempt to achieve cure while tumor burden is low. However, to date, randomized, controlled trials of postoperative adjuvant chemotherapy have not revealed definitive evidence of improved survival. Randomized trials utilizing adjuvant doxorubicin failed to demonstrate improved survival compared with surgery alone, according to Elias and Antman. The findings of randomized trials utilizing multiagent chemotherapy postoperatively are conflicting, but a recent meta-analysis by Zalupski et al. suggests that aggressive, adjuvant, multiagent chemotherapy may increase survival in patients with high-grade extremity sarcomas.

Table 7 Five-Year Survival Rates for Aggressive Soft Tissue Sarcomas

Tumor type	Survival (%)
Fibrosarcoma	39–54
Malignant fibrous histiocytoma	36–69
Liposarcoma	59–73
Leiomyosarcoma	
Retroperitoneal	0–29
Extremity	64
Rhabdomyosarcoma	26–88
Hemangioendothelioma	87 (4 yr)
Angiosarcoma	12
Synovial sarcoma	36–82
Malignant peripheral nerve sheath tumor	20–44
Neuroblastoma	60 (2 yr)
Extraskeletal Ewing's sarcoma	66
Extraskeletal myxoid chondrosarcoma	73 (10 yr)
Extraskeletal mesenchymal chondrosarcoma	55
Epitheliod sarcoma	60

Table 8 Recurrence Rates for Locally Invasive Soft Tissue Sarcoma[a]

Tumor type	Recurrence rate (%)
Dermatofibrosarcoma protuberans	18
Giant cell fibrolastoma	50
Angiomatoid fibrous histiocytoma	20
Plexiform fibrohistiocytic tumor	40
Atypical fibroxanthoma	6.4
Granular cell tumor	6.5

[a]Length of follow-up varied.

Table 9 Five-Year Survival by Tumor Size for Intermediate and High-Grade Sarcomas in Patients Treated with Surgery and Radiation

Tumor size (cm)	No. of patients	Percentage disease-free at 5 yr
<2.5	17	94
2.6–4.9	48	77
5.9–10.0	55	62
10.1–15.0	24	51
15.1–20.0	9	42
>20.0	6	17
Total	159	65

Source: Modified from Suit, et al. (1988).

Recurrence Rates for Soft Tissue Sarcomas Managed with Mohs Micrographic Surgery

Although many types of soft tissue sarcoma have been managed with Mohs micrographic surgery, the paucity of reported cases prevents reasonable estimates of recurrence rates for most tumors. However, reports of dermatofibrosarcoma protuberans (DFSP) treated with Mohs micrographic surgery now exist in larger numbers, as reviewed and expanded in the work by Gloster et al. They reported cumulative recurrence rate of only 0.6% for DFSP treated by Mohs micrographic surgery, which compares favorably to an average 18% recurrence rate after wide (>2 cm) surgical excision. This relates to the well-known capability of peripheral strands of DFSP to extend into fat and fascia well beyond the clinical margins of tumor in a haphazard fashion. Because of the impressive cure rates and opportunity for significant normal tissue sparing associated with Mohs micrographic surgery, it is considered the treatment of choice for DFSP by many authors.

In a series of 25 superficial primary and recurrent malignant fibrous histiocytomas and atypical fibroxanthomas treated with Mohs micrographic surgery, Brown and Swanson noted a 94% tumor-free survival after an average three-year follow-up. When compared with the higher recurrence rates associated with standard excisional surgery, Mohs micrographic surgery may offer a uniquely precise and controlled method for the removal of superficial malignant fibrohistiocytic neoplasms.

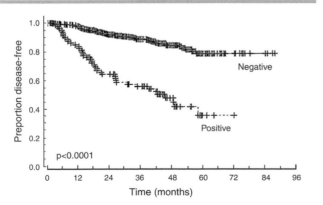

Figure 12 Survival rates for soft tissue sarcomas.

BIBLIOGRAPHY

Aebersold P, Hyatt C, Johnson S, et al. Lysis of autologous melanoma cells by tumor-infiltrating lymphocytes: association with clinical response. J Natl Cancer Inst 1993; 85:622–632.

Alpsoy E, Yilmaz E, Basaran E, Yazar S. Comparison of the effects of intralesional interferon alfa-2a, 2b and the combination of 2a and 2b in the treatment of basal cell carcinoma. J Dermatol 1996; 23:394–396.

American Joint Committee on Cancer. Cancer Staging Handbook. 6th ed. New York: Springer, 2002.

American Joint Committee on Cancer. Manual for Staging of Cancer. 2nd ed. Philadelphia: JB Lippincott, 2002.

Amonette RA, Salasche SJ, Chesney TM, Clarendon CCD, Dilawari RA. Metastatic basal-cell carcinoma. J Dermatol Surg Oncol 1981; 7:397–400.

Balch cm, Buzaid AC, Soong SJ, and et al. Final version of the American joint committee on cancer staging system for cutaneous melanoma. J Clin Oncol 2001; 19: 3635–3648.

Balch CM, Houghton AN, Peters LJ. Cutaneous melanoma. In: DeVita VT, Hellman S, Rosenberg SA, eds. Cancer: Principles and Practice of Oncology. Philadelphia: J.B. Lippincott Co., 1993:l612–1661.

Balch cm, Murad TM, Soong S-J, et al. A multifactorial analysis of melanoma. Prognostic histopathological features comparing Clark's and Breslow's staging methods. Ann Surg 1978; l88:732–742.

Balch cm, Urist mm, Karakousis CP, et al. The efficacy of 2-cm margins for intermediate-thickness melanomas (l-4mm): results of a multi-institutional randomized surgical trial. Ann Surg 1993; 218:262–267.

Balch cm, Soong S-J, Shaw HM, et al. An analysis of prognostic factors in 8500 patients with cutaneous melanoma. In: Balch cm, Houghton AN, Milton GW, et al., eds. Cutaneous Melanoma. 2nd ed. Philadelphia: J.B. Lippincott Co., 1992:165–187.

Balch cm, Soong S-J, Murad TM, et al. A multifactorial analysis of melanoma. IV. Prognostic factors in 200 melanoma patients with distant metastases (Stage III). J Clin Oncol 1983; 1:126–134.

Balch cm, Murad TM, Soong S-J, et al. Tumor thickness as a guide to surgical management of clinical stage I melanoma patients. Cancer 1979; 43:883–888.

Balch cm, Soong S-J, Murad TM, et al. A multifactorial analysis of melanoma II. Prognostic factors in patients with stage I (localized) melanoma. Surgery 1979; 86:343–351.

Balch cm, Soong S-J, Shaw HM, et al. Changing trends in the clinical and pathologic features of melanoma. In: Balch cm, Houghton AN, Milton GW, et al., eds. Cutaneous Melanoma. 2nd ed. Philadelphia: J.B. Lippincott Co., 1992:40–45.

Balch cm, Murad TM, Soong S-J, Milton GW, et al. A comparison of prognostic factors and surgical results in I, 786 patients with localized (stage I) melanoma treated in Alabama, USA, and New South Wales, Australia. Ann Surg 1982; 196:677–684.

Balch cm, Seong SJ, Bartolucci AA, et al. Efficacy of an elective regional lymph node dissection of 1- to 4-mm thick melanomas for patients 60 years of age and younger. Ann Surg 1996; 224:255–263.

Balch CM. The role of elective lymph node dissection in melanoma: rationale, results, and controversies. J Clin Oncol 1988; 6:163–172.

Barrett TL, Greenway HTJ, Massullo V, Carlson C. Treatment of basal cell carcinoma and squamous cell carcinoma with perineural invasion. Adv Dermatol 1993; 8:277–304.

Barth A, Morton DL. The role of adjuvant therapy in melanoma management. Cancer 1995; 75:726–734.

Bath-Hextall F, Bong J, Perkins W, Williams H. Interventions for basal cell carcinoma of the skin: systematic review. Br Med J 2004; 329(7468):705.

Bollag W, Holdener EE. Retinoids in cancer prevention and therapy. Ann Oncol 1992; 3:513–526.

Boztepe G, Hohenleutner S, Landthaler M, Hohenleutner U. Munich method of micrographic surgery for basal cell carcinomas: 5-year recurrence rates with life-table analysis. Acta Dermato-Venereol 2004; 84:218–222.

Breslow A, Macht SD. Optimal size of resection margin for thin cutaneous melanoma. Surg Gynecol Obstet 1977; 145: 691–692.

Breslow A. Thickness, cross-sectional areas and depth of invasion in the prognosis of cutaneous melanoma. Ann Surg 1970; 172:902–908.

Breuninger H, Black B, Rassner G. Microstaging of squamous cell carcinoma. Am J Clin Pathol 1990; 94:624–627.

Brenner S, Wolf R, Dascalu DI. Topical tretinoin treatment in basal cell carcinoma. J Dermatol Surg Oncol 1993; 19:264–266.

Broders AC, Hargrave R, Meyerding HW. Pathologic features of soft tissue fibrosarcoma with special reference to the grading of its malignancy. Surg Oynecol Obstet 1939; 69:276–280.

Brown MD, Swanson NA. Treatment of malignant fibrous histiocytoma and atypical fibrous xanthomas with micrographic surgery. J Dermatol Surg Oncol 1989; 15:1287–1292.

Brown MD, Zachary CB, Grekin RC, et al. Genital tumors: their management by micrographic surgery. J Am Acad Dermatol 1988; 18:115–122.

Cairnduff F, Stringer MR, Hudson EJ, Ash DV, Brown SB. Superficial photodynamic therapy with topical 5-amino-laevulinic acid for superficial primary and secondary skin cancer. Br J Cancer 1994; 69:605–608.

Callaway MP, Briggs JC. The incidence of late recurrence (greater than 10 years); an analysis of 536 consecutive cases of cutaneous melanoma. Br J Plast Surg 1989; 42:46–49.

Cantin J, McNeer GP, Chu FG, et al. The problem of local recurrence after treatment of soft tissue sarcoma. Ann Surg 1968; 168:47–53.

Carmichael VE, Robins RE, Wilson KS. Elective and therapeutic regional lymph node dissection for cutaneous malignant melanoma: experience of the British Columbia cancer agency. Can J Surg 1992; 35:600–604.

Cascinelli N, Van der Esch EP, Breslow A, et al. Stage I melanoma of the skin: the problem of resection margins. Eur J Cancer 1980; 16:1079–1085.

Cascinelli N, Morabita A, Santinami M, et al. Immediate or delayed dissection of regional nodes in patients with melanoma of the trunk: a randomized trial. Lancet 1998; 351:793–796.

Chang AE, Sondak VK. Clinical evaluation and treatment of soft tissue tumors. In: Enzinger FM, Weiss SW, eds. Soft Tissue Tumors. St. Louis: Mosby, 1995:17–38.

Cherpelis BS, Marcusen C, Lang PG. Prognostic factors for metastasis in squamous cell carcinoma of the skin. Dermatol Surg 2002; 28:268–273.

Childers BJ, Goldwyn RM, Ramos D, Chaffey J, Harris JR. Long-term results of irradiation for basal cell carcinoma of the skin of the nose. Plast Reconstr Surg 1994; 93:1169–1173.

Clark WH, Elder DE, Guerry D, et al. Model predicting survival in stage I melanoma based on tumor progression. J Natl Cancer Inst 1989; 81:1893–1904.

Cornell RC, Greenway HT, Tucker SB, et al. Intralesional interferon therapy for basal cell carcinoma. J Am Acad Dermatol 1990; 23:694–700.

Costa J, Wesley RA, Glatstein E, et al. The grading of soft tissue sarcomas. Results of a clinicohistopathologic correlation in a series of 163 cases. Cancer 1984; 53:530–541.

Crowley NJ, Seigler HF. Late recurrence of malignant melanoma. Analysis of 168 patients. Ann Surg 1990; 212: 173–177.

Cutler S, Ederer F. Maximum utilization of the life table method in analyzing survival. J Chron Dis 1958; 8:699–712.

Davidson LL, Frost ML, Hanke CW, et al. Primary leiomyosarcoma of the skin. J Am Acad Dermatol 1989; 21:1156–1160.

Day CL Jr, Sober AJ, Kopf AW, et al. A prognostic model for clinical stage I melanoma of the trunk: location near midline is not an independent risk factor for recurrent disease. Am J Surg 1981; 142:247–251.

Day CL Jr, Mihm MC Jr, Sober AJ, et al. Narrower margins for clinical stage I malignant melanoma. N Engl J Med 1982; 306:479–482.

Day CL Jr, Mihm MC Jr, Lew RA, et al. Prognostic factors for patients with clinical stage I melanoma of intermediate thickness (1.5–3.99 mm). A conceptual model for tumor growth and metastasis. Ann Surg 1982; 195:35–43.

Day CL Jr, Sober AJ, Kopf AW, et al. A prognostic model for clinical stage I melanoma of the lower extremity. Location on foot as independent risk factor for recurrent disease. Surgery 1981; 89:599–603.

Day CL Jr, Sober AJ, Kopf AW, et al. A prognostic model for clinical stage I melanoma of the upper extremity. The importance of anatomic subsites in predicting recurrent disease. Ann Surg 1981; 193:436–440.

Day CL, JR., Lew RA. Malignant melanoma prognostic factors: 3 surgical margins. J Dermatol Surg Oncol 1983; 9:797–801.

Day CL, Jr, Mihm MC, Jr, Lew RA, et al. Cutaneous malignant melanoma: prognostic guidelines for physicians and patients. CA Cancer J Clin 1982; 32:113–122.

Dineheart SM, Pollack SV. Metastases from squamous cell carcinoma of the skin and lip. J Am Acad Dermatol 1989; 21:241–248.

Dixon AY, Lee SH, McGregor DH. Histologic features predictive of basal cell carcinoma recurrence: results of a multivariate analysis. J Cutan Pathol 1993; 20:137–142.

Drzewiecki KT, Anderson PK. Survival with malignant melanoma, A regression analysis of prognostic factors. Cancer 1982; 49:2414–2419.

Dzubow LM, Rigel DS, Robins P. Risk factors for local recurrence of primary cutaneous squamous carcinoma. Arch Dermatol 1982; 118:900–902.

Edwards L, Berman B, Rapini RP, et al. Treatment of cutaneous squamous cell carcinomas by intralesional interferon alpha-2b therapy. Arch Dermatol 1992; 128:1486–1489.

Edwards L, Tucker SB, Perdnia D, et al. The effects of intralesional sustained-release formulation of interferon alfa-2b on basal cell carcinomas. Arch Dermatol 1990; 126: 1029–1032.

Einzig Al, Hochster J, Wiernik PH, et al. A phase II study of taxol in patients with malignant melanoma. Invest New Drugs 1991; 9:59–64.

Elder DE, Gerry D, Heigerger RM, et al. Optimal resection margin for cutaneous malignant melanoma. Plast Reconstr Surg 1983; 71:66–72.

Eldh J, Boeryd B, Peterson LE. Prognostic factors in cutaneous malignant melanoma in stage I. A clinical, morphological and multivariate analysis. Scand J Plast Reconstr Surg 1978; 12:243–255.

Elias AD, Antman KH. Adjuvant chemotherapy for soft-tissue sarcoma: a critical appraisal. Semin Surg Oncol 1988; 4:59–65.

Enneking WF. Musculoskeletal Tumor Surgery. New York: Churchill Livingstone, 1983.

Enneking WF, Spanier SS, Malawer MM. The effect of the anatomic setting on the results of surgical procedures for soft parts sarcoma of the thigh. Cancer 1981; 47:1005–1022.

Enzinger FM. Clinicopathological correlation in soft tissue sarcomas. In: Management of Soft Tissue and Bone Sarcomas. New York: Raven Press, 1986.

Enzinger FM, Weiss SW. General consideration. In: Enzinger RM, Weiss SW, eds. Soft Tissue Tumors. St. Louis: Mosby, 1995:1–16.

Falkson CU, Falkson G, Falkson HC. Improved results with the addition of interferon alpha-2b to decarbazine in the treatment of patients with metastatic malignant melanoma. J Clin Oncol 1991; 9:1403–1408.

Fewkes J, Mohs FE. Microscopically controlled surgical excision (the Mohs technique). In: Fitzpatrick TB, Eisen AZ, Wolff K, et al., eds. Dermatology in General Medicine. 3rd ed. New York: McGraw-Hill, 1987:2557–2563.

Fields IP, Helwig EB. Leiomyosarcoma of the skin and subcutaneous tissue. Cancer 1981; 47:156–169.

Fong Y, Coit DG, Woodruff JM, et al. Lymph node metastasis from soft tissue sarcoma in adults. Analysis of data from a prospective database of 1772 sarcoma patients. Ann Surg 1993; 217:72–77.

Fraunfelder FT, Zacarian SA, Wingfield DL, Limmer BL. Results of cryotherapy for eyelid malignancies. Am J Ophthalmol 1984; 97:184–188.

Frankel DH, Hanusa BH, Zitelli JA. New primary nonmelanoma skin cancer in patients with a history of squamous cell carcinoma of the skin. Implications and recommendations for follow-up. J Am Acad Dermatol 1992; 26:720–726.

Gajetta E, Di Leo A, Zampino MG, et al. Multicenter randomized trial of decarbazine alone or in combination with two different doses and schedules of interferon alpha 2a in the treatment of advanced melanoma. J Clin Oncol 1994; 12:806–811.

Geer RJ, Woodruff J, Caspar ES, et al. Management of small soft-tissue of the extremity in adults. Arch Surg 1992; 127:1285–1289.

Gershenwald JE, Thompson W, Mansfield PF, et al. Multi-institutional melanoma lymphatic mapping experience: the prognostic value of sentinel lymph node status in 612 stage I or II melanoma patients. J Clin Oncol 1999; 17:976–983.

Gloster HM, Harris KR, Roenigk RK. A comparison between Mohs micrographic surgery and wide surgical excision for the treatment of dermatofibrosarcoma protuberans. J Am Acad Dermatol 1996; 35:82–87.

Graham GF. Cryosurgery. Clin Plast Surg 1993; 20:131–147.

Griffiths RW, Feeley K, Suvarna SK. Audit of clinical and histological prognostic factors in primary squamous cell carcinoma of the skin: assessment in a minimum 5 year follow-up study after conventional excisional surgery. Br J Plast Surg 2002; 55:287–292.

Gustafson P. Soft tissue sarcoma. Epidemiology and prognosis in 508 patients. Acta Ortho Scand 1994; 259(suppl):1–31.

Guthrie TJ, Porabsky ES, Luxenberg MN, Shah KJ, Wurtz KL, Watson PR. Cisplatin-based chemotherapy in advanced basal and squamous cell carcinomas of the skin: results in 28 patients including 13 patients receiving multimodality therapy. J Clin Oncol 1990; 8:342–346.

Hafstrom L, Rudenstam cm, Blomquist E, et al. Regional hyperthermic perfusion with melphalan after surgery for recurrent malignant melanoma of the extremities. J Clin Oncol 1991; 9:2091–2094.

Hall L, Leppard BL, McGill J, et al. Treatment of basal cell carcinoma: comparison of radiotherapy and cryotherapy. Clin Radiol 1983; 37:33–34.

Hanke CW, Lee MW. Treatment of rare malignancies. In: Mikhail GR, ed. Mohs Micrographic Surgery. Philadelphia: W.B Saunders, 1991:265–267.

Hashimoto H, Diamaru Y, Takeshita S, et al. Prognostic significance of histologic parameters of soft tissue sarcomas. Cancer 1992; 70:2816–2822.

Hess KA, Hanke CW, Estes NC, et al. Chemosurgical reports: myxoid dermatofibrosarcoma protuberans. J Dermatol Surg Oncol 1985; 11:268–271.

Hill GJ II, Moss SE, Golumb FM, et al. DTIC and combination therapy for melanoma. DTIC [NSC 45388] surgical adjuvant study COG protocol 7040. Cancer 1981; 46:2557–2562.

Hobbs ER, Wheeland RG, Bailin PL, et al. Treatment of dermatofibrosarcoma protuberans with Mohs micrographic surgery. Ann Surg 1988; 207:102–107.

Holmkvist KA, Roenigk RK. Squamous cell carcinoma of the lip treated with Mohs micrographic surgery: outcome at 5 years. J Am Acad Dermatol 1998; 38:960–966.

Hruza GJ. Mohs micrographic surgery local recurrences. J Dermatol Surg Oncol 1994; 20:573–577.

Huth JF, Eilber FR. Patterns of metastatic spread following resection of extremity soft-tissue sarcomas and strategies for treatment. Semin Surg Oncol 1988; 4:20–26.

Iacobucci JJ, Stevenson TR, Swanson NA, et al. Cutaneous leiomyosarcoma. Ann Plast Surg 1987; 19:552–554.

Johnson TM, Smith JW II, Nelson BR, Chang A. Current therapy for cutaneous melanoma. J Am Acad Dermatol 1995; 32:689–707.

Johnson TM, Rowe DE, Nelson BR, Swanson NA. Squamous cell carcinoma of the skin (excluding lip and oral mucosa). J Am Acad Dermatol 1992; 26:467–484.

Joseph MG, Zulueta WP, Kennedy PJ. Squamous cell carcinoma of the skin of the trunk and limbs: the incidence of metastases and their outcome. Aust NZ J Surg 1992; 62:697–701.

Karakousis CP, Velez A, Driscoll DL, et al. Metastasectomy in malignant melanoma. Surgery 1994; 115:295–302.

Kaspar TA, Wagner RF Jr. Mohs micrographic surgery for thin stage I malignant melanoma: rationale for a modem management strategy. Cutis 1991; 50:350–351.

Koh K, Michalik E, Sober AJ, et al. Lentigo maligna melanoma has not better prognosis than other types of melanoma. J Clin Oncol 1984; 2:994–1001.

Koh KH. Cutaneous melanoma. N Engl J Med 1991; 325:171–182.

Kokoszka A, Scheinfeld N. Evidence-based review of the use of cryosurgery in treatment of basal cell carcinoma. Dermatol Surg 2003; 29:566–571.

Kuflik EG. Cryosurgery for skin cancer: 30-year experience and cure rates. Dermatol Surg 2004; 30:297–300.

Kuflik EG. Cryosurgery updated. J Am Acad Dermatol 1994; 31:925–944.

Kuflik EG, Gage AA. Cryosurgery Treatment for Skin Cancer. New York: Igaku-Shoin, 1990.

Kuflik EG, Gage AA. The five-year cure rate achieved cryosurgery for skin cancer. J Am Acad Dermatol 1991; 24:1002–1004.

Lang PG, Maize JC. Histologic evolution of recurrent basal cell carcinoma and treatment implications. J Am Dermatol 1986; 14:186–196.

Lawrence W Jr, Donegan WL, Natarajan N, et al. Adult soft tissue sarcomas. A pattern of care survey of the American College of Surgeons. Ann Surg 1987; 205:349–359.

Lawrence CM. Mohs surgery of basal cell carcinoma-a critical review. Br J Plast Surg 1993; 46:599–606.

Legha SS, Ring S, Papadopoulos N, et al. A phase II trial of taxol in patients with malignant melanoma. Cancer 1990; 65:2478–2481.

Levine H. Cutaneous carcinoma of the head and neck: management of massive and previously uncontrolled lesions. Laryngoscope 1983; 93:87–105.

Lippman SM, Parkinson DR, Itri LM, et al. 13-*cis*-Retinoic acid and interferon alpha-2a: effective combination therapy for advanced squamous cell carcinoma of the skin. J Natl Cancer Inst 1992; 84:235–241.

Little JH, Holt J, Davis N. Changing epidemiology of malignant melanoma in Queensland. Med J Aust 1980; 1:66–69.

Madsen A. Studies on basal cell epithelioma of the skin. Acta Pathol Microbiol Scand 1965; 177(suppl):1047–1049.

Mallon E, Dawbor E. Cryosurgery in the treatment of basal cell carcinoma: assessment of one or two freeze-thaw cycle schedules. Dermatol Surg 1996; 22:854–858.

Mandard AM, Chasle JC, Mandard JC, et al. The pathologist's role in a multidisciplinary approach for soft part tissue sarcoma: a reappraisal (39 cases). J Surg Oncol 1981; 17:69–81.

Mansson-Brahme E, Carstensen K, Erhardt K, et al. Prognostic factors in thin cutaneous melanoma. Cancer 1994; 73: 2324–2332.

Marmur ES, Schmults CD, Goldberg DJ. A review of laser and photodynamic therapy for the treatment of nonmelanoma skin cancer. Dermatol Surg 2004; 30(2 Pt 2):264–271.

Markhede G, Angervall L, Stener B. A multivariate analysis of the prognosis after surgical treatment of malignant soft-tissue tumors. Cancer 1982; 49:1721–1733.

Marcus SG, Merino MJ, Glatstein E, et al. Long-term outcome in 87 patients with low-grade soft tissue sarcoma. Arch Surg 1993; 128:1336–1343.

McCarthy WH, Shaw HM, Thompson JF, et al. Time and frequency of recurrence of cutaneous stage I malignant melanoma with guidelines for follow-up study. Surg Gynecol Obstet 1988; 166:497–502.

McClay EF, Mastrangelo MJ, Spradnio JD, et al. The importance of tamoxifen to a cisplatin-containing regimen in the treatment of metastatic melanoma. Cancer 1989; 63:1292–1295.

McGovern VJ, Shaw HM, Milton GW, et al. Is malignant melanoma arising in a Hutchinson's melanotic freckle a separate disease entity?. Histopathology 1980; 4:235–242.

Mehregan DA, Roenigk RK. Management of superficial squamous cell carcinoma of the lip with Mohs micrographic surgery. Cancer 1990; 66:463–468.

Mikhail GR, Kelly AP Jr. Malignant angioendothelioma of the face. J Dermatol Surg Oncol 1977; 3:181–183.

Mikhail GR, Lynn BH. Dermatofibrosarcoma protuberans. J Dermatol Surg Oncol 1978; 4:81–84.

Miller PK, Roenigk RK, Brodland DG, Randle HW. Cutaneous micrographic surgery: Mohs procedure. Mayo Clin Proc 1992; 67:971–980.

Mohs FE, Zitelli JA. Microscopically controlled surgery in the treatment of carcinoma of the scalp. Arch Dermatol 1981; 117:764–769.

Mohs F, Larson P, Iriondo M. Micrographic surgery for the microscopically controlled excision of carcinoma of the external ear. J Am Acad Dermatol 1988; 19:729–737.

Mohs FE. Fixed-tissue micrographic surgery for melanoma of the ear. Arch Otalaryngol Head Neck Surg 1988; 114: 625–631.

Mohs FE. Chemosurgery: Microscopically Controlled Surgery for Skin Cancer. Springfield, IL: Charles C Thomas, 1978.

Mohs FE, Bloom RF, Sahl WL. Chemosurgery for familial malignant melanoma. J Dermatol Surg Oncol 1979; 5:127–131.

Mohs FE. Chemosurgery. A microscopically controlled method of cancer excision. Arch Surg 1941; 44:279–295.

Myerskens FL Jr, Berdeaux DH, Parks B, et al. Cutaneous malignant melanoma (Arizona Cancer Center experience). I. Natural history and prognostic factors influencing survival in patients with stage I disease. Cancer 1988; 62:1207–1214.

Myhre Jensen O, Kaae S, Hjollund Madsen E, et al. Histopathological grading in soft-tissue tumors. Acta Pathol Microbial Immunol Scand 1983; 91A:145–150.

National Institutes of Health Consensus Development Panel on Early Melanoma. Diagnosis and treatment of early melanoma. JAMA 1992; 286:1314–1319.

Nordin P, Larko O, Stenquist B. Five-year results of curettage-cryosurgery of selected large primary basal cell carcinomas on the nose: an alternative treatment in a geographical area underserved by Mohs' surgery. Br J Dermatol 1997; 136: 180–183.

Nouri K, Rivas MP, Pedroso F, Bhatia R, Civantos F. Sentinel lymph node biopsy for high-risk cutaneous squamous cell carcinoma of the head and neck. Arch Dermatol 2004; 140:1284.

Orenberg EK, Miller BH, Greenway HT, et al. The effect of intralesional 5-fluorouracil therapeutic implant (MPI5003) for treatment of basal cell carcinoma. J Am Acad Dermatol 1992; 27:723–728.

Owens JC, Shiu MH, Smith R, et al. Soft tissue sarcomas of the hand and foot. Cancer 1985; 55:2010–2018.

Padilla RS, Shimazu C. Malignant Schwannoma treated by Mohs surgical excision. J Dermatol Surg Oncol 1991; 17:793–796.

Peabody TD, Monson D, Montag A, et al. A comparison of the prognosis for deep and subcutaneous sarcomas of the extremities. J Bone Joint Surg 1994; 76A:1167–1173.

Peck GL, DiGiovanna JJ, Sarnoff DS, et al. Treatment and prevention of basal cell carcinoma with oral isotretinoin. J Am Acad Dermatol 1988; 19:176–185.

Peters CW, Hanke CW, Pasarell HA, et al. Chemosurgical reports. Dermatofibrosarcoma protuberans of the face. J Dermatol Surg Oncol 1982; 8:823–826.

Pontikes LA, Temple WJ, Cassar SL, et al. Influence of the level and depth on recurrence rates in thin melanomas. Am J Surg 1993; l65:225–228.

Potter DA, Glenn J, Kinsella T, et al. Patterns of recurrence in patients with high-grade soft-tissue sarcomas. J Clin Oncol 1985; 3:353–366.

Potter DA, Kinsella T, Glatstein E, et al. High-grade soft tissue sarcomas of the extremities. Cancer 1986; 58:190–205.

Prade M, Bognel C, Charpentier P, et al. Malignant melanoma of the skin: prognostic factors derived from a multifactorial analysis of 239 cases. Am J Dermatopathol 1982; 4:411–412.

Preston DS, Stem RS. Nonmelanoma cancers of the skin. N Engl J Med 1992; 23:1649–1662.

Pyrohonen S, Hahka-Kemppinen M, Muhonen T. A promising interferon plus four-drug chemotherapy regimen for metastatic melanoma. J Clin Oncol 1992; 10:1919–1926.

Raszewski RL, Guyuron B. Long-term survival following nodal metastases from basal cell carcinoma. Ann Plast Surg 1990; 24:170–175.

Reintgen DS, Vollmer R, Tso CY, et al. Prognosis for recurrent stage I malignant melanoma. Arch Surg 1987; 122: 1338–1342.

Reschly MJ, Messina JL, Zaulyanov LL, Cruse W, Fenske NA. Utility of sentinel lymphadenectomy in the management of patients with high-risk cutaneous squamous cell carcinoma. Dermatol Surg 2003; 29:135–140.

Rhodes LE, de Rie M, Enstrom Y, et al. Photodynamic therapy using topical methyl aminolevulinate vs surgery for nodular basal cell carcinoma: results of a multicenter randomized prospective trial. Arch Dermatol 2004; 140(l):17–23.

Riefkohl R, Wittels B, McCarty K. Metastatic basal cell carcinoma. Ann Plast Surg 1984; 13:525–528.

Rigel DS, Robins P, Friedman RJ. Predicting recurrence of basal-cell carcinomas treated by microscopically controlled excision. J Dermatol Surg Oncol 1981; 7:807–810.

Robins P, Dzubow LM, Rigel DS. Squamous cell carcinoma treated by Mohs surgery: an experience with 414 cases in a period of 15 years. J Dermatol Surg Oncol 1981; 7: 800–801.

Robins P. Chemosurgery: my 15 years experience. J Dermatol Surg Oncol 1981; 7:779–789.

Robinson JK. Dermatofibrosarcoma protuberans resected by Mohs' surgery (chemosurgery). J Am Acad Dermatol 1985; 12:1093–1098.

Roenigk RK, Ratz JL, Bailin PL, Wheeland RG. Trends in the presentation and treatment of basal cell carcinomas. J Dermatol Surg Oncol 1986; 12:860–865.

Roenigk RK. Mohs' micrographic surgery. Mayo Clin Proc 1988; 63:175–183.

Roenigk RK, Roenigk HH Jr, eds. Surgical Dermatology. St. Louis: Mosby Year Book, 1993.

Roenigk RK, Roenigk HH Jr. Dermatologic Surgery: Principles and Practice. New York: Marcel Dekker, Inc., 1989.

Rogozinski TT, Jablonska S, Brzoska J, Michalska I, Wohr C, Gaus W. Intralesional treatment with recombinant interferon beta is an effective alternative for the treatment of basal cell carcinoma: double-blind, placebo-controlled study. Prezeglad Dermatologiczny 1997; 84:259–263.

Rosenberg SA, Suit HD, Baker LH. Sarcomas of soft tissues. In: DeVita VT, Hellman S, Rosenberg SA, eds. Cancer: Principles and Practice of Oncology . Philadelphia: J.B Lippincott, 1985:1243–1291.

Rosenberg SA, Tepper I, et al. The treatment of soft-tissue sarcomas of the extremities. Prospective randomized evaluations of (1) limb-sparing surgery plus radiation therapy compared with amputation and (2) the role of adjuvant chemotherapy. Ann Surg 1982; 196:305–315.

Rosenberg SA, Yang JC, Topalian SL, et al. Treatment of 283 consecutive patients with metastatic melanoma or renal cell cancer using high-dose bolus interleukin 2. JAMA 1994; 271:907–913.

Rowe DE, Carroll RJ, Day CL Jr. Mohs surgery is the treatment of choice for recurrent (previously treated) basal cell carcinoma. J Dermatol Surg Oncol 1989; 15:424–431.

Rowe DE, Carroll RJ, Day CL. Prognostic factors for local recurrence, metastasis, and survival rates in squamous cell carcinoma of the skin, ear, and lip. J Am Acad Dermatol 1992; 26:976–990.

Rowe DE, Carroll RJ, Day CL Jr. Long-term recurrence rates in previously untreated (primary) basal cell carcinoma: implications for patient follow-up. J Dermatol Surg Oncol 1989; 15:315–328.

Rydholm A, Gustafson P, Rooser B, et al. Limb-sparing surgery without radiotherapy based on the anatomic location of soft tissue sarcoma. J Clin Oncol 1991; 9:1757–1765.

Sadek H, Azli N, Wendling JL, et al. Treatment of advanced squamous cell carcinoma of the skin with cisplatin, 5-fluorouracil, and bleomycin. Cancer 1990; 66:1692–1696.

Sahl W, Yessenow R, Brou J, Levine N. Mohs' micrographic surgery and prompt reconstruction for basal cell carcinoma: report of 62 cases using the combined method. J Okla State Med Assoc 1994; 87:10–15.

Salasche SJ, Cheney ML, Varvares MA. Recognition and management of the high-risk cutaneous squamous cell carcinoma. Curr Probl Dermatol 1993; 5:141–192.

Salasche SJ, Amonette RA. Morpheaform basal-cell epitheliomas. J Dermatol Surg Oncol 1981; 7:387–394.

Scanlon EF, Volkmer DD, Oviedo MA, Khandekar JD, Victor TA. Metastatic basal cell carcinoma. J Surg Oncol 1980; 15: 171–180.

Schmoeckel C, Bockelbrink A, Bockelbrink H, et al. Low- and-high risk malignant melanoma-I. Evaluation of clinical and histological prognosticators in 585 cases. Eur J Cancer Clin Oncol 1983; 19:227–235.

Schmoeckel C, Bockelbrink A, Bockelbrink H, et al. Low-and-high risk malignant melanoma-IIL Prognostic significance

of resection margin. Eur J Cancer Clin Oncol 1983; 19: 245–249.

Schmoeckel C, Bockelbrink A, Bockelbrink H, et al. Low-and-high risk malignant melanoma-II. Multivariate analyses for a prognostic classification. Eur J Cancer Oncol 1983; 19:237–243.

Shea TC, Antman KH, Elder JP, et al. Malignant melanoma. Treatment with high-dose combination alkylating agent chemotherapy and autologous bone marrow transplantation. Arch Dermatol 1988; 52:1792–1802.

Shumate CR, Carlson GW, Giacco GG, et al. The prognostic implications of location for scalp melanoma. Am J Surg 1991; 162:315–319.

Silverman MK, Kopf AW, Grin CM, Bart RS, Levenstein MJ. Recurrence rates of treated basal cell carcinomas. Part 1: overview. J Dermatol Surg Oncol 1991; 17:713–718.

Silverman MK, Kopf AW, Grin CM, Bart RS, Levenstein MJ. Recurrence rates of treated basal cell carcinomas Part 4: x-ray therapy. J Dermatol Surg Oncol 1992; 18:549–554.

Silverman MK, Kopf AW, Grin CM, Bart RS, Levenstein MJ. Recurrence rates of treated basal cell carcinomas Part 3: surgical excision. J Dermatol Surg Oncol 1992; 18:471–476.

Silverman MK, Kopf AW, Grin CM, Bart RS, Levenstein MJ. Recurrence rates of treated basal cell carcinomas Part II: curettage-electrodessication. J Dermatol Surg Oncol 1991; 17:720–726.

Simon Ma, Ennekmg WF. The management of soft-tissue sarcomas of the extremities. J Bone Joint Surg 1976; 58A:317–327.

Sim FH, Taylor WF, Pritchard DJ, et al. Lymphadenectomy in the management of stage I malignant melanoma: a prospective randomized trial. Mayo Clin Proc 1986; 61:697–705.

Sim FH, Taylor WF, et al. A prospective randomized study of the efficacy of routine elective lymphadenectomy in management of malignant melanoma. Preliminary results. Cancer 1978; 41:948–956.

Slingluff CL Jr, Dodge RK, Stanley WE, et al. The annual risk of melanoma progression: implications for the concept of cure. Cancer 1992; 70:1917–1927.

Sloane JP. The value of typing basal cell carcinomas in predicting recurrence after surgical excision. Br J Dermatol 1977; 96:127–132.

Smeets NW, Kuijpers DI, Nelemans P, et al. Mohs' micrographic surgery for treatment of basal cell carcinomas of the face—results of a retrospective study and review of the literature. Br J Dermatol 2004; 151:141–147.

Soler AM, Warloe T, Berner A, Giercksky KE. A follow-up study of recurrence and cosmesis in completely responding superficial nodular basal cell carcinomas treated with methyl 5-aminoaevulinate-based photodynamic therapy along and with prior curettage. Br J Dermatol 2001; 145:467–471.

Stenquist B, Wennburg AM, Gisslen H, Larko O. Treatment of aggressive basal cell carcinoma with intralesional interferon: evaluation of efficacy by Mohs surgery. J Am Acad Dermatol 1992; 27:65–69.

Suit HD, Mankin HJ, Wood WC, et al. Treatment of the patient with stage M soft tissue sarcoma. J Clin Oncol 1988; 6: 854–862.

Tepper JE, Suit HD. Radiation therapy of soft tissue sarcomas. Cancer 1985; 55:2273–2277.

Thissen MR, Neumann MHA, Schouten LJ. A systematic review of treatment modalities for primary basal cell carcinomas. Arch Dermatol 1999; 135:1177–1183.

Thissen MR, Nieman FH, Ideler AH, Berretty PJ, Neumann HA. Cosmetic results of cryosurgery vs surgical excision for primary uncomplicated basal cell carcinomas of the head and neck. Dermatol Surg 2000; 26:759–764.

Thompson DB, Adena M, McLeod GR. Interferon alpha-2a does not improve response or survival when compared with dacarbazine in metastatic malignant melanoma: results of a multiinstitutional Australian randomized trial. Melanoma Res 1993; 3:133–138.

Thorn M, Ponten F, Berstrome, et al. Clinical and histopathologic predictors of survival in patients with malignant melanoma: a population-based study in Sweden. J Natl Cancer Inst 1994; 86:761–769.

Torre D. Cryosurgery of basal cell carcinoma. J Am Acad Dermatol 1986; 15:917–929.

Ven der Esch EP, Cascinelli N, Preda F, et al. C Stage I melanoma of the skin: evaluation of prognosis according to histologic characteristics. Cancer 1981; 48:1668–1673.

Veronesi U, Adamus J, Bandiera DC, et al. Stage I melanoma of the limbs: immediate versus delayed node dissection. Tumori 1980; 66:373–396.

Veronesi U, Adamus J, Bandiera DC, et al. Inefficacy of immediate node dissection in stage I melanoma of the limbs. N Engl J Med 1977; 297:627–630.

Veronesi U, Adamus J, Aubert C, et al. A randomized trial of adjuvant chemotherapy and immunotherapy in cutaneous melanoma. N Engl J Med 1982; 307:913–916.

Veronesi U, Cascinelli N. Narrow excision (1-cm margin): a safe procedure for thin cutaneous melanoma. Arch Surg 1991; 126:438–441.

Veronesi U, Cascinelli N, Adamus J, et al. Thin stage I primary cutaneous malignant melanoma. Comparison of excision with margins of 1 or 3 cm. N Engl J Med 1988; 318:1159–1162.

Verazin GT, Warneke JA, Driscoll DL, et al. Resection of lung metastases from soft-tissue sarcomas. Arch Surg 1992; 127:1407–1411.

Veronesi U, Adamus J, Bandiera DC, et al. Delayed regional lymph node dissection in stage I melanoma of the skin of the lower extremities. Cancer 1982; 49:2420–2430.

Vollmer RT. A multivariate analysis of prognostic factors. Pathol Ann 1989; 24:383–407.

Von Domarus H, Stevens PJ. Metastatic basal cell carcinoma. J Am Acad Dermatol 1984; 10:1043–1060.

Wang I, Bendsoe N, Klinteberg CA, et al. Photodynamic therapy vs. cryosurgery of basal cell carcinoma: results of a phase III clinical trial. Br J Dermatol 2001; 144:832–840.

Wilson BD, Mang TS, Stoll H, Jones C, Cooper M, Dougherty TJ. Photodynamic therapy for the treatment of basal cell carcinoma. Arch Dermatol 1992; 128:1597–1601.

Wilder RB, Shimrn DS, Kittelson JM, Shimm DS. Basal cell carcinoma treated with radiation therapy. Cancer 1991; 68:2134–2137.

Wilder RB, Shimrn DS, Kittelson JM, Rogoff EE, Cassady JR. Recurrent basal cell carcinoma treated with, radiation therapy. Arch Dermatol 1991; 127:1668–1672.

Wolf DJ, Zitelli JA. Surgical margins for basal cell carcinoma. Arch Dermatol 1987; 123:340–344.

Wong JH, Skinner KA, Kin KA, et al. The role of surgery in the treatment of nonregionally recurrent melanoma. Surgery 1993; 113:389–394.

Zacarian SA, ed. Cryosurgery for Skin Cancer and Cutaneous Disorders. In: St. Louis: CV Mosby, 1985.

Zeitels J, LaRossa D, Hamiliton R, et al. A comparison of local recurrence and resection margins for stage I primary cutaneous malignant melanomas. Plast Reconstr Surg 1988; 81:688–693.

Zitelli JA. Mohs surgery for melanoma. In: Mikhail GR, ed. Mohs Micrographic Surgery. Philadelphia: W.B Saunders, 1991:275–288.

Zitelli JA, Mohs FE, Snow S. Mohs micrographic surgery for melanoma. Dermatol Clin 1989; 7:833–843.

49

Skin Cancer in Organ Transplant Recipients

Clark C. Otley
Mayo Clinic, Rochester, Minnesota, U.S.A.

Henry W. Randle
Mayo Clinic, Jacksonville, Florida, U.S.A.

Stuart J. Salasche
University of Arizona Health Sciences Center, Tucson, Arizona, U.S.A.

INTRODUCTION

Organ transplantation offers the gift of life to over 25,000 patients with end-stage organ failure in the United States annually. The majority of these are renal allografts, followed by liver and heart transplants, with lesser number of multi-organ transplants and transplants of lung, pancreas, and intestine (Table 1). It is estimated that there are 150,000 organ-transplant recipients currently alive in the United States. Unfortunately, 81,262 people are on the transplant list awaiting allografts to become available and about 6000 die each year without having received an allograft. Organ donation numbers have increased only slightly over the past decade. The rise in transplantation rates is primarily due to the increased use of living related allografts from kidney and liver donors.

Patient and organ survival have increased substantially over the past two decades as a result of improved immunosuppressive regimens, better management of infectious diseases, and through the use of better human leukocyte antigen (HLA)-matched kidneys from cadaveric donors. In fact, over the past 20 years, the expected lifetime for a renal allograft has doubled. Cardiac transplantation results have drastically improved with estimated five-year survival rates of approximately 75%.

SCOPE AND ISSUES

The increased number of transplantations and improved survival translates into more patients with long-term immunosuppression for whom dermatologists will be caring. This takes the form of not only an increased number, variety and severity of skin infections, but more germane to this chapter, increased numbers and severity of the common and uncommon skin cancers. For many transplant patients, these cutaneous tumors can significantly affect their quality of life and even become fatal. The ensuing discussion will center on the causation, epidemiology, and management of these difficult tumors. Additionally, in the light of severely limited donor organs, dermatologists are being asked whether patients with preexisting skin cancers are acceptable candidates for transplantation.

Epidemiology of Skin Cancer in Organ Transplant Recipients

Organ transplant recipients have a three- to fourfold increased risk of malignancy compared with the general population. The most frequent cancers in the posttransplant setting are skin cancers as well as epithelial carcinomas of the cervix, urogenital, gastrointestinal, and upper aerodigestive tracts. Virally mediated cancers such as Kaposi's sarcoma and posttransplant lymphoproliferative disease are significantly on the increase as well.

High-quality standardized incidence ratio data quantify the increased risk of skin cancer in transplant patients (Table 2). Squamous cell carcinoma is increased 65-fold over that seen in the general population, and Kaposi's sarcoma is associated with a 84-fold increase. Squamous cell carcinoma of the lip is increased 20- to 38-fold, whereas basal cell carcinoma has a 10-fold increase and melanoma a 1.6- to 3.4-fold increase. Twenty-eight percent of transplant patients will develop skin cancer in any given year, with a mean number of squamous cell carcinomas of 1.85. Approximately 12% of transplant patients will develop greater than five squamous cell carcinomas per year, and occasional high-risk patients may develop 100 or more skin cancers per year, with a high risk of metastasis and death.

The incidence of squamous cell carcinoma is highly dependent on multiple factors including the geographic location of the patient population. Australian transplant patients have the highest rate of cutaneous carcinoma development, with 45% developing skin cancer within 10 years, whereas, patients in Holland, England, or Italy have a 10% to 15% incidence of skin cancer 10 years after transplantation. Additionally, the time to onset of skin cancer in Australia is shorter than in most temperate countries.

Well-defined phenotypic risk factors for the development of skin cancer have been identified including male gender, prior history of actinic keratosis and/or nonmelanoma skin cancer, blue or hazel eyes, birth in a tropical climate, older age, longer duration of immunosuppression, increased intensity of immunosuppression, fair skin, papilloma virus infection, and lower CD4 count. Additionally, cardiac transplant patients, being more immunosuppressed and of greater age than other patients, have a 2.9-fold

Table 1 Solid Organ Transplants in the United States, Annual Figures from United Network for Organ Sharing

Allograft type	Number of transplants
Kidney	15,138
Liver	5,671
Heart	2,057
Lung	1,085
Heart/lung	29
Intestine	116
Pancreas	502
Kidney/pancreas	870
Total	25,468

Source: From www.UNOS.org (2003).

increased risk of squamous cell carcinoma compared to renal transplant patients.

Specific subsets of patients with underlying end organ diseases that necessitated transplantation have greater susceptibility to skin cancer, including those with polycystic kidney disease, cholestatic liver disease, and cirrhosis. Patients with diabetes have a significantly lower risk of skin cancer.

The phenomenon of skin cancer in pediatric transplant patients is an emerging story. Of those transplanted at age 18 or younger, 20% had experienced skin cancer, as reported by Dr. Israel Penn. Skin cancers of the lip and melanoma were overrepresented in this young population, and the rates of metastasis and mortality were higher than that seen for skin cancer in adults.

The natural history of skin cancer in transplant patients is worse than that in non-immuno-suppressed patients. Whereas in the non-immuno-suppressed population, 3.6% of squamous cell carcinomas will metastasize within three years, in immunosuppressed transplant patients, the risk of metastatic disease from squamous cell carcinoma approximates at 7%.

Once metastasis has occurred, the prognosis is poor, with a series of 71 patients having a three-year cause-specific survival rate of 54%. In a study by Ong et al., squamous cell carcinoma in the posttransplant setting was shown to have an aggressive course, with 27% of deaths among Australian transplant patients due to skin cancer after the fourth year posttransplantation.

Pathogenetic Cofactors and Promoters

The primary pathogenetic factor responsible for the development of skin cancer in transplant-patients is ultraviolet radiation, which may act as both—an initiator as well as a promoter of skin cancer. Infection with human papilloma virus may be a cofactor that acts synergistically with ultraviolet radiation and immunosuppression to enhance development of skin cancer in transplant patients. The papilloma viruses responsible for this phenomenon are more likely to be those of the epidermodysplasia verruciformis family.

Immunosuppressive Medications

Transplantation of an allogeneic solid organ into another human-being is presently only possible with the administration of systemic immunosuppressive medications. Intense multiagent immunosuppression therapy is administered in the immediate posttransplant period to prevent acute allograft rejection by host immune mechanisms against foreign antigens in the transplanted organ. Potent induction therapy is tapered over three to six months to a lower maintenance level intended to prevent chronic rejection.

Early transplantation involved the administration of prednisone, azathioprine, and cyclophosphamide in the 1970s. With the introduction of cyclosporine in 1979, along with the use of anti-CD3 monoclonal antibody, survival rates significantly increased and have remained stable since that time. New immunosuppressants including mycophenolate mofetil, tacrolimus and sirolimus have been introduced into transplant protocols in the 1990s. The effect of these new immunosuppressive agents on skin cancer has not been as well studied as that of classic cyclosporine and azathioprine-based regimens.

Based on human and animal studies, it appears that the overall intensity of immunosuppression is more important in determining the risk of subsequent skin cancer than the use of any one particular agent is. As such, the use of triple immunosuppression with cyclosporine, azathioprine, and prednisone is associated with higher rates of skin cancer development than two-agent regimens utilizing cyclosporine and prednisone or azathioprine and prednisone. It is important to recognize, however, that al log raft survival is superior with cyclosporine-based regimens. Therefore, the effect on an allograft survival must be considered when analyzing the risk-benefit ratio of an agent in the pathogenesis of skin cancer.

The importance of intensity of immunosuppression in the pathogenesis of skin cancer is emphasized by a study by Dantal, in which patients were randomized to either low or high trough levels of cyclosporine one year after renal allograft receipt. Patients with low trough levels of cyclosporine experienced more rejection episodes, but these were all manageable, with identical overall and allograft survival rates. There were fewer overall cancers including solid tumors and lymphomas as well as skin cancers in the cohort treated with low-dose cyclosporine. Therefore, intensity of immunosuppression can directly affect the development of cancer in the posttransplant period.

The relative contributions to skin cancer pathogenesis are more difficult to decipher with the numerous new immunosuppressant medications including deoxyspergualin, leflunomide, mizoribine, and brequinar. Nevertheless, the move away from azathioprine toward mycophenolate mofetil and the move from cyclosporine to mixed cyclosporine and tacrolimus usage has been motivated by transplantation considerations but may have an effect on the incidence of skin cancer in the future. The theoretical antitumor effects of rapamycin remain to be definitively established. Steroids have a immune potentiating effect with studies by Karagas demonstrating a 2.31-fold increase in squamous cell carcinoma and a 1.49-fold increase in basal cell carcinoma in

Table 2 Standardized Incidence Ratios of Skin Cancer in Solid Organ Allograft Recipients

Tumor type	Standardized incidence ratio
Squamous cell carcinoma	65-fold increase
Squamous cell carcinoma of lip	20 to 38-fold increase
Basal cell carcinoma	10 fold increase
Melanoma	1.6 to 3.4-fold increase
Kaposi's sarcoma	84-fold increase

nontransplant patients treated with chronic systemic steroids versus controls.

Management of Transplant-Associated Skin Cancer

Before and after solid-organ transplantation, all patients should be provided with continuous educational reinforcement about the increased risk of skin cancer development and sun protective prevention practices. A randomized trial has demonstrated that repetitive physician-directed written educational reinforcement may increase the sun protective behavior of solid-organ transplant recipients. Despite this finding, noncompliance of self-examination and paucity of knowledge of skin cancer risk and preventative measures have been documented multiple times in organ transplant recipients.

In an attempt to deliver preventative measures and identify high-risk patients earlier in the transplantation process, many transplant centers have integrated dermatologic care within the structure of their transplant units. Within these transplant dermatology clinics, risk factor assessment identifies patients at an increased risk for skin cancer and intensive preventative education and administration of prophylactic medications is targeted towards high-risk patients.

Monthly self-skin examination as well as regular examination of the skin by physicians should be encouraged. The frequency of dermatologic examination should be increased in those with more advanced sun damage as outlined in the International Transplant Skin Cancer Collaborative Guidelines.

The management of individual skin cancers in the posttransplant setting is based on standard skin cancer management principles. Aggressive treatment of actinic keratosis with cryotherapy, and topical treatments such as 5-fluorouracil cream, photodynamic therapy, topical retinoids, immune-response modifiers, and diclofenac should be aggressively pursued to minimize the risk of progression into cancer. Individual tumors are managed according to traditional principles with increased diligence. Minor skin cancers can often be treated with electrodessication and curettage or curettage and cryotherapy. Some patients prefer excisional surgery due to the lesser healing time. High-risk skin cancers are optimally managed with Mohs micrographic surgery, which affords the highest cure rate and permits tissue sparing. Radiation is often reserved for particularly high-risk tumors such as those associated with perineural invasion or as adjuvant therapy for metastatic nodal disease. Guidelines for the treatment of transplant-associated skin cancer have been created by the International Transplant Skin Cancer Collaborative and are available in published form.

When confronted with accelerating cutaneous carcinogenesis manifested by the development of numerous skin cancers per year, additional considerations for therapy include reduction of immunosuppression and the administration of prophylactic systemic retinoids. The reduction of immunosuppression may provide a less hospitable environment for the development of skin cancer, and the rationale for this strategy has been outlined in a recent review. Most physicians reduce the dosage of the antimetabolite (i.e., azathioprine and mycophenolate mofetil) rather than the calcineunin inhibitor (i.e., cyclosporine and tacrolimus). However, significant reduction of immunosuppression may be associated with risks of rejection, and therefore, this strategy should only be pursued in conjunction with and directed by a patient's primary transplant physician.

The addition of systemic retinoids may effectively suppress the development of skin cancer, albeit with the potential for unpleasant adverse effects. The landmark study by Bouwes Bavinck randomized 44 renal transplant patients with extensive cancerous and precancerous changes to acitretin 30 mg per day versus placebo for six months. Eleven percent of the acitretin-treated patients developed squamous cell carcinoma versus 47% of placebo patients. There was no renal dysfunction associated with this regimen. Other studies have supported this finding, although the degrees to which patients tolerate systemic retinoids are variable. Aggressive prevention and management of mucocutaneous side effects and initiation of therapy with low-dose retinoids titrating up to efficacy and tolerance are the optimal ways to enhance compliance. Beginning therapy at 10 mg of acitretin a day and then increasing to 25 mg four days per week after one month is tolerated by the majority of patients. Daily acitretin will be more difficult for patients to tolerate, although efficacy will be greater with daily dosing. Many patients will not tolerate a dosage of 50 mg daily of acitretin for chemoprevention. Occasional laboratory abnormalities including hyperlipidemia and elevated liver function tests will be noted and often are responsive to lipid-lowering agents and reduction of dosage, with laboratory safety monitoring. Both reduction of immunosuppression and systemic retinoids are usually considered when patients develop between 5 and 10 skin cancers per year, or when confronted by metastatic skin cancer.

In some patients, catastrophic skin cancer develops, with more than 100 squamous cell carcinomas occurring annually and an associated high risk of metastasis and mortality. Reduction of immunosuppression and administration of systemic retinoids is highly encouraged in these patients, and aggressive repetitive tumor removal every two to eight weeks may be necessary. These high-risk patients may require surgical removal of large numbers of skin cancers at sessions, made easier with the administration of adjuvant sedative or analgesic medications.

Throughout the treatment of the numerous skin cancers in these patients, attention must be kept on the possibility that a single high-risk skin cancer could prove lethal. Based on the meta-analysis by Rowe et al., key features that identify high-risk squamous cell carcinomas include the presence of perineural spread, depth greater than 4 mm, size larger than 2 cm, poor differentiation, previous treatment, and location in high-risk areas such as the ear or lip. For a tumor with multiple overlapping risk factors for metastasis, consideration may be given to sentinel lymph node biopsy or adjuvant radiation.

For metastatic squamous cell carcinoma to the regional lymph nodes, surgical lymphadenectomy can be curative when involvement is limited. This highlights the importance of regular nodal examination and early intervention for metastatic disease. In cases of multiple nodal positivity or extracapsular spread, therapeutic complete lymph node dissection along with adjuvant radiation therapy offers the best chance of control. As mentioned above, reduction of immunosuppression and administration of systemic chemosuppressive retinoids should be considered in these situations.

There are multiple special clinical situations seen in transplant patients that merit emphasis. Patients may develop extensive involvement of their dorsal hands and scalp by confluent hyperkeratotic actinic keratoses with intermixed squamous cell carcinoma. Because of the confluent nature of the field neoplasia, traditional spot treatments such as cryotherapy may be relatively ineffective. In these cases, field treatments with topical 5-fluoruoracil chemotherapy cream or immune response modifiers such as imiquimod may offer a more comprehensive approach to treatment. The safety of immune-responsive modifiers in immunosuppressed transplant patients is the subject of ongoing investigations, but there have been no reported associations between their use and acute or chronic rejection. For extensively involved hands, total excision of the dorsal hand skin with thick split-thickness skin grafts can be a way to eliminate the atypia. Auricular squamous cell carcinoma may prove particularly threatening in transplant patients given the thin skin on the ears and the propensity to invade into cartilage with limited penetration. Likewise, lip carcinoma may have an increased risk of metastasis and is often associated with diffuse actinic cheilitis.

When Not to Transplant a Patient with Prior Skin Cancers

Because skin cancers are so common, patients being considered for organ transplantation not infrequently have a history of prior skin cancer. The overwhelming majority of these patients with tumors are of low risk and therefore, this incidence of previous history should not be a significant consideration for deciding as to whether or not to proceed with the transplant. Patient education and appropriate follow up monitoring after transplantation should be adequate. At the opposite extreme, candidates with active metastatic disease should not be considered for listing.

However, there is a small cohort of patients with a history of high-risk tumors who may be harboring undetectable, occult micrometastases that could potentially propagate and disseminate after institution of posttransplant immunosuppression and lead to death. Several retrospective studies have demonstrated poor outcomes from patients with a pretransplant history of high-risk skin cancer in whom there is a recurrence after transplantation.

In order to ethically distribute the limited number of donor organs, the transplant community works under the assumption that is best not to transplant someone with comorbidities that would lead to death with a functioning transplant. Some high-risk melanomas, uncommon squamous cell carcinomas, and some Merkel cell carcinomas fall into that category. A second consideration in this equation is when the tumor occurred prior to transplant, as the risk for metastasis dissipates with time. For squamous cell carcinoma, the timeframe for metastasis is relatively rapid, with 90% of the metastases occurring within three years. Therefore, after three years pass, patients who are disease-free from squanous cell carcinoma have only 10% of their metastatic risk remaining and can reasonably be reevaluated and considered for listing. Detailed Kaplan Meier survival curves are available for melanoma to guide dermatologists regarding the suitability of a given candidate based on the Breslow thickness, ulceration, level, sentinel lymph node status and when the melanoma was treated in relation to consideration for allograft.

CONCLUSION

The management of skin cancer in solid-organ transplant recipients is at once a matter of satisfaction aswell as a challenge. A true multidisciplinary approach is necessary involving the input of transplant medicine, dermatologic surgery, dermatopathology, dermatology, otorhinolaryngology, plastic surgery, ophthalmology, radiation oncology, medical oncology, and radiology. Preventative education and reinforcement is absolutely essential. Intensive sun protection measures and regular surveillance as well as aggressive treatment of precursor lesions are of paramount importance. The International Transplant Skin Cancer Collaborative, whose website is www.itscc.org., is actively pursuing research advances to enhance the care of these deserving patients.

BIBLIOGRAPHY

Adamson R, Obispo E, Dychter S, et al. High incidence and clinical course of aggressive skin cancer in heart transplant patients: a single-center study. Transplant Proc 1998; 30(4): 1124–1126.

Bavinck JN, De Boer A, Vermeer BJ, et al. Sunlight, keratotic skin lesions and skin cancer in renal transplant recipients. Br J Dermatol 1993; 129(3):242–249.

Bavinck JN, Tieben LM, Van der Woude FJ, et al. Prevention of skin cancer and reduction of keratotic skin lesions during acitretin therapy in renal transplant recipients: a double-blind, placebo-controlled study. J Clin Oncol 1995; 13(8):1933–1938.

Bellman BA, Eaglstein WH, Miller J. Low dose isotretinoin in the prophylaxis of skin cancer in renal transplant patients. Transplantation 1996; 61(1):173.

Ben-Hur H, Ben-Meir A, Hagay Z, et al. Tumor-preventive effects of the soluble p53 antigen on chemically-induced skin cancer in mice. Anticancer Res 1998; 18(6A):4237–4241.

Berg D, Otley CC. Skin cancer in organ transplant recipients: epidemiology, pathogenesis, and management. J Am Acad Dermatol 2002; 47:1–17.

Besnard V, Euvrard S, Kanitakis J, et al. Kaposi's sarcoma after liver transplantation. Dermatology 1996; 193(2):100–104.

Blohme I, Larko O. No difference in skin cancer incidence with or without cyclosporine—a 5-year perspective. Transplant Proc 1992; 24(1):313.

Bouwes Bavinck JN, Handie DR, Green A, et al. The risk of skin cancer in renal transplant recipients in Queensland, Australia. A follow-up study. Transplantation 1996; 61(5):715–721.

Bouwes Bavinck JN, Vermeer BJ, van der Woude FJ, et al. Relation between skin cancer and HLA antigens in renal-transplant recipients. N Engl J Med 1991; 325(12):843–848.

Butt A, Roberts DL. Renal transplant recipients and protection from sun: need for education. Lancet 1997; 349(9046):179–180.

Carpenter CB. Improving the success of organ transplantation. N Engl J Med 2000; 342(9):647–648.

Carucci JA, Martinez JC, Zeitouni NC, et al. In-transit metastasis from primary cutaneous squamous cell carcinoma in organ transplant recipients and nonimmunosuppressed patients: clinical characteristics, management, and outcome in a series of 21 patients. Dermatol Surg 2004; 30(4 Pt 2):651–655.

Cassisi NJ, Dickerson DR, Million RR. Squamous cell carcinoma of the skin metastatic to parotid nodes. Arch Otolaryngol 1978; 104(6):336–339.

Christenson LJ, Geusau A, Ferrandiz C, et al. Specialty clinics for the dermatologic care of solid-organ transplant recipients. Dermatol Surg 2004; 30(4 Pt 2):593–603.

Clowers-Webb HE, Christenson LJ. Phillips PK, et al. Educational outcomes regarding skin cancer in organ transplant recipients: randomized intervention of intensive vs. standard education. Arch Dermatol 2006; 142:712–718.

Cowen EW, Billingsley EM. Awareness of skin cancer by kidney transplant patients. J Am Acad Dermatol 1999; 40(5 Pt 1): 697–701.

Czarnecki D, Watkins F, Leahy S, et al. Skin cancers and HLA frequencies in renal transplant recipients. Dermatology 1992; 185(1):9–11.

Dantal J, Hourmant M, Cantarovich D, et al. Effect of long-term immunosuppression in kidney-graft recipients on cancer incidence: randomised comparison of two cyclosporin regimens. Lancet 1998; 351(9103):623–628.

De Graaf YG, Euvrard S, Bouwes Bavinck JN. Systemic and topical retinoids in the management of skin cancer in organ transplant recipients. Dermatol Surg 2004; 30(4 Pt 2):656–661.

de Jong-Tieben LM, Berkhout RJ, ter Schegget J, et al. The prevalence of human papillomavirus DNA in benign keratotic skin lesions of renal transplant recipients with and without a history of skin cancer is equally high: a clinical study to assess risk factors for keratotic skin lesions and skin cancer. Transplantation 2000; 69(1):44–49.

DiGiovanna JJ. Retinoid chemoprevention in the high-risk patient. J Am Acad Dermatol 1998; 39(2 Pt 3):S82–S85.

Dyall-Smith D, Ross JB. Cutaneous malignancies in renal transplant recipients from Nova Scotia, Canada. Australas J Dermatol 1995; 36(2):79.

Edwards NM, Rajasinghe HA, John R, Chen JM, Itescu S, Mancini DM. Cardiac transplantation in over 100 patients: a single institution experience from Columbia University. Clin Transpl 1999:249–261.

Epstein E, Epstein NN, Bragg K, Linden G. Metastases from squamous cell carcinomas of the skin. Arch Dermatol 1968; 97(3):245–251.

Espana A, Redondo P, Fernandez AL, et al. Skin cancer in heart transplant recipients. J Am Acad Dermatol 1995; 32(3):458–465.

Euvrard S, Kanitakis J, Pouteil-Noble C, et al. Aggressive squamous cell carcinomas in organ transplant recipients. Transplant Proc 1995; 27(2):1767–1768.

Euvrard S, Kanitakis J, Pouteil-Noble C, et al. Comparative epidemiologic study of premalignant and malignant epithelial cutaneous lesions developing after kidney and heart transplantation. J Am Acad Dermatol 1995; 33(2 Pt 1):222–229.

Euvrand S, Ulrich C, Lefrancois N. Immunosuppressants and skin cancer in transplant patients: focus on rapamycin. Dermatol Surg 2004; 30(4 Pt 2):628–633.

Euvrard S, Kanitakis J, Cochat P, Claudy A. Skin cancers following pediatric organ transplantation. Dermatol Surg 2004; 30(4 Pt 2):616–621.

Euvrard S, Verschoore M, Touraine JL, et al. Topical retinoids for warts and keratoses in transplant recipients. Lancet 1992; 340(8310):43–49.

Euvrard S, Kanitakis J, Claudy A. Skin cancers after organ transplantation. N Engl J Med 2003; 348:1681–1691.

Ferrandiz C, Fuente MJ, Ribera M, et al. Epidermal dysplasia and neoplasia in kidney transplant recipients. J Am Acad Dermatol 1995; 33(4):590–596.

Fortina AB, Caforio AL, Piaserico S, et al. Skin cancer in heart transplant recipients: frequency and risk factor analysis. J Heart Lung Transplant 2000; 19(3):249–255.

Frezza EE, Fung JJ, van Thiel DH. Non-lymphoid cancer after liver transplantation. Hepatogastroenterology 1997; 44(16):1172–1181.

Gjersvik P, Hansen S, Moller B, et al. Are heart transplant recipients more likely to develop skin cancer than kidney transplant recipients? Transpl Int 2000; 13(suppl 1):S380–S381.

Glover MT, Deeks JJ, Raftery MJ, Cunningham J, Leigh IM. Immunosuppression and risk of non-melanoma skin cancer in renal transplant recipients. Lancet 1997; 349(9049):398.

Glover MT, Niranjan N, Kwan JT, Leigh IM. Non-melanoma skin cancer in renal transplant recipients: the extent of the problem and a strategy for management. Br J Plast Surg 1994; 47(2):86–89.

Hartevelt MM, Bavinck JN, Kootte AM, Vermeer BJ, Vandenbroucke JP. Incidence of skin cancer after renal transplantation in The Netherlands. Transplantation 1990; 49(3):506–509.

Hariharan S, Johnson CP, Bresnahan BA, Taranto SE, Mclntosh MJ, Stablein D. Improved graft survival after renal transplantation in the United States, 1988 to 1996. N Engl J Med 2000; 342(9):605–612.

Hiesse C, Larue JR, Kriaa F, et al. Incidence and type of malignancies occurring after renal transplantation in conventionally and in cyclosporine-treated recipients: single-center analysis of a 20-year period in 1600 patients. Transplant Proc 1995; 27(4):2450–2451.

Hojo M, Morimoto T, Maluccio M, et al. Cyclosporine induces cancer progression by a cell-autonomous mechanism. Nature 1999; 397(6719):530–534.

Holmkvist KA, Roenigk RK. Squamous cell carcinoma of the lip treated with Mohs micrographic surgery: outcome at 5 years. J Am Acad Dermatol 1998; 38(6 Pt 1):960–966.

Jain AB, Yee LD, Nalesnik MA, et al. Comparative incidence of de novo nonlymphoid malignancies after liver transplantation under tacrolimus using surveillance epidemiologic end result data. Transplantation 1998; 66(9):1193–1200.

Jensen P, Hansen S, Moller B, Leivestad T, Pfeffer P, Fauchald P. Are renal transplant recipients on CsA-based immunosuppressive regimens more likely to develop skin cancer than those on azathioprine and prednisolone?. Transplant Proc 1999; 31(1–2):1120.

Jensen P, Hansen S, Moller B, et al. Skin cancer in kidney and heart transplant recipients and different long-term immunosuppressive therapy regimens. J Am Acad Dermatol 1999; 40(2 Pt 1):177–186.

Johnson TM, Rowe DE, Nelson BR, Swanson NA. Squamous cell carcinoma of the skin (excluding lip and oral mucosa). J Am Acad Dermatol 1992; 26(3 Pt 2):467–434.

Jonas S, Rayes N, Neumann U, et al. De novo malignancies after liver transplantation using tacrolimus-based protocols or cyclosporine-based quadruple immunosuppression with an interleukin-2 receptor antibody or antithymocyte globulin. Cancer 1997; 80(6):1141–1150.

Kelly GE, Meikle W, Sheil AG. Effects of immunosuppressive therapy on the induction of skin tumors by ultraviolet irradiation in hairless mice. Transplantation 1987; 44(3):429–434.

Kovach BT, Murphy G, Otley CC, et al. Oral rectinoids for chemoprevention of skin cancer in organ transplant recipients: results of a survey. Transplant Proc 2006; 38:1366–1368.

Kraemer KH, DiGiovanna JJ, Peck GL. Chemoprevention of skin cancer in xeroderma pigmentosum. J Dermatol 1992; 19(11):715–718.

Kraemer KH, DiGiovanna JJ, Moshell AN, Tarone RE, Peck GL. Prevention of skin cancer in xeroderma pigmentosum with the use of oral isotretinoin. N Engl J Med 1988; 318(25): 1633–1637.

Lampros TD, Cobanoglu A, Parker F, Ratkovec R, Norman DJ, Hershberger R. Squamous and basal cell carcinoma in heart transplant recipients. J Heart Lung Transplant 1998; 17(6):586–591.

Lennard L, Thomas S, Harrington Cl, Maddocks JL. Skin cancer in renal transplant recipients is associated with increased concentrations of 6-thioguanine nucleotide in red blood cells. Br J Dermatol 1935; 113(6):723–729.

Levine N. Role of retinoids in skin cancer treatment and prevention. J Am Acad Dermatol 1998; 39(2 Pt 3):S62–S66.

Levine N, Moon TE, Cartmel B, et al. Trial of retinol and isotretinoin in skin cancer prevention: a randomized, double-blind, controlled trial. Southwest Skin Cancer Prevention Study Group. Cancer Epidemiol Biomarkers Prev 1997; 6(11):957–961.

Lindelof B, Sigurgeirsson B, Gabel H, Stem RS. Incidence of skin cancer in 5356 patients following organ transplantation. Br J Dermatol 2000; 143(3):513–519.

Lippman SM, Parkinson DR, Itri LM, et al. 13-cis-retinoic acid and interferon alpha-2a: effective combination therapy for advanced squamous cell carcinoma of the skin. J Natl Cancer lnst 1992; 84(4):235–241.

London NJ, Farmery SM, Will EJ, Davison AM, Lodge JP. Risk of neoplasia in renal transplant patients. Lancet 1995; 346(6972):403–406.

Martinez JC, Otley CC, Euvrard S, Arpey CJ, Stasko T. Complications of systemic retinoid therapy in organ transplant recipients with squamous cell carcinoma. Dermatol Surg 2004; 30(4 Pt 2):662–666.

Marks R. Skin cancer in organ transplant patients: from a side effect of social practice to a side effect of medical practice. Dermatol Surg 2004; 30(4 Pt 2):593–594.

Martinez JC, Otley CC, Okuno SH, Foote RL, Kasperbauer JL. Chemotherapy in the management of advanced cutaneous squamous cell carcinoma in organ transplant recipients: theoretical and practical considerations. Dermatol Surg 2004; 30(4 Pt 2):679–686.

Mazariegos GV, Reyes J, Marino IR, et al. Weaning of immunosuppression in liver transplant recipients. Transplantation 1997; 63(2):243–249.

McKenna DB, Murphy GM. Skin cancer chemoprophylaxis in renal transplant recipients: 5 years of experience using low-dose acitretin. Br J Dermatol 1999; 140(4): 656–660.

McKerrow KJ, MacKie RM, Lesko MJ, Pearson C. The effect of oral retinoid therapy on the normal human immune system. Br J Dermatol 1988; 119(3):313–320.

Moloney FJ, Kelly PO, Kay EW, Conlon P, Murphy GM. Maintenance versus reduction of immunosuppression in renal transplant recipients with aggressive squamous cell carcinoma. Dermatol Surg 2004; 30(4 Pt 2):674–678.

Moon TE, Levine N, Cartmel B, et al. Effect of retinol in preventing squamous cell skin cancer in moderate-risk subjects: a randomized, double-blind, controlled trial. Southwest Skin Cancer Prevention Study Group. Cancer Epidemiol Biomarkers Prev 1997; 6(11):949–956.

Naldi L, Fortina AB, Lovati S, et al. Risk of nonmelanoma skin cancer in Italian organ transplant recipients. A registry-based study. Transplantation 2000; 70(10):1479–1484.

Naylor MF, Boyd A, Smith DW, Cameron GS, Hubbard D, Neldner KH. High sun protection factor sunscreens in the suppression of actinic neoplasia. Arch Dermatol 1995; 131(2):170–175.

Odom R. Managing actinic keratoses with retinoids. J Am Acad Dermatol 1993; 39(2 Pt 3):S74–S78.

Ong CS, Keogh AM, Kossard S, Macdonald PS, Spratt PM. Skin cancer in Australian heart transplant recipients. J Am Acad Dermatol 1999; 40(1):27–34.

Otley CC. Organization of a specialty clinic to optimize the care of organ transplant recipients at risk for skin cancer. Dermatol Surg 2000; 26(7):709–712.

Otley CC, Salasche SJ, Ulrlch C, Stockfleth E. Transplant oncology—challenges and opportunities. Dermatol Surg 2004; 30(4 Pt 2):591.

Otley CC, Maraugh SLH. Reduction of immunosuppression for transplant-associated skin cancer: rationale and evidence of efficacy. Dermatol Surg. In press.

Otley CC, Coldiron BM, Stasko T, Goldman GD. Decreased skin cancer after cessation of therapy with transplant-associated immunosuppressants. Arch Dermatol 2001; 137(4):459–463.

Penn I. Post-transplant malignancy: the role of immunosuppression. Drug Saf 2000; 23(2):101–113.

Penn I. Post-transplant malignancies in pediatric organ transplant recipients. Transplant Proc 1994; 26(5):2763–2765.

Penn I. Malignant melanoma in organ allograft recipients. Transplantation 1996; 61(2):274–278.

Penn I. The effect of immunosuppression on pre-existing cancers. Transplantation 1993; 55(4):742–747.

Ramos HC, Reyes J, Abu-Elmagd K, et al. Weaning of immunosuppression in long-term liver transplant recipients. Transplantation 1995; 59(2):212–217.

Ramsay HM, Fryer AA, Reece S, Smith AG, Harden PN. Clinical risk factors associated with nonmelanoma skin cancer in renal transplant recipients. Am J Kidney Dis 2000; 36(1): 167–176.

Randle HW. The historical link between solid-organ transplantation, immunosuppression, and skin cancer. Dermatol Surg 2004; 30(4 Pt 2):595–597.

Robinson JK. Behavior modification obtained by sun protection education coupled with removal of a skin cancer. Arch Dermatol 1990; 126(4):477–481.

Robinson JK, Rigel DS. Sun protection attitudes and behaviors of solid-organ transplant recipients. Dermatol Surg 2004; 30(4 Pt 2):610–615.

Rook AH, Jaworsky C, Nguyen T, et al. Beneficial effect of low-dose systemic retinoid in combination with topical tretinoin for the treatment and prophylaxis of premalignant and malignant skin lesions in renal transplant recipients. Transplantation 1995; 59(5):714–719.

Rowe DE, Carroil RJ, Day CL Jr. Prognostic factors for local recurrence, metastasis, and survival rates in squamous cell carcinoma of the skin, ear, and lip. Implications for treatment modality selection. J Am Acad Dermatol 1992; 26(6):976–990.

Servila KS, Burn ham DK, Daynes RA. Ability of cyclosporine to promote the growth of transplanted ultraviolet radiation-induced tumors in mice. Transplantation 1987; 44(2): 291–295.

Seukeran DC, Newstead CG, Cunlrffe WJ. The compliance of renal transplant recipients with advice about sun protection measures. Br J Dermatol 1993; 138(2):301–303.

Shamanin V, zur Hausen H, Lavergne D, et al. Human papillomavirus infections in nonmelanoma skin cancers from renal transplant recipients and nonimmunosuppressed patients. J Natl Cancer Inst 1996; 88(12):802–811.

Sheil AG, Disney AP, Mathew TH, Amiss N. De novo malignancy emerges as a major cause of morbidity and late failure in renal transplantation. Transplant Proc 1993; 25(1 Pt 2): 1333A.

Sheil AG. Development of malignancy following renal transplantation in Australia and New Zealand. Transplant Proc 1992; 24(4):1275–1279.

Shimm DS. Parotid lymph node metastases from squamous cell carcinoma of the skin. J Surg Oncol 1938; 37(1):56–59.

Shuttleworth D, Marks R, Griffin PJ, Salaman JR. Treatment of cutaneous neoplasia with etretinate in renal transplant recipients. Q J Med 1988; 63(257):717–725.

Smith KJ, Hamza S, Skelton H. Histologic features in primary cutaneous squamous cell carcinomas in immunocompromised patients focusing on organ transplant patients. Dermatol Surg 2004; 30(4 Pt 2):634–641.

Stasko T, Brown MD, Caaicci JA, et al. Guidelines for the management of squamous cell carcinoma in organ transplant recipients. Dermatol Surg 2004; 30(4 Pt 2):642–650.

Stockfleth E, Nindl I, Sterry W, et al. Human papillomaviruses in transplant-associated skin cancers. Dermatol Surg 2004; 30(4 Pt 2):604–609.

Tangrea JA, Edwards BK, Taylor PR, et al. Long-term therapy with low-dose Isotretinoin for prevention of basal cell carcinoma: a multicenter clinical trial. Isotretinoin-Basal Cell Carcinoma Study Group. J Natl Cancer Inst 1992; 84(5):328–332.

Tan SR, Tope WD. Effect of acitretin on wound healing in organ transplant recipients. Dermatol Surg 2004; 30(4 Pt 2):667–673.

Taylor BW Jr., Brant TA, Mendenhall NP, et al. Carcinoma of the skin metastatic to parotid area lymph nodes. Head Neck 1991; 13(5):427–433.

Thome EG. Long-term clinical experience with a topical retinoid. Br J Dermatol 1992; 127(suppl 41):31–36.

Transplant Patient Data Source (February 16, 2000). Richmond, VA: United Network for Organ Sharing. Retrieved August 2, 2001 from the World Wide Web: http://www.patients.unos.org/data.htm.

Ulrich C, Schmook T, Sachse MM, Sterry W, Stockfleth E. Comparative epidemiology and pathogenic factors for nonmelanoma skin cancer in organ transplant patients. Dermatol Surg 2004; 30(4 Pt 2):622–627.

United States Renal Transplant Mycophenolate Mofetil Study Group. Mycophenolate mofetil in cadaveric renal transplantation. Am J Kidney Dis 1999; 34(2):296–303.

van Zuuren EJ, Posma AN, Scholtens RE, Vermeer BJ, van der Woude FJ, Bouwes Bavinck JN. Resurfacing the back of the hand as treatment and prevention of multiple skin cancers in kidney transplant recipients. J Am Acad Dermatol 1994; 31(5 Pt 1):760–764.

Veness MJ, Quinn Dl, Ong CS, et al. Aggressive cutaneous malignancies following cardiothoracic transplantation: the Australian experience. Cancer 1999; 85(8):1753–1764.

Webb MC, Compton F, Andrews PA, Koffman CG. Skin tumours posttransplantation: a retrospective analysis of 28 years experience at a single centre. Transplant Proc 1997; 29(1–2):828–830.

www.UNOS.org.

50

Wound Healing by Second Intention

John A. Zitelli
Shadyside Medical Center, Pittsburgh, Pennsylvania, U.S.A.

INTRODUCTION

People have always searched for ways to improve wound healing, particularly to decrease pain and speed the time needed for complete healing. In ancient mythology, Aesculapius, the Greek god of healing, Ningishzida, a Babylonian god of healing, and Hermes, the Roman Mercury, were symbolized with a staff entwined with one or two snakes. The significance of the snake was its ability to repeatedly shed and regenerate its skin, a capability envied by physicians of the day.

The quest for a better understanding of wound healing has continued slowly. Some ancient methods of wound management such as wet linen wraps are similar to more modern methods of occlusive or semiocclusive dressings. Although Hippocrates advocated that wounds be kept dry, most wounds were covered with fat- or oil-based ointment after being washed in wine or vinegar. Wound management took a step backward during medieval times when it was common to treat open wounds with hot coals and caustic substances that we now recognize delay wound healing. The concept of asepsis resulted in more control of wound healing than any other approach, and as a science, wound healing became the primary interest of surgeons. However, in the last few decades, clinical and basic science research in dermatology has significantly contributed to our understanding of cutaneous wound healing so that we can better enhance this process.

NORMAL EVENTS OF WOUND HEALING

Normal wound healing is a complex series of events occurring simultaneously in the epidermis, dermis, and subcutaneous tissue. It is easy to differentiate epidermal healing from dermal healing, although it is important to remember that the events occur at the same time (Fig. 1).

Dermal Wound Healing

Wound healing begins when an injury to the skin causes bleeding. Extravasated blood clots rapidly and forms an insoluble, water-holding gel matrix of fibrin, fibronectin, and platelets as well as blood cells. Exposure of collagen to Hageman factor XII activates the coagulation pathway; fibrinogen is activated to form fibrin, and platelets are activated releasing platelet-derived growth factors and chemoattractants for connective tissue cells. For wounds created without bleeding (burns, cryosurgery), other mechanisms such as activation of complement and stimulation of the cellular immune response may participate in the first phase of wound healing.

Serum factors such as fibronectin, laminin, and vasoactive amines (i.e., kinin) are also important in attracting polymorphonuclear leukocytes (PMNs) and maintaining increased vascular permeability. Fibrin and fibronectin are very important proteins in healing wounds. As vascular permeability increases, serum proteins, including fibrin and fibronectin, enter the extravascular space. Together fibrin and fibronectin form the initial wound matrix. Fibrin in the matrix is covalently cross-linked to provide strong tensile strength. Later, as normal vascular permeability is restored, fibroblasts appear and begin synthesizing fibrin and fibronectin to maintain the integrity of the matrix while monocytes, endothelial cells, and epidermal cells migrate into the wound.

Inflammatory Phase

The inflammatory phase of wound healing is defined as the period where the effects of chemical mediators and inflammatory cells predominate. The inflammatory phase in a sutured wound may go unrecognized, lasting only four to five days with mild redness and swelling. In a clean open wound, the inflammatory phase is characterized by a copious exudate lasting 7 to 10 days, or longer in wounds complicated by the presence of denatured protein or necrotic tissue caused by infection, laser, electrosurgery, cryosurgery, topical acids, or caustics. Clinically, this is the period when an open wound is best managed with adsorbent dressings or more frequent dressing changes than those required during later stages of wound healing.

The inflammatory phase of wound healing begins when vasoactive substances are released from platelets or mononuclear cells, or when complement is activated in the initial events of healing. These signals increase vascular permeability, and with specific leukocyte chemotactic factors stimulate polymorphonuclear cell migration into the wound. Within hours, PMNs are the predominant inflammatory cell around the wound, although their function is not clear. They may play a role in preventing infection as well as debriding the wound of necrotic tissue by enzymatic digestion and phagocytosis of debris. However, it is known that wounds in neutropenic animals heal in a normal fashion and, therefore, PMNs may only be useful in complicated wounds.

Lymphocytes are also a prominent cell in the inflammatory infiltrate of wounds, first appearing after 6 to 12 hours. Although activated T-cells release factors chemotactic for fibroblasts, their role is poorly understood. Wounds in lymphopenic animals heal well also.

The most important cell orchestrating the events of wound healing is the monocyte. Unlike neutropenic or

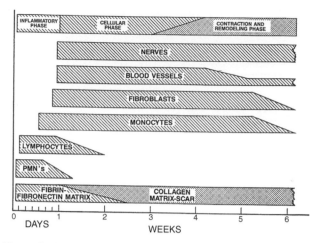

Figure 1 Normal events of dermal wound healing. *Abbreviation*: PMNs, polymorphonuclear leukocytes.

lymphopenic animals, animals depleted of monocytes do not heal normally. The monocyte comes from the blood and migrates into the wound after four to five days. The stimulus for monocyte migration includes platelet factors, cell-derived chemotactins, and fibrin. The monocyte continues many of the functions of the neutrophil including phagocytosis and debridement, but, more importantly, it releases factors (monokines) that control subsequent events in healing. Monokines attract more monocytes and fibroblasts, stimulate fibroblast replication and collagen synthesis, and stimulate angiogenesis. Under altered conditions in vitro, the monocyte can also inhibit fibroblast collagen synthesis, which suggests that monocytes may control the signal that halts wound healing as well. Clinically, any drug or condition that alters monocyte function may affect wound healing.

Cellular Phase

Transition from the inflammatory phase to the cellular phase of wound healing is characterized in a clean, open, second intention wound by a decrease in exudate as the vascular permeability returns to normal. Healthy granulation tissue appears to be composed of monocytes, fibroblasts, and numerous capillaries. This usually occurs after 7 to 10 days. In a sutured wound, this phase may also go unnoticed.

The fibroblasts, which first appear on day 5, begin to replicate under the continued stimulation of monokines. New fibroblasts continue to migrate into the wound under the stimulus of fibrin and fibronectin. Ground substance is produced and collagen synthesis occurs, peaking at six to seven days and continuing for two to four weeks. The collagen is synthesized intracellularly and is secreted extracellularly as fibrils in a random and haphazard fashion. As new collagen is formed, it is deposited on preexisting fibrin. The initial fibrin-fibronectin gel matrix is replaced and eventually transformed into a dense collagen matrix: scar tissue. As extracellular collagen cross-linking occurs, wound tensile strength slowly increases.

Monocytes also stimulate proliferation of endothelial cells, and vessel growth is stimulated by low oxygen tension and high lactate concentrations derived from cellular metabolism in the wound. This new vessel growth occurs simultaneously with fibroblast proliferation and synthesis of collagen and ground substance and allows the delivery of

oxygen and nutrients as well as disposal of toxic by-products of wound metabolism.

The cellular phase, therefore, begins as monocytes and fibroblasts, and new vessels predominate with the appearance of granulation tissue and a decrease in wound exudate. Granulation tissue expands to fill the wound. Later this is replaced with new collagen covered with epidermis, which essentially regenerates the lost skin.

Wound Contraction

Wound contraction is a phase of wound healing that overlaps the cellular phase. A decrease in the size of the wound begins after seven days but is usually not noticed clinically until 14 days. The most important cell responsible for wound contraction is the myofibroblast, a fibroblast containing large amounts of actin and myosin filaments. Granulation tissue is rich in myofibroblasts and contains as much actinomyosin per gram of tissue as the uterus from a pregnant rat. After two weeks these myofibroblasts line up end-to-end, exerting tension on the margins, pulling toward the center. This results in a decrease in the size of the wound and teleologically minimizes the area to be repaired and the time to complete wound healing.

In wounds closed primarily, ordinary synthetic fibroblasts predominate and myofibroblasts are rare. No specific biochemical or cellular stimulus has been found to account for the transformation of ordinary fibroblasts to myofibroblasts. However, some findings have pointed to inflammatory cells or by-products of inflammatory cells as the stimuli to the induction of myofibroblasts. This evidence includes the parallel, temporal relationship of inflammatory cells to myofibroblasts in the sequence of events of healing, and the finding of most myofibroblasts near to inflammatory foci of wounds. However, the stimulus to form myofibroblasts is yet to be elucidated.

The control of wound contraction is difficult. In vitro studies of collagen lattices populated with fibroblasts in Petri dishes have shown that the collagen lattices contract when fibroblasts differentiate toward myofibroblasts. This contraction may be inhibited by drugs such as dilantin, cytochalasin B, and steroids. Other drugs have also been shown to influence wound contraction, such as colchicine, smooth muscle antagonists (thiphenamil), and vinblastine. In theory, contraction might be inhibited without affecting wound healing by using a combination of steroids and vitamin A. Steroids inhibit contraction and epithelialization, while vitamin A reverses the adverse effects of epithelialization but does not reverse steroidal inhibition of contraction. However, the clinical effect of these drugs has been poor, and, other than delaying wound contraction, they seem to have no significant clinical usefulness.

Indirect methods have been used to control wound contraction. These include skin flaps and grafts because contraction of wounds repaired in this fashion is minimal. It appears that the presence of reticular dermis is important to inhibit contraction. While wounds repaired with full-thickness skin grafts contract very little, split-thickness skin grafts with very little reticular dermis will contract approximately 40%. Superficial wounds, into papillary dermis alone, which heal by second intention, contract very little, while full-thickness wounds devoid of reticular dermis contract significantly. This may be explained by the finding of myofibroblasts in the reticular dermis but not in the superficial papillary dermis.

Guiding sutures may affect this process by allowing the surgeon to control the direction of wound contraction.

(A) 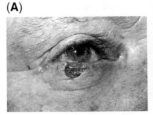 **(B)** 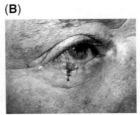 **(C)**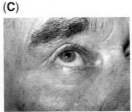

Figure 2 Guiding sutures to control wound contraction. **(A)** A full-thickness wound on the eyelid and lid margin. **(B)** Guiding absorbable sutures placed across the wound increase the laxity in the vertical direction. **(C)** Final result. An ectropion may have occurred with uncontrolled wound contraction.

Sutures pulled across the wound edges in one direction will create laxity in the direction perpendicular to the sutures and will, therefore, minimize any deformity caused by contraction in that direction. Thus, guiding sutures are useful to prevent ectropion, distortion of the brow, lip, or ala nasi (Fig. 2).

During the cellular phase of wound healing, nerve regeneration also takes place. For superficial wounds, reinnervation starts in three days from the edge and the base of the wound. After two weeks, some hyperinnervation is present, and by four to five weeks, sensation is normal. In full-thickness wounds healed by second intention, return of sensory function is slow and often incomplete, particularly in large wounds.

Wound Remodeling

Wound contraction continues through the cellular phase into the remodeling phase. Even after the wound is covered with the epidermis, contraction continues. Later, wound remodeling may correct some deformities caused by wound contraction such as ectropion, mild contractures, and distortion of adjacent structures.

Once an open wound is covered, the scar is still red from the dense network of capillaries. During the remodeling phase, these capillaries regress and the red color and mild persistent edema associated with the early scar formation diminish. Fibroblast proliferation slows and gradually the scar becomes relatively acellular. Remodeling of collagen continues for many months. Cross-linking continues, and as the original collagen is digested and replaced, bundle orientation occurs in an organized fashion, aligned parallel to the vector of stress in the skin. Thus, both cross-linking and bundle reorientation add to the slow increase in tensile strength noted over the first six months. Collagen remodeling is also responsible for some relaxation of wound contraction. When wound contraction has caused distortion of an adjacent structure, remodeling may allow partial or complete return of that structure to a normal position. This is desirable in some locations such as the ala nasi or lip. In other situations this is undesirable, such as when continued pull across a wound causes a narrow scar to widen.

Epidermal Healing

Reepithelialization begins rapidly after wounding. Within 12 hours of epidermal injury, changes in the epidermal cell morphology and function occur. Cells at the wound margin cease to form keratin and prepare for cell migration and proliferation. The earliest cells that begin to cover the wound are not newly divided cells but suprabasal cells that move over into the position of a basal cell. This migration of suprabasal to basal cell position occurs before mitosis and cell division. These migrating basal cells begin to proliferate and form new suprabasal cells that again migrate toward the center of the wound. No single cell travels across the entire wound; instead, the process of migration and mitosis allows for epidermal healing.

In full-thickness wounds, the epidermal parent cells are located only at the margin, and this leapfrog migration and mitosis must occur over the entire surface. In partial-thickness wounds, parent epidermal cells are found in transected appendages such as hair follicles and sebaceous and eccrine ducts. Thus, in partial-thickness wounds, reepithelialization begins not only at the wound margin but also at the transected pores of these appendages within the wound. This reduces the distance that epidermal cells must migrate, and allows for more rapid reepithelialization.

The factors that initiate, maintain, and halt reepithelialization are complex and poorly understood. Epithelial migration may be stimulated by serum factors such as epibolin (serum spreading factor), epidermal growth factor, and platelet-derived growth factor. In addition, it has been suggested that the epidermis is normally controlled by epidermally derived chalones, or factors that inhibit proliferation and migration. Wounding the epidermis may inhibit chalone production and release the epidermis from the inhibition. Once reepithelialization is complete, chalone synthesis resumes and proliferation is once again inhibited. Other theories suggest that epidermal injury allows circulating stratum corneum antibodies to bind to the exposed stratum corneum, activate complement, and signal the beginning of epidermal repair.

An important factor in epidermal healing is substrate. Epidermis will only migrate over substrates of type-I collagen, fibronectin, or basement membrane components such as laminin or type IV and V collagen. Epidermal cells will not migrate over a dry crust, desiccated collagen, neutrophils, and wound debris. The most important concept in epidermal wound healing is providing the proper substrate for epidermal migration. This includes a clean wound without denatured protein or necrotic debris, and a moist environment to maintain a viable substrate. An air-dried wound or a wound treated with topical alcohol, many hemostatics, caustics, lasers, electrosurgery, or cryosurgery will result in nonviable eschar. The new epidermal cells must slowly digest the eschar, wasting both energy and time required for reepithelialization.

Just as dermal wound healing continues after reepithelialization is complete, epidermal healing also continues after reepithelialization is complete. The process of contact inhibition may end epidermal migration, but epidermal maturation continues. The new epidermis is capable of rapidly forming stratum corneum, and thus the important barrier function is retained. However, new epidermis has few rete ridges and the attachment of the dermis is weak. Clinically, this is characterized by epidermal fragility, easy bruising, and blister formation. In addition, melanocyte repopulation and function is often incomplete. Partial-thickness wounds repopulate with functional melanocytes more quickly than full-thickness wounds. However, appropriate melanocyte function often lags behind repopulation. Clinically, this is seen as hypo- or hyperpigmentation, especially when the newly populated and immature melanocytes are stimulated by ultraviolet light, chemicals, or hormones (i.e., diazepam or estrogen). Full-thickness wounds do not quickly repopulate with melanocytes and, therefore, are usually hypopigmented for months, or permanently. In some patients, even large full-thickness wounds eventually repigment from the margins, but in most patients the ability of pigment to reappear is limited.

Final Result

The final result of any wound is a scar. A well-planned incision and closure should result in a fine line scar level with the skin and camouflaged by normal skin lines. If the wound is superficial (epidermis and papillary dermis only), true regeneration occurs so that clinically and histologically there is little or no evidence of scarring. The epidermis reforms its rete pegs and is quickly repopulated by melanocytes. Skin texture, color, and function all return to normal.

Deeper dermal or full-thickness second intention wounds leave a more noticeable scar with abnormal function compared to normal skin. The new dermis has disordered collagen bundles and a sparse vascular network with few or no melanocytes in the new epidermis, so that the scar appears white. The altered vascular network often results in widely dilated superficial vessels, appearing as prominent telangiectasias. Finally, the scar lacks the elastic properties and tensile strength of normal dermis. Langerhans cell function may be altered in large scars, resulting in a local immune surveillance defect that may be responsible for the higher incidence of skin cancer in old scar tissue.

Therefore, only epidermal healing is truly regenerative. Deeper dermal wounds result in new skin that has both an altered appearance and function compared with normal skin (Fig. 3).

Kinetics

Understanding the kinetics of wound healing has important clinical implications. The kinetics of sutured wounds healing by primary intention differs from open clean wounds healing by second intention. Each type of wound will be considered separately here.

Primary Intention Healing

The most important aspect of healing by primary intention is tensile strength. Reepithelialization occurs rapidly and has little clinical significance except that sutures should be removed to prevent epithelial-lined sinus tracts migrating into the dermis except around the suture.

The tensile strength of a wound develops slowly. At four to five days, when sutures are removed, collagen synthesis has not peaked and the wound edges are held together by fibrin. The tensile strength is less than 5% of normal skin. Sutures are removed at this time to prevent permanent suture marks, but there is enough strength to keep the skin edges together and everted without sutures if the wound is supported with adhesive strips and excess stress is avoided. Tensile strength is related more to collagen cross-linking than collagen synthesis. By three weeks (or longer in acral areas), 20% of normal tensile strength is present, usually enough to prevent dehiscence. In acral areas or when there is excess stress on the wound, special sutures or splinting techniques (i.e., running buried subcutaneous sutures) may be required to avoid complications. These wounds never have more than 80% of the tensile strength of normal skin, although the reduced strength of a scar is rarely a problem (Fig. 4).

Second Intention Healing

The kinetics of second intention healing are often misunderstood but are clinically important. The healing of partial-thickness wounds is related only to reepithelialization. In these superficial wounds, there are many reservoirs

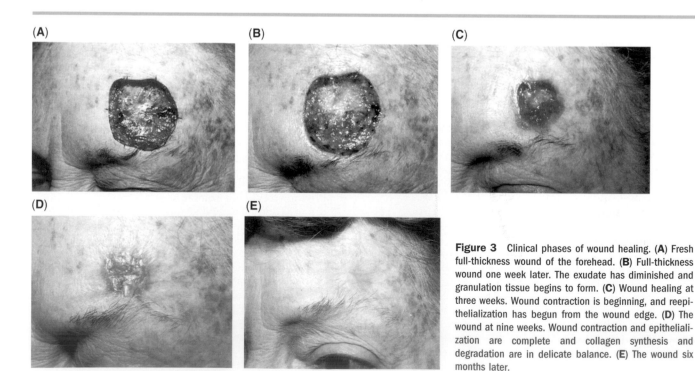

(A)　　**(B)**　　**(C)**

(D)　　**(E)**

Figure 3 Clinical phases of wound healing. **(A)** Fresh full-thickness wound of the forehead. **(B)** Full-thickness wound one week later. The exudate has diminished and granulation tissue begins to form. **(C)** Wound healing at three weeks. Wound contraction is beginning, and reepithelialization has begun from the wound edge. **(D)** The wound at nine weeks. Wound contraction and epithelialization are complete and collagen synthesis and degradation are in delicate balance. **(E)** The wound six months later.

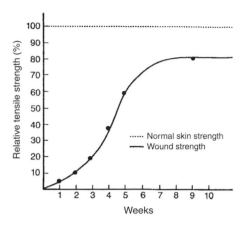

Figure 4 Wound tensile strength increases slowly after wounding, with less than 10% of normal strength present at the time of suture removal and a maximum of only 80% of the strength of normal skin. *Source*: From Zitelli (1987).

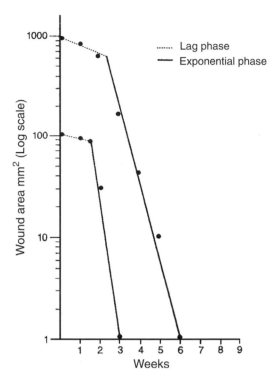

Figure 5 Healing time is proportional to the log of area, and thus large wounds often heal faster than expected. Wound size changes slowly during the first one or two weeks (lag phase) until entering the exponential phase. *Source*: From Zitelli (1987).

of epidermis in the transected adnexal structures. After an initial lag period, the rate of epidermal movement is constant as the epidermis moves from one adnexal structure to the next. Therefore, healing time is not proportional to the size of the wound, but to the density of adnexal structures. For example, large and small superficial wounds heal more quickly on the face where adnexae are close together than on the trunk or extremities where the adnexae are sparse.

For full-thickness wounds, however, a number of factors influence the healing time. During the first week of healing, there is no change in the size of the wounds. Sometimes local swelling and elastic recoil of surrounding skin actually result in the wounds enlarging. This is called the lag period and correlates with the inflammatory, exudative phase of wound healing. Later, healing occurs at a constant rate: the exponential phase.

Effect of Wound Size

One misconception is that the healing time for full-thickness wounds is directly proportional to the size of the wound. One might imagine that a 16 cm wound would take 16 times longer to heal than a 1 cm wound. However, weekly plots of wound area in full-thickness wounds document that healing time instead is related to the logarithm of the wound area; thus larger wounds take only slightly longer to heal than smaller wounds (Fig. 5). More realistically, if a 10 cm wound (10 to the first power) takes five weeks to heal, a 100 cm wound (10 to the second power) will take only twice as long—10 weeks (the log of the larger wound is twice that of the smaller wound). More simply put, because the healing time is proportional to the logarithm of the area and the area is a function of the log of the radius, the best predictor of healing time is the width of the wound. Clinically, it makes little sense to treat a 6 cm lesion in four sessions, each time destroying a 3 × 3 cm quadrant, when total wound healing time would be half as long if one treated the entire lesion at once.

Effect of Wound Shape

Other variables are important, including wound location, shape, method of wounding, and skin temperature. The effect of wound shape is often misunderstood. Hippocrates taught that circular wounds were difficult or impossible to heal. Some surgeons purposely transformed circular wounds into stellate-shaped wounds to quicken the healing time. However, their perceptions were inaccurate because the rate of wound closure is independent of wound shape. A long, thin elliptical wound will heal in less time than a circular wound of the same area only because the wound edges are closer together. Thus, although the rate of wound edge migration is the same in both shapes, the relationship of healing time to shape is best described as being dependent on the diameter of the largest circle that can be contained within the wound margins (Fig. 6). Enlarging the wound by altering its shape will not expedite healing time.

Effect of Wound Location

Location is a variable that will significantly affect healing time. Wounds of identical size, depth, and shape made on the face and leg will heal in different times. Generally, wounds in acral locations take longer to heal than more centrally located wounds, and wounds on the face heal most quickly. Although the reasons for this are unknown, it has been observed that the lag period before the exponential phase of healing is longer in acral areas (Fig. 7).

FACTORS AFFECTING WOUND HEALING

The search for better methods of managing wounds created by war or accident has led to our understanding of the importance of asepsis and improved surgical techniques. More recently, the search has continued in sophisticated laboratories for chemical factors or natural hormones that might enhance healing. While we still have no true method of enhancing wound healing, many factors, if uncontrolled, might slow wound healing.

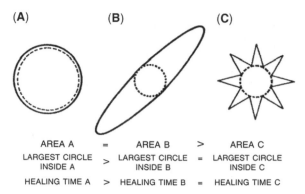

(A)   (B)   (C)

AREA A	=	AREA B	>	AREA C
LARGEST CIRCLE INSIDE A	>	LARGEST CIRCLE INSIDE B	=	LARGEST CIRCLE INSIDE C
HEALING TIME A	>	HEALING TIME B	=	HEALING TIME C

Figure 6 Healing time is related not only to wound area but also to wound shape. Healing time is best related to the diameter of the largest circle that can fit inside the wound margins. Although the area of A and B are equal, the largest circle fitting within wound A (*dotted line*) is greater than the largest circle within wound B and corresponds to the greater healing time for wound A. Similarly, although the area of wound B is larger than wound C, the diameter of the largest circle within each wound is the same, and the healing times will be similar. *Source*: From Zitelli (1987).

Method of Healing

One important variable that can be controlled is the method of wounding. The most rapid healing occurs in a wound devoid of denatured proteins, necrotic debris, or infection. Wound healing is delayed if the lag phase is prolonged while necrotic debris is digested or while epidermis migrates under a dry, denatured collagen crust. Thus, slower healing times for wounds of identical size and location will occur if the wound was created by cryosurgery, electrosurgery, laser surgery, hot cautery (Shaw scalpel), or acids. Slower healing will also occur if the wound is further

damaged by caustics, some antiseptics such as gentian violet, and many commonly used hemostatic agents. X-irradiation of the skin 24 hours before or after wounding significantly inhibits healing, although radiation of a healing wound after two weeks does not seem to retard healing.

Wound Temperature

Lower than normal temperature slows wound healing. Wounds in rabbits subjected to hypothermia or cold environments take longer to achieve expected wound tensile strength. Patients should be instructed to avoid low temperatures during the postoperative period while wound tensile strength increases.

Infection

Infection will delay healing time for an open wound and will delay the development of tensile strength in a sutured wound. Because treatment of wound infection is important, recognition of infection is also important. However, signs of infection are often confused with normal signs of healing.

Bacterial wound infection is defined as the presence of greater than 10,000 organisms/g tissue in a wound with clinical signs of infection. Organisms present at lower concentrations may represent only surface contaminants and not affect wound healing. The clinical signs of wound infection include redness more than 3 to 5 mm from the sutured wound margin, swelling, purulent discharge, pain, fever, or other systemic symptoms. Healing does not occur without inflammation, so all surgical wounds are tender. In open wounds, early signs of infection may be difficult to detect, especially if a dry crust or necrotic debris is present. When a swollen wound becomes painful, and exudate and redness are excessive, a diagnosis of infection is made. Quantitative bacteriologic study to determine if more than 10,000 organisms are present in a gram of tissue is impractical. Cultures are important only to determine the type of bacteria and antibiotic sensitivity, once the clinical diagnosis is made.

Colonization of wounds by resident flora does not interfere with wound healing. Colonization by *Staphylococcus aureus* does not adversely affect healing unless the organism is present at high levels, when a yellowish exudate is often seen. Herpes simplex infection is recognized as a complication of dermabrasion wounds. Yeasts, especially *Candida*, are often overlooked as wound pathogens and should also be considered pathogenic. Their presence should be considered in a tender, open wound that is not healing after three to five weeks with topical antibiotic ointments and semiocclusive dressings. The diagnosis can often be made by microscopic examination of the wound surface exudate, which demonstrates pseudophyphae and budding yeasts, and can be confirmed by culture. Topical antimycotic creams will allow the wound to resume normal healing.

Drugs

Steroids are probably the most potent and commonly used drugs that affect wound healing. Steroids inhibit wound healing and delay the development of tensile strength if given before or during the first three days after wounding. This is due to inhibition of migration of the important monocyte. After three days, high-dosage steroids (40 mg/day prednisone) are necessary to effect fibroplasia and collagen remodeling. Topical steroids also inhibit wound healing. Fluorinated compounds are most potent, while 1% hydrocortisone has little or no effect.

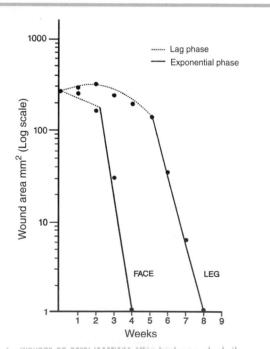

Figure 7 Wounds on acral locations often heal more slowly than wounds on the face. Once in the exponential phase, healing occurs at the same rapid rate. *Source*: From Zitelli (1987).

The inhibition of healing by steroids may be reversed by the systemic administration of vitamin A (25,000 IU/day), although the therapeutic effects of the steroid may then be affected. To reverse steroid inhibition locally, investigators have recommended the topical application of vitamin A or retinoic acid. It is curious that vitamin A administration will not reverse steroid inhibition of wound contraction, suggesting that a combination of the two drugs may be a way to control wound contraction.

One might also suspect that immunosuppressive and antineoplastic drugs would interfere with wound healing because of their role in inhibiting inflammatory cell function. Some laboratory evidence suggests that drugs such as actinomycin D, bleomycin, or BCNU are more likely to impair healing than methotrexate, 5-fluorouracil, or cyclophosphamide. However, clinical studies have shown no impairment in wound healing when resections of internal malignancies were accompanied by adjuvant chemotherapy using combinations of thiotepa, nitrogen mustard, cyclophosphamide, 5-fluorouracil, actinomycin D, or chlorambucil. The benefits of these drugs are likely to outweigh the theoretical risk of impairing wound healing.

Other drugs have been reported to have adverse effects on cell function or biochemical pathways of cells important in wound healing. Nonsteroid anti-inflammatory drugs such as aspirin and phenylbutazone decrease tensile strength of wounds in animals, but extrapolation of these findings to humans, has not been documented. It is important for patients to avoid these drugs because of their effect on platelet function, causing an increased risk of bleeding or hematoma formation.

Vitamins A, C, E, and minerals (zinc, copper, iron, and manganese) all have important functions in wound healing. Deficiencies in these substances affect collagen synthesis, collagen cross-linking, and the ability to generate superoxides to kill bacteria. Wound healing in patients who are deficient in these vitamins and minerals will be enhanced by supplementation. This is important to remember in older patients with prolonged illness. Otherwise, vitamin-mineral supplementation of otherwise healthy patients will not improve wound healing.

COMPLICATIONS

Occasionally, wound healing is complicated or influenced by systemic or external factors. If we can appropriately manage or avoid these problems, wound healing may continue in a normal course.

Seborrheic Dermatitis

The most common cause of widespread erythema and even superficial erosions surrounding the wound is acute seborrheic dermatitis. The clinical picture is similar to acute contact dermatitis because it often occurs under the dressing. Patch testing is negative, and it occurs in patients with preexisting seborrheic dermatitis. This usually occurs in locations characteristic for seborrheic dermatitis (midface, periauricular region, scalp, and upper trunk). It can also be confused with infection, but the eruption is not painful and responds quickly to topical steroids. Later, after the scar matures, seborrheic dermatitis may be localized to the scar surface itself (Fig. 8).

Excess Granulation

The formation of granulation tissue in an open wound is necessary before reepithelialization takes place. Occasionally,

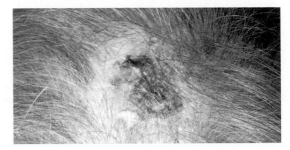

Figure 8 Seborrheic dermatitis in a scar.

however, granulation tissue continues to form unchecked until a large nodule or even a pedunculated mass accumulates on the wound bed. This is more common in wounds managed by total occlusion or stimulated by embedded hair or other foreign bodies, but often occurs for no apparent reason. Management of this complication should first be directed at removing any external stimulus such as plucking or shaving hairs and removing unnecessary suture material or other foreign bodies.

It is a common practice to remove excess granulation tissue by curettage or application of caustics such as silver nitrate, even though there is no evidence that this procedure is effective. To ascertain the value of this practice, excess granulation tissue was removed from one-half of each of five wounds. In two cases, the granulation tissue was pedunculated and hung over the healing wound edge. In both these cases, the area healed rapidly where granulation tissue was excised. In the remaining three cases, wound granulation extended above the level of the skin, but did not overhang the skin edge. In these cases, removal of half the granulation tissue did not improve the wound-healing rate (Fig. 9). If removal of granulation tissue is done, it is most reasonable to use a curet or scalpel. The capillary oozing stops rapidly with pressure. Other techniques such as silver nitrate, rewound the site and produce an eschar of denatured material that must be digested and, therefore, delays wound healing.

Hypertrophic Scars and Keloids

Hypertrophic scars and keloids are uncommon complications of superficial wounds but are not uncommon in full-thickness wounds, particularly in certain locations. The event that signals an end to wound healing is unknown, although some evidence suggests that monocytes may be involved. In any case, the cell responsible for hypertrophic and keloidal scars appears to be the myofibroblast. In sutured wounds or wounds covered with full-thickness and even split-thickness grafts, the proliferation of myofibroblasts is inhibited. In open wounds, the myofibroblast appears shortly after the fibroblasts, five days after wounding. Normally, some balance exists between fibroblasts, myofibroblasts, collagen synthesis, and collagen degradation. When this balance is altered, a keloid or hypertrophic scar may result from a more cellular, metabolically active scar. Fibroblasts cultured from keloids are similar to fibroblasts from normal skin. No conclusive difference in the characteristics of collagen has been found. Keloids have a higher density of mast cells, which may be important because histamine stimulates cell growth. It also explains the pruritus often noted in keloids and early hypertrophic scars.

(A)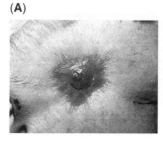

(B)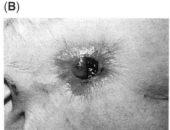

(C)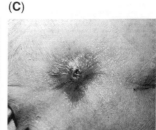

Figure 9 Excision of excess granulation tissue. **(A)** Excess granulation tissue during healing of a full-thickness wound. **(B)** Excision of the medial half with a scalpel. **(C)** Appearance one week later: no apparent effect from excision of granulation tissue. *Source:* From Zitelli (1984).

Prevention and control of keloids and hypertrophic scars are difficult. Wound location is an important factor in predicting the likelihood of keloids and hypertrophic scar formation. On the face, hypertrophic scars are most likely to occur on convex surfaces such as the cheek, chin, upper lip, or side of the nose. Keloids are most common on the earlobes, upper trunk, and deltoid areas. With this in mind, surgery in these areas should be done using techniques known to inhibit myofibroblasts such as primary closure, skin flaps, and grafts. Gentle surgical manipulation minimizes skin necrosis and inflammation. Healing by second intention encourages myofibroblast growth and should be avoided in these areas.

Controlling these complications in open wounds after myofibroblasts have appeared is more difficult. Intralesional steroids are the most effective approach. Occlusive topical dressings such as silashe sheets over prolonged periods (months) will help to resolve hypertrophic scars. Other techniques such as laser surgery have theoretical advantages but have been of little practical help. Drugs affecting fibroblast growth and collagen metabolism such as colchicine and beta-amino proprionitrile are being studied.

Wound Fragility (Blisters, Erosions, and Delayed Bleeding)

As the epidermis migrates over newly formed dermis in second intention healing, the cohesive bonds are not mature and the epidermal attachment is easily broken, resulting in blisters after epithelialization is complete or nearly complete; this may also happen in the first few months after the wound has healed. It is more likely to occur in locations where the skin is least mobile such as the forehead or scalp and is very common in the center of scars greater than 10 cm. It may be caused by very minor trauma, particularly shearing forces, or by injury from removing adhesive-backed wound dressings that adhere more strongly to the epidermis than the epidermis adheres to the dermis. It also can occur with the use of hydrogen peroxide, which releases oxygen under enough pressure to lift the epidermis. The cause of the epidermal fragility is unclear, but some evidence suggests that it may be due to the lack of anchoring fibrils and epidermal rete peg architecture. It is important to recognize this potential complication and warn patients to avoid trauma. This avoids confusion over the cause of erosions, which may easily be considered as infection or recurrence of tumor following tumor surgery.

Delayed bleeding is also related to wound fragility. Although most postoperative bleeding occurs within the first 24 hours, spontaneous bleeding may occur in sutured wounds up to one week later and is related to clot lysis in larger vessels before collagen synthesis and cross-linking seals them adequately. In open wounds, delayed bleeding may occur after the wound is epithelialized, presenting as subepidermal ecchymoses. It may also be due to fragile, immature capillaries, and small vessels that rupture with minor trauma. Recognition of these complications allows the physician to reassure the patient that no significant problem exists.

The Nonhealing Wound

The nonhealing wound is a significant problem in some patients. The mechanisms of wound healing discussed so far pertain to normal healthy tissues, but occasionally pathologic processes, either systemic or local, affect these mechanisms and cause an interruption in normal healing.

An approach to the nonhealing wound should first include a search for correctable causes. This includes evaluation and treatment of infection, including organisms often overlooked and not detected by normal bacterial culture techniques such as anerobic bacterial infection, mycobacteria, spirochetes, viruses, yeasts, fungi, and protozoa. A skin biopsy with additional studies such as immunofluorescence, if indicated, is an important tool. Allergic contact dermatitis to many topically applied wound remedies is not uncommon. The patient may also be applying agents other than those prescribed by the doctor. A careful history may reveal these home remedies. Nutritional factors in malnourished or chronically ill patients require protein and vitamin-mineral supplementation. Drugs such as glucocorticoids and penicillamine may delay wound healing, but they rarely prevent wounds from healing. Malignant and large benign tumors may ulcerate and masquerade as a nonhealing wound until skin biopsy confirms the correct diagnosis. Other diseases may produce chronic ulcers or erosions; these include pyoderma gangrenosum, Behçet's disease, and some blistering disorders. Arterial vascular occlusion may produce peripheral ulcers alone or in combination with other disorders such as scleroderma, Raynaud's disease, Buerger's disease, embolic disease, or severe vasculitis.

Two of the most common and frustrating causes of nonhealing wounds include decubitus ulcers and venous hypertension ulcers of the leg. The goal in treating decubitus ulcers is to remove the prolonged pressure on the skin that results in necrosis. Management is complex and involves treating complications such as secondary infection, nutritional deficiencies, and good wound care, which often requires tissue replacement with local flaps. Chronic leg ulcers from venous hypertension are also a frustrating problem. The mechanism of ulcer formation is unclear, but fibrin deposits around capillaries and venules that block the perfusion of oxygen and nutrients are thought to be important in the pathogenesis of these ulcers. Again, treatment is complex and requires good wound management and an attempt to reverse or prevent additional accumulation of fibrin around the vessels.

There are numerous uncorrectable disorders in which abnormal healing may occur. Atrophy and ulceration may occur in tissue deprived of pain, temperature, and light touch. This is common after transection of the trigeminal nerve but may occur after transection of other sensory nerves. In addition, inherited disorders of connective tissue may present with abnormal wound healing. However, when no apparent reason for a nonhealing wound can be found, factitial ulcers should be considered.

CLINICAL CORRELATIONS: WOUND MANAGEMENT

Applying the basics of wound healing to clinical practice minimizes complications and provides better control over wound healing. This can be translated into a number of useful guidelines for wound management in dermatologic surgery. For convenience, these guidelines are classified into primary and second intention healing even though the events of healing are similar for both types of wound management.

First Intention Healing

Wounds to be sutured are usually clean, without necrotic debris. Aseptic surgical technique reduces the chance of wound infection, which would delay healing and increase the likelihood of wound dehiscence and scar spreading. Chlorhexidine is a favorite presurgical scrub because its antiseptic action persists for days and it is active in the presence of serum or blood.

Intraoperatively, attention should be paid to careful hemostasis. Hemostasis induced by electrosurgery, cautery, or suture ligature always produces tissue necrosis. Wound healing can occur normally with small amounts of necrosis. However, if there is extensive necrosis, healing is delayed while inflammatory cells digest the necrotic tissue and replace it with granulation tissue, collagen, and scar. For dermatologic surgery, a fine-tipped needle is best, especially when applied to a dry field. Larger vessels require suture ligation rather than deep, extensive electrocoagulation. Hemostasis is also achieved with a pressure dressing applied for 24 hours. This will help to eliminate dead space until fibrin glues the tissue together. Because fibrin has little tensile strength and collagen synthesis does not peak for five days, physical activity should be restricted until the wound has stabilized by collagen cross-linking and achieved adequate tensile strength. This may take two weeks for facial wounds closed without tension, or five to six weeks on extremities, especially if the wound edge was closed with tension.

Good suturing technique is important to minimize complications and enhance both healing and the final cosmetic result. Multilayered suture techniques are more effective than a single layer of skin sutures. Buried intradermal sutures have a number of important functions. They effectively minimize dead space that leads to hematoma and seroma, and they provide prolonged wound support. Because sutures are removed five to seven days after surgery to prevent cross-hatching when the wound has only 3% of eventual tensile strength, the additional support provided by the buried sutures is important to prevent scar spread. Buried sutures also help to evert wound edges. As wound remodeling and contraction occurs, an everted wound will contract and result in a flat, unnoticeable scar. Without wound edge eversion, the scar contracts below the level of the surrounding skin, creating shadows and a more noticeable scar.

Knowledge of the events of healing is important when choosing suture material as well as timing suture removal. Wounds closed under considerable tension, or when prolonged support is needed (acral areas), or in patients taking systemic steroids, should be closed with buried sutures that are nonabsorbable (nylon, Prolene) or have prolonged tensile strength (Vicryl, Dexon, PDS). In addition, skin sutures may be left in place longer than normal. A running subcuticular suture technique can be used to minimize the chance of permanent suture marks when sutures need to be left in place for longer than one week.

After suture removal, external splinting with tape provides additional support until tensile strength increases. During this time, exercise that stretches the skin should be avoided to minimize scar spreading. Patients are usually more tolerant of red suture lines or minor distortion if they are informed that the redness will fade and slight tissue protrusions or displacements will resolve as remodeling occurs over three to six months.

Second Intention Healing

Dermatologic surgery is unique because of the various surgical techniques used to treat skin lesions. These techniques often result in wounds managed by second intention healing and include chemical destruction, cryosurgery, electrosurgery, laser surgery, punch biopsy, curettage, and tangential scalpel excision. Dermatologists also manage many nonsurgical erosive or ulcerative skin lesions for which guidelines for wound management are useful.

Today, wound management is best summarized by "wet is best." Semiocclusive dressings provide the best environment for wound healing. Even in a wound that has been allowed to air dry, a crust eventually forms, and wound healing occurs at the top of the moist portion of the wound under the crust. Of course, this slows wound healing and occurs at the expense of deepening the wound by the desiccated, denatured collagen lost when the crust is formed. Despite voluminous literature on the advantages of occlusive wound management, many physicians still recommend antiseptic tinctures, alcohol washes, and air exposure. These methods have at least three major problems: (i) enhanced tissue necrosis and deepening of the wound because of alcohol fixation and air desiccation of tissue, (ii) slow healing because the epidermis is forced to migrate under the crust, and (iii) increased pain.

Topical Agents

Topical agents are frequently applied to wounds for hemostasis, antisepsis, and to promote healing. However, many agents used for topical hemostasis delay wound healing. Ferric subsulfate (Monsel's solution) and aluminum chloride 30% both cause delays in healing and slightly larger, less cosmetically acceptable scars. Topical silver nitrate, trichloracetic acid, and oxidized cellulose, likewise, cause additional tissue damage and delay wound healing.

Topical gelatin and collagen cause little or no damage to the wound and only interfere with healing if large amounts are placed in superficial wounds. Collagen sponge matrices may enhance the healing of full-thickness wounds. A safe topical hemostatic is thrombin, but the safest is simple temporary pressure until natural hemostatic mechanisms stop bleeding.

Many popular antiseptic agents are also toxic. Chlorhexidine (0.5%), 1% povidone-iodine (Betadine), 0.5%

sodium hypochlorite (Daiken solution), 0.2% acetic acid, and 3% hydrogen peroxide are highly toxic to granulation tissue or cultured fibroblasts. More dilute solutions seriously affect the chemicals' antimicrobial activity, although povidone-iodine at dilutions of 0.001% and sodium hypochlorite 0.005% remain bactericidal while no longer damaging fibroblasts. These in vitro studies suggest that many topical antiseptics may interfere with healing, although in vitro studies have shown that hydrogen peroxide does not inhibit the growth of granulation tissue the way other toxic substances do.

Topical steroids and antibiotic ointments are also commonly applied to wounds. Potent fluorinated steroids retard epidermal resurfacing and reduce collagen biosynthesis. One percent hydrocortisone has been shown to exert little or no inhibition of wound healing. Topical nitrofurazone and a liquid detergent inhibited wound healing in pigs. Wounds treated with 70% ethanol heal as fast as air-exposed wounds. Oil and water cream, Neosporin ointment, Silvadene cream, and benzoyl peroxide lotion (10% and 20%) enhance epidermal wound healing. Topical retinoic acid, which stimulates mitoses, may enhance reepithelialization after dermabrasion if applied to intact-skin 10 days before wounding but may inhibit reepithelialization if applied to superficial wounds.

Using this information to avoid the toxic effects and minimize any inhibition of wound healing, topical antibiotic ointments may be helpful, especially if common sensitizers can be avoided (neomycin). If an anti-inflammatory topical is needed around a chronic ulcer or on damaged skin, hydrocortisone is least likely to interfere with healing.

Wound Dressings

The ideal wound dressing should enhance healing, reduce pain, absorb wound exudate, and be easy to apply and replace without causing irritation. It should protect the wound from trauma, toxins, and bacteria and not induce allergic contact dermatitis.

Many modern wound dressings available today fulfil most of these requirements. Occlusive and semiocclusive dressings provide a moist environment for the wound, preventing desiccation and, most importantly, enhancing both reepithelialization (30–45%) and collagen synthesis compared to air-exposed wound controls. This enhanced healing is seen in acute partial-thickness and full-thickness wounds as well as some chronic wounds such as leg ulcers.

Occlusive dressings also reduce the pain of surgical wounds, leg ulcers, skin graft donor sites, and dermabrasion. The moist wound bed created by these dressings is flexible. There is less inflammation in contrast to the air-dried wound with its immobile hard crust that adheres tightly to the wound and pulls with any movement. Some investigators report better cosmetic results with occlusive dressings used both on sutured wounds and wounds allowed to heal by second intention.

In the past decade, the popularity and usefulness of occlusive dressings have led to the marketing of many types of dressings. The most commonly used dressings can be classified into four main groups: (i) perforated plastic films with absorptive pad backing (band-aid, Telfa), (ii) hydrogel dressings (Vigilon, Second Skin), (iii) hydrocolloid dressings (Duoderm), and (iv) adhesive polyure-thane dressings (Op-Site, Tegaderm) (Table 1).

The most commonly used commercial dressing, and the closest to an ideal dressing, is the perforated plastic film with an absorptive pad backing. These are commercially available in many sizes, inexpensive, and easy to apply and change, and they absorb the wound exudate. Thus, they are convenient for patients and have all the advantages of occlusive dressings. For small wounds, band aids suffice as the dressing, but for larger wounds, pads must be used and cut to overlap the wound margins, and are then held in place with tape.

Hydrogel dressings are polymers of polyethylene oxide holding 96% sterile water in the form of a gelatinous sheet. This gelatin-like sheet is packaged between two thin plastic sheets. The bottom layer is usually removed before the dressing is applied so that the gelatinous layer is in direct contact with the wound and the outer plastic film prevents evaporation of the water from the gel. This dressing may also be cut to overlap the wound edges and must be held in place with tape because it is nonadhesive. This dressing feels soothing and is best for superficial, rapidly healing wounds such as dermabrasion. This dressing has been shown to selectively permit the growth of gram-negative organisms in wounds of animals and humans, resulting in an increased incidence of wound infection. A more recent improvement of this type of dressing has been the impregnation of povidone-iodine into the hydrogel to provide an antimicrobial dressing.

Some dressings have adhesive that obviates the need for additional tape. Ideally, they stick to the normal skin surrounding the wound but not the moist wound bed. Unfortunately, these adhesive dressings also stick to the newly migrated epidermis and can cause rewounding during dressing changes. For this reason, when using these dressings it can be helpful to apply a thin coat of petrolatum or antibiotic ointment over the new epidermis to prevent adherence and to change the dressing infrequently to minimize trauma. One advantage of the adhesive dressings is that they protect the wound from environmental bacterial contamination.

The hydrocolloid dressing is composed of gelatin and pectin hydrocolloid particles in a polymer. This is a thicker, more protective dressing, and is easy to cut and apply to the wound. It appears to be very effective for stimulating granulation tissue, possibly because of the low oxygen permeability. It is useful in chronic leg ulcers and decubitus ulcers. Patients should be warned that the dressing dissolves on contact with wound exudate, and the yellow mixture under the dressing often has a foul odor that should not be confused with pus or sign of infection.

Adhesive-backed polyurethane films are transparent and do not require tape, and thus are quite useful on small facial wounds where an inconspicuous dressing is desired. They are also useful for wounds after the exudative phase of healing (lag phase) because they have no absorptive capacity. In acute wounds, the exudate accumulates under the dressing, requiring frequent changes, or unpredictable leakage of the accumulated contents under the film may

Table 1 Occlusive Wound Dressings

Types	Enhances healing	Reduces pain
Perforated plastic with absorbent pad	+	+
Hydrogel		
Hydrocolloid	+	+
Polyurethane	+	+

occur. This type of dressing is often difficult to apply because it easily folds and adheres to itself. Improvements in packaging have helped somewhat.

The choice of wound dressing may depend on a number of variables. One important feature is the ability to absorb exudate. During the exudative phase of healing, an absorptive occlusive dressing such as the perforated plastic films with a pad backing is most desirable to handle the copious exudate. If protection of the wound from environmental bacterial contamination is important, one of the adhesive-backed dressings, polyurethane films, or hydrocolloid dressings may be helpful. When these dressings are used during the exudative phase, daily dressing changes are needed to clean the exudate. Later, they only need to be changed every four to five days. In chronic wounds, the hydrocolloid dressings seem to be effective in helping to debride the wound and promote the growth of granulation tissue.

Concerns about the use of occlusive dressings include oxygen permeability and the chance of infection. While some dressings are oxygen permeable (polyurethane films) and others are impermeable (hydrocolloid dressings), the rate of wound healing is similar. Thus the theoretical concern about oxygen tension under the wound dressing has little clinical application. However, bacteria do proliferate under occlusive dressings, but clinical infection is rare. The advantages of occlusive dressings outweigh the theoretical increased risk of infection. A number of factors may account for the low infection rate. Neutrophils in the exudate under occlusive dressings are active for 24 hours, actively phagocytizing and killing bacteria. The adhesive of some polyurethane films or the acid pH of the dissolved hydrocolloid dressings inhibits bacterial growth. Finally, many dressings are used in combination with antibiotic ointments.

Absorbent	Adhesive	Ease of application
+	−	+
+/−	−	+
−	+	+
−	+	−

When infection does occur, it may present differently from normal. There may be less inflammation or pain. A delay in wound healing may be the most important sign of infection to monitor.

In addition, the organisms more likely to be involved include gram-negative bacteria and yeasts as well as Staphylococcus (Fig. 10).

Wound Management

The goal of wound management is to minimize bacterial colonization, prevent desiccation of the wound, and provide a moist wound environment, all at low cost and convenience for the patient. The surgical procedure chosen should be the most effective technique that causes the least amount of necrotic tissue. If hemostasis is necessary, powdered gelatin, collagen, or topical thrombin with or without pinpoint electrocoagulation is best. Most other hemostatic agents are toxic and delay healing (i.e., Monsel's solution, aluminum chloride, silver nitrate, oxidized cellulose) and should be used only when necessary to ensure hemostasis. An occlusive dressing should be applied (i.e., perforated plastic film with an absorbent pad) and a pressure dressing if necessary. After 24 hours, patients may remove the dressing and compress the wound with tap water or 1% to 3% hydrogen peroxide. Hydrogen peroxide is used because it produces effervescence and mechanically softens and removes any crusts or blood clots. If no crusts are present, tap water cleansing is recommended to prevent epidermal blisters caused by hydrogen peroxide during the later stages of healing. A nonsensitizing antibiotic ointment is applied to the wound surface before a clean occlusive dressing is reapplied. This procedure is repeated daily until the wound is covered with epidermis.

Managing Complex Wounds

Most wounds created by dermatologic surgeons involve skin and subcutaneous tissue. The treatment plan outlined above is also effective in areas of exposed fat, muscle, and fascia. However, wounds that expose cartilage, bone, or contain necrotic tissue from disease or infection will not support epidermal migration. In these cases, additional care is needed to stimulate granulation tissue that will support epidermal migration. If small areas of bone or cartilage (<1 cm) are exposed, the only alteration from routine treatment is the more frequent and liberal use of antibiotic ointments to ensure an occlusive environment to prevent desiccation necrosis. Areas of exposed cartilage larger than 1 cm can be excised if they are located in concave areas, exposing the perichondrium from the opposite surface. This

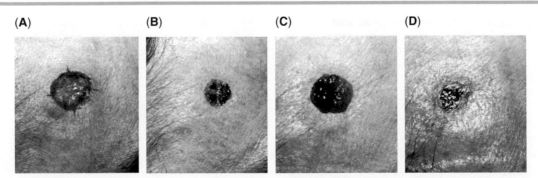

(A) **(B)** **(C)** **(D)**

Figure 10 Effect of infection on wound healing. **(A)** Full-thickness wound on the temple managed using occlusive therapy. **(B)** Appearance two weeks later shows progress as expected. **(C)** Wound six weeks after wounding shows no further healing. Culture documents infection with *Serratia marcescens*, but wound shows little surrounding redness, although it is painful. **(D)** Rapid healing one week later, after topical antibiotic is applied with occlusive dressing.

provides a good blood supply for granulation tissue and later reepithelialization. On convex surfaces (helix, antihelix, and nasal cartilages), the structural support of the cartilage must be preserved to prevent significant deformities. This may be done by removing small discs of cartilage with a 3 mm dermal punch exposing islands of perichondrium to support granulation tissue growth over the lattice of remaining cartilage (Fig. 11).

When large areas of bone are exposed, a blood supply must be obtained from the medullary portion of bone by removing a portion of the outer cortex. This may be done with a bone chisel, high-speed dental burr or drill, or carbon dioxide laser. If the need to remove bone or cartilage is in question, the decision may be delayed for three weeks to wait for the spontaneous appearance of granulation tissue from small perforating vessels. Although exposed cartilage and bone require special care, these procedures can be done quickly and painlessly on an outpatient basis; the options for wound management can be increased by adding grafts and second intention healing in addition to local flap coverage.

In wounds complicated by necrosis, control of the disease process and debridement are essential. Superficial debridement can be done with an occlusive hydrocolloid dressing or more rapidly by gentle curettage until healthy bleeding tissue is exposed. Otherwise, more aggressive debridement with a scalpel is required to remove necrotic tissue and enhance healing.

Predicting the Cosmetic Result

Dermatologic surgeons have a variety of surgical techniques at their disposal for the treatment of skin lesions. It is helpful to be able to predict the cosmetic result when choosing

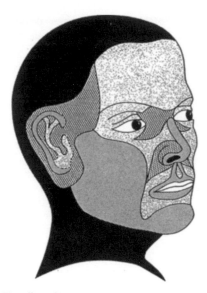

Figure 12 The effect of location on the cosmetic result of wounds managed by second intention healing. Wounds in concave areas heal well. Wounds on flat surfaces usually heal satisfactorily. Wounds on convex surfaces heal with variable cosmetic results, and deep wounds often look best if repaired surgically. *Source*: From Zitelli (1987).

between surgical repair and a method requiring healing by second intention. Although many factors influence the cosmetic result, the location of the wound is the most important factor that predicts the result after second intention healing. Wounds located in concave areas heal with excellent cosmetic results. Wounds on flat surfaces usually heal with satisfactory results, and wounds on convex surfaces often heal with a noticeable scar (Fig. 12).

Wounds in the inner canthus, crease of the nasal ala, nasolabial fold, temple, and concave areas of the ear usually heal with a cosmetic result equal or superior to the result from surgical repair (Fig. 13). Wounds on flat surfaces such as the forehead, sides of the nose, and periorbital areas may look best if a surgical repair can be designed to maintain normal tension lines and cause no distortion of important structures; otherwise they may look best if allowed to heal

(A)

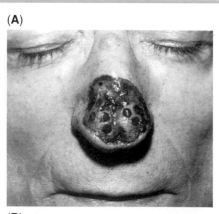

(B)

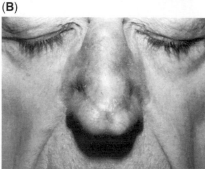

Figure 11 Excision of cartilage to promote healing. **(A)** A full-thickness wound on the nose, exposing the cartilage. Discs of cartilage (3 mm) have been removed to maintain cartilage support and promote granulation tissue growth. **(B)** Healed wound six months later. *Source*: From Zitelli (1983).

(A)   **(B)**

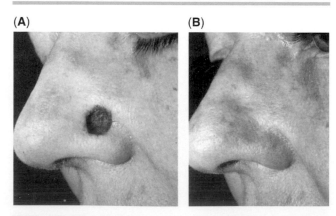

Figure 13 **(A)** A full-thickness wound on the crease of the nasal ala. **(B)** Cosmetic result six months after healing by second intention. *Source*: From Zitelli (1987)

(A) **(B)**

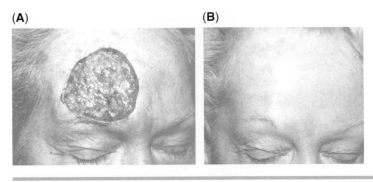

Figure 14 **(A)** A large full-thickness wound that might be managed with a skin graft. Local flaps would be likely to distort nearby landmarks. **(B)** Cosmetic result one year later after healing by second intention with guiding sutures.

(A) **(B)** **(C)**

(D) **(E)**

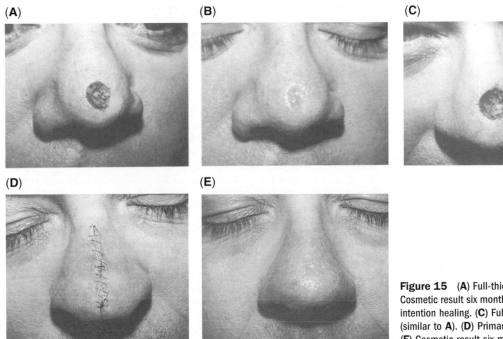

Figure 15 **(A)** Full-thickness wound on the tip of the nose. **(B)** Cosmetic result six months later with depressed scar from second intention healing. **(C)** Full-thickness wound on the tip of the nose (similar to **A**). **(D)** Primary closure without distortion of the nose. **(E)** Cosmetic result six months later. *Source*: From Zitelli (1987).

by second intention (Fig. 14). Wounds on the convex surface on the malar cheeks, tip of the nose, or vermilion border usually look best if a surgical repair is done (Fig. 15). Often wounds on the trunk or extremities look best when allowed to heal by second intention especially if wound closure is complicated or requires considerable tension.

Other factors that influence the cosmetic result include wound depth, skin color, and wound size. Skin color is an important factor to consider. Because scars from all but the most superficial wounds are hypopigmented and avascular, the healed wound will be less noticeable in light-colored skin than in darkly pigmented or telangiectatic skin (Fig. 16). Small wounds heal with better cosmetic results than large wounds, especially in older patients in whom other skin changes such as lentigines, keratoses, and wrinkles help to camouflage the scar.

BIBLIOGRAPHY

Forrest RD. Early history of wound treatment. J R Soc Med 1982; 75:198–205.

Johnston LC. Yet more, yet older, snakes (letter). JAMA 1986; 255:2445.

Dermal Wound Healing

Albright SD. Surgical gem: placement of "guiding sutures" to counteract undesirable retraction of tissues in and around functionally and cosmetically important structures. J Dermatol Surg Oncol 1981; 7:446–449.

Aldskogius H, Hermanson A, Jonsson E. Re-innervation of experimental superficial wounds in rats. Plast Reconstr Surg 1987; 79:595–599.

Clark RAF, Winn HJ, Dvorak HG, Colvin RB. Fibronectin beneath reepithelializing epidermis in vivo: sources and significance. J Invest Dermatol 1983; 80:26s–30s.

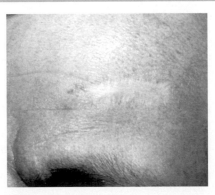

Figure 16 Hypopigmented avascular scar.

Clark YK, Stone RD, Leung D, et al. Role of macrophages in wound healing. Surg Forum 1976; 27:16.

Corps BVM. The effect of graft thickness, donor site, and graft bed on graft shrinkage in the hooded rat. Br J Plast Surg 1969; 22:125.

Eaglstein WH. The genesis of wound repair. In: Theirs B, Dobson R, eds. The Pathogenesis of Skin Disease. New York: Churchill Livingstone, 1986:617–623.

Ehrlich HP, Buttle DJ, Trelstad R, Hayashi K. Epidermolysis bullosa dystrophica recessive fibroblasts altered behaviour in a collagen matrix. J Invest Dermatol 1983; 80:56.

Ehrlich HP, Hunt TK. Effects of cortisone and vitamin A on wound healing. Ann Surg 1968; 167:324–328.

Leibovich SJ, Ross R. The role of the macrophage in wound repair: a study with hydrocortisone and antimacrophage serum. Am J Pathol 1975; 78:71.

Majno G. The story of the myofibroblasts. Am J Surg Pathol 1979; 3:535.

Majno G, Gabbiani G, Hirschel BJ, et al. Contraction of granulation tissue in vitro: similarity to smooth muscle. Science 1971; 173:548–550.

McGrath MH. Healing of the open wound. In: Rudolph R, ed. Problems in Aesthetic Surgery. St. Louis: CV Mosby, 1986: 13–48.

McGrath MH, Hundahl SA. The spatial and temporal quantification of myofibroblasts. Plast Reconstr Surg 1982; 69:975.

Postlethwaite AG, Snyderman R, Kang AH. Chemotactic attraction of human fibroblasts to a lymphocyte-derived factor. J Exp Med 1976; 144:1188.

Rudolph R. Inhibition of myofibroblasts by skin grafts. Plast Reconstr Surg 1979; 63:473.

Simpson DM, Ross R. The neutrophilic leukocyte in wound repair. A study with antineutrophil serum. J Clin Invest 1972; 51:2009–2023.

Weiss RE, Reddi AH. Role of fibronectin in collagenous matrix-induced mesenchymal cell proliferation and differentiation in vivo. Exp Cell Res 1981; 133:247–254.

Woodley DT, O'Keefe EJ, Prunieras M. Cutaneous wound healing: a model for cell-matrix interactions. J Am Acad Dermatol 1985; 12:420–433.

Zitelli JA. Secondary intention healing—an alternative to surgical repair. Clin Dermatol 1984; 2:92–106.

Epidermal Healing

Beutner EH, Binder WL, Jablonska S, et al. Nature of stratum corneum autoantibodies, antigens, and antigen conversion and their role in healing and psoriasis. In: Marks R, Christophers E, eds. The Epidermis in Disease. Philadelphia: JB Lippincott, 1981:333.

Cohen S. Isolation of a mouse submaxillary gland protein accelerating incisor eruption and eyelid opening in the newborn animal. J Biol Chem 1962; 237:1555–1562.

Dillman T, Penn J. Studies on repair of cutaneous wounds II. The healing of wounds involving loss of superficial portions of the skin. Med Proc ; 2:150–156.

Ferreira JA. Dermabrasion of the skin: prevention and/or treatment of hyperpigmentation. Aesthet Plast Surg 1978; 1:381.

Ferreira JA. The role of diazepam in skin hyperpigmentation. Aesthet Plast Surg 1980; 4:343.

Hebda PA, Alstadt SP, Hileman WT, Eaglstein WH. Support and stimulation of epidermal cell outgrowth from porcine skin explants by platelet factors. Br J Dermatol 1986; 115:529–541.

Krawczyk W. Pattern of epidermal cell migration during wound healing. J Cell Biol 1971; 49:247–263.

Stenn KS. Epibolin: a protein in human plasma that supports epithelial cell movement. Proc Natl Acad Sci USA 1981; 78:6907.

Winter GD. Epidermal regeneration studied in the domestic pig. In: Maibach HI, Rovee DT, eds. Epidermal Wound Healing. Chicago: Yearbook Medical Publishers, 1972.

Kinetics of Wound Healing

Levenson SM, Geever EF, Crowley LV, et al. The healing of rat skin wounds. Ann Surg 1965; 161:293–308.

Majno G. The Latros in the Healing Hand: Man and Wound in the Ancient World. Cambridge, MA: Harvard University Press, 1977:154–156.

McGrath MH, Simon RH. Wound geometry and the kinetics of wound contraction. Plast Reconstr Surg 1983; 72:66.

Peacock EE, Madden JW. Some studies on the effect of β-aminopropionitrile on collagen in healing wounds. Surgery 1966; 60:7–12.

Robins P, Day CL, Lew RA. A multivariate analysis of factors affecting wound healing time. J Dermatol Surg Oncol 1984; 10:219–221.

Zitelli J. Wound healing for the clinician. Adv Dermatol 1987; 2: 243–267.

Factors Affecting Wound Healing

Epstein E. Effects of tissue-destructive technics on wound healing (letter). J Am Acad Dermatol 1986; 14:1098–1099.

Grillo HC, Potsaid MS. Studies in wound healing. IV. Retardation of contraction by local x-irradiation: observations relating to the origin of fibroblasts in repair. Ann Surg 1958; 148:145.

Hell E, Lawrence JC. The initiation of epidermal wound healing in cuts and burns. Br J Exp Pathol 1979; 60:171–179.

Hunt TK. Vitamin A and wound healing. J Am Acad Dermatol 1986; 15:817–821.

Klausner JM, Lulcuk S, Inbar M, et al. The effects of perioperative fluorouracil administration on convalescence and wound healing. Arch Surg 1986; 121:239–242.

Krizek TJ, Robson MC. Evolution of quantitative bacteriology in wound management. Am J Surg 1975; 130:579–581.

Leyden JJ. Effect of bacteria on healing of superficial wounds. Clin Dermatol 1984; 2:81–85.

Lundgren C, Muren A, Zederfeldt B. Effect of cold vasoconstriction on wound healing in the rabbit. Ada Chir Scand 1959; 118:1–4.

Marks JG, Cano C, Leitzel K, et al. Inhibition of wound healing by topical steroids. J Dermatol Surg Oncol 1983; 9:819–821.

Mertz PM, Eaglstein WH. The effect of a semiocclusive dressing on the microbial population in superficial wounds. Arch Surg 1984; 119:287–289.

Mobacken H. Gentian violet and wound repair (letter). J Am Acad Dermatol 1986; 15:1303.

Moreno RA, Hebda PA, Zitelli JA, et al. Epidermal cell outgrowth from CO_2 laser- and scalpel-cut explants: implications for wound healing. J Dermatol Surg Oncol 1984; 10:863–868.

Pollack SV. Wound healing. A review III: nutritional factors affecting wound healing. J Dermatol Surg Oncol 1979; 5:615–619.

Pollack SV. Wound healing. A review IV: systemic medications affecting wound healing. J Dermatol Surg Oncol 1982; 8: 667–672.

Robson MC, Heggers JP. Delayed wound closures based on bacterial counts. J Surg Oncol 1970; 2:379–383.

Sawchuk WS, Friedman KJ, Manning T, Pinnell SR. Delayed healing in full-thickness wounds treated with aluminum chloride solution. J Am Acad Dermatol 1986; 15:982–994.

Selden ST. Candida: a common culprit. J Dermatol Surg Oncol 1985; 11:958.

Siegle RJ, Chiaramonti A, Knox DW, Pollack SV. Cutaneous candidosis as a complication of facial dermabrasion. J Dermatol Surg Oncol 1984; 10:891–895.

Sowa DE, Masterson BJ, Nealon N, von Fraunhofer JA. Effects of thermal knives on wound healing. Obstet Gynecol 1985; 66:436–439.

Spebar MJ, Pruitt BA. Candidiasis in the burned patient. J Trauma 1981; 21:237–239.

Zanini V, Viviani MA, Cava L, et al. Candida infections in the burn patients. Panminerva Med 1983; 25:163–166.

Complications

Gruber RP, Vistnes L, Pardoe R. The effect of commonly used antiseptics on wound healing. Plast Reconstr Surg 1975; 55:472–476.

Howell JB. Neurotrophic changes in the trigeminal territory. Arch Dermatol 1962; 86:442–448.

Krull EA. Chronic cutaneous ulcerations and impaired healing in human skin. J Am Acad Dermatol 1985; 12:394–401.

Murray JC, Pollack SV, Pinnell SR. Keloids and hypertrophic scars. Clin Dermatol 1984; 2:121–133.

Peacock EE. Pharmacologic control of surface scarring in human beings. Ann Surg 1981; 193:592–597.

Sproat JE, Dalcin A, Weitaver N, Robert RS. Hypertrophic sternal scars: silicone gel sheet versus Kenalog injection treatment. Plast Reconstr Surg 1992; 90:988–992.

Second Intention Healing and Special Dressings

Albom MJ. Surgical gems. J Dermatol Surg Oncol 1975; 1:60.

Alper JC, Welch EA, Ginsberg M, et al. Moist wound healing under a vapor permeable membrane. J Am Acad Dermatol 1983; 8:347–353.

Alvarez OM, Mertz PM, Eaglstein WH. The effect of occlusive dressings on collagen synthesis and re-epithelialization in superficial wounds. J Surg Res 1983; 35:142–148.

Ariyan S, Krizek TJ. In defense of the open wound. Arch Surg 1976; 111:293–296.

Eaglstein WH, Mertz P, Alvarez OM. Effect of topically applied agents on healing wounds. Clin Dermatol 1984; 2(3):112–115.

Eaton AC. A controlled trial to evaluate and compare a sutureless skin closure technique (Op-Site skin closure) with conventional skin suturing and clipping in abdominal surgery. Br J Surg 1980; 67:857–860.

Field LM. Letter to the editor. J Dermatol Surg Oncol 1981; 7:597.

Fox SA, Beard C. Spontaneous lid repair. Am J Ophthamol 1964; 58:947–952.

Geronemus RG, Robins P. The effects of two new dressings on epidermal wound healing. J Dermatol Surg Oncol 1982; 8:850–852.

Goldwyn RM. Value of healing by secondary intention seconded (letter). Ann Plast Surg 1980; 4:435.

Holland KT, Davis W, Ingham E, Gowland G. A comparison of the in-vitro antibacterial and complement activating effect of 'OpSite' and 'Tegaderm' dressings. J Hosp Infect 1984; 5:323–328.

James JH, Watson CH. The use of Op-Site, a vapor permeable dressing, on skin graft donor sites. Br J Plast Surg 1975; 28:107–110.

Katz S, McGinley K, Leyden JJ. Semipermeable occlusive dressings. Arch Dermatol 1986; 122:58–62.

Lineaweaver W, McMorris S, Soucy D, Howard R. Cellular and bacterial toxicities of topical antimicrobials. Plast Reconstr Surg 1985; 75:394–396.

Linsky CB, Rovee DT, Dow T. Effect of dressing on wound inflammation and scar tissue. In: Dineen P, Hildick-Smith G, eds. The Surgical Wound. Philadelphia: Lea & Febiger, 1981:191–205.

Mandy SH. A new primary wound dressing made of polyethylene oxide gel. J Dermatol Surg Oncol 1983; 9:153–155.

Mandy SH. Tretinoin in the preoperative and postoperative management of dermabrasion. J Am Acad Dermatol 1986; 15:878–879.

Mehta HK. Surgical management of carcinoma of eyelids and periorbital skin. Br J Ophthalmol 1979; 63:578–585.

Mertz PM, Marshall DA, Eaglstein WH. Occlusive wound dressings to prevent bacterial invasion and wound infection. J Am Acad Dermatol 1985; 12:662–668.

Mertz PM, Marshall DA, Kuglar MA. Povidone-iodine in polyethylene oxide hydrogel dressing. Arch Dermatol 1986; 122:1133–1138.

Mohs FE, Zitelli JA. Microscopically controlled surgery in the treatment of carcinoma of the scalp. Arch Dermatol 1981; 117:764–769.

Niedner R, Schöpf E. Inhibition of wound healing by antiseptics. Br J Dermatol 1986; 115(suppl 31):41–44.

Silverberg B, Smoot CE, Landa SJF, Parsons RW. Hidradenitis suppurativa: patient satisfaction with wound healing by secondary intention. Plast Reconstr Surg 1987; 79:555–559.

Vanderveen EG, Stoner JG, Swanson NA. Chiseling of exposed bone to stimulate granulation tissue after Mohs surgery. J Dermatol Surg Oncol 1983; 9:925–928.

Varghese MC, Balin AK, Carter M, Caldwell D. Local environment of chronic wounds under synthetic dressings. Arch Dermatol 1986; 122:52–57.

Winter GD. Formation of scab and the rate of epithelization of superficial wounds in the skin of the young domestic pig. Nature (London) 1962; 193:293–294.

Zitelli JA. Delayed wound healing with adhesive wound dressings. J Dermatol Surg Oncol 1984; 10:709–710.

Zitelli JA. Wound healing by secondary intention, a cosmetic appraisal. J Am Acad Dermatol 1983; 9:407–415.

51

Complex Closures

Ali Hendi

Department of Dermatology, Mayo Clinic, Jacksonville, Florida, U.S.A.

David G. Brodland

*Departments of Dermatology and Otolaryngology, University of Pittsburgh Medical Center,
Pittsburgh, Pennsylvania, U.S.A.*

Z-PLASTY

Background

Z-plasty is one of the oldest flaps used in dermatologic surgery. The traditional Z-plasty is essentially two transposition flaps in which there is no defect, and the movement of tissue is performed to realign and move the scar or to increase the tissue length of a closure in a desired direction. Many variations of Z-plasty have been created and used.

Preoperative Plan

First, the surgeon needs to determine the purpose for performing a Z-plasty. The Z-plasty is often used to perform a scar revision on an unfavorably oriented scar and change its direction. After the decision has been made to perform a Z-plasty, the surgeon should plan and draw the incision lines on the areas involved in the operation. With this planning, the surgeon should be able to visualize tissue movement in a predictable manner.

Technique

The classic Z-plasty consists of three separate limbs that form two triangular flaps which, when interposed, change the direction of the middle limb. Essentially, this completely reorients a scar line at the expense of creating two new scar lines. This needs to be weighed against the potential enhancement of the cosmetic outcome. The movement of tissue in a classic Z-plasty is shown in Figure 1. Z-plasty can also be performed in a series to break up a long conspicuous scar. This is often useful for a scar line that is placed counter to the relaxed skin tension lines (RSTLs) and would improve with reorientation using a single Z-plasty (Fig. 2A) or Z-plasties in series (Fig. 2B). This will afford the placement of some of the scar lines within the RSTLs and make the scar less conspicuous. In multiple-flap Z-plasty, the angles of a classic Z-plasty are bisected and the flaps are interposed between each other (Fig. 3).

Another use for Z-plasty is to lengthen a scar line. By lengthening a scar on a convex area, the surgeon minimizes the possibility of a depressed scar, which may be the result of a straight-line closure after scar contraction occurs. This is commonly used in the repair of bifid or torn earlobes. In repairing a torn earlobe with Z-plasty, the surgeon increases the length of the scar along which contraction will occur

as the myofibroblasts move into the healing tissue. This redistribution and lengthening of the scar minimizes notching on convex surfaces such as the earlobe. The variations of Z-plasty that can be performed to repair a torn earlobe are discussed elsewhere in this book.

Z-plasty is a useful tool that should be mastered by the dermatologic surgeon. Its uses include lengthening of a closure line to prevent notching over a convex surface area, reorienting an unfavorably placed scar line, and, when performed in series, camouflaging and breaking up a long scar line.

W-PLASTY

Background

Although W-plasty may seem similar to Z-plasties in series, it is inherently different. Its design and tissue dynamics are uniquely useful to dermatologic surgeons.

Preoperative Plan and Technique

W-plasty is a simple excision in which the edges of the closure are saw-toothed in shape and the opposing wound edges are complementary. This provides a broken-line closure, which is thought to provide scar camouflage, compared with a straight-line closure. The manner of scar excision in a W-plasty is planned so that the angulated sawtooth-shaped broken-line closure is planned with half of the lines oriented along RSTLs. Because the scar line is lengthened by the complementary interdigitating skin edges and the tension vectors are directed in many directions, there is less likelihood of a depressed scar (Fig. 4). In planning for a W-plasty, the surgeon must ensure that the wound edges fit precisely, as in a puzzle. The preoperative planning and undertaking of a W-plasty require considerable time and diligence.

A simplified method to plan and execute a W-plasty is to draw an equilateral 60° triangle at the base of the W-plasty. From the base of this triangle, which is perpendicular to the scar line to be excised, parallel lines, equal in length, are drawn in a zigzagging pattern on each side (Fig. 5).

A W-plasty can also be used to revise a curvilinear scar. In performing such a revision, the angles of the skin edges on the inside of the arc of the excision are more acute than those on the outside (Fig. 6).

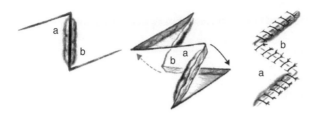

Figure 1 Classic 60° Z-plasty with interposition or transposition of flaps *a* and *b*. Notice net gain in length in the vertical direction along line from *a* to *b*. *Source*: From Brodland (1998).

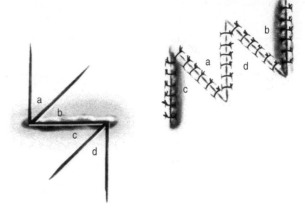

Figure 3 Multiple Z-plasty. Two 90° angles are bisected resulting in flaps *a*, *b*, *c*, and *d*. Flaps *a* and *c* are interposed, and *b* and *d* are interposed, resulting in an accordian-like configuration and a large net gain of tissue in the horizontal direction. *Source*: From Brodland (1998).

In conclusion, W-plasty is a useful technique for dermatologic surgeons. It allows complete removal and camouflage of a scar by a zigzagging excision. It allows for the excision of a scar that is oblique to RSTLs and placement of every other limb of the incision within RSTLs. However, this potential benefit should be weighed against the possibility of producing a longer zigzagging scar and the increased surgical time necessary to perform a W-plasty closure.

V-Y-PLASTY

Background

The use of the V to Y repair preceded the island pedicle flap (IPF) and has much in common with it. The principles and vectors of tissue movement for these two closures are very similar. A triangular flap is moved in the direction of its base and away from its apex for both flaps. The V-Y-plasty flap is useful in repositioning displaced anatomic structures and has a dermal blood supply. The IPF is used to reconstruct a loss of tissue and derives its blood supply from a subcutaneous pedicle.

Preoperative Plan

The V-Y flap is most useful in the repair of retracted or malpositioned tissue resulting from scar retraction. This type of scar most commonly occurs in association with free margins such as the lip, alar rim, and eyelid. For example, an eclabion can appear from scar contraction displacing the vermilion border of the lip upward. The preoperative plan is crucial for a V-Y flap. The amount of tissue movement needed is measured precisely in repairing an eclabion. The position of the normal vermilion border must be determined by comparing it with the opposite side. This line can be drawn in ink. The distance from the drawn vermilion border to the malpositioned vermilion border is measured. (A V-shaped incision is made, with the open mouth of the V coinciding with the width of the distorted tissue being pulled.) The incised tissue is advanced the distance that is equivalent to the distance measured preoperatively from the distorted

vermilion border to its desired position (Fig. 7). Once the position of the flap is adequate, the flap is sutured into place, resulting in a suture line resembling a Y, hence the name, "V-Y flap." Undermining of the surrounding tissue improves mobilization, closure, and proper wound eversion.

The best way to ensure precise advancement of the tissue is to suture the apex of the flap at a distance away from the apex of the donor site that is exactly the same as the distance of the preoperatively measured deformity. The V-Y flap is versatile and useful in repairing retraction of free and mobile skin edges, such as the lip (Fig. 8).

S-SHAPED CLOSURE

Background

The S-shaped closure is a variation of the primary elliptical style closure in which the line of closure is lengthened. This lengthening is obtained by adding curvature to an otherwise straight closure line. The curved closure resembles a lazy S. It is sometimes mistakenly referred to as "S-plasty." However, S-plasty is a variant of Z-plasty that interposes two lobes, much like the two triangular flaps of a Z-plasty. There is no transposition in an S-shaped closure, only a curvilinear configuration.

Preoperative Plan and Technique

The S-shaped closure is often performed on convex areas such as the extremities to minimize the inverted, depressed

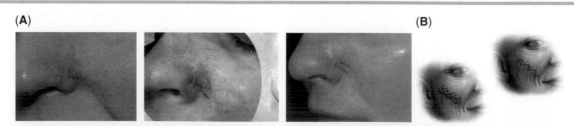

(A)   **(B)**

Figure 2 **(A)** Single Z-plasty used to reorient a scar extending from the cheek to the ala (*left*); scar extending from the cheek to the ala (*middle*); (ii) Z-plasty incisions made; and (*right*) Z-plasty after excision of scar and transposition of triangular flaps. **(B)** Series of Z-plasties along a scar that is long and oriented against the relaxed skin tension line. *Source*: **(B)**: From Brodland (1998).

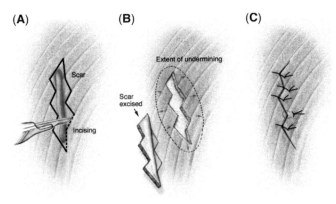

Figure 4 W-plasty designed to form a zigzag line in which half of the lines are oriented in the relaxed skin tension lines. *Source*: From Brodland (1998).

scar that can occur with contracture of a straight scar crossing a convex surface. The inherent flexibility of an S-shaped closure lessens the tendency for a scar on a convex area to become depressed. When an S-shaped closure is performed in the process of excising a lesion, the desired margins should be drawn around the lesion in a circular fashion. Two techniques can be used to draw an S-shaped closure. The first technique is to draw a curvilinear line that intersects the midpoint of the circular defect or lesion and forms an S. With this in place, the curvilinear lines can be drawn from the apex to the tangent of the circle on each side (Fig. 9A). The second technique is to draw a relatively straight line in the superior and the contralateral inferior aspects of the defect or lesion. These two lines should be parallel and the same length. Next, curved lines are drawn on the opposite sides of the straight lines. These two lines on opposite sides of the defect should be curved and the same length (Fig. 9B). On the extremities, the proximal tip of the S-shaped closure points proximally on the limb and the distal tip points distally (Fig. 9C). RSTLs on an extremity can be difficult to delineate. The direction of hair growth on an extremity can be used to define the most desirable RSTLs for closure. On the midcheek, however, the superior tip of an S-shaped closure should always point superior and perpendicular to the lid or toward the medial canthus and the inferior tip should follow the RSTLs along the cheek. With

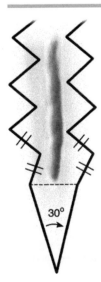

Figure 5 A simplified method to plan the terminal portion of a W-plasty. The base of the 30° equilateral triangle serves as the starting point for the complementary parallel lines. *Source*: From Brodland (1998).

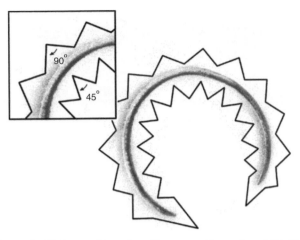

Figure 6 W-plasty revision of curvilinear scar. The angles of the inner incision are slightly more acute (inset), but the length of the sides of the angles are approximately the same as in the outer incision. *Source*: From Brodland (1998).

an S-shaped closure and careful eversion of the wound edge, the surgeon can prevent an undesirable depressed scar across convex surfaces, for example, the cheek (Fig. 10).

M-PLASTY
Background
M-plasty is a closure technique that in effect decreases the linear length of a scar line by dividing the tip of an elliptical closure into two acute-angled triangles (Fig. 11). It is a modification of a simple ellipse that can be used to prevent pushing on or violating certain anatomic borders.

Preoperative Plan
In deciding whether to perform an M-plasty, the surgeon should consider the benefits it provides over the cosmetic outcome of the closure as well as the increased surgical time. M-plasty is desired for areas in which certain anatomic margins are best not violated. The best examples are the eyelid margin and perhaps the nasal sill or alar rim. The difficulty with extending an elliptical excision beyond the nasal sill is the challenge of placing sutures intranasally and reducing the size of the nasal aperature. Many surgeons consider the vermilion border an anatomic border that should not be violated; however, in contrast to surgical dogma, excisions can be extended beyond this border and onto the mucosal surface of the lip, with a good cosmetic outcome (Fig. 12).

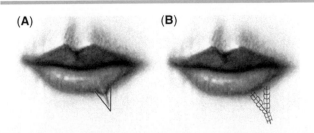

Figure 7 V-Y flap. The extent of the defect is measured preoperatively (A) and should be the same as the advancement of the apex of the flap. The "stem" of the "Y" (B) should equal the height of the tissue defect being corrected. *Source*: From Brodland (1998).

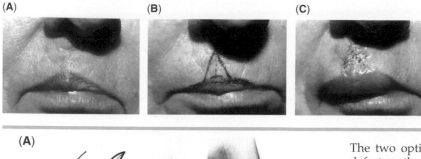

Figure 8 **(A)** Eclabion of right upper lip. **(B)** Surgical markings for V-Y flap. **(C)** V-Y flap immediately postoperatively. Tissue edema is due to local anesthetic.

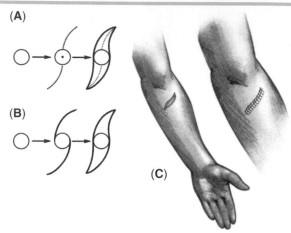

Figure 9 **(A and B)** Simplified techniques for drawing S-shaped closure. **(C)** Orientation of S-shaped closure on an extremity. *Source*: **(C)**: From Brodland (1998).

The eyebrow is often considered an inviolable surgical margin; however, an excision can be extended across the eyebrow and onto the eyelid without causing much distortion of the eyebrow if care is taken not to transect the acutely angled hair follicles (Fig. 13). It should be kept in mind that it is difficult to maintain the scars of an M-plasty within the RSTLs. As such, M-plasty closures may be more visible than a simple straight-line scar kept within the RSTLs. This disadvantage diminishes the use of an M-plasty to shorten a scar. However, it may be performed if the extension of the incision beyond a certain anatomic point would cause an unacceptable cosmetic outcome.

When the apex of a fusiform defect abuts free margins such as the vermilion border or other mobile anatomic borders, a push or displacement of the margin often occurs, resulting in distortion of the anatomic landmark. An M-plasty is a feasible option to shorten the linear length of the scar and to prevent pushing on a free margin (Fig. 14).

The two options that the surgeon has when faced with a defect on the cutaneous lip are to extend the fusiform excision beyond the vermilion border or to perform an M-plasty to shorten the linear length of a scar and to prevent pushing of the vermilion border.

Technique

The easiest way to plan an M-plasty is to draw the standard elliptical excision. The tip of the closure, which needs to be shortened, is addressed by inverting the apex of the triangle away from its drawn position and toward the defect or the center of the ellipse. This effectively breaks the single 30° angle apex into two smaller 30° angled Burow triangles (Fig. 15). This leaves a triangular peninsula between the two smaller triangles.

The net effect of an M-plasty is to shorten the linear length of the closure by 10% if a single M-plasty is performed. However, the overall length of the sutured area remains approximately the same.

GEOMETRIC BROKEN-LINE CLOSURE
Background

The geometric broken-line closure (GBLC) is a wound closure technique that is used to take advantage of the concept that a series of short, unpatterned lines is more inconspicuous than a single straight line. GBLC is a series of geometric shapes with a complementary pattern on the opposite side of the wound edge. These mirror-image shapes fit together like the pieces of a puzzle. This type of closure is used most commonly to revise depressed linear scars or scars that are aesthetically unacceptable (Fig. 16).

The geometric figures used in designing a GBLC include triangles, rectangles, squares, and half circles. Each of these components should be smaller than 5 mm because larger components may be more conspicuous than smaller ones. This technique is typically used for scar revision; thus, it is drawn to include the scar to be removed. The incisions are made with a no. 11 blade, which allows easy maneuverability and sharp-angle incisions. As with all excisions, care should be taken that the incisions are made at a 90° angle to

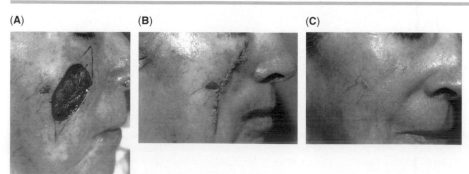

Figure 10 **(A, B)** Curvilinear, S-shaped closure on the convex surface of the cheek. **(C)** Six-month follow-up.

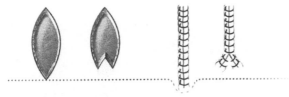

Figure 11 M-plasty used to obtain shorter vertical scar length. *Source:* From Brodland (1998).

the skin. Suturing a GBLC is time-consuming and requires meticulous suturing of the sharp angles and edges. Because of the complexity and time required for this closure, it is not performed frequently.

POSTOPERATIVE MANAGEMENT

The postoperative management of complex closures is not different from that of any routine closure. However, because of the sharp angles in some of the closures described herein (Z-plasty, W-plasty, and GBLC), it is important that the sutured area not be disturbed. This will prevent disruption of the small and angulated borders, which may not have been sutured in certain areas, for example, the tips. Postoperative bandages are discussed elsewhere in this book. The authors prefer to apply Steri-Strips and flesh-colored tape directly on the closure line for support. This is followed by the application of a pressure dressing of fluffed gauze

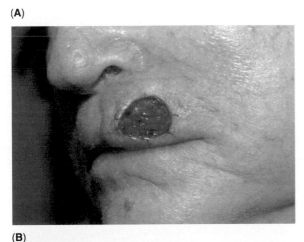

Figure 12 Primary closure of lip defect. Incisions cross the vermilion border into the mucosal surface of the lip. **(A)** Preoperative and **(B)** postoperative.

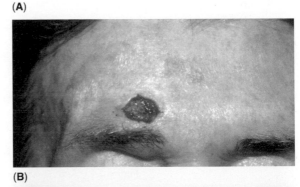

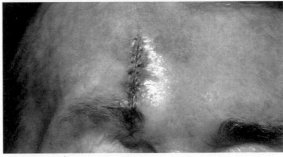

Figure 13 Primary closure of brow defect. Note vertical orientation of closure to avoid pull on the eyebrow. **(A)** Preoperative and **(B)** postoperative.

secured in place with tape. Pressure dressing is used to minimize the risk of hematoma and bleeding. The fluffed gauze should cover the entire undermined area. The pressure dressing is kept intact for one to two days. For patients receiving anticoagulant or antiplatelet agents, two days is preferred. The patient removes the pressure dressing, but the Steri-Strips and flesh-colored tape are kept in place, intact, and dry for one week and then replaced with a similar dressing at the one-week postoperative visit. During this visit, the wound is examined for signs of infection, hematoma, or dehiscence. Steri-Strips and flesh-colored tape are applied, and the patient is instructed again to keep the dressing dry and intact for a second week.

ADVERSE SEQUELAE AND COMPLICATIONS OF COMPLEX CLOSURES

Adverse sequelae of complex closures are not different from those of any other surgical closure of the skin. These sequelae include depressed scar, hypertrophic or keloidal scar, hyperpigmented or hypopigmented scar, and telangiectasia. Depressed scars can often be avoided by meticulous suture technique and wound eversion. Eversion is best accomplished with the use of the buried vertical mattress suture technique. Also, meticulous reapproximation of the wound edges with both buried and superficial sutures is important. The surgeon should attempt to have near-perfect approximation of the skin edges with the buried sutures alone. The epidermal sutures should only be relied on to keep the wound edges in contact with each other and to make slight adjustments in discrepancies of the level of the wound edges.

Such adverse sequelae as telangiectasias may improve with time. If not, these neovascularized areas can be treated with a vascular laser. Hypertrophic scars can be treated with firm massage 10 to 20 times daily. The massage should be in a firm circular motion, and each session can be as short as 30

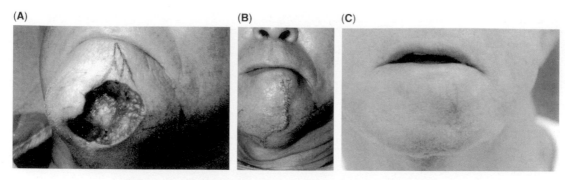

Figure 14 (A–C) M-plasty performed to avoid crossing vermilion border.

to 60 seconds. For larger hypertrophic scars and ones recalcitrant to massage, intralesional corticosteroids will expedite the reduction of scar tissue, but this has the risk of further neovascularization and atrophy. Pigmentary changes often resolve within a year. Hyperpigmentation is more likely to resolve than hypopigmentation postoperatively. Sun avoidance, use of a sun block with a high sun protection factor, and bleaching creams can be used to expedite the resolution of hyperpigmentation.

Complications of complex closures are similar to those of cutaneous surgical procedures. Although rare, hematoma is one of the more common complications. This complication can be minimized by meticulous intraoperative hemostasis. Hemostasis of the undermined surfaces depends on the surgeon being able to visualize the entire area, including the most remote edges of the undermined area. To facilitate hemostasis, the assistant should use two skin hooks to raise and reflect the undermined skin to better visualize any potential pinpoint bleeding.

The management of a hematoma depends on size and timing. Acute and enlarging hematomas need to be evacuated and hemostasis obtained for any bleeding vessels. Hematomas that are discovered later (i.e., one to two weeks postoperatively) and are not enlarging become organized and can be observed. The clot will resolve in several months. Venous hematomas usually stop enlarging because of the tamponade effect of the hematoma. Patients with hematomas should be treated with one to two weeks of antibiotics for infection prophylaxis because nonviable tissue, as in a resolving hematoma, can be a nidus for infection. Causes of

postoperative hematoma include inadequate hemostasis secondary to inadequate visualization of all undermined surfaces. Incomplete hemostasis may also be due to the vasoconstrictive effects of epinephrine, which can mask subsequent bleeding sites.

Patients who resume vigorous activity shortly after the operation can experience bleeding. Patients should be specifically instructed to avoid vigorous activity, especially for the first 48 hours postoperatively. An accidental bump to the sutured area can cause a rupture of deep sutures and bleeding. Patients also should be warned against bearing down or straining, which can increase venous pressure and cause bleeding. For patients who are at high risk for postoperative bleeding, a bolster dressing may be applied, similar to holsters used for skin grafts. With meticulous hemostasis, good surgical technique, and good dressings and postoperative instructions, postoperative hematomas can be minimized.

Another relatively common complication is wound infection. This typically becomes evident three to seven days after the operation. The most common signs of wound infection are increasing erythema, tenderness, and warmth with or without purulent exudates. The most obvious measure for preventing a wound infection is sterile operative technique, which is reviewed elsewhere in this book. Other factors that promote infections include the presence of devitalized tissue such as a hematoma or seroma. Proper surgical technique can minimize postoperative wound infections. This means avoiding tissue trauma as much as possible intraoperatively. A common source of tissue trauma is crush injury from the use of forceps during suturing. To reduce this, surgeons should use only the first two or three fingers to handle forceps or, preferably, use skin hooks instead of forceps. Tissue devitalization from excessive

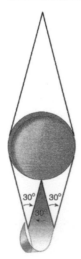

Figure 15 Design of M-plasty closure by inverting the apex of the fusiform closure toward the center. *Source*: From Brodland (1998).

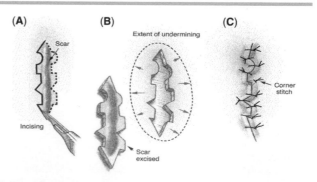

Figure 16 (A–C) Geometric broken-line closure. Note complementary pattern of excision.

intraoperative electrodesiccation should be avoided by the use of precise and focused hemostatic technique. Proper undermining can also reduce the likelihood of wound infection by minimizing tension on the wound edges and by not disturbing the blood supply to wound edges or flap tips.

When a wound infection is suspected, the exudate should be cultured and empiric antibiotic therapy should be initiated while awaiting the antimicrobial susceptibility profile. Surgical evacuation of an abscessed wound can be decided on a case-by-case basis. An alternative to complete takedown of a sutured wound is removal of one or two buried sutures to allow any purulence to drain. A pressure dressing is then reapplied to minimize the reaccumulation of pus. The decision to pack a wound that has been opened and drained can be made on an individual basis. Smaller, early wound infections can be treated with antibiotics, with or without the removal of sutures.

BIBLIOGRAPHY

Borges AF. Linear scar revision technique: Z-plasty and W-plasty. In: Borges AF, ed. Elective Incisions and Scar Revision. Boston: Little Brown, 1973:45.

Borges AF. Surgical incisions of choice. In: Borges AF, ed. Elective Incisions and Scar Revision. Boston: Little, Brown, 1973:91.

Borges AF. W-plasty. In: Thomas JR, Hold GR, eds. Facial Scars, Incision, Revision, and Camouflage. St. Louis: CV Mosby, 1989:150.

Boyer JD, Zitelli JA, Brodland DG. Undermining in cutaneous surgery. Dematologic Surgery 2001; 27(1):75–78.

Brodland D. Complex closures. In: Ratz JL, ed. Textbook of Dermatologic Surgery. Philadelphia: Lippincott-Raven Publishers, 1998:183–200.

Davis WE, Renner GJ. Z-plasty and scar revision. In: Thomas JR, Hold DR, eds. Facial Scars: Incision, Revision and Camouflage. St. Louis, MO: CV Mosby, 1989:137.

Frodel JL, Wang TD. Z-plasty. In: Baker SR, Swanson NA, eds. Local Flaps in Facial Reconstruction. St. Louis: CV Mosby, 1995:131.

McCarthy JG. Introduction to plastic surgery. In: McCarthy JG, ed. Plastic Surgery. Philadelphia: WB Saunders, 1990:1.

Thomas JR. Geometric broken-line closure. In: Thomas JR, Hold GR, eds. Facial Scars: Incision, Revision and Camouflage. St. Louis, MO: CV Mosby, 1989:160.

Wheeland RG. Random pattern flaps. In: Roenigk RK, Roenigk HH Jr, eds. Dermatologic Surgery: Principles and Practice. New York: Marcel Dekker, 1989:265.

Zitelli JA. Tips for wound closure Pears for minimizing dog-ears. and applications of periosteal sutures. Dermatologic Clinics 1989; 7(1):123–128.

Zitelli JA, Moy RL. Buried vertical mattress suture. J Dermatol Surg Oncol 1989; 15(1):17–19.

52

Skin Grafts

Ronald G. Wheeland
University of Arizona College of Medicine, Tucson, Arizona, U.S.A.

HISTORY

The first skin graft was performed in India nearly 3000 years ago. The Hindus reconstructed nasal defects with full-thickness skin grafts. It was not until 1869 that Reverdin published his experience with small pinch grafts in the treatment of a variety of cutaneous defects. In 1870, Lawson used full-thickness skin grafts to repair defects of the eyelid, and von Esmarck later used full-thickness skin grafts in other areas of the body. Thiersch reported the first use of split-thickness skin grafts in 1886. Since that time, the technique has improved. The dermatologic surgeon should be able to place several different types of skin grafts in order to treat the patient with a cutaneous defect most satisfactorily.

USE

Skin grafts are used when primary repair is impossible due to size, location, or tension on the wound. They are also indicated when repair with a flap would result in significant disfigurement or morbidity. Skin grafts are typically used to protect deeper vital structures such as bone or cartilage and keep them from becoming desiccated. Skin graft may reduce wound contraction of soft issue. This is helpful when the defect is around the facial orifices such as the eyelids or lips. Skin grafts speed healing time compared to the time required for second intention healing. Lastly, skin grafts may provide temporary coverage for a defect after oncologic surgery. This warrants careful evaluation of the wound for evidence of recurrent tumor.

TYPES

There are essentially three types of skin grafts (Table 1). The split-thickness skin graft (Fig. 1) consists of full-thickness epidermis and partial-thickness dermis. One type of split-thickness skin graft is the pinch graft, which was described more than a century ago. The full-thickness skin graft consists of epidermis and a complete thickness of dermis. One type of full-thickness skin graft is the dog-ear graft. The composite graft is composed of skin and some other appendage such as hair or cartilage. Hair transplant autografts consist of both skin and hair follicle structures used for hair replacement.

SPLIT-THICKNESS SKIN GRAFTS
Pinch Graft

The pinch graft is the simplest type of split-thickness skin graft. It is used in the treatment of stasis ulceration, decubitus ulcers, slowly healing traumatic or burn wounds, or ulcers of chronic radiodermatitis. The benefit of this technique is largely its safety and simplicity. Pinch grafting can be performed by surgeons with little experience in skin grafting. It can be used for patients who have significant medical problems or who are on medication that might typically interfere with normal wound healing. No special instrumentation is required.

This procedure can be performed on an outpatient basis in most situations. The grafts are highly successful because they have exceedingly low metabolic demands. For this reason, this type of graft is often successful when other grafts fail. Pinch grafts are capable of surviving in areas of decreased blood flow or in the presence of bacterial colonization. Functional results can be expected and grafting can be repeated as needed because the donor site is not permanently damaged.

A major disadvantage is that pinch grafting can be time-consuming. In addition, the small donor scars are obvious and may be difficult to hide. Most importantly, however, the ulcers that are treated have a typical cobblestone appearance (Fig. 2). This may be cosmetically unacceptable in spite of the fact that they are functionally acceptable.

The ulcer bed must be clean, well vascularized, and devoid of necrotic debris. This can be done in several ways, the most expeditious being blunt surgical debridement. Other approaches include enzymatic debridement, application of synthetic membrane dressings, topical benzoyl peroxide, dextranomer granules, whirlpool baths, and antibacterial ointments. If the patient is to be treated at home, an effective way to obtain a clean ulcer bed is to use an oral hygiene device such as WaterPik.

Once the ulcer bed is ready for grafting, wheals, approximately 1 cm in diameter, are raised on the donor site (Fig. 3A), which is typically the anterior thigh, by the intradermal injection of lidocaine 1%. The grafts are taken by shaving the top off each wheal using a #11 Bard-Parker blade (Fig. 3B) or sterile razor blade (Fig. 3C) at the level of the papillary dermis. These grafts are then placed in the ulcer bed spaced 1 to 2 mm apart (Fig. 3D). The grafted ulcer is then covered with a sheet of sterile transparent polyurethane (Fig. 3E) (Op-Site, Tegaderm, Bioclusive, or Ensure It). This membrane should overlap the ulcer bed by 2 to 3 cm onto the adjacent normal skin. A cotton-ball stent is placed on top of the polyurethane membrane to compress the grafts into the base of the ulcer. The grafted site is then immobilized and dressed with an elastic wrap, which is left in place for seven to eight days.

The donor site is treated in a similar fashion. This permits rapid wound healing by second intention. The polyurethane membrane is allowed to separate within 12 to

Table 1 Comparison of Skin Grafts

	Full thickness	Split thickness	Composite
Nutritional requirements	High	Low	High
Color	Good	Poor	Good
Contraction	Low	High	Low
Durability	Fair	Poor	Fair
Sensation	Good	Fair	Fair
Appendageal functions (hair, eccrine, sebaceous)	Excellent	Poor	Good

14 days after reepithelialization is complete (Fig. 3F). Pooling of blood or exudative fluids can be drained by puncturing the membrane with an 18-gauge needle. This puncture site can be repaired with a small piece of polyurethane membrane so that desiccation will not occur. If incomplete wound healing of the ulcer bed has not occurred in six weeks, these portions can be regrafted (Fig. 3G). While the patient may ambulate somewhat, walking should be kept to a minimum to avoid dislodging the grafts.

Classification

A split-thickness skin graft is the free transfer of epidermis and a portion of the dermis from one site to another. Split-thickness skin grafts are classified according to the thickness and are typically classified as thin (0.0006–0.0012 in.), intermediate (0.0012–0.0018 in.), or thick (0.0018–0.0024 in.) (Fig. 1).

Split-thickness skin grafts are used to cover large defects. After tumor surgery, they permit observation of the wound for evidence of tumor recurrence, while a more definitive repair is planned at a later date. Split-thickness skin grafts can also be used to cover the secondary defect from a flap or to line composite grafts.

The benefit of split-thickness skin grafts is that there is almost no limitation to the size of the defect that can be treated, and virtually no part of the body cannot be used as a donor site (Fig. 4). The success rate is relatively high, especially with thinner split-thickness grafts. While these skin grafts do not prevent wound contraction, they will reduce what would normally occur. At the same time, split-thickness skin grafts will speed wound healing compared to healing by second intention.

To apply properly, a split-thickness skin graft requires more meticulous technique than pinch grafts. In addition, special equipment and assistance are necessary. While the

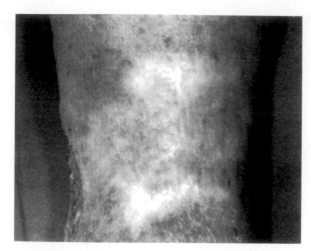

Figure 2 The irregular cobblestone appearance of a healed pinch-grafted site is obvious long after the wound has healed.

appearance of the final cosmetic wound following split-thickness skin grafting is acceptable, it is not excellent, because in most cases there are both alopecia and differences in texture and color of the skin (Fig. 5A and B). In addition, split-thickness skin grafts may not recover normal sensation. The donor site heals by second intention and may be the source of postoperative pain as well as permanent disfigurement.

Instrumentation

Several devices are available to harvest grafts of split thickness. The oldest are hand-operated knives, which are inexpensive but limited in the quality of grafts obtained. With the surgeon's increased experience, these instruments are capable of providing split-thickness skin grafts of sufficient length and width to cover most wounds (Fig. 6A).

More popular today are the power dermatomes such as the Brown, Padgett, and Castroviejo types (Fig. 6B and C). These instruments are capable of providing minute variability in the thickness and width of split-thickness skin grafts. They are expensive but relatively easy to operate. The Simon-Davol battery-powered dermatome (Fig. 6D and E) is less expensive. It has only one setting—1 to 5/16 in. wide and 0.015 in. thick—but it is light, convenient, and the head is disposable.

Technique

The typical donor sites used include the anterior thigh, buttocks, abdomen, and back. The scalp can be used because the hair will hide the donor site once it has regrown. For young patients who like to wear swimsuits, the pubic area has also been used as a donor site.

On the day of surgery, the donor site is shaved and prepped. The tissue to be harvested is marked at least 10% to 25% larger than the defect because contraction of the graft can be expected. Local anesthesia is obtained with lidocaine 1%. Hyaluronidase may be added to this solution to decrease the number of injections required.

A liberal amount of sterile lubricant is applied to the surface of the donor site. With the donor skin pulled taut, the dermatome is pushed with even pressure over the skin. Another technique used to make harvesting easier is to apply a sheet of sterile polyurethane to the donor site prior to cutting the graft. This makes the skin more rigid and

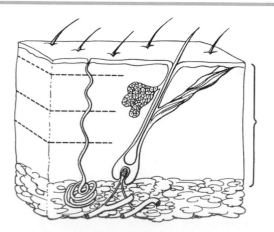

Figure 1 Various thickness of skin grafts; split thickness (thin, medium, and thick) on left, full thickness on right.

(A)   **(B)**   **(C)**   **(D)**

(E)   **(F)**   **(G)**

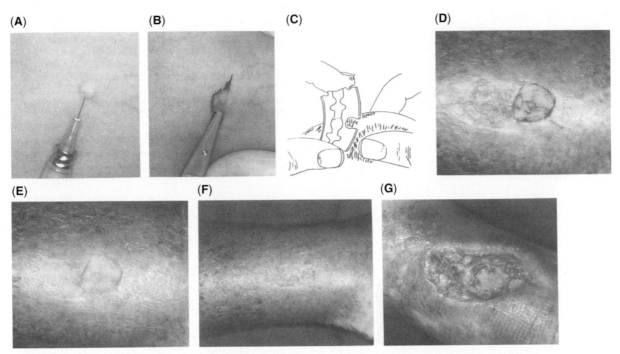

Figure 3 **(A)** Creation of a wheal by the intradermal injection of 1% plain lidocaine. **(B)** Harvesting a thin pinch-graft with a sawing motion and a #11 Bard-Parker scalpel blade, **(C)** alternative method for harvesting pinch grafts using a razor blade, **(D)** immediate postoperative appearance of a small stasis ulcer with pinch-grafts placed in the ulcer bed. **(E)** Stasis ulcer with translucent polyurethane membrane in place to assist healing and protect grafts. **(F)** Healed stasis ulcer six weeks postoperatively. **(G)** Large stasis ulcer with partial take of pinch grafts; complete healing can still occur by second intention after pinch-graft procedure.

allows the dermatome to harvest the graft uniformly. These membranes are all approximately 0.002 in. thick; so this must be considered when setting thickness on the dermatome. The polyurethane membrane remains adherent to the harvested graft. The graft is then lifted off the dermatome and draped loosely into the wound. Precise placement of the graft is not important because excess at the edges of the wound will undergo necrosis and shed (Fig. 7A). The edges are then sutured or stapled into place. A basting stitch may be required for larger wounds to ensure attachment to the base. If excessive exudate is

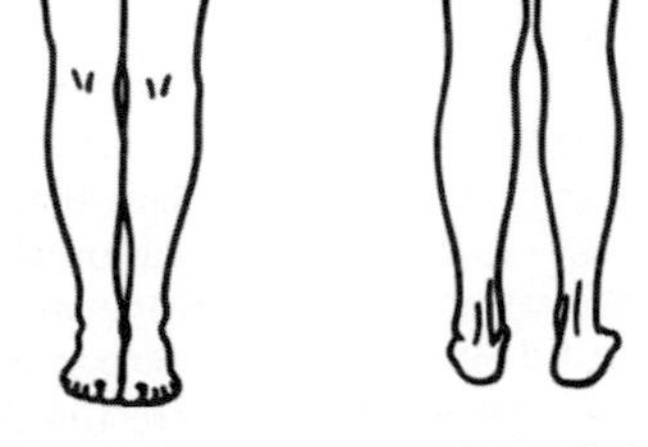

expected, fenestrations are made in the graft to permit drainage (Fig. 7B and C). The defect is then irrigated under the graft with chilled saline and an immobilizing pressure dressing is applied.

After bleeding has stopped at the donor site, it is covered with a sheet of sterile polyurethane or hydrocolloid synthetic dressing material. If fluid accumulates beneath these membranes, it may be drained by puncturing the membrane with an 18-gauge needle.

Both graft and donor sites are reexamined at 24 to 48 hours to be sure that no excess fluid has accumulated beneath the graft or the membrane at the donor site. If so, this is drained by puncturing the membrane with an 18-gauge needle and patching the puncture site with a small piece of the adhesive membrane. Graft adhesion is typically satisfactory within two to three weeks. Maturation may take many months. Dermabrasion may be considered at 6 to 12 weeks to even out the edges of the grafted site.

Meshed Split-Thickness Skin Grafts

Meshing a split-thickness skin graft is done when donor tissue is limited or the wound is relatively large (Fig. 8). Meshing allows the graft to expand like an accordion due to slits made by a mechanical mesher. A standard split-thickness skin graft placed through this meshing device can increase the area of coverage from 100% to 900%. The mesh graft is particularly beneficial for anatomic areas that are highly mobile such as the knee, scrotum, or axillae because it easily fits irregular body folds.

The meshed graft allows drainage of exudate and blood without disruption of the healing process. The meshed spaces heal by second intention, which results in a slightly more irregular surface. However, the wound

Figure 4 Typical split-thickness skin graft donor sites.

(A) **(B)**

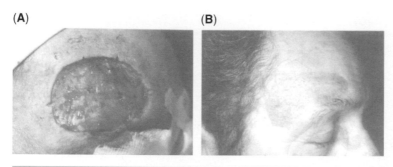

Figure 5 **(A)** Large defect on the forehead immediately following Mohs micrographic surgery. **(B)** Final appearance of treatment site six months after repair of wound with a split-thickness skin graft; note hyperpigmentation of grafted tissue compared to surrounding normal issue.

maintains its durability and healing time is not substantially different from that of the traditional split-thickness skin graft.

FULL-THICKNESS SKIN GRAFTS

A full-thickness skin graft involves the free transfer of epidermis and the complete thickness of dermis from one site to another with disruption of the vascular supply. This type of graft is used for small- to medium-sized defects where primary closure is not possible or where local skin flap surgery would create an undesirable effect and maximal cosmetic results are desired.

The primary benefit of this graft is that it prevents wound contraction in up to 80% of the cases. At the same time, the cosmetic appearance is maximized because the tissue color, texture, and thickness match better than an STSE. This graft allows excellent wound durability and is typically associated with less morbidity than local flaps. An additional advantage is that this procedure can be performed with standard surgical instruments without the need for new or expensive instrumentation.

A disadvantage of full-thickness skin grafts is that there are only a limited number of donor sites available, and the donor site must match closely with the tissue surrounding the defect. As an example, for facial defects, the donor site must be superior to the blush line, which is typically the clavicle or nipple, so that the vessels in the graft will dilate when appropriate. The metabolic demands of this graft are relatively high and failure is not uncommon. As a consequence, grafts of this type are limited in size.

The recipient site for full-thickness grafts must be clean and well vascularized. Full-thickness skin grafts should not be placed directly on exposed bone, cartilage, tendon, or fat, which lack sufficient vascular supply. In spite of this, failure of the graft may occur due to either hematoma or seroma formation; so meticulous hemostasis is important.

Donor Site

Several areas of facial tissue excess are more likely to provide a graft that has good color and texture, matching the tissue adjacent to the defect. Typical donor areas (Fig. 9A) are the superior retroauricular area or upper eyelid used for the lower eyelid; lower retroauricular area used for defects on the cheek and temple; the preauricular area and lower lateral neck for the mid-cheek and chin; the supraclavicular area for both the medial canthus and lower eyelid; the upper lateral neck for the helix; and the glabella for

(A) **(B)**

(C) **(D)** **(E)**

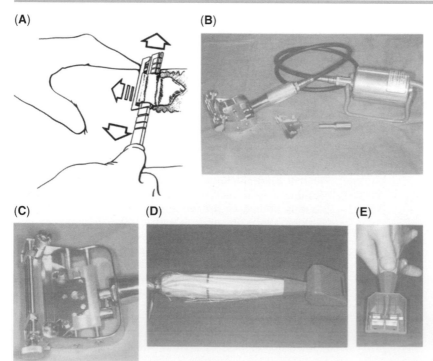

Figure 6 **(A)** Free-hand blade harvesting split-thickness skin graft. **(B)** Brown dermatome with its electric motor. **(C)** Close-up of head of Brown dermatome. **(D)** Profile view of Simon-Davol dermatome with disposable sterile head in place and handle containing battery pack within sterile plastic bag, ready for use. **(E)** Frontal appearance of Simon-Davol dermatome.

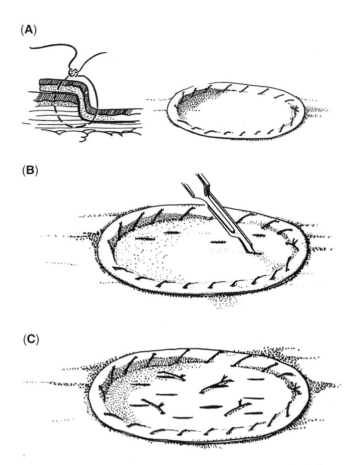

(A)

(B)

(C)

Figure 7 **(A)** Suturing technique for split-thickness skin graft, **(B)** fenestrations made in split-thickness skin graft to permit egress of exudate. **(C)** Basting sutures in center of graft to provide maximum attachment of graft to base.

the chin, forehead, and nose. The upper back in the area of the trapezius muscle (Fig. 9B) is good for defects on the nasal tip because the thickness of this tissue allows it to be sculptured to fit properly around the alar cartilages. The nasolabial fold may be sufficiently redundant to harvest a small graft for the nose as well (Fig. 9A). The inguinal fold and the antecubital fossa are used for defects on the hand (Fig. 9B).

Technique

First, the recipient site must be healthy, clean, well-vascularized, and not contaminated with necrotic debris or microorganisms. There should be little subcutaneous fat on the base of the graft. A template that matches the defect can be made to harvest a graft of appropriate size and shape. This is only a rough approximation because the graft contracts 20% to 40% after harvesting. Once the size of the graft has been determined, the best donor site is selected according to color, texture, thickness, and presence or absence of appendageal structures such as hair follicles. The graft is harvested and all fat is stripped from the base (Fig. 10A). It is then cut to fit the defect, so that it may be placed without tension or excess tissue at any margin.

The graft is sutured into position. Alternate sutures are left long to support a tie-over dressing (Fig. 10B). For larger grafts, a basting stitch may be placed through the graft to the wound bed. The space under the graft is then irrigated with chilled saline to flush out residual blood or debris.

Many different dressings have been used successfully, to immobilize and support a skin graft. An interpositional membrane, such as N-terface, is placed between the graft and the dressing. This membrane permits easy removal of the dressing by preventing crust from adhering to the gauze stent. A nonadherent gauze pad is cut slightly larger than the graft so that the compression is outward and downward and not directly on the sutures themselves. A bulky cotton stent is placed over the gauze to absorb exudate and act as a buffer from external trauma. A button-foam dressing may be used instead of the cotton stent. After the cotton stein is applied, the long sutures used to anchor the graft into position are tied over the stent (Fig. 10B). A bulky protective dressing is then placed over this. While not required, antibiotics are given to most patients for one week.

To minimize interference with wound healing, the graft is not examined for five to seven days. At that time, the dressing is soaked with either sterile saline or hydrogen peroxide. The graft is typically cyanotic, and there may be epidermal blistering (Fig. 11C). This tissue should be left in place. An antibiotic ointment is applied to the surface of the graft, and a smaller protective dressing is applied, to be changed daily for an additional week. Within several days, depending on the location, the epidermal crusting will disappear and revascularization of the graft can be expected (Fig. 11D). Dermabrasion can be considered in 6 to 12 weeks to smooth the edges and help blend the graft in with the surrounding skin.

Dog-Ear (Burow's Triangle) Grafts

When full-thickness defects are created on the inelastic, thick skin such as the forehead, sometimes only partial linear closure is possible. In these situations, the superfluous tissue that forms at one or both ends of the closure, commonly called "dog-ear" deformities, can sometimes be utilized advantageously as free full-thickness skin grafts to provide wound closure without the need to create a second donor defect elsewhere. These dog-ear or Burow's triangle grafts provide excellent color and texture match because they are obtained from the immediately adjacent area. The technique used for placement of these grafts is identical to that employed for more traditional full-thickness grafts, and either one or both of the excised Burow's triangles can be placed in the central defect and sutured in place (Fig. 12A). A stent dressing is applied (Fig. 12B), and standard wound care is followed. If the defect is not entirely covered by the combined use of primary closure and Burow's triangle grafts, the remaining portion can be allowed to heal by second intention (Fig. 12C) with anticipated good cosmetic results. Because these grafts contribute a substantial amount of tissue to the overall repair of the wound, the time required for complete healing is reduced over that normally necessary for total healing by second intention.

Composite Grafts

Composite grafts are composed of more than one tissue type. These are typically used for defects on the alae, auricles, or eyelids (Fig. 13) that have free edge and no base. Hair transplants are a type of composite graft because they are composed of both skin and hair.

(A)   **(B)**

(C)   **(D)**

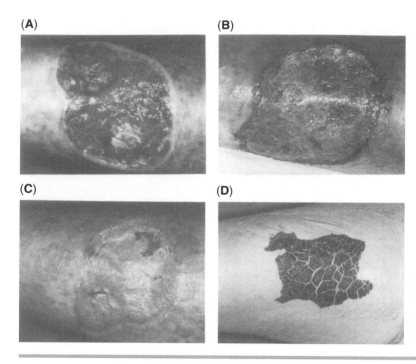

Figure 8 (A) Defect of the lower leg following removal of squamous cell carcinoma with Mohs micrographic surgery, (B) meshed split-thickness skin graft in place, (C) one month postoperatively: irregular texture and color, (D) donor site on anterior thigh with translucent polyurethane membrane placed; dried serosanguineous fluid is present beneath.

The main disadvantage of composite grafts is the higher failure rate due to their increased metabolic demands. This is especially true if the graft is greater than 1 cm in diameter. The ear is the typical donor site for many composite grafts; so there may be some distortion of the donor area. The technique varies significantly from one surgeon to another. Some allow the initial wound to heal by second intention before proceeding with the graft. Others will proceed with immediate repair.

The size of the defect is determined and marked on the anterior crus of the helix of the ear (Fig. 13). This zone is typically chosen because it has the proper contour for defects of the nasal alae and has similar texture, color, and thickness. The donor area is harvested as an excision, and the graft is lined with either a mucosal flap from the nose or a split-thickness skin graft. This is then sutured into place with great care to prevent injury to the vascular structures. Survival of the composite graft depends on circulation from the periphery and perfusing centrally. The donor site on the ear is then repaired typically with an interior-based preauricular advancement flap.

Cultured Epithelial Autografts

Nearly 25 years ago, initial laboratory techniques were developed for the cultivation of animal and human keratinocytes. Within a few years, the technique had been sufficiently perfected to allow the growth of cultured keratinocytes in large enough quantities to permit their use as a type of skin graft known as a cultured epithelial autograft (CEA). This type of skin graft has now proven useful as a functional skin replacement and has been used experimentally at split-thickness skin graft donor sites as well as to treat wounds produced by Mohs micrographic surgery, carbon dioxide laser vaporization, or electrosurgery. CEAs are also routinely used in the management of patients with severe burns and to speed the healing of certain chronic wounds, like stasis and decubitus ulcers.

CEAs have been used for skin replacement after the excision of giant congenital nevi, but because these grafts are typically applied without any fibrous dermal component,

(A)

(B)

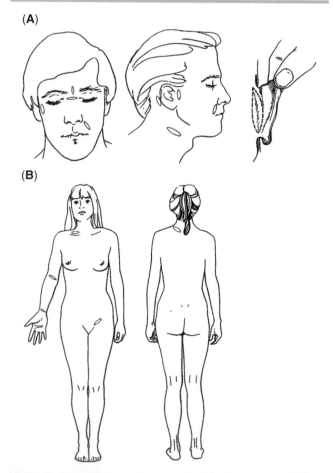

Figure 9 Donor sites available for (A) full-thickness skin grafts on the face and neck; (B) full-thickness skin grafts on trunk and extremities.

(A)

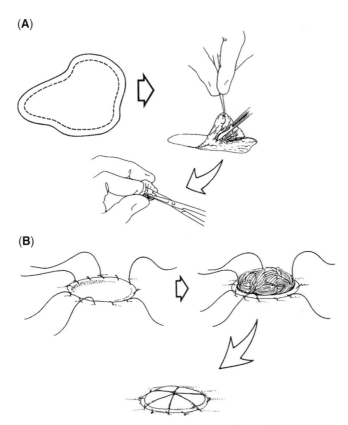

(B)

(A)   **(B)**

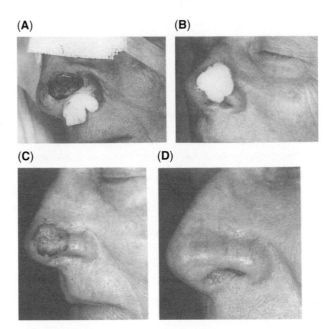

(C)   **(D)**

Figure 11 **(A)** Wound on the ala after removal of a basal cell carcinoma by Mohs micrographic surgery, **(B)** tie-over stent dressing holding full-thickness skin graft compressed and immobile, **(C)** full-thickness graft one week postoperatively shows epidermal crust and cyanosis, **(D)** full-thickness skin graft two months postoperatively. Preservation of normal contours and good color match.

Figure 10 **(A)** Graft harvesting is planned 10% to 20% larger than defect (*upper left*); graft harvested in the subcutaneous plane (*upper right*); removal of subcutaneous fat prior to graft placement (*bottom*), **(B)** graft sutured into place. Alternate sutures left long (*upper left*), cotton stem, or bolus applied on top of full-thickness skin graft (*tipper right*), with tie-over suture (*bottom*).

they often appear atrophic. For that reason, when used as a sheet of epithelium, they are of only limited usefulness for most cosmetic problems. However, in order to improve the cosmetic results, a number of artificial tissues known as living skin equivalents have been developed, which employ autologous cultured keratinocytes suspended on a dermal substitute composed of an acellular, synthetic, porous membrane of cross-linked collagen, glycosaminoglycans, and autologous cultured fibroblasts or a bovine collagen gel to provide both dermal and epidermal components to the graft. Although additional clinical experience is required to substantiate the benefits these skin equivalents may provide, their promise seems substantial. A new delivery system for cultured epithelial cells using an aerosol mist has recently been developed in Australia for the treatment of large wounds or extensive burns. Known as "CellSpray ReCell," this product has dramatically changed the way patients with burns, chronic wounds, and scars are managed.

Overgrafting

Overgrafting is the serial application of split-thickness skin grafts applied to increase thickness. A split-thickness skin graft is placed on a wound and allowed to heal. Then the epidermis is removed by dermabrasion down to the papillary dermis. Another split-thickness graft is applied to the surface. This may be repeated two or three times to increase the thickness of a defect. This technique is also

not commonly performed today because a variety of alternative flaps may be more appropriate. Also, because full-thickness skin grafts can be harvested from donor sites with a thicker dermis, there is little use for overgrafting. The occurrence of small cysts is typical because appendageal structures may be left intact and buried beneath the layers of grafted skin.

Delayed Grafting

Ceilley has reported that defects need not be repaired immediately. Instead, the wound is managed as if allowed to heal by second intention. This is done for 10 to 14 days, which allows removal of necrotic debris and the development of sufficient vascular supply and granulation issue to support a graft. Because contraction of the wound may occur during this time, the small proof advancing epithelium should be excised prior to performing the final closure. The main advantage of this technique, in addition to improving circulation, is that the depth of the wound may fill in significantly with granulation tissue during this delay period, which decreases the required thickness of grafted tissue. This will also improve the final cosmetic appearance by eliminating some of the irregular contours.

Substitutes for Human Skin

Several products are now available for use in place of the autologous skin graft. While they are traditionally used for larger wounds such as severe thermal injuries, knowledge of these materials is important. One of the original grafts used for burn wounds is the porcine xenograft. This material is used as a temporary dressing until sufficient donor tissue can be harvested or cultured from the patient. In this same fashion, chorioamnion biologic membrane can be used as a temporary covering. It also serves to demonstrate the ability of the body

(A)   **(B)**   **(C)**

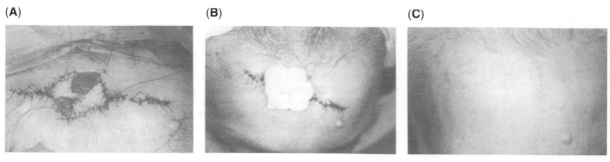

Figure 12 **(A)** Partial primary closure of a Mohs micrographic surgery defect; the dog-ears have been used as full-thickness skin grafts. A portion of the defect is allowed to heal by second intention, **(B)** stent dressing is placed over the dog-ear grafts for stability, **(C)** postoperative result at one year.

to accept a permanent graft according to the quantity and quality of the vascular supply generated.

CAUSES OF GRAFT FAILURE AND THEIR TREATMENT

General Causes

While there are many reasons (Table 2) for a graft to fail, the most common cause is disruption of the newly formed blood vessels by movement or shearing forces. For this reason, a variety of different dressing suturing patterns, and basting stitches have been used to minimize disruption of the healing wound. Another reason grafts are lost is secondary infection, especially due to *Staphylococcus, Streptococcus,* and *Pseudomonas.* The temporary impairment of circulation after injury or surgery predisposes to contamination, colonization, and necrosis.

Both hematoma and seroma are also causes of graft failure. Hematomas interfere with neovascularization to the graft, and it appears that breakdown products of the blood clot are toxic. In a similar fashion, seromas may predispose to wound infection. For this reason, the wound must be meticulously examined for hemostasis prior to application of the grafts and then be sufficiently compressed into the defect by sutures or dressings to minimize the collection of serum or blood beneath the graft.

Another common reason that grafts fail is that they are placed on an inappropriate recipient site. Exposed bone, cartilage, and tendons do not provide enough vascularity to support a graft. In these circumstances, if primary closure is possible, it is preferred. If a flap is not possible and yet, because of the size or location of the defect, wound closure is desirable, sufficient time should be allowed for development of a well-vascularized wound bed to ensure graft

survival. Many find that subcutaneous fat is not adequately vascularized for grafting and recommend that the fat be removed and the graft applied to the underlying fascia or muscle to improve graft survival. If a full-thickness graft is being used to repair a defect, all fat on the base of the graft should be removed. This serves to minimize the chance of secondary infection and maximize the chance for graft survival.

Excessive tension on a graft further impairs vascular supply because the caliber of the vessels within the graft is decreased by tension across the surface caused by wound closure. In this way, tension not only decreases the chance for survival but also predisposes to graft failure by increasing the risk of secondary infection.

Treatment of Failed Grafts or Grafts with Poor Cosmetic Results

It is important to be patient when performing graft surgery. Epidermal necrosis and cyanosis almost always occur with full-thickness skin grafts. The surgeon should expect these and warn the patient that they are not a sign of graft failure and provide sufficient emotional support for the patient during the healing process. Wound care, such as mild debridement during the postoperative period done at the office, is helpful. In many cases even when the graft appears to be nonviable, complete and satisfactory wound healing will still occur.

For the pinch graft, it appears that sufficient numbers of epidermal cells are transferred with this technique to allow the wound to heal despite apparent total graft failure. In a similar fashion, a split-thickness skin graft may provide a stimulus for wound healing in spite of the fact that the graft may have been lost entirely. Thus, if a graft fails, it does not necessarily represent an intrinsic problem with the

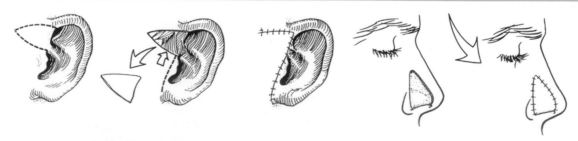

Figure 13 Composite graft from the ear is transferred to a full-thickness defect of the ala.

Table 2 Causes of Graft Failure

Technical errors
  Improper size or thickness
  Tension
  Incomplete hemostasis resulting in hematoma
  Error in timing of surgical repair
  Improper dressing: too tight; not immobilizing
Improper patient care
  Dependent position
  Motion
Insufficient bed vascularity
  Improper bed (fat. bone, cartilage, tendon)
  Necrotic debris
  Hematoma
  Seroma
Infection
  Staphylococcus
  Streptococcus
  Pseudomonas
Trauma
Motion
Systemic disease
  Diabetes
  Immunologic dysfunction

procedure, anatomic location, or patient. Instead, once a new vascularized base has developed, regrafting should be attempted if necessary.

Spontaneous improvement in the texture or color of grafted tissue can be expected over a period of 6 to 12 weeks. Because improvement may be substantial over this period of time, patience is a necessity. If after 6 to 12 weeks the results have been less than optimal, dermabrasion may be performed to help blend the color with the surrounding tissue and improve the texture of the grafted site.

BIBLIOGRAPHY

Bell E, Erlich HP, Slier S, et al. Development and use of a living skin equivalent. Plast Reconstr Surg 1981; 67:386–392.

Boyee ST, Hansbrough JF. Biologic attachment, growth, and differentiation of cultured human epidermal keratinocytes on a graftable collagen and chondroitin-6-sulfate substrate. Surgery 1987; 103:421–431.

Ceilley RI, Burnsted RM, Panje WR. Delayed skin grafting. J Dermatol Surg Oncol 1983; 9:288–293.

Fatah MF, Ward CM. The morbidity of split-skin graft donor sites in the elderly: The case for mesh-grafting the donor site. Br J Plast Surg 1984; 37:184–190.

Field LM. Nasal alar rim reconstruction utilizing the crus of the helix, with several alternatives for donor site closure. J Dermatol Surg Oncol 1986; 12:253–255.

Gallico GG III, O'Connor NE, Compton CC, et al. Cultured epithelial autografts for giant congenital nevi. Plast Reconstr Surg 1989; 84:1–9.

Gallico GG III, O'Connor NE, Compton CC, et al. Permanent coverage of large burn wounds with autologous cultured human epithelium. N Engl J Med 1984; 311:448–451.

Gilmore WA, Wheeland RG. Treatment of ulcers on legs by pinch grafts and a supportive dressing of polyurethane. J Dermatol Surg Oncol 1982; 8:177–183.

Hansbrough JF, Boyce ST, Cooper ML, Foreman TJ. Bum wound closure with cultured autologous keratinocytes and fibroblasts attached to a collagen-glycosaminoglycan substrate. J Am Med Assoc 1989; 262:2125–2130.

Harris DR. Healing of the surgical wound. J Am Acad Dermatol 1979; 1:208–215.

Hefton JM, Caldwell D, Biozes DG, et al. Grafting of skin ulcers with cultured autologous epidermal ceils. J Am Acad Dermatol 1986; 14:399–405.

Hill TG. A simplified method for closure of full-thickness skin grafts. J Dermatol Surg Oncol 1980; 6:892–893.

Hill TG. Enhancing the survival of full-thickness grafts. J Dermatol Surg Oncol 1984; 10:639–642.

Hill TG. Reconstruction of nasal defects using full-thickness skin grafts: A personal reappraisal. J Dermatol Surg Oncol 1983; 9:995–1001.

Hull BE, Finley RK, Miller SF. Coverage of full-thickness burns with bilayered skin equivalents: A preliminary clinical trial. Surgery 1989; 107:496–502.

Igel HJ, Freeman AE, Boecfonan CR, Kleinfeld KL. A new method for covering large surface area wounds with autografts. II. Surgical application of tissue culture and expanded rabbit skin autografts. Arch Surg 1974; 108:724–729.

James JH, Watson ACH, The use of Op-site, a vapour permeable dressing, on skin graft donor sites. Br J Plast Surg 1975; 28:107–110.

Johnson TM, Racner D, Nelson BR. Soft tissue reconstruction with skin grafting. J Am Acad Dermatol 1992; 27:151–165.

Leigh IM, Purkis PE. Culture grafted leg ulcers. Clin Exp Dermatol 1986; 11:650–652.

Mareclo CL, Kim YG, Kaine JL, Voorhees JJ. Stratification, specialization and proliferation of primary keratinocyte cultures. J Cell Biol 1978; 79:356–370.

Petry JJ, Wortham KA. Contraction and growth of wounds covered by meshed and nonmeshed split-thickness skin grafts. Br J Plast Surg 1986; 39:478–482.

Phillips TJ, Gilchrest BA. Cultured allogenic keratinocyte graft in the management of wound healing: Prognostic factors. J Dermatol Surg Oncol 1989; 15:1169–1176.

Phillips TJ, Kehinde O, Green H, Gilchrest BA. Treatment of skin ulcers with cultured epidermal allografts. J Am Acad Dermatol 1989; 21:191–199.

Porter JM, Griffiths RW, McNeill DC. The surgical management of intractable venous ulceration in the lower limbs: Excision, decompression of the limb, and split-skin grafting. Br J Plast Surg 1984; 37:I79–183.

Robinson JK. Improvement of the appearance of full-thickness skin grafts with dermabrasion. Arch Dermatol 1987; 123:1340–1345.

Silfverskiold KL. A new pressure device for securing skin grafts. Br J Plast Surg 1986; 39:567–569.

Stal S, Spira M. Mons pubis as a donor site for split-thickness skin grafts. Plast Reconstr Surg 1985; 75:906–910.

Swanson NA, Tromovitch TA, Stegman SJ. Glogau RG. Skin grafting: The split-thickness graft in 1980. J Dermatol Surg Oncol 1980; 6:524–526.

Wheeland RG. The Technique and current status of Pinch Grafting. J Dermatol Surg Oncol 1987; 13:873–880.

Wood F. Hand craft rays off. Chamer 2005; 76:26–30.

Wright JK, Brawer MK. Survival of full-thickness skin grafts over avascular defects. Plast Reconstr Surg 1980; 66:428–431.

Yuspa SH, Morgan DL, Walker RJ, Bates RR. The growth of fetal mouse skin in cell culture and transplantation to F1 mice. J Invest Dermatol 1970; 55:379–389.

Zitelli JA. Burow's grafts. J Am Acad Dermatol 1987; 17:271–279.

53

Rotation Flaps

William J. Grabski

Brooke Army Medical Center, Fort Sam Houston, Houston, Texas, U.S.A.

Stuart J. Salasche

University of Arizona Health Sciences Center, Tucson, Arizona, U.S.A.

THE CLASSIC ROTATION FLAP

Rotation flap, one of the three main types of random-pattern flaps, is named after the method of tissue movement. The classic rotation flap can be conceptualized as a triangular defect closed by the rotation of skin around a pivot point (Fig. 1A). In reality, as the primary defect is closed by the rotation of tissue, a secondary defect is created along the curvilinear arc of the flap (Fig. 1B). This longer and narrower secondary defect contains the same surface area as the primary defect but can often be closed by a combination of simple advancement of the curvilinear arc as well as secondary advancement of the surrounding skin (Fig. 1C). As will be discussed later, a dog-ear usually forms along the outer curvilinear arc.

FLAP DESIGN

The design of the rotation flap is not complex in conception or execution. It consists of incising along the curvilinear arc drawn away from the defect, usually in a relaxed skin tension line (RSTL) or a junction line between cosmetic units. If possible, it is best to base the flap inferiorly and laterally to help with drainage and cosmesis because the new scar line will be displaced away from the midline (Fig. 2).

Unfortunately, the rotation flap is a relatively inefficient method of recruiting tissue, because a long incision is often required. The arc may need to be three to four times the length of the primary defect. In selected situations, a rotation flap with a short curvilinear arc can be utilized as a method of either changing the closure tension vector or moving redundant skin (dog-ears) to a more advantageous location around a defect than could otherwise be accomplished by a side-to-side closure. The maneuver of creating a rotation flap also effectively shortens the scar line. This not only allows for closure without extension into an adjoining cosmetic unit, it also breaks up the scar line. Two short incision lines have a cosmetic advantage over a single long one.

When required, there are two methods of increasing flap mobility. Each has the advantage of allowing less tension on the distal flap; however, both confer viability disadvantages. First, the curvilinear arc is successively lengthened until mobility is sufficiently increased to allow tension-free closure of the flap tip (Fig. 3A). In addition, a longer, narrower secondary defect is created, which also closes under less tension (Fig. 3B). The disadvantage of this lengthening maneuver is that a longer scar is created and vascular pedicle width decreases relative to the length of the flap. In a random-pattern flap, blood must reach the most distal portion of the flap via the subdermal plexus. Lengthening the distance that blood must travel may put this area at risk of insufficient perfusion.

The second method of increasing flap mobility is to perform a back-cut incision into the vascular pedicle at the far end of the curvilinear arc (Fig. 4). A back-cut is an efficient maneuver to change the pivot point with a short incision and hence increase mobility. This contrasts with the much longer continuation of the curvilinear arc required to produce the same increase in flap movement. Unfortunately, the back-cut also decreases the pedicle width just as the lengthening of the curvilinear arc decreases the pedicle width relative to the length of the flap. In general, rotation flaps are designed with wide, thick vascular pedicles, which can tolerate either a back-cut or lengthening of the arc. The gain in tissue mobility and decrease in tension from these maneuvers often more than compensate for the decrease in blood supply to the flap tip. Only clinical experience will help the surgeon decide how wide a vascular pedicle must be in order to supply the flap tip and how much tension can be tolerated.

There are two common errors in the design of a rotation flap. Both involve selection of the beginning point of the curvilinear arc. The first consists of starting this point too low around the defect. This does not compensate for the inevitable loss of height that occurs during the actual rotation of the flap. Tension is required to pull the flap tip into place, and the surgeon must often resort to either lengthening the arc or back-cutting the pedicle. It is easier to account for the expected loss of height and raise the leading edge of the flap beforehand (Fig. 5). The flap then drapes into place with little or no vertical tension on the flap tip. The blood supply to the tip is not compromised, and vertical tension on important anatomic structures (i.e., eyelid or lip) is avoided.

The second error involves round or oval defects where the tip designed is too narrow. When pulled into place, it is obvious this small triangle will not fit in or survive. This, in effect, shortens the flap and the same problems as indicated above are created. A better design would be to widen and raise the take-off point of the curvilinear arc (Fig. 6).

CLINICAL FLAP DESIGN

Although the classic rotation flap is conceptualized as beginning as a triangular defect, most cutaneous surgical defects tend to be circular or oval. Triangulating the defect

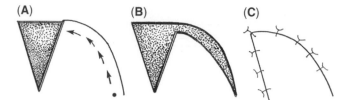

Figure 1 (A) Triangular defect and rotation flap design. (B) Creation of secondary defect after incision of flap. (C) Idealized closure of primary and secondary defects.

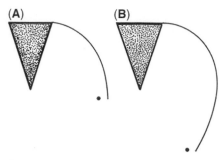

Figure 3 (A) Initial rotation flap design. (B) Flap lengthened to increase mobility. Area of secondary defect also increased.

is unnecessary and only creates a larger defect. The rotation flap should be designed and executed utilizing the original shape of the defect, with redundant tissue eliminated only as necessary. As stated earlier, the curvilinear arc of the flap should be designed so that it can be hidden in a junction line or a RSTL for best cosmesis. The length of the flap can initially be incised to a conservative length (one or two times the diameter of the primary defect) and then widely undermined. Undermining should include the tissue surrounding the flap to ensure good secondary movement, but should not extend too far under the pedicle to prevent compromising blood flow to the tip (Fig. 6C). The flap is undermined at the deepest safe level possible for that given anatomic site, but must always include at least some subcutaneous fat in order to include the subdermal plexus. The thicker the flap can be designed, the better the blood supply to the flap tip.

Once elevated, the flap can be pulled into place with a skin hook to test for the ease of flap mobility and the degree of closure tension. If an increase in flap mobility is required to fill the primary defect, an appropriate adjustment of arc

lengthening or back-cutting can be made at this time. Once an adequate amount of flap tissue has been recruited to fill the defect, the flap tip can be tacked into place with a temporary suture. Placement of the tip is the key stitch in a rotation flap as the tension vector of closure runs through this point (Fig. 7). Placement of the tip stitch defines how much of the primary defect will be filled with the flap and how much by secondary movement of the surrounding skin. If there is an important anatomic structure adjacent to the primary defect that should not be distorted, the flap should be draped in to fill the whole defect. This creates a larger secondary defect and produces more pronounced dog-ears. More often, it is advantageous to partially close the primary defect, which creates two similar wounds that are easier to close and have less pronounced dog-ears.

The actual closure consists of placing buried dermal absorbable sutures along the curvilinear arc (secondary

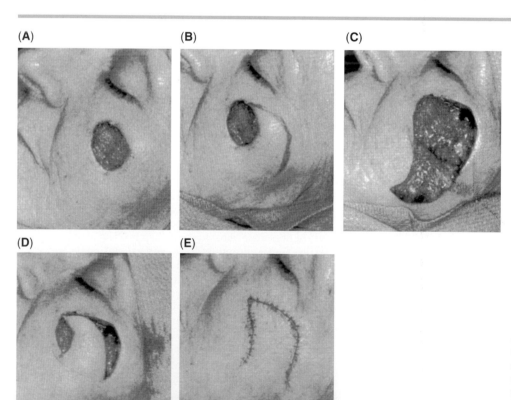

Figure 2 (A) A surgical defect of the malar cheek. (B) Inferior/lateral based rotation flap. The proposed incision is in the curvilinear RSTLs of the cheek. (C) The body of the flap is draped back. Undermining around primary and secondary defect already accomplished. (D) The key stitch is placed, partially closing the primary defect and creating a longer, narrower secondary defect. (E) After closure both incision lines parallel the RSTLs of the cheek.

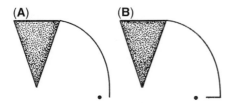

Figure 4 (**A**) Initial rotation flap design. (**B**) Back-cut changes pivot point and increases flap mobility.

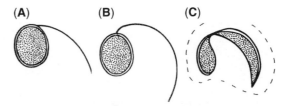

Figure 6 (**A**) Initial flap design. (**B**) Improved flap design. (**C**) Flap incised. Extent of undermining indicated.

defect) to relieve the tension on the tip stitch. They are arranged in a tangential manner across the defect so that they pull the flap into place and distribute the tension to several points away from the tip (Fig. 7). Buried sutures are also placed in the primary defect not so much to decrease tension but to spread out and arrange the flap placement. If the flap tip forms a narrow angle, it is often best to trim a small amount off to create a better fit and avoid tip necrosis.

Two areas of tissue redundancy can be expected whenever a rotation flap is done to close a circular or oval defect (Fig. 8A). A symmetrical dog-ear develops as the primary defect closes because it contains an angle greater than 30°. The tissue redundancy should be resected in a direction that does not narrow the vascular pedicle of the flap (Fig. 8B). An asymmetric dog-ear occurs along the closure of the secondary defect because of the difference in length of the two sides of the curvilinear arc. This dog-ear can be removed anywhere along the arc, but classically it is resected at the distal end in a "hockey stick" manner. Nonabsorbable surface sutures are then placed to approximate the epidermal edges in a slightly everted manner. A simple running suture is often a quick and efficient way to complete the closure.

SPECIAL DESIGN MODIFICATIONS

Bilateral rotation flaps can be designed in selected situations to recruit tissue from both sides of a defect, thus creating two smaller secondary defects rather than one larger one (Fig. 9). This becomes cosmetically advantageous when curvilinear junction lines or RSTLs are available on both sides of the primary defect. Bilateral rotation flaps may allow closure of a defect within a single cosmetic unit and obviate the need to cross over into the next cosmetic unit. The flap design is actually a rotational modification of an A-to-T or an O-to-T closure. The latter is considered advancement rather than rotation flaps.

Another variation is the O-to-Z flap (Fig. 10). This flap also borrows skin bilaterally. However, in this instance, the

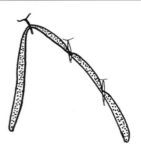

Figure 7 Placement of key stitch and tension reducing subcuticular stitches along secondary defect.

two curvilinear incisions are designed on opposite sides of the wound and arc away from each other rather than toward each other as in the standard bilateral rotation flap. This flap has limited application because of the resultant Z-shaped scar, which is not easily camouflaged, especially in one area where it is often attempted—the forehead. The vertex of the scalp is one area where this modification has proven useful.

REGIONAL APPLICATIONS

The rotation flap is one of the simpler random-pattern flaps, but one that requires careful planning and design as well as good surgical technique to obtain the best cosmetic results. This flap exploits the adjacent tissue elasticity along the curvilinear arc of the incision and has the potential to mobilize large volumes of tissue. One major advantage of the rotation flap is that it has a broad base. Thus, it contains a good vascular supply and has a low incidence of necrosis. It is usually designed as an inferiorly based flap, which results in better venous and lymphatic drainage (Fig. 2). The rotation flap is best utilized in areas where the incision lines can be camouflaged in a curvilinear junction line or RSTL.

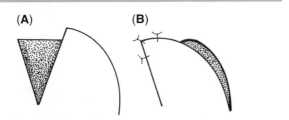

Figure 5 (**A**) Step-up design raises the lead edge of the flap. (**B**) The flap falls easily into place without tension.

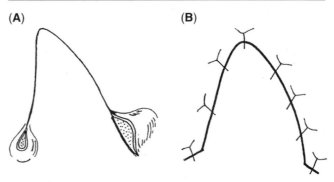

Figure 8 (**A**) Dog-ears form predictably in rotations flaps. (**B**) After excision of dog-ears.

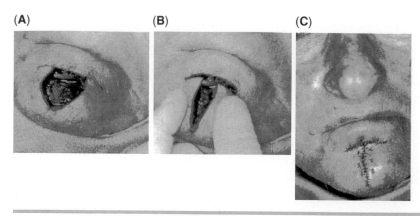

Figure 9 **(A)** Bilateral rotation flap created by paired incisions along mentolabial crease. **(B)** The two flaps rotate to meet each other in the midline. **(C)** The final closure is confined to the chin. Scar lines confined to the mentolabial crease and midline chin.

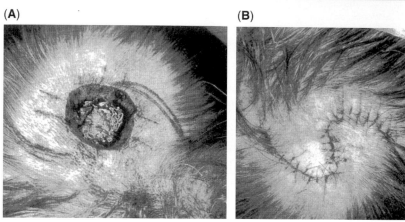

Figure 10 **(A)** An O-to-Z flap is created by two curvilinear incisions on opposite sides of a scalp defect. **(B)** The final closure after rotation toward the center.

The cheek and temple are particularly receptive to repairs by rotation flap (Fig. 11). Temple and lateral cheek rotation flaps can be designed with the curvilinear incisions placed along the temporal hairline or the preauricular junction. The lateral dog-ear repair can be hidden in the hairline or just inferior to the earlobe. These flaps take advantage of the lax tissue of the cheek, preauricular area, jowls, and neck.

Defects of the central cheek can be repaired effectively with inferolaterally based flaps. This is probably the

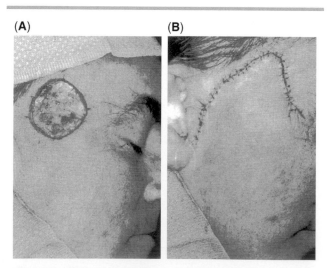

Figure 11 **(A)** A surgical defect of the temple, **(B)** Repair utilizing a lateral/inferior-based rotation flap. Arc incised along the hairline and the preauricular junction.

"cleanest" indication for this flap. Wounds can be closed away from the central portion of the face. The superior dog-ear that would form with a side-to-side closure and run onto the convex malar eminence is avoided. Finally, a long scar is broken up and camouflaged in the lateral cheek RSTL or preauricular folds.

Similarly, infraorbital cheek defects are especially challenging because of the need to avoid pull on the lower eyelid. The flap incision should arc superiorly along the infraorbital crease to compensate for the loss of flap height during rotation (Fig. 12). This allows the flap to drape across rather than having to be pulled up into place. Downward tension on the eyelid is avoided and ectropion prevented. A long flap is frequently required to mobilize sufficient tissue to minimize vertical tension upon closure of the secondary defect.

If small defects of the infraorbital cheek were closed in a side-to-side fashion, removal of the superior dog-ear would carry the scar line onto the lower eyelid. This can be avoided by performing an inferolaterally based rotation flap. The tissue redundancy is repositioned to the inferior poles of the closure and the repair can be completed within the cheek cosmetic unit.

Medially displaced cheek wounds can also be repaired with a rotation flap. In these instances, the flap is incised in the melolabial fold to tap into the lax, excessive skin of the inferior portion of the fold (Fig. 13). Often, more efficient or more cosmetic flaps such as the subcutaneous pedicle flaps or the perialar advancement flaps are chosen for repair of defects in this region.

Surgical defects of the middle to upper portion of the cutaneous upper lip can also be repaired by designing a rotation flap with the curvilinear arc incised along the

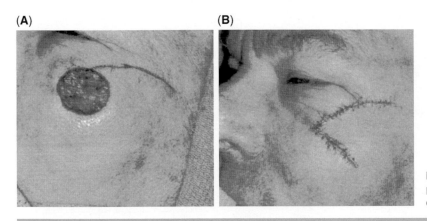

(A) **(B)**

Figure 12 **(A)** The proposed flap arcs superiorly to compensate for loss of height during rotation. **(B)** The final closure without downward tension on the eyelid.

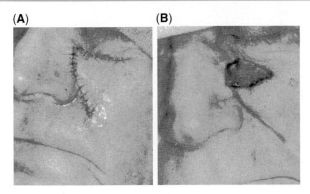

(A) **(B)**

Figure 13 **(A)** Inferior based rotation flap designed in melolabial fold. **(B)** The key stitch tacks the flap tip to the medial aspect of the defect to avoid downward pull on the eyelid.

melolabial fold (Fig. 14). There must be sufficient lax skin to fill the wound but not pull up the labial commissure.

Rotation flaps have proven useful in the repair of small defects of the distal nose only in special situations where recruitment of only a few millimeters of tissue is required and there is sufficient lax skin in the nasal sidewall to allow it. The arc is designed superiorly into the RSTL, radiating down from the medial canthus. Unfortunately, if the defect is large or near the nostril rim, the tension vector will be directed to pull up on this free margin. In these situations, a transposition flap that changes the tension vector

transversely would be a better choice to avoid unsightly elevation of the nostril.

Another useful repair for small-to-moderately sized defects of the distal nose is the dorsal nasal flap (Fig. 15). This is essentially a rotation flap with a back-cut built into the design. A curvilinear design is initiated from the lateral portion of the defect superiorly into the nasofacial sulcus and continuing into the ipsilateral glabellar frown line. The back-cut is continued into the contralateral frown line. The flap is widely undermined below the muscle plane at the level of the periosteum and the perichondrium. The flap is then draped into place to fill the defect. The secondary defect of the glabella is closed in a V-to-Y manner, which tends to push the flap further into place. The remaining closure lines are injunction lines and normal creases.

Bilateral rotation flaps are useful for larger repairs of the chin (Fig. 9). Curvilinear arcs fit nicely into the curved mentolabial crease. Tissue is recruited bilaterally and closure of the defect is completed within one cosmetic unit without extension onto the cutaneous lower lip. The glabella is another location that may be amenable to repair by a superiorly based bilateral rotation flap.

The O-to-Z bilateral rotation flap is a very useful flap for repairs on the hair-bearing scalp (Fig. 10). In this region, the Z-shaped scar is well camouflaged. It may be the ideal repair for defects of the vertex of the scalp because it results in a normal whorled configuration of the hair in this region.

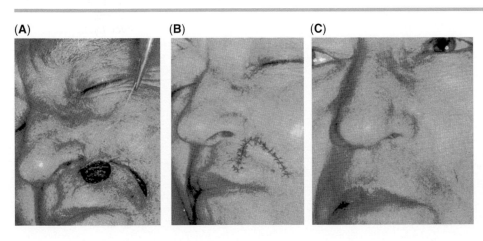

(A) **(B)** **(C)**

Figure 14 **(A)** Upper lip defect repaired with rotation flaps placed in melolabial fold. **(B)** Final closure. Incisions confirmed to RSTL of lip and melolabial fold. **(C)** At two-month follow-up.

(A)   (B)

(C)   (D)

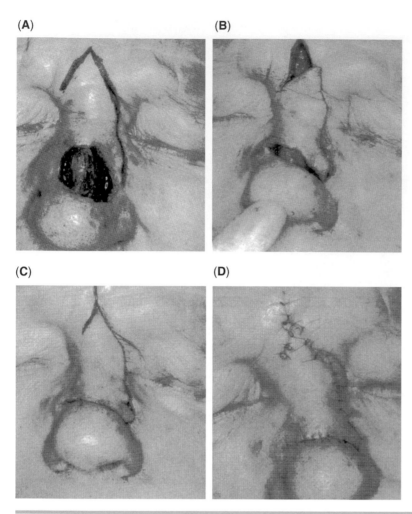

Figure 15 (A) Defect of nasal dorsum with back-cut rotation flap design. (B) Incisions confined to nasofacial junction and glabellar frown lines. (C) Flap rotated and advanced to fill primary defect. Secondary defect closed in a V-to-Y manner. (D) The final closure at 5 days.

BIBLIOGRAPHY

Albom MJ. Repair of large scalp defect by bilateral rotation flaps. J Dermatol Surg Oncol 1978; 4:906–907.

Baron JL, Reynaud JP, Gary-Bobo A, Maya M. Specificity of hatchet flaps in the laterofacial region. Ann Chir Plast Esthet 1990; 35:47–52.

Cook TA, Israel JM, Wang TD, Murakami CS, Brownrigg PJ. Cervical rotation flaps for midface resurfacing. Arch Otolaryngol Head Neck Surg 1991; 117:77–82.

Crow ML, Crow FJ. Resurfacing large cheek defects with rotation flaps from the cheek. Plast Reconstr Surg 1976; 58:196–199.

Dzubow LM. The dynamics of flap movement: the effect of pivotal restraint on flap rotation and transposition. J Dermatol Surg Oncol 1987; 13:1348–1353.

Golomb FM. Closure of the circular defect with double rotation flaps and Z-plastics. Plast Reconstr Surg 1984; 74:813–816.

Hardaway RM. The useful rotation flaps. Am J Surg 1955; 90:1013–1019.

Larrabee WR Jr., Sutton D. The biomechanics of advancement in rotation flaps. Laryngoscope 1981; 91:726–734.

Snow SN, Mohs FE, Olansky DC. Nasal tip reconstruction: the horizontal "J" rotation flap using skin from the lower lateral bridge and cheek. J Dermatol Surg Oncol 1990; 16:727–732.

Stark RB, Kaplan JM. Rotation flaps, neck to cheek. Plast Reconstr Surg 1972; 50:230–235.

Winton GB, Salasche SJ. Use of rotation flaps to repair small surgical defects on the ala nasi. J Dermatol Surg Oncol 1986; 12:154–158.

54

Transposition Flaps

Holly L. F. Christman and Roy C. Grekin
University of California, San Francisco, California, U.S.A.

INTRODUCTION

In the preceding chapters, the principles of flap surgery have been well covered. These serve as a good basis for understanding transposition flaps, which are conceptually the most difficult flaps to design and execute. In this chapter, we will present some general concepts about transposition flaps and then discuss specific examples. Finally, we will cover anatomic sites where they are most commonly used.

CLASSIFICATION

Flaps may be classified by a number of systems. Most flaps used in dermatologic surgery are local, indicating that they come from the same or adjacent cosmetic units. They usually have a blood supply, which is a random pattern, i.e., not based on a specific artery but nourished by the network of the deep dermal plexus. They are most successful therefore in richly vascularized areas such as the head and neck, or in other areas if they are small in size.

These principles apply to the transposition flaps most commonly used by dermatologic surgeons and the ones we will be considering in this chapter. There are transposition flaps that are harvested from more than one cosmetic unit away and performed as staged or pedicle flap, and they will be covered in the next chapter. There are also transposition flaps based on specific arteries, such as the many variations on the temperoparietal–occipital flap used in hair-replacement surgery, but we shall not discuss these specialized examples.

Flaps are also classified according to their type of movement. Advancement and rotation flaps are sliding flaps, but transposition flaps are not. Rather, they are cut, lifted, and rotated over intervening tissue into the primary defect.

DEFINITION OF TRANSPOSITION

To transpose means to change the place without destroying the basic structure. The key concept in transposition flap design is that the vectors of the wound closure are transposed by 45° to 120°. Often a primary defect cannot be closed along a certain axis, either because there is not enough tissue or in so doing it will distort some adjacent structure. If there is a tissue available 45° to 120° from the defect, the surgeon can make use of this excess skin to create a transposition flap (Fig. 1).

The basic structure of the flap that is moved into place is maintained in transposition flaps, which are generally cut to fit the size and shape of the defect. In contrast, for sliding flaps (e.g., advancement and rotation flaps) the skin is stretched (pulled) into place.

ADVANTAGES OF TRANSPOSITION FLAPS

Efficient Use of Tissue

Because the flap is essentially the same size as the defect, transposition flaps are small compared to advancement and rotation flaps. The latter have 3:1 to 4:1 flap size–to–defect size ratios, making transposition flaps economical in their tissue use.

Transferring Tension

The key suture in a flap is generally the first suture placed when moving a flap into position. It both aligns the flap over the primary defect and redirects the tension of the closure toward the secondary defect. In sliding flaps such as rotation and advancement flaps, the key suture closes the primary defect and the tension is maintained across that primary site.

Transposition flaps are unique in that the key suture is the one that closes the secondary defect, i.e., the defect is 45° to 120° away from the primary defect. In so doing, all of the tension is transferred to the secondary defect, allowing the flap to be "pushed" into place, rather than pulled, so that it drapes over the primary defect without any tension. Thus, transposition flaps are very useful for the closure of defects near free margins such as the nasal alae or lower eyelids, where transfer of the tension can prevent distortion of those structures (Figs. 1 and 2).

Broken-Line Appearance

Long-term camouflage of scars is an important goal in dermatologic surgery. Our specialty teaches that hiding scars in skin tension lines (STLs), or at the junction of cosmetic units aid in camouflage.

Another cosmetic principle is that a viewer's eye follows the lines of a linear scar more easily than the irregular pattern of a geometric design. Therefore, in certain areas, the geometric, broken-line scars that a transposition flap creates are preferred (Fig. 2).

SECONDARY DEFECT

In determining from where to elevate a transposition flap, several factors must be considered. First, in dealing with noncircular wounds, the flaps should always be designed off the short axis of the defect. Harvesting a transposition flap off the long axis results in a long, narrow-pedicled flap. This configuration also requires excessive rotation of the flap, placing increased tension on the pedicle and further limiting blood supply.

The next factor, and possibly the most important, is placement of the secondary defect in relation to surrounding

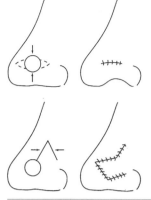

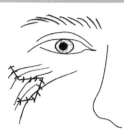

Figure 1 Schematic representation of transposition flap. Note direction of closure of secondary defect as compared to a side-to-side repair of this defect. Size of flap is approximately the same as the size of the defect.

Figure 2 Transposition flaps have utility near free anatomic margins as the tension of the closure is directed across closure of the secondary defect, allowing the flap to "drape" into the primary defect in a tension-free manner. Proper flap design and placement of the secondary defect is essential to achieve this effect. Note that due to the rotation of a transposition flap, at least one incision line will traverse relaxed skin tension lines.

anatomy. Because the tension of this repair is across the secondary defect, the donor site must be situated such that the tensions of its closure parallel free margins (Figs. 1 and 2).

The third factor is camouflage. The multiple geometric broken lines and the small flap size facilitate camouflage. However, this can be maximized by using cosmetic borders and aligning these flaps as much as possible within STLs. It is inherent in transposition flaps due to their 45° to 120° rotations that at least one closure line will cross rather than parallel STLs (Fig. 2).

TYPES OF TRANSPOSITION FLAPS

Banner Flap

The classic transposition flap is the banner flap—a finger-shaped flap—that rotates from 45° to 120° over intervening tissue into the primary defect (Fig. 3A). The flap width is the same size as the primary defect. Its length should be designed by determining the rotation point at the base of the flap and measuring from there to the most distal point of the primary defect. The novice surgeon will often be surprised by just how long the flap must be made. This is because of the effective shortening that occurs with rotation of the flap, and it is always prudent to add yet a few more millimeters to the measured length. These can always be trimmed if not needed, but it is difficult to salvage the situation if a flap is cut too short.

Once the flap is cut and elevated, the tissue surrounding the secondary defect is undermined to facilitate its closure. Undermining around the primary defect is controversial; some believe it may lessen the chance of the flap becoming bulky or "pincushioning." The key suture is then placed to close the secondary defect. With this one suture,

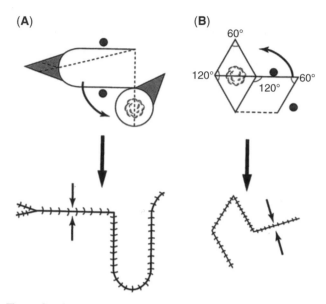

Figure 3 (A) Classic banner transposition flap. (B) Rhombic transposition flap. *Note:* • indicates key suture placement; →←— indicates secondary tension.

the genius of the transposition flap is evident—the tension is transferred from the primary defect to the secondary defect and the flap, without tension, drapes into place. The flap is then sutured into place, trimmed as required, and the rest of the secondary defect is closed. All transposition flaps will follow this basic pattern.

Dog-ears are constant in all transposition flaps (Fig. 3A). One occurs at the point of rotation at the base of the primary defect. This redundant tissue, created by rotation of the flap into the primary defect, can be removed by excision of a triangle of tissue, called removal by "triangulation." Some surgeons design the removal of this as a part of the flap. We prefer to remove it once the flap is in place to better determine the exact location and amount of excess skin to be removed. There are situations where removing this would decrease the size of the base of the flap and compromise its blood supply, therefore it can be left. In several weeks or months, it may disappear or a small second procedure to remove it can be performed once the flap's blood supply is firmly established.

The second dog-ear occurs at the superior aspect of the closure of the secondary defect and is dependent on the shape of the flap. If the flap has a rounded appearance or an angle of 60° or greater, there will be a dog-ear. Often the flap can be redesigned with a 30° angle or an M-plasty to prevent this. The M-plasty not only shortens the length of this secondary defect but confers upon the scar even more of a broken-line appearance (Fig. 3A).

Rhombic Flap

In contrast to the banner flap, the rhombic flap is designed with sharp angles.[a] This design capitalizes on the concept presented earlier that sharp angles and zigzagging lines are less perceptible to the viewer's eye.

The first step in designing a rhombic flap is to draw a rhombus around the outer edges of the defect.[b] It is not

---

[a] Due to technical definitions in geometry, these flaps are properly referred to as rhombic, but rhomboid is also in common use.
[b] Note that this is a parallelogram.

necessary to cut the defect into this shape. The flap is usually designed off the short axis of the rhombus so it extends out from one of the obtuse angles (Fig. 3B). One side of the rhombus is measured and a diameter extended through one of the obtuse angles for a distance equal to the rhombus side length. At the end of this length, a 60° angle is made and another line of the same length, which parallels the near side of the rhombic defect, is drawn (Fig. 3B).

At first glance, it seems that only a triangle has been drawn, and novice surgeons see only that shape. If one uses the mind's eye to extend yet another line parallel to the initial line drawn out from the obtuse angle to the near acute angle, it will be clear that actually a parallelogram, specifically a rhombus, has been formed, of exactly the same measurement as the defect (Fig. 3B).

The flap is cut as designed and undermined, and as with the classic banner flap, the secondary defect will be closed first, allowing the flap to rotate into place without tension. Note that this transposes the vector of closure approximately 90° from the primary defect. Again there will be dog-ears to repair; this could be predicted because 60° angles are not favorable closure angles, and these exist at the base of the rhombic primary defect and at the superior tip of the rhombic secondary defect. The dog-ear at the base of the rhombic primary defect can sometimes be designed out of the flap by extending the base to create a 30° angle. This sacrifices a lot of normal skin; therefore some surgeons prefer to design it as an M-plasty, but this can diminish the base of the flap. As discussed with the banner flap, one can wait until the flap is rotated into place and remove the dog-ear by triangulation or leave the protrusion for correction at a later date.

When the rhombic flap is rotated into the primary defect, either it can be trimmed to fit the shape of the defect or the defect enlarged to accommodate the flap. Both options maintain the broken-line appearance, although the former does spare more normal tissue.

The 30° Angle Flap

The 30° angle flap is a refinement of the rhombic flap designed to provide more favorable closure angles and thus eliminate the dog-ear repairs. It does so by converting the 60° angles of the rhombic flap into 30° angles. The design, however, is predicated on the ability to close some of the primary defect by side-to-side motion; thus it loses the advantage of being able to transfer all the tension of the closure away from the primary defect. It follows that it is not a good choice for a primary defect located near a free margin. Because the tension of the closure is shared between the primary and secondary defect, it has the advantage of distributing tension over a larger area. Additionally, a smaller flap is required, because not all of the closure of the primary defect has to come from the flap.

This flap is designed by creating a rhombus out of the primary defect, with 60° angles top and bottom and 120° side angles. In the classic rhombic flap, the flap was designed by extending a line out that bisected the obtuse angle. Here, in contrast, a "plumb line" is drawn extending one side of the rhombus (Fig. 4A). This line serves as a base for design of the flap. The primary defect is measured across its short axis and one-half of this width is taken to draw out the base of the flap along the plumb line starting from the obtuse angle. Then, using the measure of one side of the diamond, an isosceles triangle is created with the plumb line as its base. Thus, the isosceles triangle has its two long legs equal to a side of the primary defect, and its base is half

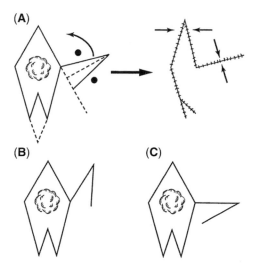

Figure 4 (A) Design and movement of a 30° angle flap. Note that the flap is one-half the width of the defect and drawn off a "plumb line" created by extending one side of the defect downward. Tension is shared equally across both the primary and secondary defects. *Note:* ● indicates key suture; →← indicates secondary tension. (B and C) Inappropriate designs for 30° angle flap.

the width. Because the flap is half the width of the primary defect, it closes half the defect, and the remaining closure is side to side (Fig. 4A).

This flap can be hard to visualize, and two mistakes are commonly made in its design. One is to have the flap arise at too acute an angle from the plumb line (Fig. 4B). When this flap is closed, its vectors of closure are oriented in the same direction as those of the primary defect, and therefore there is no sharing of the tension and thus no advantage to the flap. If the angle is too obtuse, i.e., greater than 90° because of the 30° angle at the tip of the flap and its small size, the flap base will be narrowed and its blood supply compromised (Fig. 4C). This flap can be modified by converting the angle at the bottom of the rhombus into an M-plasty, thereby shortening the wound (Fig. 4A).

It is important, with both the classic rhombic and the 30° angle flaps, to understand the appearance of the final incision lines. Because of the geometric pattern of this flap, clearly all lines will not be in relaxed STLs. In fact, some lines will go against the relaxed skin tension lines (RSTLs). The flap, however, can be pivoted to maximize its conformation to the RSTLs and thus its final cosmetic appearance (Fig. 2).

Bilobed Flap

The bilobed flap is another variation on the basic transposition flap (Fig. 5). It is considered when a transposition flap with all its advantages is desired but there is insufficient tissue movement immediately adjacent to the primary defect to close a secondary defect. By adding a second lobe to the flap, one "walks" the excess tissue from the more distant site so that the defect immediately adjacent to the primary defect can be closed. In this case, the key suture is placed to close the tertiary defect, which is the harvest site of the secondary lobe. As with all transposition flaps, the tension is transferred to this site at closure so that the flap drapes into place.

The actual size of the two lobes of the flap is dependent on how much secondary movement one can rely on

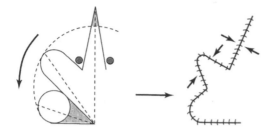

Figure 5 Schematic of the bilobed flap. Note the similarity to a rotation flap in its movement as well as its broad base. However, less tissue is moved than with a rotation flap, the geometric broken lines aid in camouflage, and tension is directed away from the primary defect. *Note:* • indicates key suture; →← indicates secondary tension.

from the surrounding skin. The first lobe is designed to be 75% to 100% of the size of the primary defect. For instance, if the flap is to be used to repair a nasal alar defect, and no closure is wanted to derive from the primary defect so as not to pull up the alar rim, one designs the lobe at 100%. If some closure of the primary defect is acceptable, then the size of the lobe can be closer to 75%. The second lobe is usually one-half the size of the first, relying on movement of the surrounding tissue to facilitate closure.

The two lobes may be designed with 30° angle tips to obviate dog-ear repair. The primary lobe is generally rounded, as it is often closing a circular defect, and it will be closed by transfer of the secondary lobe into it. Some surgeons feel, however, that there is less pincushioning and better geometric line appearance if the primary lobe is designed with a 30° angle. It has also been stated that undermining of the area around the primary defect will help prevent pincushioning.

The overall rotation of the flap may vary from 90° to 180° depending on the location of excess tissue. The greater the angle of rotation, the more tissue protrusion there will be at the point of rotation. It is very important that each lobe rotates the same number of degrees or there will be "buckling" at the base of the lobe that has rotated to a greater degree.

Determining the length of the lobes is critical, and perhaps is the trickiest task involved with transposition flaps. As with the classic banner flap, one must determine the point of rotation of the flap and remember that the length of the lobes will be effectively shortened in their rotation. If the lobe is made too short, it will not fit the primary defect and therefore the use of a flap will have been for naught; it is better to err by making the lobe several millimeters too long.

Once the tertiary defect is closed, allowing the flap to drape into place, and the flap is anchored, the dog-ear created by the rotation may be excised by triangulation. As stated earlier, some surgeons prefer to design this into the flap, but we believe it is important to remove excess tissue only once the flap is in place. It can always be removed later—after the flap's blood supply is established.

Postoperatively, the appearance of the bilobed transposition flap is often compromised by the pincushioning discussed above. This can occur in both the primary and secondary lobes. Pincushioning can often be treated by the injection of steroids intralesionally beginning at four to eight weeks postoperatively. We usually use triamcinolone acetonide 5 to 10 mg/cc, depending on the amount of bulkiness, and inject at three- to four-week intervals for a total of one to three injections. This will often result in a surprising reduction in bulkiness. Occasionally, we need to go back and revise the flap by incising the lobes, lifting them up, and paring down their undersurface. We would wait several months postoperatively before doing this, as time may result in a reduction in bulkiness. Dermabrasion 6 to 10 weeks postoperative aids in both camouflaging incision lines and debulking the flap.

AREAS OF UTILITY FOR TRANSPOSITION FLAPS

Because of their economy of size and the nature of their movement, transposition flaps can be used almost anywhere, particularly for facial defects. The main limitations relate to the ability to close secondary defects primarily without compromising local anatomy and obtaining optimum camouflage within RSTLs and cosmetic borders.

Because transposition flaps are pushed into the primary defect, creating little or no tension at that site, they are ideally suited for closures near free margins. In these areas the secondary motion of an advancement or rotation flap may pull down on an eyelid or elevate a nasal ala. Flaps particularly useful on the nasal ala include the rhombic, bilobed, or nasolabial fold (Figs. 6–8). The decision to use one or the other of these depends on the size of the defect, the amount and location of donor tissue, and the precise location of the defect in respect to the alar rim, nasal tip, or alar groove. On the lower eyelid, defects can be repaired by a rhombic flap harvested from lateral canthal skin (Fig. 9). or a banner-type flap transposing upper eyelid skin to the lower lid. While cheek skin may be transposed superiorly to close a lower lid defect, this skin is much thicker than eyelid skin, and its weight may cause an ectropion.

Transposition flaps may be used around the free margins of the lips, but the nature of the incision lines and

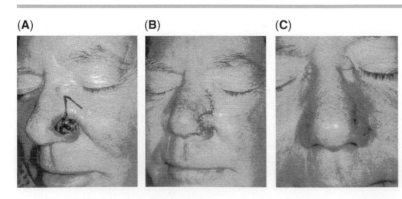

Figure 6 Rhombic flap on nasal ala: **(A)** defect; **(B)** closure; **(C)** long-term follow-up.

(A)   (B)   (C)

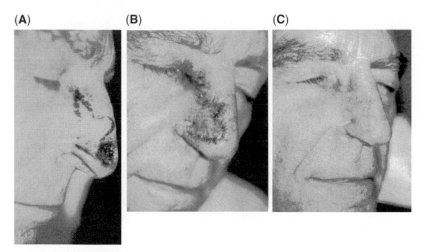

Figure 7 Bilobed flap on nasal ala: (**A**) defect; (**B**) closure; (**C**) long-term follow-up.

(A)   (B)   (C)

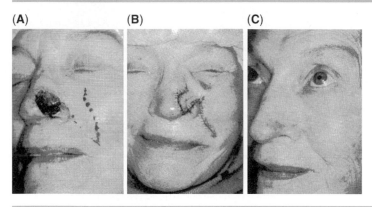

Figure 8 Nasolabial fold flap on nasal ala: (**A**) defect; (**B**) closure; (**C**) long-term follow-up.

tissue movement inherent in these flaps will usually result in at least one scar cutting across rather than paralleling RSTL. Advancement and rotation flaps generally work better on the lips.

A banner-type flap may be raised from the glabella to repair nasal root or medial canthal defects. The surgeon must be sure that the closure of the secondary defect does not draw the eyebrows too close together. Also, the glabellar skin is considerably thicker than that of the lateral nasal root and may create a bulky appearance (Fig. 10). Another use for the banner flap is in repair of superior helical defects. A superiorly based flap may be raised from preauricular skin with secondary defect closure hiding well within the preauricular crease. The flap is then transposed onto the superior helix providing excellent coverage, cosmetic appearance, and more reliable take than a graft.

Transposition flaps have utility for repair of cheek defects. They are most useful for lateral and mid-cheek repairs where ample and extensible skin is available. They are less useful for medial cheek repairs where closure of the secondary defect may distort the eyelids or position of the melolabial fold. Also, camouflage with RSTLs is more difficult in the medial cheek. For lateral and mid-cheek repairs, a medially or inferiorly based rhombic flap should be designed to facilitate outflow drainage and lessen edema and flap thickening (i.e., pincushioning). A 30° angle flap is useful in this region because of good skin extensibility and the lack of nearby important anatomic structures. Bilobed flaps are neither necessary nor cosmetically advantageous on the cheek.

Rhombic flaps can be used for closure of wounds on the temple. However, they must usually be superiorly based, which may affect drainage of blood and lymph from

(A)   (B)   (C)

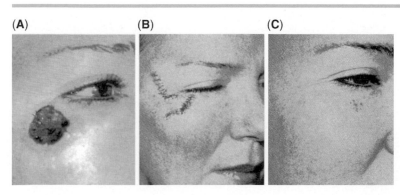

Figure 9 Rhombic flap repairing lower eyelid defect: (**A**) defect; (**B**) closure; (**C**) long-term follow-up.

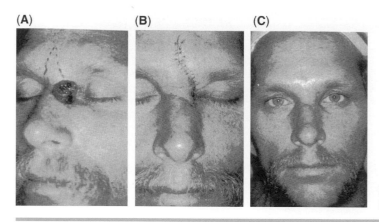

(A) **(B)** **(C)**

Figure 10 Banner transposition flap used to close a medial canthal-lateral nasal root defect: **(A)** defect, **(B)** closure; **(C)** one-month follow-up.

the flap and in men may remove hair-bearing cheek skin into this nonglabrous area.

The forehead skin is considered an extension of the scalp. As such it is thick and inelastic, making closure of the secondary defect created by a transposition flap difficult. This, combined with the well-defined horizontal STLs, makes the region less amenable for use of transposition flaps. However, in patients with lax forehead skin, a rhombic or banner-type flap may be useful for closure of lateral or superolateral forehead defects.

BIBLIOGRAPHY

Arnold AT, Bennett RG. The bilateral dog-ear transposition flap. J Dermatol Surg Oncol 1990; 16:667–672.

Borges AF. The rhombic flap. Plast Reconstr Surg 1981; 67: 458–466.

Davidson TM, Webster R, Gordon BR. The Principles and Dynamics of Local Skin Flaps. Alexandria: American Academy of Otolaryngology-Head and Neck Surgery Foundation Inc., 1988.

Dzubow LM. Design of an appropriate rhombic flap for a circular defect created by Mohs microscopically controlled surgery. J Dermatol Surg Oncol 1988; 14:126–128.

Field LM. Design concepts for the nasolabial fold flap (letter). Plast Reconstr Surg 1983; 71:283–285.

Field LM. Peripheral tissue undermining is not the final answer to prevent trapdooring in transposition flaps (letter). J Dermatol Surg Oncol 1993; 19:1131–1132.

Gormley DE. A brief analysis of the Burrow's wedge/triangular principle. J Dermatol Surg Oncol 1985; 11:121–123.

Holt PJ, Motley RJ. A modified rhombic transposition and its application in dermatology. J Dermatol Surg Oncol 1991; 17:287–292.

Jackson IT. Local Flaps in Head and Neck Reconstruction. St. Louis: CV Mosby Co., 1985.

Kaufman AJ, Kiene KL, Moy RL. Role of tissue undermining in the trapdoor effect of transposition flaps. J Dermatol Surg Oncol 1993; 19:128–132.

Kolbusz RV, Goldberg LH. The labial-ala transposition flap. Arch Dermatol 1994; 130:162–164.

Larrabee WF, Trachy R, Sutton D, Cox K. Rhomboid flap dynamics. Arch Otolaryngol 1981; 107:755–757.

Masson JK, Mendelsohn BC. The banner flap. Am J Surg 1977; 134:419–423.

McGregor JC, Soutar DS. A critical assessment of the bilobed flap. Br J Plast Surg 1981; 34:197–205.

Monheit GD. The rhomboid flap. In: Dermatologic Surgery. CV Mosby Co.St. Louis1988.

Moy RL. In: Atlas of Cutaneous Facial Flaps and Grafts—a Differential Diagnosis of Wound Closures. Philadelphia: Lea & Febiger, 1990.

Robinson JK, Horan DB. Modified nasolabial transposition flap provides vestibular lining and cover of alar defect with intact rim. Arch Dermatol 1990; 126:1425–1427.

Salasche SJ, Bernstein G, Senkarik M. Surgical Anatomy of the Skin. Norwalk: CT, 1988.

Salasche SJ, Grabski WJ. Grekin RC, ed. Flaps for the Central Face. New York: Churchill Livingstone, 1990.

Summers BK, Siegle RJ. Facial cutaneous reconstructive surgery: general aesthetic principles. J Am Acad Dermatol 1993; 29:669–681.

Summers BK, Siegle, RJ. Facial cutaneous reconstructive surgery: facial flaps. J Am Acad Dermatol 1993; 29:917–941.

Swanson NA. Atlas of Cutaneous Surgery. Boston: Little Brown and Co., 1987:1–177.

Tromovitch TA, Stegmen SJ, Glogau RG. Flaps and Grafts in Dermatologic Surgery. Chicago: Mosby Year Book, 1989.

Walkinshaw M, Caffee HH. The Nasolabial Flap: a Problem and its correction. Plast Reconstr Surg 1982; 69:30–34.

Webster RC, Davidson TM, Smith TC. The thirty-degree transposition flap. Laryngoscope 1978; 88:85–94.

Zitelli JA. The bilobed flap for nasal reconstruction. Arch Dermatol 1989; 125:957–959.

Zitelli JA. The nasolabial fold flap as a single-stage procedure. Arch Dermatol 1990; 126:1445–1448.

Zitelli JA, ed. Special issue: local flaps. J Dermatol Surg Oncol 1991; 17:112–204.

55

Pedicle Flaps

J. Ramsey Mellette, Jr.
University of Colorado Health Sciences Center, Denver, Colorado, U.S.A.

THE PARAMEDIAN FOREHEAD PEDICLE FLAP FOR NASAL RECONSTRUCTION

In the 27th edition of Dorland's Illustrated Medical Dictionary, a pedicle flap is defined as "a flap consisting of full thickness of skin and the subcutaneous tissue attached by tissue through which it achieves its blood supply." In practice, most pedicle flaps remain attached to their source for a period of several days to a few weeks. Viability is thus assured by establishment of a blood supply in the recipient bed. In dermatologic surgery, the three most common pedicle flaps utilized are the paramedian forehead flaps for nasal reconstruction, the superiorly based naso-labial pedicle flap for extensive defects of the ear. This chapter will present applications of the forehead pedicle flap for nasal reconstruction. (RKR also commonly prefers the subcutaneous island pedicle flap, especially for upper lip defects, as discussed in Chapter 25).

HISTORICAL NOTES

The forehead flap for nasal reconstruction was known to have been performed by the Kanghiara family of India as early as 1440 A.D. and may well has been performed as early as 1000 B.C. The more modern reports on the forehead flaps extend back at least 150 years. In the last 40 years, most practitioners have utilized either "the precise midline" forehead flap or the "paramedian" forehead flap. Both of these variations have been employed successfully with excellent aesthetic results; however, the paramedian version will be emphasized here.

GENERAL

The vascular supply for the pedicle forehead flap is provided primarily by the supratrochlear vessel system, which emanates from the supratrochlear foramen inferior to the medial orbital rim.

When based on both supratrochlear vessels, this flap is usually described as "midline;" when based on one of the paired supratrochlear vessels, it is described as "paramedian."

Although the paramedian flap appears to be have been utilized by Labat in the 1830s, Millard is generally credited with revealing it in the current reconstructive literature beginning in the 1960s. Burget and Menick, along with Millard, have provided much of the literature detailing the technique and its applications.

It is clear that the paramedian flap with its single-vessel system is equal in reliability to the two-vessel midline flap and offers significant advantages, which includes the following:

1. A narrow pedicle of approximately 1 cm at its origin, with the result that there is less possibility of strangulation of the pedicle. This narrow pedicle can be amputated at its origin in the glabella with the defect closed simply side to side.
2. A longer flap is possible, because the incisions at its origins can be extended below the level of the brow in the area of the medial canthus and into the nasal bridge medially.
3. The opposite side can be utilized as a backup should there be a recurrence of skin cancer or other indications for forehead flap reconstruction.

The paramedian flap is unusually versatile. It can be used to reconstruct the entire surface of the nose and, when properly lined, can be used to repair full-thickness defects. Two procedures are necessary. The first requires insertion of the pedicle into the defect. The second involves division of the pedicle once its blood supply in the recipient area is assured, usually within 14 to 21 days. In many cases it can be done in the outpatient operatory under local anesthesia or local combined with regional block anesthesia.

ANATOMIC CONSIDERATIONS

McCarthy et al. have demonstrated that the forehead has a rich blood supply from the supraorbital, supratrochlear, infratrochlear, dorsal nasal, and angular branches of the facial artery (Fig. 1). Anastomoses among these vessels ensure more than adequate profusion of forehead flaps, but the supratrochlear vessel is the branch most important to the paramedian flap. It originates from the supratrochlear foramen medially beneath the orbital rim, where it lies between the corrugator and frontalis muscle. The corrugator frontal crease (the glabellar crease) serves as a landmark of the location of the supratrochlear vessel in this area. One can dissect over the orbital rim beneath the muscle without injury to the vessel. The flap origin can therefore be inferior to the level of the brow, which, as previously stated, provides extra length.

Consideration must be given to the length of tissue available from the forehead. The height from the glabella to the hairline varies significantly. One would see as ideal a male with a receded hairline with unlimited vertical height, but is not infrequently faced with a patient whose eyebrows seem to join his or her hairline (Fig. 2). In the case of short vertical height, there are two possible solutions.

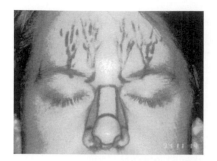

Figure 1 Extensive anastomoses of supratrochlear (medial brow) and supraorbital (mid-brow) vessels.

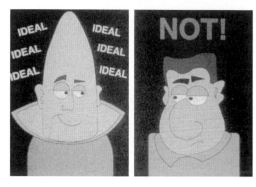

Figure 2 Vertical height of forehead will influence flap design.

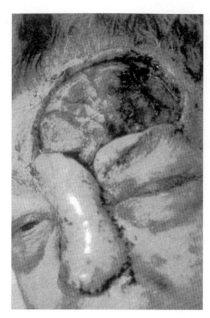

Figure 4 Forehead flap arched to provide necessary length.

One is to extend the flap into the hairline. This soon-to-be-distal portion of the flap can be thinned extensively with an attended attempt to transect the hair bulbs. Another solution is to arch the flap horizontally along the forehead. This may present problems with healing of the forehead defect. However, due at least in part to the extensive anastomotic connections previously mentioned, even lengthy horizontal extensions have not compromised flap viability (Figs. 3–9).

The patient pictured presented an extreme case of an unusually short vertical forehead and the need for a long and wide forehead flap. The defect included the surface of the nose, the full thickness of the nasal ala and a portion of adjacent cheek (Fig. 3). The cheek was advanced to the nasal sidewall, and the forehead flap was utilized to resurface the nasal defect (Fig. 4). The aforementioned technique of extending the incision inferior to the orbital rim would have provided additional length and has been routinely employed in subsequent cases. There was minimal ecchymoses at the tip (Fig. 5), but no significant impediment to flap viability. After two weeks the pedicle was divided, the stump of the pedicle returned to the forehead, and the

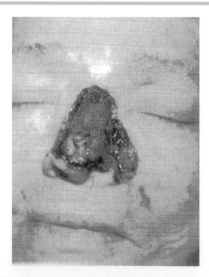

Figure 3 Extensive nasal and cheek defect following Mohs micrographic surgery. Note short vertical height of forehead.

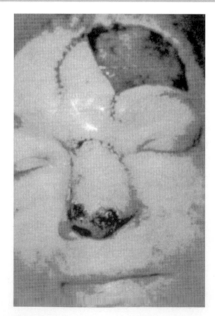

Figure 5 Stump of pedicle returned to forehead. Remainder of defect to receive full-thickness graft.

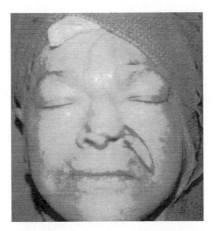

Figure 6   Design of superiorly based naso-labial fold flap to recreate nasal ala.

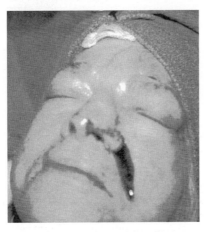

Figure 7   Naso-labial fold flap attached. Flap division planned in two weeks.

remainder of the forehead defect repaired with a full-thickness graft (Figs. 5 and 8). A superiorly based naso-labial flap was utilized to reconstruct the nasal ala (Figs. 6 and 7) with the long-term result as seen in Figure 9. An auricular composite graft to further reconstruct the inferior lateral alar was offered but refused by the patient.

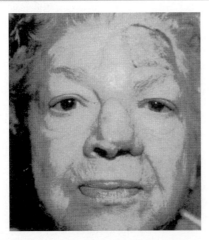

Figure 8   Six-week follow-up of full-thickness graft to forehead and naso-labial fold flap to alar rim.

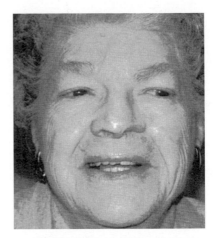

Figure 9   Result at one year.

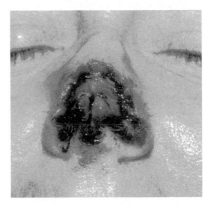

Figure 10   Extensive nasal tip and alar defect.

THE TECHNIQUE

The technique for the usual case is developed as follows:

The forehead and nasal defect area are injected with 1% lidocaine 1:100,000 epinephrine buffered with 1:10 sodium bicarbonate. A template of the defect (Figs. 10–12)

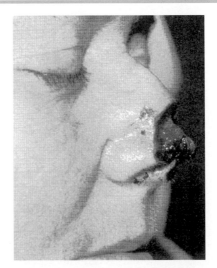

Figure 11   Right lateral view of defect.

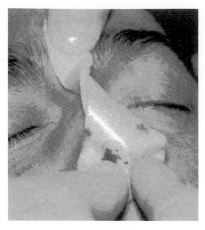

Figure 12 Dressing pad template including excess to allow for enfolding to reconstruct alar rims.

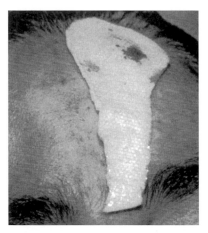

Figure 13 Precise placement of template.

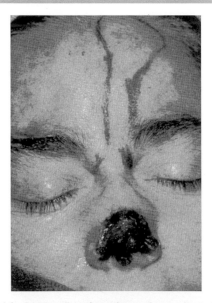

Figure 14 Inked outline of template and approximate location.

is made utilizing nonadherent pads (alternatively, aluminum foil or the metal wrapping of sutures may suffice).

The length of the flap is carefully measured from the area of the chosen supratrochlear vessels to the lower limits

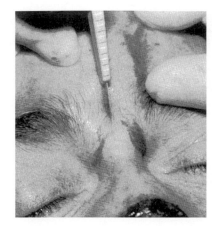

Figure 15 Mid-glabella incision. Note accurately estimated location of supratrochlear vessels.

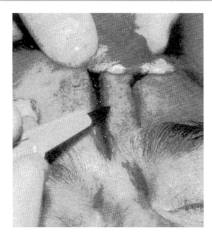

Figure 16 Incision to medial eyebrow.

of the defect (Fig. 12). A Doppler may be used to precisely identify the supratrochlear blood flow; however, no complications have been encountered in identifying the vessel location by anatomic landmarks. The template is applied to the forehead and outlined with a sterile marking pen (Figs. 13 and 14). The length and fit are verified. An incision (Fig. 15) is begun in the mid-glabella between the eyebrows. This incision is taken deep through the subcutaneous tissues down to the periosteum and is extended upward in the forehead precisely along the inked margins. The incision is then continued downward toward the area of the medial eyebrow (Fig. 16). At a point just superior to the medial brow, the incision is made shallow through the epidermis and dermis until the flap can be fully elevated. At this point, the flap is retracted away from the forehead, the incision is extended slightly inferior to the brow, and with good visualization the remaining attachment of the flap is bluntly dissected (Fig. 17). This dissection can be carried along and below the orbital rim. The raised flap is held in the hand and the tip of the flap is thinned of fascia and muscle with serrated iris scissors (Fig. 18). It is advisable to leave enough fat for additional vascularity (presumably provided in the fat by the subdermal plexus) but not so much as to compromise good wound apposition. The flap is then rotated inward on its axis and the tip placed in the

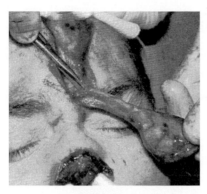

Figure 17 Scissor dissection of flap. For added length, the incision can be extended below the brow.

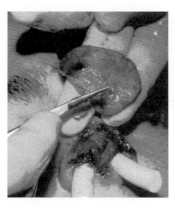

Figure 18 Scissor removal of fascia and muscle from the distal flap.

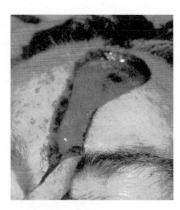

Figure 19 Inward 180° rotation of flap.

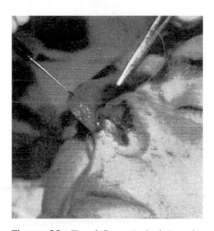

Figure 20 Tip of flap attached to columella.

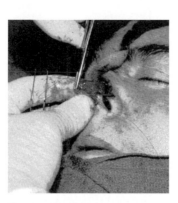

Figure 21 The suture needle is placed near the distal rim and exited 5 mm proximal.

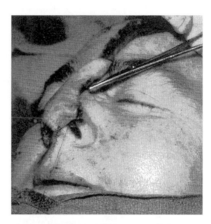

Figure 22 With the suture tied, the alar rim is recreated. This was repeated on the opposite side.

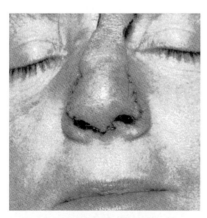

Figure 23 Flap is sutured with simple and vertical mattress suture.

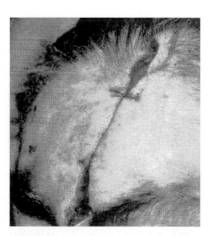

Figure 24 Partial closure of defect. Dog-ear was rotated into defect to close widest part in hairline.

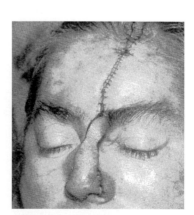

Figure 25 Complete closure of forehead defect.

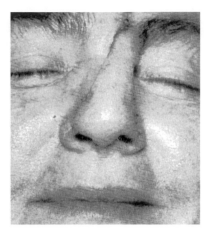

Figure 26   At two weeks flap viability is assured.

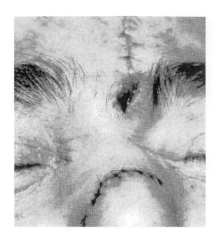

Figure 28   Amputated pedicle stump.

defect (Figs. 19 and 20). Exceptionally, due to eccentric location of the defect, an outward rotation of the flap may be desirable. In Figures 21 and 22, the flap is infolded with absorbable suture to recreate the alar rims. The wound edges are approximated with 5–0 nylon or other suitable suture material (23). Due partly to wound contracture, there is a tendency for wound inversion at the point of attachment. Vertical mattress sutures to evert the wound edge may be helpful in preventing this tendency (Fig. 23).

With a properly designed flap, the pedicle width at its origin in the medial brow area generally need not be more than 1 cm wide; therefore, the lower part of the forehead defect can usually be closed side to side (Figs. 24 and 25). The undermining plane for the forehead closure lies above the periosteum in a manner similar to that employed for scalp reductions. The upper part of the forehead defect may be broad enough to require repair by flap (Fig. 24) or graft or to provide for healing by second intention.

The flap will be left attached to its pedicle for a period of two to three weeks. The stump is dressed with a moist dressing usually consisting of Vaseline-impregnated gauze, antibiotic or a moisturizing ointment, nonadherent pads, and gauze. Within the first 24 hours, the wound is inspected in the office and is usually cleaned with saline

or diluted hydrogen peroxide (1/2 hydrogen peroxide diluted with water) and redressed. The dressing is generally changed once or twice a week. If necessary, the dressing can be changed at home by family members or home care assistants.

After two weeks (rarely three), the pedicle is ready to be divided (Fig. 26). Viability may be confirmed by compressing the stump with a Penrose drain. There will be a slight blanching because there tends to be some hyperemia at the tip, but failure to adequately vascularize at this point has not been encountered. With sterile technique and under local anesthesia, the flap is divided at the superior point of insertion in the defect (Fig. 27). The proposed division should offer generous excess of tissue, which will be trimmed to assure appropriate wound apposition. It is again helpful to apply eversion techniques to decrease the tendency for a crease to form along the line of closure. The pedicle is then amputated in the glabella area (Fig. 28). Electrocautery is generally sufficient to seal the remaining supratrochlear vessels. There is usually sufficient tissue laxity to allow for simple side-to-side closure of the defect left by the amputated stump (Fig. 29). At six months, the outstanding bulk and color match of the forehead flap can be appreciated (Figs. 30–33).

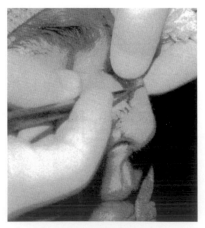

Figure 27   Division of pedicle.

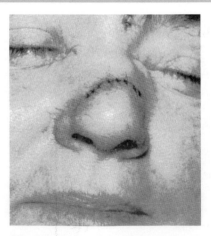

Figure 29   Completed closure of flap insertion and stump.

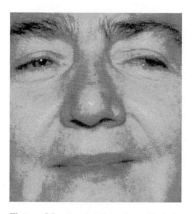

Figure 30 Frontal view of result at six months.

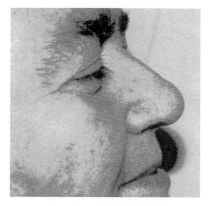

Figure 31 Result of reconstruction of right alar rim.

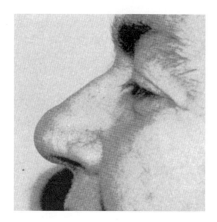

Figure 32 Result of reconstruct of left alar rim.

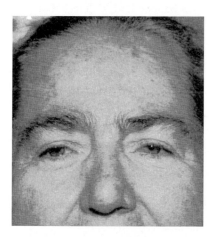

Figure 33 Acceptable forehead scar.

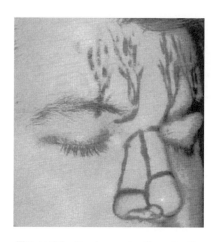

Figure 34 Nasal reconstructive subunits.

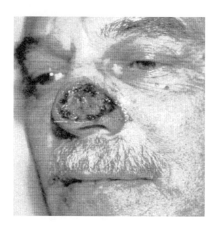

Figure 35 Nasal tip alar defect.

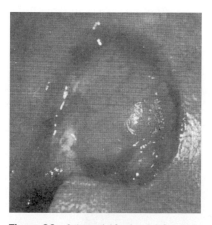

Figure 36 Substantial forehead defect. Note very thick "sebaceous" skin.

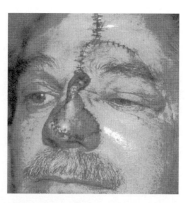

Figure 37 Primary closure accomplished by combination side-to-side and advancement flap.

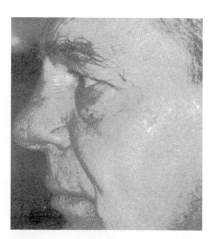

Figure 38 Side view of result of reconstruction of patient in Figure 35.

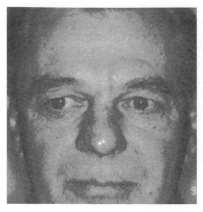

Figure 39   Frontal view of result of reconstruction of patient in Figure 35.

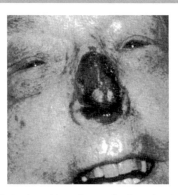

Figure 40   Defect enlarged to replace entire tip and part of nasal dorsum.

CONSIDERATION OF REGIONAL OR TOPOGRAPHIC SUBUNITS

Gonzales-Ulloa is generally credited with advancing the concept of reconstruction of regional or topographic subunits. This has been expanded and emphasized in recent articles by various reconstructive surgeons, most notably Burget and Menick, and is covered in detail elsewhere in this text (see Chapter 22). The concept is that the nose is considered an aesthetic unit of the face. The smaller parts of the nose are then designated topographic subunits (Fig. 34). When a significant part of a subunit or subunits has been lost, it is often advisable to replace the entire subunit or units. This is a valid consideration, and attempts are always made to adhere to its principals. On occasion, the potential size of the forehead

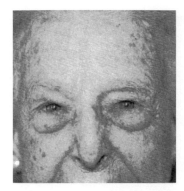

Figure 42   Six-month result of defects in Figures 41 and 42.

defect—which should always be secondary in consideration of the nasal reconstruction—will require that the surgeon not follow these principals absolutely. Particularly in the case of some males, a less than perfect nasal reconstruction may be preferable to a very undesirable forehead scar.

A middle-aged male patient had a defect that was full-thickness beneath the alar rim (Fig. 35). His life-long style was to comb his hair backward away from the forehead. In consideration of reconstructive subunits, it would have been appropriate to extend the defect at least to the midline of the tip and to the lateral extent of the alar (in some cases the entire tip and ala are removed and replaced). Because of the anticipated forehead scar, a more conservative reconstruction was planned, resulting in a more manageable forehead defect (Figs. 36 and 37). Added length to the flap was achieved by extending the pedicle below the level of the brow (Fig. 37). The long-term result reveals an acceptable reconstruction of the nose and forehead (Figs. 38 and 39).

An elderly female patient (Fig. 40) offers a significant contrast to the male patient seen in Figure 35. Her defect following Mohs micrographic surgery was enlarged to provide replacement of the entire tip and adjacent nasal dorsum. The anticipated large forehead defect (Fig. 41) could not be closed and was allowed to heal by second intention (Fig. 42). Very acceptable results were achieved on the forehead as well as the nose (Figs. 42 and 43).

An attractive middle-aged female patient had a full-thickness defect of the alar rim following Mohs micrographic surgery for a recurrent basal cell carcinoma (Fig. 44). Consideration was given to extending the defect to replace the

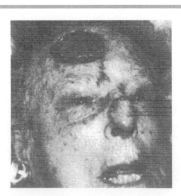

Figure 41   Forehead flap with large donor defect.

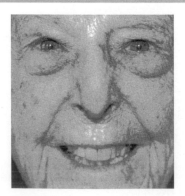

Figure 43   Close-up of forehead flap repair of defect in Figure 40.

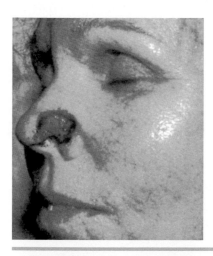

Figure 44 Deep defect including full thickness loss of mid-alar rim.

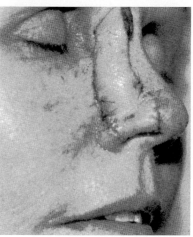

Figure 45 Alar rim recreated by enfolding flap. Note pexing suture.

lateral nasal tip and ala with a composite cartilage graft. Ultimately it was decided that a less complicated approach involving infolding of the forehead flap to recreate the alar rim would provide an acceptable aesthetic result (Figs. 45 and 46). A pexing suture (Fig. 45) was utilized to assist in recreating the superior alar crease. Approximately 1.5 cm of added length for the flap was achieved by extending the incisions below the brow (Figs. 46). The long-term result is seen in Figures 47 and 48. The forehead defect

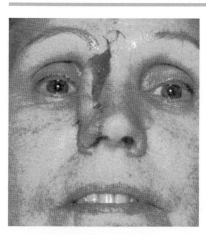

Figure 46 Frontal view of attached flap. Note pedicle origin inferior to brow.

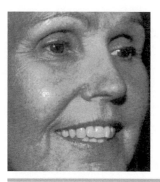

Figure 47 The alar rim is recreated.

was closed side to side. The resulting scar was minimally visible (Fig. 48).

CONSIDERATIONS

The richly vascularized paramedian forehead flap is exceptionally suited for nasal reconstruction and can be done safely and reliably in the outpatient setting under local anesthesia. In bulk and color, it more closely resembles normal nasal tissue than any other flap or graft. This technique may be used to reconstruct the entire surface of the nose and provides especially elegant tissue for replacement of the nasal tip and ala. Even if the vertical height of the forehead is short, a flap of sufficient length will be possible. Added length is obtained by incising over the orbital rim to a point just inferior to the medial brow. In exceptional circumstances, the flap may extend vertically into the hairline, or it may be arched horizontally. With added flap length, the full-thickness defects, especially along the alar rim, tip, and columella, can be repaired by inward folding of the distal edge. More extensive full-thickness defects will require lining and support with various combinations of skin and cartilage grafts and adjacent tissue flap.

Difficulties and complications in utilizing these flaps have been minimal. Bleeding from the pedicle has occurred in three of 35 cases, developing in each case within the first 24 hours. One episode was the result of direct trauma four hours postoperative. The patient stumbled and fell against the bedpost. The other two cases were detected at the time of initial dressing change 24 hours postoperative and were controlled by electrocautery under local anesthesia. There have been no flap failures.

Prophylactic antibiotics are not routinely prescribed. In cases of long duration and/or if a break in sterile technique is known or suspected, antibiotics are given for 7 to 10 days. Infection has not been encountered. The forehead scar, especially the upper part, may rarely be significant. Intralesional steroids prove useful in softening

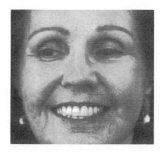

Figure 48 Acceptable long-term result with minimal forehead scar.

these scars and hairstyling techniques may provide camouflage. Not uncommonly, the flaps may have too much bulk. Revision, especially thinning, may be necessary to achieve optimal results.

BIBLIOGRAPHY

Antia NH, Daver BM. Reconstructive surgery for nasal defects. Clin Plast Surg 1981; 8(3):535–563.

Burget GC. Aesthetic reconstruction of the nose. Clin Plast Surg 1985; 12(3):463–480.

Burget GC, Menick FJ. Aesthetic Reconstruction of the Nose. St. Louis: Mosby, 1994.

Burget GC, Menick FJ. The subunit principal in nasal reconstruction. Plast Reconstr Surg 1985; 76(2):239–247.

Dorland's Illustrated Medical Dictionary. 27th ed. Philadelphia, WB Saunders Co., 1988.

Gaze NR. Reconstructing the nasal tip with a midline forehead flap. Br J Plast Surg 1980; 33:122–126.

Gonzales-Ulloa M. Restoration of the face covering by means of selected skin in regional aesthetic units. Br J Plast Surg 1957; 9(3):212.

Gonzalez-Ulloa M. Reconstruction of the nose and forehead by means of regional aesthetic units. Br J Plast Surg 1961; 13(4):305.

Kotler R. The midline forehead flap for resurfacing the nose. J Dermatol Surg Oncol 1981; 7(1):57–66.

McCarthy JG, Lorene ZD, et al. The median forehead flap revisited: The blood supply. Plast Reconstr Surg 1985; 76:866.

Menick FJ. Aesthetic refinements in use of forehead for nasal reconstruction: The paramedian forehead flap. Clin Plast Surg 1990; 17(4):607–622.

Millard DR Jr. Hemirrhinoplasty. Plast Reconstr Surg 1967; 40:440.

Millard DR Jr. Reconstructive rhinoplasty for the lower half of a nose. Plast Reconstr Surg 1974; 53:133–139.

Millard DR Jr. Reconstructive rhinoplasty for the lower two-thirds of the nose. Plast Reconstr Surg 1978; 57: 722–728.

Shumrick K. Arterial circulation of the forehead. Its importance in nasal reconstruction. In: Burgett CG, Menick FJ, eds. Aesthetic Reconstruction of the Nose. St. Louis: Mosby, 1994:62.

Tardy ME Jr, Sykes S, Kron T. The precise midline forehead flap in reconstruction of the nose. Clin Plast Surg 1985; 12(3): 481–494.

Thomas R, Griner N, Cook TA. The precise midline forehead flap as a musculocutaneous flap. Arch Otolaryngol Head Neck Surg 1988; 114:79–84.

56

Interpolation Flaps

Michael J. Fazio
Department of Dermatology, Skin Cancer Surgery Center, University of California Davis, Sacramento, California, U.S.A.

John A. Zitelli
Shadyside Medical Center, Pittsburgh, Pennsylvania, U.S.A.

INTRODUCTION

As our sophistication in skin cancer surgery has markedly improved with the advent of Mohs micrographic surgery, so has the demand for more esthetic reconstructive surgery. Prior to Mohs surgery, it was not uncommon for the surgeon to remove entire cosmetic subunits to assure complete tumor extirpation. This approach usually necessitated a larger or more complex reconstructive surgery. Mohs micrographic surgery has allowed for removal of the entire tumor, with the highest cure rate, while conserving the maximum amount of normal tissue. The tissue-sparing properties of Mohs micrographic surgery has markedly influenced how the surgeon approaches the reconstructive surgery. Not all nasal tip tumors require extensive grafting or forehead flaps to repair entire cosmetic units. Likewise, not all vermilion defects require mucosal advancement repairs. The advent of Mohs micrographic surgery has afforded the reconstructive surgeon to consider the entire spectrum of reconstructive options, with the added assurance of a tumor-free defect.

Unlike the cosmetic surgeon, whose goal is to improve upon normal anatomy, the challenge before the reconstructive surgeon is to restore normal function and anatomy after significant loss of tissue. The reconstructive options (many are discussed in other chapters of this book) consist of secondary intention healing, primary closures, local flaps, skin grafts, distant flaps (interpolation and pedicled flaps), or a combination of these procedures. It is incumbent upon the reconstructive surgeon to consider the entire armamentarium of reconstructive options before beginning the restoration process. The experienced surgeon will always choose the simplest procedure that provides the optimal outcome.

An Interpolation flap is a two-stage tissue flap in which the base of the flap is not directly adjacent to the recipient site. These flaps are reserved for reconstruction of complex wounds that often result from facial cancer surgery. The interpolation flaps are invaluable options for the reconstructive surgeons on certain facial wounds where the size, depth, and location preclude secondary intention healing, local flaps, or graft closure. Interpolation flaps allow for recruitment of distant, thick vascular-rich tissue, which is often similar in texture and color to the recipient wound site. The most common interpolation flaps used in cutaneous surgery are the melolabial interpolation flap, the preauricular interpolation flap, the postauricular interpolation flap, and the subcutaneous interpolation flap. The forehead flap is a specific type of interpolation flap, which is pedicled upon the supratrochlear vascular bundle, and has been discussed in another chapter of this book. In this chapter, we will review the most common utilization and indications of interpolation flaps in facial reconstructive surgery.

NASAL RECONSTRUCTION

Nasal reconstruction provides many challenges for even the most seasoned reconstructive surgeon. The desire to obtain a perfect esthetic outcome must be paralled with due diligence in maintaining a normal patent nasal airway. Centrally situated, the nose is one of the most important cosmetic structures on the face. The multitude of tissue types constituting the nose, including skin, cartilage, bone, and mucosa must be individually considered when designing the optimal functional and esthetic reconstructive procedure. The distal third of the nose has a unique sebaceous and vascular quality, which is difficult to match and must be carefully considered in all reconstructive procedures. The lack of tissue mobility and elasticity in the lower third of the nose often precludes local flaps for larger defects because of the tendency for distortion of free tissue margins of the nasal tip and ala.

Topographic anatomy of the nasal ala is especially intricate (Fig. 1). Superiorly, the ala is bounded by the prominent alar grove, which separates the lateral sidewall. The lateral alar groove helps form the superior apex of the melolabial fold. Medially, the ala abuts the soft triangle and the nasal tip. Inferiorly, the entire ala is a free tissue margin.

When the surgeon is evaluating a complex nasal alar wound that is too deep for skin grafting and too large for local flap coverage, there are basically two reservoirs of tissue, the forehead and the medial cheek. Because the forehead flap is discussed in another chapter, we will emphasize our experience with different types of cheek flaps utilized to repair alar wounds: (i) single-staged nasolabial flap, (ii) melolabial interpolation flap, and (iii) melolabial subcutaneous interpolation flap (Spear) (Table 1).

Single-Staged Nasolabial Flap

Questions often arise as to the value of a single-stage nasolabial flap verses a two-stage melolabial interpolation flap.

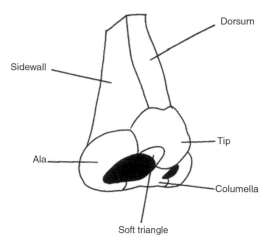

Figure 1 Topographic anatomy of the nose.

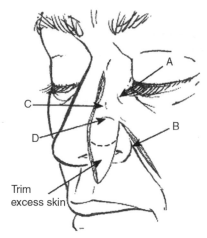

Figure 2 Key subcutaneous sutures for the single-staged nasolabial flap. **(A)** Base of the superior/lateral aspect of the flap sutured to the ascending process of the maxilla to recreate the nasofacial sulcus. **(B)** Lateral/superior aspect of the donor site sutured to the pyriform aperture of the maxilla to recreate the melolabial fold. **(C)** Subcutaneous suture placed to properly direct the vector pf tension horizontally and prevent upward displacement of the nasal tip and ala. **(D)** Deep suspension suture to reform the alar groove.

In our experience, both of these reconstructive procedures are invaluable and used often. The single-stage nasolabial flap is best suited for wounds on the lower lateral sidewall and ala. It is not well suited for very wide defects (>2.0 cm), defects limited to the ala alone, and medial defects involving the tip and ala. Although trap-door deformity and blunting of the alar groove have been cited as some of the drawbacks of this flap, we have previously published modifications to the original design of the single-stage nasolabial flap to help remedy these complications and facilitate a simplified single-stage procedure. The important modifications include (i) removal of a Burow's triangle from the nasal sidewall at the pivot point of the flap; (ii) use of the periosteal sutures to recreate the nasofacial sulcus, the melolabial fold, and a deep suspension suture to reform the alar groove. These sutures also minimize tension and pull on the alar rim and nasal tip; (iii) wide undermining of the flap, donor site, and wound edges to create a plate-like scar and minimize trap-door deformity; (iv) aggressive thinning (defatting) of the flap so the flap is inset and concave from the wound edges; and (v) meticulous trimming of the flap to recreate the original preincisional skin tension across the flap after suturing.

Movement of tissue across the nasofacial sulcus or melolabial fold often results in tenting or blunting of the normal contour. The placement of four key subcutaneous sutures will optimize the esthetic outcome (Fig. 2). First, a subcutaneous suture connects the undersurface of the lateral aspect of the donor cheek wound to the lateral alar crease in the area of the triangular isthmus of the upper lip. The underside of the flap is suspended from the periosteum of the pyriform aperture of the maxilla. This suture

reforms the contour of the melolabial fold and relieves tension on closure of the donor site. This suture also prevents lateral displacement of the ala. Second, the cheek skin is advanced by a periosteal suture in the nasofacial sulcus. The underside of the flap is suspended to the periosteum overlying the ascending process of the maxilla in the nasofacial sulcus. This suture must be high enough to maintain the normal convex contour above the melolabial fold as it continues into the alar groove. This suture also prevents tenting, and reforms the normal contour of the nasofacial sulcus. Another critical function of this suture is to lessen tension of the flap to minimize distortion of the distal aspect of the nose. The remainder of the donor site is then closed in a standard layered fashion. At this point, the flap should be carefully thinned and defatted, so the flap can be sutured into place slightly concave and inset from the surrounding wound edges. The fat left on the underside of the flap will fibrose and contract during normal wound healing, which can contribute to trap-door deformity. A third key subcutaneous suture is placed at the anterior distal aspect of the flap directed toward the nasal tip. The purpose of this stitch is to direct wound tension horizontally and to minimize upward pull and distortion of the alar rim. The fourth key subcutaneous suture is placed at the undersurface of the central aspect of the flap and is connected to the central aspect of

Table 1 Flaps for Alar Reconstruction

Single-staged nasolabial flap	Melolabial interpolation flap	Subcutaneous melolabial interpolation flap
Indications		
Vertically oriented, tall narrow wounds of the lateral nasal ala and nasal sidewall	Horizontally oriented, short wide, deep alar wounds not extending more than 2 mm above alar groove	Extensive alar wounds with loss of lateral alar crease
Alar wounds crossing the alar groove		
Wounds no greater than 2 cm		
Potential disadvantages		
Blunting nasofacial sulcus	Two-stage procedure	Thick alar rim
Blunting alar groove	Blunting of alar groove	Flattening melolabial fold
Flattening melolabial fold	Flattening of melolabial fold	
Trap-door deformity		

(A)   **(B)**   **(C)**

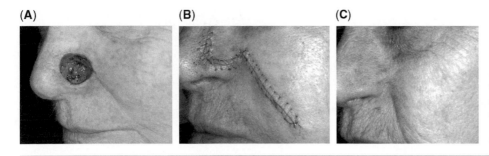

Figure 3 **(A)** A deep vertically oriented wound of the ala and extending onto the nasal sidewall. **(B)** Closure using the four key subcutaneous sutures and a single-staged nasolabial flap. **(C)** Result three months after surgery.

the alar crease. This will recreate the normal contour of the alar groove. This stitch will also close the dead space between the alar crease and the flap, and will give support to the underlying nasal mucosa. Once these four key subcutaneous sutures have been placed, the distal aspect of the flap can be carefully amputated to the shape of the defect, and the flap sutured in a normal layered fashion. Because of the thickness and quality of the melolabial tissue, cartilage grafts are usually unnecessary (Fig. 3A–C).

Melolabial Interpolation Flap

While the single-stage melolabial flap is useful for defects involving both the nasal sidewall and the ala, the melolabial interpolation flap is best suited for deep, wide defects limited to the ala alone, or involving the lateral tip and ala (Table 1). Often these wounds involve more than 50% of the alar lobule where the complexity of the wound precludes a simpler procedure such as a single-stage nasolabial flap or skin grafting.

The esthetic outcome of the melolabial interpolation flap is far superior when the design is for reconstruction of the entire alar subunit. The soft, pliable melolabial tissue, when transposed onto the nose, undergoes normal and expected wound contraction. If only a portion of the ala is reconstructed, contraction can result in an asymmetrical, uneven bulbous appearance of the flap (Fig. 4). But when the entire cosmetic subunit is replaced, the normal flap contraction can actually improve the cosmetic appearance by restoring the normal curvature of the ala. It is important that the melolabial interpolation flap not be used for vertically oriented wounds extending more than 2 to 3 mm superior of the alar crease as this will likely result in an unnatural and uneven fullness of the alar crease. For wounds extending higher on the nasal sidewall, a single-stage nasolabial flap or a forehead flap may be more appropriate. Another limitation for the melolabial interpolation flap is a wound extending more distally onto the nasal tip and columella.

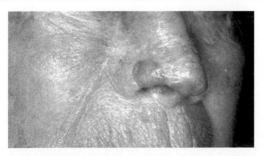

Figure 4 Subtotal alar reconstruction resulting in uneven bulbous appearance of the melolabial interpolation flap.

Complex wounds, with significant involvement of the nasal tip, will best be managed with other reconstructive options such as the forehead flap.

Two other considerations prior to undertaking the melolabial interpolation flap are (i) the need for cartilage grafting and (ii) restoring any mucosal defect. Even though the normal anatomy of the alar lobule is devoid of cartilage, the restoration process prior to the melolabial interpolation flap often includes cartilage grafting. The cartilage graft can serve as a structural support to maintain the convex surface of the alar rim during wound contraction and maintain a patent nasal airway. The most common donor site for the cartilage graft is the naturally curved cartilage of the concha of the ear.

Mucosal defects also need to be addressed prior to performing a melolabial interpolation flap. Options for reconstruction of mucosal defects include (i) a mucosal flap, (ii) skin grafting the backside of the melolabial interpolation flap, (iii) a turn-down Burow's hinge flap, and (iv) turning under of the melolabial interpolation flap.

Because of the symmetry of the nose, the contralateral ala provides a superb "normal" model to provide a copy to help restore the deformed ala (Fig. 5A–D). Therefore, foil from the suture packet is placed over the contralateral ala to form a three-dimensional template. The perimeter of the foil template should be 1 mm larger than the defect to allow for wound contraction. The foil template of the normal ala is then flattened into a two-dimensional template, reversed and placed on the melolabial fold below the deformed ala. The template is situated so that the most medial aspect of the foil touches the medial aspect of the melolabial fold, just above the oral commissure. Superior of the template, a triangle is tapered to the most superior aspect of the melolabial fold. Once dissected, this will serve as the vascular pedicle. Inferior of the template, a standard Burow's triangle is designed with enough length to prevent dog-ear formation. This will assure that the donor site suture line is esthetically situated along the melolabial fold. Preparation of the recipient site includes repairing any bevel and the remainder of the deformed ala cosmetic subunit, leaving approximately 2 to 3 mm of normal tissue at the base of the alar. This allows for the most esthetic recreation of the lateral alar crease. Once the defect has been properly prepared and the melolabial flap designed, supportive cartilage grafts should be considered. It has been our experience that cartilage grafting is not always necessary. Partial-thickness wounds, which do not impinge upon the alar rim, often do very well with only flap reconstruction. However, if the entire alar surface is replaced, cartilage support will maintain the normal curvature of the rim much better than reconstruction without cartilage.

Prior to harvesting the flap, it is always a good idea to use stretched gauze to assure proper flap length. The flap is

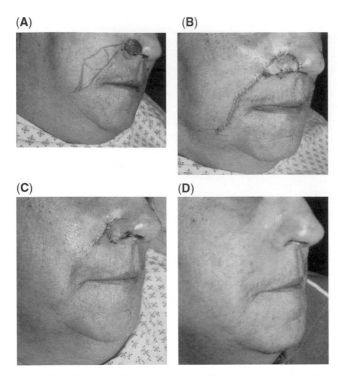

Figure 5 (**A**) Horizontally oriented wound of the ala and planning of the two-staged melolabial interpolation flap. (**B**) Interpolation of the melolabial flap on its pedicle, and flap sutured to the alar defect. (**C**) Three weeks after the surgery, the pedicle is transected and the alar crease is reconstructed. (**D**) Results six months after surgery *Note*: No cartilage replacement was necessary.

to approximately 1 to 2 mm in thickness. A small pocket is created proximally (nasal tip) and laterally (alar base), with a scalpel blade to help secure the batten cartilage graft. The cartilage is further secured with 5-0 subcutaneous sutures and should be placed as close to the alar rim as possible to prevent retraction. A small gauge suture needle should be used to minimize traumatic breaking of the cartilage graft. Also, light scoring of the cartilage with the scalpel blade can facilitate contouring to the alar curvature.

The second stage of the melolabial interpolation flap is usually done approximately three weeks after the first stage (Figs. 5, 6D and E). The base of the pedicle is simply incised at the superior aspect of the melolabial fold in a fusiform fashion, and meticulously closed in a layered fashion exactly along the melolabial fold. The alar wound edge is freshened to the crease. The lateral aspect of the pedicle flap, attached to the alar base, is sharply dissected approximately 1.0 cm and carefully thinned to recontour the alar lobule. The flap is then inset to the lateral alar base and secured with 6-0 buried and 6-0 fast absorbing gut.

Further surgery is rarely needed. If the original wound extended above the alar crease, a second thinning procedure may be necessary three to six months postoperatively to reestablish a normal crease. Occasionally, scar abrasion may be useful to help soften the scar lines, especially on the nose. This is also best performed approximately three months postoperatively because early visible lines often disappear in the first three months. Interestingly, procedures, which repair only a portion of a cosmetic unit, are more likely to need dermabrasion to soften the scar. Alternatively, procedures, which replace entire cosmetic subunits, rarely require a blending procedure such as scar abrasion. Two other potential complications include blunting of the alar crease and flattening of the melolabial fold.

Subcutaneous Melolabial Interpolation Flap

Another specialized flap to consider when reconstructing extensive alar defects is the reverse melolabial (nasolabial) subcutaneous interpolation flap as described by Spear (Fig. 7A–E). The flap is ideally suited for large full-thickness defects involving loss of the alar base or lateral alar crease. The design is similar to the single-stage nasolabial flap or the melolabial interpolation flap. When performing the reverse melolabial flap, it is important to carefully dissect to a vascular-rich muscular pedicle, approximately 2 mm lateral of the alar defect. The flap is meticulously trimmed and the excess fat globules are removed. The flap is turned on its vascular pedicle to form the lateral alar crease and inner nasal lining. The nasal mucosa is sutured to the cutaneous surface of the flap using 5-0 chromic gut sutures. Once the lining has been secured, the flap is turned up upon itself to reform the alar rim. The cutaneous portion of the flap should be sutured to the cutaneous portion of the defect in a standard layered fashion. The donor site is closed in a standard layered fashion. If a dog-ear forms along the superior portion of the nasal wound, a triangular excision can be made in this area to flatten the surrounding tissue. Because this is a subcutaneous interpolation flap, there is usually no need for a secondary procedure or for cartilage support.

Other miscellaneous interpolation flaps are described using the forehead and cheek as donor sites and tunneling the flap under a bridge of skin to reach the nose. In reality, those flaps frequently leave unnatural tissue bridges at the tunneled site and require a second stage to debulk the unnatural bridge of tissue. They are no better and often more troublesome than the one- and two-staged procedures

harvested starting at the most distal aspect and carefully dissecting in the superficial subcutaneous plane. The most distal aspect of the flap is aggressively thinned of fat so as to allow for proper insetting. Once undermining reaches the proximal part of the flap, the path of dissection should extend deeper into the muscle and should be performed bluntly to minimize vascular disruption. The proximal pedicle should have a widely based muscular and subcutaneous pedicle. The proximal cutaneous pedicle is not necessary, and cutting through the skin allows for greater flap mobility. Dissection of the proximal pedicle should be very superficial in the subcutaneous plane. The donor site is undermined in the usual manner. The flap is then rotated on its subcutaneous muscular pedicle (approximately 150°). The flap is rotated from the inferior aspect, clockwise for the left ala and counter clockwise for the right ala. Once adequate flap coverage is assured, the distal Burow's triangle can be amputated and discarded, and the proximal triangle supports the flap, which is sutured into the donor wound. The flap is secured using 5-0 or 6-0 buried, subcutaneous vertical mattress sutures and 6-0 fast absorbing gut. The donor site is then sutured in a similar manner. With larger defects, 4-0 buried, subcutaneous vertical mattress sutures may be necessary to close the donor site.

When dealing with deeper, more extensive wounds, a cartilage batten graft is essential for support (Fig. 6A–F). The normal foil template can be used to harvest the conchal cartilage. The anterior approach to the conchal bowl is preferred. Posterior harvesting of the cartilage cuts through muscle and involves more bleeding than the anterior approach. The cartilage is meticulously trimmed and thinned

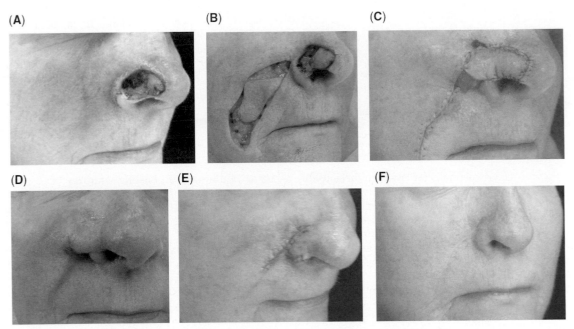

Figure 6 (A) Extensive, deep, horizontally oriented alar defect with cartilage loss. (B) Formation of a cartilage lattice structure of the ala using conchal cartilage. Dissection of the melolabial interpolation flap and amputation of the distal Burow's triangle. (C) Interpolation flap is rotated counterclockwise on its vascular pedicle and sutured to the alar wound. (D) Three weeks after surgery prior to transaction of the pedicle. (E) Transection of pedicle, reforming of the apex of the melolabial flap and insetting of the interpolation flap on the lateral ala. (F) Results six months after surgery. *Note:* The entire alar subunit is replaced.

described above. Occasionally, these flaps may be useful to reach more medially situated wounds (Fig. 8A–C).

AURICULAR RECONSTRUCTION

Our zest for perfection in reconstructive surgery must be tempered by the patient's desire for perfection. Patients are often far less fastidious about the esthetic result of auricular reconstruction compared to the nose or other more centrally situated wounds. The lateral, less conspicuous location of the ears, combined with the fact that hair commonly covers them, frequently leads to ambivalence in patients with regard to complex reconstruction of the ear. It is not uncommon for a patient to be concerned only about having a place for their hearing aid or to hang their glasses. We cringe at the thought of a patient walking around with a deformed "Spock" style ear with our name attached as their reconstructive surgeon. Nevertheless, if the patient is satisfied, we should fight the temptation to over-repair. With that in mind, it makes sense that the number of interpolation flaps

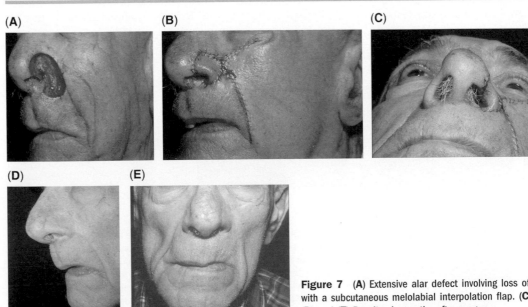

Figure 7 (A) Extensive alar defect involving loss of the alar base. (B) Reconstruction with a subcutaneous melolabial interpolation flap. (C) Inferior view of the turnover flap. (D) and (E) Results six months after surgery.

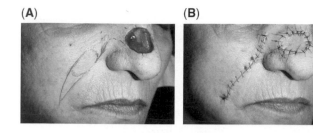
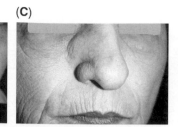

(A) **(B)** **(C)**

Figure 8 (A) Deep, medially situated wound of the nasal sidewall and dorsum. Planning of a subcutaneous melolabial interpolation flap. (B) Reconstruction of the defect and donor site after tunneling the subcutaneous pedicle under the intervening island of normal tissue in the nasofacial sulcus. (C) Unnatural bridging of the nasofacial sulcus at the tunneled site.

we use in auricular reconstruction is far less than those used in nasal reconstruction. In the patients who demand perfection, auricular interpolation flaps often deliver good results.

Topographic anatomy of the auricle consists of a thin vascular cutaneous layer enveloping the rigid auricular cartilage. Because the perimeter of the auricle is essentially a free tissue margin, second intention healing of larger wounds often leads to cicatricial deformity. The taughtness of the skin overlying the cartilage often prevents local flap reconstruction. Therefore, auricular interpolation flaps are commonly utilized to recruit distant tissue to reconstruct the ear.

AURICULAR INTERPOLATION FLAPS

The most commonly used interpolation flap for reconstruction of the ear is the postauricular interpolation flap (Fig. 9A–E). This flap is richly vascularized, based on the perforators of the retroauricular artery. The height of flap parallels the height of the wound. The length of the flap largely depends on the extent of the wound. The donor site of the flap starts from the posterior aspect of the wound and extends posterior to the retroauricular sulcus and on to the mastoid, widening slightly as it extends posterior to account for contraction of the width of the flap. The flap is dissected to the perichondrium at the distal aspect, while the base is dissected to the fascia. The only preparation of the defect involves squaring-off of the wound edges at the helical rim. This preparation allows for a more natural appearing junction with the flap tissue. The postauricular interpolation flap is then draped over the wound and secured with 6-0 subcutaneous sutures and 6-0 fast absorbing gut. A very important procedure to enhance the final result consists of

using quilting or basting sutures (5-0 chromic) to recreate contours of the helical groove. Occasionally, a postauricular interpolation flap without cartilage grafting can lead to uneven contraction, resulting in flattening of the helical rim.

More extensive auricular wounds with significant cartilage loss will likely require cartilage grafting to optimize esthetic outcome (Fig. 10A–D). For small defects, the ipsilateral conchal bowl can be used as the donor site, but for large wounds, the contralateral ear can be used as the donor site to minimize interfering with the vascular supply to the flap. In these situations, a foil template is made of the defect and utilized to harvest conchal cartilage. The cartilage can be lightly scored to increase mobility. The cartilage is secured to the defect using 5-0 subcutaneous suture. The template is then used to mark the size of the postauricular flap. The flap is harvested as outlined above. A bolster dressing is constructed using cardboard or plastic batten cut from the suture package and this is secured using 4-0 suture to recreate the helical rim and sulcus.

A variant of the postauricular interpolation flap is the postauricular pull-through interpolation flap. This may be useful for extensive defects of the antihelix, scapha, concha, and triangular fossa in which the helical rim is intact. Applications of this flap are best suited for larger defects of the above-mentioned areas where skin grafting would not survive, and second intention contraction may lead to unacceptable deformity.

In all of the postauricular interpolation flaps, the second stage of the procedure is performed at approximately three weeks postoperatively (Fig. 9C and D). The base of the flap is transected, thinned, and folded to cover the posterior portion of the wound. The donor site often heals fine by

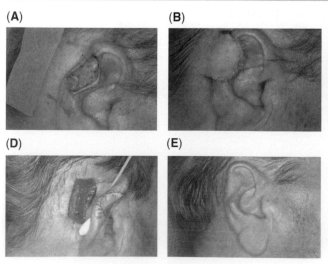
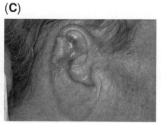

(A) **(B)** **(C)**

(D) **(E)**

Figure 9 (A) Deep, medially situated wound of the nasal sidewall and dorsum. Planning of a subcutaneous melolabial interpolation flap. (B) Suturing of the postauricular interpolation flap without cartilage grafting (patient's request). (C) Insetting of the postauricular interpolation flap three weeks after the original surgery. (D) Postauricular donor site is relatively small and will heal fine by second intention. (E) Results three months after surgery. The mild flattening of the helical rim may have been improved with cartilage grafting.

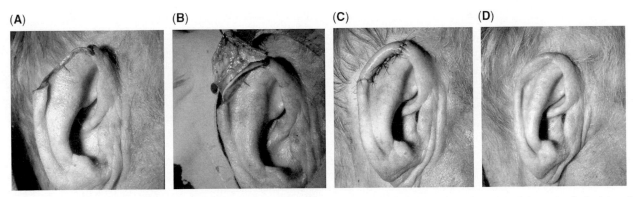

Figure 10 (**A**) Large full-thickness defect of the auricle. (**B**) Cartilage grafting from the ipsilateral conchal and dissection of the postauricular interpolation flap. (**C**) Insetting of the postauricular interpolation flap. The second stage of the procedure is preformed as previously described three weeks after the original surgery (no photos). (**D**) Results six months after surgery.

second intention. A skin graft may be needed to repair larger donor defects involving both the posterior ear and the mastoid, which would otherwise heal with unnatural tethering to the scalp.

Finally, another variant of the auricular interpolation flap is the preauricular interpolation flap (Fig. 11A–D). This reconstruction is best suited for defects of the superior helical rim. A strip of tissue approximately the width of the wound is incised and dissected from the preauricular crease on which the pedicle is based superiorly. The flap is transposed and draped over the superior helix. Preparation of the defect consists of squaring the portions of the wound along the helical rim. The preauricular interpolation flap is commonly completed in a single stage.

LIP RECONSTRUCTION

Because the lips are devoid of any cartilaginous or bony supporting structures, they are capable of a wide range of motion and multiple functions including verbal and nonverbal communication, oral continence, and proper deglutition. Therefore, any choice in reconstructive surgery must also not only be esthetically pleasing but must also maintain or restore a competent oral aperture including a satisfactory range of motion.

SUBCUTANEOUS MELOLABIAL INTERPOLATION FLAP

Because the vermilion-cutaneous junction is a free tissue margin, second intention healing of larger wounds can often

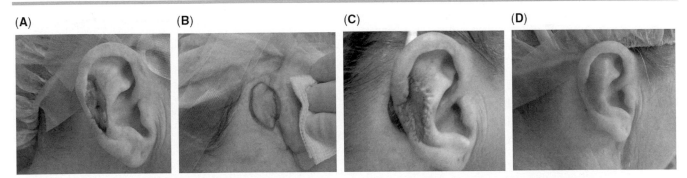

Figure 11 (**A**) Partial full-thickness defect of the left antihelix with an intact helical rim. (**B**) Dissection of postauricular interpolation flap. (**C**) The postauricular pedicle flap is pulled through a small slit and sutured into place. (**D**) Three weeks after the first stage, prior to the second-stage surgery.

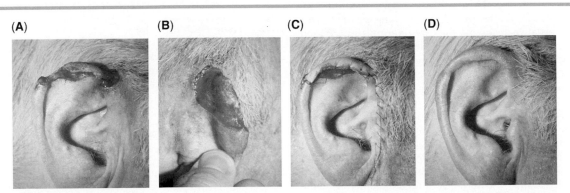

Figure 12 (**A**) Defect of the superior auricular. The cartilage is mostly intact, but is denuded. (**B**) Reconstruction with a preauricular interpolation flap. (**C**) Results six months after surgery.

(A)   (B)   (C)   (D)

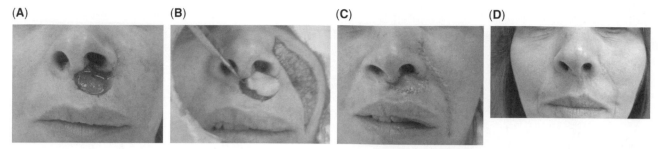

Figure 13   **(A)** Defect of the upper lip and nasal sill. **(B)** Intraoperative view after tunneling the subcutaneous melolabial interpolation flap under the intervening normal tissue of the cutaneous lip. Donor site dissection of the donor site along the nasofacial sulcus and melolabial flap. **(C)** Immediately after reconstruction. The donor site is closed in a lazy S-shape. **(D)** Results two months after surgery.

lead to eclabium formation. Occasionally, defects of the lip are situated such that standard advancement, rotation, transposition, or island pedicle flap would lead to unacceptable blunting of the melolabial fold or pulling of the vermilion. These types of defects are ideally suited for a subcutaneous melolabial interpolation flap (Fig. 12A–C). The concept is similar as outlined in the melolabial interpolation flap. A foil template is formed of the defect and placed in the ipsilateral melolabial flap. Burow's triangles are removed superior and inferior of the template. These incisions are carefully placed in a lazy S-like fashion so that the donor scar is meticulously situated in the melolabial fold. The subcutaneous melolabial interpolation flap is carefully dissected to a central vascular pedicle based on the underlying muscular perforators. The normal intervening tissue between the subcutaneous interpolation flap and the defect is sharply undermined. The subcutaneous interpolation flap is then tunneled under the intervening island of normal tissue and placed into the defect. Upon closing the donor site in the standard layered fashion, the flap should be under minimal tension. The subcutaneous interpolation flap is then sutured in a layered fashion. Because the interpolation is all subcutaneous, no second stage is necessary.

POSTOPERATIVE CONSIDERATIONS

A perfect reconstructive procedure does not always result in a perfect outcome. Communication is critical to prevent many avoidable complications. Frequently, patients have preconceived and unrealistic expectations of the healing process. Although with most interpolation flaps, a second-stage repair is expected, we believe it is prudent to prepare the patient that the healing process may take three to six months. We prefer typed wound care instructions that also outline expected changes during the healing process. This reinforces verbal instructions that are often misunderstood or forgotten once the patient leaves the office.

In our experience, postoperative scar revision is not commonly needed (<10%). When revision is necessary, it is usually only minor revision such as scar abrasion to blend the wound, which is best performed at approximately three months postoperatively. Scar abrasion is usually only necessary on the nose. In wounds involving thick sebaceous skin over the distal nose, tangential excision with the scalpel at three months may be used to level uneven edges. Medium, sterile, aluminum oxide sandpaper (80–100 grit) can be used to feather the edges for minor contour adjustments of the nasal scars. More extensive surgical scar revision to reform the natural alar crease may be necessary for trap-door

deformity and depressed scars, or cicatricial changes should be delayed until the wound has completely healed. These more extensive surgical revisions are probably best preformed approximately six months postoperatively, unless it is certain that natural healing will not be sufficient to provide a satisfactory result.

BIBLIOGRAPHY

Baker SR. Internal lining. In: Baker SR, Naficy S, eds. Principles of Nasal Reconstruction. St. Louis: Mosby, 2002:31–46.

Baker SR, Johnson TM, Nelson BR. The importance of maintaining the alar-facial sulcus in nasal reconstruction. Arch Otolaryngol Head Neck Surg 1995; 121:617–22.

Baker SR, Swanson NA. Local Flaps in Facial Reconstruction. St. Louis: CV Mosby, 1995.

Bennett RG. Fundamentals of cutaneous surgery. St. Louis: CV Mosby, 1988.

Brodland DG. Fundamentals of flaps and graft wound closure in cutaneous surgery. Cutis 1994; 53:192.

Brodland DG, Zitelli JA. Surgical margins for squamous cell carcinoma. J Am Acad Dermatol 1992; 27:241.

Burget GC, Menick FJ. Aesthetic Reconstruction of the Nose. St. Louis: CV Mosby, 1994.

Byrd Dr, Otley CC, Nguyen TH. Alar batten cartilage grafting in nasal reconstruction: functional and cosmetic results. J Am Acad Dermatol 2000; 43(5 Pt 1):833–836.

Dzubow LM. Facial Flaps: Biomechanics and Regional Application. Norwalk, CT: Appleton & Lange, 1990.

Fader DJ, Baker SR, Johnson TM. The staged cheek-to-nose interpolation flap for reconstruction of the nasal alar rim/lobule. J Am Acad Dermatol 1997; 37:614–619.

Fazio MJ, Zitelli JA. Principles of reconstruction following excision of nonmelanoma skin cancer. Clin Dermatol 1995; 13:601.

Fazio MJ, Zetelli JA. The single-staged nasolabial flap. Operative Tech in Plast Reconstr Surg 1998; 5:50–58.

Jackson IT. Local Flaps in Head and Neck Reconstruction. St. Louis: CV Mosby, 1985.

Lask GP, Moy RL. In: Principles and Techniques of Cutaneous Surgery. New York: McGraw-Hill, 1996.

Menick FJ. The two-staged nasolabial flap for subunit reconstruction of the ala. Operative Tech in Plast Reconstr Surg 1998; 5:59–64.

Mikhail GR. Mohs Micrographic Surgery. Philadelphia: W.B. Saunders, 1991.

Moy RL. Atlas of cutaneous facial flaps and grafts: a differential diagnosis of wound closure. Philadelphia: Lea & Febiger, 1990.

Salasche SJ, Bernstein G, Senkarik M. Surgical Anatomy of the Skin. Norwalk: CT: Appleton & Lange, 1988.

Salasche SJ, Jarchow R, Feldman BD, et al. The suspension suture. J Dermatol Surg Oncol 1987; 13:973.

Skouge JW. Upper-lip repair: the subcutaneous island pedicle flap. J Dermatol Surg Oncol 1990; 16:63.

Spears SL, Kroll SS, Romm S. N new twist to the nasolabial flap for reconstruction of lateral alar defect. Plast Reconstr Surg 1987; 79:915–920.

Wolf DJ, Zitelli JA. Surgical margins for basal cell carcinomas. Arch Dermatol 1987; 123:340.

Zitelli JA. Mohs micrographic surgery for skin cancer. In: DeVita VT Jr., Hellman S, Roseberg SA, eds. Principles and Practice of Oncology. Philadelphia: J.B. Lippincott, 1992:1.

Zitelli JA. The nasolabial flap as a single-stage procedure. Arch Dermotal 1990; 126:1445.

Zitelli JA. Tips for wound closure: pearls for minimizing dog-ears and applications of periosteal sutures. Dermatol Clin 1989; 7:123.

Zitelli, JA. Wound healing for secondary intention. J Am Acad Dermatol 1983; 9:407.

Zitelli JA, Fazio MJ. Reconstruction of the nose with local flaps. J Dermatol Surg Oncol 1991; 17:184.

Zitelli JA, Moy RL. Buried vertical mattress suture. J Dermatol Surg Oncol 1989; 15:17.

57

Random Pattern Flaps

Ronald G. Wheeland

University of Arizona College of Medicine, Tucson, Arizona, U.S.A.

INTRODUCTION

A skilled dermatologic surgeon quickly learns that the simplest and easiest repair for a cutaneous wound frequently results in fewer complications, faster healing, and minimal scarring. Yet there are many cases in which simple primary closure would fail to yield a desirable result because of the size of the wound or its anatomic location. In these circumstances, more complex repairs with the use of local random pattern flaps may be required to obtain the most satisfactory functional and cosmetic result. It is important to understand the appropriate applications of the different types of local random pattern cutaneous flaps. This greatly expands the number of surgical therapeutic options available to best repair a cutaneous defect. The basic concepts and principles of local flap repair and various clinical applications will be discussed.

A flap is defined as skin and its subcutaneous tissue with its own intact vascular supply moved from its original location to another. Movement of this type is possible due to the elasticity or redundancy of the skin. The terminology used to describe different types of flaps is confusing because many different names have been used to describe the same type of flap.

In general, flaps are named according to their proximity to the defect: local or distant (Table 1). Most local flaps are random pattern flaps because the vascularity is not based on a single blood vessel that arises from the deep dermal plexus. Local random pattern flaps are named according to the prevailing motion they make to fill the adjacent defect (sliding, stretching, or pivoting). All local flaps present some combination of these basic types of movement. Typically, these flaps are divided into advancement or sliding flap, rotational flaps that pivot in an arc about a point, or transpositional flaps.

A second major type of flap is known as the regional flap. It is moved into the wound from the same general anatomic area as the defect; however, this flap is based on a specific artery. This may also be called an axial pattern flap. The name of the blood vessel that supplies the flap is typically used to name the flap. The temporal artery flap is an example of a regional flap that allows tissue from the temple to be mobilized to fill a defect on the forehead. These flaps are also known as interpolation or pedicle flaps because the intact pedicle that contains the arterial supply crosses normal skin. Once circulation has been established from the tissue surrounding the defect, the pedicle is divided and the wound revised.

A third major group of flaps includes distant flaps. These flaps are located at a significant distance from the anatomic location of the defect. Most distant flaps require a series of staged procedures to improve flap survival by augmenting circulation through the newly created pedicle. These flaps are typically tubed to bridge the normal skin surrounding the defect.

A different classification of flaps divides them into simple or compound. The simple flap is composed of epidermis, dermis, and its attached subcutaneous tissue. The compound flap used for major reconstructive surgery is composed of skin, subcutaneous fat, and bone, muscle, or cartilage. Flaps used by dermatologic surgeons are almost exclusively the local random pattern type, and this discussion will be limited to them.

REPAIR OF WOUNDS WITH UNEQUAL LENGTH

To use flaps, special suturing and wound closure techniques must be understood because flaps often result in a wound of unequal sides. The first special technique is closure for wounds of unequal length. The simplest method for repairing a wound of this type is by "the rule of halves" (Fig. 1A). The incision on the longer side is spread out evenly over the entire length of the wound. This is done by placing the first stitch at the center of the excision. Then, the remaining halves are sutured half again to help spread out the excess tissue on the longer side over the remaining length of the wound. This process is repeated until the wound has been closed and all excess tissue has been distributed evenly over the length of the incision.

Burow's Triangle

A second way to close a wound of unequal sides is to remove a small triangular piece of tissue—Burow's triangle—from the longer side, thus decreasing its length (Fig. 1B). This triangular excision can be done anywhere along the longer side of the excision (Fig. 1C). If one recognizes this, the linear closure that results from this triangular excision can frequently be hidden in an adjacent anatomic line, crease, fold, or hairline and does not add to the cosmetic deformity.

Dog-Ear (Tricone Deformity) Repair

Another technique to remove excess tissue from one side of an unequal wound that puckers is the dog ear repair or a Tricone. Dog ears generally result when a wound is closed primarily but the angles at the ends of the incision are greater than 30°. Repair may be done in a number of ways, all of which yield an excellent cosmetic result. The simplest technique (Fig. 2) is to use a skin hook placed in the tip of the dog ear and to pull the tissue to one side. This side is incised

Table 1 Type of Flap

Local: random pattern flaps	Distant:
Advancement (sliding) flap	Bridging flap
Rotational (pivotal) flap	Tubed flap
Transposition flap	Simple flaps
Regional: axial pattern flaps	Epidermis
Temporal artery flap	Dermis
Deltopectoral flap	Subcutaneous tissue
	Compound:
	Skin
	Subcutaneous tissue
	Bone (or) cartilage (or) muscle

with a scalpel, extending the original incision. The partially transected piece of tissue is pulled to the opposite side of the suture line and completely incised in the same fashion. The triangular piece of tissue is discarded and the wound closed in a linear fashion.

Another technique is simply to excise the redundant tissue as a new ellipse (Fig. 3). This further extends the length of the original incision line but keeps it oriented in the same direction.

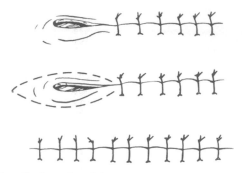

Figure 3 Correction of dog-ear deformity by simple excision.

Dog ears can also be removed by creating two small triangles, dividing the apex of the dog ear in half with a scalpel. The redundant tissue from each side is then pulled over the incision line and cut off. Two small triangular pieces of

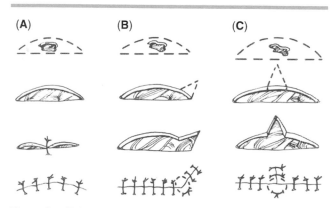

Figure 1 **(A)** Closing a wound of unequal sides by halves. **(B)** Closing a wound of unequal sides with a Burow's triangle. **(C)** Placement of the Burow's triangle at any position on long side.

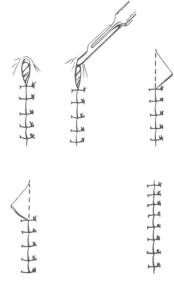

Figure 4 Correction of dog-ear deformity by division of the dog-ear in half and excision of two small triangular pieces of tissue.

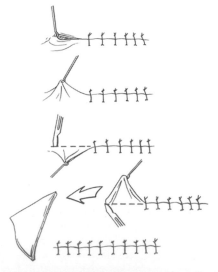

Figure 2 Repair of dog-ear deformity by pulling excess tissue to each side of the incision line and removing a single triangular piece of excess tissue.

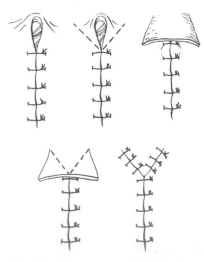

Figure 5 Correction of dog-ear deformity with M-plasty.

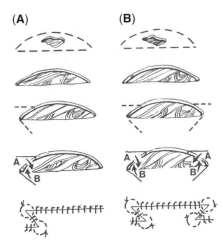

(A) **(B)**

Figure 6 **(A)** Repair of anticipated dog ear from a wound of unequal sides by a single Z-plasty. **(B)** Repair of a wound of unequal sides with anticipated dog-ear deformity with two Z-plasties.

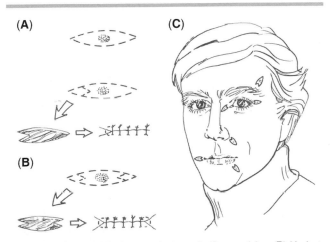

(A) **(C)**

(B)

Figure 7 **(A)** Single M-plasty to shorten a fusiform excision. **(B)** M-plasty at both ends of excision. **(C)** M-plasty used at anatomic borders.

redirects the orientation of the incision at the end and has particular advantages when one is excising close to natural free margins such as the lips or eye.

The Z-plasty may be used to equalize wound margins of different lengths as well. This technique will be discussed in greater detail later in this chapter. One (Fig. 6A) or two Z-plasties (Fig. 6B) can be done at the ends of the long margin of an excision to shorten its effective length.

M-Plasty

The M-plasty is used to shorten the overall length of an incision and is used most typically when one is performing a fusiform excision to a vital anatomic structure, natural body fold, or crease. It is also known as a crown closure because of the shape at the end of the wound. The M-plasty may be performed at one (Fig. 7A) or both ends (Fig. 7B) of an excision. Typically, a standard fusiform excision with 30° angles is drawn on the skin. Then two smaller 30° angles are drawn within the angle to form an M. These two lines at 30° angles are inset into the apex of the excision to form a rhomboid of equal sides with alternating 30 and 150° angles. The M-plasty may be used to remove a dog ear, as previously discussed, but is more typically used to shorten an excision. This is desirable when the excision is near areas such as the ocuclar canthi or the oral commissures (Fig. 7C). This helps to preserve the symmetry of anatomic structures by creating lines that fit into the natural folds.

Corner Stitch or Three Point Tie

The technique used most often to suture triangular defects is a half-buried horizontal mattress suture. This is also known as a corner stitch or three-point tie. This stitch is crucial to learn because many of the flaps that will be discussed later rely on it. If standard closures are performed, impairment of vascular flow to the tip of the flap may result in necrosis. In addition, if standard simple interrupted suturing techniques are used to close a triangular defect, this may result in depression or elevation of the flaptip, which that may need to be revised later.

The corner stitch begins as the needle is inserted in the surrounding skin and exits at the middermis (Fig. 8A). The tip of the flap is then punctured with the needle oriented horizontal entirely within the mid-dermis. This is carried across the tip in buried fashion and emerges from the tip at the same depth as its point of entrance. The needle is then rotated back to the traditional position and inserted in the mid-dermis of the adjacent side. It exits on the skin surface and is tied. This stitch results in minimal vascular impairment of the tip and maintains the proper alignment with the surrounding skin. A four-corner stitch is typically used with double advancement flaps, where two rectangles of tissue meet in the middle of the wound. The procedure (Fig. 8B) is similar to that of the

tissue are removed, and the wound is repaired by simple linear closure (Fig. 4).

Another technique is the M-plasty (Fig. 5) for repair of dog ears. Curvilinear incisions are made on each side of the redundant tissue. The tissue is then unfolded and allowed to lie flat on top of the wound edge. The excess tissue is excised with a scalpel or sharp scissors as two small triangular pieces. This results in the creation of an M at the end of the incision line. The advantage of this technique is that normal tissue is spared. This results in a shorter incision. It also

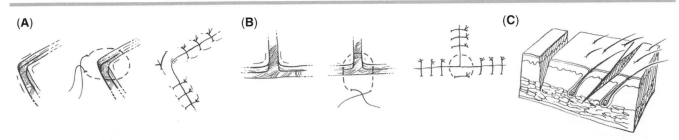

(A) **(B)** **(C)**

Figure 8 **(A)** Half-buried mattress suture as corner stitch. **(B)** Half-buried mattress suture as two-corner stitch. **(C)** Proper alignment of incision with the direction of hair growth.

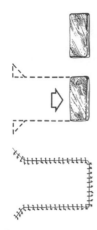

Figure 9   Single advancement U-flap.

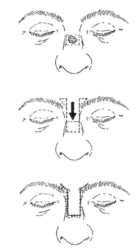

Figure 10   Advancement of Rintala flap along the bridge of the nose.

three-point stitch except that the additional flap tip is included in the buried horizontal segment.

Undermining

Proper undermining of flaps is important so that the tissue can move appropriately. The vascular supply for random pattern flaps is based on the deep dermal plexus. Consequently, the risk of injury to this vascular supply must be minimized. Blunt undermining with scissors and a skin hook is best done at the level of the upper subcutaneous tissue, especially when the location is the face. On the scalp, undermining is in the subgaleal plane, and, for the extremities, undermining is performed within the subcutaneous tissue or fascial plane.

PLANNING WOUND CLOSURE

The next preliminary consideration that must be paramount to the surgeon considering the use of a flap for repair of a defect is the relationship of the size and shape of the wound to the adjacent donor tissue. Careful planning should begin with an evaluation of the vascular supply for a proposed flap. Vascular supply on the head and neck is usually good, but the length-to-width ratio of the proposed flap must always be considered. Also, elasticity of the adjacent donor

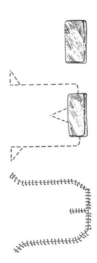

Figure 11   Peng variant of the single advancement flap to increase the base of the pedicle.

tissue must be evaluated for its ability to tolerate tension. In addition, the effect tension from the flap will have on adjacent anatomic structures must be considered. It is important to remember that in addition to the primary defect from removal of the lesion, a secondary defect is also created as the flap is moved. Also, tissue surrounding both the flap and the defect moves in the opposite direction. This movement is known as the secondary motion.

Skin chosen for the flap should be evaluated for color, texture, and the presence or absence of hair. To obtain the best cosmetic result, tissue that most closely matches the original tissue should be used.

To obtain the best cosmetic and functional result, when considering wound closure options in the reconstruction

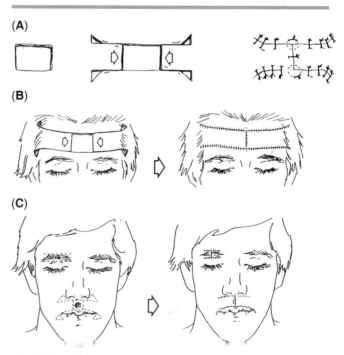

Figure 12   (A) Double advancement H-flap. (B) H-flap to repair forehead defect. (C) H-flap to repair midbrow defect and upper lip defect.

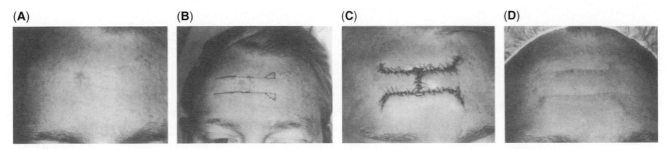

Figure 13 (**A**) Scar following curettage and electrodesiccation. (**B**) Double advancement flap planned. (**C**) Immediately after closure. (**D**) Double advancement flap two months postoperative.

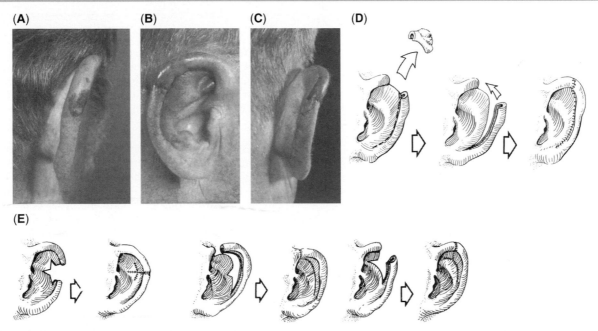

Figure 14 (**A**) Lentigo maligna melanoma (**B** and **C**) Wide excision and closure with a double advancement flap. (**D**) Advancement flap of helix. (**E**) Burow's triangles to reduce ear distortion. *Source*: Courtesy of Randall K. Roenigk.

of facial defects, several general aesthetic concepts must not be overlooked. It is always important to first carefully examine the patient's skin to identify the existing tension lines, creases, and natural folds. This will allow the surgeon to make incisions so that the resulting scars can be effectively camouflaged by normal facial lines. These lines, also known as Langer's lines, vary from one patient to another but are typically perpendicular to the underlying muscles of facial expression. The skin tension lines, which may be present at rest or with motion, can also be utilized to help properly orient the planned repair of the wound or defect. However, if the potential donor reservoir of tissue is of insufficient quantity to permit tensionless wound closure, then all of the preliminary planning will prove to be inadequate and the cosmetic and functional result impaired. The potential reservoirs of donor tissue for local flap reconstructive surgery vary from patient to patient and also with age and the amount of solar damage. However, common donor sites include the glabella, temple, cheek nasolabial folds, neck, and preauricular area.

Children and teenagers may not have obvious skin tension lines. In this case, remove the lesion as clinically appropriate (usually in a circle). Then undermine the margins; by checking for tension in various directions with skin hooks, the most appropriate direction of closure can be chosen. Ask the patient to smile, frown, or purse the lips, and the natural creases may become more pronounced.

When incisions are to be made in or adjacent to hair-bearing skin, avoid advancing hair-bearing tissue into non–hair-bearing skin. It is also important, especially around the eyebrows or side-burns, that the incision be angled parallel to the hair shafts and not perpendicular to the surface as is typically performed (Fig. 8C). This will minimize transection or injury to hair follicle structures that may result in a permanent patch of alopecia.

TYPES OF RANDOM PATTERN FLAPS

In order to understand local random pattern flaps, remember that while each flap is named for the primary motion used to position it into the defect, there is always secondary motion. In fact, flaps involve combinations of various types of motion. Illustrations used to represent flap sure use idealized squares, circles, triangles, or other geometric shapes. In fact, many flaps can be modified to fill a defect without converting it into a stylized geometric shape. In general, flaps can be characterized by their primary motion as advancement, rotation, or transposition.

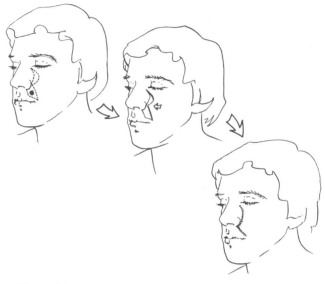

Figure 15 Perialar crescent-shaped advancement flap schematic.

Advancement Flap

The advancement flap is one with which most dermatologic surgeons are familiar. The simplest fusiform excision can be viewed as a double advancement flap when wide undermining is necessary to permit tensionless closure. Because tissue from both sides of the excision is advanced to fill the defect, this can be considered a simple type of advancement flap.

Advancement flaps traditionally move in a straight line. This type of movement is possible due to the elasticity of the flap and the adjacent tissue. When, one is creating an advancement flap, the tissue is stretched over the defect and the unequal sides of the wound are closed using techniques previously described. Flaps included in this category are the H-flap, U-flap, O–T flap, V–Y flap, and the Burow's triangle flap.

U-Flap

The U-flap, also known as the O–U repair, trapdoor flap, or single advancement flap, is one of the simplest flaps to use because the geometric pattern (Fig. 9) and incision lines can easily be oriented to fit natural folds. In general, this flap should have a length-to-width ratio of no more than 3:1 in order to maintain sufficient vascular supply to nourish the tip of the flap. There are several ways to modify this flap so that even moderate-sized defects can be repaired.

One U-flap that is useful for defects of the nasal tip is the Rintala flap (Fig. 10). This flap, also known as the median glabellar flap, is used to advance glabellar skin in a straight line down the nasal bridge to cover defects of the nasal bridge and tip. The dog ears are excised just above the medial ends of the eyebrows to help hide the scars.

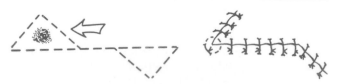

Figure 16 Burow's triangle flap.

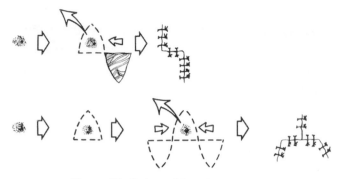

Figure 17 Variants of Burow's triangle flap.

A modified U-flap proposed by Peng (Fig. 11) increases the pedicle size to improve flap survival. This flap is designed to advance into and around a defect, and the dog ear is repaired centrally. The large flap pedicle with improved vascular supply has a greater chance of survival.

H-Flap

Synonyms for the H-flap include the double-U, double tab, or doubled advancement flap (Fig. 12A). This flap is commonly used to repair defects on the forehead (Fig. 12B), within the eyebrow (Fig. 12C), because it permits the remaining hair-bearing portion of the brow to be approximated to avoid alopecia, and on the upper lip (Fig. 12C). Burow's triangles are removed wherever excess tissue is present along the edge of the incision. This incision should be hidden as inconspicuously as possible. Redundant tissue may be distributed evenly along the closure, with suturing by the rule of halves, previously described, to avoid the formation of a Burow's triangle.

For a defect in the midline of the upper lip, tissue can be advanced from both lip margins. The Burow's triangles are removed within the nasolabial line (Fig. 12C). The forehead lends itself well to this closure because the incision lines can be placed within the natural folds (Fig. 13). Relatively large amounts of tissue can be mobilized with this flap.

Another location successfully repaired with an advancement flap is the helical rim of the ear (Figs. 14A–C). The helical sulcus is incised to the superior edge of the lobule. Because the lobe of the ear is mobile, it allows the helix to be

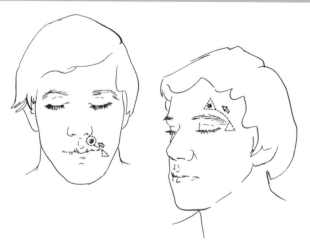

Figure 18 Locations where Burow's triangle flap is useful.

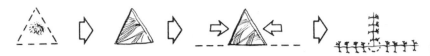

Figure 19 A–T flap used to close a wound.

advanced upward (Fig. 14D). Removal of a Burow's triangle permits advancement without significant distortion of the ear. The Burow's triangle may include full-thickness cartilage to permit the helical rim to advance without difficulty. A second advancement flap can be created using the superior pole of the helical rim if needed (Fig. 14E).

Defects around the nose or upper lip can frequently be closed with a crescent-shaped advancement flap. Redundant tissue from the cheek is advanced medially and closed along the nasolabial fold (Fig. 15). Large defects may be closed without deforming the base of the ala or the lip. Redundant tissue is removed at the junction of the nose and face at the nasofacial sulcus. A dog ear is excised, tissue from the medial portion of the cheek is undermined, and the triangular flap is advanced.

Burow's Triangle Flap

The Burow's triangle flap can be used to close a defect with tissue mobilized from areas some distance from the wound (Fig. 16). This flap can be visualized as a simple elliptical closure; however, part of the ellipse is separated from the remainder of the ellipse by a distance. This permits redundant tissue from nearby to be moved into the defect. The size of the defect dictates the size of the Burow's triangle and whether or not two triangles are used (Fig. 17). The distance between the defect and where the Burow's triangle is removed is a function of the anatomic location and degree of skin laxity. This versatile flap can be used in a number of areas but is especially useful when natural folds can be incorporated into the motion of the flap.

The flap can be modified by increasing or decreasing the distance between the defect and the Burow's triangle to take advantage of excess skin. By placing the Burow's triangle some distance from the defect, distortion of an important structure such as the upper lip or eyebrow is minimized. The secondary defect can be repaired in a less conspicuous tension line (Fig. 18). When two lesions are immediately adjacent to one another and are to be removed in one session, the Burow's triangle flap may be used to close both defects at once by advancing the tissue between them.

O–T or A–T Flap

The O–T or A–T flap is a bilateral advancement flap with incisions made at one end of the defect (Fig. 19). By extending the incision from the base of a triangular defect or the top or bottom of a circular defect, the adjacent tissue can be advanced and sutured in a straight line (Fig. 20). Removal of Burow's triangles are often necessary to accommodate secondary movement. The two pedicles advanced are broad based, and there is little risk of vascular impairment. Furthermore, this closure is especially useful to shorten the final length of an ellipse that might otherwise extend across a vital anatomic structure such as vermilion border of the lip, eyebrow, or natural crease or fold such as the chin crease or nasolabial fold (Fig. 21). Placing the limbs of the T within a natural fold makes them inconspicuous (Fig. 22). Closure requires the use of a four-corner stitch or the half-buried mattress suture previously discussed.

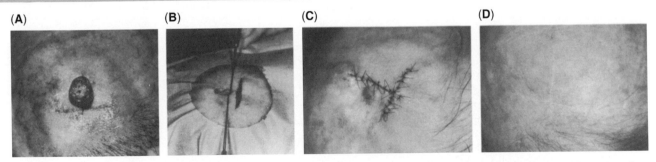

Figure 20 (A) Circular defect of scalp after Mohs surgery. (B) Anticipated closure. (C) Postoperative appearance. (D) Two months postoperative.

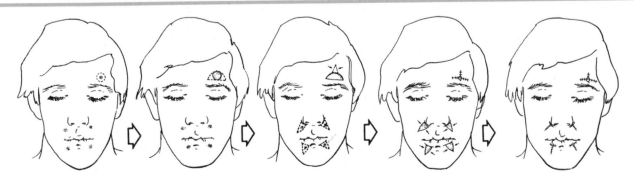

Figure 21 Clinical uses of O–T and A–T advancement flaps.

(A)   **(B)**

(C)   **(D)**

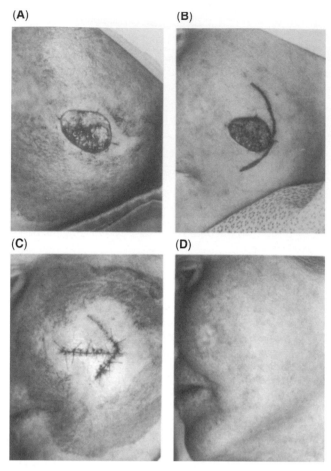

Figure 22   (**A**) Oval defect following Mohs surgery. (**B**) Curvilinear incisions to create the O–T flap. (**C**) Immediately postoperative. (**D**) Two months postoperative.

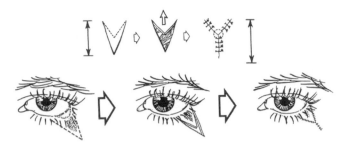

Figure 23   The V–Y flap used to lengthen a scar.

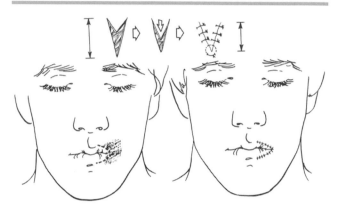

Figure 24   The Y–V flap used to shorten a scar.

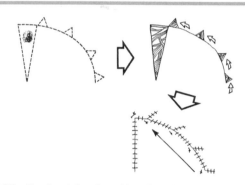

Figure 25   Classic rotation flap with various dog-ear correction options. The line of maximal tension shown.

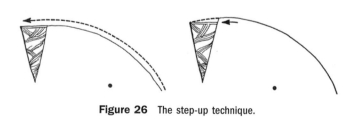

Figure 26   The step-up technique.

V–Y or Y–V Advancement Flap

The V–Y advancement flap (Fig. 23) is created by initially making a V-shaped incision and advancing the triangular portion of the flap in a straight line toward its base. The wound is closed in the shape of a Y. This technique increases the overall length of the wound and is beneficial for the correction of wounds that have contracted around the eye or mouth. The lengthening of the scar depends on the size of the V. As a consequence, this may be limited in order to keep the incision as short as possible. The flap is closed with a three-point suture to avoid lip necrosis.

The Y–V incision is made in a Y-shape, and the tip of the triangular flap is advanced. This variation of the V–Y flap is used to move the oral commissures laterally when some defect has pulled the commissure toward the midline (Fig. 24).

Rotation Flap

The rotation flap is one of the simpler types of random pattern flaps. It uses lateral movement of tissue while at the same time rotating about a pivot point (Figs. 25 and 26). This flap exploits the elasticity of adjacent skin along the curved portion of the incision line to permit advancement of rather large flaps (Fig. 27). Safety is one major advantage of the rotation flap because it has a broad base and a good vascular supply. Another advantage is that large amounts of tissue from virtually any side of a wound may be moved to close

even large defects (Fig. 28). In general, the curved incision lines inherent with the rotation flap are easier to disguise and yield a better cosmetic result than the straight lines that result from repairs with some other flaps. This flap is typically used on the cheek and based inferiorly with advancement and rotation in a forward, medial direction (Fig. 29). By placing the curved incision within relaxed skin tension lines, this flap is relatively easy to camouflage.

The rotation flap is classically shown as a way to close triangular defects (Fig. 30), but it can be used successfully to

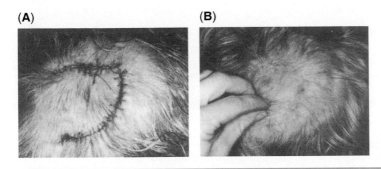

Figure 27 **(A)** Rotation flap of the scalp, immediately postoperative. **(B)** Six weeks postoperative.

close round and square defects as well (Fig. 31). Conversion of a round wound into a triangular defect is often not required.

To plan the rotation flap properly, the broad base pedicle should be inferior whenever possible. This maximizes gravitational assistance for both venous and lymphatic drainage. The pivot point, through which lies the line of maximum tension, determines the length of the advancing edge. The leading edge should he slightly longer than the length of the distal edge of the defect (Fig. 26). This is especially important for locations where the tissue is thick, inelastic, or immobile. If the wound is closed with excess tension, the flap may become ischemic.

Back Cut

In some circumstances, when closing a defect in inelastic tissue, a small back cut is made into the pedicle. This will release tissue for easier closure. The back cut is a relaxing incision (Fig. 32) that helps facilitate rotation. However, this incision may compromise vascularity of the flap

because the pedicle has been made narrower; so caution must be exercised.

Secondary movement adjacent to the flap may result in a dog ear. This redundant tissue can be excised at any point along the arc of the flap. Placement of this triangular excision should be planned so that it can be hidden in a natural hairline or skin tension line.

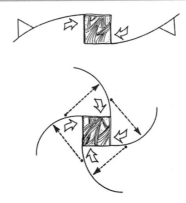

Figure 30 Rotation flaps used for closure of a triangular defect.

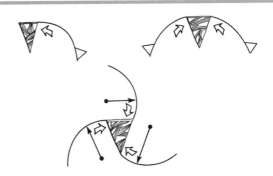

Figure 31 Closure of a square defect with rotation flaps.

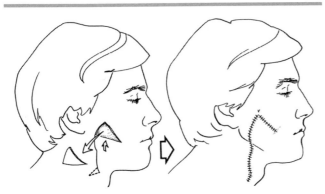

Figure 28 Large rotation flap of inferior cheek.

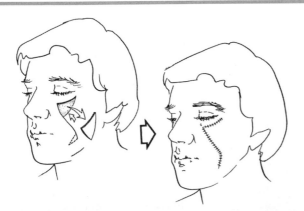

Figure 29 Large inferiorly based rotation flap for superior cheek defect.

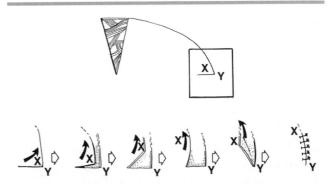

Figure 32 Lengthening of the arc of a rotation flap with a back cut.

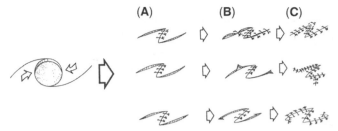

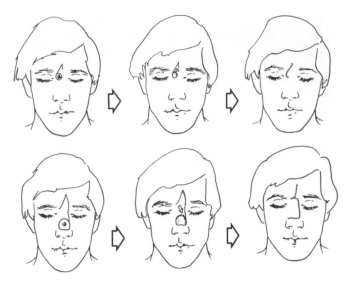

Figure 33 (**A**) O–Z closure of a circular defect: unequal edges are closed with the halving technique. (**B**) O–Z flap with Burow's triangles used to close uneven edges. (**C**) O–Z flap with Z-plasties to close unequal sides.

Figure 36 Banner flap variants of rotation flap used to repair a nasal defect: small (*top*) and large (*bottom*).

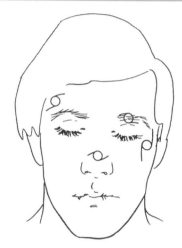

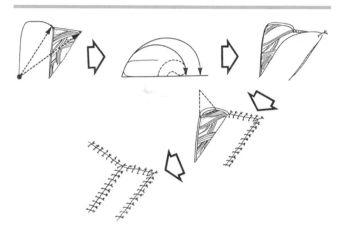

Figure 34 Various uses of O–Z flaps at different anatomic sites.

Figure 37 Classic transposition flap movement.

O–Z Closure

Many variations on the simple rotation flap can be used for wound closure. One of the more common variants is the O–Z closure. This consists of two rotation flaps, one on each side of the defect. Both flaps are rotated into the defect and closed side to side (Fig. 33A). Burow's triangles may be placed anywhere along the incision (Fig. 33B). The O–Z flap is traditionally used to decrease distortion of the anatomy at sites where loose tissue is limited (Fig. 34), on the face or trunk (Fig. 35). Because it does not excise the complete ellipse, the O–Z flap is a method for conserving tissue; approximately one-half of the ellipse is not removed. Furthermore, the tension on this closure is parallel to the limbs of the Z. Therefore, this flap can be used when a traditional fusiform excision would distort the adjacent structure. It is a commonly used adjacent to the eyebrow where one limb of the Z can be hidden within the hairline. It can also be used

along the nasal bridge, adjacent to the free eyelid margin or near the outer canthus.

Globellar, Anvil, or Banner Flap

This variant of the rotation flap is known as a glabellar flap. Synonyms are the anvil flap, dorsal nasal flap, or Banner flap. Movement of tissue uses excess skin in the glabellar area of the forehead. It is a rotation flap with a prominent back cut (Fig. 36). Tissue from the glabella can be rotated to fill defects of the inner canthus or the nasal root.

(A)   **(B)**

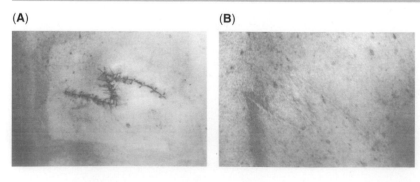

Figure 35 (**A**) Repair of a defect on the back with O–Z flap. (**B**) Six months postoperative.

(A)

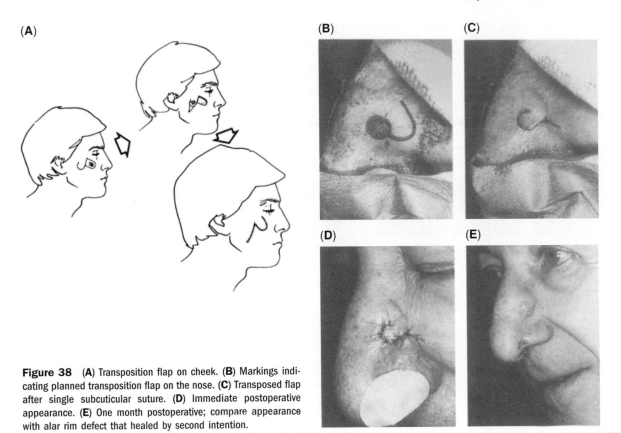

(B)　　**(C)**

(D)　　**(E)**

Figure 38 **(A)** Transposition flap on cheek. **(B)** Markings indicating planned transposition flap on the nose. **(C)** Transposed flap after single subcuticular suture. **(D)** Immediate postoperative appearance. **(E)** One month postoperative; compare appearance with alar rim defect that healed by second intention.

Transposition Flap

The transposition flap combines advancement and rotation to pivot about a given point (Fig. 37) without stretching the flap. An advantage of this flap is that the secondary defect can be placed away from the primary wound. The flap can be lifted over a zone of normal skin and moved into a new position (Fig. 38). The main disadvantage of this flap is that it may be difficult to turn a transposition flap more than 90°. Many different transposition flaps will be discussed separately, including the rhombic or Limberg flap, the nasolabial flap, the labial-ala flap, the bilobed-flap, and the Z-plasty.

Rhombic Flap

The rhombic flap is one of the most popular transposition flaps because of its versatility; with proper planning, any one of eight individual flaps can be devised for closure of

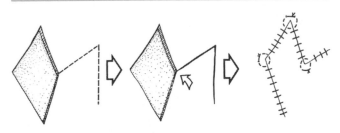

Figure 40 Closure of the rhomboid flap.

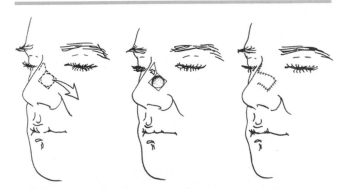

Figure 41 Rhombic flap for closure of defect on the side of the nose.

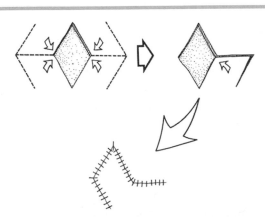

Figure 39 Schematic diagram shows four options available for the repair of a rhomboid defect. Four more can be created with incisions from the other two points in the rhombus.

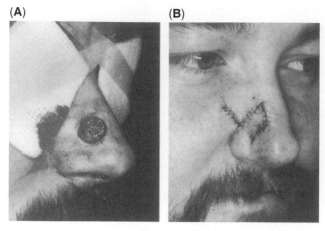

Figure 42 (A) Defect on the side of the nose. (B) Rhombic flap to repair this defect.

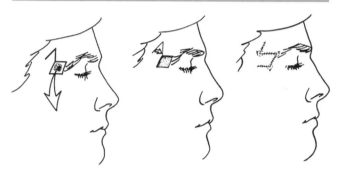

Figure 43 Rhombic flap for temple defect.

a given defect (Fig. 39). To design these flaps to allow proper closure, a precise geometric pattern is created. The defect is made into a rhombus, or equilateral parallelogram, with angles of 60° and 120°. An incision is extended perpendicularly, usually from the point of the 120° angle. The length of this line is equal to the length of the other sides of the rhombus. Another incision of similar length is made at 60°, parallel to one side of the rhombus. The flap and adjacent tissue are undermined and the flap is then transposed into the primary defect (Fig. 40). This closes not only the original defect but also the secondary defect (Fig. 41) created to develop this flap. The line of maximum tension occurs at the closure point of the secondary defect; so this is where the first stitch is placed.

This flap can actually be used to transpose tissue in any direction (Fig. 42). This allows unlimited possibilities; so excess skin and the tension lines can be maximally considered. Rather than change the defect into a rhombus, a circular defect is maintained. The first incision is made perpendicular to the defect at an appropriate point for closure on the basis of the location of the defect. The length of the incision is approximately equal to the radius of the circle. The second incision is of the same length and at a 60° angle. After appropriate undermining, the flap is transposed and the circle trimmed and molded to fit the flap. In this way, this transposition flap can be very versatile and valuable (Fig. 43).

DuFourmental Flap

A modification of the rhomboid flap is the DuFourmental variation (Fig. 44). This flap is constructed by decreasing the angle of the first incision from the defect. This facilitates both transposition of the flap and closure of the secondary defect.

Webster 30° Transposition Flap

Another variation on the rhomboid flap is the Webster 30° transposition flap (Fig. 45). The incision is made at a very narrow angle from the 120° angle of the defect. The normal 60° angle of the rhomboid defect is elongated into a 30° angle. This creates an uneven rhomboid that is closed with the transposed flap and an M-plasty.

W-Plasty or Double Rhomboid Flap

Another variant uses two rhombic flaps to close one wound. This may be useful for the closure of long defects. Two rhombic flaps (Fig. 46) are placed end to end. This can be applied to circular defects that may be closed with three rhombic flaps. The defect is converted into a hexagon that can be repaired using flaps planned from the 120° angles (Fig. 47).

The temple is an area where closure of a defect with a rhombic flap is common. The area between the eyebrow and the anterior hairline is easily narrowed and distorted by many closure techniques. To minimize distortion, it is essential to maintain the distance between these two hair-bearing points. A rhombic flap moved into such an area can maintain the relationship between these two hair-bearing structures and close the defect without significant tension. Excess tissue is utilized from the preauricular area. Closure of small defects on the bridge or side of the nose can also be done with a small rhombic flap. Excess tissue comes from the glabella or lateral to the nasofacial sulcus.

Nasolabial Flap

The nasolabial flap is a transposition flap used to repair defects on the side of the nose or upper lip (Fig. 48).

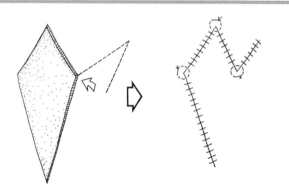

Figure 44 DuFourmental flap.

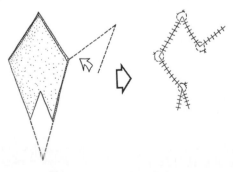

Figure 45 Webster 30° flap.

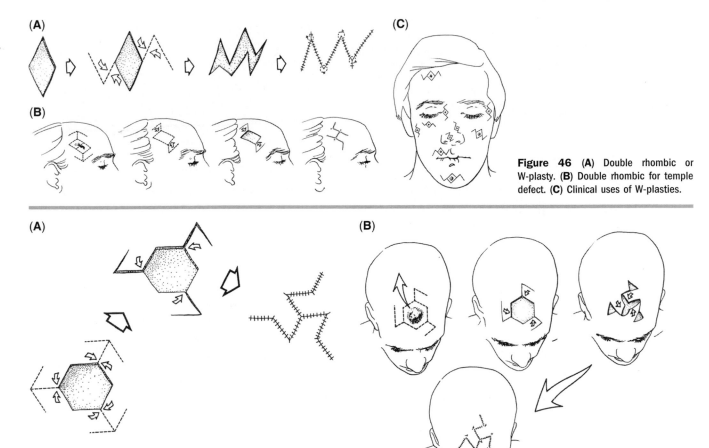

Figure 46 **(A)** Double rhombic or W-plasty. **(B)** Double rhombic for temple defect. **(C)** Clinical uses of W-plasties.

Figure 47 **(A)** Three rhombic flaps are used to close the hexagonal defect. **(B)** Scalp closure.

This flap utilizes excess tissue typically available from the nasolabial area. The pedicle of this flap can be based either superiorly or inferiorly. The vascular supply in this location is excellent.

The nasolabial flap is traditionally based in a superior fashion and extended down the nasolabial fold (Fig. 49). The secondary defect is primarily closed along the nasolabial fold. A narrow bridge of normal skin may separate the defect from the base of the flap. It is beneficial to excise this tissue and close it along with the original defect because this will help avoid the need for a second procedure later to revise the wound. Once the flap is mobilized, the distal end is trimmed to fit the defect. The wound is then sutured in place.

While color and texture match are good, the main disadvantage of this flap is that the skin of the ala is thicker than skin from the medial cheek. This may result in irregularities in the margins of the flap. There also may be some blunting of the nasofacial sulcus at the side of nose. If this blunting is.unacceptable and shows no tendency to resolve with time, a revision may be done after the vascular supply has been established from the surrounding skin. A deformity may occur with contraction around the distal end of the flap (Fig. 50). This deformity may resolve with time. Use of intralesional steroids (Fig. 51A and B) or correction with small Z-plasties (Fig. 51C) may help. When using this flap, remember not to transfer hair-bearing tissue onto the nose.

When the nasolabial flap is used to repair defects on the lip, it can be based either superiorly or inferiorly (Fig. 52). The greater the angle the flap turns, the

more likely is distortion of an inferiorly based flap. Nevertheless, this flap is useful for closure of defects in this area.

Labial-Ala Flap

Another transposition flap, the labial-ala flap, can also be used to repair small defects (lesser 1 cm) on the nasal ala. This superiorly based flap has an advantage over the traditional nasolabial flap as the donor tissue is developed inferior to the nasal rim and does not cross or otherwise distort the nasofacial sulcus. In addition, the healed incision scars are easily hidden under the nasal sill rather that being present in the more visible melolabial fold. Pin cushioning may occur as with any transposition flap, but this can be easily corrected using standard techniques.

Traditional Transposition Flaps

Another use of the transposition flaps is for the correction of defects of the lower eyelids. This is known as the Tripier flap and is constructed with excess tissue from the upper eyelid (Fig. 53). The flap is elevated with its pedicle based laterally. The defect on the lower lid is closed when the flap is transposed. The secondary defect is closed in a primary fashion. Often a small amount of orbicularis oculi muscle is transposed with the flap to ensure vascularity.

Glabellar Transposition Flap

This flap is used to repair defects (Fig. 54) of the nasal root and inner canthus. Tissue from the glabella is transposed approximately 90°. The secondary defect is closed primarily and the

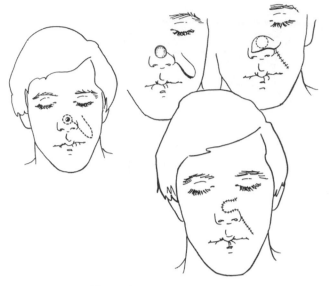

Figure 48   Nasolabial fold flap.

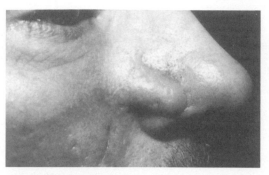

Figure 50   Six weeks postoperative—trapdoor deformity.

flap trimmed to fit the defect exactly. Glabellar skin is thicker than that of the nasal root or inner canthus so all subcutaneous fat must be removed to prevent bulging. Care must be taken to minimize transposition of hair-bearing tissue into this area.

Bilobed Flap

The bilobed flap, also known as a double rotation flap, is used when a defect is in thick or inelastic tissue but adjacent to relatively loose tissue. This flap permits tissue transfer 180° away from the donor area. The first lobe of the flap is constructed slightly smaller than the primary defect, and the second lobe is slightly smaller than the secondary defect (Fig. 55). This permits a gradual decrease in the donor defect; so tension on the adjacent tissue is spread between both lobes of the flap. The bilobed flap is used to

repair defects of the nose with tissue from the glabella (Fig. 56). Because these flaps are round, there is some potential for the development of a trapdoor deformity. Correction with Z-plasties or other modifications frequently leaves a good result but will require a delayed second procedure. Despite being useful for wounds with little adjacent donor skin, this flap is typically limited to inelastic areas on the face.

Hinged Turnover Flap

When a full thickness defect is produced on the alar rim, a special variant of the transposition flap, known as the hinged turnover flap, may be used for a one-stage reconstruction. Using this flap requires that the tissue superior to the defect be incised first and draped into the wound and then turned over onto itself to recreate the alar∗∗∗

Z-Plasty

The Z-plasty is another transposition flap used to lengthen scars, decrease tension, change direction, or reorient a preexisting scar (Fig. 57) to improve the cosmetic appearance.

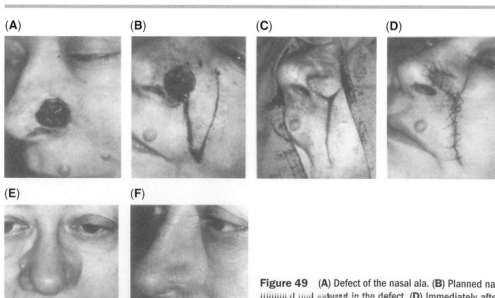

(A)   **(B)**   **(C)**   **(D)**

(E)   **(F)**

Figure 49   (**A**) Defect of the nasal ala. (**B**) Planned nasolabial transposition flap. (**C**) The flap is trimmed and sutured in the defect. (**D**) Immediately after surgery. (**E**) Frontal view demonstrating the blunting of the left nasofacial sulcus. (**F**) Three months following surgery the flap is thinner, conforming with the nasofacial sulcus.

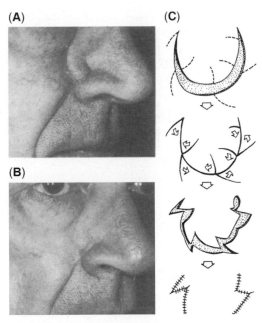

Figure 51 (**A**) Trapdoor defect after nasolabial flap repair for the alar defect. (**B**) Improvement six weeks after injection of intralesional steroids. (**C**) Correction of the trapdoor with multiple Z-plasties.

It is also used to prevent contraction of a straight line scar in a site of frequent motion.

The Z-plasty is usually designed at 60° angles with limbs of sufficient length to move tissue on either side of the central arm of the incision. The two flaps are transposed and sutured together in a new position. At 60° angles, this will result in a 75% increase in length. If more acute angles are utilized, the net increase in length will be less (Fig. 58). For practical purposes, angles greater than 60° are not used because the tension created would be unacceptable for flap closure.

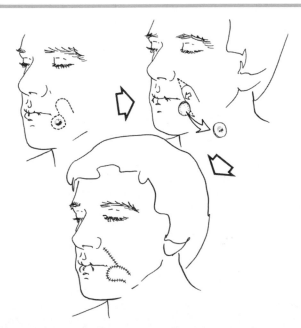

Figure 52 Inferiorly based nasolabial flap to repair defect on the lip.

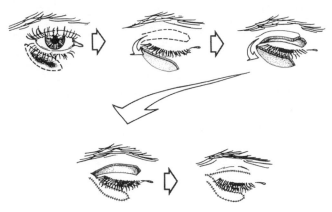

Figure 53 Tripier transposition flap for repair of a lower lid defect.

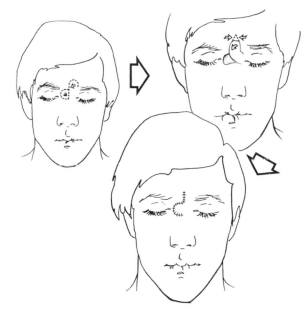

Figure 54 Glabellar transposition flap for defects of the nasal root and inner canthus.

Subcutaneous Island Pedicle Flap

The most elastic component of a skin flap is the subcutaneous tissue. The most inelastic component is the dermis. The subcutaneous pedicle flap or kite flap permits advancement of tissue from the ends of a fusiform excision without

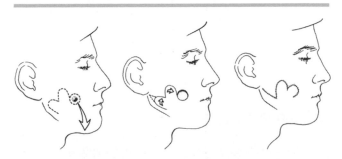

Figure 55 Bilobed flap for midcheek defect.

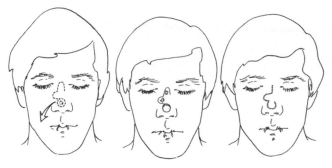

Figure 56 Bilobed flap repair on the nose.

(A)

(B)

(C)

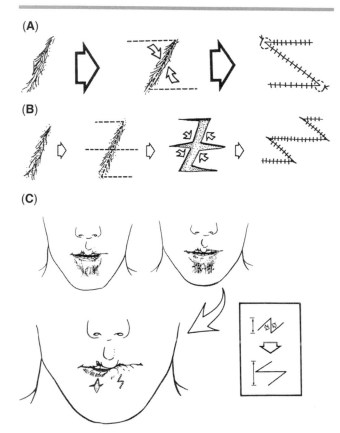

Figure 57 (**A**) Z-plasty changes the direction of a scar. (**B**) Z-plasty reorients a scar. (**C**) Z-plasty lengthens a scar to release a contracture.

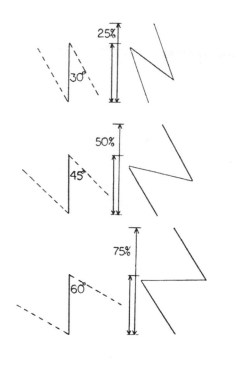

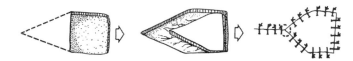

Figure 59 Single subcutaneous pedicle flap.

wasting normal tissue to close a wound and minimize tension. One or two island pedicle flaps may be advanced from the ends of an excision or from one end of a square defect (Figs. 59–61). Because the subcutaneous fat is left intact, there is sufficient vascular supply for the flap. The dermis is incised to the subcutaneous fat but is left attached. This permits skin to be shifted in the direction of the defect (Fig. 62). Sometimes, the defect must be made deeper to accommodate the advancing pedicle, otherwise the flap meets resistance when advanced or will bulge.

EVALUATING THE FLAP

Once a flap has been created, the vascular supply should be evaluated prior to final closure and application of the dressing. Typically, flaps should be either pink or slightly cyanotic. They tend to blanch slightly with light pressure and rapidly return to normal color. If the distal tip appears white, the flap should be released and an alternative closure considered.

Maximizing Flap Survival

To minimize interference with the circulation, close the flap with as few sutures as possible. The flap tissue should be handled with as much care as possible. Prior to suturing, complete hemostasis must be obtained. Hematoma formation will separate the flap from its base and predispose it to secondary infection. Secondary infection, although rare, may occur after flap surgery because at least some diminution of the normal vascular supply exists. As a consequence, a strict aseptic technique should be utilized during flap surgery, and any dead space created should be closed. Tension on the flap must be avoided because this also impairs circulation and decreases survival. The postoperative dressing should lightly compress and immobilize the wound to permit rapid healing. External pressure should not be excessive as this will further impair the circulation to the flap. Epidermal blistering is a sign of unpaired vascularity and occurs within several days after surgery.

Revising the Flap

All patients who undergo flap repair of a cutaneous wound or defect should be advised in advance that secondary procedures are often necessary to improve the result from the flap. This may be a debulking or defatting procedure,

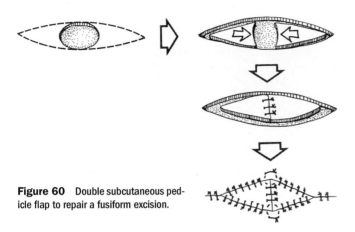

Figure 60 Double subcutaneous pedicle flap to repair a fusiform excision.

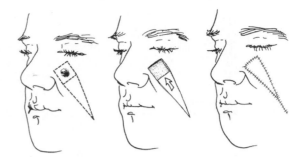

Figure 62 Large subcutaneous pedicle flap for medial cheek defect.

dog ear tricone repair at the point of pivot, dermabrasion of suture, lines, or possibly injection of collagen to build up a depressed wound.

ADVANTAGES OF RANDOM PATTERN FLAP SURGERY

The advantages of flap surgery include a better chance of survival compared to skin grafting. This, of course, is due to the uninterrupted blood supply of the flap. In addition, the aesthetic appearance is usually better than a graft because tissue of similar color, texture, and thickness is used. The functional result of flap surgery compared to skin graft surgery is substantially better as well, because flaps tend to show greater durability than grafts and generally undergo less scar contracture. Normal function of sweat glands and oil glands and hair growth function can be expected with flaps, especially if care is taken not to transect hair follicles. There may be a delay, however, of several months before normal sensation returns within flap tissue.

DISADVANTAGES OF RANDOM PATTERN FLAP SURGERY

One of the disadvantages of flap surgery is that while success rates are usually very high, failure can occur. If this happens, all of the adjacent donor skin is usually gone; so repeated procedures are difficult to perform. Flap failure often requires coverage of the defect with a skin graft. Flap surgery is more difficult to perform in children because

their skin is tight and does not lend itself well to stretching, and their scars tend to hypertrophy. Also, proper planning of a flap in a child may be difficult because natural creases and body lines may not have formed. Flap surgery may be associated with some anatomic distortion or asymmetry between sides of the face. Careful planning is the key to success.

COMPLICATIONS

Most complications with local random pattern flaps are due to an error in planning or execution of the flap. One main cause is poor design. When an incorrect method of closure is utilized, tension may result in necrosis. Flaps designed with insufficient length for closure may require a back cut that may impair the vascular supply, which will result in flap failure. A hematoma or seroma after flap surgery can disrupt vascular supply, predispose to infection (Fig. 63), and subsequently result in loss of the flap. The flap must be handled delicately since inadvertent injury to the vascular supply may result in necrosis.

Failure to use an inferiorly based flap, when possible, to improve venous return and limit lymphatic congestion can result in flap necrosis. This is a more common cause of flap failure than deficient arterial supply. Disruption of blood flow can result from seroma formation as well; if a seroma should develop beneath a flap, it should be evacuated as soon as possible. The trapdoor defect typically occurs with U- or V-shaped flaps. This is secondary to scar contracture around the distal end of the flap. Much of this deformity improves spontaneously in about six months. Intralesional steroids injected into the base of the wound may improve this. Alternatively, this flap can be incised and excess fibrotic material or subcutaneous tissue removed. If this is not satisfactory, a series of small Z-plasties can be performed (Fig. 51C).

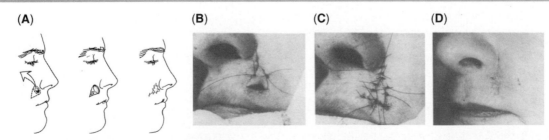

Figure 61 **(A)** Subcutaneous pedicle flap on the upper lip. **(B)** Subcutaneous pedicle flap mobilized from the nasofacial sulcus into the defect of the upper lip; primary closure of the superior portion has been performed. **(C)** Postoperatively, closure obtained without crossing the vermilion border. **(D)** One month postoperative no upward pull or distortion of the vermilion border.

(A)   (B)   (C)

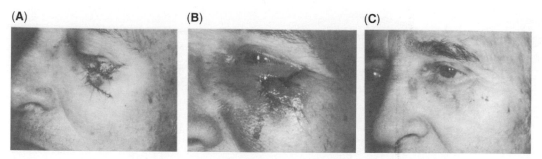

Figure 63   **(A)** Transposition flap immediately after repair. **(B)** Hematoma 48 hours postoperative and ecchymosis of the cheek. **(C)** Six weeks after evacuation of the hematoma.

Systemic Diseases and Flap Failure

Internal disease may also predispose to flap failure. Individuals with a bleeding diathesis or on anticoagulant medication are more likely to develop postoperative hematoma and associated complications. Diabetes, neoplasia, immunosuppressive therapy, and a variety of connective tissue diseases increase the risk of secondary infection and also result in slowed wound healing. Systemic or topical corticosteroid therapy may result in thinning of the skin such that poor wound healing or a flap failure may occur.

Infection

Infection is relatively uncommon with local random pattern flaps. Use of strict aseptic technique is important, however. Meticulous preparation with preoperative antiseptic scrubs, sterile instruments, and a sterile operating field are required. Prophylactic systemic antibiotics may be indicated if a large, complicated flap is performed. If infection should develop, appropriate measures include obtaining cultures and sensitivities to guide antibiotic therapy, draining any abscess formation, and debridement of necrotic tissue.

DRESSINGS

Immobilizing dressings that do not exert excess pressure to limit blood flow are beneficial. Instruction to the patient in proper postoperative care to minimize injury that might otherwise occur is also very important. Frequent follow-up visits are worthwhile.

BIBLIOGRAPHY

Asken S. A modified M-plasty. J Dermatol Surg Oncol 1986; 12:369–373.

Becker FF. Local tissue flaps in reconstructive facial plastic surgery. South Med J 1977; 70:677–680.

Becker FF. Rhomboid flap in facial reconstruction. Arch Otolaryngol 1979; 105:5 69–573.

Becker H. The rhomboid-to-W technique for excision of some skin lesions and closure. Plast Reconstr Surg 1979; 64:444–447.

Bennett RG. Local skin flaps on the cheeks. J Dermatol Surg Oncol 1991; 17:161–165.

Borges AF. The rhombic flap. Plast Reconstr Surg 1931; 67: 458–466.

Borges AF. Pitfalls in flap design. Ann Plast Surg 1982; 9: 201–209.

Borges AF. Relaxed skin tension lines (RSTL) versus other skin lines. Plast Reconstr Surg 1984; 73:144–150.

Bray DA, Eichel BS, Kaplan HJ. The dorsal nasal flap. Arch Otolaryngol 1981; 107:765–766.

Cameron RR, Latham WD, Dowling JA. Reconstructions of the nose and upper lip with nasolabial flaps. Plast Reconstr Surg 1973; 52:145–150.

Dzubow LM. Subcutaneous island pedicle flaps. J Dermatol Surg Oncol 1986; 12:591–596.

Dzubow LM, Zack L. The principle of cosmetic junctions as applied to reconstruction of defects following Mohs surgery. J Dermatol Surg Oncol 1990; 16:353–355.

Field LM. Design concepts for the nasolabial flap (letter). Plast Reconstr Surg 1983; 71:283–285.

Gormley DE. A brief analysis of the Burow's wedge/triangle principle. J Dermatol Surg Oncol 1985; 11: 121–123.

Hallock GG, Trevaskis AE. Refinements of the subcutaneous pedicle flap for closure of forehead and scalp defects. Plast Reconstr Surg 1985; 75:903–905.

Johnson TM, Baker S, Brown MD, Nelson BR. Utility of the subcutaneous hinge flap in nasal reconstruction. J Am Acad Dermatol 1994; 30:459–466.

Kara AE, Grande DJ. Check-neck advancement-rotation flaps following Mohs excision of skin malignancies. J Dermmol Surg Oncol 1986; 12:949–955.

Kolbusz RV, Goldberg LH. The labial-ala transposition flap. Arch Dermatol 1994; 130:162–164.

Koranda FC, Webster RC. Trapdoor effect in nasolabial flaps. Arch Otolaryngol 1985; 111:421–424.

Kraissl CJ. The selection of appropriate lines for elective surgical incisions. Plast Reconstr Surg 1951; 8:1–28.

Lee KK, Gorman AK, Swanson NA. Hinged turnover flap: A one-stage reconstruction of a full-thickness nasal ala defect. Dermatol Surg 2004; 30:479–400.

Mandy SH. The practical use of Z-ptasry. Dermatol Surg 1975; 1:57–60.

McGregor LA. Local skin flaps in facial reconstruction. Otolaryngol Clin North Am 1982; 15:77–98.

Mellette JR. Ear reconstruction with local flaps. J Dermatol Surg Oncol 1991; 17:176–182.

Monheit GD. The rhomboid transposition flap reevaluated. J Dermatol Surg Oncol 1980; 6:464–471.

Rubin LR. Langers lines and facial scars. Plast Reconstr Surg 1948; 3:147–155.

Salasche SJ, Grabski WJ. Complications of flaps. J Dermatol Surg Oncol 1991; 17:132–140.

Salasche SJ, Roberts LC. Dog-ear correction by M-plasty. J Dermatol Surg Oncol 1984; 10:478–482.

Sicgle RJ. Forehead reconstruction. J Dermatol Surg Oncol 1991; 17:200–204.

Simmonds WL. Reflections on dermatologic surgery and the management of perioral and labial lesions. J Dermatol Surg Oncol 1978; 4:383–389.

Spicer TE. Techniques of facial lesion excision and closure. J Dermatol Surg Oncol 1982; 8:551–556.

Stegman SJ. Fifteen ways to close surgical wounds. J Dermatol Surg 1975; 1:25–31.

Stegman SJ. Planning closure of a surgical wound. J Dermatol Surg Oncol 1978; 4:390–393.

Summers BK, Siegle RJ. Facial cutaneous reconstructive surgery: General aesthetic principles. J Am Acad Dermatol 1993; 29:669–681.

Summers BK, Siegle RJ. Facial cutaneous reconstructive surgery: Facial flaps. J Am Acad Dermatol 1993; 29:917–941.

Walkinshaw MD, Chaffee HH. The nasolabial flap: a problem and its correction. Plast Reconstr Surg 1982; 69:30–34.

Webster RC, Davidson TM, Smith RC. The thirty degree transposition flap. Laryngoscope 1978; 88:85–94.

Wheeland RG. Reconstruction of the lower Up and chin using local and random-pattern flaps. J Dermatol Surg Oncol 1991; 17:605–615.

Win GB, Sato SJ. Use of rotation flaps to repair small surgical defect on the ala nasi. J Dermatol Surg Oncol 1986; 12:154–158.

Yanai A, Nagata S, Okabe K. The Z in Z-plasty must have a long trunk. Br J Plast Surg 1986; 39:390–394.

Zimany A. The bi-loped flap. Plast Reconstr Surg 1952; 11:424–434.

Zitelli JA. The nasolabial flap as a single stage procedure. Arch Dermatol 1990; 126:1445–1448.

Zitelli JA. A regional approach to reconstruction of the upper lip. J Dermatol Surg Oncol 1991; 17:143–148.

Zitelli JA, Fazio MJ. Reconstruction of the nose with local flaps. J Dermatol Surg Oncol 1991; 17:184–189.

58

Scar Revision

Dana Wolfe, Wesley Low, and Terence M. Davidson
University of California, School of Medicine, San Diego, California, U.S.A.

PRINCIPLES OF WOUND HEALING AND SCAR FORMATION

A complete understanding of scar revision is possible only if one has a good grasp of the basic principles of wound healing and scar formation. Any wound that penetrates more deeply than the epidermis, whether inflicted by biologic, chemical, or physical injury, results in healing by scar formation. Initially an intense inflammatory reaction involves histamine, prostaglandins, complement, lymphokines, lipid peroxidases, the release of lysosomal enzymes, and numerous other cellular chemotactic substances. The cells that are attracted to the site of injury, particularly macrophages, produce substances that stimulate fibroblastic activity. The fibroblasts and epithelial cells then migrate along a scaffolding of fibrin strands constructed from coagulation and thrombus formation. Collagen is subsequently deposited in this matrix.

After extrusion from the fibroblasts and deposition in the matrix, collagen molecules aggregate into large fibrillar complexes by weak cohesive forces. Intra- and intermolecular covalent cross-links gradually form between reactive aldehyde groups, stabilizing the collagen complex and increasing the tensile strength of the matrix. The strength and integrity of the final repair are dependent upon this process.

After the initial period of wound healing, scar remodeling begins, a process that continues for years. As the collagen polymerizes, scar density increases. Wound contracture develops, usually weeks to months after the original injury, and may be disfiguring or disabling.

Several factors influence the remodeling process and affect the appearance of the final scar. Tension on a wound stimulates fibroblasts to secrete more collagenous proteins into the extracellular space, thereby increasing the scar size. If the noxious agent that originally produced the wound and induced the fibroproliferative inflammation is not absorbed or eliminated but remains as a source of chronic irritation, propagation of scar will result. Similarly, infection will prolong the inflammatory process, resulting in a less favorable scar. Hypoxia stimulates the synthesis and deposition of collagen, so poor oxygenation also impacts adversely on scar formation. Age and genetic factors also come into play.

It is becoming evident that cutaneous wound healing is a complex interaction of many cell types and growth factors. Wound healing has classically been divided into an inflammatory phase, a proliferation phase, and a remodeling phase. The growth factors have been shown to be intimately involved in each phase of wound healing. It has been learned that protein growth factors regulate processes crucial for normal wound healing. The healing wound contains protein growth factors and their levels change during wound healing. In experimental studies, wound healing has been impaired by inhibitors of growth factors. In experimental and clinical studies, chronic wounds have been shown to have low levels of growth factors, and treatment with growth factors has promoted healing of chronic wounds.

A growth factor is a polypeptide molecule that binds to a specific receptor to effect multiple intracellular processes. Growth factors have mitotic, morphogenic, and chemotactic effects. Binding to specific receptors causes changes in gene transcription and expression, protein synthesis, and protein modification. The effects of a growth factor depend on the cell types and the cell cycle stage. The major growth factor families include fibroblast growth factor (FGF), epidermal growth factor (EGF), transforming growth factor (TGF), platelet-derived growth factor (PDGD), nerve growth factor, and insulin-like growth factor (IGF).

Inflammatory Phase

Following cutaneous wounding, the first biologic response involves the clotting cascade, platelet aggregation, and degranulation. The platelets not only form the initial hemostatic platelet clot, but they also release peptide-regulating factors or "growth factors" that have a profound effect on healing. The platelets release TGF-α, TGF-β, EGF, and PDGD. Tissue injury initiates the clotting cascade to form thrombin. The thrombin causes fibrin formation, which stimulates platelet degranulation of α-particles, which contain growth factors PDGF, TGF-β, TGF-α, and FGF. These growth factors modulate cellular responses, cellular proliferation, and chemotaxis. In the early inflammatory phase neutrophils migrate into the wound to remove bacteria. In three to five days macrophages in the wound site release TGF-β, basic FGF (bFGF), and PDGF to facilitate the wound-healing process. The macrophages play a vital role in wound healing with their phagocytic properties and as sources of regulating growth factors. Patients who are neutropenic will be able to heal, but patients with macrophage dysfunction have great difficulty. It is believed that TGF-β plays a suppressor role in macrophage production of superoxides, and it also appears to regulate PDGF, TGF-α, EGF, and bFGF. The migration of epithelial cells from the wound edges begin within hours after injury, possibly under the chemotactic and mitogenetic effects of EGF and TGF-α.

Proliferative Phase

The proliferation phase lasts for several weeks and is characterized by increasing number of fibroblasts, endothelial cells, and keratinocytes. The fibroblasts secrete IGF-I, bFGF, TGF-β, and PDGF, all of which contribute to synthesis of extracellular matrix protein (i.e., collagen) and neovascularization. These growth factors also have different effects in transforming fibroblasts to myofibroblasts. FGF stimulates angiogenesis and neovascularization in the healing wound.

Remodeling Phase

Major restructuring of the extracellular matrix must be accomplished in the conversion of granulation tissue during scar formation and remodeling. TGF stimulates collagen production and proteinase inhibitors. It also enhances contraction of the collagen matrix.

Chronic Wounds

Fluid from healing wounds contains higher levels of growth factors than fluid from chronic wounds. Chronic wounds have been shown to have increased levels of protease activity (125 X), which can degrade growth factors. The molecular environment of chronic wounds may impair the ability of endogenous growth factors to stimulate healing. EGF and EGF receptors are degraded in chronic wounds.

CLINICAL APPLICATION

In a clinical trial, Brown reported that topical treatment of skin graft donor sites with EGF accelerated the rate of epithelial regeneration by an average of 1.5 days. The improved result in normal healing was small, but in impaired healing models, such as genetically diabetic mice, treatment with PDGF or bFGF significantly decreased the time to wound closure and increased the number of fibroblasts and capillaries in the wound bed. Increased wound healing was noted in clinical trials of chronic wounds and pressure ulcers treated with EGF and PDGF. EGF has been shown to have beneficial effects on corneal wound healing. EGF has mitotic effects on corneal endothelial cells, which may have promising prospects for corneal healing. In animal models, EGF has been shown to improve tympanic perforation healing.

Peptide growth factors clearly play a major role in wound healing. In the future, we anticipate improving impaired wound healing with growth factor application and may even be able to modulate normal wound healing.

GENERAL TECHNICAL CONSIDERATIONS

Probably the most important physician-controlled factor in obtaining good wound closure is correct subcutaneous stitch placement. Properly performed, the following objectives will be achieved:

1. Elimination of deadspace. This will prevent hematoma formation and minimize wound infection.
2. Proper alignment of skin edges. This facilitates an accurate skin closure, providing the best opportunity for an aesthetically acceptable scar.
3. Elimination of wound edge tension. Wounds heal with less scarring when tension is minimal. In addition, much finer suture material may be used, resulting in less wound edge trauma and scar formation, when its only role is the precise alignment of the epidermal margins when the margins are already approximated. Skin suture removal may be safely performed sooner after surgery (ideally after three to four days), minimizing epithelial ingrowth and permanent suture marks.

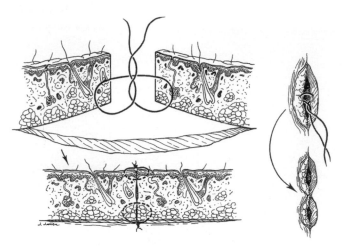

Figure 1   Classic subcutaneous stitch placement. *Source*: From Davidson (1978).

4. Promotion of skin edge eversion. Mild eversion of the epidermal wound edges enhances optimal healing.

Traditionally, subcutaneous suture placement incorporates a small bite of dermis in a loop of fine absorbable suture (such as 5–0 Vicryl), repeated many times along the wound edge. An alternative and preferable technique requires that the wound edges be undermined for about 1 cm, followed by eversion of the edges and placement of the subcutaneous suture 8 to 10 mm back on each side. Because it is placed back from the wound edge, each stitch exerts its influence over a greater distance. Therefore, with this method fewer stitches are required, the local blood supply at the wound edge is less likely to be compromised, and a greater degree of eversion is obtained. All these factors contribute to more favorable wound healing. Figures 1 and 2 illustrate the difference between these two techniques for subcutaneous stitch placement.

The epidermal closure can be performed with permanent sutures (i.e., 5–0 or 6–0 nylon or Prolene) or with rapidly absorbing 6–0 chromic sutures. Running simple and running subcuticular stitches are probably most frequently used for cosmetic closures, and results are excellent for both if used properly. Interrupted stitches can also be used but

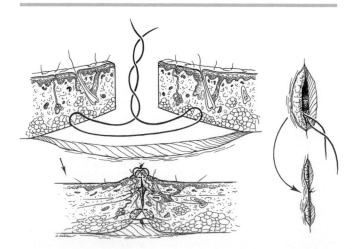

Figure 2   Modified subcutaneous stitch placement demonstrating the additional eversion produced. *Source*: From Davidson (1978).

take longer to place and are more difficult to remove. Whatever technique is employed, small superficial bites should be taken, including only 25% to 50% of the total skin thickness, except where the skin is very thin, in which case deeper bites are used. Sutures should be snug, but not tight, to prevent tissue strangulation. Throughout wound closure, the tissues must be handled as gently and as infrequently as possible to avoid unnecessary tissue trauma.

After closure is complete, a wound dressing should be applied. Semiocclusive dressings are advised for several reasons. First, they maintain a moist, warm environment at the wound surface, thus preventing superficial dehydration and tissue loss. They also allow gas exchange to occur, while providing a physical barrier against microbial ingress. In addition, the use of semiocclusive dressings appears to reduce the inflammatory infiltrate in healing wounds, presumably due to a diminution of inflammation-inciting necrotic elements, thereby keeping fibroblast proliferation and fibrogenesis to a minimum.

PLACEMENT AND ORIENTATION OF INCISIONS

Before proceeding with a description of specific scar revision techniques, mention should be made of the basic principles of incision placement and orientation for optimum scar appearance and healing. In general, there are four favorable sites for incision placement:

1. Inside an orifice such as the nose, mouth, or ear
2. In hair-bearing skin
3. At the junction of two aesthetic areas
4. In or paralleling favorable skin tension lines (FSTL)

The first two sites, although quite desirable, are rarely useful in scar revision unless a scar can gradually be moved from an unfavorable site into an orifice or the hairline (i.e., by serial excision). It is also sometimes possible to move a scar into the junction of one aesthetic area with another, such as the junction of the forehead with the nose, the forehead with the temple, the temple with the cheek, the temple and cheek with the eyelid, the cheek with the nose, the cheek with the lip, the cheek with the chin, and the chin with the lip. Even though they are out in the open, such incisions are difficult to discern—much more so than scars that are only one or two millimeters away from the exact boundary or junction between the two areas. Figure 3 illustrates the main aesthetic areas of the human face.

If unable to place an incision into one of these areas, it should be kept in or parallel to the FSTL. These lines are easy to find in older patients, for they correspond to the natural creases and wrinkles. In younger patients who have not yet developed wrinkles, one must predict where they will eventually form by having them frown, squinch their nose, smile, squint, etc. In areas other than the face one may discern the FSTL by pinching the skin and observing the ease and size of the furrows and ridges thus formed. Figure 4 demonstrates typical FSTL of the human face, exhibited as wrinkles produced by aging as depicted in Figure 3.

These FSTL are generally parallel to the directional orientation of dermal collagen, which tends to grow in a plane perpendicular to the underlying muscle pull. Since the collagen that forms in scars basically parallels the long axis of the incision, incisions placed perpendicular to the underlying muscle pull (parallel to the FSTL) will heal with collagen fibers parallel to the predominant orientation of the dermal collagen, resulting in a scar that is merely an

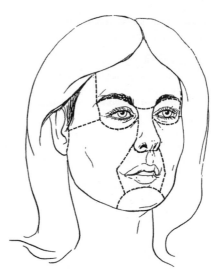

Figure 3 The major aesthetic areas of the human face.

accentuation of the normal pattern. Incisions placed parallel to the underlying muscle pull (perpendicular to the FSTL) will heal with collagen fibers disrupting the directional orientation of the normal dermal collagen, resulting in a more obvious scar that is prone to distort normal anatomy and function.

CASE SELECTION
Physical Characteristics

Any scar that is 2 cm or more in length or wider than 1 to 2 mm may be improved with scar revision. Other unfavorable scar characteristics prompting revision include disturbance of function, a nonparallel orientation to the FSTL, significant degrees of widening, depression, elevation, or poor color match with surrounding tissues, and scar hypertrophy or frank keloid formation. However, remember that these are generalities and not absolute indications; some very long, mature scars that parallel the FSTL or lie in the junction of two aesthetic areas are truly inconspicuous and cosmetically

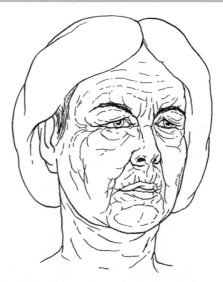

Figure 4 Wrinkles produced by aging of the human face depicted in Figure 3. Such wrinkles tend to parallel favorable skin tension lines.

quite acceptable—they need not be revised on the basis of length alone.

Timing Considerations

Since scars usually take at least six months to one year to mature, they should usually not be revised prior to this time, in spite of the patient's insistence. Because of the ongoing maturation process, scars that might require surgery at three months may heal quite satisfactorily if given more time.

As some scars require multiple revision procedures spread out over several years, it is sometimes acceptable to operate sooner when it is clear that a revision will be necessary. Such scars may be operated on as soon as the patient is psychologically ready and after the acute inflammation of the original injury has subsided—generally at least 6 to 12 weeks posttrauma.

Psychological Factors

In our culture, scars, particularly facial scars, are considered unattractive. Because of this, patients are often not happy with whomever they perceive as being responsible for their scar, whether it was inflicted in a fight, in an accident, or in surgery. The anger and self-pity such patients feel will not be resolved until (1) the event is completely erased and their skin is returned to its original state or (2) they resolve their anger and come to some realistic acceptance of their disfigurement. Since the first option is clearly impossible, every effort must be made to help these patients understand their anger so that they can accept their deformity. It is only then that they can think clearly about realistic improvement goals. As long as they are still angry, there is a significant risk that their anger will be redirected toward their current surgeon, even after a successful scar revision, as it is unlikely that they will be pleased with anything less than a perfect result.

In addition to the angry patient, the surgeon must also avoid patients who expect surgery to solve other emotional or social problems. For example, patients with underlying psychiatric disease who blame their deformity for their psychological difficulties are not good candidates for surgery. Similarly patients who are soon to be married, or patients who are involved in litigation related to their scar, are poor surgical candidates.

SIMPLE FUSIFORM EXCISION

Simple excision is the most basic scar-revision technique, but it is rarely the procedure of choice. It is sometimes useful for small, round, elliptical, or stellate scars that lie within a hairline or at the junction of two aesthetic areas or that parallel the FSTL. The scar is simply excised in a fusiform manner, and the wound edges undermined and closed. The fusiform and resultant closure need not be perfectly straight—they can be curved as necessary to better conform with the local FSTL. Figures 5 and 6 demonstrate two ways in which simple fusiform excisions can be used to revise relatively short scars.

Serial Excision

Serial excision is a powerful tool for scar revision and is based on the tremendous ability of the skin to stretch with time. One use of this technique is the removal of lesions with a larger surface area (such as burn scars, skin grafts, large hairy nevi, etc.) by serially excising them in several operations. An incision is made near one edge of the lesion, a portion of the lesion excised, and the wound edges undermined and then closed under moderate tension. After 6 to 12 weeks, the skin will stretch sufficiently to allow repetition of the procedure. All incisions and closures must be made within the lesion until the last operation, when normal, healthy tissue is approximated on both sides.

Serial excision can also be employed to move scars into more favorable locations (such as into a hairline, into the junction of two aesthetic areas, or to a less visible site). In the first operation the scar is excised along with enough normal adjacent tissue (on the side toward which the scar is to be moved) so the wound can be closed under a moderate amount of tension. A narrow "cuff" of scar tissue should be preserved along the edge of the normal tissue that is being advanced (so you do not suture normal skin). In 6 to 12 weeks the skin will stretch enough to allow the procedure to be repeated. This is continued until the scar is brought into its final position. At this point the cuff of scar tissue along the advancing margin is finally excised and healthy skin approximated.

TISSUE EXPANDERS

Tissue expansion is a new surgical concept that involves the implantation of one or several inflatable silicone bags in the subcutaneous plane. A small dome connected by tubing is buried in the same plane and is injected with saline on a weekly basis, progressively stretching the overlying skin. Once sufficient excess skin has been obtained in this manner, the expander is removed and the lesion excised. The stretched skin (along with the underlying "capsule" that

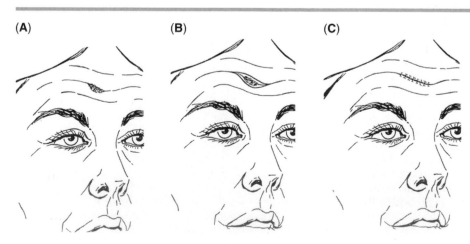

(A)   **(B)**   **(C)**

Figure 5 Simple fusiform excision demonstrating how the directional orientation of both ends of the excision can be modified so that the final scar will lie completely within a prominent skin crease.

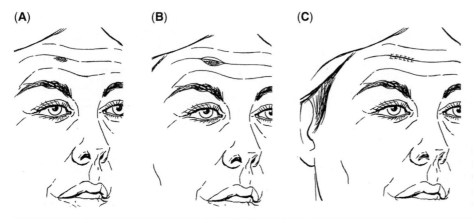

(A) **(B)** **(C)**

Figure 6 Simple fusiform excision demonstrating how equal amounts of skin can be excised from either side of a prominent skin crease producing a final scar that lies completely within that crease.

has formed around the expander) is advanced in a single stage to close the defect.

Expanders are therefore potentially useful for some of the same lesions as serial excision and may decrease the number of procedures required. However, careful preoperative planning is necessary, and the expander must be properly placed at the initial operation. There is also some risk of infection and extrusion. A separate incision is often required for placement of the expander, and the incision must be away from the area to be expanded. It is recommended that the placement incision be in nonscarred skin to minimize the risk of exposure and extrusion.

M-PLASTY

One problem that arises when excising broad scars is how to keep the resultant scar length to a minimum. In order to prevent protrusions or dog ears at either end, the lines of excision must be gradually tapered together so that they meet at an angle not exceeding 30°. In some cases this may result in an unacceptably long, straight scar and require excision by a large amount of normal skin.

By using an M-plasty, two small side-by-side 30° triangles of normal skin are excised, thereby reducing the total amount of skin to be removed and minimizing tissue protrusion. If the triangle of tissue in the middle of the M is then advanced centrally in a "Y-to-V" maneuver, the total central axis incisional length is further reduced. In addition, advancing these triangles centrally results in less overall tissue distortion with wound closure, since skin is being borrowed from both the longitudinal plane and the transverse plane (with respect to the central incision) (Fig. 7).

In addition to keeping incisions shorter while preventing tissue protrusions and distortions, M-plasties also camouflage. This concept is based on the ability of the eye to quickly perceive a straight line when even a portion of it is seen. If the line is broken into a series of short segments oriented in different directions, it is much more difficult for the eye to follow, even if the total length is now longer. This concept is the basis for more sophisticated scar-revision techniques.

Z-PLASTY

Z-plasty was one of the original techniques used for scar revision and is still the technique of choice for lengthening scars and altering their direction. It is ideal when used for linear scars that cross the junction of two aesthetic areas or are perpendicular to important FSTL, especially when

the natural tissues are concave or convex, since this results in contracture formation and webbing or creasing.

A Z-plasty is basically two transposition flaps transposed over one another. In so doing, tissue is borrowed from an area of excess and transposed into an area of deficiency. The orientation of the scar is redirected by about 90°. First the scar is excised. This becomes the central limb of the Z. Two separate incisions are then made, beginning at each end of the central limb, which parallel each other at identical angles with the central limb. These incisions are called the lateral limbs, and the angles they make with the central limb define the Z-plasty (i.e., 60° Z-plasty, 30° Z-plasty, etc.)

The triangular flaps and the surrounding tissues are undermined and the flaps transposed. The additional length obtained is a function of the angle of the Z-plasty; the greater the angle, the greater the lengthening, but also the greater the amount of tissue distortion and protrusion. For this reason, surgeons rarely use Z-plasties of more than 60°.

Figure 8 illustrates the basic concept of Z-plasty. In planning and designing Z-plasties, one must pay careful

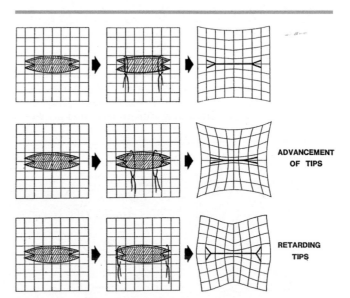

ADVANCEMENT
OF TIPS

RETARDING
TIPS

Figure 7 A fusiform wound closed with M-plasties at each end. Note that advancement of the M-plasty tips reduces tissue distortion in the vertical axis at the expense of additional distortion in the horizontal plane. When the tips are retarded the tissues become bunched at either end of the wound, and as more tissue must be borrowed from the vertical axis for closure, distortion is maximized in this direction.

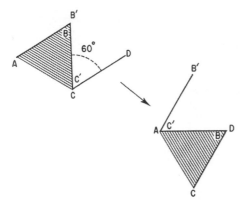

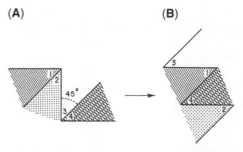

Figure 8 Simple 60° Z-plasty. Note that the orientation of the central incision is changed by 90° and that the orientation of the lateral limb incisions remains the same.

Figure 10 Compound Z-plasty. Two 45° lateral limb incisions are created at either end of the central axis, and when the triangular tissue flaps are transposed, a zig-zag scar results.

attention to the lateral limb orientation, since the final scar orientation will be the same. As there are four different possible designs for the lateral limbs of any given Z-plasty, the one in which the lateral limbs most closely parallel the FSTL should be chosen. Figure 9 illustrates this point, showing both a correct and an incorrect choice of lateral limb placement.

Compound Z-Plasty

Sometimes more lengthening is necessary than can be obtained with a simple Z-plasty. The compound Z-plasty is done to avoid transposing very large flaps, resulting in long scars and substantial tissue distortion and protrusion. Several lateral limbs can be created, forming a number of triangular flaps, which can then be transposed. Four- and even six-flap Z-plasties can be interdigitated in this manner, resulting in a "zig-zag" type of scar (Fig. 10).

While not ideal for facial surgery, such compound Z-plasties can be useful in other areas of the body where significant lengthening is needed and appearance is less important. The tissue compressions and protrusions created by this method generally flatten with time.

Serial Z-Plasty

An alternative to the compound Z-plasty for lengthening markedly contracted scars is the serial Z-plasty. First, two simple Z-plasty lateral limb incisions are made. Then several more incisions are made on either side of the central limb, parallel to the lateral limb incisions at the ends. Again, a zig-zag type of scar results after transposing the flaps (Fig. 11).

In addition to increasing the length along the long axis of an unfavorably oriented scar (while simultaneously changing the direction of that scar), this Z-plasty technique also camouflages long, straight scars by breaking them into several shorter segments. However, it does so at the expense of multiple incisions and possible tissue protrusion and distortion. For this reason, other techniques have been devised for revising scars by breaking them into smaller pieces without lengthening or distorting surrounding tissues.

RUNNING W-PLASTY

The rationale for running W-plasty scar revision is the concept of scar camouflaging by breaking the scar into short segments connected by acute angles. The scar is excised with a minimum of normal tissue, and a series of small side-by-side triangular flaps or serrations are cut into each wound edge. After undermining, the edges are advanced together with several deep, interrupted subcutaneous stitches placed at least 5 mm back from the edges. The triangular tips on one side are then interdigitated with the triangular notches on the opposing side. The skin closure is most expeditiously performed using rapidly absorbable 6–0 chromic suture as a running, locked stitch. First, all flap tips on one side are

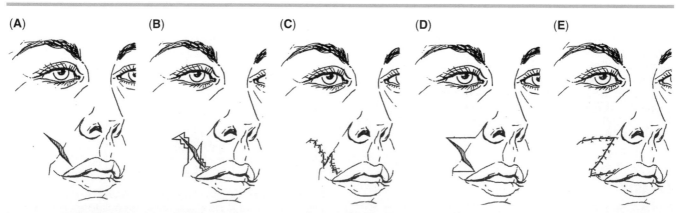

Figure 9 **(A)** Theoretical facial scar crossing an aesthetic border. **(B and C)** Appropriate way to deal with the scar using a running W-plasty. A Z-plasty is utilized at the site where the scar crosses the aesthetic border in order to change its directional orientation to conform to that of the border itself. **(D and E)** Incorrect way to deal with this scar. Although the central axis of the scar is changed to correspond to the direction of the aesthetic border, the lateral limb incisions are unacceptably long and do not parallel the favorable skin tension lines.

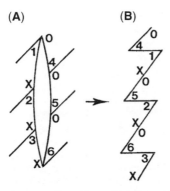

(A) **(B)**

Figure 11 Serial Z-plasty. Note that multiple lateral limb incisions are created along the length of the central axis, and again a zigzag scar is produced when the resultant tissue flaps are transposed as shown.

GEOMETRIC BROKEN LINE

This technique is a natural progression of the running W-plasty that, instead of a series of nearly identical triangular flaps, consists of a random pattern of constantly changing flaps, all variable in shape and size. It has the advantage of avoiding an easily recognized pattern. Once the eye has followed two or three zig-zags, the remainder of the scar can be easily detected and more readily perceived.

As with the running W-plasty, no segment should exceed 5 mm in length and all should parallel FSTL whenever possible. It is important that rectangular and square flaps be identical in size and shape to their respective recipient sites, so triangular flaps are superior along curved segments of scar.

The scar is excised and the flaps cut as a single step using a #11 blade. The edges are undermined, and wound closure is performed in the same manner as for running W-plasty.

The geometric broken-line technique can be used for straight, curved, short, or very long scars and is an effective camouflaging method. The surgery requires precise planning and accurate flap design to ensure an even mesh of the two wound edges when the flaps are interdigitated. This planning is best done prior to anesthetic injections, which distort and blanch the tissues.

Figures 15 and 16 show two examples of geometric broken-line revisions. The actual techniques are superbly demonstrated on the videotapes *The San Diego Classics in Soft Tissue Surgery*.

sutured into position, then, crossing over, all the flap tips on the other side are similarly stitched into place. The result is an aesthetically favorable, zig-zag type scar. If desired, M-plasties can be used on the ends of these closures to minimize their length.

Properly done, no line should exceed 5 mm in length and no angle should exceed 90°. The eye tends to lose this type of scar at each corner as it goes off into healthy, non-scarred skin. As long as the angles are acute, the eye does not readily follow from one broken segment to the next. The camouflage thus produced results in a less visible scar despite an increase in the actual scar length.

This technique may be used for excision of thin scars, wide scars, or curved scars. Two important technical points are:

1. Keep as many of the short segments as possible parallel to the FSTL.
2. When cutting the flaps on a curved scar, make the flaps on the outside of the curve broader based and less acutely angled in order to keep the number of flaps on each side equal.

The resultant disparity between flap size and their corresponding notches will become insignificant as the skin stretches and contracts during healing. If more flaps are accidently created on one side of the excision than on the other, one of the flaps on the deficient side is simply bisected, creating one additional flap and one additional notch, and the size disparity will dissipate with time (Figs. 12–14).

KELOIDS AND HYPERTROPHIC SCARS

These scars are caused by an imbalance between collagen deposition and degradation and probably represent different points along a continuum of excessive scar formation. Hypertrophic scars are thick and raised but generally remain within the boundaries of the original wound and often regress with time. Keloids extend beyond the boundaries of the original wound, invade surrounding tissues, and often recur after surgical removal.

Both are characterized histologically by an overabundant deposition of dermal collagen and biochemically by extremely high levels of proline hydroxylase activity and an increase in collagenase inhibitors. They are more likely to occur in younger patients and from wounds in thick skin, closed under tension. Keloids are more prevalent in the darker-skinned races, particularly in blacks.

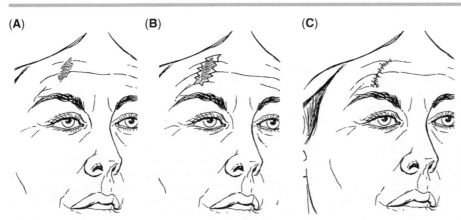

(A) **(B)** **(C)**

Figure 12 Running W-plasty. Note that a small M-plasty was utilized for closure at the inferior end of the wound.

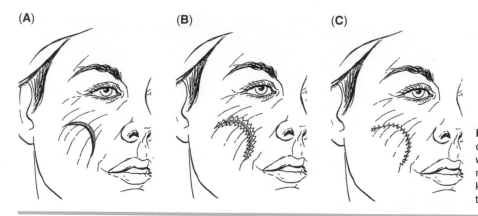

Figure 13 Running W-plasty. Note how the directional orientation and size of the triangles were altered in order to maintain an identical number of triangles on either side, and also to keep all incisions as parallel to the favorable skin tension lines as possible.

Because of their tendency to recur, treatment of keloids is problematic. A wide range of treatment modalities have been advocated and several novel approaches are now being investigated, but at present it is unlikely that single modality treatment will render satisfactory results—combination therapy is generally more effective. In addition, a long period of frequent observation is mandatory, probably for at least two years following treatment, with additional intervention at the first sign of recurrence.

Surgical Excision

Many surgeons are reluctant to excise keloids because of a recurrence rate of about 55% following surgery alone. However, if certain general principles are adhered to and adjunctive modalities employed, results can be quite satisfactory. These general principles include sharp, minimally traumatic dissection technique, wound closure under minimal or no tension and good wound edge eversion, and use of nonabsorbable sutures which are removed as soon as possible after surgery. The use of tension-reducing measures, such as Z-plasty, or of camouflaging techniques is to be avoided, as they are likely to cause extension of the keloid. If necessary, it is acceptable to "core out" keloids and save part of the overlying skin if the wound cannot otherwise be closed without tension.

Corticosteroids

Intralesional corticosteroids can be used alone or in combination with surgery or other techniques, both to shrink and to prevent the recurrence of keloids. Corticosteroids are felt to work both by decreasing collagen synthesis and by increasing collagen degradation by decreasing the level of collagenase inhibitors.

Triamcinolone (Kenalog) is the most commonly used drug for this purpose, and it can be administered either with a needle and syringe or with a Dermajet. For many small keloids and most hypertrophic scars, a few Dermajet treatments repeated at two-week intervals is all that is required. For some larger keloids, serial injections with a needle and syringe are necessary to deliver a sufficient steroid volume. In some cases up to 20 or 30 injections may be necessary to resolve the keloid. Often one is left with a large pouch of wrinkled, redundant skin, which can then be excised.

When used as an adjunct to surgery, presurgical intralesional injections should be performed about a month preoperatively with close follow-up after surgery. Injections should be continued at two-week intervals at the first sign of recurrence. The maximum monthly dose of injected Kenalog is 120 mg for adults, 80 mg for children 6 to 10 years of age, and 40 mg for children one to five years of age. It is important that injections be made directly into the scar or keloid itself and not into the surrounding skin. Excessive use of steroids can result in thinning, atrophy, telangiectasias, and depigmentation and must be avoided. At the first signs of local steroid toxicity, further injections must be withheld.

Pressure Devices

The use of pressure devices and garments is another method for preventing the development of hypertrophic scar and keloid. There are several theories on-mechanisms responsible for the effect of pressure on maturing scars, but as yet it has not been fully elucidated.

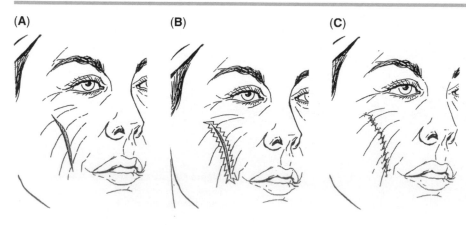

Figure 14 Running W-plasty. This again demonstrates how the orientation of the triangles is altered along the length of the scar to maintain a parallel orientation of the triangular incisions to the favorable skin tension lines. An M-plasty is used to facilitate closure at the inferior end of the wound.

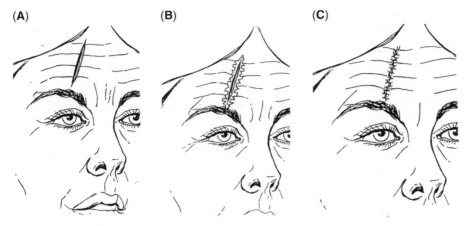

Figure 15 Geometric broken-line closure.

Custom-tailored nylon compression garments have been used to prevent the development of excessive scarring and contracture in burn patients. Polyurethane sponges, foam splints, and polymethylmethacrylate molded splints have also been used to prevent keloid recurrence after treatment. These devices particularly lend themselves to use on the ear lobes following keloid excision but must remain in continuous use for at least 18 months to 2 years following surgery.

Radiation Therapy

Administration of external beam radiation therapy is the perioperative and postoperative period, up to a total dose of 1500 to 2000 rads, has been advocated to prevent postsurgical keloid recurrence. Its efficacy is probably due to the inhibitory effect on both fibroplasia and endothelial vascular budding.

Extreme caution must be exercised when giving radiation to keloids. There is a small but definite risk of developing cutaneous, thyroid, and other malignancies following its use. Some clinicians feel that it is never indicated for the treatment of benign conditions such as keloids. It probably never should be used in children or for abdominal or pelvic lesions in women of childbearing age.

Cryotherapy

Although cryotherapy is not an accepted first-line treatment for keloids, some provocative case reports have recorded impressive results with cryotherapy. However, others have reported poor results using this technique. In addition, cryotherapy is very prone to cause depigmentation due to the melanocytes' sensitivity to cold. At present it appears that cryotherapy may be a useful procedure in situations where other available modalities are contraindicated or ineffective, with great caution taken in non-Caucasian patients because of possible depigmentation.

Laser Surgery

Use of the CO_2 laser to excise keloids, alone or followed by intralesional corticosteroid injections, has produced good results in several preliminary studies and deserves further evaluation as a treatment for keloids. Theoretical advantages include sterilization, sealing of blood vessels up to 0.5 mm as it cuts, minimal necrosis of surrounding tissues, and sealing of nerve endings. The Nd:YAG laser may also prove to be useful in this regard.

Medical Therapy

Several medications, applied topically, orally, or injected locally, have been investigated and hold varying degrees of promise as either adjunctive or first-line models of therapy for keloids. These include oral tetrahydroquinone, oral asiatic acid (Medecassol), topical 0.05% fetinoid acid solution, topical ZnO_2, oral β-amino propionitrile fumarate (BAPN) or penicillamine combined with colchicine, and antineoplastic agents such as nitrogen mustard, thio-TEPA, and methotrexate. Obviously, there is considerable potential for side effects and long-term toxicity with several of these

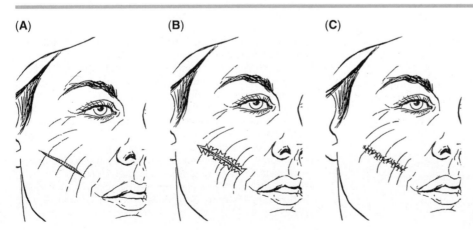

Figure 16 Geometric broken-line closure.

agents, and these issues must be addressed and clarified before such agents can be used routinely in keloid therapy.

DERMABRASION

Even after a well-performed scar revision there are frequently minor irregularities which detract from an ideal result. Examples include fine scars which are not quite flush with the surrounding skin and the presence of subtle differences in texture and color from scar to healthy skin. In these situations, further improvement may be obtained by one, two, or occasionally more dermabrasions. Dermabrasion works to level out contour irregularities by bringing the level of healthy adjacent tissue down to the level of the scar. This also reduces color mismatch.

Before considering the use of dermabrasion, one must be certain that full maturation of the scar has occurred. This means a wait of at least six months, and often one to two years, following the last scar revision. However, some have gotten nice results with dermabrasion as early as six weeks postoperatively. Depressed scars, mild-to-moderate acne pitting, and fine wrinkles are all indications for dermabrasion. Raised, hypertrophic scars and otherwise normal but elevated scars are not appropriate for dermabrasion. Hypertrophic scars only proliferate more actively if abraded. Since dermabrasion is only good for lowering the height of normal tissue down to the level of a scar and not vice versa, treatment of elevated scars will only produce excessive thinning of the already very thin dermal and epidermal layers, with very little chance for satisfactory improvement.

Dermabrasion is the mechanical removal of the epidermis and some, but not all, of the dermis, leaving the skin appendages and the depths of the rete pegs intact. New epidermal cells then migrate across the exposed dermis within three to seven days. A progressive thickening of the dermis and epidermis occurs over the next several months, but the original thickness is never attained—thus the effect of the dermabrasion is maintained. Areas of thick skin that are rich in skin appendages are therefore most amenable to dermabrading.

Before starting, the deepest portions of the scar are marked with ink or dye. After anesthesia (local or general) and freezing (with Freon, to provide a firm surface against which to work and to facilitate consistency in depth of abrasion), the skin is dermabraded down to the level of the inked marks, until the inked scar is just removed. At the edges, the level of planing is made progressively more superficial and careful feathering is performed peripherally to ensure a smooth transition to normal skin. Hemostasis is obtained with pressure (never cautery), a semiocclusive dressing is applied, and at 7 to 10 days the eschar will fall off and the skin can be washed.

BIBLIOGRAPHY

Amoils CP, Jackler RK, Lustig LR. Repair of chronic tympanic membrane perforations using epidermal growth factors. Otolaryngol Head Neck Surg 1992; 107(5):669–683.

Bennett NT, Schultz GS. Growth factors and wound healing: biochemical properties of growth factors and their receptors. Am J Surg 1993; 165:728–737.

Bennett NT, Schultz GS. Growth factors and wound healing: part II. Role in normal and chronic wound healing. Am J Surg 1993; 166:74–81.

Boucek RJ. Factors affecting wound healing. Otolaryngol Clin North Am 1984; 17:243–264.

Brown GL, Curtsinger LJ, Jurkiewicz M, et al. Stimulation of healing of chronic wounds by epidermal growth factor. Plast Reconstr Surg 1991; 88(2):189–194.

Brown GL, Curtsinger LJ, White M, et al. Acceleration of tensile strength of incisions treated with EGF and TGF-α. Ann Surg 1988; 208(6):788–794.

Brown GL, Nanney LB, Griffen J, et al. Enhancement of wound healing by topical treatment with epidermal growth factor. N Engl J Med 1989; 321:76–79.

Brown LA, Pierce HE. Keloids: scar revision. J Dermatol Surg Oncol 1986; 12:51–56.

Carr-Collins JA. Pressure techniques for the Prevention of hypertrophic scar. Clin Plast Surg 1992; 19(3):733–743.

Carrico TJ, Mehrhof AI Jr, Cohen IK. Biology of wound healing. Surg Clin North Am 1984; 64:721–733.

Chvapil M, Koopmann CF. Scar formation: physiology and pathological states. Otolaryngol Clin North Am 1984; 17: 265–272.

Davidson TM. Lacerations and scar revisions. In: Cummings CW et al., eds. Otolaryngology—Head and Neck Surgery. St. Louis: C.V. Mosby Co., 1986:289–311.

Davidson TM, Webster RC, Gordon BR. The principles and dynamics of local skin flaps. A self-instructional package from the Committee on Continuing Education in Otolaryngology (SIPAC). Am Acad Otolaryngol 1979; 1–93.

Davidson TM, Webster RC. Scar revision. A self-instructional package from the Committee on Continuing Education in Otolaryngology (SIPAC). Am Acad Ophthal Otolaryngol 1977; 1–97.

Davidson TM. Subcutaneous suture placement. Laryngoscope 1987; 97:501–504.

Davies DM. Scars, hypertrophic scars, and keloids. Br Med J 1985; 290:1056–1058.

Fina M, Baird A, Ryan A. Direct application of basic fibroblast growth factor improves tympanic membrane perforation healing. Laryngoscopy 1993; 103(7):804–809.

Ketchum LD, Smith J, Robinson DW, et al. Treatment of hypertrophic scar keloid and scar contracture by triamcinolone acetonide. Plast Reconstr Surg 1966; 38:209.

Kischer CW. The microvessels in hypertrophic scars, keloids and related lesions: a review. J Submicrosc Cytol Pathol 1992; 24(2):281–296.

Mcgee G, Davidson J, Buckley A, et al. Recombinant basic fibroblast growth factor accelerates wound healing. J Surg Res 1998; 45:145–153.

Nanney LB. Biochemical and physiologic aspects of wound healing. In: RG Wheeland, ed. Cutaneous Surgery: Basic Surgical Concepts and Procedures. Philadelphia: W.B. Saunders, 1994:113–121.

Pastor JC, Calonge M. Epidermal growth factor and corneal wound healing. Cornea 1992; 11(4):311–314.

Petroutsos G, Guinmaraes R, Pouliquen D, et al. Comparison of the effects of EGF, pFGF, and EDGF on corneal epithelium wound healing. Curr Eye Res 1984; 3(4): 593–598.

Pollack SV. Wound healing 1985: an update. J Dermatol Surg Oncol 1985; 11:296–300.

Robson M, Phillips L, Thomason A, et al. Platelet-derived growth factor for the treatment of chronic pressure ulcers. Lancet 1992; 339:23–25.

Schultz G, Cipolla L, Whithouse A, et al. Growth factors and corneal endothelial cells: Stimulation of adult human corneal endothelial cells mitosis in vitro by defined mitogenic agents. Cornea 1992; 11(l):20–27.

Tritto M, Kanat IO. Management of keloids and hypertrophic scars. Am Podiatr Med Assoc 1991; 81(11):601–605.

Webster RC, Davidson TM, Nahum AM. The San Diego Classics in Soft Tissue Surgery. Scar Revision, Parts I, II, and III. 1977 (Videotape).

59

CO$_2$ Laser Resurfacing Scar Revision

Christopher B. Kruse
Advanced Dermatology Surgery Center, Tinton Falls, New Jersey, U.S.A.

John Louis Ratz
Center for Dermatology and Skin Cancer, Tampa, Florida, U.S.A.

While the conventional CO$_2$ laser has been used to treat acne scarring in the past, the Ultra-Pulse^R CO$_2$ laser is now a much safer and effective tool for improving the appearance of surgical, traumatic, and acne scars. It may also have a role in the resurfacing of some hypertrophic scars and in flaps or grafts that have pin-cushioned. The precise control and hemostasis of the laser make it technically easier to use when compared to dermabrasion. History and examination of the patient should address the duration of the scarring, mechanism of injury, and any previous treatments. It should also evaluate for an active or previous herpes simplex infection. No resurfacing should be performed while there is an active infection, herpetic or otherwise, on the skin. Prophylactic antiviral medication is advised if there is a history of herpes simplex eruptions. One regimen is Famciclovir 500 mg b.i.d. for one week, or Valcyclovir 125 mg b.i.d. for one week, starting either the day before or the morning of the procedure. Preoperative photographs should also be taken and are useful to demonstrate the results to the patient, as well as to provide good documentation.

Preoperative counseling is important to educate the patient on the procedure, immediate postoperative appearance and care, and expected degree of benefit. Experience and photographs of typical outcomes are useful for this purpose. Potential complications including persistent erythema, dyspigmentation, infection, and the possibility of not attaining the expected degree of improvement should be discussed. If the patient is unable or unwilling to properly manage the wound postoperatively, treatment should not be offered.

In the treatment of acne scarring, it is best to delay resurfacing until the acne is under good control or, better yet, resolved. If isotretinoin was used, resurfacing should not be performed for at least 6 to 12 months after its discontinuation because of an increased risk of hypertrophic scarring. In patients with a history of keloid formation, it is prudent to wait two years after the isotretinoin has been discontinued and possibly treat an isolated test area first. One should also consider excising, subcising, or punch elevating scars if amenable and of sufficient depth that resurfacing alone is unlikely to provide an adequate result. For some patients, beginning with a test area can allow the patient to view results in an isolated area (Figs. 1–3). This may also help the surgeon identify nonresponsive scarring. Laser resurfacing can be done simultaneously or within the ensuing two to three months to blend these revisions.

However, and in general, best results are usually attained when resurfacing is carried out at least three months after the causative incident when erythema has faded or has started to fade. A good way to start is by beginning with the forehead moving on to one cheek then on to the next cheek followed by the muzzle area and finally the periocular area.

This resurfacing procedure is probably not very effective with large hypertrophic scars or keloids, but can produce excellent results with traumatic and postsurgical scars of the face. For scars of this type, anesthesia is accomplished by direct infiltration or nerve blocks. Nerve blocks are preferred because there is little or no distortion of the skin to be resurfaced. Patients requiring full face resurfacing because of extensive scarring may require deep sedation or general anesthesia. The individual depressions and elevations should be treated initially in an attempt to bring all areas to the same level. Once this is accomplished, full face resurfacing is performed. The skin must be prepped with antiseptic and draped sterilely using damp towels, making sure to cover inflammable material such as hair. Proper eye protection must be worn by everyone in the room.

The goal of the procedure is to smooth the skin contour by bringing scar tissue and the surrounding normal tissue to the same level and carefully feathering the edges to soften the overall surface of the treated area. This removes sharply contrasting tissue depressions and elevations, thus eliminating the shadows these areas cast which, magnify the appearance of scarring.

The areas of elevation and depression in the skin should be determined. Elevated scars need to be treated with the laser until flattened. Because depressed areas cannot be raised with the laser, the elevated tissue needs to be carefully vaporized so that there is a smooth transition from the elevated to the normal skin. The laser should be set to the equivalent of 300 to 400 mJ and 10 W with repeat pulsing. The scar size, location, and configuration determine the size and shape of the pattern selected. Perhaps the most useful shape is the hexagon as hexagonal impacts can be linked together for minimal overlap when needed and untreated or "dead" spots can be avoided. For elevated scars, a single pass is made with 10% to 20% overlap and the desiccated tissue is removed with cotton swabs or gauze moistened with either sterile saline or sterile water. The size of the pattern used in the initial passes is generally the smallest usable for the particular scar being treated. This is commonly the second smallest size for any particular

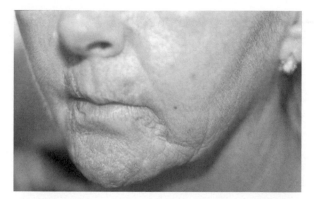

Figure 1   Acne type scarring test area prior to resurfacing.

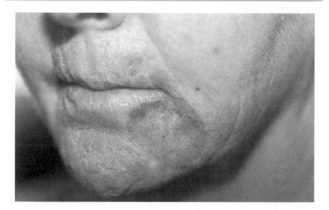

Figure 2   Same test area immediately after resurfacing.

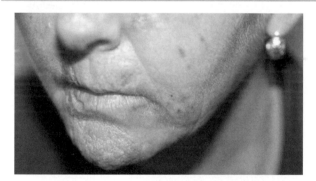

Figure 3   Test area three weeks after resurfacing.

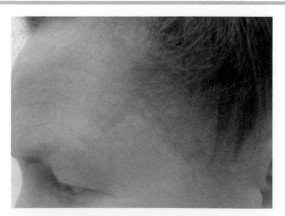

Figure 4   Patient three months post-Mohs with a depressed scar of the forehead following healing by second intention.

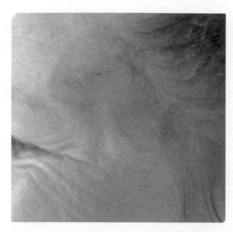

Figure 5   Patient (same as in Fig. 4) immediately following resurfacing.

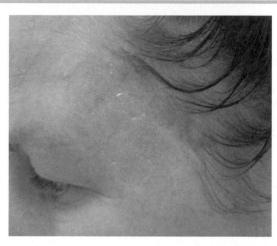

Figure 6   After re-epithelialization, the resurfaced area is smooth, flat, and still erythematous.

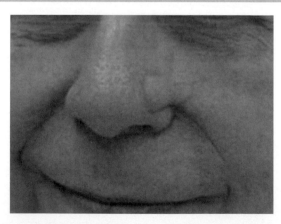

Figure 7   Patient with a significant pin cushioning of a cheek flap repair of a Mohs surgical wound.

pattern, although the smallest size can be useful in treating thready or stellate scars. Palpate and assess the appearance. Additional passes are usually necessary, followed by removing the char and reassessing contour. This is repeated until the elevated scar has been reduced to a satisfactory level. The pattern size is then made larger so that it covers both

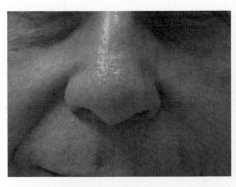
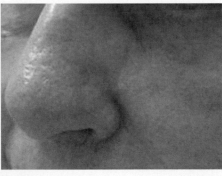

Figure 8 Patient (same as in Fig. 7) two weeks after re-surfacing.

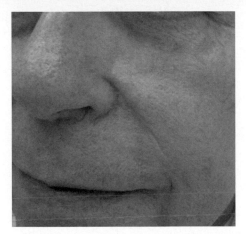

Figure 9 Patient (same as in Fig. 7) four months after resurfacing.

the previously treated site and a margin of surrounding tissue. This is followed by as many pattern size increases necessary to soften the overall appearance. A final pass is made using a larger spot size that covers the treated site and a margin of surrounding skin to feather the appearance. The wound created will be substantially larger than the pre-treated scar—something the patient needs to be advised of prior to the resurfacing; however, treatment of an entire cosmetic unit is often not necessary.

Treating a depressed scar begins with small concentric rings of ablation of normal skin surrounding the depression, followed by passes with ever-increasing pattern sizes until the scar and adjacent tissue feel and appear smooth. After each pass, the char is removed and the progress assessed. As with treatment of an elevated area, a final pass is made using a larger spot size that covers the treated site and a margin of normal surrounding skin to feather the appearance. The desiccated tissue from the final pass can be removed or left in place as a biologic dressing. Although such

a wound still needs to re-epithelialize, the improvement in appearance can be appreciated immediately following the procedure (Figs. 4–6).

When treating a graft or flap that has pin cushioned, consideration must be given to bridged areas such as can be obtained in flaps crossing the alar groove or crease. It may be prudent to excise such "bridges" and follow with the appropriate resurfacing technique. Resurfacing this type of wound is time consuming but improvement is noted immediately after the procedure, and further improvement is noted after re-epithelialization has been completed (Figs. 7–9).

The resurfaced wound can be dressed with a hydrocolloid such as Vigilon[R], or petrolatum ointment and a nonstick bandage. The area should be cleaned twice daily with cotton-tipped applicators and sterile normal saline, followed by the application of sufficient petrolatum to prevent crusting. The treated area should be kept covered at all times, except for cleaning, until the wound has totally healed. The wounds generally re-epithelialize in 7 to 10 days but may take up to two weeks for large surfaces. Makeup should not be applied until the treated area has healed. Erythema usually resolves by six weeks but can persist longer. Proper sun protection is mandatory.

BIBLIOGRAPHY

Alster TS. Cutaneous resurfacing with CO2 and erbium:YAG lasers: preoperative, intraoperative and postoperative considerations. Plastic Reconstr Surg 1999; 103:619–632.

Alster TS, Lupton JR. Complications of laser skin resurfacing. Facial Plast Surg Clin N Am 2000; 8:163–172.

Garrett AB, Dufresne RG, Ratz JL, et al. Carbon dioxide laser treatment of pitted acne scarring. J Dernatol Surg Oncol 1990; 16:737–740.

Lupton JR, Alster TS. Laser scar revision. Dermatol Clin 2002; 20(1):55–65.

60

Nonablative Laser Revision of Scars and Striae

Tina S. Alster
Department of Dermatology, Georgetown University Medical Center, Washington, D.C., U.S.A.

Divya Railan
Colby Skincare, San Jose, California, U.S.A.

INTRODUCTION

Many patients seek treatment for scars and striae, which they consider to be cosmetically disfiguring. Over the past decade, refinements in laser technology and techniques have enabled dermatologic surgeons to define the most appropriate laser systems to be used for many types of scars and striae, without the adverse sequelae and recurrence rates noted with older surgical revision and continuous wave laser techniques. In order to optimize the clinical outcome of laser treatment, patient selection, scar and striae evaluation, laser parameters, specific treatment protocols, and management of possible adverse effects should be considered.

PREOPERATIVE CONSIDERATIONS

Patient Evaluation

Patients with darker skin tones (Fitzpatrick phototype IV or higher) have a greater amount of epidermal melanin that can potentially absorb laser light, thereby reducing the amount of energy effectively delivered to the dermal tissue. As a result, the efficacy of laser scar treatment in patients with dark skin may be reduced, and potential epidermal melanin destruction may eventuate in postoperative hypopigmentation.

Patients presenting with facial hypertrophic scars or keloids commonly also display similar scars in other areas (e.g., knees, elbows, and hands). In addition to evaluating these trauma-prone regions, patients should be made aware that future trauma or surgery could also potentially lead to abnormal scarring. Patients with the propensity to scar are excellent candidates for early or prophylactic laser treatment in an effort to deter scar formation. Laser irradiation of skin during or soon after cutaneous wounding or repair has been shown to reduce or even prevent scar formation in patients at high risk of scar development.

Treatment of patients with infectious or inflammatory disease should be delayed until the condition has resolved. Koebnerization secondary to laser irradiation is a valid concern in the setting of bacterial or viral infection, such as impetigo, herpes simplex, or verrucae. Inflammatory skin disorders such as cystic acne, atopic dermatitis, or psoriasis may be exacerbated with laser treatment, and postoperative healing and clinical effect delayed due to dermal inflammation.

A discussion with the patient should take place to determine the patient's expectations. Patients must be counseled regarding the improvement to be expected after each treatment, the anticipated number of treatment sessions, and final clinical outcome. Patients who expect total disappearance of their scars or striae following laser treatment will be uniformly disappointed, regardless of the clinical improvement observed in most cases. If the patient has unrealistic expectations, laser treatment should not be pursued.

Scar Characteristics

Proper scar classification is important because differences in clinical scar characteristics determine the laser selection and treatment protocol. Scar characteristics such as color, texture, and morphology, as well as previously applied treatments, will affect the choice of laser parameters and ultimate number of treatment sessions required for optimal improvement (Table 1).

Hypertrophic scars are raised, firm erythematous scars formed as the result of overzealous collagen synthesis coupled with limited collagen lysis during the remodeling phase of wound healing. The result is the formation of thick, hyalinized collagen bundles consisting of fibroblasts and fibrocytes. Despite the obvious tissue proliferation, hypertrophic scars remain within the confines of original integument injury and may regress with time.

Keloids are raised, reddish-purple, nodular scars that are palpably firmer than hypertrophic scars. Keloids exhibit a prolonged, proliferative phase resulting in the appearance of thick hyalinized collagen bundles similar to those produced by hypertrophic scars. Unlike hypertrophic scars, however, keloids extend beyond the borders of the inciting wound and do not regress over time. Although they can be seen in any skin type, keloids appear most frequently in patients with darker skin.

Atrophic scars are dermal depressions most commonly caused by collagen destruction during the course of an inflammatory skin disease such as cystic acne or varicella. Scarring after inflammatory or cystic acne can manifest as atrophic, saucerized, ice pick, or boxcar scars. While ice pick and boxcar scars are typically treated with dermal filler augmentation or punch excision, atrophic scars usually respond best to laser therapy.

Scar History

The duration of the scar and its etiology should also be ascertained. Young scars present for less than one year are typically more erythematous than older scars. Although these younger scars are amenable to vascular-specific pulsed dye laser (PDL) irradiation, they may not necessitate laser treatment, as some degree of spontaneous improvement is expected over the first 12 months. In patients whose scars

Table 1 Nonablative Laser Selection for Different Scar Types

Scar type	Clinical characteristics	Preferred nonablative laser
Hypertrophic	Raised	585 nm PDL
	Pink–red	
	Limited to site of original trauma	
Keloid	Raised	585 nm PDL
	Deep red–purple	
	Extend beyond original border	
Atrophic	Saucerized/ice-pick indentations	LP 1450 nm diode
	Flesh-colored or white	LP 1320 nm Nd:YAG

Abbreviations: PDL, pulsed dye laser; LP, long-pulsed; Nd:YAG, neodymium: yttrium-aluminum-garnet.

continue to worsen, it is best to advise early laser intervention in order to arrest further abnormal scar growth and attain more rapid improvement. Hypertrophic scars secondary to thermal burn injury can be treated effectively with 585 nm PDL irradiation, whereas periocular burn scars causing ectropion often requires surgical reconstruction.

Increased scar fibrosis may be seen in the setting of failed surgical scar excision, making the scar even more difficult to treat, Dermabrasion of atrophic scars may result in dermal thickening, thereby rendering the scar less amenable to laser vaporization and potentially reducing the final clinical response. History of intralesional injections of corticosteroids (for hypertrophic scars and keloids, in particular) should not influence the scar's responsiveness to subsequent PDL treatment.

LASER TREATMENT FOR HYPERTROPHIC SCARS AND KELOIDS

Progress in laser technology and refinements in technique have made laser therapy a preferred treatment choice for hypertrophic scars and keloids. Studies published using the vascular-specific 585 nm PDL have demonstrated striking improvements in scar erythema, pliability, bulk, and dysesthesia with minimal side effects and treatment discomfort. These observations have been substantiated by skin surface textural analysis, erythema reflectance spectrometry readings, scar height measurements, and pliability scores. Patients with pruritic hypertrophic scars and keloids requiring the use of oral antihistamines, often report the antihistamines as unnecessary after PDL irradiation of their scars. While significant improvement in hypertrophic scars is generally noted after PDL treatment alone, thick keloids or proliferative hypertrophic scars can be further enhanced with the simultaneous use of intralesional corticosteroid or 5-fluorouracil injections.

Adjacent, nonoverlapping 585 nm PDL pulses at fluences ranging 6.0 to 7.5 J/cm^2 (7 mm spot) or 4.5 to 5.5 J/cm^2 (10 mm spot) should be applied over the entire surface of the scar. Energy densities are decreased by 10% in patients with darker skin phototypes or for scars in delicate body locations (e.g., neck, anterior chest). With PDL irradiation, the patient experiences a snapping sensation similar to that of a rubber band. Posttreatment, a mild sunburn-like heating of the skin is experienced for 15 to 30 minutes that is generally well tolerated; however, some patients may require application of an ice pack. Patients are evaluated at six to eight weeks to determine the response to treatment. If the initial treatment session produced satisfactory results, the energy setting generally remains the same at the next treatment session. However, if only minimal results were achieved, the treatment fluences can be increased by 5% to 10%.

LASER TREATMENT FOR ATROPHIC SCARS

As a consequence of the risks associated with ablative (CO_2 and erbium) laser resurfacing, great interest has been shown for less invasive methods to effectively treat atrophic facial scars. Several nonablative laser devices have demonstrated efficacy in the treatment of atrophic facial scars; however, the most popular and widely used are long-pulsed infrared lasers (e.g., 1320 nm Neodymium:Yttrium-Aluminum-Garnet or Nd:YAG and 1450 nm diode). Each system combines epidermal surface cooling with deeply penetrating infrared wavelengths that selectively target water-containing tissue, thereby creating a discrete thermal injury in the dermis without damage to the epidermis. Protocols for treatment often include three consecutive monthly laser sessions with the greatest clinical improvement noted three to six months after the final laser procedure. Improvement of scars by 40% to 50% has been observed after 1320 nm Nd:YAG or 1450 nm diode laser treatment, with results substantiated by clinical assessments, patient satisfaction surveys, histologic evaluation, and skin surface texture (optical profilometry) measurements. Although a series of nonablative laser treatments can effect modest improvement in atrophic scars with minimal side effects, the degree of clinical improvement does not equal the success of ablative laser resurfacing. Therefore, it is critical to identify those patients best suited for nonablative procedures in order to optimize patient satisfaction.

LASER TREATMENT OF STRIAE DISTENSAE
Striae Distensae Characteristics

Striae distensae are linear bands of atrophic or wrinkled skin, which result from rapid change in body weight or growth. New striae have a pinkish–purplish hue due to underlying dermal inflammation and dilated capillaries. With time, the striae become more fibrotic and hypopigmented. The pathogenesis of striae has not been fully elucidated, but is hypothesized to be the result of several factors including mechanical forces causing elastin fiber damage, hormones (particularly estrogen), and mast cell degranulation with secondary elastolysis.

Striae represent a common problem for which satisfactory treatments are limited. The laser of choice in the treatment of striae is the 585 nm PDL (Table 2). Striae are treated in a manner similar to hypertrophic scars and keloids, but using more conservative fluences of 3.0 to 3.5 J/cm^2 (10 mm spot). The most significant improvement has been observed in treatment of early erythematous striae, whereas only minimal to modest effects have been observed in mature hypopigmented striae. Due to the lower fluences used, irradiated striae do not exhibit the characteristic purpura seen after PDL treatment of hypertrophic scars and keloids. Mild transient erythema of the treatment site is expected due to postoperative tissue hyperemia and edema; however, signs of vesiculation and crusting indicate that improper fluence (too high) or technique (pulse stacking) may have been used. Desired results are typically obtained after one or two treatment sessions at six-week or longer time intervals.

Table 2 Categorization of Striae Distensae

Striae type	Clinical characteristics	Preferred nonablative laser
Early	Pink, lavender, and purple	585 nm PDL
	Wrinkled	
Late	White	585 nm PDL
	Fibrotic	

Abbreviation: PDL, pulsed dye laser.

POSTOPERATIVE MANAGEMENT

During the initial purpuric or erythematous healing phase, an antibiotic or healing ointment should be applied daily. Showers are permitted but the lased skin should not be scrubbed. The areas can then be gently patted dry. During the secondary healing phase (6–8 weeks) after laser irradiation, care should be taken to prevent sun exposure to the area. If a tan is present, it becomes more difficult to identify the degree of improvement achieved from the previous laser treatment. In addition, the efficacy of subsequent laser treatment may be hindered by limited dermal penetration of the 585 nm laser light through the increased epidermal pigment of sun-exposed skin.

MANAGEMENT OF COMPLICATIONS

Pulsed Dye Laser

While complications of PDL treatment are rare, vesiculation, crusting, dyspigmentation, and scarring has been reported with use of excessive fluences, overlapping or stacking of laser spots, or in treatment of darker skin tones. Postoperative purpura is the most commonly experienced side effect of 585 nm PDL treatment and can persist for several days. With the development of PDL systems with extended pulse durations and epidermal cooling devices, the incidence and severity of postoperative purpura has been reduced. Swelling of treated skin may occur immediately after laser irradiation, but generally subsides within 48 hours. Strict sun precautions should be practiced between treatment sessions in order to avoid stimulating pigment production in the treated areas. Subsequent laser sessions should be postponed until any excess pigment has resolved, so that the presence of epidermal melanin does not compromise the effectiveness of the laser. Topical bleaching agents may be applied to hasten pigment resolution. Treatments are typically delivered at six- to eight-week intervals; however, longer treatment intervals may be necessary for adequate healing in patients with darker skin phototypes or in scars located in slower-healing areas (e.g., extremities) that have a higher tendency for postoperative hyperpigmentation.

NONABLATIVE (LONG-PULSED INFRARED) LASER SKIN REMODELING

Side effects and complications of long-pulsed infrared laser treatment of atrophic facial scars are generally mild. Transient posttreatment erythema is a typical event and resolves within 24 hours. Blistering, crusting, and scarring are rare and, although the risk of postinflammatory hyperpigmentation is substantially reduced with nonablative laser treatment (compared to ablative CO_2 or Er:YAG laser skin resurfacing), it is still possible—particularly in patients with darker skin tones. The postinflammatory hyperpigmentation observed, however,

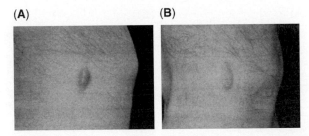

Figure 2 Keloid scar on the elbow before **(A)** and after **(B)** two treatments with concomitant intralesional corticosteroid injections and 585 nm PDL irradiation.

is typically mild and responds well to topical lightening agents combined with sun protection.

CASE REPORTS

Case 1: Hypertrophic Scars

A 24-year-old woman presented with hypertrophic scars on her neck six months after thyroid surgery (Fig. 1A). No prior treatments had been obtained for the asymptomatic scars, but she was concerned about their obvious appearance and desired treatment. Treatment plan included 585 nm PDL treatments at six- to eight-week time intervals at fluences ranging 4.5 to 5.0 J/cm^2 (10 mm spot, 1.5 msec pulse duration). Nonoverlapping laser pulses were applied to the length of each scar. Two months after three PDL treatments, improvement of scars was evident (Fig. 1B).

Case 2: Keloid Scars

A 14-year-old boy presented with a keloid on his elbow, which appeared after minor trauma. He complained of intense itching within the scar. Prior injections of intralesional corticosteroids had resulted in temporary cessation of symptoms but no reduction in the scar's height or bulk (Fig. 2A). Treatment plan included 585 nm PDL treatment of the keloid with concomitant intralesional corticosteroid injections (triamcinolone acetate 20 mg/cc) at four- to six-week intervals. After two treatments at a fluence of 6.0 J/cm^2 (7 mm spot, 1.5 msec pulse), the keloid showed marked improvement in size, symptoms, and pliability (Fig. 2B).

Case 3

A 46-year-old man presented with atrophic facial scars secondary to acne, which had required oral antibiotics and two separate courses of isotretinoin (last course was five years

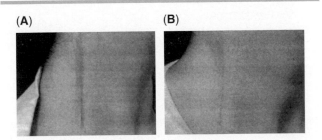

Figure 1 Hypertrophic scar on the neck before **(A)** and 2 months after **(B)** third 585 nm PDL treatment.

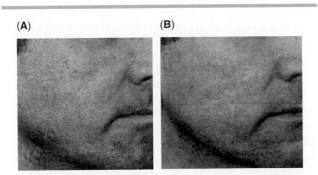

Figure 3 Atrophic acne scars before **(A)** and after **(B)** three long-pulsed 1450 nm diode laser treatments.

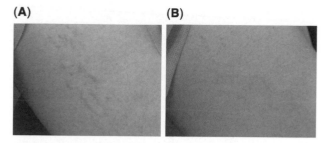

Figure 4 Striae distensae before **(A)** and 2 months after **(B)** second 585 nm PDL treatment.

prior to presentation) (Fig. 3A). He had undergone prior dermabrasion with a 50% reduction in the severity of his scars as well as erbium laser skin resurfacing, which resulted in further scar improvement. He desired additional treatment, but was not interested in undergoing a procedure, which would require a prolonged recovery period. Treatment plan included a series of monthly nonablative long-pulsed 1450 nm diode laser treatments (12–14 J/cm^2, 6 mm spot). Improvement was evident three months after the third treatment (Fig. 3B).

Case 4

A 12-year-old girl complained of stretch marks on her thighs and buttocks that occurred during a recent growth spurt and 15 pound weight gain (Fig. 4A). She had not received any prior treatments. A 585 nm PDL was used at low fluences (3.0–3.5 J/cm^2, 10 mm spot, 1.5 msec pulse) to treat the striae. Two months after the second PDL treatment, marked improvement in the clinical appearance of the striae was noted (Fig. 4B).

LATEST DEVELOPMENTS

The newest approach in the treatment of acne and atrophic scarring includes a nonablative radiofrequency device. Unlike a laser, which uses light energy to generate heat in targeted chromophores based on the theory of selective photothermolysis, radiofrequency technology produces an electric current that generates heat through resistance in the dermis and subcutaneous tissue, thus stimulating neocollagenesis and collagen remodeling. Preliminary studies demonstrate promise in the treatment of acne and, potentially, acne scarring. Further investigation is warranted to determine the role of this novel device in the treatment of atrophic facial scars.

FUTURE DIRECTION

Current laser technology permits successful treatment of various types of scars and striae. It order to achieve optimal results, it is imperative that laser selection be preceded by careful and complete lesional and patient evaluations. The 585 nm PDL is best used to treat hypertrophic scars, keloids, and striae. Nonablative infrared lasers such as the long-pulsed diode or Nd:YAG systems can be used in a series of treatments to remodel atrophic scars through induction of neocollagenesis. Future laser technologic advances, as well as concomitant use of other treatment modalities, may serve to further enhance clinical results.

BIBLIOGRAPHY

Alster TS, Greenberg HL. Laser treatment of scars and striae, hi. In: Kauvar ANB, Hruza G (eds). Principles and Practices in Cutaneous Laser Surgery. New York: Marcel Decker, Inc., 2005:625–641.

Alster TS, Handrick C. Laser treatment of hypertrophic scars, keloids, and striae. Semin Cutan Med Surg 2000; 19: 287–292.

Alster TS. Laser scar revision: comparison study of 585 nm pulsed dye laser with and without intralesional corticosteroids. Dermatol Surg 2003; 29:25–29.

Alster TS, Tanzi EL. Hypertrophic scars and keloids: etiology and management. Am J Clin Dermatol 2003; 4:235–243.

Alster TS, Williams CM. Treatment of keloid sternotomy scars with 585 nm flashlamp pulsed dye laser. Lancet 1995; 345:1198–2000.

Alster TS. Improvement of erythematous and hypertrophic scars by the 585 nm flashlamp-pumped pulsed dye laser. Ann Plast Surg 1994; 32:186–190.

Alster TS, Nanni CA. Pulsed dye laser treatment of hypertrophic bum scars. Plast Reconstr Surg 1998; 102:2190–2195.

Dierickx C, Goldman MP, Fitzpatrick RE. Laser treatment of erythematous/hypertrophic and pigmented scars in 26 patients. Plast Reconstr Surg 1995; 95:84–90.

Fiskerstrand EJ, Svaasand LO$_3$ Volden G. Pigmentary changes after pulsed dye laser treatment in 125 Northern European patients with port wine stains. Br J Dermatol 1998; 138:477–479.

Fitzpatrick RE. Treatment of inflamed hypertrophic scars using intralesional 5-FU. Dermatol Surg 1999; 25:224–232.

Gaston DA, Clark DP. Facial hypertrophic scarring from pulsed dye laser. Dermatol Surg 1998; 24:523–525.

Groover I, Alster TS. Laser scar revision of scars and striae. Dermatol Ther 2000; 13:50–59.

Jacob CI, Dover JS, Kaminer MS. Acne scarring: a classification system and review of treatment options. J Am Acad Dermatol 2001; 45:109–117.

Lupton JR, Alster TS. Laser scar revision. Dermatol Clin 2002; 20:55–65.

Macedo O, Alster TS. Laser treatment of darker skin tones: a practical approach. Dermatol Ther 2000; 13:114–126.

McCraw JB, McCraw JA, McMellin A, et al. Prevention of unfavorable scars using early pulse dye laser treatments: a preliminary report. Ann Plast Surg 1999; 42:7–13.

Nehal KS, Lichtenstein DA, Kamino H, Levine VJ, Ashinoff R. Treatment of mature striae with the pulsed dye laser. J Cutan Laser Ther 1999; 1:41–44.

Nigam PK. Striae cutis distensae. Int J Dermatol 1989; 28:426–431.

Nouri K, Romagosa R, Chartier T, Bowes L, Spencer JM. Comparison of the 585 nm pulsed dye laser and the short pulsed CO$_2$ laser in the treatment of striae distensae in skin types IV and VI. Dermatol Surg 1999; 25:368–370.

Nouri K, Jimenez GP, Harrison-Balestra C, et al. 585-nm pulsed dye laser in the treatment of surgical scars starting on the suture removal day. Dermatol Surg 2003; 29:65–73.

Rogachefsky AS, Hussain M, Goldberg DJ. Atrophic and mixed pattern of acne scars with a 1320 nm Nd:YAG laser. Dermatol Surg 2003; 29:904–908.

Ruiz-Esparza J, Gomez JB. Nonablative radiofrequency for active acne vulgaris: the use of deep dermal heat in the treatment of moderate to severe active acne vulgaris (thermotherapy): a report in 22 patients. Dermatol Surg 2003; 29:333–339.

Sommer S, Sheehan-Dare RA. Atrophie blanche-like scarring after pulsed dye laser treatment. J Am Acad Dermatol 1999; 41:100–102.

Tanzi EL, Alster TS. Comparison of a 1450 nm diode laser and a 1320 nm Nd:YAG laser in the treatment of atrophic facial scars: a prospective clinical and histological study. Dermatol Surg 2004; 30:152–157.

Tanzi EL, Lupton JR, Alster TS. Review of lasers in dermatology: four decades of progress. J Am Acad Dermatol 2003; 49:1–31.

Zheng P, Lavker RM, Kligman AM. Anatomy of striae. Br J Dermatol 1985; 112:185–190.

61

Basic Laser Physics

Timothy J. Rosio

Anew Skin^{TM} Dermatology, Folsom-Auburn, California, U.S.A.

INTRODUCTION

Just a few years ago, dermatologic lasers were primarily employed by a handful of laser cognoscenti, who had made a serious academic and financial commitment to understanding their use. Rarely was one of the few existing laser types available to general, private dermatologists or residents. Today, increasing numbers and types of specialized lasers are accessible to a majority of practicing and training dermatologists through purchase, lease, hospitals, rental, and other arrangements.

This laser windfall breeds enthusiasm as well as high expectations on the part of patients and practitioners, and is often followed by confusion and disappointment; and the latter may be costly. Many newer lasers employ multiple wavelengths and high-intensity physical principles that appear easier to use but that place patients, staff, and physicians at higher risk of serious eye or other injury. Also, patients may be subjected to multiple, unsuccessful treatments when laser treatment, in general, or the particular wavelength or settings are inappropriate. Education is the key. A lack of background in laser physics impairs the reasoned application of lasers, purchase of the most cost-effective option by a practice or institution, and safe use by practitioners.

As a physician laser user (and decision maker or owner), you will be partially or largely responsible for practical, financial, and technical choices including selection, maintenance, growth, life cycle, and safety involving laser instruments; these and many other questions require a passing knowledge of "what's in the laser box." Since a single ideal laser does not yet exist, limited resources are a practical reality. This requires the laser user to decide on whether to use available laser hardware on a tissue structure, pigment, vessel size, depth, or anatomic location to be treated.

On the other hand, the dilemma may be which laser is to be purchased first and which one next. The fact that the features of some lasers overlap to a degree, allowing, for example, a laser marketed for pigmented lesions to be promoted for vascular problems or the "catch all" category "rejuvenation," makes this decision more complicated. An increased number of accessories available either as integral or as "add-ons" have become an important part of laser operation and purchase. These include scanners and a plethora of externally applied cooling devices. Therefore, knowledge of laser physics and safety is cost-effective and practical in fiscal, therapeutic, and safety terms. One must first apply a standard nomenclature and an organized approach to the settings and application of laser operations, and modify it as new parameters become available.

STANDARDIZED LASER THERAPY NOMENCLATURE

- Type of laser used and spectral distribution
- Irradiance: Watts/cm^2
- Laser beam cross-sectional area and shape at tissue surface
- Laser pulse duration or exposure time in seconds
- Energy in Joules; energy density in J/cm^2
- Pulse or exposure repetition rate per second
- Treatment time segments and intervals between treatment times
- Total treated skin area in cm^2
- Total number of applied laser pulses of exposures
- Degree of overlap or superimposition or exposures
- Cooling mechanism, temperature, phase, duration, time to equilibrate

LIGHT VS. LASER: NATURE'S FIRST "PERMANENT WAVE"

To understand lasers, one must first appreciate that matter, energy, and light are unified. Beginning 200 years ago, a series of concepts, experiments, and theories comprising the foundation of quantum mechanics were put forth by the following: in 1805, physician scientist Thomas Young established the wave nature of light; in 1900, Max Planck described the quantum nature of energy; Einstein explained light and energy interactions with his description of the photon and the quantum unit of light and photovoltaic theory in 1905, for which he later received the Nobel prize; Neil Bohr supported his model of the atom with quantum theory showing the spectral signature of hydrogen in 1913; and Louis de Broglie's proposal in 1927 that matter can exhibit wave characteristics, and energy can also behave as matter.

Thus the basic material building blocks of our universe are subatomic particles, grouped as a nucleus and its orbiting electron(s) and operating under quantum mechanic principles. Atoms, ions, and molecules exist predominantly in their minimal energy, resting or nonexcited state but may exist temporarily in discretely higher-energy, excited states specified by units of energy characteristic of that atom (Fig. 1).

In the excited state, electrons store energy and inhabit specific higher-energy orbitals until the additional quantum of transitional energy is released as a photon of electromagnetic radiation (EMR), and the atom returns to its original resting state. This spontaneous energy emission is in the form of a photon, whose wavelength or "color" and energy is characteristic for the type of atom. First envisioned by

Photon excitation, followed by spontaneous photon emission

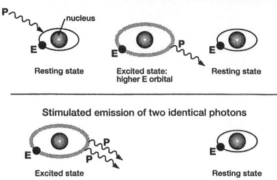

E = electron   P = photon

Figure 1 Spontaneous and stimulated photon emission. In the excited state, electrons store the energy and inhabit specific higher energy orbitals until the additional quantum of transitional energy is released as a photon and the atom returns to its original resting state. This spontaneous energy emission is in the form of a photon, whose wavelength is characteristic for the type of atom. If an already excited atom is stimulated further by sufficient additional energy, the atom will immediately return to resting state by releasing identical photons at the same moment. These photons are the same wavelength, in the same direction and spatial orientation (i.e., in phase) as the original stimulating beam.

Albert Einstein at the turn of the century, spontaneous light emission returns the atom to its usual resting state, analogous to a battery discharging all its stored energy.

Quantum theory was described by Neils Bohr in an equation:

$$E_e - E_r = hf_{er}$$

where E_e is the energy of the excited system, from which is subtracted the energy of the system at rest (E_r), and h is Planck's constant $= 6.6 \times 10^{-34}$ J/sec. The difference between the two transitional energy states results in a photon of frequency f_{er}. Wavelength is related to frequency by the equation $\lambda f = c$, where the speed of light $c = 3 \times 10^{10}$ cm/sec. If an already excited atom is stimulated further by sufficient additional energy, the atom will immediately return to the resting state by releasing identical photons at the same moment. In other words, these photons are of the same wavelength in the same direction and spatial orientation ("in phase") as the original stimulating beam (imagine a pair of nested spoons!). This stimulated emission of radiation phenomenon underlies the production of laser energy. Laser light (more correctly termed laser energy) does not exist in nature. It is a specialized form of light that is produced by amplifying, concentrating, and channeling stimulated emission photons. An acronym, Laser defines a high concentration of light amplified by stimulated emission of radiation. The wavelength produced is characteristic for the specific type of atom or molecule, known as the lasing medium (e.g., $CO_2 = 10,600$ nm; Ar $= 488,514$ nm; YAG $= 1064$ nm).

The lasing medium may be a gas, liquid, crystal, or ionized metal. Examples of commonly used lasing media include Argon, He-Neon, or CO_2 gas, which may be diluted in an inert gas such as nitrogen; a ruby or YAG crystal; an organic dye such as rhodamine used in tunable and flash-lamp-excited dye lasers (FEDLs); diode lasers that depend

on layers or arrays of semiconducting rare earth elements like gallium aluminum arsenide; and metals as in copper or gold vapor lasers.

In our prototypical system, the atoms or molecules constituting the lasing medium are confined within the lasing "optical cavity," which generally has a reflective surface at opposite ends; the mirrors, lasing medium, and optical cavity when taken together constitute an "optical resonator," a place for photons to "bounce" or resonate back and forth. A power source pumps energy to the atoms in this closed system, which may be via electricity, radiofrequency waves, a flashlamp (photons), chemical, or even mechanical means (Fig. 2). The disproportionately high average energy level achieved by the atoms is referred to as a "population inversion," since normally very few atoms are present in that state.

An increasing percentage of highly energetic atoms in the population continue to undergo repeated stimulated emissions as continuous energy pumps them to a completely amplified state. The reflected photons travel parallel to the long axis of the optical cavity, and so do the stimulated photon emissions they provoke in turn. Therefore, laser light is propagated in a highly directional manner. The optical resonator releases the laser light through one end of the reflectors, which is partially transmissive, through the delivery system. The type of laser, the pattern of energy pumping, and the delivery system determine whether the laser beam is a brief burst or a continuous wave (CW) as well as the waveform of the output (magnitude vs. time).

Electromagnetic Radiation

The photon is the smallest structural unit of EMR which describes a basic form of energy possessing both wave and particle characteristics. All photons travel at the same fixed rate: 186,000 miles/sec or 3×10^{10} cm/sec. The energy possessed by a photon is proportional to and determines the wave frequency, i.e., the more energetic the photon, the higher its frequency and the shorter the distance between corresponding wave segments, i.e., the wavelength. The lower the photon's energy, the longer is the wavelength.

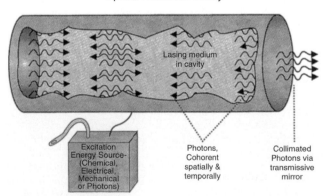

Optical Resonator Cavity

Figure 2 Schematic laser diagram. The lasing medium is confined within an optical cavity or resonator that has reflective mirrors on opposing ends. A power supply excites resting state atoms to a high-energy state known as a "population inversion." The laser power supply "pumps" still more energy into the system in the form of either direct current, radiofrequency, light, or other means. The result of energy pumping and continued stimulated emissions is "amplification," producing an extremely intense laser beam, a percentage of which exits through the partially transmissive mirror.

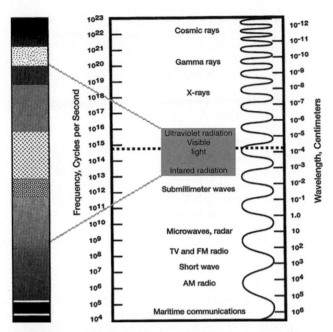

Figure 3 Electromagnetic radiation spectrum with visible wavelengths and frequencies. Visible light is only a small part of the electromagnetic spectrum, sandwiched in between the most energetic ionizing gamma rays at one end and the low-energy radio and microwaves at the other. Wavelength = 1/frequency × (c).

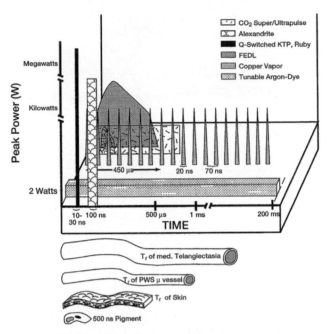

Figure 4 Thermal relaxation time related to power and exposure times of selected cutaneous lasers. Peak power (W) and temporal delivery of the laser's energy result in characteristic energy profiles, which are superimposed here on a graphic plane, together with pictogram representation of relative thermal relaxation times (T) for small microvessels, moderate telangiectasias, skin, and pigment (melanosomes and small pigment granules). Exposures approximating T_r for the target selectively destroy it, and spatially confine damage to the target zone. Lower fluences with much longer exposures than T_r cause coagulation but also allow heat conduction to surrounding tissue, resulting in nonspecific epidermal and dermal damage (and possible visible scarring). Very brief (nanosecond) low-power pulses closely spaced (e.g., 2–5 kHz) are "quasi-continuous," e.g., copper vapor and non–Q-switched KTP lasers. The total energy contained in an individual pulse (area under the curve) is low despite a moderate peak power due to brief duration. *Abbreviation*: FEDL, flashlamp-excited dye laser.

The formula $\lambda = 186,000$ miles/sec $\times 1/f$ describes the photon's fixed rate of the speed of light and the inverse relationship between wavelength and frequency. Visible light constitutes only a small segment of the wide range of EMR, sandwiched in between the most energetic ionizing gamma rays and x-rays at one end and the low-energy radio and microwaves (Fig. 3). The term "light" refers to the visible part of the EMR spectrum but will be used interchangeably with EMR for convenience.

Laser Light Production

Laser production begins with a collection of specific atoms or molecules (lasing medium) confined within an optical cavity or resonator with reflective mirrors on opposing ends. A power supply furnishes energy to the predominantly resting state atoms, exciting the majority to a state known as a "population inversion," since excited-state atoms now predominate. Laser energy emission resonates back and forth, building up within the laser tube, continuing to stimulate more laser emissions. These stimulated emissions generate ever-increasing photons traveling in the same direction as the propagating beam and are therefore summated. Meanwhile, the laser power supply pumps still more energy into the system in the form of direct current, or radio frequency, or light, or through other means. The result of energy pumping and continued stimulated emissions is amplification, producing an extremely intense laser beam. One mirror is partially transmissive, allowing egress of a percentage of the beam. Lasers with similar average power and wavelength output may differ radically in power output versus time (temporal emission or mode) (Fig. 4). The mode dramatically influences the laser's effects on chromophores. The laser mode depends on the type of power supply used for excitation and the lasing medium. CW lasers (e.g., argon) provide a constant power output over time.

Quasi-continuous lasers deliver extremely short (nanosecond), weak pulses (low fluences) that must be summated over hundreds of thousands of milliseconds to have a clinical effect.

Quasi-CW mode lasers have clinical effects comparable to CW lasers of similar average power. Pulsed lasers deliver moderately high fluences over milliseconds or microseconds (e.g., flashlamp dye lasers). Q-switched lasers produce extremely high fluences in milliseconds to nanoseconds, resulting in photomechanical effects, which can disrupt tattoo or melanocytic pigments.

Three Properties of Laser Energy

Ordinary light consists of photons with a variety of energies (frequencies or 1/wavelengths) traveling in multiple directions (Fig. 5); photons of the same wavelength are not synchronized either in space or time (out of phase). Conversely, laser light photons are monochromatic (same wavelength and energies), travel in exactly the same direction with minimal divergence (highly collimated), and wave peaks and valleys are coherent (synchronized in time and space like a marching band, i.e., in phase). These three properties define laser light, conferring capabilities impossible for ordinary light. Monochromaticity provides opportunity for strategic absorption selectivity (Fig. 6) via

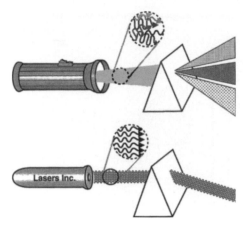

Figure 5 Laser versus incoherent light source characteristics. Ordinary light consists of photons with a variety of energies (frequencies or 1/wavelengths) traveling in multiple directions, out of phase. Conversely, laser light photons are monochromatic (same wavelength, therefore refracted in the prism to the same degree), travel in exactly the same direction with minimal divergence (highly collimated), and wave "peaks and valleys" are coherent, i.e., in phase. These three properties define laser light, conferring capabilities impossible for ordinary light.

distances, such as from the earth to the moon, and still be detectable. Directionality also makes spatial precision possible, such that tissues near the intended target may be avoided.

Coherence describes the synchronization of the electromagnetic waves that characterize laser light. Coherence underlies laser wave propagation and makes possible, for example, holography.

Laser Beam Spatial Configuration
Transverse Electromagnetic Mode
Beam shape is critical to the dermatologic surgeon because it influences the power density that may be applied and the precision available. Is the curette a reasonable incisional tool? Conversely, would you choose a scalpel to ablate tissue? These questions highlight that for surgical lasers, similar to other surgical instruments, laser beam profile influences resurfacing, recontouring, and incisional surgery functions. The spatial intensity distribution (profile) of a laser beam at the source depends on details of the optical resonator that produced it—mirror radius, spacing, or curvature—and lasing medium dimensions. Note that the beam profile at the target tissue may be similar to that at the source, or it may have undergone significant changes by the delivery system. The three most commonly encountered spatial beam modes or configurations in dermatologic laser surgery are transverse electromagnetic mode (TEM_{00}) (gaussian, fundamental), TEM_{01} (doughnut), and multimode (Fig. 7).

The spot size of a radially symmetric (gaussian) beam is defined as that radius, r_{00}, which transmits 86 of the gaussian beam energy (Fig. 8):

$$r_{00} = 0.9\lambda \times f_L/D$$

where f_L, is the focal length of the lens and D is the diameter of the laser beam perpendicular to the axis of propagation (prior to lens transmission). Short-focal-length lenses, smaller-original-beam diameters, and shorter wavelengths all favor production of small spot sizes.

matching of laser wavelengths to desired chromophore targets and relative avoidance of other chromophores. Furthermore, ordinary polychromatic light wavelengths are refracted ("bent") to varying degrees as they pass through an interface to a medium of different optical density, e.g., air to water or glass. Thus, differential refraction results in a spread beam with diminished intensity (e.g., prisms and rainbows), while laser light maintains its directional focus and intensity all the way to the target.

Collimation emphasizes the high degree to which all photons are traveling in the same direction, allowing the intensity of the laser light to be maintained. This characteristic makes possible a beam that can travel immense

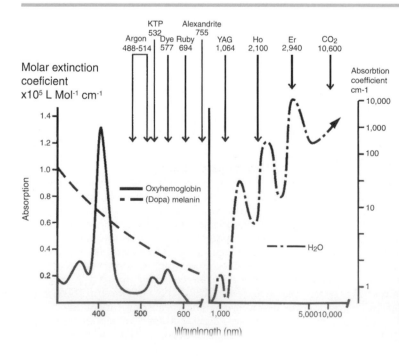

Figure 6 Laser and skin chromophore absorption. Laser photons encountering skin undergo absorption, transmission, reflection, and scattering. The relative probabilities of these continuous events depend on the tissue transmissibility and absorption efficiencies of the chosen wavelength and target tissues' competing chromophores. Depicted are the absorption profiles of the dominant skin chromophores and the main cutaneous laser wavelengths. *Abbreviation:* TEM, transverse electromagnetic modes.

Sagittal Sections of Beams' Power Densities

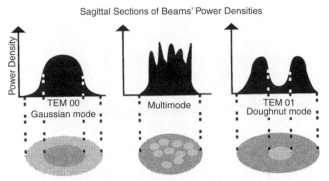

Power Densities across beam profiles at the target

Figure 7 Transverse electromagnetic modes (TEM). Beam shape is critical to the dermatologic surgeon because it influences the power density that may be applied and the precision available. The three most commonly encountered spatial beam modes or configurations in dermatologic laser surgery are TEM_{00} (gaussian, fundamental), TEM_{01} (doughnut) and multimode.

The gaussian beam profile allows the smallest spot size, and therefore the highest peak power density, and is preferable for incisional work. In contrast, the TEM_{01} mode results in approximately 30% larger spot sizes, and thus a ratio of 0.56 of the power density available from the gaussian beam ($1{:}1.33^2 = 0.56$). For ablation at the same working distance, the cooler central spot of the doughnut beam and larger spot area may be partially compensated for by doubling the power output and scanning the beam with rapid, overlapping hand movements similar to the way in which one prevents grooving from the peripheral "tails" of the gaussian beam (Fig. 9). Lasers may also produce more complex spatial beam patterns, such as multimode, characterized by many small rarefactions alternating with higher-power densities. Multimode, as in TEM_{01}, results in a slightly larger minimum spot size and may be seen in some solid-state lasers, e.g., YAG or ruby. However, the YAG laser is normally used with larger spot sizes and lower-power densities for coagulation or with an energy-intensifying contact fiber or sapphire tip for incisional work. Also, the Q-switched ruby and Q-switched YAG are used for delivery

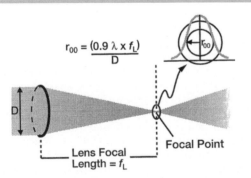

$$r_{00} = \frac{(0.9\ \lambda \times f_L)}{D}$$

Lens Focal Length = f_L

Focal Point

Figure 8 Laser spot size. The spot size of a radially symmetric (gaussian) beam is defined as that radius, r_{00}, which transmits 86% of the gaussian beam energy, $r_{00} = (0.9\ 1 \times f_L)/D$, where f_L is the focal length of the lens and D is the diameter of the laser beam perpendicular to the axis of propagation (prior to lens transmission). Short-focal-length lenses, smaller original beam diameters, and shorter wavelengths favor production of small spot sizes.

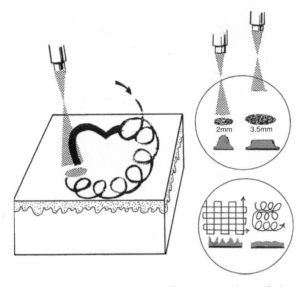

Figure 9 Depth control and tissue uniformity vary with resurfacing and recontouring technique. Different power profiles related to spot size are obtained from different hand piece-to-tissue distances. Tissue injury or removal uniformity is related to both beam profile and hand speed and direction of movement. Flat beam profiles, overlapping circles, and rapid scanning with alternating direction of highly regular, rapid hand movements are keys to excellent cosmetic laser surgery.

of large-spot-size pulses for photodisruption, as will be discussed later.

Delivery Methods

The spatial intensity distribution of the beam at tissue may be strongly influenced by the delivery system responsible for conduction of the beam from the laser source. These include items such as mirrors, lenses, optical fibers, and waveguides. Mirrors in articulated armatures, when correctly aligned, come closest to maintaining the original beam configuration. Optical fibers and waveguides result in a loss of collimation and produce a blunted spatial beam profile more similar to multimode, but which diverges much more rapidly. The laser surgeon should analyze data available on the beam profile at tissue, since alterations of the beam's spatial mode may result from delivery system attachments planned for use.

Basic Tissue Optics and Lasers

Four Fates for Laser Energy

Laser photons encountering skin are variably subjected to four fates: absorption, transmission, reflection, and scattering (Fig. 10). The relative probabilities of these continuous events depend on the transmissibility and absorption efficiencies of the chosen wavelength in the target tissues' competing chromophores (Fig. 6). In addition to absorption, variable scattering of wavelengths also influences outcome; highly energetic short wavelengths (290–400 nm) undergo strong scattering, while long wavelengths (600–1200 nm) are highly transmitted to depths of 2 mm or more. A primary principle of photomedicine is that photon absorption must occur for a reaction to take place. But how deep will the photon travel? We know that the probability of sufficient photons being absorbed at the intended target declines exponentially with depth in a tissue because of attenuation. This is described qualitatively in Figure 11, which displays

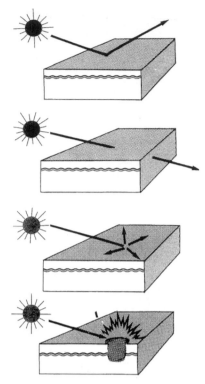

Figure 10 Four fates for laser energy. Photons and tissue interaction result in four potential outcomes: absorption, transmission, reflection, and scattering. The relative probabilities of these continuous events depend on the transmissibility and absorption efficiencies of the chosen wavelength in target tissues' competing chromophores. *Abbreviations*: PLDL, pigmented lesion dye laser; CVL, copper vapor laser; ADL, argon dye laser; FEDL, flash-lamp-excited dye laser.

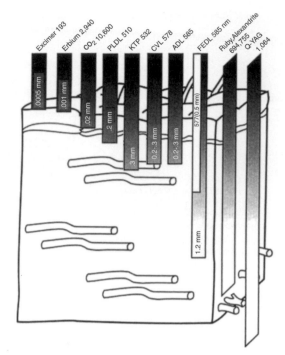

Figure 11 Relative laser wavelength penetration depths. The probability of sufficient photons being absorbed at the intended target declines exponentially with depth in a tissue because of attenuation. Approximate relative penetration depths for common wavelengths are displayed. Calculated absorption values for infrared and ultraviolet wavelengths are used where absorption dominates, and histologic research observations are combined that consider selective clinical effects for more complicated visible wavelengths (scattering significant and many tissue variables).

approximate relative penetration depths and combines calculated absorption values for infrared (IR) and ultraviolet (UV) wavelengths with histologic research observations for more complicated visible wavelengths that consider selective clinical effects.

Beer's Law

Photon absorption is described quantitatively by Beer's law, which shows that a fixed percentage of a beam of a given wavelength is absorbed per length as it travels through an ideally uniform (isotropic) tissue. Two common measures of a substance's absorption strength of a specific wavelength are (i) absorption length, or the distance wherein 63% of an incident beam is absorbed, and (ii) extinction length, or the distance wherein 90% is absorbed. One extinction length is approximately 2.3 times the absorption length. The first 90% of a beam is absorbed in one extinction length; the remaining 10% undergoes 90% absorption in the second extinction length, etc. Experience has shown that minimum achievable tissue damage is between 1 and 2.3 times the absorption length for a specific wavelength. Beer's law is written as follows:

$$I_{(x)} = I_{(0)} \times 10^{\alpha x}$$

where, $I_{(x)}$ is the transmitted intensity, α is the extinction length, and x is the depth (cm) of penetration in the tissue. The absorption coefficient is commonly used to display relative absorbance by substances at varying wavelengths;

it is derived from 1 divided by the absorption length (cm) and named μa or given as absorbance (cm^{-1}).

An Optical Model of the Skin

A simple optical model has been used by Anderson and Parrish in efforts to explain and predict clinical laser-tissue interactions. This and other models are helpful gross approximations, since complex interrelationships between variables exist. The author have depicted numerous facts with a layered model of the skin that helps visualize these experimental findings simultaneously by juxtaposing the skin's nonmelanin major chromophore absorption spectra as a relative absorbing and scattering wall, with an optical window representing minimal absorption and less scatter and reflection from 600 to 1200 nm (Fig. 12).

Optical skin compartments and their effects upon particular wavelengths fall into three categories: (i) those with high absorption coefficients for a wavelength (absorption dominates), (ii) compartments with low absorption coefficients for a wavelength (dominant scattering, transmission, and some reflection), and (iii) particularly with visible wavelengths, compartments where much complicated photo-medicine takes place with a balance of absorption and scattering present. Notably, the wavelength range (600–1200 nm) may be considered as an "optical window" due to the paucity of absorption efficiency across these wavelengths by skin chromophores in all four compartments.

One may vary the skin model by assuming vitiliginous skin, or various melanized clinical conditions, with four layered compartments of varying thicknesses. stratum corneum (10 μm), epidermis (100 μm), papillary

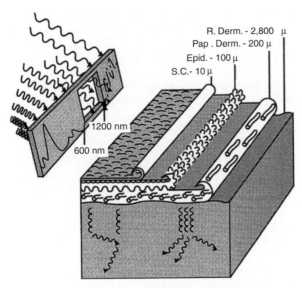

Figure 12 Four-compartment optical skin model. A four-compartment model of the skin, juxtaposed with the skin's major chromophores absorption spectra, is illustrated together with an optical window with minimal absorption from 600 to 1200 nm in all four compartments. Compartments and particular wavelengths fall into three categories: absorption dominant, transmissive/scattering dominant, and mixed. Most photomedicine takes place in the visible spectrum across multiple compartments where a mixture of absorption and scattering occurs.

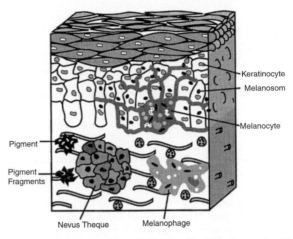

Figure 13 Pigmented optical model of the skin. Melanin may be distributed in the epidermal compartment in the basal layer as melanocytes and in the basal and suprabasal keratinocytes as transferred melanosomes. Superficial to deep dermal pigments include, for example, melanin in melanophages, compound and dermal nevi found alone or in theques, organic carbon, or other tattoo pigments. Any of these cells or pigment granules may be broken into smaller fragments by Q-switched photomechanical laser impulses.

dermis (200 μm), and reticular dermis (2800 μm). The stratum corneum, by virtue of this thinness and lack of visible-range chromophores, transmits 95% of the entire visible spectra (only 5% remittance) for both white and black skin, unless it is excessively thickened as in psoriasis.

Epidermal Compartment

In the epidermal compartment, melanin is the only strong broadband broadband absorber of visible light from 400 to 600 nm (dramatically less and decreasing between 600 and 1200 nm). Melanin is responsible for three orders of magnitude variation in 400 to 600 nm light transmission between fair and darkly pigmented skin types. Melanin may be found in the epidermal compartment in basal layer melanocytes and in the basal and suprabasal keratinocytes as transferred melanosomes (Fig. 13). Clinical examples of this superficial melanized compartment are found in ephelides (freckles), lentigos, junctional nevi, postinflammatory hyperpigmentation, superficial types of melasma (chloasma), and superficial café au lait macules. Junctional nevi overlap into the third (papillary dermal) compartment, in that they may have theques or nests of nevus cells below the basal layer as well as melanosomes in keratinocytes above. Postinflammatory hyperpigmentation may possess melanophages in the papillary dermis as well as hemosiderin.

Superficial Pigment and Vascular Lasers

Superficial pigment and vascular lasers include all the green and yellow light laser systems, including the argon (488 and 514 nm), the KTP (532 nm), copper vapor (511 and 578 nm), the continuous-wave argon pumped dye laser, the flashlamp-excited green dye laser or pigmented lesion dye laser (PLDL: 510 nm), and the FEDL (577, 585, and 595 nm). These laser wavelengths transmit through water but penetrate the skin poorly, absorbed on average at a level of less than

0.1 mm in the epidermis by melanin predominantly in melanosomes, or 0.02 to 0.5 mm in the papillary dermis by blood and to a lesser degree other tissue constituents. Higher absorption efficiency by melanin at shorter wavelengths causes highly specific melanosome destruction in the epidermal compartment. More efficient absorption at shorter wavelengths required lower effective energy densities at 355 nm vs. 532 nm vs. 1064 nm to disrupt superficial melanosomes. Deeper penetrating pigment lasers include the ruby (694 nm), alexandrite (755 nm), and the YAG (1064 nm). They may also be used to treat superficial pigment, and will be discussed further.

Long temporal high fluence exposure to the wavelengths from any of these lasers coagulates tissue widely. Short intense exposures of the order of nanoseconds to hundreds of microseconds allows thermal spatial confinement to superficial melanin and hemoglobin targets in the epidermis and papillary dermis.

If one assumes that no melanin is in the epidermis, the vast majority of all visible light would be transmitted or forward-scattered to the next compartments—the papillary and reticular dermis. Melanin in dermal nevi or incontinent free or macrophage bound may be found here. Non-visible light spectra that are highly absorbed in tissue proteins or water will be mentioned below.

Papillary Dermis Compartment

The third compartment, representing the papillary dermis, has circulating soluble pigments in blood vessels that selectively absorb visible wavelength bands at 400 to 500 nm (bilirubin and carotenes) and at 400 and 520 to 600 nm (hemoglobins). These absorption bands are used to selectively thermolyze (heat-coagulate) the blood vessels, while sparing adjacent, poorly absorbing tissues, as mentioned above.

Papillary and Reticular Dermis Compartments

The papillary and reticular dermis comprising the third and fourth compartments is made of collagen fibers, which variably scatter visible wavelengths forward to a degree

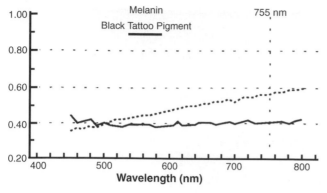

Figure 14 Reflectance spectra of melanin and organic carbon pigments. Reflectance spectra of melanin and black tattoo pigments reveal a rough correspondence in absorption profiles, but with melanin showing less absorption over a range of wavelengths, particularly toward the longer end of the far-red and near-IR spectrum. *Source*: Courtesy of Candela Laser Corp.

inversely proportional to wavelength (i.e., shorter wavelengths scatter more than longer wavelengths). Optical scatter explains why blue nevi—and the sky—appear blue. As photons of wavelengths less than 600 nm are scattered or absorbed to such a degree few will be transmitted past the superficial dermis. Conversely, wavelengths in the "optical window" are both absorbed less and scattered less. Therefore, approximately 1% of photons with wavelengths from 605 to 850 nm will be transmitted through chest wall dermis. This percentage may seem miniscule, but, recalling that tissue effects are time and energy dependent, if enough photons are delivered with high intensity in a short enough time period, they may be sufficient to have a dramatic effect on a selectively absorbing chromophore, even deep within the dermis. Examples of this are photo-disruption of melanocytic or tattoo pigment (decorative or traumatic).

Returning to a pigmented version of our optical skin model (Fig. 13), superficial to deep dermal pigments comprise of: melanin in melanophages, compound and dermal nevi, nevus of Ota, organic carbon, or other tattoo pigments. Reflectance spectra of melanin and black tattoo pigments suggest a rough correspondence in absorption profiles, with melanin showing less absorption over a range of wavelengths, particularly toward the longer end of the far-red and near-IR spectrum (Fig. 14). Professional tattoo pigments show a much greater variability in reflectance/absorption profiles associated with particular colors, most commonly

reds, greens, and bright blues. The highest absorption (lowest reflectance) for reds is at 550 to 600 nm, while greens absorb best around 675 to 775 nm (Fig. 15). Hemosiderin poorly absorbs these deeper penetrating wavelengths.

Near-IR, Nd-YAG Wavelengths: Deep Pigment Lasers

The lasers used to treat tattoos and melanin pigments located in the dermis are characterized by longer wavelengths in the far red to near-IR range. For pigment treatment, they are used at extremely high intensity and extremely short pulse duration, i.e., high fluence in the nanosecond domain. This intensity-duration requires operation in Q-switched mode, and is commonly performed with the ruby, neodymium and erbium YAGs, and alexandrite lasers. Q-switching (special pulsing) uses a Pockels cell that act like a capacitor, that stores and suddenly releases laser light. This results in extremely high-intensity, nanosecond photomechanical effects (fragmentation) to deeper tissue targets (Fig. 13). Surrounding tissues are protected from thermal injury. This occurs because delivery of the photons takes place over a period shorter than the thermal relaxation time of the target (Fig. 4), i.e., before significant heat dissipation can occur. Selective photothermolysis can occur in any chromophores that absorb these wavelengths efficiently enough, which includes most tattoo pigments over a broad range and, to some lesser degree, melanin pigment. The far-red and near-IR wavelengths of these lasers are capable of penetrating several millimeters through the skin because of long-wavelength transmission and poor absorption by other chromophores. The YAG IR wavelength is less efficiently absorbed by melanin than shorter wavelengths (only 10% that of the ruby laser), however, transmission efficiency is considerably greater so that a greater percentage of energy reaches the target.

YAG (1064 nm) is minimally absorbed by any skin chromophore, including melanin; therefore, it is one of the most deeply penetrating wavelengths, being transmitted and scattered through all four compartments. Water absorbs minimal IR energy up to wavelengths close to 1200 nm as demonstrated in the skin model. The low absorptive affinity of the skin for YAG energy is demonstrated by the skin thickness (3 mm) required to absorb 90% of the beam energy, or the extinction length. Virtually all laser energy is absorbed within three extinction lengths within a tissue. The large extinction length for the YAG is borne out by observation that the beam expands three times after passing through just 2 mm of mucosa, resulting in a ninefold reduction in power density. The poor absorption of the beam prevents targeting

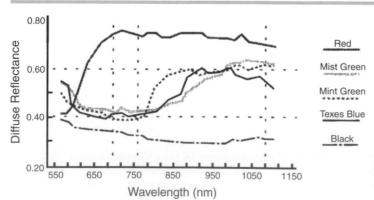

Figure 15 Reflectance spectra of colored professional tattoo pigments. Professional tattoo pigments show a much greater diversity in reflectance/absorption profiles for various colors, most notably reds, greens, and bright blues. Highest absorption (lowest reflectance) for reds is at 550 to 600 nm, while greens absorb best around 675 to 775 nm. *Source*: Courtesy of Candela Laser Corp.

a precise or small amount of tissue. The YAG energy is thus scattered throughout a tissue volume 300 to 900 times larger than CO_2 energy. Therefore compared to the ruby and alexandrite lasers the Nd-YAG is less likely to damage darker pigmented skin, but may require more treatments and show somewhat less efficacy for the same number of treatments, especially with non-black colors versus the other lasers.

Longer non–Q-switched pulses ("normal mode") exposures of 10 to 50 msec may be effective and spatial damage confined when a highly absorbing larger target such as blood vessel or hair retains more heat from far red/near-IR photons, while rapid epidermal heat dissipation and cooling prevents injury to the epidermis. The deeper pigment category of lasers comprising the long pulsed ruby, alexandrite, 810 diode, and Nd-YAG is, therefore, ideal for treating these structures below the epidermal compartment.

Far-UV, Mid-IR, Far-IR

On both sides of the spectrum further outside the visible range lie the far-UV (e.g., 193 Excimer), mid-IR (1320 CoolTouch, 1450 Diode, 2100 Holmium and 2940 Erbium YAGs, 1540 Erbium Glass), and far-IR (10,600 nm CO_2) laser wavelengths. The Excimer, Er-YAG, and CO_2 lasers are all exceptionally well absorbed in tissue, allowing them to be used for precise cutting or ablation tools. Far-UV is absorbed with such extreme efficiency by tissue proteins that it is stopped at the surface of the first compartment with no thermal effect on the epidermal compartment (0.5–2 μm). The Far-IR CO_2 wavelength is so efficiently absorbed that its extinction length is only 0.03 mm in tissue, 30 to 100 times less than the 3 mm for YAG in tissue water, which additionally undergoes marked scattering. The Erbium YAG laser wavelength coincides with the greatest absorption peak of water at 2940 and therefore is absorbed 16 times more efficiently than CO_2 and with one-tenth the thermal injury zone. Erbium and CO_2 have thus found excellent utility in resurfacing, with the caveat that the Erbium requires extended pulsing to achieve a modicum of coagulation.

The remaining mid-IR laser wavelengths are absorbed in water too with moderate efficiencies, much better than Nd-YAG, however with less efficiency than Erbium and CO_2 because they fall off the absorption peaks of water. The Holmium-YAG wavelength at 2100 nm falls at an absorption trough for water such that it penetrates 200 μm, the same as argon at 488 nm. This moderate water transmission, without absorption by hemoglobin, allows it to be used as an ablative tool capable of achieving hemostasis in a bloody fluid medium (e.g., joint surgery). More common dermatologic lasers in this category include the 1320, 1450, and 1540 nm (CoolTouch, SmoothBeam, Er-Glass, e.g., Fraxel) used for milder diffuse fibroblastic injury/stimulation for tightening/rejuvenation, or more focused lesional ablation for scar remodeling, and in sebaceous hyperplasia.

Spot Size

Spot size is another significant tissue optics variable. Optical scattering of visible light at small spot sizes diminishes dermal penetration depth when wavelength is held constant. A broad beam of photons undergoes random scatter such that the center portion of the beam may be slightly intensified relative to the average energy across the beam and may result in a slightly increased effective penetration depth. This phenomenon has been referred to as "tissue-lensing." Meanwhile, photon density at the periphery of the beam is diminished or less intense. Small spot sizes with radii less than the wavelength's 50% penetration depth suffer

markedly reduced penetration depth. For visible wavelength lasers, this effect is most notable at beam diameters of 1 mm or less. Penetration depth for visible spectra lasers is not significantly augmented at beam diameters greater than 3 mm.

Application of Basic Tissue Optics

In selective cutaneous laser surgery, we consider the simplified skin model just presented and find the degree to which specific targeting "fits" the pathology of our individual patients. It is then our objective to deliver light with chromatic, spatial, and temporal characteristics suggested by the model of sufficient magnitude to effect the desired change and minimize risk of unintended or undesirable side effects.

FORMULAS FOR QUANTIFYING LASER ENERGY

A number of terms and their mathematical expressions are crucial to quantify laser energy and its delivery in time and space. The physical importance of these definitions is that, for any given wavelength, the result of light-tissue interactions is both time and energy dependent. Use of a common, standard nomenclature helps us specify laser techniques and parameters that are reproducible, which facilitates research, communication, and practice.

Characterizing the physics of a laser delivery system and its tissue effects includes identifying wavelength, output power, power density, fluence, temporal and spatial beam profile, and finally optical-thermal interactions with tissue (reflection, transmission, absorption, scattering) with subsequent biological responses (damage and healing). See Figure 4 for the major types of laser energy output and temporal profiles.

Power

Power is the rate of photon output of the laser, described as watts equivalent to joules per 1 second, which may be likened to a liquid flow rate past a fixed point, e.g., liters per second. The formula for deriving power is:

$$Power = Watts\ (W) = J/sec$$
$$i.e.,\ Power = Energy/Time$$

Joules, or Total Beam Energy

The joule is the common unit used to quantify light energy. Joules relate to the number of photons in a beam, analogous to moles, which specify the number of particles in chemistry. Joules describe the total energy of a beam by the product of the photon flow rate (power in watts) and the amount of time in seconds. The formula for deriving joules is:

$$Joules = Watts\ (W) \times Seconds = Total\ beam\ energy$$
$$i.e.,\ Energy = Power \times Time$$

Power Density (Irradiance)

Power density or irradiance is the degree of photon concentration, intensity, or density in a spot size in mm^2 at a given rate of delivery (Fig. 16). The more concentrated the photons, the more rapidly they will affect the tissue target. Returning to our liquid analogy, water may flow from a large hose opening or be sprayed under pressure through a smaller opening at the same rate. The higher-pressure (more intense) spray will concentrate more water molecules upon its smallest target surface area (spot size). Similarly, a

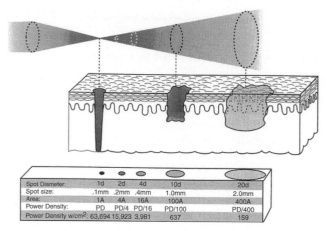

Spot Diameter:	1d	2d	4d	10d	20d
Spot size:	.1mm	.2mm	.4mm	1.0mm	2.0mm
Area:	1A	4A	16A	100A	400A
Power Density:	PD	PD/4	PD/16	PD/100	PD/400
Power Density w/cm²:	63,694	15,923	3,981	637	159

Figure 16 Spot size, power density, and tissue effect. The more concentrated the photons, the more rapidly they will affect the tissue target. The formula for power density, also known as irradiance, relates the flow rate of photons (W) per unit surface area of a circular spot of size (πr^2). Since area is a squared function, doubling the radius leads to a fourfold decrease in power density. Conversely, small decreases in spot size markedly increase power density, suitable for incisions or drilling (0.1-mm spot size). Defocusing to 1- to 3-mm spot size achieves ablation-sized spot tools and intermediate power densities. A very defocused beam of 4 to 6 mm achieves lower power densities suitable for coagulation.

higher-power density beam is capable of doing more work on the smaller surface area. The formula for power density, also known as irradiance, relates the flow rate of photons per unit surface area of a circular spot of size (πr^2). Since area is a squared function, small increases in radius lead to marked decreases in power density. Conversely, small decreases in spot size markedly increase power density. The formula for deriving power density is:

$$\text{Power density} = \text{W/cm}^2 = \text{Power (W)}$$
$$\times (100 \, \text{mm}^2/\text{cm}^2) - \pi r^2 \, \text{mm}^2$$

i.e., Power density = Power/Circular beam area.

Fluence, Energy Density, or Energy "Dose"

Fluence may be thought of as the concentration of laser energy, i.e., total dose of beam energy related to the target surface area. In other words, it is the product of power density and time. Since tissue effects are time and power-density dependent, one must know the independent terms, not just the final product; for example, a laser beam fluence = 100 J/cm² may be derived from either 100 W/cm² × 1 sec or 1 W/cm² × 100 sec. The former would vaporize tissue, while the latter would barely be perceived as warm. The formula for deriving energy density is:

$$\text{Fluence} = \text{J/cm}^2 = \text{W} \times \text{T/cm}^2$$
$$= \text{Power density (W/cm}^2) \times \text{Time}$$

i.e., Fluence = Power × Time/Area.

Average Power, Peak Power, and Duty Cycle

$$\text{Average power} = \text{Output power} \times \text{Duty cycle(\%)}$$
$$\text{Duty cycle} = \text{Laser"on-time"/Total time}$$

i.e., Laser on Plus laser off time.

Some of laser surgery's significant advances in recent years relate to achieving precise, reproducible, energy delivery in

sufficiently short time periods to spatially confine damage to tissue targets while sparing adjacent tissue. Even expert surgeons' manual control of laser exposure time and energy has been shown to vary by orders of magnitude in vitro. Greater precision has been accomplished with a variety of laser hardware strategies to make laser exposure duration very predictable. Laser types and designs vary dramatically in their basic power output, irradiance, and temporal delivery profiles. Power supplies and other electronic means may generate brief, extremely intense peak beam powers. Delivery systems may also interrupt the beam en route to the patient with electromechanical shutters to alter the quantity and temporal delivery of light. The most common terms used to describe these differences are shuttering and chopping, pulsing, superpulsing, and Q-switching (Fig. 4). The basic terms used to describe temporally interrupted beams are total power, average power, exposure duration, interval, and duty cycle. A noninterrupted CW beam has a total power = average power. If the beam is interrupted by an interval time:

$$\text{Total on-time} = T_{\text{total}} = T_{\text{on}} + T_{\text{off}}$$

Until the beginning of the next exposure. Duty cycle can be calculated as follows:

$$\text{Duty cycle} = \frac{T_{\text{total}} - T_{\text{off}} \times 100\%}{T_{\text{total}}}$$

The average power of a periodically interrupted beam is the product of peak power × duty cycle, e.g., 20 W × 25% duty cycle = 5 W average power. Note that the same average power may be obtained from markedly different combinations of peak powers and duty cycles. An average power of 5 W may be obtained from 200 W × 2.5% duty cycle, 100 W × 5% duty cycle, etc. Thus, the total or average power delivered by interrupted beams, whether they are shuttered or superpulsed, is a fraction derived from the percentage on-time multiplied by the peak power.

MANIPULATING POWER AND TIME PARAMETERS TO ACHIEVE SPECIFIC TISSUE EFFECTS

Shuttering or Chopping

Low- to moderate-power, moderate-duration exposures of 0.1 to 2.0 seconds are most correctly referred to as shuttered, chopped, or gated exposures. Average power is reduced by the fraction of laser "on-time" or duty cycle that any time energy flow is cyclically interrupted. It is important to recognize the many clinically significant benefits achievable with conventional lasers operating in the shuttered mode. Reproducible, more precise laser effects are achievable, often with less patient discomfort and greater physician control. 20 W CO_2 lasers shuttered at 0.05 seconds can achieve vaporization with spatial confinement of irreversible peripheral tissue damage to four to five times the CO_2 wavelength penetration depth of 20 μm. This approximates the benefits achieved with superpulsed lasers at a lower cost. Trade-offs may be less flexibility, slower working speed, and smaller spot size.

Pulsing

The term "pulsed" is reserved for extremely short laser emissions with very high peak energies orders of magnitude higher than its average power (e.g., FEDL). However, even expert users will occasionally lapse into applying the term

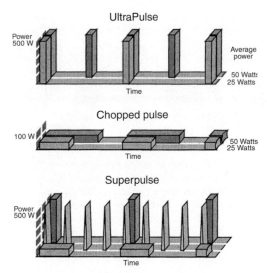

Figure 17 Chopped vs. superpulse vs. UltraPulse™. Three variables are used to characterize noncontinuous pulses of CO_2 laser energy as chopped, superpulsed, or UltraPulse: peak power, duration, and fluence. For a fluence capable of vaporizing 1 cm² of skin, the chopped mode must have the longest duration exposure because of its low peak power; the superpulse has a much higher peak power, therefore an equivalent fluence is reached with an extremely brief pulse duration repeated several times; the UltraPulse sustains the high peak power of the superpulse four to five times longer, obtaining the equivalent fluence in the fewest pulses. *Source*: Courtesy of Coherent Laser Corp.

pulsed to describe low- to moderate-power, shuttered brief exposures on CW lasers. Laser manufacturers have frequently called timed exposures "pulses" on the controls of their CW argon, krypton, tunable-dye, and other lasers. Three variables are used to characterize noncontinuous pulses of CO_2 laser energy as shuttered or chopped, superpulsed, or UltraPulse™, peak power, duration, and fluence (Fig. 17). For a fluence capable of vaporizing 1 cm² of skin, the chopped mode must have the longest-duration exposure because of its low peak power. The superpulse has a much higher peak power, therefore an equivalent fluence is reached with an extremely brief pulse duration repeated several times. The UltraPulse sustains the high peak power of the superpulse four to five times longer, obtaining the equivalent fluence in the fewest pulses.

Superpulsing

Superpulse is a term usually reserved for CO_2 lasers with brief, rapid microsecond pulses (hundreds to a thousand Hertz), capable of achieving ≥ 10 times higher peak powers than non-superpulsed lasers. CW-like results occur at rates approaching 1000 Hz, but at slower repetition rates in the hundreds of Hertz, minimal hemostasis and spatially confined thermal damage plus slower controlled working speeds are features of this type of system. Generally, small spot sizes (1 mm and less) ensure sufficient energy densities to achieve instant vaporization and spatial confinement of thermal damage to 100 µm (0.1 mm) or less, allowing char-free tissue incision or ablation.

A high-energy, radiofrequency-excited CO_2 laser dubbed the UltraPulse achieves spot sizes notably larger (3 mm) while delivering the 5 J/cm² critical energy density needed to achieve vaporization within the skin's thermal

relaxation time (estimated at 600 µsec), or preferably within 1000 µsec (1 msec), are required to vaporize 1 g of water and, therefore, approximately the same for cutaneous tissue, which is 85% water. Note in Figure 4 the relative total energies (~1:5) ratio, areas under the curves of the superimposed superpulse, and UltraPulse waveforms. Both waveforms rise sharply; the superpulse falls off slightly, then drops rapidly to zero. UltraPulse laser waveforms deliver more energy in one pulse, are more flattened indicating longer sustained peak power, until dropping to zero (Fig. 17).

Superpulsed lasers may be applied to wider area ablations, resurfacing similar to the UltraPulse, by employing several strategies, including mechanically scanning a small spot size at impact sites, just slightly offsetting the impulses, or using a larger spot size but superimposing several superpulses in less than the skin's longest thermal relaxation time of 1 msec.

Scanning

The principle of working at or above tissue vaporization threshold to minimize thermal injury is crucial to the application of laser resurfacing. At the time of writing this, the freehand use of miniscule spot sizes with individual pulses makes uniform controlled-depth, large-scale ablation difficult to achieve. However, small spot sizes in CW mode combined with rapid scanning is another practical approach to resurfacing and ablation discussed here.

So currently, two approaches offer an enhanced margin of safety and uniformity relative to traditional freehand CW resurfacing. The two methods are high-energy-density pulses up to several mm in diameter, or scanning a high-power 0.2-mm CW beam very rapidly over the skin (i.e., SilkTouch™ Flashscan, Sharplan); the latter rapid scanning method allows brief tissue exposures and has reliably and practically obtained uniform ablation required for laser resurfacing. Both pulsing and scanning methods are capable in a single exposure of vaporizing 3 mm of tissue to a depth of 50 to 100 µm, with a limited zone of thermal necrosis of 50 to 150 µm. The SilkTouch scans the 0.2-mm beam through a 2- to 5-mm circular area in 0.2 sec (Fig. 18). Since software controls the scan area and shape, elliptical or other shapes

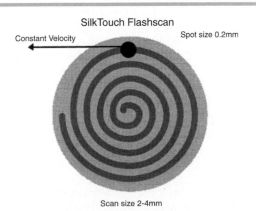

Figure 18 High-intensity scanning for resurfacing. A high-intensity copper vapor laser beam is capable in a single exposure of vaporizing 3 mm of tissue to a depth of 50 to 100 µm, with a limited zone of thermal necrosis of less than 50 µm. The SilkTouch™ scans the 0.2-mm beam through a 2- to 5-mm circular area in 0.2 seconds. *Source*: Courtesy of Sharplan Lasers Corp.

and sizes are possible, facilitating hair transplant-recipient sites and other procedures.

Q-Switching

Q-switching produces extremely high photon intensities (mega to gigawatt peak powers) in extremely short durations (nanoseconds). This is accomplished by using a Pockels cell (polarizing gate) within the laser optical cavity to build up huge quantities of photons, which are suddenly released. Examples are the Q-switched ruby, alexandrite, and YAG lasers. The resultant massive power density results in photo-disruption or photomechanical destruction of small objects with appropriate absorption coefficients and thermal relaxation times.

LASER-TISSUE INTERACTION CATEGORIES: FROM FUNCTIONAL TO ANATOMIC

Clinical effects of lasers occur by the interaction of laser fluence, time, and the relative absorption efficiencies of target chromophores operating under the principles discussed earlier. The physical changes that occur after photon absorption may be classified in three nonlinear functional categories: photochemical (low fluence), photothermal (moderate fluence), or photomechanical (very brief exposure, high fluence). The majority of past laser treatments have been of moderate fluence and poorly selective photothermal nature. Applications of very selective photo-thermolysis, photomechanical (e.g., pigment and lithotripters), and photochemical [e.g., photodynamic therapy (PDT)] mechanisms have increased recently.

Photochemical Principles

The chemical bonds of a tremendous number of common molecules are capable of absorbing a visible-range photon whose energy matches that needed to move the material's electrons to the next energy level (orbital). The total amount of energy therefore is exceedingly low. PDT exploits this principle by using a chemical photosensitizer as an intermediary to maximize the reaction while selectively localizing the effect to specific target sites. The transitional energy is used to generate singlet oxygen, which is highly reactive and therefore exerts a destructive effect on cellular membranes. Lasers are used to generate monochromatic light. Large quantities of it are consistent and may be easily quantified and delivered to varying delimited areas, if necessary via optical fibers. Milder "bio-stimulation" may accelerate, stimulate, or inhibit directly or enzymatically catalyzed processes. While poorly understood and difficult to reproducibly demonstrate, proponents have purportedly utilized light emitting diodes (LEDs) as lasers or noncoherent light to speed healing or stimulate skin for esthetic improvement.

Photothermal Principles

Photothermal effects range on a continuum from protein denaturation and coagulation (>50°C) to vaporization (>100°C), depending on the amount of energy, the delivery rate, and target size. However, very high-power (megawatt) and rapid (≤ nanoseconds) pulsed energy delivery induces nonlinear photomechanical target disruption typified by Q-switched lasers. Cutaneous tissue may recover from brief exposures in excess of 50°C temperatures, thereby decreasing the likelihood or quantity of fibrosis. Absolute temperature and duration are both important in determining reversible laser thermal injuries. Selective photothermolysis spatially confines irreversible thermal injury to the target tissue

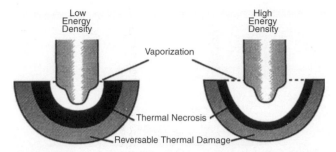

Figure 19   Thermal damage related to fluence and time. Slow heat delivery achieves lower peak temperatures and conducts the heat injury to a broader area around the target before vaporization occurs. Conversely, high-intensity rapid delivery of energy reaches much higher temperatures for shorter periods of time and confines thermal injury closer to the target. Therefore, the surgeon attempting to work at lower energy densities beneath the threshold for vaporization will cause greater thermal necrosis; working at higher power densities restricts damage to the narrowest zone.

(e.g., vessels or pigment) while limiting heat diffusion injury to the surrounding stromal tissue (e.g., collagen, adnexal structures). Inadequate energy delivery or insufficient depth leads to treatment failure, whereas excessive energy delivery may result in scarring and pigmentary and textural changes. Selective photothermolysis surgery techniques operate either in the photothermal or photomechanical realm.

Photothermal effects on tissue depend upon the tissue temperature achieved (and total time): temperatures of less than 50°C for brief periods may cause reversible thermal injury. Temperatures from 50°C to 70°C cause irreversible thermal injury and coagulation; cells reaching 100°C vaporize when their tissue water boils. Prolonged or repeated subvaporization laser exposure over time heats and desiccates tissue and reduces it to carbon. The carbon residue cannot vaporize. It does absorb laser radiation and conducts heat, potentially damaging surrounding tissue and leading to a wider zone of thermal necrosis.

The time course of the elevated temperature is important too. Slow heat delivery achieves lower peak temperatures and conducts the heat injury to a broader area around the target before vaporization occurs. Conversely, high-intensity rapid delivery of energy reaches much higher temperatures for shorter periods of time and confines thermal injury closer to the target. Therefore, the surgeon attempting to work at lower energy densities beneath the threshold for vaporization will cause greater thermal necrosis; working at higher power densities restricts damage to the narrowest zone (Fig. 19).

Selective Photothermolysis and Thermal Relaxation Time

Among the first laser variables to be manipulated for a given laser wavelength was power density. In the 1980s, the emphasis turned to raising peak powers of selectively absorbed wavelengths and limiting exposure time; this strategy delivers photothermal energy to the target in less time than that required to lose 50% of the acquired heat, thus confining thermal damage. In the 1990s, the strategy of combining externally applied cooling to reduce nonselective injury from conduction and competing chromophore absorption was made practical with a wide array of devices. See *Thermal Sparing by Externally Applied Cooling below.*

In brief, absorption of sufficiently concentrated photons during periods equal to or less than a structure's

Table 1 Selected Cutaneous Target Thermal Relaxation Time (T_r) Values

Target	Diameter (μm)	T (nsec)
Melanosome	1	200
Erythrocyte	5	5000
Microvessel	20	140,000
Microvessel (enlarged)	100	3,600,000

thermal relaxation time minimizes thermal loss from conduction to its surroundings. Therefore, peak temperature is reached more quickly at a lower total energy, and less energy is wasted damaging nontarget tissues. Conduction dominates as the mechanism of heat transfer for tissue objects. Surface area is the prime determinant of conductive losses, confirming our experience that small objects exchange heat much faster than large objects (e.g., children gain or lose heat much faster than adults). These physical principles allow calculation of thermal relaxation time T_r, which varies most dramatically by the structure's diameter or thickness D (a squared function) (Table 1). Other terms include the ease of heat diffusion and constants. Note the marked difference in T_r for modest changes in structure size.

$$T_r = G(D^2C)/K$$

Thermal relaxation (cooling time) is proportional to the square of the vessel diameter. Essentially, T_r describes the period required for a structure to lose 50% of its elevated temperature, i.e., the absorbed photothermal laser energy. The FEDL was one of the first laser tools to specifically utilize this principle in tissue (Fig. 20). Subsequently, design of other lasers was based upon this principle for treating other problems with different chromophores, with radically different T_r values.

Photomechanical Disruption

Extremely high-intensity, very short pulses (e.g., nanoseconds) produce photomechanical effects resulting in disintegration of the target and minimal damage to surrounding tissues.

For e.g., ruby, alexandrite, or Q-switched KTP-YAG laser photodisrupting tattoo pigment particles or melanocytes by highly efficient absorption of massive quantities of

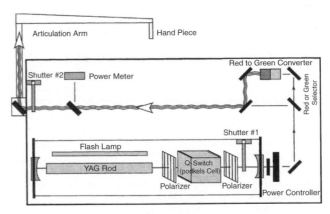

Figure 21 Q-switched KTP-YAG. Q-KTP-YAG adds a "Q-switch" mechanism and frequency-doubling crystal to a basic YAG laser. Similar to the well-known ruby laser, Q-KTP-YAG provides thousands of times greater peak energy in brief delivery time intervals (millions of watts equivalence, 10 nsec) providing selective photothermolysis capabilities, at 1064 or 532 nm, versus the ruby's 694 nm. The Q-switch polarizing Pockels cell mechanism interrupts the optical path, allows a massive photon buildup and then sudden energy release, resulting in high peak power, short pulse width.

photons (Fig. 21). This abrupt photothermal transfer generates nonlinear physical effects, including plasma formation (removal of atomic particle's electrons) and rapid expansion followed by contraction, that propagate mechanical forces (pressure wave) capable of fragmenting the absorbing particle. If the wavelength chosen is very selective for the absorbing chromophore, virtually complete spatial confinement of tissue injury to the target is possible.

Laser-Tissue Interaction: Three Anatomic Categories

In contrast to the functional laser-tissue interaction categories just discussed, analyzing the physics of laser-tissue interaction allows applications to be viewed in three anatomic-level categories: whole organ, tissue-specific surgical lasers, and cell or subcellular specific.

Organ Level

Water is the predominant organ of the skin. Lasers such as the CO_2 and YAG (at moderate energy densities) are similar in affecting many different tissues indiscriminately by raising intracellular and extracellular water temperatures. Depending on the power density and beam size, the same laser may coagulate, cut, or vaporize large or small tissue volumes.

Tissue Level

Tissue-level laser treatments utilize selectively absorbed wavelengths in aspecific tissue, such as vascular tissue, collagen, or an adnexal structure like hair, at moderate peak powers medium exposure durations in the microsecond and millisecond domain. Dissimilar tissues nearby are relatively unaffected by coagulation injury due to either poor absorption of that wavelength, or much shorter thermal relaxation times.

Cell or Subcellular Level

Extremely brief, high energy densities with specific wavelength matching to cell or subcellular organelles allow selective destruction on the cellular or subcellular level. Individual macrophage and pigment particle destruction

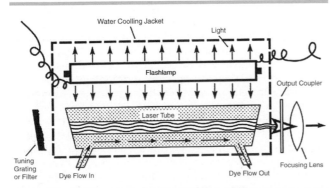

Figure 20 Flashlamp-excited dye laser (FEDLs). FEDLs operate by storing high quantities of energy in a capacitor; sudden energy release powers a very brief intense flashlamp burst to excite laser production in rhodamine dye contained within the laser tube. Filters and resonators may be adjusted in series with the optical cavity to restrict wavelength and extend duration output from the original 450 μsec and 577 nm to the currently desired 585 to 595 nm, 1.5 to 40 msec.

in tattoos or melanosomes in pigmented cells exemplifies the most precise functional category of laser treatment.

Thermal Sparing by Externally Applied Cooling

Externally applied cooling is often valuable and sometimes necessary for patient safety and comfort in laser applications, particularly larger and deeper vascular, hair, and diffused collagen stimulation treatments. Photothermolysis selectivity is not as perfect when clinically applied as it is presented mathematically. Reduced selectivity is often due to competing chromophores in the epidermis; longer exposure times are used to treat a heterogenous group of target sizes, depths, absorption characteristics and to reduce purpura, e.g., vessels; longer exposure times and higher total fluences are used to allow weaker devices to be used, and increase effective treatment percentages in heterogenous hair target colors and depths. Furthermore, rapid pulsing systems and hand-piece design may result in greater risk of overlapping treatment zones injury. Cooling increases the threshold for epidermal injury by reducing the superficial peak temperature and duration in nearby structures and tissues at risk. Caution and proper device and setting selection is still crucial. So far, cooling has not proven sufficient to prevent epidermal damage in darker skin types when paired with shorter IR wavelengths, i.e. 694 to 755 nm. Therefore 1064 to 810 nm is predominately utilized in skin types IV to VI.

Cooling Variables

Cooling mechanisms and the strategies they employ, temperatures reached, phase of cooling, duration, and time to equilibrate are all important variables to be considered when evaluating cooling devices. In-depth physics of cooling mechanisms is beyond the scope of this chapter. However appreciating cooling devices' crucial role in many of today's lasers applications and observing the differences between these devices is important. Too little or too late cooling may impair patient safety and comfort, while excessive cooling may defeat the success of the treatment or even injure the patient.

Cooling Mechanisms

Cooling mechanisms employ the following strategies:

1. Evaporative and conductive cooling used with cold air chillers, cryogenic sprays, hydrogels
2. Conductive contact cooling with hydrogels, cold packs, coolant flow through chilling plate, and piezogenic chilling plate such as sapphire

MECHANISMS AND PHYSICS OF BASIC LASER TYPES

The comparative mechanisms by which current classical lasers and more recent arrivals function can be briefly illustrated by drawings and discussion of four lasers: the tunable argon dye laser (ADL), the FEDL, the metal vapor laser, and the Q-switched KTP-YAG laser. These four lasers illustrate a wide range of various modes of function, including temporal output (CW, quasi-continuous, microsecond pulse, and extremely short Q-switched nanosecond pulse), lasing medium (gas ions, metal vapor ions, organic dye, and solid-state rare earth mineral-doped crystal), and means of excitation (direct current, secondary laser pumping, flashlamp). Two lasers exhibit very different methods of obtaining alternative wave-lengths: the tunable dye laser, with multiple-wavelength secondary laser output, and the

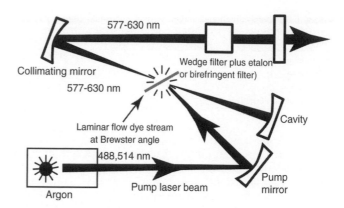

Figure 22 Tunable argon dye laser. The argon laser is used as an optical energy pumping source to excite organic rhodamine dye molecules. The rhodamine dye in turn emits a secondary laser light in the yellow to red range.

KTP-YAG, using frequency doubling to achieve a single alternate wavelength one-half that of the original.

Tunable ADL

The ADL begins with a basic gas tube laser mechanism—similar to the carbon dioxide laser, with argon ions constituting the lasing medium in an optical resonator containing inert gases—and is excited by direct current (Fig. 22). The resultant CW green beam contains both 488 nm blue and 514 nm green laser photons produced by argon. The argon laser is used as an optical energy-pumping source to excite a mixture of organic rhodamine dye molecules. The rhodamine dye mixture in turn emits secondary laser light in the yellow-to-red range. The yellow-range beam (577–585 nm) more closely matches the β-absorption peak of oxyhemoglobin and achieves deeper penetration. The specific mixture of rhodamine has been designed to emit a range of laser wavelengths (577–630 nm) when stimulated by the blue-green laser light. The precise wavelength is selected by adjusting the refraction angle of an optical crystal in the laser light path. The laser surgeon may "tune" or select any wavelength and time exposure within the range of the laser at any time, hence the designation tunable dye. This is in contrast to fixed-wavelength and fixed-pulse-duration dye lasers of the FEDL type, changeable only with major factory servicing modifications to the dye mixture, software, and possibly hardware.

The ADL produces laser light at modest power (1–3 W) as a CW. Electromechanical timed shuttering (comparable to a camera) allows user-selectable exposure times ranging from 2.0 to 0.02 seconds. In laser terminology, low-power brief exposures are most correctly referred to as "shuttered" or "gated" exposures.

The blue-green or yellow-to-red laser light is delivered through an optical fiber or cable. Commonly this is coupled to a hand-piece with interchangeable fixed-focal-length lenses to achieve different spot sizes; even more useful is a focusing hand-piece that can produce spot sizes from 0.05 to 6 mm. Optical cavity alignment is crucial to obtain normal power output. Significant movement of the laser may require a service call for mirror alignment or for replacement of very expensive light-conduction cables that may break when bumped or stretched. Dye replacement may only be necessary every 2 to 3 years, depending on usage, although a replacement every 6 to 12 months is advised by the vendor. This much less frequent dye-replacement rate (compared to FEDL systems) is due to less dye photodegradation at relatively low power argon laser pumping. The longevity, stability, relative simplicity, and large installed base of argon lasers make the cost of purchase, operation, and maintenance moderate compared to other lasers. Tunability allows use in PDT but may require a different dye mixture for optimization of power and prolonged 630 nm output.

FEDL and PLDL

FEDLs operate by storing high quantities of energy in a capacitor; sudden energy release powers a very brief intense flashlamp burst to excite laser production in rhodamine dye (Fig. 20). The rhodamine group allows selection of a dye with a specified wavelength output range. Filters and optical resonators may be adjusted in series with the optical cavity to restrict wavelength and along with multiple combined pulses extend macro pulse duration output to the currently desired 585 to 595 nm, 450 μsec to 1.5 msec to 40 msec. The selection of these parameters depends on whether small superficial oxygenated microvessels or deeper, larger, and more deoxygenated multiply pulsed targets. An approximate 4 to 12 kW peak output is produced. Two main flashlamp designs (linear vs. coaxial) are available in clinical systems. Linear flashlamps excite the dye mainly from one direction, possibly aided by reflecting surfaces. A patented design claimed to be more efficient utilizes a coaxial flashlamp, which surrounds the dye medium with more uniform light. A variation on the FEDL vascular layer used for treating superficial pigmented lesions is PLDL, with parameters of 510 nm, 400 nsec pulse width, 0.5 to 1 Hz, and output of 3 to 5 J/cm². The latter parameters are suitable for some very superficial melanocytic lesions or red tattoo pigments.

The treatment beam is delivered by an optical fiber coupled to a fixed-focal-length handpiece with a 5-mm spot size at a rate of 0.5 to 1 Hz. A 2-mm handpiece and a finger-activated control (alternative to the standard foot pedal) are available. Newer models supply energy more rapidly, with a 7- to 10-mm spot size. Software systems and electronic controls are used to assure safe and accurate energy densities. Software, hardware, or simultaneous problems can cause prolonged treatment interruptions and downtime ranging from 30 minutes to several days. Therefore, the more expensive service contracts with these lasers are indispensable. Long downtimes were common in early models (occasionally several per month). This is very disruptive to patient and physician scheduling. Current models are much more reliable, and scheduled preventative maintenance visits greatly reduce to a manageable level the frequency and severity of downtime. The much higher peak energies used in FEDLs to excite the dye medium cause rapid photodegradation, requiring fresh dye to maintain output levels. Replacement of dye containers should be considered, along with flashlamp replacement and maintenance visits. Competition in the marketplace has stimulated less frequent dye replacement, changes to the hardware, slightly lowering cost and increasing efficiency.

Quasi-CW, Low-Average-Power, Metal Vapor Ion Laser; Excimer Laser

Copper vapor lasers (CVL) (Fig. 23) emit two harmonic wavelengths: 510.6 nm (green) and 578.2 nm (yellow) light. The yellow beam matches the β-absorption peak of oxyhemoglobin. The CVL uses vaporized copper ions as its lasing medium, generated from metal beads in a vaporization

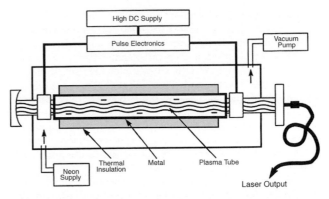

Figure 23 Metal vapor laser. The copper vapor laser uses vaporized copper ions as its lasing media. Electrical energy pumping leads to stimulated emission of extremely brief, very rapidly repeating, moderately high peak power, but low average power pulses. The minimal energy contained in any one 20-nsec pulse, together with the very rapid repetition rate, result in the classification of this as a "quasi-continuous" beam, with clinical effects comparable to continuous wave lasers of similar wavelength.

chamber. Electrical energy pumping leads to stimulated emission of extremely brief, very rapidly repeating, moderately high peak power, but low average power pulses. Power output is 2 to 3 W. Typical pulses have a duration of 15 to 20 nsec, frequency of 15 kHz (15,000/sec), interval of 70 nsec, peak energy of 90 μJ and a peak power of 5 kW. The minimal energy contained in any one brief pulse, together with the very rapid repetition rate, result in the classification of this beam as "quasi-continuous." Shuttered operation allows exposures from 0.05 to 2.0 seconds. Variable-spot-size handpieces allow beam diameters from less than 0.5 mm to greater than 5 mm. Fiberoptic delivery is standard.

Metal vapor lasers must raise the temperature of the lasing medium. This has historically required long warm-up times, commonly 45 minutes. Interruption of the vaporization during treatment may require shorter but noticeable delays to resume treatment. Recently, Cu-Br systems have decreased these drawbacks. The system is not truly tunable but allows switching from yellow to green wavelength for treatment of epidermal melanocytic lesions. Another possibility is substitution of vaporization chamber components (at significant cost) to use a gold tube and produce 628 nm red light suitable for PDT. The Excimer (Excited Dimer) laser uses electron beam pumping of rare gas or halides such as Xenon-Fluoride to produce UV wavelengths used in stimulating repigmentation.

Solid-State Lasers: Q-Switched KTP-YAG and Semiconductor Diode

The Ruby, Erbium, and many other IR lasers function is exemplified by the Nd-YAG (Fig. 21). The Nd-YAG has at its core a crystalline rod composed of an yttrium-aluminum-garnet crystal, doped (incorporated) with a rare earth element known as neodymium (Nd). When the Nd is excited by a high-intensity optical pumping source such as a xenon flashlamp, 1064 nm laser light is generated. The YAG wavelength may be used as is or may be halved [by either a frequency doubling potassium titanyl phosphate (KTP) crystal or a photo-acoustic method], resulting in 532-nm beam output. The green 532-nm beam comes close to the α-absorption peak of oxyhemoglobin. The KTP beam is quasi-continuous, similar to the CVL. Average power peak outputs may be from 5 to 20 W, and minor variations on the following beam specifications occur depending on the make and model. Typical beams have continuous appearing power peaks with duration of 150 nsec, frequency of 5 kHz (5000/sec), and interval of 200 nsec. While the intervals between pulses are three times longer than the CVL, thereby allowing some thermal relaxation, the total energy per pulse is insufficient to accomplish coagulation. Therefore, like the CVL, the energy from a train of pulses must be combined to achieve sufficient temperature for coagulation.

Shuttering and delivery aspects are similar to those for the CVL and ADL. Nd-YAG lasers are touted as solid-state lasers with few moving parts and minimal consumables. No dyes are used. Only the flashlamp-pumping source will need replacement based on use. Many systems are now primarily air-cooled, advantageous where plumbing difficulties exist or mobility is a factor. However, heat generation could be undesirable in smaller rooms or ones with less generous air-exchange and cooling rates. Stability and performance are felt to be strong due to infrequent alignment problems and service requirements. Robotized scanners may be attached for treating large areas with a point-by-point technique.

Q-switched KTP-YAG lasers (Q-YAG) begin with a frequency-doubled KTP-YAG laser; the addition of a Q-switch mechanism provides thousands of times greater peak energy delivery over much shorter time intervals (millions of watts equivalence, 10 nsec) providing selective photothermolysis capabilities at 1064 nm or 532 nm. The Q-switch Pockels cell mechanism interrupts the optical path by rotating the polarity of the laser light as long as power is supplied to the switch. A polarizing filter oriented 90° out of phase with the powered Pockels cell prevents release of optical laser beam. Deactivating the Pockels cell suddenly allows transmission of all of the now-parallel-phase laser energy through the polarizing filter in nanoseconds.

Delivery is through an articulated arm system, with a 2-mm spot size and repetition rate of 1 to 10 Hz. The Nd-YAG laser foundation makes this a solid-state laser with few moving parts without consumables. The flashlamp-pumping source will need replacement based on use, and due to the very high intensity of the beam, optics (chiefly lenses and their coatings) should be regularly inspected. This system is air-cooled, with a liquid radiator heat exchanger. Stability and performance are felt to be strong due to infrequent alignment problems, a stable crystal, and claimed infrequent service requirements.

Diode lasers: Solid-state silicon lasers are produced by precisely aligning a positive and negative "P-N" junction formed by two doped gallium arsenide layers, i.e., a dipole. The N layer donates electrons to the P layer resulting in a unidirectional or forward flow, thus creating ions in the junction region (Fig. 24). The layers need to be optically flat and parallel, with one end mirrored and one partially reflective. The length of the junction must be precisely related to the wavelength of the light to be emitted. The recombination process releases light (electroluminescence) as in the LED (incoherent). At higher current induced energies however, the photons moving parallel to the junction can stimulate emission and initiate laser action. Individual diodes produce low levels of laser energy. But precisely fused arrays can reach much higher cumulative energies. Frequency doubling may be applied to achieve shorter wavelengths. A problem develops when diodes in the array cease functioning and energy output may drop precipitously, since individual diodes in the array cannot be switched. Minimum and mean times to diode failures are critical milestones in anyone considering a diode laser, though reliability and life span of these devices has improved dramatically.

The last five years has seen a greater increase in types of lasers and development of their safe and effective applications than the preceding 35 years. The future is now and has just ushered in "fiber lasers" with multiple optical fibers comprising the optical resonator. This design is already providing for certain mid-IR lasers a 10-fold greater efficiency in laser light generation, much smaller power supplies, and greater stability in optical alignment. Our lasers are also getting "smarter" with auto-sensing of temperature levels, geographic treatment zone recognition and automatic adjustment with feedback to the operator. An understanding of the physics of these proliferating devices makes their selection, use, and proper care safer and more cost effective.

BIBLIOGRAPHY

Alam M, Hsu TS, Dover JS, et al. Nonablative laser and light treatments: histology and tissue effects—a review. Lasers Surg Med 2003; 33(1):30–39.

Anderson RR, Margolis RJ, Watenabe S, et al. Selective photothermolysis of cutaneous pigmentation by Q-switched Nd: YAG laser pulses at 1064, 532, and 355 nm. J Invest Dermatol 1989; 93(1):28–32.

Anderson RR, Parrish JA. Microvasculature can be selectively damaged using dye lasers: a basic theory and experimental evidence in human skin. Lasers Surg Med 1981.

Anvari B, Milner TE, Tanenbaum BS, et al. Selective cooling of biological tissues: application for thermally mediated therapeutic procedures. Phys Med Biol 1995; 40(2):241–252.

Anvari B, Tanenbaum BS, Hoffman W, et al. Nd:YAG laser irradiation in conjunction with cryogen spray cooling induces deep and spatially selective photocoagulation in animal models. Phys Med Biol 1997; 42(2):265–282.

Anvari B, Tanenbaum BS, Milner TE, et al. A theoretical study of the thermal response of skin to cryogen spray cooling and pulsed laser irradiation: implications for treatment of port wine stain birthmarks. Phys Med Biol 1995; 40(9):1451–1465.

Anvari B, Milner TE, Tanenbaum BS, et al. A comparative study of human skin thermal response to sapphire contact and cryogen spray cooling. IEEE Trans Biomed Eng 1998; 45(7):934–941.

Arndt KA, Noe JM, Northam DB, et al. Laser therapy. Basic concepts and nomenclature. J Am Acad Dermatol 1981; 5(6):649–654.

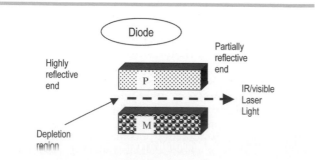

Figure 24 Diode laser. Electrons flow from N to P semiconductor layers creating laser light.

Baumler W, Eibler ET, Hohenleutner U, et al. Q-switch laser and tattoo pigments: first results of the chemical and photophysical analysis of 41 compounds. Lasers Surg Med 2000; 26(1):13–21.

Ben-Baruch G, Fidler JP, Wessler T, et al. Comparison of wound healing between chopped mode-superpulse mode CO_2 laser and steel knife incision. Lasers Surg Med 1988; 8(6):596–599.

Black JF, Wade N, Barton JK. Mechanistic comparison of blood undergoing laser photocoagulation at 532 and 1,064 nm. Lasers Surg Med 2005; 36(2):155–165.

Brunner F, Hafner R, Giovanoli R, et al. Removal of tattoos with the Nd:YAG laser. Hautarzt 1987; 38(10):610–614.

Chang CJ, Anvari B, Nelson JS. Cryogen spray cooling for spatially selective photocoagulation of hemangiomas: a new methodology with preliminary clinical reports. Plast Reconstr Surg 1998; 102(2):459–463.

Chang CJ, Nelson JS. Cryogen spray cooling and higher fluence pulsed dye laser treatment improve port-wine stain clearance while minimizing epidermal damage. Dermatol Surg 1999; 25(10):767–772.

Chernoff G, Slatkine M, Zair E, et al. SilkTouch: a new technology for skin resurfacing in aesthetic surgery. J Clin Laser Med Surg 1995; 13(2):97–100.

Dahan S, Lagarde JM, Turlier V, et al. Treatment of neck lines and forehead rhytids with a nonablative 1540-nm Er:glass laser: a controlled clinical study combined with the measurement of the thickness and the mechanical properties of the skin. Dermatol Surg 2004; 30(6):872–879; discussion 879–880.

Dai T, Pikkula BM, Wang LV, et al. Comparison of human skin opto-thermal response to near-infrared and visible laser irradiations: a theoretical investigation. Phys Med Biol 2004; 49(21):4861–4877.

Dang YY, Ren QS, Liu HX, et al. Comparison of histologic, biochemical, and mechanical properties of murine skin treated with the 1064-nm and 1320-nm Nd:YAG lasers. Exp Dermatol 2005; 14(12):876–882.

Dang Y, Ren Q, Hoecker S, et al. Biophysical, histological and biochemical changes after non-ablative treatments with the 595 and 1320 nm lasers: a comparative study. Photodermatol Photoimmunol Photomed 2005; 21(4):204–209.

Dover JS, Margolis RJ, Polla LL, et al. Pigmented guinea pig skin irradiated with Q-switched ruby laser pulses. Morphologic and histologic findings. Arch Dermatol 1989; 125(1):43–49.

Drnovsek-Olup B, Beltram M, Pizem J. Repetitive Er:YAG laser irradiation of human skin: a histological evaluation. Lasers Surg Med 2004; 35(2):146–151.

Fitzpatrick RE, Ruiz-Esparza J, Goldman MP. The depth of thermal necrosis using the CO2 laser: a comparison of the superpulsed mode and conventional mode. J Dermatol Surg Oncol 1991; 17(4):340–344.

Fitzpatrick RE, Goldman MP, Ruiz-Esparza J. Clinical advantage of the CO2 laser superpulsed mode. Treatment of verruca vulgaris, seborrheic keratoses, lentigines, and actinic cheilitis. J Dermatol Surg Oncol 1994; 20(7):449–456.

Gilchrest BA, Rosen S, Noe JM. Chilling port wine stains improves the response to argon laser therapy. Plast Reconstr Surg 1982; 69(2):278–283.

Greenwald J, Rosen S, Anderson RR, et al. Comparative histological studies of the tunable dye (at 577 nm) laser and argon laser: the specific vascular effects of the dye laser. J Invest Dermatol 1981; 77(3):305–310.

Green HA, Burd EE, Nishioka NS, et al. Skin graft take and healing following 193-nm excimer, continuous-wave carbon dioxide (CO2), pulsed CO2, or pulsed holmium:YAG laser ablation of the graft bed. Arch Dermatol 1993; 129(8):979–988.

Grevelink JM, Duke D, van Leeuwen RL, et al. Laser treatment of tattoos in darkly pigmented patients: efficacy and side effects. J Am Acad Dermatol 1996; 34(4):653–656.

Hammes S, Raulin C. Evaluation of different temperatures in cold air cooling with pulsed-dye laser treatment of facial telangiectasia. Lasers Surg Med 2005; 36(2):136–140.

Ho DD, London R, Zimmerman GB, et al. Laser-tattoo removal—a study of the mechanism and the optimal treatment strategy via computer simulations. Lasers Surg Med 2002; 30(5):389–397.

Hobbs ER, Bailin PL, Wheeland RG, et al. Superpulsed lasers: minimizing thermal damage with short duration, high irradiance pulses. J Dermatol Surg Oncol 1987; 13(9):955–964.

Hoffman WL, Anvari B, Said S, et al. Cryogen spray cooling during Nd:YAG laser treatment of hemangiomas. A preliminary animal model study. Dermatol Surg 1997; 23(8):635–641.

Hohenleutner S, Koellner K, Lorenz S, et al. Results of nonablative wrinkle reduction with a 1,450-nm diode laser: difficulties in the assessment of "subtle changes". Lasers Surg Med 2005; 37(1):14–18.

Hulsbergen Henning JP, van Gemert MJ. Port wine stain coagulation experiments with a 540-nm continuous wave dye-laser. Lasers Surg Med 1983; 2(3):205–210.

Kaufmann R, Hartmann A, Hibst R. Cutting and skin-ablative properties of pulsed mid-infrared laser surgery. J Dermatol Surg Oncol 1994; 20(2):112–118.

Kaufmann R, Hibst R. Pulsed 2.94-microns erbium-YAG laser skin ablation—experimental results and first clinical application. Clin Exp Dermatol 1990; 15(5):389–393.

Kauvar AN. The role of lasers in the treatment of leg veins. Semin Cutan Med Surg 2000; 19(4):245–252.

Kauvar AN, Khrom T. Laser treatment of leg veins. Semin Cutan Med Surg 2005; 24(4):184–192.

Keijzer M, Jacques SL, Prahl SA, et al. Light distributions in artery tissue: Monte Carlo simulations for finite-diameter laser beams. Lasers Surg Med 1989; 9(2):148–154.

Keijzer M, Pickering JW, van Gemert MJ. Laser beam diameter for port wine stain treatment. Lasers Surg Med 1991; 11(6):601–605.

Khan MH, Sink RK, Manstein D, et al. Intradermally focused infrared laser pulses: thermal effects at defined tissue depths. Lasers Surg Med 2005; 36(4):270–280.

Khatri KA, Ross V, Grevelink JM, et al. Comparison of erbium:YAG and carbon dioxide lasers in resurfacing of facial rhytides. Arch Dermatol 1999; 135(4):391–397.

Kilmer SL, Lee MS, Grevelink JM, et al. The Q-switched Nd:YAG laser effectively treats tattoos. A controlled, dose-response study. Arch Dermatol 1993; 129(8):971–978.

Klavuhn KG, Green D. Importance of cutaneous cooling during photothermal epilation: theoretical and practical considerations. Lasers Surg Med 2002; 31(2):97–105.

Lahaye CT, van Gemert MJ. Optimal laser parameters for port wine stain therapy: a theoretical approach. Phys Med Biol 1985; 30(6):573–587.

Lanzafame RJ, Naim JO, Rogers DW, et al. Comparison of continuous-wave, chop-wave, and super pulse laser wounds. Lasers Surg Med 1988; 8(2):119–124.

Laub DR, Yules RB, Arras M, et al. Preliminary histopathological observation of Q-switched ruby laser radiation on dermal tattoo pigment in man. J Surg Res 1968; 8(5):220–224.

Leuenberger ML, Mulas MW, Hata TR, et al. Comparison of the Q-switched alexandrite, Nd:YAG, and ruby lasers in treating blue-black tattoos. Dermatol Surg 1999; 25(1):10–14.

Lupton JR, Williams CM, Alster TS. Nonablative laser skin resurfacing using a 1540 nm erbium glass laser: a clinical and histologic analysis. Dermatol Surg 2002; 28(9):833–835.

McKenzie AL. How far does thermal damage extend beneath the surface of CO2 laser incisions? Phys Med Biol 1983; 28(8):905–912.

Nanni CA, Alster TS. Complications of carbon dioxide laser resurfacing. An evaluation of 500 patients. Dermatol Surg 1998; 24(3):315–320.

Nelson JS, Milner TE, Anvari B, et al. Dynamic epidermal cooling during pulsed laser treatment of port-wine stain. A new methodology with preliminary clinical evaluation. Arch Dermatol 1995; 131(6):695–700.

Nelson JS, Milner TE, Anvari B, et al. Dynamic epidermal cooling in conjunction with laser-induced photothermolysis of port wine stain blood vessels. Lasers Surg Med 1996; 19(2):224–229.

Pikkula BM, Tunnell JW, Anvari B. Methodology for characterizing heat removal mechanism in human skin during cryogen spray cooling. Ann Biomed Eng 2003; 31(5): 493–504.

Pikkula BM, Tunnell JW, Chang DW, et al. Effects of droplet velocity, diameter, and film height on heat removal during cryogen spray cooling. Ann Biomed Eng 2004; 32(8): 1131–1140.

Polla LL, Margolis RJ, Dover JS, et al. Melanosomes are a primary target of Q-switched ruby laser irradiation in guinea pig skin. J Invest Dermatol 1987; 89(3):281–286.

Ramirez-San-Juan JC, Aguilar G, Tuqan AT, et al. Skin model surface temperatures during single and multiple cryogen spurts used in laser dermatologic surgery. Lasers Surg Med 2005; 36(2):141–146.

Ramli R, Chung CC, Fried NM, et al. Subsurface tissue lesions created using an Nd:YAG laser and a sapphire contact cooling probe. Lasers Surg Med 2004; 35(5):392–396.

Rokhsar CK, Fitzpatrick RE. The treatment of melasma with fractional photothermolysis: a pilot study. Dermatol Surg 2005; 31(12):1645–1650.

Ross EV, Sajben FP, Hsia J, et al. Nonablative skin remodeling: selective dermal heating with a mid-infrared laser and contact cooling combination. Lasers Surg Med 2000; 26(2):186–195.

Ross EV. Extended theory of selective photothermolysis: a new recipe for hair cooking? Lasers Surg Med 2001; 29(5):413–415.

Schomacker KT, Walsh JT Jr., Flotte TJ, et al. Thermal damage produced by high-irradiance continuous wave CO2 laser cutting of tissue. Lasers Surg Med 1990; 10(1):74–84.

Sherwood KA, Murray S, Kurban AK, et al. Effect of wavelength on cutaneous pigment using pulsed irradiation. J Invest Dermatol 1989; 92(5):717–720.

Stafford TJ, Lizek R, Tan OT. Role of the Alexandrite laser for removal of tattoos. Lasers Surg Med 1995; 17(1):32–38.

Tan OT, Kerschmann R, Parrish JA. The effect of epidermal pigmentation on selective vascular effects of pulsed laser. Lasers Surg Med 1984; 4(4):365–374.

Tan OT, Murray S, Kurban AK. Action spectrum of vascular specific injury using pulsed irradiation. J Invest Dermatol 1989; 92(6):868–871.

Tannous ZS, Astner S. Utilizing fractional resurfacing in the treatment of therapy-resistant melasma. J Cosmet Laser Ther 2005; 7(1):39–43.

Taylor CR, Gange RW, Dover JS, et al. Treatment of tattoos by Q-switched ruby laser. A dose-response study. Arch Dermatol 1990; 126(7):893–899.

Taylor CR, Anderson RR, Gange RW, et al. Light and electron microscopic analysis of tattoos treated by Q-switched ruby laser. J Invest Dermatol 1991; 97(1):131–136.

Tunnell JW, Torres JH, Anvari B. Methodology for estimation of time-dependent surface heat flux due to cryogen spray cooling. Ann Biomed Eng 2002; 30(1):19–33.

Tunnell JW, Chang DW, Johnston C, et al. Effects of cryogen spray cooling and high radiant exposures on selective vascular injury during laser irradiation of human skin. Arch Dermatol 2003; 139(6):743–750.

van Gemert MJ, Jacques SL, Sterenborg HJ, et al. Skin optics. IEEE Trans Biomed Eng 1989; 36(12):1146–1154.

Venugopalan V, Nishioka NS, Mikic BB. The effect of laser parameters on the zone of thermal injury produced by laser ablation of biological tissue. J Biomech Eng 1994; 116(1):62–70.

Venugopalan V, Nishioka NS, Mikic BB. The effect of CO2 laser pulse repetition rate on tissue ablation rate and thermal damage. IEEE Trans Biomed Eng 1991; 38(10):1049–1052.

Waldorf HA, Alster TS, McMillan K, et al. Effect of dynamic cooling on 585-nm pulsed dye laser treatment of port-wine stain birthmarks. Dermatol Surg 1997; 23(8):657–662.

Walsh JT Jr., Flotte TJ, Anderson RR, et al. Pulsed CO2 laser tissue ablation: effect of tissue type and pulse duration on thermal damage. Lasers Surg Med 1988; 8(2):108–118.

Walsh JT Jr., Deutsch TF. Pulsed CO2 laser tissue ablation: measurement of the ablation rate. Lasers Surg Med 1988; 8(3): 264–275.

Weiss RA, McDaniel DH, Geronemus RG, et al. Clinical trial of a novel non-thermal LED array for reversal of photoaging: clinical, histologic, and surface profilometric results. Lasers Surg Med 2005; 36(2):85–91.

Wheeland RG. Clinical uses of lasers in dermatology. Lasers Surg Med 1995; 16(1):2–23.

Yaghmai D, Garden JM, Bakus AD, et al. Comparison of a 1,064 nm laser and a 1,320 nm laser for the nonablative treatment of acne scars. Dermatol Surg 2005; 31(8 Pt 1):903–909.

Yules RB, Laub DR, Honey R, et al. The effect of Q-switched ruby laser radiation on dermal tattoo pigment in man. Arch Surg 1967; 95(2):179–180.

Zachary CB. Modulating the Er:YAG laser. Lasers Surg Med 2000; 26(2):223–226.

Zelickson BD, Mehregan DA, Zarrin AA, et al. Clinical, histologic, and ultrastructural evaluation of tattoos treated with three laser systems. Lasers Surg Med 1994; 15(4):364–372.

Zweig AD, Meierhofer B, Muller OM, et al. Lateral thermal damage along pulsed laser incisions. Lasers Surg Med 1990; 10(3):262–274.

62

Basic Laser Safety

Timothy J. Rosio

Anew Skin^{TM} Dermatology, Folsom-Auburn, California, U.S.A.

INTRODUCTION

Safety—The Great Intangible

This chapter begins with the question: How does one achieve, or even describe, the intangible "safety" with lasers? Safety describes a nonevent, or the absence of an adverse occurrence. Accident rates or injury risk are described in statistics or probabilities, but as the saying goes, it's 100% if the complication happens to you! Is a 5% occurrence of minor laser injury (e.g., finger burns) less safe than a 0.1% occurrence of severe injuries (e.g., partial blindness) Unfortunately, severe injuries such as blindness often occur to the individual under circumstances very similar to those that have never caused that particular user an injury or complication before. According to a British national study, 67% of injuries are caused by "operator error". Ironically, these low-probability, high-impact events occur at both ends of the experience spectrum: because expert users are lulled into disregarding safety standards or conversely because inexperienced personnel (e.g., students in research facilities) are unaware of proper protection. Dermatology has a rich founding history for medical applications of lasers and leadership in their safe use in the outpatient setting, thanks to the father of laser medicine and surgery being one of our own. Yet, increasing competition in healthcare and regulatory legislation threatens to limit office surgery, the very birthplace of most laser usage, citing flawed safety data. So it is contingent upon us to learn about and use these tools safely, and contribute to studies verifying our track record. Because the public has been conditioned by the media and marketing to expect miracles, and this may lead to dissatisfaction even with a reasonable result, we must also help our patients develop realistic expectations and obtain informed consent, and analyze likely sources of litigation for negligence or less than perfect outcomes.

Entire books have been written on laser safety and it may be discussed from a myriad of perspectives. To summarize, laser injury prevention and minimization relies on a multifactorial interaction between vendors, regulation standards, users, patients, staff, and facilities. But no hardware, regulation, or protocol provides complete safety. Laser safety is only achieved by a continuous state of safety-mindedness on top of safety mechanisms. Safety begins with knowledge. Knowledge of basic laser physics and tissue interaction, preferably obtained in a hands-on laser course, followed by a preceptorship with wavelengths and procedures to be used in practice. We will first look at background information on laser safety standards, followed by laser hazards and organs at risk, dealing with the methods of laser injury and prevention. Then the procedural and technical steps to achieve and maintain a safe operating environment will be summarized, including eye, skin, respiratory, infection, respiratory, mutagenicity, and surgical safety.

LASER SAFETY STANDARDS AND GUIDELINES

Laser Device Hazard Classification

Lasers can be categorized in four main groups and a few subgroups, based on risk of injury potential from the beam. The criteria for classifying lasers into classes I, II, III, or IV are "the capability of the radiant energy of the laser system to injure health care personnel or the patient's body area other than the intended treatment sites, the environment in which the laser system is used, the personnel who may use, or be exposed to, laser radiation, and the nonemission hazard associated with the laser."

It is important to note that safe limits have been defined partially through research on specific wavelengths under specific conditions and partially through calculation and extrapolation of an enormous number of combinations. Safe limits are associated with the term maximum permissible exposure (MPE), based on observations and calculations, plus a safety factor. It may be possible under certain extreme circumstances to cause injury with a certain laser despite meeting safety criteria from its laser hazard class. This includes the aiming beam or ubiquitous laser pointer used in our lectures!.

Class I lasers are safe for viewing even for prolonged periods under normal circumstances. Normal circumstances preclude any additional beam intensification. Class II lasers are of visible wavelength and low-output power that does not exceed the safe limits of radiation within 0.25 seconds, the critical time period required for a nonsedated healthy person to blink or avert their gaze. Certain medical conditions or medications may impair the healthy aversion reflex, leading to the potential for visual damage. Such patients near these sources should be monitored and provided with well-secured passive eye protection, such as opaque corneal shields, goggles, or tape-fixed dressings.

Class II laser examples include the helium–neon (He–Ne) aiming beams on most CO_2 lasers and some radiotherapy devices. Class III lasers must produce less than 0.5 W continuous energy, or for pulsed lasers less than 10 J/cm^2 in 0.25 seconds. Class III lasers must not be capable of causing injuries from diffuse reflected beams. Subclass III-a could cause eye injury if further concentrated by additional optical attachments, e.g., parabolic mirrors or microscopes. Subclass III-b could cause eye injury by direct intra-beam viewing or nonconcentrating reflections.

Most lasers used therapeutically in dermatology are Class IV lasers that comprise lasers with greater than 0.5 W power in 0.25 seconds, or greater than 10 J/cm² or having a potential for eye damage from diffuse reflection. Unconcentrated beams are capable of causing severe eye injury from intra-beam viewing or combustion of materials in or near the operative field.

Regulation and Standards Agencies

A variety of organizations are involved in regulating laser safety standards or issuing safety guidelines. The American National Standards Institute (ANSI) has produced a periodically updated comprehensive guide to medical laser safety, referred to as Z136.3. Institutions are responsible for producing their own laser safety plan, which is customarily overseen by their representative laser safety committee, which in turn is charged with demonstrating effective compliance with the accepted standards of the Joint Commission for Accreditation of Health Care Organizations (JCAHO). Standards emphasize documentation of all aspects of the plan, including physician credentialing and education with specific lasers and procedures, safety protocols, and a quality assurance program reviewing outcomes and indicators. Demonstrations may be demanded onsite to prove effectiveness and familiarity with safety protocols.

The Food and Drug Administration (FDA) governs the approval of laser hardware and procedures and through the Center for Devices and Radiological Health (CDRH) regulates the manufacture of these devices. FDA maintains a list of approved laser wavelengths and applications. Similar to medications, companies are not allowed to promote a laser for an unapproved application (e.g., vascular treatment) despite other approved applications for the same laser (e.g., hair or melanin pigment).

The Occupational Safety and Health Administration (OSHA) deals with work safety hazards such as laser plume, chemical dyes used in certain lasers, etc. Review of this information is mandatory by law for the protection of employees and must be available to them in the form of Material Safety Data Sheets at any time. Additionally, local regulations are derived by individual states. One must check with the appropriate state government office for variable policies comprising registration, facility certification, site specifications and inspections, training and operating requirements, and reporting mandates to responsible agencies. The American Society for Laser Medicine and Surgery (ASLMS) has produced guidelines on training and practice, which have influenced or been significantly incorporated into the published standards of the JCAHO and World Health Organization. ASLMS guidelines are available from the society, which is located in Wausau, Wisconsin.

Documentation and Quality Assurance

"If it isn't documented, it wasn't done" is the JCAHO maxim. Compliance with institutional and regulatory agency requirements is made feasible by series of checklists to ensure documentation and consistency with safety policies. Administrative and safety checklists may be grouped into categories and column headings, such as installation and in-service, credentials and privileges, and preoperative, operative, and postoperative. Much of this information should be cross-referenced for accessibility and accuracy between the patient's medical record, quality assurance reports, laser safety committee reports, and the essential laser logbook.

Laser Logbook

Information recorded should include the following:

- procedure time and date
- assistants and observers present
- pertinent health history and diagnosis
- laser wavelength and type
- average power
- temporal mode (CW, shuttered, pulsed, chopped, Q-switched, etc.)
- power density
- fluence, spot size
- spot profile at tissue (TEM mode)
- delivery system and accessories (fiber, arm, waveguide, etc.)
- pattern of beam application (e.g., superimposed or overlapping spots, number of impulses, CW)
- time duration of treatment (laser on-time)
- cryogen or cooling method and settings (temperature, duration, pre/during/post cycles)
- complications, etc.
- Documentation of the informed consent, photographs, post-op instructions, and entry of information that laser log and checklists were completed, when, and by whom.

Outcome information should be routinely recorded on the chart. Complications should be recorded and quality assurance informed with all pertinent information to facilitate quality improvement. Opportunities for procedural, technical, and hardware improvement can be realized from cumulating and analyzing quality assurance/improvement data.

LASER SAFETY HAZARDS AND CONCERNS

Basic laser safety hazards and concerns comprise the following:

- Protection of the eye and skin
- Avoidance of electrical shock
- Fire hazards, toxic gases, or infectious particles in the plume
- Avoidance of potential chemical injuries due to toxic or carcinogenic substances used in the operation of some lasers
- Laser safety hazards will be discussed individually below

Eye and Skin Damage
Mechanisms of Eye and Skin Injury

The eye is more susceptible to harm in the course of using lasers than is any other organ or tissue. The relative risk to the eye exceeds all others due to its tremendous photon-concentrating ability upon the posterior segment. A 1 W laser beam forms an image 100,000 times brighter than the sun on the retina. The greatest focusing ability derives from the cornea and together with the 25% lens contribution multiplies light intensity 100,000 times! Even aphakic individuals are at risk, because 75% of light concentration occurs at the air-corneal interface. So small amounts of divergent or reflected laser energy, too weak to harm the skin, may nevertheless cause temporary or permanent damage to vision.

Retina

The visible and near-infrared spectrum (400–1400 nm) is mostly transmitted through the cornea, anterior chamber, lens, and vitreous, finally to be efficiently absorbed in the retinal pigment epithelium (Fig. 1). The rate of energy absorption and total quantity will determine whether injury will occur and the severity. A substantial amount of 1060 nm radiation may be tolerated at a low-energy density by the lens due to its relative transparency to that wavelength, and therefore, with minimal risk to it. However, it is the pigmented and vascular layers of the retina that are likely to absorb harmful energy densities, due to the combined focus of the cornea and lens, and the absorption efficiency of melanin and hemoglobin proximal to the delicate photoreceptors. Keep in mind that an injury in a 10° arc near the macula damages the fovea centralis, the central area responsible for visual acuity. Serious acute or subacute retinal injuries include retinal membrane formation, macular contraction, bleeding from rupture of retinal or choroidal vessels, nerve fiber damage, retinal hole with consequent scotoma (visual field defect), and retinal detachment, and any or all may lead to permanent blindness. Disruption of Bruch's membrane (Fig. 1) can cause acute retinal bleeding and detachment, or it may impair vision with neovascularization, similar to the uncontrolled blood vessel growth in severe diabetes. This is particularly dangerous with intense Q-switched exposures due the additional injury of the shockwave.

Chronic intense blue light exposure, too weak to cause acute injury, has been documented to destroy components of color vision. A photochemical breakdown of visual receptor pigments is the mechanism. Note that intense blue light is emitted from heating of char material by infrared lasers, which some believe should be filtered by tinted eye shields instead of completely clear lenses, yet another reason for good technique, including char removal during CO_2 surgery.

Cornea and Lens

The opposite ends of the spectrum, ultraviolet, and far-infrared, are highly absorbed by protein and water, respectively, with potential for injuring the cornea and lens in the anterior half of the eye. The cornea is at acute risk from brief exposure to CO_2, holmium-YAG, erbium-YAG, and excimer lasers, with 10,600, 2000, 3000, and 193–351 nm, respectively. Corneal burns are very painful but usually heal rapidly. More severe burns may leave permanent scars, interfering with vision.

Less severe injuries for both the cornea and lens include acute keratitis (welder's flash), which is briefly painful and may cause enough pain, tearing, and swelling to disable a person for several days. Chronic effects of these wavelengths, and also argon, on the lens may induce cataracts.

Skin Injury and Possible Mutagenicity

Acute burns of the skin may occur from either direct or reflected energy. This may occur at any wavelength, while the depth and severity depends on the effects of wavelength, irradiance, and exposure time. Risk reduction is achieved by use of preset laser shuttered modes, correct power or energy settings, and operative safety protocols. The mutagenicity of certain excimer wavelengths has been researched. KrF, at 248 nm is excluded for human use due to this property. Several excimer wavelengths such as 308 nm for psoriasis and vitiligo theoretically also have some risk but are believed to be less hazardous.

Eye Protection

Of the many factors considered for laser eye protection, wavelength absorption and optical density (OD) are paramount. Historically, the color of eyeglasses could be correlated with the wavelength they are protected against. New materials have led to many lenses that are clear or of

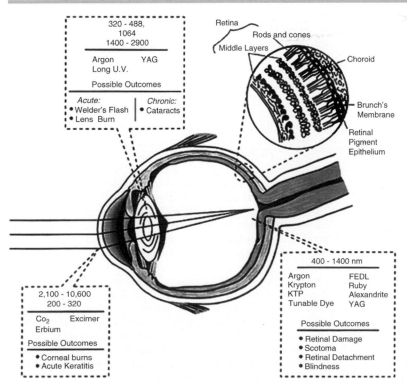

Figure 1 The specific sites of laser-induced ocular damage, listed by wavelength.

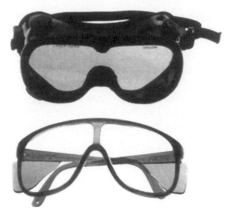

Figure 2 One should never assume the wavelength or optical density of laser safety glasses. Color is not a reliable indicator of wavelength protection. Values should be inscribed on the glasses indelibly.

slight and variable tints. Lasers have increased in power or energy density. Therefore, one must read the inscribed wavelength range of protection and OD (Fig. 2).

OD is expressed in a logarithmic scale indexed to the decrease in transmitted light by a factor of 10 for each increase in the OD. For example, a lens with an OD of two reduces ambient light for the specified wavelength 100-fold; one with an OD of three reduces it one thousand times. MPE data are available for common wavelengths and are ordinarily determined for the worst-case scenario and an additional safety factor added. With increasing availability of multiwavelength lasers, many ask, why not produce glasses that protect against all common wavelengths? More is not always better. If the wavelength range is too broad, vision may be compromised, which is also dangerous.

Correct fit considers coverage from all angles. Gaps in the frame or between the frame and the face may allow damaging beam access to the eyes. Side shields may be added to many glasses to improve protection. Some adjustable lenses or larger goggles fit over prescription lenses to maintain corrected vision. All lenses should be routinely inspected for clarity and defects, including cracks and incipient breaks at temple joints and fixation of lens to frame. Many standard prescription lenses are adequate frontal protection for CO_2 lasers of low to average power. Note that even moderate power CO_2 lasers can burn through plastic lenses in an instant when focused and that contact lenses are inadequate protection.

Patients may be allowed to wear glasses or goggles, particularly if the area of the body treated is away from the face and the wavelength is in the far infrared range. Because much laser surgery is accomplished near the patient's face, opaque goggles, wet gauze, or corneal shields after topical anesthetic is preferred (Fig. 3). Opacity is safer because the eye of the patient is likely to be nearer the focal point of the beam, beam deflection angles are more likely to be toward the patient, and the patient is less likely to be startled by any visual stimulus. However, corneal shields can themselves cause injury through pressure, corneal abrasion directly, or through dried cellulose irregularities, and may become dislodged by cryogenic sprays and other maneuvers.

Eye Examinations and Treatment of Eye Injuries

Eye examinations for personnel working with lasers have been the subject of much controversy. Complications

abound in attempting to differentiate laser-induced lesions from those of other causes; people may have congenital defects or suffer mild injuries without being aware of pain or visual field defects. Focal defects may go undetected by careful ophthalmologic testing even if the central field of vision corresponding to the macula is affected. Furthermore, except for serious injuries, which are immediately recognizable by the patient, no treatment is available. But what about mild cumulative exposures over a long period? Ophthalmologists were discovered to have decreased color sensitivity due to chronic unprotected slit lamp exposure to higher energy blue wavelengths, which caused photobleaching of their cone photoreceptors. This can been prevented by switching to a softer green wavelength. No other group is exposed without eye protection in this manner.

Current recommendations vary by institution, with most following the World Health Organization guideline that no exam is needed unless there is an accidental exposure. An alternative approach recommended by Epstein Photomedicine Institute at Marshfield Clinic is to obtain a baseline eye exam of personnel who will work directly around lasers in operation and repeat the exam on termination or transfer as well as if an incident is reported. The eye exam consists of visual acuity, Amsler grid, anterior segment exam (cornea, iris, lens), and dilated fundus exam (retina). The Amsler grid utilizes very finely spaced lines, which help identify scotomas or defects in the central visual field, which could be caused by endogenous as well as exogenous injuries.

Figure 1 shows eye structures with potential injury sites affected by specific lasers and wavelengths in current use. Many of the newer lasers, for all their ease of use, are potentially more dangerous to the eye than their lower-energy-density predecessors. Clearly, knowledge of injury potential and precautions is required for all who work around lasers. Serious injuries have repeatedly occurred in laboratory settings where safety procedures are not known or followed by the primary personnel or part-time employees and visitors. Keep in mind that lower-power lasers can be as great a threat as high-power ones. Even a 1 W direct hit can damage the eye, in some cases through approved safety lenses!

Recent studies have quantified safety parameters and the likelihood of eye injury from CO_2 beams reflected off surgical instruments. Friedman et al. found that "without the use of eye protection or anodized instruments, there is extreme irreversible ocular hazard . . . within 12 cm of the eye" and a "potential for grade III irreversible corneal damage at reflected beam distances of 30 cm." Anodized instruments decreased the power of reflected laser beam 700 times. Friedman's assumptions of injury likelihood are based on ocular damage studies performed by Borland, in 1971, on CO_2 wavelength injuries to rabbits. Mild injury causing temporary opalescence of the cornea (grade I) similar to welder's flash and snow blindness resolved in 24 hours. This may be treated with lubricants, anti-inflammatory drugs, and cool compresses. Grade II injuries caused epithelial coagulation and loss, requiring seven days to resolve without scarring. Such an injury may require topical steroids and lubricants with an antibiotic, along with compresses, and close follow-up. Grade III injuries were burns involving the substantia propria, which healed with full-thickness scar and visual loss. Treatment of this kind of injury would require corneal transplant after keratectomy.

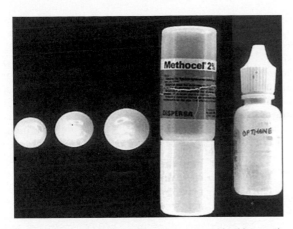

Figure 3 Corneal protectors used in laser surgery should cover the cornea, be opaque, and fit comfortably and snugly under the lids without migrating. They are placed after using topical anesthetic drops (e.g., Opthaine™) and lubrication with viscous methocellulose.

Physical Safety Measures

Fire Prevention and Control

Preparedness is the key to fire prevention and control, because a large variety of items in or near the operative field may be ignited by contact with the beam. All items such should be either fireproof or fire-resistant, and prepared or dealt with in such a way as to minimize and contain flammability. This includes during routine treatment of flashlamp excited dye lasers for port-wine stain birthmarks, especially in the presence of supplementary oxygen.

Flammable substances include patient and staff clothing, hair and operating room hair bonnets, drapes, gauze, cotton applicator sticks, prep solutions containing alcohols, acetone, or other combustible substances, plastics, ointments, oils (including certain makeups), hair preparations (many even when dry, e.g., sprays, mousses), oxygen and many anesthetic gas mixtures, tubing used for endotracheal tubes, intravenous lines, and monitoring equipment. Methane bowel gas is of concern for intra-abdominal or deeper rectal closed spaces, but generally is not a hazard for cutaneous surgeons operating in the peri-rectal area. Preventive steps include restricting all but necessary clothing, drapes, and monitoring tubing, making sure that they are snug fitting and secured next to the body of staff and patients by tucking in, taping, securing with Velcro, snaps, or elastic bands. Flame-retardant materials should be employed in drapes and personnel clothing. Anesthesia and operating room personnel should know the surgeon's preference and operative field approach to locate materials and tubes unobtrusively. Thorough wetting of drapes and gauze adjacent to and underneath the target tissue field should be standard procedure. A basin of water or saline solution should be kept on the tray for rewetting of drapes, packing materials, etc., and for emergencies, along with a fire extinguisher rated for all types of potential fires (electrical, chemical, etc.). Hair near the operative field should be either trimmed or restrained and preferably wet as often as needed with wet Telfa™ or saturated drapes. Even wet gauze can cause a flash fire in the presence of oxygen; therefore, for eyes, wet Telfa is preferable to wet gauze. I have found use of oil-free water-based gels (e.g., K-Y™) valuable in sticking down flyaway hair and maintaining protective moisture. Trimming or shaving hair avoids burning it and

improves visualization and laser penetration to target. You may treat vascular lesions through gel applied to the eyebrow or frontal hairline margin without shaving. Certain hair products such as pomades and sprays containing petroleum-based vinyls and other coating substances are surprisingly flammable. I have seen a miniscule flash ignite a few hairs, which burned to the scalp such as a fast-burning fuse!

Lightly wash hair and scalp on the operating table and wipe with towels to remove these residues.

Masks, endotracheal, and other tubing. Laser-resistant endotracheal tubes and wrapping materials are available, and literature should be reviewed before using them. Clear masks, cannulae, and airway materials are not ignitable with visible light laser even in a 100% oxygen-enriched atmosphere; however, green and other colored airway devices can be ignited in the presence of oxygen. The most likely places for oxygen leaks are near the eye region, where a nose-sealing mask is used, near the nose when nasal cannulae are used, and near the mouth when using endotracheal tubes. Research has established the order of decreasing flammability as polyvinyl Chloride (PVC) tubing (149°F) greater than red rubber (intermediate) greater than Silastic tubing (700°F). Newer flame-retardant plastics are under investigation for their combination of greater stiffness and burning temperature than Silastic. Preferences and application demands prevent unanimity as to the ideal endotracheal tube. Laser-resistant taping is advocated for nonmetallic tubes applied with one-half overlap; an inflatable cuff filled with methylene-blue or other visible nontoxic dye in sterile water provides a tight seal, decompression early warning, and ignition extinguishment.

An oxygen concentration of less than 30% after dilution by mixture with compressed air and nonflammable anesthetic gas is safest; also, flow rate should not be in excess of what is required. Nitrous oxide is an example of a gas as flammable as oxygen in effective concentrations, and halothane burns at high temperatures. The stream of escaping O_2 or other gases should be scavenged or at least diverted away from the operative field, if possible, to minimize support of ignition.

I frequently pack the rectum proximal to my removal of intra- or peri-rectal warts, more to gain control of mucosal walls, as backstop provision, and to prevent entrance of fecal material into the field than from concern about methane gas. Rectal packing material (combustible) should be thoroughly wet before use and lubricated only with oil-free substances (e.g., K-Y gel). The distal portion and retrieval string will need remoistening. Ebonized or "brushed" diffuse reflectance instruments should be utilized in the operative field to minimize ricochet burns and potential ignition of combustible materials nearby. The laser should be placed on standby mode or turned off when not in immediate use.

Infectious and Toxic Airborne Hazards: Protection and Evacuation

Laser surgery hazards include toxic and infectious substances, which become airborne safety risks by vaporization and splatter, constituting the laser plume. Most of these irritating, toxic, potentially infectious, mutagenic, or carcinogenic foreign substances are produced by high temperatures or liberated by physical forces produced by lasers and electrocautery units. A few of the better-known chemical substances are also found in cigarette smoke and include benzene, carbon monoxide, creosols, formaldehyde, free radicals, ammonia, xylene, and hydrocyanide. Carbon particulate matter in smoke, often referred to as soot and causative in black lung, must also be considered. Tomita and Mihaski put laser smoke inhalation risk into perspective by noting that 1 g of CO_2 laser vaporized tissue inhaled is equivalent to smoking three cigarettes (six for electrocautery smoke). Tissue particles from laser treatments may result from vaporization or ejection. Smoke evacuators (with adequate suction and filtration) held within 1 cm of the laser impact site may achieve greater than 98 efficiency in plume removal, but efficiency drops to 50 at 2 cm. Splattered or ejected particles traveling near sonic speeds are caused by rapid thermal expansion or pressure waves. Plume or ejected particles may contain intact DNA, and some studies have demonstrated transfer of viable microorganisms. However, the incidence of warts in CO_2 laser users is no greater than in the general population, indicating that the risks of viral transmission maybe nil if precautions are taken. Clearly, multistep and universal precautions must be taken to protect against airborne and fomite-contactant exposures to potentially harmful substances associated with laser use. Safety points will be further elaborated in the following material.

Smoke Evacuators

The smoke evacuator is the first-line protection against airborne substances. Doubling the distance from 1 to 2 cm from the laser site reduces evacuation efficiency by 50%. Proper integration and use of the following four components including maintenance is also required: vacuum unit, high-efficiency particulate air (HEPA) filter, ultralow particulate air (ULPA) filter, and charcoal filter (Fig. 4). The vacuum must be set high enough to capture all plume, yet not exceed the capacity of the filter series to capture airborne substances. HEPA filters describe first-stage glass fiberglass or glass wool used to trap 0.3-μ particles and water vapor by physical blockage (interception and impaction) with greater than 99.97 efficiency. ULPA filters achieve trapping of particles of 0.1-μ size, but efficiency may vary depending on flow rate, and industry definitions appear up in the air. The activated charcoal filter is used for toxic chemical and noxious odor absorption. Note that charcoal becomes useless once saturated or if air flow rate exceeds its capacity. I noted large

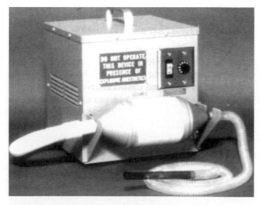

Figure 4 The laser filter should be specifically designed to fit the type of evacuator, rated for the airflow range of the evacuator, and hours of use safely also marked on the filter. This classic smoke evacuator with high-efficiency particulate air and charcoal filter has been superseded by the addition of an ultralow particulate air filter, which increased filtering efficiency rating from 0.3 to 0.1 μm.

particles or pieces of tissue and fluid were generated early in many cases; and frequently along with gauze squares were sucked into the tubing. A procedure I developed in the early days of CO_2 lasers prevents case interruption from accidental suctioning of gauze pads into the apparatus while protecting and extending the life of the filters. I secured a thin layer of 4×4 gauze over the mouth of the suction tubing wand, held tautly by an elastic band or a plastic bar-stool leg cover. I cut off the end of the cover producing a short cylinder with a slightly larger inner diameter than the wand. The short cylindrical cover fit tightly over the suction tubing wand, making a quick attach/release for disposing of inexpensive gauze as a prefilter. Shortly after seeing this, a few companies began marketing similar disposable accessories.

Smoke evacuator filters must be replaced prior to the weakest link becoming saturated, increasing resistance or reducing effectiveness. Units may be rated by time of use, which should be documented on the filter or by sensors that monitor components of the filter. Beware of excessively long tubing, folds, or kinks in the tubing, and filter saturation from particularly high-plume volume cases, which increases resistance and decreases flow rate. Either situation may be manifested by the need to increase vacuum motor settings higher than 50% to 75% speed to maintain adequate plume evacuation. When in doubt, change the filter. You may request an exchange unit while yours is being serviced and evaluated.

Masks

Filtering efficiency means that little if most air flows around (not through) a mask. Moldable nosepiece and flexible side panels that mold to the jaw and cheeks are required for a snug fit. Additional surface area provided by pleating and billowing the mask fabric greatly lowers breathing resistance through the mask. Comfortable fabric surfaces prevent irritation and encourage compliance, along with antifog and moisture-resistant features (Fig. 5). Masks designed for laser use combine electrostatically charged synthetic fibers with traditional filtering mechanics of diffusion, interception, and inertial impaction to achieve 0.1 μ and smaller particle clearance. Combining these mechanisms increases efficiency and decreases breathing resistance. The laser surgeon and staff must understand that multiple factors govern mask-filtering function, and the safety benefits of a mask may not be realized without optimizing snug fit, contour, surface area, comfort, and moisture saturation. It is important that masks be changed between cases or if inadvertently splashed or wet; even during prolonged cases, when the mask may be moistened from respiration or sweating. Electrostatic charge filtering by mask fibers is eliminated when they are wet, thus lowering safety protection of the mask.

Tissue and Fluid Splatter

Lasers may splatter tissue fragments or fluid particles up to sonic velocities, especially the high-energy pulsed lasers increasingly used in removing pigment or resurfacing applications. Smoke evacuators, masks, goggles, and clothing are essential for protection. But manufacturers and users have offered or devised additional products to reduce risk from flying particles, including acrylic tubes, screens, and cones, which largely contain splatter or screen the user from direct flying fragments. Tubes and cones offer more complete protection than screens but should be pressed against the skin to seal. Dressings may be applied prior to treatment. I have seen fragments penetrate through thin membrane materials

(A)   **(B)**

(C)   **(D)**

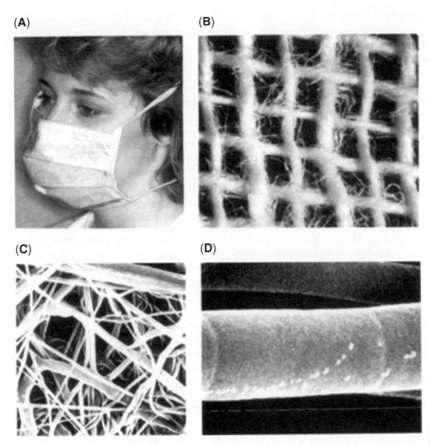

Figure 5 **(A)** The laser mask should fit snugly and comfortably at nose, cheeks, and jaw with no gaps for airflow around the mask. **(B)** Cloth mask II: ordinary cloth fiber masks have large spaces filtering only the largest debris and splatter. **(C)** Laser mask III: 500 x enlargement of laser mask shows densely packed fibers capable of filtering 0.3-um particles. **(D)** Laser mask IV: 10,000 x enlargement of laser mask shows fiber capable of capturing 0.I-μ particles via electrostatic forces, which is dominant for charged particles of extremely low mass.

such as Tegaderm™ and Opsite™. Thicker gel membranes, e.g., Vigilon™, are more effective, particularly with the splatter-prone Q-switched YAG treatments. Despite some reduction in target visualization and energy density results.

Universal Precautions With Biohazard Contaminants

Cleaning, handling, and disposal of areas treated and items used during laser surgery is well outlined by OSHA and professional society guidelines. Specific attention should be paid to surfaces closest to the operative field, such as laser handpieces, protective clothing, lights, and light handles.

STEPS TO CONSISTENT RESULTS AND SAFETY

Environmental Design, Management, Maintenance, and Safety

Room and Door Location, Access, Keys

Selection of rooms in which to use lasers should allow implementation or modifications to achieve the many essential safety factors discussed throughout this chapter, including room access, warning signs, window protection, operating and traffic space, lighting sources, freedom from unexpected visitors and interruptions, fire prevention and burn treatment facilities, and smoke evacuation. Laser rooms are preferably located in controlled-access locations or at least in low-traffic areas. Solitary doors to laser rooms are best to minimize possible entry points. Doors may open inward, outward, or recess or fold. However, laser-location

planning should preclude the surgeon, patient, laser, or ancillary equipment from being struck by an abruptly opened door.

Locks on operating room doors are recognized as a potential hazard to the patient and staff. Therefore, interlocks that prevent laser operating room doors from opening while lasers are in use are seldom installed or employed. Rooms may be locked when not in use, and laser keys are best stored at a separate site rather than with the laser. Such steps control access to expensive and hazardous equipment, preventing unauthorized use and injury.

Space, Equipment, Foot Pedal Arrangement, and Clutter

Adequate space must be allocated for laser procedures. Handpiece, laser arm, or fiberoptic equipment must be able to move freely so as not to obstruct the surgeon during the procedure.

Foot pedals operating power tables, suction, cautery, dermabraders, etc., must not be confused with the laser and vice versa. Rolling stools and chairs must not be capable of activating the laser foot pedal. A metal housing that restricts access to a carefully placed foot pedal is excellent insurance.

Operative Personnel and Observers

Just as nonessential equipment should be aggressively cleared from the perioperative area, so should observers. Each person present is subject to general risks of ocular, pulmonary, and cutaneous injury. Moreover, observers or operative personnel frequently lean on the surgical table or patient, in their efforts to watch the procedure, or may bump or startle the personnel. Changing the relative position of equipment, operator, or laser target may lead to unintended tissue destruction, ricochets, or other hazard to patient or medical staff members. If an emergency occurs, then the less crowded the perioperative area, the faster and more organized the response will be, whether rescue, evacuation, or both are needed.

Laser Warning Signs

Clear, uniform, laser warnings signs with adequate information are crucial to prevent personnel from entering an area with a potential vision hazard. Sign dimensions, letter size, color, etc., shall be in accordance with American National Standard Specification for Accident Prevention Signs (ANSI A35.1). Signs must display the word "Danger" prominently at the top and specify which wavelength is being used, and correct eyewear protection should be located near the sign. This practical consideration lessens the likelihood of personnel knocking on the door and then peeking around the door to ask for protective lenses.

Window Covers

Wavelengths transmissible through window glass must be prevented from leaving the operatory, placing passersby at risk. Therefore, removable or fixed opaque shades or coverings need to be installed on internal or external windows for any rooms posing this type of risk. Removal of focusing lenses or other measures resulting in delivery of collimated beams dramatically increases the degree of risk, even at distance. Operatories several stories above the ground must still consider the presence of nearby rooms with facing unshielded windows as well as the possibility of a window washer.

Lighting

Lighting should be adequate for visualizing the operating field and all other areas of the room. Lights and armatures should not interfere with the laser armature or operator and assistants.

Electrical and Fiber-Optic Hookups and Inspections

Lasers are electrically powered devices storing large amounts of energy capable of discharging even hours after all electrical sources are disconnected. This stored energy has been a source of electrocution of experienced operators inappropriately attempting to investigate or fix their laser, and even authorized repair personnel have been injured.

Proper connections require wiring up to electrical code wall receptacles, grounding, and laser device wiring and plugs. The enormous amount of current some lasers draw requires special wiring specified by the manufacturer, of which most laser users are unaware. Thus, moving some lasers may not be feasible without rewiring or at least determining wiring and receptacles to be compatible with device requirements.

Any defects in electrical wiring or worn spots should be reported and replaced. Areas of frequent bending or pressure from wheeled stools and the like beg for preventive maintenance. Small cracks may continue to function normally until meeting a metal surface or being dragged through a small puddle of water dripping from an instrument stand. Ground fault protection circuits and periodic electrical device leakage testing by trained personnel is insurance against unnoticed or invisible problems.

External fiberoptics from laser devices to handpieces are subjected to similar stresses as electrical wiring. Fibers more commonly cause a loss of delivered laser energy or a loss of precise pattern, which may lead to unintended target exposure when damaged. However, damaged connectors or fibers occasionally lead to potentially injurious laser exposure. If a disconnect leads to a collimated beam being loosed, the potential injury radius (nominal hazard zone) may be much greater than the usual treatment beam, which is strongly defocused after passing through the handpiece lens. Therefore, connectors with the handpiece and fiberoptic junctions with the laser device should be routinely inspected. We have found it helpful with some of our lasers to build an additional protection box to shield the fiber from physical trauma at its exit point.

Water Hoses and Connections

Many laser systems generate considerable heat during operation. This heat is either dissipated by external water cooling or through an internal heat exchanger to air. External water-cooled systems demand a critical volume and flow rate to function properly. Dangers include ruptures, leaks, disconnects, drain backups, sediment plugging internal or external to the laser, and interruptions in water delivery; any of these may lead to electrocution, short-circuit fire damage, water damage to electronics, overheating damage to key components resulting in fires, and physical injury from slipping. Quick-disconnect fittings tested for pressures and type of use at hand are indicated.

Minimum water flow pressure should be guaranteed; otherwise, laser protection circuits may shut down the system when someone on the same plumbing system uses water. Cleaning personnel should be warned against stressing electrical of plumbing connections or, for many laser systems, the laser system itself in any way. Preferably, water supplied for cooling is already sediment poor. However, filters and drains should be inspected periodically to prevent occlusion by debris or sediment.

Communications Devices

Hands-free communications should be incorporated into the laser operatory, allowing surgeons or other personnel to respond to questions without opening the door and to give clear instructions if and when entry is permitted as well as to confirm safety precautions. Convenient communication into the operatory prevents garbled communications through or around the door.

The Laser Safety Officer

Who oversees and troubleshoots the broad variety of safety issues described here while the physician is concentrating on treating the individual patient? The laser safety officer (LSO) is an individual physician, nurse, or technician designated to monitor and manage the safe use of the laser in any particular case and who has the authority to discontinue laser use in a procedure if laser safety or standard of care requirements are not met. There may be several LSOs, who may be designated by the physician or operating room supervisor at the beginning of a case.

The LSO should be thoroughly familiar with all basic principles concerning lasers and laser safety and must accept responsibility for additional administrative duties. LSO administrative duties include reviewing all laser policies and procedures for adequacy and updating as required, documenting implementation and compliance with laser practice standard of care, instituting or updating a continuing staff laser education program, including in-services for new or modified equipment, and monitoring calibration, maintenance, and repair schedules.

Operative Procedures and Techniques

Prep Solutions

Prep solutions should be nonalcohol-based or allowed to dry completely. Iodophors may flash at high temperatures, especially if pooled near the operative site. I recommend removal of chlorhexidine scrub solutions with a water wash or blot due to a report of prolonged tracheobronchitis in laser surgery staff and physician who vaporized a surface area with this prep.

Nonreflective Instruments

Instruments used in the laser operative field (Fig. 6) should be brush finished, which adds many microsurfaces at varying angles; this prevents a concentrated beam from reflecting to nearby tissue with a high-power density. Better than brushed finishes is ebonization, which combines a roughened black finish to avoid specular reflections of the beam. Note that a smooth black finish alone may still reflect far-infrared beams without significant absorption. Businesses provide new or refinish currently owned instruments with these specifications.

Spatulae or other flat, curved, and variable-shaped instruments may be used as backstops (Fig. 7) and tissue-controlling or protective tools. By placing a blocking instrument adjacent to or behind tissue to be excised or ablated, nearby tissue is protected.

Backstops and Heat Sinks

A wet dental roll or gauze may be placed in the naris or labial gingival sulcus overlapping the teeth to protect nearby structures such as nasal mucosa or tooth enamel during laser surgery. Wet large or small cotton-tipped applicators likewise provide a backstop function, which is easily manipulated, offer better tissue traction than metal or plastic instruments, and are more comfortable for the patient in unanesthetized areas. Packing material may be saturated with water, and then coated with a water-based lubricant (no oil allowed!). Curettes are invaluable on the tray to remove charred tissue and to assess tissue character and depth, e.g., when treating warts.

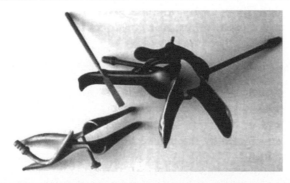

Figure 6 Instruments used in the laser operative field should be brush finish or, better yet, ebonized with a rough black finish to avoid specular reflections of the beam. Businesses provide new or refinished previously owned instruments with these specifications.

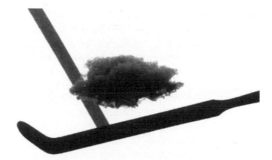

Figure 7 Laser excision with spatula backstop: nearby tissue is protected by a blocking instrument adjacent to or behind tissue to be excised or ablated.

Laser Calibration, Aiming Beam Coaxial Alignment Check, and Fiber Tips

Coaxial alignment checks of invisible beam lasers together with their aiming beams should be performed each day and whenever a laser has been moved from its previous location or sustained a jar or impact to the laser. A tongue blade with a safe, light-colored backstop is regularly used with our CO_2 laser set at 20 W and 0.05-second single pulse. If alignment is correct, the aiming beam travels through the tongue blade burn hole to reveal itself on the underlying backstop. If alignment is incorrect, the aiming beam remains on the anterior surface of the blade surface, somewhere adjacent to the entry hole. Fiber-tipped lasers should be checked at low-aiming beam power on a light-colored surface and defocused. Significant beam asymmetry reveals the need to score and break, then clean the fiber. Q-switched lasers may use burn paper to examine their impact profile.

Lens Focal Length

Short-focal-length lenses reduce power and energy densities in much shorter distances, thereby decreasing the zone of potential injury and severity of injury within a given distance in the operative field. Longer-focal-length lenses make it easier to maintain consistent beam size and power density while excising or ablating tissue.

Equipment and Operator Settings

Laser personnel are advised to use laser equipment whenever feasible in shuttered modes, to practice hand movements with the laser in standby prior to excising or ablating, and thereby to gain better control. Should the patient move or observers jar the surgeon, equipment, or patient, damage control will already have been initiated by the limited exposure.

Smoke Evacuator Methodology

The smoke evacuator should be maintained within 1 cm of the laser treatment site. Tubes should be as short and straight as possible, the filter adequate for the procedure scheduled, and the vacuum setting in the medium range.

Physician and Staff Education

All laser-using physicians and staff members working around or with lasers should have a basic education in relevant laser biophysics and tissue effects, laser systems and their hazard classification, and laser safety protocols to prevent harm to themselves, other health-care providers, and the patient.

Physician Education

Recommended ANSI and ASLMS standards of practice for physician use of lasers in medicine and surgery include both training and experience, which may be obtained in a combination of settings, including residency training, postgraduate training in courses and preceptorships, literature, and audio-visual learning aids. Comprehensive coverage of laser topics, the necessity of hand-eye coordination, and development of clinical judgment are considered so vital to good outcomes and safety that the total education should include (i) courses devoted to laser principles and safety, including physics, tissue interaction, clinical specialty topics, and hands-on experience with lasers (for a minimum total of 8–10 hr) and (ii) a laser preceptorship with a minimum of six to eitht hours of observation with an expert and some hands-on involvement. Documentation of actual cases is very important.

Staff Education

Hospital and clinic nonphysician staff responsible for performing or assisting in laser procedures need a basic understanding of laser physics and tissue interaction; even more, they need in-services on laser hazards, accident prevention, adherence to principles of operatory environmental design, management, and safety as well as practice with safety protocols. In addition to organized didactic information, the following hands-on in-services/courses are vital: demonstrating laser systems to be used; connection, disconnection, cleaning, and maintenance of laser accessories (handpieces, lenses, scopes); gas tank or dye canister-handling and gauge interpretation; set-up and tear-down procedures; calibration; smoke evacuator use and filter changes; sterile and nonsterile draping of the laser for clean versus truly sterile procedures.

The Laser Safety Officer

LSO's duties have been described above. Frequent laser and safety education updates are needed by the LSO to remain current with new technology, be aware of new regulatory guidelines, fulfill staff education duties, and work with quality assurance personnel to ensure compliance with institutional requirements. The LSO should be thoroughly familiar with all basic principles concerning lasers and laser safety and must accept responsibility for additional administrative duties as outlined above.

BIBLIOGRAPHY

Administration. OSHA. Publications of OSHA standards online.

AlHaddad S, Brenner J. Helium and lower oxygen concentration do not prolong tracheal tube ignition time during potassium titanyl phosphate laser use. Anesthesiology 1994; 80(4):936–938.

Anderson RR. Lasers in dermatology—a critical update. J Dermatol 2000; 27(11):700–705.

Baggish MS, Baltoyannis P, Sze E. Protection of the rat lung from the harmful effects of laser smoke. Lasers Surg Med 1988; 8(3):248–253.

Baggish MS, Elbakry M. The effects of laser smoke on the lungs of rats. Am J Obstet Gynecol 1987; 156(5):1260–1265.

Baggish MS, Poiesz BJ, Joret D, et al. Presence of human immunodeficiency virus DNA in laser smoke. Lasers Surg Med 1991; 11(3):197–203.

Bonner RF, Meyers SM, Gaasterland DE. Threshold for retinal damage associated with the use of high power neodymium YAG

lasers in the vitreous. Am J Ophthalmol 1983; 96(2):153–159.

Borland RG, Brennan DH, Nicholson AN. Threshold levels for damage of the cornea following irradiation by a continuous wave carbon dioxide (10.6 millimicron) laser. Nature 1971; 234(5325):151–152.

Cadwell GHJ. A Brief History of the Modern ULPA Filter. Institute of Environmental Sciences. Las Vegas, 1985.

Canestri F. The fluidodynamics of potentially neoplastic plumes produced by medical lasers: first quantitative non-tissue-specific measurements using PMMA samples (phase I). J Clin Laser Med Surg 1999; 17(5):199–203.

Canestri F. Sudden and unpredictable below-surface ablation pattern changes by CO_2 laser beams: a qualitative description of five macroscopic cases observed in PMMA with high probability to occur during surgery in low-water-content tissues. J Clin Laser Med Surg 2002; 20(6):335–339.

Chen SK, Vesley D, Brosseau LM, Vincent JH. Evaluation of single-use masks and respirators for protection of health care workers against mycobacterial aerosols. Am J Infect Control 1994; 22(2):65–74.

Davi SK. Pulsed laser damage thresholds and laser treatment energy parameters, in vivo, of human aphakic intraocular membranes. Lasers Surg Med 1986; 6(5):449–458.

Davis RK, Simpson GT, 2nd. Safety with the carbon dioxide laser. Otolaryngol Clin North Am 1983; 16(4):801–813.

Driver I, Taylor C. The effect of surface finish on the reflection of CO_2 laser beams from specula. Phys Med Biol 1987; 32(2):22735.

Ediger MN, Matchette LS. In vitro production of viable bacteriophage in a laser plume. Lasers Surg Med 1989; 9(3):296–299.

Epstein RH, Brummett RR Jr., Lask GP. Incendiary potential of the flash-lamp pumped 585-nm tunable dye laser. Anesth Analg 1990; 71(2):171–175.

Epstein RH, Halmi BH. Oxygen leakage around the laryngeal mask airway during laser treatment of port-wine stains in children. Anesth Analg 1994; 78(3):486–489.

F.D.A. US. Website for FDA Government Regulations and Information on Laser and Light Devices: http://www.fda.gov/cdrh/comp/eprc.html. U.S. F.D.A. Electronic Product Radiation Control.

Forster W, Scheid W, Weber J, et al. Fluence and mutagenic side effects of excimer laser radiation applied in ophthalmology in human lymphocytes in vitro. Acta Ophthalmol Scand 1997; 75(2):124–127.

Frenz M, Mathezloic F, Stoffel MH, et al. Transport of biologically active material in laser cutting. Lasers Surg Med 1988; 8(6):562–566.

Friedman NR, Saleeby ER, Rubin MG, et al. Safety parameters for avoiding acute ocular damage from the reflected CO2 (10.6 microns) laser beam. J Am Acad Dermatol 1987; 17(5 Pt 1):815–818.

Garden JM, O'Banion MK, Shelnitz LS, et al. Papillomavirus in the vapor of carbon dioxide laser-treated verrucae. Jama 1988; 259(8):1199–1202.

Gloster HM Jr., Roenigk RK. Risk of acquiring human papillomavirus from the plume produced by the carbon dioxide laser in the treatment of warts. J Am Acad Dermatol 1995; 32(3):436–441.

Goldberg DJ. Legal issues in laser operation. Clin Dermatol 2006; 24(1):56–59.

Goldman L. Optical Radiation Hazards to the Skin. In: Safety with Lasers and Other Optical Sources: A Comprehensive Handbook. New York: Plenum Press, 1983.

Goldman L. Plans and goals of the Laser Safety Conference. Arch Environ Health 1970; 20(2):148.

Goldman L. Progress in laser safety in biomedical installations. Arch Environ Health 1970; 20(2):193–196.

Goldman L. Safety programs for current high output laser systems and new systems. Am J Public Health 1974; 64(8):812–813.

Hancox JG, Venkat AP, Coldiron B, et al. The safety of office-based surgery: review of recent literature from several disciplines. Arch Dermatol 2004; 140(11):1379–1382.

Hancox JG, Venkat AP, Hill A, et al. Why are there differences in the perceived safety of office-based surgery? Dermatol Surg 2004; 30(11):1377–1379.

Institute AANS. Standards for lasers and light devices: Z136: http://www.z136.org/.

Khodadoust AA, Arkfeld DF, Caprioli J, Sears ML. Ocular effect of neodymium-YAG laser. Am J Ophthalmol 1984; 98(2):144–152.

Laser safety eyewear. Health Devices 1993; 22(4):159–204.

Laser use and safety. Health Devices 1992; 21(9):306–310.

Liu B, Rubow KL, et al. Performance of HEPA and ULPA Filters. Institute of Environmental Sciences. Las Vegas, 1955.

Mainster MA. Damage mechanisms, instrument design, and safety. Ophthalmology 1983; 90:973.

Mainster MA, Sliney DH, Belcher CD, Buzney SM. Laser photodisruptors. Damage mechanisms, instrument design and safety. Ophthalmology 1983; 90(8):973–991.

Matchette LS, Faaland RW, Royston DD, Ediger MN. In vitro production of viable bacteriophage in carbon dioxide and argon laser plumes. Lasers Surg Med 1991; 11(4):380–384.

Matchette LS, Vegella TJ, Faaland RW. Viable bacteriophage in CO_2 laser plume: aerodynamic size distribution. Lasers Surg Med 1993; 13(1):18–22.

Matsumoto T, Yoshida D, Tomita H. Determination of mutagens, amino-alpha-carbolines in grilled foods and cigarette smoke condensate. Cancer Lett 1981; 12(1–2):105–110.

McBurney EI. Side effects and complications of laser therapy. Dermatol Clin 2002; 20(1):165–176.

McCullough NV, Brosseau LM, Vesley D. Collection of three bacterial aerosols by respirator and surgical mask filters under varying conditions of flow and relative humidity. Ann Occup Hyg 1997; 41(6):677–90.

McCullough NV, Brosseau LM, Vesley D, Vincent JH. Improved methods for generation, sampling, and recovery of biological aerosols in filter challenge tests. Am Ind Hyg Assoc J 1998; 59(4):234–241.

McGhee CN, Craig JP, Moseley H. Laser pointers can cause permanent retinal injury if used inappropriately. Br J Ophthalmol 2000; 84(2):229–230.

Mohr RM, McDonnell BC, Unger M, Mauer TP. Safety considerations and safety protocol for laser surgery. Surg Clin North Am 1984; 64(5):851–859.

Moseley H. Operator error is the key factor contributing to medical laser accidents. Lasers Med Sci 2004; 19(2):105–111.

Moseley H. Ultraviolet and laser radiation safety. Phys Med Biol 1994; 39(11):1765–1799.

Moseley H, Davison M, Allan D. Beam divergence of medical lasers. Phys Med Biol 1985; 30(8):853–857.

Organizations JCAHO. website: http://www.jcaho.org/.

Pahlajani N, Katz BJ, Lozano AM, et al. Comparison of the efficacy and safety of the 308 nm excimer laser for the treatment of localized psoriasis in adults and in children: a pilot study. Pediatr Dermatol 2005; 22(2):161–165.

Passeron T, Ortonne JP. Use of the 308-nm excimer laser for psoriasis and vitiligo. Clin Dermatol 2006; 24(1):33–42.

Patel K, Hicks JN. Prevention of fire hazards associated with use of CO_2 lasers. Anesth Anal 1981; 60:885–888.

Prendiville PL, McDonnell PJ. Complications of laser surgery. Int Ophthalmol Clin 1992; 32(4):179–204.

Raulin C, Grema H. Psoriasis vulgaris. An indication for lasers? Hautarzt 2003; 54(3):242–247.

Rodriguez JG, Sattin RW. Injuries as an adverse reaction to clinically used laser devices. Lasers Surg Med 1987; 7(6): 457–460.

Rose RF, Yeung SR, Sheehan-Dare R. Deflection of an eye shield by the cryogen cooling spray causing a cryogen-induced conjunctivitis in a patient receiving treatment with the pulsed dye laser. Lasers Surg Med 2005; 36(1):1.

Rupke G. Vigilance, education are keys to overcoming laser safety complacency. Aorn J 1992; 56(3):523–525.

Sliney DH. Laser safety. Lasers Surg Med 1995; 16(3): 215–225.

Sliney DH, Mainster MA. Potential laser hazards to the clinician during photocoagulation. Am J Ophthalmol 1987; 103(6): 758–760.

Sliney DH. Neodymium: YAG laser safety considerations. Int Ophthalmol Clin 1985; 25(3):151–157.

Sosis MB. Evaluation of a new laser-resistant operating room drape, eye shield, and anesthesia circuit protector. J Clin Laser Med Surg 1993; 11(5):255–257.

Sosis MB, Braverman B. Advantage of rubber over plastic endotracheal tubes for rapid extubation in a laser fire. J Clin Laser Med Surg 1996; 14(2):93–95.

Surgery AASoLMa. Standards of Practice, Care, Training, Courses. Link to ASLMS home page.

Thach AB, Lopez PF, Snady-McCoy LC, et al. Accidental Nd:YAG laser injuries to the macula. Am J Ophthalmol 1995; 119(6):767–773.

Tomita Y, Mihashi S, Nagata K, et al. Mutagenicity of smoke condensates induced by CO_2-laser irradiation and electrocauterization. Mutat Res 1981; 89(2):145–149.

Toon S. Doctors using lasers risk problems without proper training, protection. Occup Health Saf 1988; 57(7):30.

Vassiliadis A. Ocular Damage from Laser Radiation. New York: Plenum Press 1971.

Wheeland RG. The pitfalls of regulating office-based surgery by state legislatures and boards of medical examiners. Semin Cutan Med Surg 2005; 24(3):124–127.

Wheeland R, Bailin PL, et al. Use of scleral eye shields for periorbital laser surgery. J Dermatol Surg Oncol 1987; 13(2):156–158.

Willey A, Anderson RR, Azpiazu JL, et al. Complications of laser dermatologic surgery. Lasers Surg Med 2006; 38(1):1–15.

63

CO₂ Laser Treatment of Epidermal and Dermal Lesions

Leslie C. Lucchina

Department of Dermatology, Brigham and Women's Hospital and Harvard Medical School, Boston, Massachusetts, U.S.A.

Suzanne M. Olbricht

Department of Dermatology, Lahey Clinic, Burlington, Massachusetts and Department of Dermatology, Harvard Medical School, Boston, Massachusetts, U.S.A.

BACKGROUND

The use of the CO_2 laser in dermatology has greatly altered the path by which we treat many skin diseases and understand wound-healing processes. The CO_2 laser emits far-infrared light at a wavelength of 10,600 nm and is absorbed by water. Directing CO_2 laser light energy on skin results in a heating and vaporization of intracellular water resulting in tissue vaporization. This tissue interaction can be harnessed by mechanical and/or manual manipulations of the beam, allowing for predictable vaporization. CO_2 laser systems have been shown to be quite useful in the successful treatment of many epidermal and dermal skin lesions where there is no specific target chromophore other than water.

The earliest CO_2 lasers, used clinically since 1960s, delivered the energy as a continuous wave beam. At that time, it was appreciated that if the energy of the CO_2 laser is emitted as a tightly focused beam with very high power densities, highly localized thermal destruction is produced which can be precisely directed using a terminal attachment to produce cutting. If the beam is unfocused and of a lower power density, it can be directed with precision to ablate cutaneous lesions. Ablation produced by the CO_2 laser occurs through vaporization and coagulative necrosis and is modified by wound healing.

Further studies defined the nature of thermal damage created by CO_2 laser energy. Although the energy of continuous wave CO_2 lasers is absorbed in the upper 20 mm of a layer of water, skin absorption and evidence of thermal damage is affected by several factors: scatter of the laser energy in the tissue, spot size of the laser beam at the tissue surface, duration of exposure, and the amount of water within the tissue. Early instrumentation allowed for mechanical control of power output; however, spot size was controlled manually. As a prism in the hand piece focused the beam, holding the hand piece closer or farther from the skin could create effective spot sizes from 0.1 to 6 mm in diameter with varying power densities at the tissue surface. In addition, power density was affected by duration of exposure which was controlled by a mechanical shutter, foot pedal, or manual movement of the energy across the tissue surface. Despite these variables, for most clinical uses,

it is assumed that continuous wave or shuttered pulsed CO_2 laser energy penetrates tissue 1 mm. In a guinea pig model, a laser beam with a power density of 10 kW/cm², easily obtained with a 30 W commercially available CO_2 laser, takes 12.5 ms to penetrate 1 mm of skin in vivo. A laser beam with a power density of 1 kW/cm² takes 125 ms to do so. The duration of energy delivery affects both vaporization and adjacent thermal damage. The volume of tissue vaporized varies directly with the power density at the tissue level. The width of the zone of thermal damage of the adjacent tissue (coagulation) is directly proportional to the duration of exposure. If exposure times are shorter than the time it takes the heated tissue to cool (termed thermal relaxation time), adjacent thermal damage is minimized, because there is no excessive heat energy available for diffusion. Therefore, a short laser exposure time with a high power density vaporizes the same volume of tissue as a longer exposure at a lower power density, but with much less adjacent thermal damage. Tissue damaging temperature elevations have been recorded as far as 2 mm from the wound edge. The area of adjacent thermal damage largely determines the extent of the wound and subsequent healing processes.

During 1990s, CO_2 lasers with very short pulses (1 ms) and high peak powers sometimes attached to rapid scanners were developed using the earlier principles. Pulsed and rapid beam scanner CO_2 lasers allow the rapid and precise ablation of tissue (20 mm of skin) with minimal residual thermal damage (50–150 mm) because the thermal relaxation time of the target tissue is 1 ms, a time, that is, slightly longer than the pulse duration of the laser. The development of mechanical means to control duration of exposure to laser energy opened up new applications for the use of CO_2 lasers such as resurfacing (Chapter 29). However, many of the techniques used in the 1980s remain useful in the treatment of some skin lesions.

CLINICAL INDICATIONS

Table 1 identifies cutaneous disorders that may be successfully treated with the CO_2 laser. Laser treatment is the first

Table 1 Epidermal Skin Lesions that May Be Treated by Ablation with the CO_2 Laser

Actinic keratosis
Condyloma acuminatum
Epidermal nevus
Inflammatory linear verrucous epidermal nevus
Familial benign pemphigus (Hailey-Hailey disease)
Keratosis follicularis (Darier-White disease)
Lichen sclerosis
Porokeratosis
Verruca plantaris
Verruca vulgaris

choice for some of the disorders because of the ease of the procedure, effectiveness, and minimal amount of surrounding tissue damage. The CO_2 laser may also be used as an alternative method of treatment for other cutaneous disorders in which the laser treatment achieves clinical results similar to results obtained by more conventional means, but facilitates the procedure, making it easier for the patient and the surgeon. The CO_2 laser may offer an additional therapeutic option for some patients with lesions that have not responded to conventional medical or surgical therapies.

In the past 30 years, there have been many reports of skin disease treated with the CO_2 laser. Over this time period, many new lasers have been developed that have been shown to yield better results in the treatment of many skin lesions such as vascular lesions, lentigines, and tattoos. Frequent use of the laser for some procedures has also redefined its utility. For example, there have been reports of using the CO_2 laser in the cutting mode for the removal of simple lesions such as a pilar cyst or keloid. It is now appreciated that the ease of treatment and results are not different than the use of cold steel scalpel excision. Although superpulse and ultrapulse capabilities have broadened the utility of the CO_2 laser, some procedures are still more effective when done with a continuous wave beam or shuttered continuous wave beam. Ablating a wart successfully requires vaporizing and coagulating a large volume of tissue, which is more quickly produced by a continuous wave laser. If a CO_2 laser is being used for its hemostatic properties for cutting or ablation, a continuous wave or long pulse CO_2 laser should be used.

Epidermal and Mucosal Lesions

Epidermal and mucosal lesions are easily accessible to treatment by the CO_2 laser. CO_2 laser ablation is the treatment of choice for actinic cheilitis. Secondary to excessive sun exposure, actinic cheilitis is characterized histopathologically as atypical epidermal cells that are confined to the squamatizing mucosa of the lower lip. The CO_2 laser is used to ablate rapidly and precisely a thin layer of mucosal lower lip. The coagulated tissue and thermal debris separate in three to seven days. Re-epithelialization occurs within four weeks. Morbidity is minimal and results are excellent. Cytologic atypia is absent at six months. Scarring is usually not seen. The incidence of charring is minimized by the selection of laser parameters that result in vaporization and not charring. With experience and dexterity, the surgeon can use the continuous wave beam for this procedure. The use of the superpulse laser has also been described and may allow for faster healing. It is useful to

note that a very superficial wound will heal quickly but may not be sufficient for cure.

Other epidermal processes for which the CO_2 laser is an effective treatment include squamous cell carcinoma in situ of the penis (erythroplasia of Queyrat) and vulva. Also reported is the use of the continuous wave CO_2 laser in the treatment of squamous cell in situ of the fingers. At these anatomically difficult surgical sites where there is a lack of hair follicles allowing extension of atypical cells more deeply in the tissue, superficial ablation of the lesion with surrounding wide margins is produced quickly and heals well. Balanitis xerotica obliterans, Zoon's balanitis, oral florid papillomatosis, oral leukoplakia, and sublin-gual keratoses may be treated in a similar fashion. The CO_2 laser has also been used to treat epidermal diseases that have failed medical therapy or are not amenable to conventional surgical excision, although the mechanism by which improvement occurs is not clear. These diseases usually have a superficial dermal component, and successful ablation probably extends to at least some coagulative changes at that tissue level. Disorders in this category include epidermal nevus, inflammatory linear verrucous epidermal nevus, porokeratosis of Mibelli, lesions of familial benign pemphigus (Hailey-Hailey disease), keratosis follicu-laris (Darier-White disease), and lichen sclerosus et atrophicus. Paget's disease of the skin often located in the genitalia can be treated this way though the patients need to be followed closely as extension occurs along adnexal structures and may give rise to reoccurrence if the coagulative changes do not extend to that level.

Human Papillomavirus Disease

The CO_2 laser has been used extensively in the treatment of the manifestations of human papillomavirus (HPV) infection, verruca vulgaris, verruca plantaris, condy-loma acuminatum, and Bowenoid papulosis. HPV is a family of at least 70 known subtypes that cause epithelial or mucosal hyperplasia and may cause squamous cell atypia as is best described for Bowenoid papulosis. For some subtypes, evidence has mounted for the progression to frank carcinoma in cervical and anogenital lesions, in immunosuppressed patients, and even in otherwise healthy patients. Given that the pathologic process resides on the surface, it appeared that treatment using the CO_2 laser would be effective; however, cure rates vary from 32% to 70% with the lower figures in studies of recurrent warts. The significant recurrence rate of warts after treatment with the CO_2 laser is not entirely clear. However, it may be related to the persistence of the virus in clinically adjacent uninvolved skin. In a study of women with vulvar warts, the HPV was found a centimeter from lesional skin.

There is considerable morbidity associated with the carbon laser treatment of warts located on glabrous skin. The wound healing time is two to three weeks for wounds on the hands and three to six weeks for wounds on the feet. Complications include significant post-operative pain, temporary loss of function, atrophic scarring, and rarely infection and hypertrophic scarring. For patients with mucosal or anogenital lesions, the morbidity may be less than for other means to treat the lesions and scarring is usually not seen. Given these considerations, CO_2 laser treatment of warts may be best reserved for those warts recalcitrant to other means of treatment, warts that are particularly large and bulky, or warts that are anatomically located where the use of the CO_2 laser may facilitate treatment.

In particular, extensive areas of involvement in the ano-genital skin can be treated easily. For large, exophytic and bulky warts, the CO_2 laser may be used to first cut excessive tissue followed by vaporization.

As the rate of recurrence is high, the patient should be aware that the HPV would probably not be eradicated and long-term observation must be done in treated patients where there is potential for malignant degeneration.

Dermal Lesions

Dermal lesions that are extensive and at least partially extrude above the surrounding normal epidermal surface are particularly well suited for treatment with CO_2 vaporization. In comparison to standard surgical excision and closure or electrosurgery, the use of the CO_2 laser allows for faster removal of a greater number of lesions. Even atrophic scarring after treatment of multiple or confluent tumors may be a marked cosmetic improvement. Good results are reported for the treatment of adenoma sebaceum and angiofibromas in tuberous sclerosis, apocrine hidrocysto-mas, cylindromas, leiomyomas, neurofibromas, syringomas, trichilemmomas of Cowden's disease, pearly penile papules and tricho-epitheliomas. Other dermal lesions that have been treated successfully with the CO_2 laser include chondrodermatitis nodularis helicis, granuloma faciale, hidradenitis suppurativa, myxoid cyst, nodular amyloidosis, pyogenic granuloma, xanthomas, and xanthelasma (Table 2). The CO_2 laser may add another therapeutic choice in difficult to treat diseases such as lichen sclerosis. While lymphangioma circumscriptum has been treated with relative success, the process is usually fed by deep vascular abnormalities and may recur at some point.

The first laser treatment of tattoos was with the CO_2 laser used to vaporize overlying epidermis, then the pigment was removed in part by vaporization and in the slough of tissue that was coagulated. At best, a thin atrophic scar resulted when healing was complete. Most tattoos are treated now with Q-switched wavelengths that are specific for the pigment and do little damage to the epidermis, although the complete

Xanthoma or nearly complete removal of pigment commonly requires six to eight treatments. There remain, however, some indications for the use of the CO_2 laser, for example, Q-switched laser resistant tattoos or tattoo pigment that darkens when treated with a Q-switched laser, and tattoos complicated by reactions to the pigment. In addition, the CO_2 laser generally removes the tattoo in one treatment though wound care is required for several weeks. It is, therefore, a satisfactory treatment for patients who prefer minimal number of treatments and do not mind the formation of a scar.

Rhinophyma is hypertrophy of the sebaceous glands of the nose commonly associated with rosacea in middle aged to elderly men. It is easily treated with the CO_2 laser. The excess tissue is first removed by cutting with the CO_2 laser and the nose is then reshaped by ablation of the surface. Re-epithelialization occurs rapidly, within three to four weeks, thought to be from epidermal cells at the base of the hair follicles. The surface is often somewhat shiny and atrophic; however, when the entire cosmetic unit of the nose is treated, it blends in well. Care must be taken when treating the ala because over-treatment causes contraction and distortion of both the ala and the nostril opening which is often somewhat spatulous even before treatment.

Treatment of dermal lesions requires careful attention to the intended volume of tissue destruction, taking into account vaporized tissue as well as coagulative necrosis that sloughs post-treatment. Enough tissue has to be vaporized or coagulated for the lesion to be ablated. Generally this means that a scar is produced, although in some areas where the skin heals very well, such as the eyelid, the scar may not be apparent. Scarring may be minimized when a pulsed or rapidly scanned CO_2 laser system is used; however, an experienced operator will be able to produce the same result more quickly using a continuous wave beam manipulated manually.

Advantages and Limitations

In the appropriate clinical setting, the use of the CO_2 laser has many advantages. Tissue can be vaporized rapidly and precisely with effective hemostasis. A sterile wound bed is created. Hyperkeratotic debris and nail may be ablated more easily than with other destructive modalities. Bone can also be ablated, although significant charring is produced. The laser does not interfere with pacemakers or monitoring devices.

There are limitations to using the CO_2 laser for treatment of epidermal and dermal lesions. Reproducibility of technique and results is limited because of variables such as nonuniform size and shape of lesions as well as the changing thickness of tissue compartments depending on anatomic site. For ablative procedures, it is not possible to precisely calculate power densities and duration of exposure for each treatment. Of particular note, when the CO_2 laser is used for ablation, no tissue specimen is available for evaluation by the dermatopathologist. Hence, any lesion of questionable diagnosis should be biopsied and sent for histopathologic evaluation prior to treatment with the CO_2 laser. When the laser is used for cutting, the specimen obtained may be sent to pathology and it is generally possible to evaluate all but the last 0.5 to 1 mm of the margins for residual tumor.

CO₂ Laser Safety

All personnel within the laser workspace must be trained in the safety procedures and policies regarding the use of the CO_2 laser. Each office or institution should have training and credentialling processes prior to personnel assisting in surgery utilizing a laser.

The room in which the CO_2 laser is used must have several safety features that vary from a usual procedure room. The door must be posted with warning signs. There should be as few reflective surfaces as possible and any reflective surfaces present including windows must be covered. Fire extinguishers must be readily available. Surgical tools should be nonreflective or have a black coating to prevent deflection of the laser beam.

During a laser procedure, the door must be closed and posted for active laser use. Some safety officers recommend

Table 2   Dermal Lesions that May Be Treated by Ablation with the CO_2 Laser

Adenoma sebaceum	Neurofibroma
Angiofibromas	Pearly penile papules
Angiokeratoma	Pyogenic granuloma
Apocrine hidrocystoma	Sebaceous hyperplasia
Chondrodermatitis nodularis helices	Syringoma
Granuloma faciale	Trichoepithelioma
Hidradenitis suppurativa	Tricholemmoma
Lymphangioma circumscriptum	Xanthelasma
Myxoid cyst	

that the room be locked from within. All personnel in the laser treatment room must wear laser surgical masks which filter particles as small as 0.1 mm. For the treatment of lesions of infectious etiology, such as verruca vulgaris, the patient must also wear a mask. When a CO_2 laser is used, all personnel and the patient must wear clear plastic or glass safety goggles to avoid corneal damage. CO_2 laser treatment around the eyes requires nonreflective metal eye shields to be placed over the patient's sclerae. The patient or personnel should not wear jewelry. No flammable materials, such as alcohol, should be used or located within the workspace. There should be no dry sponges in the treatment field. Normal saline or sterile water soaked sponges and drapes should be placed around the treatment area. Water must be readily available. A high efficiency smoke evacuator that filters particles as small as 0.1 mm should always be used with the suction hose within 1 cm of the treatment area.

Unfortunately, reports of unintentional burns to the personnel or the patient, fire, and laryngitis secondary to a failed smoke evacuator system have all been reported.

TECHNIQUE

The surgeon relies on visual inspection of the treatment site after each pass of the laser and wiping the site with wet then dry sponges in order to determine the extent of the lesion and surrounding tissue damage. The surgeon may need to alter the laser parameters as the treatment progresses depending on the clinical results. The power density may be varied by changing the power output, beam configuration, spot size, movement speed of hand piece, or shuttering the laser beam. These changes may be done either by hand or with the use of a mechanical scanning device.

Clinically, during the first pass with a CO_2 laser, vaporization of skin results in a white and slightly scaly surface. Once the treated area is gently wiped with a wet sponge, the epidermis may still be visible if the treated lesion is particularly thick or the power density was very low and the speed of movement was very fast. If the epidermis is thin and a greater power density is delivered, the superficial dermis is seen with normal dermatoglyphic markings. When the dermis is heated or vaporized, visible collagen contraction is noted. If coarse and woven collagen bundles are seen, the tissue has been ablated into the deep dermis. If ablation is continued further, subcutaneous fat will be obvious. If charring is seen, there has been slow tissue burning at very high temperatures resulting in heat diffusion to surrounding tissues rather than tissue ablation. Charring is therefore not desired.

Optimal use of the CO_2 as an ablative instrument includes many steps. First, the laser surgeon must determine the desired clinical end point which varies depending on the lesion treated. Actinic cheilitis is successfully treated when the end point of coagulation or white discoloration of the entire external lower mucosal (Table 3) lip is seen. The clinical end point for the treatment of an epidermal nevus is evidence of some coagulation in the dermis under the ablated area. The clinical end point for the treatment of a plantar wart is the presence of normal dermis under the visible wart as well as 5 to 10 mm surrounding it.

The clinical end point for the treatment of small appendageal tumors of the face includes vaporization of epidermis and dermis to a depth just beneath the surrounding uninvolved skin.

Table 3 Mucosal Lesions that May Be Treated by Ablation with the CO_2 Laser

Actinic cheilitis
Balanitis xerotica obliterans
Bowenoid papulosis
Squamous cell carcinoma of the penis (erythroplasia of Queryat)
Oral florid papillomatosis
Oral leukoplakia
Sublingual keratosis
Zoon's balanitis

With a surgical marking pen, the lesion(s) is outlined with appropriate margins. Anesthesia is administered and may include local infiltration, regional blocks, or sedation. After reviewing a list of laser safety procedures and testing the beam on an inaminate object such as a tongue blade, the laser surgeon focuses the laser beam at the treatment site and the procedure is begun. Air brush-like movements with the defocused laser beam of the continuous wave CO_2 laser or discrete pulses of the pulsed or rapidly scanned CO_2 laser create visible vaporization and/or coagulation. At the completion of the first pass with the laser beam, the treatment site is gently wiped with a normal saline or sterile water soaked sponge to remove tissue fragments, char, or coagulum after which the area is blotted dry with a sterile sponge. A judgement is then made by the laser surgeon to continue with the same laser parameters or to modify them. Each individual site and lesion to be treated will vary, even within the same site or lesion, in many characteristics affecting the laser injury including thickness of normal skin, thickness of lesion, amount of tissue fluid, and amount of tumescence from anesthesia. Skilled laser technique means being aware of and utilizing these differences, and constantly modifying the energy parameters for an optimal result. Vaporization and debridement are then repeated until the desired clinical end point has been achieved.

The quantity of tissue ablated depends on the power output, exposure duration and spot size diameter at the skin surface, and movement speed of the hand piece. When using

Table 4 Technique for the Treatment of Plantar Warts

Surgical plan—end point is the ablation of the plantar wart and 5–10 mm of surrounding uninvolved epidermis.
Demarcation—treatment margins are outlined with a surgical marking pen.
Anesthesia—local infiltration of 1% lidocaine with epinephrine into the treatment area. Regional block may also be useful.
Preparation—place normal saline or sterile water soaked sponges and drapes around treatment area.
Set laser parameters—power output 15–25 W, waveform (continuous wave, pulsed or scanned), spot size (defocused beam with spot size of 3–5 mm at skin surface).
Vaporization—move hand piece with air brush-like movements over wart and surrounding epidermis to margins.
Debridement—curettage large pieces of desiccated wart from surface. Wipe treated area with a normal saline or sterile water soaked sponge then blot with dry sponge.
Repeat vaporization and debridement as necessary until normal dermis is identified.
Dressing—bacitracin ointment, sterile nonadherent dressing, and tape.
Post-operative instructions—wash area with soap and water, apply bacitracin and dressing twice daily. Elevation of foot, post-operative shoe, and crutches may be necessary to avoid weight bearing.

(A) **(B)**

(C) **(D)**

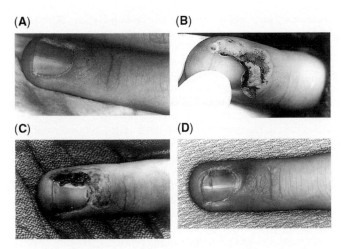

Figure 1 **(A)** Periungal wart, preoperative view, **(B)** periungal wart, immediately after ablation, with coagulation of surface and some char visible, **(C)** periungal wart, immediately post-procedure, and **(D)** periungal wart, eight-week followup.

the CO_2 laser in the continuous wave mode, a defocused beam is maintained by keeping the hand piece further away from the skin than the focal length of the lens. In doing so, the spot size is increased thereby delivering the same amount of power to a greater surface area. This results in less tissue damage. The use of the CO_2 laser in the continuous wave mode with a defocused beam is demonstrated in the treatment of a plantar wart. An epidermal lesion, the plantar wart requires extensive ablation to prevent recurrence (Table 4, Fig. 1). This is in comparison to the treatment of the syringomata. A dermal lesion, the syringoma is small, well circumscribed, and typically located on the face where the skin is consistently thin. Treatment of the syringomata includes using a pulsed or rapidly scanned CO_2 laser system that uses very short pulses of energy to precisely ablate the lesion (Table 5). When treating a superficial mucosal lesion such as actinic cheilitis, continuous wave with a

defocused beam, pulsed or rapidly scanned CO_2 lasers may be used. Treatment includes ablating a very superficial layer of mucosa (Table 6).

The CO_2 laser is also used in the cutting mode followed by vaporization to treat extensive epidermal and dermal lesions. This treatment is commonly used in the treatment of rhinophyma, where the focused CO_2 laser beam is used to excise the nodular portion of the nose followed by the defocused CO_2 laser beam to reshape the nose

Table 6 Technique for the Treatment of Actinic Cheilitis

Surgical plan—end point is the coagulation or white discoloration of the entire external lower mucosal lip.

Demarcation—vermilion border is outlined with a surgical marking pen.

Anesthesia—mental block with 2% lidocaine, local infiltration into the superficial submucosa, particularly at lateral commissures with 1% lidocaine with epinephrine.

Preparation—place a normal saline or sterile water soaked sponge over teeth and cutaneous lower lip.

Set laser parameters—power 15 W, waveform (continuous wave, pulsed or scanned beam), spot size (defocused beam with spot size of 4–5 mm at skin surface).

Vaporization—quickly, move the hand piece with air brush-like quality along the lower lip, starting within the mouth and proceeding to the vermilion border. The epidermis will "bubble." One or two slightly overlapping passes are typically sufficient. The hand piece is being moved too slowly if char is noted. Debridement—wipe treated area with a normal saline or sterile water soaked sponge then blot with a dry sponge.

Repeat vaporization and debridement if thick or scaly areas persist.

Dressing—bacitracin ointment.

Post-operative instructions—wash area twice daily with soap and water, apply bacitracin several times daily while awake.

Table 7 Technique for the Treatment of Rhinophyma

Surgical plan—the endpoint is a sculpted nose, with ablation deep or superficial of the entire nasal unit. Nodules may be aggressively obliterated, treatment of ala and tip should be a less aggressive as contraction will occur with healing.

Demarcation—nodular areas are outlined with a surgical marking pen.

Anesthesia—paranasal sensory nerve block with 2% lidocaine, local infiltration into the nose with 1% lidocaine with epinephrine as needed.

Preparation—place normal saline or sterile water soaked sponges and drapes around treatment area.

Set laser parameters for the initial excision of nodular areas with the focused CO_2 laser beam—power 20–25 W, waveform (continuous wave, pulsed or scanned beam), spot size at focal point.

Excision—direct the beam parallel to the surface of the nose to excise the nodular and pedunculated areas on the nose. Grabbing the nodules with forceps or towel clamps may facilitate cutting.

Debridement—wipe treated area with a normal saline or sterile water soaked sponge then blot with a dry sponge.

Set laser parameters for the vaporization of the nose with the defocused CO_2 laser beam—power 20–25 W, waveform (continuous wave, pulsed or scanned beam), spot size 3–5 mm.

Vaporization—quickly, move the hand piece with air brush-like quality over the nose.

Debridement—wipe treated area with a normal saline or sterile water soaked sponge then blot with a dry sponge.

Repeat vaporization until the contour is appropriate and the surface is smooth, taking into account the postlaser coagulum slough. Sebaceous glands or their oily products may be visible in the wound bed. Dressing—bacitracin ointment, sterile nonadherent dressing, and tape.

Post-operative instructions—wash area twice daily with soap and water and reapply bandage.

Table 5 Technique for the Treatment of Syringomas

Surgical plan—end point is the ablation of syringoma to a depth just beneath the surrounding uninvolved skin surface.

Demarcation—syringoma is outlined with a surgical marking pen.

Anesthesia—local infiltration into the superficial dermis (just enough to raise a bleb) with 1% lidocaine with epinephrine.

Preparation—place normal saline or sterile water soaked sponges and drapes around the treatment area.

Set laser parameters—power 15 W, waveform (shuttered continuous wave, pulsed or scanned beam at 0.1–0.2 sec), spot size (defocused beam with spot size of 2–3 mm at skin surface). The spot size may be adjusted manually with the diameter of the lesion.

Vaporization—direct the shuttered beam to the lesion with 1 or 2 pulses.

Debridement—wipe treated area with a normal saline or sterile water soaked sponge then blot with dry sponge.

Repeat vaporization and debridement, as necessary to reach desired end point.

The remaining eyelid epidermis may be superficially vaporized in order to blend any pigment changes caused by the treatment.

Dressing—bacitracin ointment.

Post-operative instructions—wash area with soap and water then apply bacitracin twice daily.

(A)   **(B)**

(C)   **(D)**

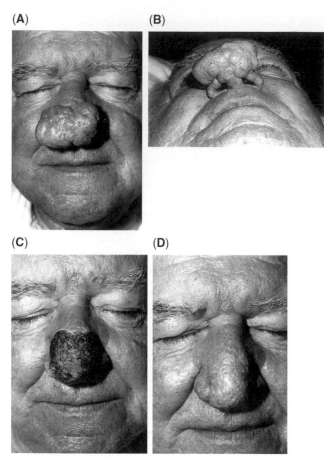

Figure 2   (**A**) Rhinophyma, preoperative view, (**B**) rhinophyma, preoperative view, (**C**) rhinophyma, immediately post-procedure, and (**D**) rhinophyma, 6 months followup.

(Table 7, Fig. 2). It is of utmost importance that the laser surgeon be conservative in the amount of tissue removed from the site in order to minimize the risk of hypertrophic scarring and unilateral alar lift.

Large and bulky veruccae may be treated in a similar fashion. However, as described in the treatment of warts (Table 4), it is important to ablate an area of clinically normal appearing skin around the wart lesions (Table 6).

Wounds created by vaporization with a CO_2 laser heal by secondary intention with a time frame dependent on the anatomic location and the depth of the treatment. A surgical dressing is selected, that is, appropriate for the size and anatomic location of the wound. Written wound care instructions are always reviewed and given to the patient.

COMPLICATIONS

The most frequently noted complication of CO_2 laser treatment is the development of a scar that may be either atrophic or hypertrophic. In addition, intraoperative or post-operative hemorrhage, excessive pain, prolonged healing, and infection can occur. Events reported rarely include reactive tissue processes post-operatively such as excess granulation tissue, pyogenic granuloma, and lip mucocele.

To hasten wound healing and minimize scarring, the laser surgeon must select the appropriate CO_2 laser waveform and laser parameters, pay attention to surgical technique and apply appropriate wound care. Although CO_2 laser wounds heal by secondary intention, excellent wound care is essential. The wounds are cleansed twice daily with soap and water, rinsed well, and patted dry. An antibacterial ointment is applied followed by a sterile nonadherent dressing and sponge that are taped in place. A bio-occlusive dressing such as Vigilon (CR Bard, Murray Hill, New Jersey, U.S.A.) or Duoderm (Convatec, Princeton, New Jersey, U.S.A.) may be used as an alternative for wounds not on the face and may speed re-epithelialization. Topical care is continued until complete re-epithelialization occurs which may be as long as six weeks depending on the anatomic location and the size and depth of the wound. Wound care should be continued beyond re-epithelialization to minimize scar tissue formation. This includes moisturizing and massaging the wound area. Constant pressure items such as compression earrings, tailor-made pressure garments as well as splints may deter hypertrophic scarring.

CONCLUSION

The CO_2 laser is useful for the treatment of many epidermal and dermal lesions where there is no specific target chromophore other than water. The relevant issues in the treatment of epidermal and dermal lesions with the CO_2 laser include maintenance of safety procedures, knowledge of the clinical end point of treatment, selection of appropriate laser waveform and laser parameters, and optimal wound care.

BIBLIOGRAPHY

Adamson R, Obispo E, Dychter S, et al. High incidence and clinical course of aggressive skin cancer in heart transplant patients: a single-center study. Transplant Proc 1998; 30:1124–1126.

Alora, Anderson RR. Recent developments in cutaneous lasers. Lasers Surg Med 2000; 26:108–118.

Anderson RR, Parrish JA. Selective photothermolysis: precise microsurgery by selective absorption of pulsed radiation. Science 1983; 220:524–527.

Apfelberg DB, Druber D, Maser MR, et al. Benefits of the carbon dioxide laser for verruca resistant to other modalities of treatment. J Dermatol Surg Oncol 1989; 15:371–375.

Baggish MS. CO_2 laser surgery for condyloma acuminata venereal infection. Obstet Gynecol 1980; 55:711–715.

Baldwin HE, Geronemus RG. The treatment of Zoon's balanitis with the carbon dioxide laser. J Dermatol Surg Oncol 1989; 15:491–494.

Bar-Am A, Shilon M, Peyser MR, et al. Treatment of male genital condylomatous lesions by carbon dioxide laser after failure of previous non-laser methods. J Am Acad Dermatol 1991; 24:87–89.

Becker DW. Use of the carbon dioxide laser in treating multiple cutaneous neurofibromas. Ann Plast Surg 1991; 26:582–586.

Bellina JH. The use of the carbon dioxide laser in management of condyloma acuminata with eight-year follow-up. Am J Obstet Gynecol 1983; 147:375–378.

Bickley LK, Goldberg DL, Imaeda S, et al. Treatment of multiple apocrine hidrocystomas with the carbon dioxide laser. J Dermatol Surg Oncol 1989; 15:599–602.

Boyce S, Alster TS. CO_2 laser treatment of epidermal nevi: long-term success. Dermatol Surg 2002; 28:611–614.

Bragg JW, Ratner D. HPV type 2 in a squamous cell carcinoma of the finger. Dermatol Surg 2003; 29:766–768.

Calkins JW, Masterson BJ, Magrina JE, et al. Management of condyloma acuminata with the carbon dioxide laser. Obstet Gynecol 1982; 59:105–108.

Carpo BG, Grevelink S V, Brady S, et al. Treatment of cutaneous lesions of xanthoma dissemi-natum with a carbon dioxide laser. Dermatol Surg 1999; 25:751–754.

Christenson LJ, Smith K, Arpey CJ. Treatment of multiple cutaneous leiomyomas with carbon dioxide laser ablation. Dermatol Surg 2000; 26:319–322.

Christian MM, Moy RL. Treatment of Hailey-Hailey disease (or benign familial pemphigus) using short pulsed and short dwell time carbon dioxide lasers. Dermatol Surg 1999; 25:661–663.

David LM. Laser vermilion ablation for actinic cheilitis. J Dermatol Surg Oncol 1985; 11:605–609.

Del Mistro A, Chieco Bianchi L. HPV-related neoplasias in HIV-infected individuals. Eur J Cancer 2001; 37:1227–1235.

Dover JS, Arndt KA, Geronemus RG, et al. Illustrated cutaneous laser surgery. A Practitioner's Guide. East Norwalk, CT: Appleton & Lange, 1990:98–104.

Dover JS, Arndt KA, Geronemus RG, et al. Illustrated cutaneous laser surgery. A Practitioner's Guide. East Norwalk, CT: Appleton & Lange, 1990:21–73.

Dufresne RG, Garett AB, Bailin PL, et al. Carbon dioxide laser treatment of chronic actinic cheilitis. J Am Acad Dermatol 1988; 19:876–878.

Dufresne RG Jr., Garrett B, Bailin PL, et al. Carbon dioxide laser treatment of traumatic tattoos. J Am Acad Dermatol 1989; 20:137–138.

Eliezri YD. The toluidine blue test: an aid to the diagnosis and treatment of early squamous cell carcinoma of mucous membranes. J Am Acad Dermatol 1988; 18:1339–1349.

Ewing TL. Paget's disease of the vulva treated by combined surgery and laser. Gynecol Oncol 1991; 43:137–140.

Fader DJ, Ratner D. Principles of carbon dioxide and erbium laser safety. Dermatol Surg 2000; 26:235–239.

Finley EM, Ratz JL. Treatment of hidradenitis suppurativa with carbon dioxide laser excision and second intention healing. J Am Acad Dermatol 1996; 34:465–469.

Fitzpatrick RE, Goldman MP. Carbon dioxide laser surgery. In: Goldman MP, Fitzpatrick RE, eds. Cutaneous Laser Surgery: The Art and Science of Selective Photothermolysis. St. Louis: Mosby, 1994:198–258.

Frame JW. Treatment of sublingual keratosis with the carbon dioxide laser. Br Dent J 1984; 156:243–246.

Fulton JE, Shitabata PK. Carbon dioxide laser physics and tissue interaction in skin. Lasers Surg Med 1999; 24:113–121.

Greenbaum SS, Glogau R, Stegman SJ, et al. Carbon dioxide laser treatment of erythroplasia of Queyrat. J Dermatol Surg Oncol 1989; 15:747–750.

Haas AF, Narurkar VA. Recalcitrant breast lymphangioma circumscriptum treated by ultra-pulse carbon dioxide laser. Dermatol Surg 1998; 24:893–895.

Hamzavi I, Lui H. Excess tissue friability during carbon dioxide laser vaporization of nodular amyloidosis. Dermatol Surg 1999; 25:726–728.

Hernandez-Hernandez DM, Omlas-Barnal D, Guido-Jimenez M, et al. Association between high-risk human papillomavirus DNA load and precursor lesions of cervical cancer in Mexican women. Gynecol Oncol 2003; 90:310–317.

Hrebinko RL. Circumferential laser vaporization for severe metal stenosis secondary to balanitis xerotica obliterans. J Urol 1996; 156:1735–1736.

Hruza GJ. Laser treatment of warts and other epidermal and dermal lesions. Dermatol Clin 1997; 15:487–506.

Huilgol SC, Neill S, Barlow RJ. CO₂ laser of vulvar lymphangioma circumscriptum. Dermatol Surg 2002; 28:575–577.

Janniger CK, Goldberg DJ. Angiofibromas in tuberous sclerosis comparison of treatment by carbon dioxide and argon laser. J Dermatol Surg Oncol 1990; 16:37–320.

Jensen P, Hansen S, Moller B, et al. Skin cancer in kidney and heart transplant recipients and different long-term immunosuppressive therapy regimens. J Am Acad Dermatol 1999; 40:177–186.

Johnson PJ, Mirzai TH, Bentz ML. Carbon dioxide laser ablation of anogenital condyloma acuminata in pediatric patients. Ann Plast Surg 1997; 39:578–582.

Johnson TM, Sebastien TS, Lowe L, et al. Carbon dioxide laser treatment of actinic cheilitis: clinicohistopathologic correlation to determine the optimal depth of destruction. J Am Acad Dermatol 1992; 27:737–745.

Kang WH, Kim NS, Kim YB, Shim WC. A new treatment for syringoma. Combination of carbon dioxide laser and trichloracetic acid. Dermatol Surg 1998; 24:1370–1374.

Karim AM, Streitmann MJ. Excision of rhinophyma with the carbon dioxide laser: a ten-year experience. Ann Otol Rhinol Laryngol 1997; 106:952–955.

Kartamaa M, Reitamo S. Treatment of lichen sclerosis with carbon dioxide laser vaporization. Br J Dermatol 1997; 13: 356–359.

Leshin B, Whitaker DC. Carbon dioxide laser matrixectomy. J Dermatol Surg Oncol 1988; 14:608–611.

Logan RA, Zachary CB. Outcome of carbon dioxide laser therapy for persistent cutaneous viral warts. Br J Dermatol 1989; 121:99–105.

Magid M, Garden JM. Pearly penile papules: treatment with the carbon dioxide laser. J Dermatol Surg Oncol 1989; 15:552–554.

Malek RS. Laser treatment of squamous cell lesions of the penis. Lasers Surg Med 1992; 12:246–249.

McElroy JA, Mehregan DA, Roenigk RK. Carbon dioxide laser vaporization of recalcitrant symptomatic plaques of Hailey-Hailey disease and Darier's disease. J Am Acad Dermatol 1990; 23:893–897.

McKinlay JR, Graham BS, Ross EV. The clinical superiority of continuous exposure versus short-pulsed carbon dioxide laser exposures for the treatment of pearly penile papules. Dermatol Surg 1999; 25:124–126.

Molin L, Sarhammar G. Perivulvar inflammatory linear verrucous epidermal nevus treated with CO₂ laser. J Cutan Laser Ther 1999; 1:53–56.

Nanni CA, Alster TS. Complications of cutaneous laser surgery. A review. Dermatol Surg 1998; 24:209–219.

Olbricht SM, Tang SV, Stern RS, et al. Complications of cutaneous laser surgery: a survey. Arch Dermatol 1987; 123:345–349.

Persley MS. Carbon dioxide laser treatment of oral florid papillomatosis. J Dermatol Surg Oncol 1984; 10:64–66.

Rabbin PE, Baldwin HE. Treatment of porokeratosis of Mibelli with carbon dioxide laser vaporization versus surgical excision with split-thickness skin graft. A comparison. J Dermatol Surg Oncol 1993; 19:199–202.

Ratz JL. Carbon dioxide laser treatment of balanitis xerotica obliterans. J Am Acad Dermatol 1984; 10:925–928.

Raulin C, Schoenermark MP, Werner S, Greve B. Xanthelasma palpebrarum: treatment with the ultra-pulsed carbon dioxide laser. Lasers Surg Med 1999; 24:122–127.

Roodenburg JL, Panders AK, Vermey A. Carbon dioxide laser surgery of oral leukoplakia. Oral Surg Oral Med Oral Pathol 1991; 71:670–674.

Rosenbach A, Alster TS. Multiple trichoepitheliomas successfully treated with a high energy, pulsed carbon dioxide laser. Dermatol Surg 1997; 23:708–710.

Sajben FP, Ross EV. The use of the 1.0 mm handpiece in the high energy, pulsed carbon dioxide laser destruction of facial adnexal tumors. Dermatol Surg 1999; 25:41–44.

Sanders PL, Reinisch L. Wound healing and collagen thermal damage in 7.5-microsec pulsed carbon dioxide laser skin incisions. Lasers Surg Med 2000; 26:22–32.

Sawchuk WS, Heald PW. Carbon dioxide laser treatment of trichoepithelioma with focused and defocused beam. J Dermatol Surg Oncol 1984; 10:905–907.

Schiffman M, Kjaer SK. Natural history of anogenital human papillomavirus infection and neoplasia. J Natl Cancer Inst Monograph 2003; 3–13.

Schomacker KT, Walsh JT, Flotte TJ, Deutsch TF. Thermal damage produced by high-irradiance continuous wave carbon dioxide laser cutting of tissue. Lasers Surg Med 1990; 10:74–84.

Song MG, Park KB, Lee ES. Resurfacing of facial angiofibromas in tuberous sclerosis patients using carbon dioxide laser with flash scanner. Dermatol Surg 1999; 25:970–973.

Sood S, Hurza GJ. Treatment of verruca vulgaris and condyloma acuminatum with lasers. Dermatol Ther 2000; 13:90–101.

Stanley TH, Roenigk RK. The carbon dioxide laser treatment of actinic cheilitis. Mayo Clin Proc 1988; 63:230–235.

Stoner MF, Hobbs ER. Treatment of multiple dermal cylindromas with the carbon dioxide laser. J Dermatol Surg Oncol 1988; 14:1263–1267.

Street ML, Roenigk RK. Recalcitrant periungual verrucae: the role of carbon dioxide laser vaporization. J Am Acad Dermatol 1990; 23:115–120.

Tanitikun N. Treatment of Bowen's disease of the digit with carbon dioxide laser. J Am Acad Dermatol 2000; 43:1080–1083.

Taylor MB. Chondrodermatitis nodularis chronica helicis. Successful treatment with the carbon dioxide laser. J Dermatol Surg Oncol 1991; 17:862–864.

Walsh JT, Flotte TJ, Anderson RR, Deutsch TF. Pulsed carbon dioxide laser tissue ablation: effect of tissue type and pulse duration on thermal damage. Lasers Surg Med 1988; 8: 108–118.

Wang JI, Roenigk HH Jr. Treatment of multiple facial syringomas with the carbon dioxide laser. Dermatol Surg 1999; 25:136–139.

Wheeland RG, Ashley JR, Snick DA, et al. Carbon dioxide laser treatment of granuloma faciale. J Dermatol Surg Oncol 1984; 10:730–733.

Wheeland RG, McGillis ST. Cowden's disease—treatment of cutaneous lesions using carbon dioxide laser vaporization. J Dermatol Surg Oncol 1989; 15:1055–1059.

Whitaker DC. Microscopically proven cure of actinic cheilitis by carbon dioxide laser. Lasers Surg Med 1987; 7:520–523.

Windahl T, Hellstens. Carbon dioxide laser treatment of lichen sclerosus et atrophicus. J Urol 1993; 150:868–870.

Zelickson BD, Roenigk RK. Actinic cheilitis. Treatment with the carbon dioxide laser. Cancer 1990; 65:1307–1311.

64

Laser Surgery and Cosmetic Enhancement: Other Sources

Melissa A. Bogle
Laser and Cosmetic Surgery Center of Houston, Houston, Texas, U.S.A.

Michael S. Kaminer and Jeffrey S. Dover
SkinCare Physicians, Chestnut Hill, Massachusetts, U.S.A.

INTRODUCTION

Over the past decade, there has been increasing research and development in the field of laser, light, radiofrequency, and other similar technologies to treat conditions related to the skin and aging. This chapter will discuss some of the most prominent non-laser modalities including intense pulsed light (IPL), radiofrequency, combined radiofrequency and optical energy sources, light-emitting diodes (LEDs), and plasmakinetic skin resurfacing.

INTENSE PULSED LIGHT

Background

Intense pulsed light sources use high-intensity flashlamps which emit non-coherent light in a broad wavelength spectrum from approximately 515 to 1200 nm. Polychromatic light was first described for use in the treatment of capillary hemangiomas and port-wine stains in 1976. The first commercially available device became available in 1994 (PhotoDerm VL; Lumenis Ltd, Yokneam, Israel). Currently there are a wide variety of devices available with varying wavelengths, spot sizes, pulse durations, pulse delays, and maximal fluences allowing for great variability in selecting individual treatment parameters to suit different skin types and indications. The most common uses are the treatment of photodamage, benign vascular conditions, pigmentary disorders such as lentigines, and hair removal. Devices delivering IPL combined with radiofrequency energy have been recently added to the therapeutic armamentarium and will be discussed later in the chapter.

The mechanism of action of IPL systems follows the principles of selective photothermolysis. This principle states that target chromophores in the skin preferentially absorb certain wavelengths of light. By limiting the exposure of the light energy to a time shorter than the target's thermal relaxation time, the energy is contained in the selected chromophore and collateral damage to surrounding tissue is limited. One of the primary hemoglobin absorption peaks is at 577 nm, while melanin absorbs light in the range of 300 to 750 nm. Longer wavelengths penetrate deeper into the skin, so optical cutoff filters from 515 to 715 nm can be used to eliminate shorter wavelengths and control the depth of penetration and target deeper structures such as hair follicles or blood vessels. Similarly, cutoff filters can be used

to reduce the absorption of melanin in tanned or dark skinned patients to avoid erythema, burns, and dyspigmentation. Generally, the 515, 550, 560, 570 and 590 nm filters are used for vascular lesions as inclusion of some of the shorter wavelengths is necessary to ensure absorption in vessels. The 615, 645 and 755 nm filters cut off more yellow light (577–597 nm) and are commonly used for hair removal and possibly improvement in superficial rhytids through fibroblast stimulation and increased collagen production.

Similar to lasers, the pulse duration of IPL systems are set to be approximately equal to the thermal relaxation time of the target structure to appropriately damage the target without heating the surrounding tissue. The thermal relaxation time is defined as the time required for the temperature of a tissue or target to cool as a result of heat conductivity. IPL devices currently on the market have pulse durations between 0.5 and 88.5 msec. Pulses can be delivered as single, double or triple pulses, and the time interval between pulses can be set between 1 and 300 msec. When using high fluences, it is often a good idea to split the energy into multiple pulses. The delay between pulses gives the epidermis and surrounding tissue a chance to cool while keeping heat confined to the target area. In treating blood vessels, multiple pulsing may be of benefit as oxygenated hemoglobin is converted to methemoglobin during the first pulse of the sequential pulsing. Methemoglobin has a high absorption coefficient throughout the 600 to 750 nm range where oxyhemoglobin has a high absorption coefficient up to 630 nm with a second peak near 900 nm. Larger blood vessels (>0.3 mm in diameter) require delay times spaced 10 msec or longer to allow adequate cooling of the epidermis and surrounding structures. Single pulses and short pulse durations are appropriate for smaller diameter vessels as heat is assumed to occur instantaneously. Darker skinned individuals (types IV–V) should be treated with caution using the highest available optical filter (755 nm) and long delay times of 50 to 100 msec to sufficiently allow the skin to cool and prevent thermal damage. A general list of treatment parameters for IPL can be found in Table 1.

One of the most effective uses of IPL is the treatment of poikiloderma. In a previous study, the device was found to improve both telangiectasia and hyperpigmentation on the neck and chest by over 75%. Treatment parameters included use of the 515 or 550 nm filters, pulse durations of

Table 1 General Treatment Parameters for Intense Pulsed Light

Target	Optical filter (nm)	Fluence (J/cm^2)	Pulse duration (msec)	Pulse mode	Pulse delay (msec)
Essential telangiectasias	515, 550, 570, 590	21.5–50	2.5–6	1, 2, 3	10–30
Hemangiomas	550, 570, 590	36–45	2.5–6	3	20–30
Leg telangiectasias	515, 550, 570, 590	22–70	2.4–7.7	1, 2, 3	10–100
Port-wine stains	515, 550, 570	20–70	2.5–5	1, 2, 3	Not stated
Venous malformations	515, 550, 570, 590	30–90	0.5–25	1, 2, 3	10–500
Hair	590, 615, 645, 690, 695	18–55	1.5–10	2, 3, 4, 5	1.5–50
Solar lentigines	560	20–24	2.6–5	2, 3	20
Rhytids	645, 590, 755	40–70	3–7	3	20–60
Poikiloderma of Civatte	515, 550, 570	20–34	2–4	1, 2	10
Photodamage	550, 560, 570, 645	23–50	2.4–7	2, 3	10–60

Source: From Raulin, Greve, Grema (2003).

2 to 4 msec, fluences of 20 to 40 J/cm^2, and either single or double pulses with a 10-msec delay between pulses. The device has also been shown to be useful in the reduction of rhytids, although other modalities may be better suited for this indication. One study has demonstrated an 18% increase in type I collagen transcripts with IPL treatments (vs. 23% for the pulsed dye laser), with over 85% of patients getting an increase in types I and III collagen, elastin, and collagenase. Histological studies after five treatments using the 570 to 645 nm filters, 25 to 42 J/cm^2, 2.4 to 6.0 msec, double pulse with a 20-msec delay revealed epidermal thickening of 100 to 300 µm, improved cellular polarity, dermal neocollagenosis, decreased elastosis, and new rete ridge formation.

Equipment

The IPL device includes a flashlamp housed in an optical treatment head with water-cooled reflective mirrors. Spot sizes vary with different devices but most have a rectangular treatment crystal measuring roughly 8 × 35 mm (Fig. 1). An internal filter covers the flashlamp to cutoff wavelengths less than 500 nm. Optical coated quartz filters can be placed over the treatment head to cutoff wavelengths shorter than 500 nm to control the depth of penetration and the absorption of melanin (Table 2). Metal collars with chilled, circulating water at 1°C are also available to fit over the treatment crystal in devices without an internal cooling mechanism within the tip. Newer models have computerized treatment programs with pre-set parameters making the device easier to use; however, at least with some IPL devices, the full selection of parameter options can be somewhat limiting for expert users.

A water-based gel is required to optically couple the treatment head to the skin. The coupling gel (i) increases the optical transmission of light by decreasing the index of refraction of light to the skin, (ii) minimizes reflection, and (iii) enhances cooling by absorbing heat given off by the epidermis. The gel may also act as a partial filter for potentially damaging near-infrared wavelengths as water absorbs wavelengths longer than 1000 nm.

Procedure

Before beginning the procedure, the patient's skin should be closely examined as there are many factors which may affect outcome and the risk for side effects including skin type, degree of tanning, skin tone and thickness, sensitivity, and relative number of sebaceous glands on the particular part of the body being treated. If necessary, a test area should be treated in advance of the full procedure. In addition, the patient's skin should be re-examined before each treatment session to determine if alterations need to be made to the treatment parameters because of an interim change such as an increase in the degree of tan or reaction to a previous treatment. While most patients tolerate the procedure well, patients with low pain thresholds may want to arrive 45 minutes to one hour before the procedure for application of a topical anesthetic cream such as LMX-5 (Lidocaine 5% cream; Ferndale Laboratories, Ferndale, Michigan, U.S.A.). Topical anesthetics containing prilocaine are generally not recommended because of vasoconstriction and a decreased vascular target.

After the parameters have been selected and the patient's skin has been cleansed, protective eyewear should be donned and a thick layer of cool gel is applied over the area to be treated. If the handpiece does not have an integrated cooling mechanism within the tip, it is important to lift up on the handpiece several millimeters to create a space between the crystal and the skin to protect the epidermis from excessive heat while the pulse is being delivered. When using newer devices with a chilled tip, the crystal is

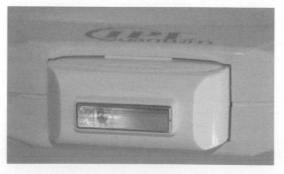

Figure 1 Rectangular treatment crystal of the intense pulsed light device (IPL Quantum, Lumenis Inc., Santa Clara, California, U.S.A.)

Table 2 Available Cutoff Filters for the Intense Pulsed Light Device. Wavelengths Below the Cutoff Filter Do Not Pass Through the Treatment Head

Wavelength (nm)	
515	615
550	645
560	690
570	755
590	

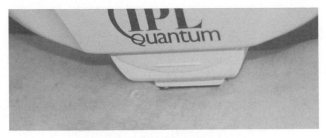

Figure 2 During treatment with the intense pulsed light the crystal floats lightly on a layer of cool gel (IPL Quantum).

rested lightly on the skin when the pulse is delivered (Fig. 2). The device should not be used without the coupling gel as blisters from excessive thermal damage may occur on the skin. Patients will feel a burning or stinging sensation with each pulse, especially at higher fluences. Pulses should be delivered in a parallel fashion as close together as possible over the entire treatment area. Normally, men should only be treated from the beard line up as photoepilation effects from the IPL device may cause unwanted loss of beard or moustache hair.

The initial treatment series consists of four to six treatment sessions carried out at 3- to 4-week intervals. Fluences may be increased by approximately 10% per treatment session as needed to achieve the desired results. In the second treatment, the handpiece should be held perpendicular to the way it was held in the first treatment to avoid stripes. Patients should be instructed that maintenance treatments are an integral part of any photorejuvenation series with continued treatments at 6-month intervals for photodamaged skin and 3-month intervals for inflammatory disorders such as rosacea (Fig. 3).

Complications

Because of the wide variety of wavelengths, pulse durations, frequencies, and fluences that can be chosen to treat a particular condition or skin type, any operator of an IPL system should be fully trained to perform the procedure. The most common effect occurring after IPL treatments is transient erythema which may be accompanied by edema. This usually resolves within several hours but may last up to two days. Mild edema of the cheeks occurs in approximately 25% of full-face treatments, tends to be most prominent after the initial treatment, and resolves within 1 to 3 days.

High fluences or short pulse widths may cause transient purpura, blisters, or crusting. Purpura often occurs with scattered, isolated pulses, particularly when the 515 nm

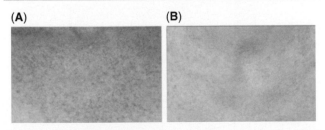

(A)   **(B)**

Figure 3 Photodamaged chest before **(A)** and after **(B)** four treatments with intense pulsed light. *Source*: Photos courtesy Drs. Robert and Margaret Weiss, Baltimore, Maryland.

cutoff filter is used or when the pulse duration is very short. Patients who are tan or of darker skin type are prone to blisters, crusting, and hypo- or hyperpigmentation. Light-skin patients are most likely to develop crusts over curved body areas such as the neck over the sternocleidomastoid muscle prominence. Blisters or crusts should be actively treated with diligent wound care using bland ointment several times a day. Scarring, necrosis, and permanent changes in pigmentation are rare.

RADIOFREQUENCY

Background

Radiofrequency energy has been used in many areas of medicine including cardiology, urology, and sleep medicine. In dermatology the technology has been used for electrocoagulation, hemostasis, endovenous closure, and skin rejuvenation. In esthetic dermatology, radiofrequency systems have been used for skin resurfacing and improvement of facial laxity.

The first radiofrequency device on the market was the Visage unit for skin resurfacing (ArthroCare Corp., Sunnyvale, California, U.S.A.). It introduced a process called coblation ("cold ablation") in which bipolar radiofrequency energy rather than heat is used for skin resurfacing. The concept is that radiofrequency energy is applied to a conductive medium (saline), forming a plasma field of highly ionized particles with sufficient energy to break molecular bonds within the skin. The 1.0-cm stylet contains three flush gold active electrodes on the tip with integrated gold return electrodes on each side. A saline drip port is incorporated into the tip of the stylet to permit a constant supply of the conductive medium. The device operates between 70 and 90°C. Because there is no cooling, epidermal damage ensues and tissue is removed in successive layers with each pass of the stylet through low-temperature molecular disintegration. Simultaneous hemostasis allows a bloodless procedure. The most common side effects are erythema, edema, crusting, pain, and hyperpigmentation. The first large-scale prospective study to evaluate radiofrequency resurfacing for the treatment of perioral and periorbital rhytids used two to three passes of 125 to 139 V. Patients and investigators determined a positive mean improvement in both periorbital and perioral treatment sites using the Fitzpatrick wrinkle assessment scale. An independent panel thought the periorbital region improved a mean 0.7 points and the perioral region a mean 0.7 points on the Fitzpatrick scale at six months.

The first device to use monopolar radiofrequency energy for skin tightening was the ThermaCool device (Thermage, Inc., Haywood, California, U.S.A.). Radiofrequency differs from laser/light energy in that laser energy tends to scatter or absorb in the upper layers of the skin, making it difficult to deliver sufficient energy to the deep dermis without causing damage. Certain lasers such as those in the infrared spectrum are able to affect upper dermal collagen and improve fine wrinkles and textural irregularities, however to date they are unable to address the problem of skin laxity.

Monopolar radiofrequency devices can deliver uniform heating at controlled depths to the deep dermis and subdermal layers of the skin, causing immediate collagen contraction and subsequent remodeling over the course of months. This differs from laser and light sources, which heat tissue targets in accordance with the principles of selective photothermolysis. With the ThermaCool device, it is thought that volumetric heating of the dermis causes direct tissue tightening by breaking hydrogen bonds in the collagen triple helix, causing contraction. Electron microscopic evaluation of skin immediately post-treatment supports a morphological change in individual collagen fibrils with contracted, partially denatured collagen in the mid to deep dermis. Studies have also found selective contraction of fibrous septae in the subcutaneous fat which is thought to be responsible for the inward (Z-dimension) tightening. This gives the patient immediate, visible improvement the day of the procedure with continued improvement over the course of 4 to 6 months from a delayed wound healing response.

A study using the original 1.0-cm tips in the treatment of cheek, jawline, and neck laxity revealed clinical improvement of nasolabial and mesolabial folds in 28 of 30 patients, with peak improvement occurring 1 month after treatment, measuring approximately 35% to 40% by independent subjective evaluation. In the same study, improvement in submandibular and neck laxity was observed in 17 of 20 patients, with peak improvement occurring three months after treatment, measuring approximately 30% to 35%. Average treatment fluences were $130\,J/cm^2$ on the cheek and $110\,J/cm^2$ on the neck. A split-face study analyzing changes to the brow and superior palpebral crease using treatment fluences of 97 to $143\,J/cm^2$ revealed an average 4.3 mm brow elevation and 1.9 mm superior palpebral crease elevation along the midpupillary line, and an average 2.4 mm brow elevation along the lateral canthal line. The same study also attempted to measure jowl surface area changes during split-face treatment of the cheek and found a mean decrease of 22.6% on the treated side. No improvements in either region were noted on the untreated side.

Equipment

The ThermaCool radiofrequency skin tightening device consists of a radiofrequency generator, processing computer, cooling component, handpiece, and single use treatment tip. The radiofrequency generator produces a 6-MHz alternating current that creates an electric field through the skin. The electric field shifts polarity six million times per second, causing a change in orientation of charged particles within the electric field. Tissue resistance to this particle movement generates heat. Thus, heat is generated by the skin's resistance to the flow of current within an electric field, not by photon absorption as with a laser (Fig. 4).

Contact cooling from cryogen spray on the inner surface of the treatment tip occurs before, during and after each energy pulse to protect the epidermis and create a reverse energy gradient where temperatures are highest in the deep dermis and coolest near the epidermis. A computer within the device receives and displays real-time data from a microprocessor in the treatment tip on pressure, current flow, and skin temperature. Internal monitors will not permit a complete radiofrequency pulse if any parameters fall outside preprogrammed limits. Thus, feedback from the treatment tip to the computer in the radiofrequency generator regulates the amount of energy applied to the tissue. Treatment tips are disposable, intended for single-patient use, and come programmed with a limited number of pulses within a certain period of time (Fig. 5).

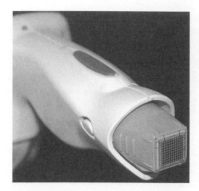

Figure 5   ThermaCool 1.5-cm treatment tip containing a microprocessor which sends data on pressure, current flow, and skin temperature back to the device. *Source*: Thermage, Inc., Haywood, California, U.S.A.

Procedure

To perform the procedure, it is useful to have the patient arrive at the office about an hour before the scheduled treatment time for preliminary preparations. Because the procedure can cause significant discomfort, some physicians recommend one of several forms of analgesia. Patient pain feedback to the operator is the basis used to choose the appropriate energy for a particular treatment area in a given individual. Anesthetic options include topical anesthetic cream and/or additional analgesics such as lorazepam 1 to 2 mg by mouth an hour prior to the procedure, and demerol 75 mg intramuscularly (IM) 15 minutes prior to the procedure. Use of nerve blocks and intravenous sedation, however, are not recommended as some degree of pain feedback from the patient is necessary to limit side effects and enhance patient safety. Local infiltration anesthesia should never be used as it alters the tissue impedance and can increase adverse effects and decrease treatment efficacy. Topical anesthetic must be meticulously removed before the procedure begins so that contact between the treatment tip membrane and skin surface is not altered in any way.

When the skin is thoroughly cleansed, a grid is applied to the treatment area using either dye transfer paper or freehand with a marking pen (Fig. 6). While we recommend using the provided grid, a red, fine point permanent

$$\text{Energy (joules)} = I^2 \times Z \times t$$

Figure 4   Ohm's law states the impedance (Z) to the movement of electrons creates heat relative to the amount of current (*I*) and time (*t*).

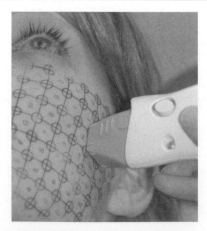

Figure 6   ThermaCool treatment session illustrating the importance of the grid in positioning of the treatment tip for the initial passes. *Source*: Thermage, Inc., Haywood, California, U.S.A.

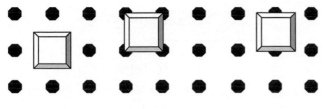

Pass 1: on the dots   Pass 2: in the squares   Pass 3: between dots

Figure 7 Position of handpiece on grid in first three passes to ensure even coverage.

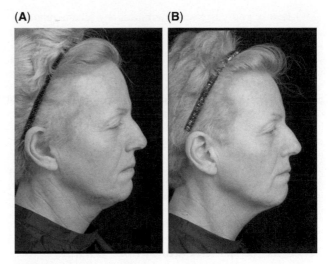

Figure 8 Patient before (**A**) and 2 months after (**B**) treatment with the ThermaCool monopolar radiofrequency device using the low fluence, multiple-pass technique.

marker works well as it stays visible throughout the treatment session yet is easily removed afterward with an alcohol swab. The grid will need to be spaced depending on the size of the treatment tip used, currently either 1 cm for the original tips or 1.5 cm for the newer fast tips. Additional tip sizes are being developed for use in small areas such as the eyelids or to efficiently cover larger areas of the body such as the thighs, abdomen, or posterior arms. When the grid is complete, a return pad must be attached to the patient and hooked up to the machine. The return pad provides a low resistance path for current to flow to complete the electrical circuit. It is important to use the proper return pad and to make sure it is applied correctly. If the pad is too small or inaccurately applied, a burn can occur at the site of the pad from unintended high resistance to current.

Coupling fluid should be applied generously to all treatment areas and will need to be reapplied as needed during the procedure. As a general rule, the first three passes are carried out over the entire grid to ensure even heating of the skin (Fig. 7). Individual pulses should never be stacked or overlapped, and the operator should wait at least two full minutes between passes before re-treating an area to allow adequate cooling. To achieve maximal results with minimal side effects, the treatment strategy should be to use multiple passes at low to moderate temperature settings until a desired endpoint of visual tightening is seen (Table 3). Patients should be asked continually throughout the treatment about their level of pain on a scale of 1 to 10. The goal is to calibrate temperature settings to keep the pain level below 5 or 6. Greater pain levels mean the temperature is too high and should be turned down to reduce the risk of side effects. In addition, persistent erythema, localized swelling or hives are all indicators that the tissue has not had sufficient time to cool before additional passes can be considered.

After the first three passes are complete, the remaining passes should be concentrated on improving the patient's desired trouble spots, with careful attention to the most appropriate placement of each pulse to achieve not only tightening in the XY-axis along the surface of the

face, but also along the three-dimensional inward Z-axis. Newer 1.5 cm treatment tips are programmed with up to 900 pulses, allowing up to eight or nine passes if needed. The endpoint of treatment is visual skin tightening in the desired areas.

After the treatment is complete, the face should be gently cleansed with water to remove excess coupling fluid and any remaining grid. The patient should be carefully inspected for areas of persistent erythema, localized swelling, or hives. If such areas are found, it may be of help to apply a mid- to high-potency topical corticosteroid cream immediately after the procedure to reduce the incidence of crusts or pigment alteration (Fig. 8).

Complications

The most common potential problems with radiofrequency skin tightening are pain during the procedure, temporary postoperative surface irregularities, postoperative changes in sensation, and unrealistic patient expectations. Patient pain may be mitigated by topical, oral or IM analgesics as discussed above, however it is best to keep sensation as intact as possible so that the pain feedback calibration system for temperature settings is secure. If in doubt, it is safest to use the lowest possible treatment settings. The incidence of both postoperative surface irregularities and changes in sensation has decreased dramatically with the introduction of the newer fast tips. Surface irregularities are often described as small nodules or lumps that patients feel but rarely see on casual inspection. They are most common over thin-skinned areas such as the neck and self-resolve within a few weeks. Changes in sensation may include itching or numbness and occur most commonly along the preauricular area, jawline, temples, and forehead. Symptoms are usually mild and resolve completely in days to weeks.

Unrealistic patient expectations should be managed at the initial consultation. Patients should be aware that radiofrequency skin tightening is not a substitute for a facelift and should not be marketed as such. Explain that results can be modest and a small group of patients perceive no improvement at all. Patients should also understand that radiofrequency alone is not effective for the textural aspects of photoaging including wrinkles and pigmentary alterations.

Table 3 Maximum Settings for Thermage Radiofrequency Procedures of the Face

	Pass 1	Pass 2	Pass 3	Subsequent passes
Forehead	63	63	62.5	62
Temples	62	Not recommended		
Lower face	64	63.5	63	62
Upper lip	61	Not recommended		

Rarely, patients may experience side effects related to overly aggressive treatment approaches such as burns, indentations, scars, or changes in pigmentation. The overall incidence of such problems is 0.15% of patients treated. Indentations are thought to occur when high-energy settings overheat fat lobules and fibrous septa. This is extremely unlikely to happen at settings below 64 on the ThermaCool dial with the 1.5-cm tip. Thirty percent of depressions have occurred in patients using topical anesthesia and may be related to the incomplete removal of the product before the procedure. There also appears to be a higher incidence of side effects in patients using local infiltrative anesthesia, nerve blocks, or general anesthesia. Again, this is likely due to overly aggressive treatments as the patient feedback loop is cut off.

COMBINED ELECTRICAL AND OPTICAL ENERGY

Background

Selective electro-thermolysis is a newly developed technology combining radiofrequency energy with optical energy from laser or light sources. This technology has shown efficacy in hair removal for all hair colors and skin types, wrinkle reduction, and the treatment of both pigment and vascular disorders. Whereas tightening devices delivering radiofrequency energy alone to the skin use monopolar electrodes, the radiofrequency component of the combined electrical and optical energy units currently available uses bipolar electrodes (Fig. 9). In a bipolar system, the electrical current passes between two electrodes at a fixed distance over the skin rather than through a single electrode with a grounding pad attached to the patient.

The flow of current between two electrodes in a bipolar system is illustrated in Figure 10. Current (I) flows between two electrodes perpendicular to an electromagnetic field (E). In electromagnetic theory the penetration depth of energy into any material, rather it be a metal or human tissue, is called the skin depth. While the skin depth is influenced by the type of tissue serving as the conductor, temperature, and the frequency of electrical current applied to the conductor, this number is generally equal to the depth at which the current density is reduced by a factor of $1/e$, where e is the base of the natural log (2.72...). At the skin depth, roughly two-thirds of the current ($1 - 1/e$) will be flowing above the line and one-third ($1/e$) below. If one plots the current density as a function of the penetration depth for different distances between electrodes, one finds that at the point where the current density falls to $1/e$, the penetration depth equals approximately half the distance between the

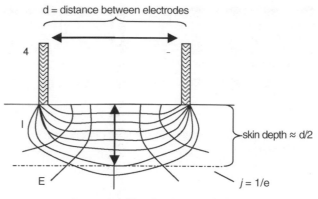

d = distance between electrodes

I = current; E = electromagnetic field;
j = current density; skin depth ≈ d/2;
*e is base of the natural log, 2.72.

Figure 10   Schematic diagram illustrating the distribution of current density between electrodes in a bipolar system. Current (I) can be seen flowing between the two electrodes perpendicular to the electromagnetic field (E). The penetration depth of the energy into the tissue is roughly half the distance between electrodes.

electrodes. Thus, the penetration depth of the energy into the tissue is roughly half the distance between electrodes.

Electrical conductivity varies among different types of tissue (Table 4). Blood has the highest electrical conductivity, while fat, bone, and dry skin have low conductivities such that current tends to flow around these structures rather than passing through them. Wet skin has a higher electrical conductivity allowing greater penetration of current. This may explain the improved results seen with generous amounts of coupling fluid and increased hydration of skin in the Thermage procedure.

Tissue conductivity is also influenced by temperature, and the distribution of electrical current can be influenced by pre-heating or cooling selected targets within the field. Every 1°C increase in temperature lowers the skin impedance by 2%. Mathematically, this is expressed by the thermal coefficient of skin conductivity (α), roughly equal to 2% per °C. In theory, target structures that have been pre-warmed with optical energy will have greater conductivity, less resistance, and greater selective heating by the radiofrequency current. Similarly, surface cooling will increase resistance to the electrical field near the epidermis, driving

Table 4   The Dielectric Properties of Human Tissue at 1 MHz, Room Temperature

Tissue	Electrical Conductivity (Siemens/m)
Air	0.00
Bone	0.02
Nail	0.02
Fat	0.03
Dry skin	0.03
Nerve	0.13
Cartilage	0.23
Wet skin	0.22
Mucosa	0.22
Muscle	0.50
Lymphatics	0.60
Thyroid	0.60
Blood	0.70

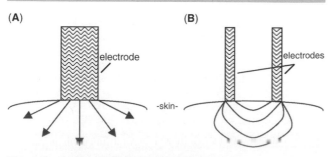

Figure 9   The flow of electrical current through the skin using a **(A)** monopolar electrode system and **(B)** bipolar electrode system.

the radiofrequency current into the tissue and increasing the penetration depth. The precise impact of these theoretical constructs on the clinical application of these devices is currently under investigation.

A study evaluating the effect of combined optical and radiofrequency energy on adult women with blond or white facial hair using 15 to 30 J/cm^2 light energy and 10 to 20 J/cm^3 radiofrequency energy in four treatments 8 to 12 weeks apart revealed hair clearance of 40% to 60%. As with other technologies, hair removal efficacy appears to be greater in patients with darker hair (mean clearance 80–85%). A series of three to five treatments on photoaged skin revealed a 70% improvement in erythema and telangiectasia, a 78% improvement in lentigines, and a 60% improvement in skin texture as determined by subject satisfaction levels.

Equipment

There are several devices currently on the market using combined radiofrequency and laser or light technology including the Aurora, Polaris, and Galaxy systems (Syneron Medical Ltd, Yokneam, Israel). The Aurora uses combined radiofrequency and IPL with systems available for hair removal, skin rejuvenation, and acne treatment. The Polaris uses combined radiofrequency and a 900-nm diode laser with systems available for wrinkle reduction and leg vein/vascular lesions. The Galaxy incorporates the Aurora and Polaris in a single device. For skin rejuvenation, the theoretical advantage to this technology is that the radiofrequency component will penetrate into the skin, limited to a depth of one half the distance between the bipolar electrodes, potentially heating deeper tissues than standard non-ablative lasers. The laser component will address superficial lentigines and telangiectasias which radiofrequency alone cannot treat. For hair removal and the treatment of vascular lesions, the goal is to heat the target to a sufficient temperature that causes permanent injury. The two forms of energy act synergistically to generate heat at the target. Radiofrequency energy is preferentially absorbed by the target structure as higher temperatures correlate with decreased impedance and electrical current likes to follow the path of least resistance.

In all of these systems, the radiofrequency energy is applied through electrodes located in the handpiece at an appropriate distance from each other to provide the optimal penetration depth for whatever the indication (Fig. 11). The handpiece also contains a fiber delivering optical energy

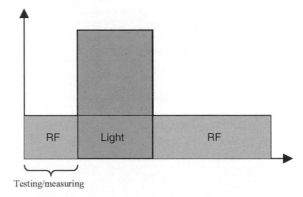

Testing/measuring

Figure 12 Pulse sequence of combined radiofrequency and optical energy devices. The initial RF pulse is for calibration by the device; then pulses of optical and radiofrequency energy are initiated at the same time, with the radiofrequency pulse having a longer duration.

to the skin and an internal contact cooling mechanism to protect the epidermis. When the tip is brought into contact with the skin surface, pulses of optical and radiofrequency energy are initiated at the same time, but the radiofrequency pulse has a longer duration (Fig. 12). This ensures that the optical component preheats the target, allowing the radiofrequency constituent to be preferentially absorbed by it. The tip measures changes in the skin impedance, allowing active dermal monitoring.

Procedure

Before the procedure, the treatment area should be thoroughly cleansed and hydrated with a clear conductive gel. A thicker layer of gel should be applied over bony areas such as the forehead and periorbital regions. In determining the therapeutic energy it is important to take into account the patient's skin type and the anatomic location being treated. General treatment guidelines can be found in Table 5. It is a good idea to perform a test spot treatment at the start of every treatment session. If there are any signs of epidermal injury after waiting five minutes (intense erythema, blisters, or blanching skin), the optical fluence should be decreased by increments of 2 J/cm^2. Likewise, if optimal endpoints are not observed (mild erythema and subtle edema), consider increasing the optical fluence by 1 J/cm^2.

When performing the actual treatment, the applicator tip should be placed onto the skin with slight pressure (Fig. 13). The trigger must then be depressed one pulse at a time, ensuring even contact of the applicator tip and both electrodes before each pulse. Slight overlap is acceptable, however pulses should never be stacked. In this fashion, the entire treatment area should be treated with a single pass when using the combined IPL-RF unit and at least three to four passes when using the combined diode-RF unit for wrinkle reduction. With the diode-RF unit, deep folds and rhytids may require up to six passes to show the clinical endpoint of mild erythema and subtle edema, while fine rhytids in thin-skinned areas may require only two to three passes. Treatment of the nasal area and tissue inside the bony orbit should be avoided. Similarly, hair bearing areas such as the eyebrows or beard area in men should be avoided as permanent hair loss can occur (Table 6).

Optical and radiofrequency fluences may be increased by 10% to 15% in subsequent treatments if no adverse effects

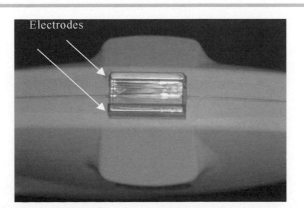

Figure 11 Combined radiofrequency and intense pulsed light treatment head illustrating bipolar electrodes between which an electrical current passes. *Source*: Syneron Medical Ltd., Yokneam, Israel.

Table 5 General Treatment Parameters for Combined Radiofrequency Plus Intense Pulsed Light

Skin type	Optical energy (J/cm^2)	Radiofrequency energy (J/cm^3)		Pulse type[a]	ISL (%)[b]
		Bony areas	Soft tissue		
I, II	24–26	18	25	Short	30
III	22–24	18	25	Short	30
IV	18–20	18	25	Short	30

[a]Long pulse mode is recommended for patients with a very deep or extensive vascular component.
[b]ISL is the impedance safety limit which provides a closed loop feedback system to automatically shut off the RF pulse to prevent tissue overheating.

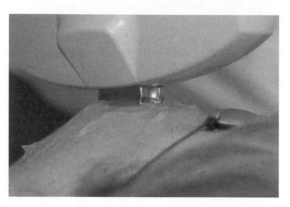

Figure 13 Combined radiofrequency and intense pulsed light treatment with the applicator placed on the skin with slight pressure over a layer of conductive gel. *Source*: Syneron Medical Ltd., Richmond Hall, Ontario, Canada.

have occurred. Caution should be used in treating darker-skin types or tanned skin because of the IPL component. Optical fluences should be lowered by at least 20% when treating darkly pigmented lesions or dense pigment irregularity, even in light skinned patients.

Complications

Side effects associated with combined electrical–optical energy are minimal. This may be because the synergistic effects of the two forms of energy allow lower levels of each to be used than with either component alone. The most common occurrence appears to be mild transient erythema after the procedure, usually resolving in several hours. Patients tolerate the procedure well without need for analgesics. Crusting, blisters, pigmentary change, and scarring are uncommon.

LIGHT-EMITTING DIODE TECHNOLOGY

Background

Light-emitting diodes have been touted to be of use in a variety of conditions including photoaging, acne, rosacea, facial erythema, skin tone/texture, and rhytids. The theory behind the technology is similar to that of plant cells and photosynthesis. Low-intensity light photons of the proper parameters interact with sub-cellular chromophores to activate cells to induce or inhibit activity in a non-thermal, non-ablative fashion.

Table 6 General Treatment Parameters for Combined Radiofrequency Plus Diode Laser

	Optical energy (J/cm^2)	Radiofrequency energy (J/cm^3)
Bony areas	Skin type I–III: 36–40	60–75
Soft tissue	Skin type IV: 24–40	75–100

Blue (407–420 nm) and red light (633–660 nm) have shown some efficacy in the treatment of mild to moderate inflammatory acne. Ashkenazi et al. have shown that the viability of *Propioniobacterium acnes* bacteria in vitro is reduced by four orders of magnitude after two illuminations with intense blue light. A randomized controlled trial evaluating blue light and mixed blue-red light therapy found a 76% decrease in inflammatory acne lesions with daily mixed blue-red light therapy for three months.

Red light at 633 nm is thought to accelerate mast cell degranulation and increase the synthesis of fibroblast growth factors. In addition, it has been shown that irradiation with red light at 660 nm induces the release of growth factors from macrophages in vitro and clinically improves healing of ulcers and postoperative wounds. The effects of red light on mast cells may also be of use for anti-aging treatments by increasing fibroblast growth factors and enhancing angiogenesis.

Yellow light (588 nm) is thought to act in a similar manner in anti-aging therapy through the preferential degranulation of mast cells, release of glycosaminoglycans, promotion of epithelial remodeling, and stimulation of fibroblasts to produce collagen. Results of a 12-month, multi-site clinical trial of photodamaged facial skin showed an increase in type I collagen and a decrease in enzymes leading to collagen breakdown such as collagenase and matrix metalloproteins after eight treatments at intervals of 2 to 5 days. Eighty-five percent of subjects improved by at least one grade in the Fitzpatrick scale of periorbital wrinkles. Histological studies after treatment with pulsed yellow light at 588 nm have documented new collagen formation.

Equipment

Most LED-based devices use either a panel or handpiece containing an array of focused diodes (Fig. 14). The diodes

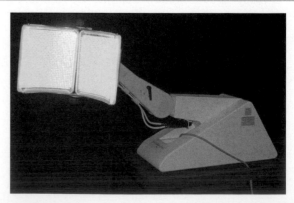

Figure 14 LED device with a split panel containing an array of diodes emitting pulsed yellow light. *Source*: Gentlewaves; Light Bioscience, Virginia Beach, Virginia, U.S.A.

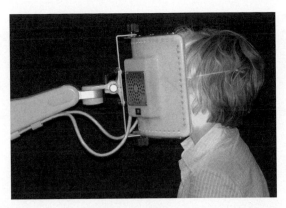

Figure 15 Patient undergoing treatment with an LED device. *Source*: Gentlewaves; Light Bioscience, Virginia Beach, Virginia, U.S.A.

Table 7 Tissue Effect of Various Fluences with Plasmakinetic Resurfacing

Fluence (J)	Equivalent technology
1–1.5	Non-ablative laser rejuvenation, IPL
2–3	Moderate depth chemical peel
3–4	Single pass CO_2 resurfacing

can either emit light in a pulsed fashion or in a non-pulsed, continuous wave. Some devices emit light of a single color while others are polychromatic to maximize particular therapeutic strategies (for example, red and blue LEDs for the treatment of acne).

Procedure

Before undergoing the LED procedure the treatment area should be cleansed of all makeup and sunscreen, and the patient should don opaque eyewear protection. The treatment area is then placed in close proximity to the LED device and exposed for one to several minutes, depending on the condition and device. The treatment is painless and requires no aftercare. Systems with larger panels of diodes are ideal for quickly and easily treating diffuse areas such as the sun-damaged chest.

The procedure must be repeated for a series of treatments, however clinical studies have not yet been done to determine the most effective schedule for rejuvenation or the treatment of particular skin disorders. LED treatments may be of use immediately following non-ablative laser or light therapies to theoretically enhance collagen formation or incorporated into treatments such as microdermabrasion or chemical peels to theoretically reduce post-procedure erythema and inflammation by decreasing matrix metalloproteinases and inflammatory mediators (Fig. 15).

Complications

Low-intensity LED devices have shown no significant side effects. As there is yet little clinical evidence to support the theoretical claims, patient expectations should be managed to avoid dissatisfaction.

PLASMA SKIN REGENERATION TECHNOLOGY
Background

Plasma skin regeneration technology uses energy delivered from plasma rather than light or radiofrequency. Plasma is the fourth state of matter in which electrons are stripped from atoms to form an ionized gas. The plasma is emitted in a millisecond pulse to deliver energy to target tissue upon contact without reliance on skin chromophores.

The technology can be used at varying energies for different depths of effect, from superficial epidermal sloughing similar to microdermabrasion to deeper dermal heating similar to CO_2 resurfacing (Table 7). At fluences of less than

2.5 J, the thermal energy is generally limited to above the dermal–epidermal junction. At fluences greater than 2.5 J, the thermal effect enters the dermis causing collagen heating and contraction. The operator must, however, keep in mind that depth of effect is also dependent upon skin hydration. Epidermal hydration influences the amount of energy that is absorbed and the depth of thermal insult. In a study presented at the 2005 Meeting of the American Society of Laser Medicine and Surgery, hydration of the epidermis and the delay in applying energy after removing the local anesthetic both provided variables to the depth of thermal insult achieved.

Equipment

The device consists of an ultra high frequency radiofrequency generator which excites a tuned resonator and imparts energy to a flow of inert nitrogen gas within the handpiece. The activated, ionized gas is termed plasma and has an optical emission spectrum with peaks in the visible (mainly indigo/violet) and near infrared range. Nitrogen is used for the gaseous source because it is able to purge oxygen from the surface of the skin, minimizing the risk of unpredictable hot spots, charring, and scar formation. Upon formation, the plasma is directed through a quartz nozzle out of the tip of the handpiece and onto the skin. The plasma appears as a characteristic lilac glow which transitions to a yellowish light called a Lewis–Raleigh afterglow (Fig. 16). A 4-J N_2 plasma pulse delivers 10 mJ of optical energy with its strongest output at 420 nm in the indigo/violet spectrum of visible light, explaining the lilac color of the early afterglow. As the plasma hits the skin, energy is rapidly transferred to the skin surface causing instantaneous heating in a controlled, uniform manner, without an explosive effect on tissue or epidermal removal. The depth and area of thermal effect are determined by the energy setting and spot size of the handpiece. The energy can be adjusted from 1 to 4 J per pulse. There is a self-calibration feature within the generator that verifies the

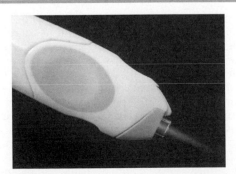

Figure 16 Plasma resurfacing handpiece demonstrating the characteristic lilac glow of the plasma as it transitions to a yellowish light. *Source*: Lewis-Raleigh Afterglow, PSR; Rhytec, Inc., Waltham, Massachusetts, U.S.A.

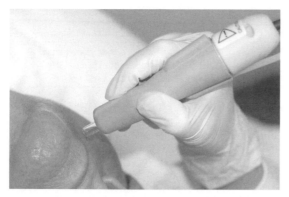

Figure 17 When performing plasmakinetic resurfacing, the tip of the handpiece should be held approximately 5 mm from the skin's surface, and pulses should be delivered in a paintbrush fashion across the treatment area. *Source*: Rhytec, Inc., Wattham, Massachusetts, U.S.A.

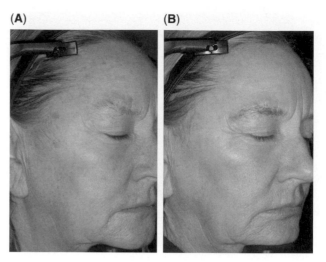

Figure 18 Patient before (**A**) and 3 months after (**B**) three low energy plasma skin regeneration treatments.

energy delivered matches the preset level. The frequency of pulses can be varied from 1 to 4 Hz.

The handpiece contains a tungsten resonator within a quartz tube for plasma generation. High temperatures during each pulse erode the resonator so the handpiece must be replaced at periodic intervals automatically indicated by the generator.

Procedure

The first step in treatment is to assess the patient and determine the goals of treatment. Very superficial treatments which remove only the stratum corneum can normally be performed under local anesthesia with a topical agent. For mid to higher fluences, patients will require adjunctive oral anesthesia such as meperidine or a codeine derivative in addition to a topical agent. Patients should arrive at least an hour beforehand so that the topical anesthetic cream can be applied and left on for approximately one hour. Oral anesthesia should be administered 30 to 45 minutes before the procedure begins. To avoid unexpected downtime, it is important for the physician to develop a standard protocol for removal of topical anesthesia and delay time before starting the procedure. Hydration of the epidermis influences the amount of energy that is absorbed and the depth of thermal insult achieved with drier tissue absorbing more energy.

Generally, it is a good idea to work in aesthetic segments of the face (i.e., forehead, nose, cheek, chin, etc.) removing the anesthetic cream for each area immediately before treating that area rather than removing the cream for the entire face at once. This helps to standardize the delay time between anesthetic removal and treatment. Anesthetic should be gently wiped off with dry gauze. Again, it is not necessary to use water- or alcohol-soaked gauze as this will change the hydration properties of the skin.

Once a facial segment is ready for treatment, the tip of the handpiece should be held approximately 5 mm from the skin's surface (Fig. 17). The pulses are delivered in a paintbrush fashion across the treatment area. Pulses should not be overlapped, although histologic studies indicate that the thermal damage is self-limited with pulse stacking or a second pass. To avoid lines of demarcation, the borders of the treatment area should be feathered by increasing the distance of the nozzle from the surface of the skin to about 1 cm. Feathering can also be achieved by holding the handpiece nozzle at an angle with respect to the skin

surface or reducing the power setting. Full face treatments should be feathered along the neck and hairline.

Patients should be instructed to avoid sun-exposure and apply a bland ointment to the face at frequent intervals after the procedure while the skin is healing. Very low fluence treatments may cause only erythema for 2 to 3 days. Mid-level treatments will cause erythema and a "dirty" look to the skin which will resolve in 4 to 7 days as re-epithelialization occurs and the photodamaged epidermis sloughs off. It is important for patients not to manually pick at the peeling skin to avoid prolonged erythema or scarring. High fluences may have 7 to 10 days of downtime similar to that in the mid-level group (Fig. 18).

Complications

Side effects include erythema, edema, epidermal de-epithelialization, scarring and dyspigmentation. Erythema and edema are common post-procedure, usually resolving in several days. Edema can be decreased by the application of ice post-procedure. Epidermal de-epithelialization is a risk at higher fluences and should be treated with appropriate wound care and liberal application of a bland ointment. Temporary dyspigmentation has been reported at mid to high fluence treatments. Scarring is rare.

BIBLIOGRAPHY

Alster T, Tanzi E. Improvement of neck and cheek laxity with a nonablative radiofrequency device: a lifting experience. Dermatol Surg 2004; 30:503–507.

Ashkenazi H, Malik Z, Harth Y, Nitzan Y. Eradication of Propionium acnes by its endogenic porphyrins after illumination with high intensity blue light. FEMS Immunol Med Microbiol 2003; 35:17–24.

Bitter P Jr., Mulholland RS. Report of a new technique for enhanced non-invasive skin rejuvenation using a dual mode pulsed light and radiofrequency energy source: selective radiothermolysis. J Cosmet Dermatol 2002; 1:142–145.

Chess C. Prospective study on combination diode laser and radiofrequency energies (ELOS) for the treatment of leg veins. J Cosmet Laser Ther 2004; 6:86–90.

Duck FA. Physical Properties of Tissue. New York, NY: Academic Press Limited, 1990.

Gabriel S, Lau RW, Gabriel C. The dielectric properties of biological tissues: III. Parametric models for the dielectric spectrum of tissues. Phys Med Biol 1996; 41:2271–2293.

Grekin RC, Tope WD, Yarborough JM, et al. Electrosurgical facial resurfacing: a prospective multicenter study of efficacy and safety. Arch Dermatol 2000; 136:1309–1316.

Hernandez-Perez E, Ibiett EV. Gross and microscopic finding in patients submitted to nonablative full face resurfacing using intense pulsed light. Dermatol Surg 2002; 28:651–655.

Hsu TS, Kaminer MS. The use of nonablative radiofrequency technology to tighten the lower face and neck. Semin Cutan Med Surg 2003; 22:115–123.

Iusim M, Kimchy J, Pillar T, et al. Evaluation of the degree of effectiveness of Biobeam (low level narrow band light on the treatment of skin ulcers and delayed post-operative wound healing. Orthopedics 1992; 15:1023–1026.

Muhlbauer W, Nath G, Kreitmair A. Treatment of capillary hemangiomas and nevi flammei with light. Langenbecks Arch Chir 1976; 343:91–94.

Nahm WK, Su TT, Rotunda AM, Moy RL. Objective changes in brow position, superior palpebral crease, peak angle of the eyebrow, and jowl surface area after volumetric radiofrequency treatments to half of the face. Dermatol Surg 2004; 30:922–928.

Narins DJ, Narins RS. Non-surgical radiofrequency facelift. J Drugs Dermatol 2003; 2:495–500.

Papageorgiou P, Katsambas A, Chu A. Phototherapy with blue (415 nm) and red (660 nm) light in the treatment of acne vulgaris. Br J Dermatol 2000; 142:973–978.

Penny K, Sibbons P, Andrews P, Southgate A. A histopathologic evaluation of the effects of hydration on the absorption of plasma skin regeneration energy (PSR) in an animal model. Presented at the 2005 Meeting of the American Society of Laser Medicine and Surgery, Orlando, FL.

Pope K, Levinson M, Ross EV. Selective Fibrous Tissue Heating: An Additional Mechanism for Capacitively Coupled Monopolar Radiofrequency. Vol. 2. Haywood, CA: Thermage, Inc., 2005.

Raulin C, Greve B, Grema H. IPL technology: a review. Lasers Surg Med 2003; 32:78–87.

Sadick NS, Laughlin SA. Effective epilation of white and blond hair using combined radiofrequency and optical energy. J Cosmet Laser Ther 2004; 6:27–31.

Sadick NS, Makino Y. Selective electro-thermolysis in aesthetic medicine: a review. Lasers Surg Med 2004; 34:91–97.

Sadick NS, Shaoul J. Hair removal using a combination of conducted radiofrequency and optical energies—an 18-month follow-up. J Cosmet Laser Ther 2004; 6:21–26.

Trelles MA, Rigau J, Velez M. LLLT and *in vivo* effects on mast cells. In: Simunovic Z, ed. Lasers in Medicine and Dentistry. Croatia: Vitagraf, 2000:169–186.

Waldman A, Kreindle M. New technology in aesthetic medicine: ELOS electro optical synergy. J Cosmet Laser Ther 2003; 5:204–206.

Weiss RA, Goldman MP, Weiss MA. Treatment of Poikiloderma of Civatte with an intense pulsed light source. Dermatol Surg 2000; 26:823–827.

Weiss RA, McDaniel DH, Geronemus RG. Review of nonablative photorejuvenation: reversal of the aging effects of the sun and environmental damage using laser and light sources. Semin Cutan Med Surg 2003; 22:93–106.

Weiss RA, McDaniel DH, Geronemus RG, Weiss MA. Clinical trial of a novel non-thermal LED array for reversal of photoaging: clinical, histologic, and surface profilometric results. Lasers Surg Med 2005; 36:85–91.

Young S, Bolton P, Dyson M, et al. Macrophage responsiveness to light therapy. Lasers Surg Med 1989; 9:497–505.

Zelickson B, Kist D. Effect of pulse dye laser and intense pulsed light source on the dermal extracellular matrix remodeling. Lasers Surg Med Abstract Suppl 2000; 12:17.

Zelickson B, Kist D, Bernstein E, et al. Histological and ultrastructural evaluation of the effects of a radiofrequency-based nonablative dermal remodeling device: a pilot study. Arch Dermatol 2004; 140:204–209.

65

Laser Treatment of Tattoos and Pigmented Lesions

Arielle N. B. Kauvar

New York Laser and Skin Care and New York University School of Medicine, New York,
New York, and SUNY Downstate Medical Center, Brooklyn, New York, U.S.A.

Tatiana Khrom

SUNY Downstate Medical Center, Brooklyn, New York, U.S.A.

INTRODUCTION

Lasers were first applied for the treatment of pigmented lesions and tattoos by Goldman and colleagues in the early 1960s. Goldman and colleagues investigated both a normal-mode and Q-switched ruby laser (QSRL). They found that the QSRL, using nanosecond-domain pulses, was more effective at clearing epidermal pigment and dark tattoo ink without producing the non-specific thermal necrosis observed with the millisecond-range pulses of the normal-mode ruby laser. Others soon confirmed these early results, but work on the QSRL was then abandoned for some 15 years, while attention was focused on the development of the argon and carbon dioxide (CO_2) lasers.

In the 1970s and early 1980s, the argon and CO_2 lasers were used to treat pigmented lesions and tattoos. The argon laser emitted at 488 to 514 nm in a continuous wave mode, and was later adapted to deliver millisecond-range pulses by shuttering the light. Melanin and tattoo ink absorbed well in this spectrum, but the long exposure times produced non-specific thermal damage and often led to hypertrophic scarring. The continuous wave CO_2 laser was used to produce direct vaporization of tissue. For superficial epidermal lesions, acceptable clinical results could be achieved with proper technique, but deeper vaporization of tissue performed for tattoo removal resulted in fibrosis and visible scar formation (Fig. 1). The development of the principles of selective photothermolysis in the 1980s stimulated the development and investigation of lasers that produce selective rupture of melanosomes and tattoo ink particles without damaging the surrounding tissue.

Today, two main classes of light-based devices are used for treating melanocytic lesions. The major class of light-based devices includes pulsed lasers and filtered xenon flashlamps, known as intense pulse light sources (IPLs), that selectively destroy melanin-containing targets inside the skin. These devices are further classified into long-pulse (millisecond devices) and short-pulse (Q-switched, nanosecond) lasers. The long-pulse devices are best at targeting larger pigmented structures such as nests of nevus cells or hair follicles, and are also useful for treating benign epidermal pigmented lesions. Only the nanosecond lasers can target individual pigmented cells or tattoo ink particles, and they are used for the treatment of both epidermal and dermal pigmented lesions. Q-switched lasers remain the treatment of choice for all types of tattoos and pigmented lesions characterized by "non-nested" dermal melanocytes such as the nevus of Ota.

Mid- and far-infrared resurfacing lasers are the other group of lasers used for pigmented skin lesions. They are sometimes useful for treating the epidermal and superficial dermal component of pigmented lesions such as café-au-lait macules (CALM), refractory melasma, the superficial component of congenital melanocytic nevi, and flesh-colored tattoo inks at risk for idiosyncratic darkening with pulsed laser treatment. The CO_2 (10,600 nm) and erbium (2940 nm) resurfacing lasers emit wavelengths strongly absorbed by water and produce precise vaporization of tissue.

LASER–TISSUE INTERACTIONS
Selective Photothermolysis

The theory of selective photothermolysis, conceived by Anderson and Parrish in 1983, and more recently refined, describes the requirements to produce site-specific, thermally mediated damage of pigmented structures in biological tissues. Wavelengths of light are chosen that are preferentially absorbed by the target (which, for pigmented lesions, requires strong pigment absorption and weak absorption by the skin's other natural occurring chromophores—hemoglobin and water). Laser or light-induced thermal damage is confined to the structure, without diffusion of heat to the surrounding skin, when the pulse duration or exposure time of the light is less than or equal to the structures' thermal relaxation time (*trt*). The *trt* is the time required for significant cooling of a small target structure and is proportional to the square of its size. The calculated *trt* for melanosomes, which measure 0.5 to 1 μm is 250 to 1000 nsec, and the *trt* for tattoo ink particles, measuring in the range of 40 nm, is less than 10 nsec. Wavelengths of light are also chosen based on their ability to sufficiently penetrate the skin to reach the target. Lastly, sufficient energy density is provided to produce irreversible damage of the structure.

Selective photothermolysis requires that pulse durations less than 1 μsec be used for selective damage of melanosomes. This was demonstrated first with a 20-nsec, 351-nm XeF excimer laser, and subsequently with a 300- to 750-nsec, 435- to 750-nm tunable dye laser, a 40-ns QSRL, and a 5- to 10-nsec Q-switched neodymium:yttrium-aluminum-garnet (Nd:YAG) laser. Electron microscopic studies showed selective, dose-dependent disruption of

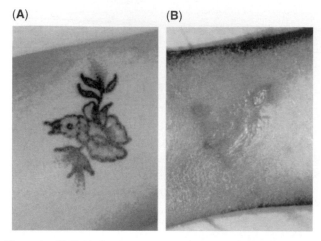

Figure 1 **(A)** Multicolored tattoo, prior to treatment. **(B)** Hypertrophic scar after treatment with the carbon dioxide laser.

melanosomes in melanocytes and keratinocytes following Q-switched laser pulses. Q-switched or "quality switched" refers to the ability to store large amounts of energy in the laser cavity using an optical shutter. Extremely high-power pulses, on the order of 100 W, are released when the laser fires with an ultrashort, nanosecond-domain pulse. Pigment particles or melanosomes are heated to 10 million degrees per second and explode. Mechanical damage from acoustic shock waves destroys the pigment-laden cells. Electron microscopic studies of the Q-switched laser-treated skin show cellular vacuolization, condensation of pigment and nuclear material at the cell periphery and subepidermal vesiculation at the level of the lamina lucida.

Clinically, at threshold fluences, Q-switched lasers produce an immediate ash-white discoloration of the skin at the laser impact site, which lasts approximately 30 minutes. This is thought to be caused by the scattering of visible light by steam cavities formed in melanosomes. Suprathreshold fluences will cause the ejection of fragments of tissue and pinpoint bleeding.

Pulse Duration

The optimal pulse duration for laser or light-based destruction of pigmented lesions is governed by the concentration and spatial distribution of the pigment. When the target for laser destruction is a homogeneous structure, the theory of selective photothermolysis applies. The goal is to irreversibly damage the target while keeping the surrounding tissue intact. Nevus of Ota, for example, consists of individual melanocytes dispersed singly through the dermis, and tattoos consist of pigment-laden phagocytes scattered in the dermis. Melanosomes and tattoo ink granules are submicrometer, intracellular particles with *trt* of 250 to 1000 and < 10 nsec, respectively. Only Q-switched lasers deliver sufficiently high-peak-power pulses in suitably short (nanosecond) pulses to produce explosive rupture of these dispersed pigment cells without harm to the surrounding dermis. Pulsewidths exceeding the *trt* of melanosomes do not create melanosomal disruption, even at exposure levels that cause gross injury. Instead, there is generalized damage to the surrounding organelles and cells. In addition, higher radiant exposures are required for lesions of lower pigment concentration. Treatment of pigmented lesions characterized by scattered, submicrometer chromophores

with a millisecond-duration laser or IPL would therefore require higher exposure and increase the risk of non-specific damage and scarring.

The use of such a short pulsewidth becomes ineffective when the absorbing chromophore is non-uniform or portions of the target structure exhibit weak or no absorption. The hair follicle and melanocytic nevi are examples of such cases. The light-absorbing structures in the hair follicle are the pigmented hair shaft and matrix cells. With sub-microsecond pulses, there would be minimal heat transfer to the stem cells and living outer root sheath, which must be damaged for permanent hair removal. Melanocytic nevi are composed of nests of melanocytes, including a subset of non-melanized cells, which must also be destroyed to prevent regrowth of the lesions. The extended theory of selective photothermolysis describes the requirements for longer pulsewidths when non-uniformly pigmented structures are targeted. Long (millisecond) pulses are therefore used for permanent hair removal and the treatment of melanocytic nevi, where diffusion of thermal energy from absorbing to non-absorbing regions of the target is required.

Almost any dermatologic laser or light source, when used properly, can safely remove benign epidermal lesions such as lentigines due to the impressive capacity for epidermal regeneration. Millisecond, pulsed green and yellow light lasers and IPLs generate thermal damage in pigmented lesions via direct pigment absorption. Ablative lasers such as the CO_2 and erbium, can be used to literally peel away such lesions. Treatment induces focal, confined epidermal necrosis. A fine crust forms and the skin reepithelializes without sequelae after approximately 1 week.

Melanin and Melanosomes

Melanin is normally present in the epidermis and hair follicles. Melanocytes synthesize melanin in melanosomes, and these structures are present in cells at various stages of pigmentation. Melanosomes are bound to cytoplasmic cytoskeletal proteins, and are transferred to keratinocytes in membrane-bound phagosomes. Melanin has a broad absorption spectrum which is most intense in the ultraviolet region, and slowly drops off throughout the visible to near-infrared spectra. In general, the red and near-infrared regions (approximately 600–1100 nm) are the best wavelengths for treating pigmented lesions. This band provides the most selective absorption by melanin (with minimal competition from hemoglobin) and the deepest skin penetration. While longer wavelengths provide deeper penetration, the absorption coefficient for melanin decreases with increasing wavelength. Consequently, the threshold dose for melanosome disruption (which correlates clinically with tissue whitening), is greater with longer wavelengths. Green and yellow sources are absorbed strongly by both hemoglobin and melanin, but their depth of penetration is more limited. Devices emitting in this range are used to treat superficial pigmented lesions.

Tattoo Ink

Professional tattoo inks consist mainly of insoluble metal salts, oxides, or organic complexes. Amateur tattoos are usually composed of India ink, graphite, or ash. Following the intradermal injection of tattoo ink, nanometer-sized insoluble ink particles are taken up by phagocytic cells. Over time, tattoos may slowly fade owing to the limited migration of phagocytic skin cells.

Goldman et al. were the first to demonstrate clearance of tattoos with a normal-mode ruby laser. QSRLs were successfully used by Laub et al. in 1968 and by Reid et al. in 1983 to remove tattoos. Dose–response and ultrastructural studies of the interaction of Q-switched laser pulses with tattooed skin, performed by Taylor and colleagues in 1990, stimulated great interest in the use of ultrashort-pulsed lasers to remove tattoos. Electron microscopic studies show that Q-switched laser treatment fractures the ink particles into 10 to 100 smaller fragments, which are present extracellularly, presumably via rupture of phagocytic cells. Small ink particles are evident in phagocytes weeks after treatment, and may be present histologically even when there is no longer evidence of residual tattoo.

Tattoo ink pigmentation is present in the draining lymph nodes of tattooed skin. It is likely that this is the fate of much of the ink following laser treatment, other than the small amount that is extruded in the scale crust after treatment. The exact mechanism of tattoo ink removal by Q-switched lasers remains largely unknown, but the process is thought to involve the following steps: (i) fragmentation of ink particles, (ii) release of ink particles into the extracellular space, (iii) loss of some ink via transepidermal elimination with scale-crust sloughing, (iv) elimination into the lymphatics, and (v) rephagocytosis of the smaller particles.

Unlike melanin, which absorbs broadly throughout the visible to near-infrared region, absorption of light by tattoo ink relates to their color. Reflectance data for tattoo inks help determine the best wavelengths for treatment. Absorption for the blue and green pigments is greatest at 600 to 800 nm, red absorbs best below 575 nm, tan below 560 nm, cream below 535 nm and yellow below 520 nm. The wavelengths currently available to treat tattoos in the nanosecond range are 532, 694, 755, and 1064 nm. The 532-nm wavelength can be converted to 585 or 650 nm with dye-impregnated handpieces, but the available fluence is quite low.

LASERS AND LIGHT SOURCES FOR PIGMENTED LESIONS AND TATTOOS
Pigment-Selective Lasers: Pulsed Lasers and IPLs
Q-Switched Laser Group
The QSRL has a wavelength of 694 nm and pulsewidth of approximately 30 nsec. Light is delivered through an articulated arm, and available systems pulse at about 1 Hz. Pigment absorption and depth of penetration are excellent at this wavelength. The QSRL effectively lightens black, blue, and green tattoo pigments, epidermal lesions (lentigines, freckles, and CALM), and dermal melanocytic lesions [nevus of Ota, Ito, blue nevi, acquired bilateral nevus of Ota-like macule (ABNOM, Hori's nevus), and congenital nevi].

The Q-switched alexandrite laser (QSAL) emits at 755 nm and has a pulsewidth of 100 to 300 nsec. Light is delivered through an articulated arm or a fiberoptic cable. Treatment applications of the QSAL are similar to those of the QSRL. The Q-switched YAG laser (QSYL) also operating through an articulated arm with a wavelength of 1064 nm and pulsewidth of 5 to 10 nsec, can remove black, but not blue or green tattoo pigments. It is effective for nevi of Ota, blue nevi, and ABNOM, but less so for superficial pigmented lesions, such as lentigines or freckles. The QSYL is especially effective for the treatment of tattoos or dermal pigmentation in darker phototype skin due to its longer absorption coefficient for melanin and lower risk of altering the skin pigment. The frequency-doubled QSYL emits at 532 nm. The wavelength is halved by placing a potassium-titanyl-phosphate (KTP) crystal in the path of the 1064-nm light. This laser is most effective for red ink and less so for orange, pink, and yellow pigments. With its short penetration depth, the Q-switched 532-nm laser is mainly used for epidermal pigmentation. Treatment results in purpura and pinpoint bleeding due to the strong hemoglobin absorption at this wavelength (Table 1).

Long-Pulse Laser Group
Millisecond-domain KTP lasers, emitting in the green (532 nm) spectrum, which are commonly used to treat vascular lesions, are also effective for treating superficial pigmented lesions, such as lentigines, macular seborrheic keratosis, and photodamage-associated dyschromia. These longer pulsewidths do not produce selective disruption of melanosomes, but rather impart thermal damage to the entire lesion, which crusts and rapidly reepithelializes. The yellow-light-pulse dye lasers with pulsewidths of 1.5 to 6 msec can similarly be used to treat superficial pigmented lesions. A new 595-nm laser was recently developed for this purpose. A specialized compression handpiece is used during treatment of pigmented lesions to propel blood away from the treatment site during light delivery and prevent purpura formation, even when pulsewidths as low as 1.5 msec are used. Due to the relatively short penetration depth at the green and yellow wavelengths, and the lack of melanosomal selectivity, these lasers cannot be used to treat dermal pigmentation.

The long-pulsed ruby (694 nm), alexandrite (755 nm), diode (800 nm), and Nd:YAG (1064 nm) lasers are widely used for laser hair removal where millisecond-domain pulses are required. The long-pulsed ruby and alexandrite lasers can be used to treat epidermal pigmentation, but not dermal lesions, where single cells predominate. The long-pulsed ruby and alexandrite lasers are also employed

Table 1 Response of Tattoo Colors to Pulsed Laser Therapy

	Q-switched ruby (694 nm)	Q-switched Nd:YAG (694 nm)	Q-switched Nd:YAG (532 nm)	Q-switched alexandrite (755 nm)	Pulsed green dye (510 nm)
Black-amateur	++	++	−	++	−
Black-professional	++	++	−	++	−
Blue	++	+	−	++	−
Green	++	−	−	++	−
Brown	++	+	−	++	−
Red	−	−	++	−	++
Yellow	+	+	+	+	+
Orange	+	+	+	+	+
Purple	+	+	+	+	+

++, Excellent response; +, moderate response; −, poor response.

to treat congenital melanocytic nevi, where the longer pulse durations are required to target nests of nevus cells.

Intense pulse light sources are high-intensity light sources that emit polychromatic light with millisecond-pulse durations. Depending on the unit, they may emit non-coherent light over a broad spectrum from 400 to 1200 nm. A series of cut-off filters are used to narrow down the spectrum, to increase selectivity for specific chromophore and/or depth of tissue penetration. Since melanin absorbs strongly throughout the visible light spectrum, the IPLs are useful for epidermal pigment and laser hair removal. The longer millisecond-pulse durations and lack of selectivity for dermal melanocytes and ink particles preclude their use for tattoo treatment and nevi of Ota.

Ablative Devices: CO$_2$ and Erbium Lasers

The CO$_2$ (10,600 nm) and erbium:YAG (2940 nm) lasers are pigment non-selective, but can ablate epidermal and dermal tissue because of their ability to target water. The CO$_2$ laser vaporizes tissue in a bloodless field by producing 100- to 150-μm zones of thermal coagulation as it ablates. The erbium laser ablates tissue with minimal residual damage, and will produce bleeding upon reaching the level of the papillary dermal plexus. Some newer erbium lasers permit simultaneous ablation and coagulation by means of combining supra-ablative and sub-ablative pulses. With appropriate techniques, these lasers can selectively remove epidermal lesions atraumatically. This is covered more extensively elsewhere in this text. Ablative lasers are also used to remove the superficial portions of congenital melanocytic nevi and for the treatment of tattoos comprised of pigment at risk for immediate darkening.

TREATMENT INDICATIONS
Epidermal Pigmented Lesions
Lentigo

Simple lentigo, solar lentigo (Fig. 2), labial lentigo (Fig. 3), and ephelides are easily removed with the QSRL, QSAL, and 532-nm QSYL in one to two treatment sessions. Histologically, theses lesions are characterized by an increased number of melanocytes in the basal layer with elongated rete ridges. Transient hypopigmentation is more common with the 532-nm QSYL and QSRL because of the increased

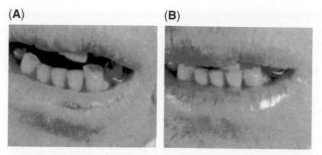

Figure 3 (A) Labial lentigo, prior to treatment. (B) Complete clearance after treatment with the argon laser.

absorption by melanin at these wavelengths. Treatment should therefore be limited to fair-skinned individuals without a sun tan. The 532-nm QSYL may also produce purpura with treatment due to the strong hemoglobin absorption. There is increased crusting and post-treatment erythema with this laser compared with the 694- and 755-nm wavelengths. The purpura may be minimized with the use of a glass microscope slide used to compress the blood away from the area during laser treatment. The 1064-nm QSYL is often less effective, particularly for faintly pigmented lesions, because of the lower absorption by melanin. The desired clinical endpoint is lesional whitening without purpura and ablation. The lesions crust for approximately 1 week. Lentigines may also be treated with IPLs and long-pulsed lasers, including the pulsed KTP and pulsed dye lasers, used with millisecond-pulse durations. Treatment efficacy is comparable to the Q-switched lasers. A compression handpiece now available for use with the pulsed dye laser and, along with a new micro-pulse sequence, preclude the development of purpura. The desired endpoint with millisecond-duration devices is lesional darkening without vesiculation or skin whitening, which signify epidermal necrosis. These short- and long-pulse laser and light devices produce similar results for lentigines associated with Peutz-Jegher, Moynahan, and Leopard syndromes.

Café-au-lait macule

CALM are tan to brown macules or patches that occur with an incidence of up to 14% in the population. These lesions are typically an isolated finding, but may be associated with a variety of neurocutaneous syndromes, including Von Recklinghausen disease, Albright syndrome, and Marfan syndrome. CALM may be treated with any of the Q-switched lasers, but the 1064-nm QSYL is least effective due to its lower absorption coefficient for melanin. Approximately one-third of CALM hyperpigment before clearing, and one-third recur after treatment. When they do respond to laser therapy, several treatments are usually required (Fig. 4).

Becker's Nevus

Becker's nevi are tan to brown patches, ranging from 2 to 40 cm in diameter, that appear during childhood or early adulthood, and are usually associated with hypertrichosis that becomes apparent after puberty. Histologically, these hamartomatous lesions are comprised of basal layer hyperpigmentation and with an increased number of melanocytes, sebaceous gland hyperplasia, and enlarged pilar apparati. Similar to the CALM, Becker's nevi respond variably to treatment with the Q-switched lasers.

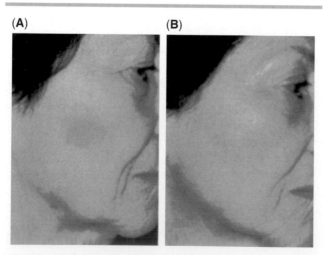

Figure 2 (A) Solar lentigo on the cheek of a woman. (B) Complete clearance after treatment with the Q-switched ruby laser.

(A)   **(B)**

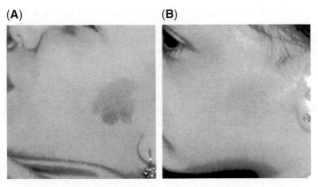

Figure 4 (A) Café-au-lait macule on the cheek of an infant, prior to treatment. (B) Approximately 90% lightening after five treatments with the Q-switched ruby laser.

Dermal Pigmented Lesions
Nevus of Ota

Nevus of Ota is a benign congenital blue–black discoloration of the face in the distribution of the first and second branches of the trigeminal nerve, which is often associated with pigmentation of the ipsilateral sclera. The lesion is usually present at birth but may darken after puberty with stimulation of the dermal melanocytes. These lesions occur most commonly in Asians, with an estimated incidence of 1% to 2% in the Japanese population, and other races are variably affected. Nevi of Ota fall within the spectrum of blue nevi, and are characterized histologically by elongated, bipolar melanocytes scattered throughout the upper half of the dermis. The shorter-wavelength green light lasers are ineffective in lightening these lesions since the light does not penetrate far enough into the dermis. Excellent results with complete or partial clearing without scarring are obtained using the QSRL (Fig. 5), the QSAL and the 1064-nm QSYL. Nevus of Ito is a lesion that clinically and histologically resembles the nevus of Ota, but is found on the shoulder or upper arm in the distribution of the supraclavicular and lateral brachial cutaneous nerves. Nevi of Ito, blue nevi, mongolian spots, and the pigmented patches in phakomatosis pigmentovascularis also respond well to treatment with the QSRL, QSAL, and QSYL.

(A)   **(B)**

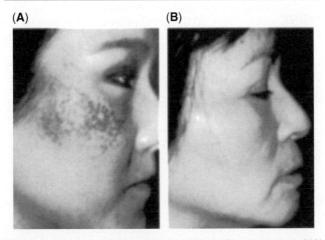

Figure 5 (A) Nevus of Ota, prior to treatment. (B) Approximately 90% lightening after five treatments with the Q-switched ruby laser.

Q-switched lasers remain the treatment of choice for nevi of Ota and other blue nevi. The presence of single, non-nested dermal melanocytes in these lesions requires selective heating and rupture of melanosomes to lighten these lesions without risking damage to the surrounding skin, as described above. Treatment is usually associated with 1-week period of crusting. The QSRL has the greatest potential for transient hypopigmentation, and the QSYL is safest in the darker phototypes. Transient hyperpigmentation may occur after treatment, and responds well to hydroquinone and sunscreen. ABNOM or Hori's nevus consists of epidermal and dermal pigmentation that responds to a combination of Q-switched laser treatment and bleaching creams. These patients usually have coincident melasma.

Melanocytic Nevi

Removal of benign melanocytic nevi is often sought for cosmesis. Laser eradication of melanocytic nevi without scarring offers considerable advantages over conventional surgical techniques, particularly for lesions located in cosmetically sensitive locations. Common acquired nevi usually appear after the first 6 months of life, and most develop in adolescence and early adulthood, during which time crops of new lesions may arise.

Histologically, melanocytic nevi are composed of collections of melanocytes present in the epidermis (junctional nevi), dermis (intradermal nevi), or both (compound nevi). The shorter-wavelength green light lasers are ineffective modalities for treating lesions with dermal melanocytes. The 694-nm QSRL was reported to be effective in removing 12% (9 of 74) of benign melanocytic nevi in a Japanese population. Histologic evaluation revealed that lesions with junctional nests responded well, while nevi with mid-dermal nests failed to respond to the QSRL. A preliminary histological study of nevi treated with the QSRL in eight patients showed no evidence of residual nevus cells in two nevi, a decreased number of nevus cells in five nevi, and no change in the number of nevus cells in one nevus. The QSRL and QSAL are capable of removing junctional nevi and some thin compound nevi. When laser treatment results in partial removal of the nevus, repigmentation remains possible. Since partial removal of common acquired melanocytic nevi is routinely performed using conventional surgical techniques, laser treatment remains an acceptable alternative to lightening clinically benign appearing junctional and compound nevi. While junctional nevi are removed in one or two sessions, compound nevi may require a greater number of treatments.

Dysplastic Nevi and Melanoma-In-Situ

Acquired dysplastic melanocytic nevi should not be treated because these lesions are potential histogenic precursors of melanoma and markers of increased melanoma risk. Continuous wave lasers and the QSRL have been used to treat melanoma-in-situ, but there are several reports of melanoma-in-situ recurring after laser treatment. This is likely a result of persistence of the atypical melanocytes in the deeper portions of the adnexal structures that repopulate the epidermis. There are also anecdotal reports of recurrence of amelanotic melanoma-in-situ after QSRL, likely due to expansion of non-melanized clones of cells that could not be targeted with the pigment-specific laser. Laser treatment should not be considered as a potential curative procedure for melanoma-in-situ. In rare instances, it has been used as a palliative procedure in elderly patients who are inoperable.

These considerations must be explained in detail to anyone considering this intervention.

Congenital Melanocytic Nevi

Laser treatment of congenital nevi remains a controversial topic. Small congenital nevi have a diameter of 1 to 3 cm and occur in approximately 1/100 births. These lesions are present with a greater than normal frequency in patients with malignant melanoma. Large congenital nevi are usually 5 to 20 cm in diameter, but may involve larger surface areas of the body. When most of the trunk is involved, the lesion is called a giant hairy bathing-trunk nevus. Although the incidence of malignant melanoma arising in large congenital nevi is unknown, the lifetime risk has been reported to vary from 4% to 20%. Since congenital nevi extend into the deep reticular dermis, it is unlikely that treatment with either Q-switched or long-pulsed lasers could destroy all the nevus cells. Laser treatment, therefore, is unlikely to prevent the development of melanoma in these lesions. Nonetheless, for purposes of cosmesis, partial surgical excision or dermabrasion of large lesions is routinely performed. It may be argued that laser treatment of congenital nevi poses similar risks by partially removing the nevus cells, but the cosmetic outcome is likely to be superior, with less chance of permanent scarring or textural change. Laser treatment always leaves some residual nevus cells, and one must also consider the possibility that laser may inadvertently stimulate transformation of nevus to melanoma (although no evidence exists to substantiate this concern). Complete surgical excision remains the treatment of choice, and laser must be considered a secondary alternative. The risks and benefits of laser treatment in the context of other treatment alternatives must be candidly discussed with patients, and the informed consent should be well documented. While controversial, laser treatment of small congenital nevi or portions of large congenital nevi that are located in cosmetically important areas may be an appropriate modality in cases when surgical excision is an impractical consideration.

Most of the experience using lasers to treat congenital nevi comes from Japan. Ueda and Imayama first reported on the successful clinical resolution of congenital nevi after a series of high-fluence long-pulse ruby laser treatments. Histological examination of these lesions suggested that the formation of a superficial layer of fibrosis served to "hide" the residual layer of deep nevus cells. Kono et al. achieved improved responses by combining Q-switched and long-pulse laser treatment of congenital nevi. The rationale was that these lesions are comprised of both nests of nevus cells and isolated nevo-melanocytes, the former being more susceptible to long-pulse irradiation, and the latter to Q-switched pulses. Any of the Q-switched lasers can be used in combination with the long-pulse lasers that are routinely used for hair removal (ruby, alexandrite, diode, or Nd:YAG) or IPLs. Improved results are achieved when the epidermis is removed at the time of laser treatment. The Q-switched lasers, at high fluence, or the ablative lasers (CO_2 or erbium) are used to strip the epidermis prior to long-pulse irradiation. The long-pulse lasers are used with bulk cooling to avoid gross thermal injury and scarring. Local or general anesthesia is required for these procedures.

Nevus Spilus

Nevus spilus is a pigmented lesion comprised of junctional or compound nevi within a background field of macular café-au-lait pigmentation. The response of these lesions to pulsed and Q-switched lasers is not predictable, and multiple treatment sessions are necessary when they do respond to laser therapy.

Melasma

Melasma is an acquired hypermelanosis of the face usually associated with pregnancy or oral contraceptive therapy. Two types of melasma are found on histologic examination and can be clinically differentiated by Wood's light examination. The epidermal type is characterized by highly melanized melanosomes in the basilar and suprabasilar layers. In the dermal type, melanophages are scattered throughout the dermis in addition to the epidermal hyperpigmentation. Although the Q-switched lasers, IPLs, and ablative lasers have all been reported to clear melasma, repigmentation is common. Post-inflammatory hyperpigmentation and hemosiderin deposition usually responds to treatment with the QSRL or QSAL in combination with an aggressive topical bleaching regimen and sun protection.

Drug Deposits

A variety of systemic medications may produce dermal deposits that clinically present with skin pigmentation. Minocycline may produce focal gray (type I) or generalized blue–brown (type II) pigmentation. Melanophages and siderophages are present in the dermis. The QSRL and the 532-nm QSYL are effective in treating this pigmentation, but variable responses are seen with the 1064-nm QSYL. Other dermal deposits that are responsive to Q-switched laser therapy include amiodarone pigmentation, pigmentation due to antimalarial agents, imipramine, and dental agents such as amalgam. Iron deposits leave a brownish discoloration in the skin. This phenomenon can be observed after intramuscular iron injections and has been successfully treated with Q-switched lasers (Table 2).

Certain medications may result in paradoxical skin pigmentation following treatment with Q-switched lasers. The QSRL has been reported to induce chrysiasis in a number of patients on long-term gold therapy. Laser-induced chrysiasis appears to be irradiance dependent, either due to mechanical alteration of the aurosome particles or due to a chemical change. One group of investigators proposes that the high irradiances may promote multiphoton events responsible for this change. These authors found that pulse-widths >1 msec did not induce chrysiasis, and successfully treated their patient with a long-pulse ruby laser.

Tattoos

Tattooing is a common behavior is the Western world among people of all ages, social classes, and occupations. Three percent to 9% of the general population and 16% of adolescents are reported to have at last one decorative tattoo. Decorative tattoos are applied with a wide variety of pigments, including metal oxides, metal salts, and organometallic complexes. Crude, amateur tattoos are often self-inflicted or forced by gangs, prisoners, military personnel, or adolescents using pins or needles with charcoal, India ink, soot, or mascara. Traumatic tattoos may result from asphalt abrasions, gunpowder explosions, or lead pencil impregnation. Cosmetic tattoos are placed as permanent makeup applications (e.g., lip liner, eyeliner, eyebrows, or blush), or to camouflage scars or birthmarks.

Multiple modalities have been used in the past to remove tattoos, including excisional surgery, acid applications, cryosurgery, dermabrasion and salabrasion, but they

Table 2 Treatment of Drug-Induced Pigmentation

Drug	Distribution	Histology	Treatment
Antimalarials	Bluish pigmentation shins, face, oral mucosa, nail bed, cartilage, joints	Increase in melanin and hemosiderin in lower epidermis and dermis	Q-switched ruby
Imipramine	Blue to slate-gray hyperpigmentation in sun-exposed areas	Brown granules (drug-melanosome complexes) free in the dermis, within macrophages and along the basement membrane zone	Q-switched ruby, alexandrite
Amiodarone	Slate-blue discoloration of sun-exposed areas	Yellow-brown granules within histiocytes of the upper dermis (presumably composed of drug, lipofuscin, and melanin)	Q-switched ruby
Minocycline	Blue–black pigment in areas of inflammation or scarring	Hemosiderin associated with macrophages	Q-switched ruby, alexandrite, YAG
	Blue–gray pigmentation of shins	Iron (possibly complexed with drug)	
	Diffuse muddy brown pigmentation	Increased melanin of the basal cell layer and within dermal macrophages	
Gold	Blue–gray discoloration in sun-exposed areas	Gold granules within histiocytes or in the dermis	Long-pulsed ruby laser. Avoid Q-switched laser therapy
Silver	Slate-blue pigmentation in sun-exposed areas, oral mucosa, conjunctivae	Silver granules within histiocytes; silver granules and melanin within dermis	?
Amalgam	Dark gray or blue macule adjacent to a restored tooth. Most are located on the gingiva and alveolar mucosa followed by the buccal mucosa and the floor of the mouth	Irregular dark, solid fragments of metal or numerous, discrete fine, brown or black granules dispersed along collagen bundles and around small blood vessels and nerves. In most lesions, it is presented in both forms	Q-switched alexandrite
Iron	Injection sites	Hemosiderin	Q-switched Nd:YAG and/or Q-switched ruby, alexandrite

Source: From Buchner (2004); Derpurp (2110); Elder (1997).

all result in undesirable scarring. Treatment of tattoos with continuous wave lasers, including the ruby, argon, and CO_2, produced poor results with a high incidence of hypertrophic scarring. CO_2 laser treatment of tattoos produces direct vaporization of pigment-containing tissue as well as thermal necrosis of adjacent tissue, and often leads to hypertrophic scarring. Scarring was only somewhat improved with the use of superpulsed CO_2 lasers and ablative "resurfacing" lasers that produce more precise vaporization and limit non-specific thermal damage.

Q-Switched Lasers

Goldman and colleagues studied the response of a tattoo to a microsecond and nanosecond ruby laser in the 1960s. The QSRL produced a "peculiar" whitening of the skin, and the tattoo faded with continued monitoring. Few others confirmed these results over a period of some 20 years with little interest in the subject. Detailed dose–response studies performed by Taylor and colleagues demonstrated 78% clearance of amateur tattoos, but only 23% clearance of professional tattoos using a 40- to 80-ns QSRL at 1.5 to 4.0 J/cm^2. There was also a 39% to 46% incidence of

Table 3 Red, Yellow, Orange, Purple Tattoos

Shorter-wavelength lasers	Longer-near-infrared-wavelength lasers
Red, yellow, orange, purple tattoos	Green, black tattoos
Seborrheic keratosis	Congenital nevi
Café-au-lait macules	Lentigines
	Nevus of Ota, nevus of Ito
Becker's nevus	Mongolian spots
	Café-au-lait macules
Melasma	Becker's nevus
	Melasma

hypopigmentation, depending on the fluence used. Improved results were achieved with higher fluences and shorter pulsewidths.

The QSRL is best at removing black and green inks, and less so with blue ink. Multiple treatment sessions are required, usually four to six for amateur (Fig. 6) and 6 to 12, but sometimes more for professional tattoos (Fig. 7). Laser treatment is usually performed at 6- to 12-week intervals. Even after multiple treatment sessions, a "ghost" of the tattoo may remain, and patients should be warned of this possibility. Treatment is somewhat painful, and most patients prefer local intradermal anesthesia over topical lidocaine creams. The treatment endpoint should be immediate skin whitening without bleeding or ablation, and the fluence is adjusted to achieve this result. Healing consists of crusting and serosanguinous drainage lasts up to 10 to 14 days. The healing site is cleansed and dressed with bacitracin or polysporin ointment and a dry dressing twice daily.

The QSYL at 1064 nm was next explored with the thought that its increased dermal penetration and decreased melanin absorption would improve tattoo clearance with fewer side effects. Observations from multiple reports indicate that the QSYL is equally effective as the QSRL for the removal of black and blue–black tattoos, but less effective for green pigments. Higher fluences produce increased pigment clearance. There is less hyperpigmentation and hypopigmentation than with the QSRL, and this wavelength is safer in darker phototypes. As with the QSRL, other colors do not respond to the 1064-nm QSYL. The 1064-nm QSYL can be converted to 532 nm using a frequency doubling KTP crystal. The green light is well absorbed by melanin, hemoglobin, red inks, less so by purple, orange inks, and has minimal absorption by yellow pigment. Due to coincident absorption by melanin and hemoglobin, purpura, pinpoint bleeding and blistering frequently occur. The

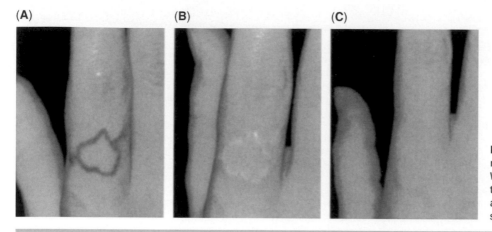

Figure 6 (**A**) Amateur tattoo, prior to treatment with the Q-switched ruby laser. (**B**) Whitening of tattoo immediately following a treatment session. (**C**) Complete clearance after four treatment sessions with the Q-switched ruby laser.

number of required treatments, the treatment intervals, and pre- and postoperative care are the same as with the QSRL. The 510-nm pulsed dye laser was another green light laser developed for treating epidermal pigmentation and red tattoo pigment. This laser had a pulse duration of 300 nsec, and was effective for red, and less so for purple, orange, and yellow inks. This system is no longer commercially available.

The QSAL at 755 nm, with pulse durations of 50 to 100 nsec, was the next system developed for the treatment of tattoos and pigmented lesions. As would be expected from its wavelength, it behaves very similarly to the QSRL at 694 nm. Black, blue–black and green tattoo pigments respond well, while other colors do not. There is less transient pigmentary alteration observed with the QSAL than the QSRL, but the QSYL remains the safest laser for darker phototypes. Again, the same treatment guidelines apply for this Q-switched laser.

At present, no one laser can remove all tattoos colors well (Fig. 8). Several studies have compared the relative efficacy of different Q-switched lasers in treating the same tattoos. Although in many of these studies sample sizes were too small for accurate comparisons, certain trends have emerged from these investigations. The QSRL, QSYL, and

QSAL are equally effective in removing black pigment. The QSRL and QSAL are more effective in the removal of green ink than the QSYL. The 532-nm QSYL is best at removing red ink, but less so for purple, orange, and yellow pigments. These results were confirmed with an in vitro agarose gel assay developed by one author (ANBK) to test the responsiveness of various color tattoo inks to Q-switched laser treatment. A study comparing a picosecond to a nanosecond Nd:YAG laser showed improved clearance of tattoo pigment with the picosecond pulses, presumably due to the higher peak temperatures achievable with these shorter pulsewidths. Unfortunately, high-energy picosecond pulses are difficult and expensive to produce, and the commercial development of such a system is not a viable option.

Several generalizations can be made concerning the treatment of tattoos with all of the Q-switched lasers. Although some patients can tolerate laser therapy of their tattoos without anesthesia, many patients desire local anesthesia which is administered with injections of 1% lidocaine with epinephrine. For large tattoos, the author performs tumescent anesthesia using 0.3% lidocaine to decrease the total dose of lidocaine delivered. Amateur tattoos generally require fewer treatment sessions than professional tattoos. The carbon-based and India ink pigments found in amateur tattoos appear to clear more easily than the organic

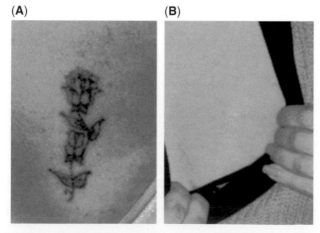

Figure 7 (**A**) Professional tattoo on a woman's chest, prior to treatment. The red areas were treated with the 532-nm Q-switched Nd:YAG, and the black and green areas were treated with the 694-nm Q-switched ruby laser. (**B**) Complete clearance with transient hypopigmentation following seven treatment sessions.

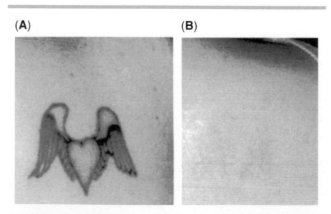

Figure 8 (**A**) Multicolored, professional tattoo prior to treatment. (**B**) Approximately 90% lightening after six treatment sessions with the Q-switched ruby laser for the black pigment and the Q-switched YAG laser for the red pigment.

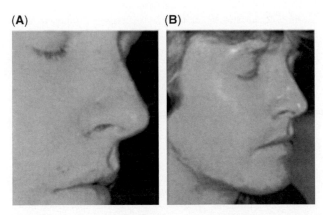

(A) **(B)**

Figure 9 **(A)** Traumatic tattoo, prior to treatment. **(B)** Approximately 90% lightening after four treatment sessions with the Q-switched ruby laser.

dyes in professional tattoos. The Q-switched lasers are also used to remove tattoos applied for marking purposes (e.g., radiation ports), and traumatic tattoos comprised of gunpowder (Fig. 9), asphalt, or lead pencil. The greater density of ink placed in professional tattoos may also be a factor. Green inks, fluorescent inks, and those with "brighteners" are the most difficult to remove. Older tattoos usually require fewer treatments than newer tattoos, presumably owing to greater uptake in phagocytes, and distally placed tattoos are slower to respond than more proximal tattoos. These phenomena may relate to tattoo ink dispersion over time and the relative efficiency of lymphatic drainage in different anatomic locations.

Adverse Effects

Laser removal of cosmetic tattoos, especially those with skin-colored pink, tan, or white pigments, should be approached with caution. Immediate, irreversible darkening of cosmetic tattoos following Q-switched and pulsed nano-second laser treatment has recently been described (Fig. 10). Irreversible ink darkening has been documented to occur with the QSRL, QSYL, and pulsed green dye (510 nm) lasers, but may occur with any high-energy, short-pulse duration laser operating in the visible through near-infrared wavelengths. In only some cases is removal of the darkened ink possible with subsequent laser treatments. Patients who seek laser removal of cosmetic tattoos must be forewarned of this possible complication, and test sites should be performed before embarking on treatment of a large area.

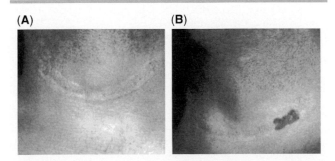

(A) **(B)**

Figure 10 **(A)** A white cosmetic tattoo on the anterior neck applied to cover a thyroidectomy scar. **(B)** Immediate tattoo blackening was noted after Q-switched ruby laser exposure in a test area.

Although the chemical mechanism of tattoo ink darkening is unknown, it is likely that conversion of ferric oxide (Fe_2O_3) to ferrous oxide (FeO) and/or other iron compounds is involved. Extreme temperatures, pressures, and free charge carriers induced by high-peak power laser pulses presumably cause this conversion to ferrous oxide. In vitro tests have demonstrated the conversion of white, yellow, red, and brown pigments, composed of ferric oxide, to a gray–black color immediately following exposure to QSRL, QSYL, and QSAL.

A similar phenomenon may be involved in white and other iron-free pigments. Ross et al. demonstrated that titanium is present in higher concentrations in laser-resistant tattoos, and may be the cause of poor response to treatment. In untreated tattoos, titanium is present as titanium dioxide (TiO_2), which is bright white. High-intensity laser irradiation reduces Ti^{4+} to Ti^{3+}, which turns a blue color. Titanium is commonly added to green and flesh color pigments to "brighten" them, but may be added any color ink. Some green pigments are comprised of as much as 30% titanium. This may explain the relative resistance of green inks, in particular, to laser treatment.

Cosmetic tattoos can be safely removed with resurfacing CO_2 and erbium lasers in a staged procedure. An ablative procedure is performed to the level of the papillary dermis, not to the depth of the pigment. The wound is kept moist with frequent soaks and ointment application until reepithelialization at approximately one week. The pigment is removed via transepidermal elimination. Three to six treatment sessions may be required, at approximately 6- to 8-week intervals.

As mentioned previously, hypertrophic scarring is a phenomenon of the past, now that continuous wave lasers are no longer used. When treating tattoos, the lowest possible fluence inducing an adequate clinical response consisting of skin whitening in the treated areas should be used to minimize trauma to the skin. Only Q-switched lasers should be used for the treatment of tattoos. Anecdotally, hypertrophic scarring has been observed with the use of some IPLs for treatment of tattoos.

Tattoo pigments may produce localized immediate or delayed hypersensitivity reactions, and treatment with high-energy lasers may induce several types of allergic response. One is a local reaction consisting of an urticarial or id-like reaction. The other is a systemic immediate hypersensitivity reaction. If a local allergic reaction is present, laser treatment may induce a generalized allergic reaction. Pretreatment with 3 days of prednisone and anti-histamines has been reported to prevent generalized allergic reactions in such individuals.

The potential transmission of infectious particles is another concern during Q-switched laser treatment of tattoos. The high energy, nanosecond pulses often produce ejection of tissue fragments. When tissue ejection is observed the fluence should be lowered. All personnel involved in the laser treatment should use appropriate protective barriers.

CONCLUSION

The tremendous advancements made in the development of lasers in the past decades have produced novel therapies for both tattoos and a wide variety of benign pigmented lesions. With the emergence of the concept of selective photothermolysis, high-peak-power, short-pulse duration lasers were developed that could direct preferential injury to pigment particles and melanosomes, thereby minimizing the risk of damage to the surrounding skin. It has recently been shown that long-pulse lasers can also clear epidermal lesions by imparting localized thermal damage. Excellent clearing of multicolored tattoos can be obtained using a combination of Q-switched lasers. Pigmented lesions that can be safely and effectively treated with lasers include ephelides, solar lentigines, and the nevus of Ota. Many café-au-lait macules, Becker's nevi, and melanocytic nevi are successfully cleared with lasers. Post-inflammatory pigmentation and melasma respond variably to laser therapy.

BIBLIOGRAPHY

Alster TS. Q-switched alexandrite laser treatment (755 nm) of professional and amateur tattoos. J Am Acad Dermatol 1995; 33(1):69–73.

Altshuler GB, Anderson RR, Manstein D, Zenzie HH, Smirnov MZ. Extended theory of selective photothermolysis. Lasers Surg Med 2001; 29:416–432.

Amrstrong ML, Murphy KP. Tattooing: another adolescent risk behavior warranting health education. Appl Nurs Res 1997; 10:181–189.

Anderson RR, Margolis RJ, Watanabe S et al. Selective photothermolysis of cutaneous pigmentation by Q-switched Nd:YAG laser pulses at 1064, 532 and 355 nm. J Invest Dermatol 1989; 93:28–30.

Anderson RR, Margolis RJ, Watanabe S, Flotte T, Hruza GJ, Dover JS. Selective photothermolysis of cutaneous pigmentation by Q-switched Nd:YAG laser pulses at 1064, 532, and 355 nm. J Invest Dermatol 1989; 93:28–32.

Anderson RR, Parrish RR. Selective photothermolysis: precise microsurgery by selective absorption of pulsed radiation. Science 1983; 220:524–527.

Anderson RR. Tattooing should be regulated (letter). N Engl J Med 1992; 326:207.

Apfelberg DB, Maser MR, Lash H et al. The argon laser for cutaneous lesions. JAMA 1981; 245:2073–2075.

Apfelberg DB, Rivers J, Maser MR et al. Update on laser usage in treatment of decorative tattoos. Lasers Surg Med 1982; 2: 169–177.

Apfelberg DB, Maser MR, Lash R et al. Comparison of argon and carbon dioxide laser treatment of decorative tattoos: a preliminary report. Ann Plast Surg 1985; 14:6–8.

Apfelberg DB, Maser MR, Lash R et al. Comparison of argon and carbon dioxide laser treatment of decorative tattoos: a preliminary report. Ann Plast Surg 1985; 14:6–8.

Apfelberg DB, Manchester GH. Decorative and traumatic tattoo biophysics and removal. Clin Plast Surg 243–251.

Ara G, Anderson RR, Mandel KG, Onesen M, Oseroff AR. Irradiation of pigmented melanoma cells with high intensity pulsed radiation generates acoustic waves and kills cells. Laser Surg Med 1990; 10:52–59.

Argenyi ZB, Finelli L, Bergfeld WF et al. Mincocycline-related cutaneous hyperpigmentation as demonstrated by light microscopy, electron microscopy and X-ray energy spectroscopy. J Cutan Pathol 1987; 14:176–180.

Armstrong ML, McConnell C. Tattooing in adolescents: more common than you think—the phenomenon and risks. J Sch Nurs 1994; 10:22–29.

Armstrong ML, Stuppy DJ, Gabriel DC, Anderson RR. Motivation for tattoo removal. Arch Dermatol 1996; 132(4): 412–416.

Arndt KA. Argon laser treatment of lentigo maligna. J Am Acad Dermatol 1984; 10:953–957.

Arndt KA. New pigmented macule appearing 4 years after argon laser treatment of lentigo maligna. J Am Acad Dermatol 1986; 14:1092.

Ashinoff R, Levine VJ, Soter NA. Allergic reactions to tattoo pigment after laser treatment. Dermatol Surg 1995; 21(40): 291–294.

Ashinoff R, Levine V, Tse Y et al. Removal of pigmented lesions: comparison of the Q-switched ruby and neodynium:YAG lasers (abstr). Laser Surg Med 1994; 14(suppl 6):50.

Atkin DH, Fitzpatrick RF. Laser treatment of imipramine-induced hyperpigmentation. JAAD 2000; 4:77.

Bailin PL, Ratz JL, Levine HL. Removal of tattoos by CO_2 laser. J Dermatol Surg Oncol 1980; 6:997.

Bailin PL, Ratz JL, Levine HL. Removal of tattoos by CO_2 laser. J Dermatol Surg Oncol 1980; 6:997–1001.

Bailin PL, Ratz JL, Levine HL. Removal of tattoos by CO_2 laser. J Dermatol Surg Oncol 1980; 6:997–1001.

Ballin DB. Cutaneous hypersensitivity to mercury from tattooing: report of case. Arch Dermatol Symph 1933; 27:292.

Beacon JP, Ellis H. Surgical removal of tattoos by carbon dioxide laser. J Roy Soc Med 1980; 73:298–301.

Beacon JP, Ellis H. Surgical removal of tattoos by carbon dioxide laser. J Roy Soc Med 1980; 73:298–300.

Beacon JP, Ellis H. Surgical removal of tattoos by carbon dioxide laser. J Roy Soc Med 1980; 73:298–300.

Beacon JP, Ellis H. Surgical removal of tattoos by carbon dioxide laser. J Roy Soc Med 1980; 73:298–301.

Becker-Wegerich PM, Kuhn A, Malek L et al. Treatment of non-melanotic hyperpigmentation with the Q-switched ruby laser. JAAD 2000; 43:272.

Bjornberg A. Reactions to light in yellow tattoos from cadmium sulfide. Arch Dermatol 1963; 88:267.

Bjornberg A. Allergic reactions to chrome in green tattoo markings. Acta Derm Venereal 1959; 39:23.

Bonnell JA, Russell B. Skin reactions at sites of green and red tattoo marks. Proc R Soc Med 1956; 49:823.

Brady SC, Blokmanis A, Jewett L. Tattoo removal with the carbon dioxide laser. Ann Plast Surg 1978; 2:482–484.

Brady SC, Blokmanis A, Jewett L. Tattoo removal with the carbon dioxide laser. Ann Plast Surg 1978; 2:482–484.

Buchner A. Amalgam tatoo (amalgam pigmentation) of the oral mucosa: clinical manifestations, diagnosis and treatment [republished]. Refuat Hapeh Vehashinayim 2004; 21(2):19–22.

Buncke HJ Jr., Conway H. Surgery of decorative and traumatic tattoos. Plast Reconstr Surg 1957; 20:67–69.

Chai KB. The decorative tattoo: its removal by dermabrasion. Plast Reconstr Surg 1963; 32:559–563.

Chang CJ, Nelson JS, Achauer BM. Q-switched ruby laser treatment of oculodermal melanosis (nevus of Ota). Plast Reconstr Surg 1996; 98(5):784–790.

Clabaugh W. Removal of tattoos by superficial dermabrasion. Arch Dermatol 1968; 98:515–521.

Collins P, Cotterill JA. Minocycline-induced pigmentation resolves after treatment with the Q-switched ruby laser. Br J Dermatol 1996; 135:317–319.

DeCoste SD, Anderson RR. Comparison of Q-switched ruby and Q-switched Nd:YAG laser treatment of tattoos. Lasers Surg Med 1991; (suppl 3):64.

Dereure O. Drug-induced skin pigmentation. Am J Clin Dermatol 2110; 2(4):253–262.

Dixon J. Laser treatment of decorative tattoos. In: Arndt KA, Noe JM, Rosen S, eds. Cutaneous Laser Therapy: Principles and Methods. New York: John Wiley and Sons, 1983:201–211.

Dover JS, Polla LL, Margolis RJ et al. Pulsewidth dependence of pigment cell damage at 694 nm in guinea pig skin. In: Scott RS, Parrish JA, Jaffe N, eds. Lasers in Medicine. Proceedings of SPIE , 1986.

Dover JS, Margolis RJ, Polla LL, et al. Pigmented guinea pig skin irradiated with Q-switched ruby laser pulses. Arch Dermatol 1989; 125:43–49.

Dover JS, Smoller BR, Stein RS. Low-fluence carbon dioxide laser irradiation of lentigines. Arch Dermatol 1988; 124:1219–1224.

Ee HL, Goh CL, Khoo LS, Chan EY, Ang P. Treatment of acquired bilateral nevus of Ota-like macules (Hori's nevus) with a combination of the 532 nm Q-switched Nd:YAG laser followed by the 1,064 nm Q-switched Nd:YAG is more effective: prospective study. Dermatol Surg 2006; 32(1):34–40.

Elder D, Elenitsas R, Jaworsky C, Johnson B. Lever's Clinical Histopathology. 8thn. Philadelphia: Lippincott-Raven, 1997.

England RW, Vogel P, Hagan L. Immediate cutaneous hypersensitivity after treatment of tattoo with Nd:YAG laser: a case report and review of the literature. Ann Allergy Asthma Immunol 2002; 89(2):215–217.

Everett MA. Tattoos: abnormalities of pigmentation. In: Clinical Dermatology. Vol. 2. Hagerston, MD: Harper & Row, 1980: 11–21.

Ferguson JE, August PJ. Evaluation of the Nd:YAG laser for treatment of amateur and professional tattoos. Br J Dermatol 1996; 135(4):586–591.

Fitzpatrick RE, Goldman MP. Tattoo removal using the alexandrite lasers. Arch Dermatol 1994; 130(12):1508–1514.

Fitzpatrick RE, Goldman MP, Ruiz-Esparza J. The use of the alexandrite laser (755 nm, 100 msec) for tattoo pigment removal in an animal model. J Am Acad Dermatol 1993; 28:745.

Fitzpatrick RE, Goldman MP, Ruiz-Esparza J. Laser treatment of benign pigmented epidermal lesions using a 300 nsec pulse and 510 nm wavelength. J Dermatol Surg Oncol 1993; 18:341–347.

Geronemus RG, Ashinoff R. Use of the Q-switched ruby laser to treat tattoos and benign pigmented lesions of the skin. Lasers Surg Med 1991; (suppl 3):64.

Geronemus RG. Q-switched ruby laser therapy of nevus of Ota. Arch Dermatol 1992; 128(12):1618–1622.

Goldman L, Rockwell RJ, Meyer R et al. Laser treatment of tattoos. J Am Med Assoc 1967; 201:163.

Goldman L, Wilson RG, Hornby P et al. Radiation from a Q-switched ruby laser. J Invest Dermatol 1965; 44:69.

Goldman MP, Fitzpatrick RE. Treatment of benign pigmented cutaneous lesions. In: Cutaneous Laser Surgery: The Art and Science of Selective Photothermolysis. St Louis, MO: Mosby, 1994:106–141.

Goldberg D. Benign pigmented lesions of the skin, treatment with the Q-switched ruby laser. J Dermatol Surg Oncol 1993; 19:376–379.

Goldman L, Blaney DJ, Kindel DJ et al. Effect of the laser beam on the skin: preliminary report. J Invest Dermatol 1963; 40:121.

Goldstein N, Penoff J, Price N et al. Techniques of removal of tattoos. J Dermatol Surg Oncol 1979; 5:901–910.

Goldman L et al. Laser treatment of tattoos: a preliminary survey of three years' clinical experience. J Am Med Assoc 1967; 201:841.

Goldstein N. Complications for tattoos. J Dermatol Surg Oncol 1979; 5:869.

Goldman L, Blaney DJ, Kindel DJ et al. Pathology of the effect of the laser beam on the skin. Nature 1965; 197:912.

Goldberg D. Treatment of pigmented and vascular lesions of the skin with the Q-switched Nd:YAG laser. Lasers Surg Med 1993; 13(suppl 5):55.

Grekin RC, Shelton RM, Geisse JK et al. 510-nm pigmented lesion dye laser: itch characteristics and clinical uses. J Dermatol Surg Oncol 1993; 19:380.

Grekin RC, Shelton RM, Geisse JK et al. 510 nm pigmented lesion dye laser. J Dermatol Surg Oncol 1993; 19:380–387.

Grevelink JM, Duke D, Van Leeuwen RL, Gonzalez E, DeCoste SD, Anderson RR. Laser treatment of tattoos in darkly pigmented patients: efficacy and side effects. J Am Acad Dermatol 1996; 34(4):653–656.

Grossman MC, Nderson RR, Farinelli W, Flotte TJ, Grevelink JM. Treatment of cafe au lait macules with lasers. A clinicopathologic correlation. Arch Dermatol 1995; 131(12): 1416–1420.

Hodersdal M, Bech-Thomsen N, Wulf HC. Skin reflectance-guided laser selections for treatment of decorative tattoos. Arch Dermatol 1996; 132:403.

Hruza GJ, Dover JS, Flotte TJ, Watanabe S, Anderson RR. Q-switched ruby laser irradiation of normal human skin. Arch Dermatol 1991; 127:1799–1805.

Imayama S, Ueda S. Long and short-term histological observations of congenital nevi treated with the normal-mode ruby laser. Arch Dermatol 1999; 135:1211–1218.

Jones A, Roddey P, Orengo I, Rosen T. The Q-switched Nd:YAG laser effectively treats tattoos in darkly pigmented skin. Dermatol Surg 1996; 22(12):999–1001.

Karrer S, Hohenleutner U, Szeimies RM, Landthaler M. Amiodarone-induced pigmentation resolves after treatment with the Q-switched ruby laser. Arch Dermatol 1999; 135(3):251–253.

Kasai K, Notodihardjo HW. Analysis of 200 nevus of Ota patients who underwent Q-switched Nd:YAG laser treatment (abstr). Laser Surg Med 1994; 14(suppl 6):50.

Kauvar ANB, Geronemus R. Histology of laser resurfacing. Dermatol Clin 1997; 15(3):459–469.

Kauvar AN. Laser skin resurfacing: perspective at the millennium. Dermatol Surg 2000; 26(2):174–177.

Kilmer SL, Farinelli WF, Tearney G, Anderson RR. Use of a larger spot size for the treatment of tattoos increases clinical efficacy and decreases potential side effects. J Lasers Surg Med 1994(suppl 6):51.

Kilmer SL, Anderson RR. Clinical use of the Q-switched ruby and the Q-switched Nd:YAG (1064 nm and 532 nm) lasers for treatment of tattoos. J Dermatol Surg Oncol 1993; 19:330.

Kilmer SL, Wheeland RG, Golderg KJ, Anderson RR. Treatment of epidermal pigmented lesions with the frequency-doubled Q-switched Nd:YAG laser. A controlled, single-impact, dose-response, multicenter trial. Arch Dermatol 1994; 130(12):1515–1519.

Kilmer SL, Lee M, Farinelli W, Grevelink JM et al. Q-switched Nd:YAG laser (1064 nm) effectively treats Q-switched ruby laser resistant tattoos. Lasers Surg Med 1992; (suppl 4):72.

Kilmer SL, Lee MS, Grevelink JM et al. The Q-switched Nd:YAG laser (1064 nm) effectively treats tattoos: a controlled, dose-response study. Arch Dermatol 1992; 129(8):971.

Kilmer SL, Lee MS, Adnerson RR. Treatment of multi-colored tattoos with the frequency-doubled Q-switched Nd:YAG laser (532 nm): a dose–response study with comparison to the Q-switched ruby laser. Lasers Surg Med Suppl 1993; 5:54.

Kono T, Ercocen AR, Chan HH, Kikuchi Y, Nozaki M. Effectiveness of the normal-mode ruby laser and the combined (normal-mode plus ! -switched) ruby laser in the treatment of congenital melanocytic nevi: a comparative study. Ann Plast Surg 2002; 49:476–485.

Kopera D. Treatment of lentigo maligna with the carbon dioxide laser. Arch Dermatol 1995; 131:735–736.

Landthalder M, Haina D, Waidelich W et al. A three-year experience with the argon laser in dermatotherapy. J Dermatol Surg Oncol 1984; 10:456–461.

Laub DR., Yules RB, Arras M et al. Preliminary histopathological observation of Q-switched ruby laser radiation on dermal tattoo pigment in man. J Surg Res 1968; 5(8):220.

Lee PK, Rosenberg CN, Tsao H, Sober AJ. Failure of Q-switched ruby laser to eradicate atypical-appearing solar lentigo: report of two cases. J Am Acad Dermatol 1998; 38: 314–317.

Levins PC, Anderson RR. Q-switched ruby laser for the treatment of pigmented lesions and tattoos. Clin Dermatol 1995; 13:75–79.

Levy JL, Mordon S, Pizzi-Anselme M. Treatment of individual café-au-lait macules with the Q-switched Nd:YAG: a clinicopathologic correlation. J Cutan Laser Ther 1999; 1(4):217–223.

Loewenthal LJA. Reactions in green tattoos: the significance of valence state of chromium. Arch Dermatol 1960; 82:237.

Lowe NJ et al. Q-switched ruby treatment of professional tattoos. Lasers Surg Med 1993; (suppl 5):54.

Lu Z, Fang L, Jiao S, Huang W, Chen J, Wang X. Treatment of 522 patients with Nevus of Ota with Q-switched Alexandrite laser. Chin Med J 2003; 116(2):226–230.

Mafong EA, Kauvar AN, Geronemus RG. Surgical pearl: removal of cosmetic lipliner tattoo with the pulsed carbon dioxide laser. J Am Acad Dermatol 2003; 48(2):271–272.

Margolis RJ, Dover JS, Polla LL, et al. Visible action spectrum for melanin-specific selective photothermolysis. Laser Surg Med 1989; 9:389–397.

Margolis RJ, Dover JS, Polla LL et al. Visible action spectrum for melanin-specific selective photothermolysis. Lasers Surg Med 1989; 9:389–391.

McBurney EL. Carbon dioxide laser treatment of dermatologic lesions. South Med J 1978; 71:795–798.

McBurney EL. Carbon dioxide laser treatment of dermatologic lesions. South Med J 1978; 71:795–798.

Murphy GP, Shepard RS, Paul DS, Menkes A, Anderson RR, Parrish JA. Organelle-specific injury to melanin-containing cells in human skin by pulsed laser irradiation. Lab Invest 1983; 49:680–685.

Murphy GF, Shepard RS, Paul BS et al. Organelle-specific injury to melanin-containing cells in human skin by pulsed laser irradiation. Lab Invest 1983; 49:680–683.

Novy FG. A generalized mercurial (cinnabar) reaction following tattooing. Arch Dermatol 1944; 49:172.

Ozawa T, Fujiwara M, Harada T, Muraoka M, Ishii M. Q-switched alexandrite laser therapy for pigmentation of the lips owing to Laugier–Huziker syndrome. Dermatol Surg 2005; 31(6):709–712.

Papadavid E, Walker NP. Q-switched alexandrite laser in the treatment of pigmented macules in Laugier–Hunziker syndrome. J Eur Acad Dermatol Venereol 2001; 15(5): 468–469.

Piggot TA, Norris RW. The treatment of tattoos with trichloracetic acid: experience with 670 patients. Br J Plast Surg 1988; 41:112–117.

Polla LL, Margolis DR, Dover JS, Whitaker D Murphy GF, Jacques SL, Anderson RR. Melanosomes are a primary target of Q-switched ruby laser irradiation in guinea pig skin. J Invest Dermatol 1987; 89:281–286.

Raulin C, Werner S, Greve B. Circumscripted pigmentations after iron injections—treatment with Q-switched laser systems. Laser Surg Med 2001; 28:456–460.

Reid R, Muller S. Tattoo removal by CO₂ laser dermabrasion. Plast Reconstr Surg 1980; 65:717–719.

Reid WH, McLeod PJ, Ritchie et al. Q-switched ruby laser treatment of black tattoos. Br J Plast Surg 1983; 36:455.

Reid R, Muller S. Tattoo removal by CO₂ laser dermabrasion. Plast Reconstr Surg 1980; 65:717–719.

Ross EV, Yashar S, Michaud N, et al. Tattoo darkening and nonresponse after laser treatment: a possible role for titanium dioxide. Arch Dermatol 2001; 137(1):33–37.

Ross V, Naseef G, Lin G, et al. Comparison of responses of tattoos to picosecond and nanosecond q-switched neodymium: YAG lasers. Arch Dermatol 1998; 134(2):167–171.

Ross EV, Naseef G, Lin C, et al. Comparison of responses of tattoos to picosecond and nanosecond Q-switched Neodymium:YAG lasers. Arch Dermatol 1998; 134:167–171.

Rostenberg A, Brown RA, Caro MR. Discussion of tattoo reactions with report of a case showing a reaction to a green color. Arch Dermatol Symph 1950; 62:540.

Scheibner A, Kenny G, White W et al. A superior method of tattoo removal using the Q-switched ruby laser. J Dermatol Surg Oncol 1990; 16:1091.

Shah G, Alster TS. Treatment of an amalgam tattoo with a Q-switched alexandrite (755 nm) laser. Dermatol Surg 2002; 28:1180.

Sherwood KA, Murray S, Kurban AK, Tan OT. Effect of wavelength on cutaneous pigment using pulsed irradiation. J Invest Dermatol 1989; 92:717–720.

Sherwood KA, Murray S, Kurban AK et al. Effect of wavelength on cutaneous pigment using pulsed irradiation. J Invest Dermatol 1989; 92:717–720.

Sherwood KA, Murray S, Kurban AK et al. Effect of wavelength on cutaneous pigment using pulsed irradiation. J Invest Dermatol 1989; 92:717.

Shimashi T, Kamide R, Hashimoto T. Long-term follow-up in treatment of solar lentigo and cafe-au-lait macules with Q-switched ruby laser. Aesthetic Plast Surg 1997; 21(6):445–448.

Stafford TJ, Lizek R, Tan OT. Role of the alexandrite laser for removal of tattoos. Lasers Surg Med 1995; 17(1):32–38.

Suh DH, Han KH, Chung JH. Clinical use of the Q-switched Nd:YAG laser for the treatment of acquired bilateral nevus of Ota-like macules (ABNOMs) in Koreans. J Dermatol Treat 2001; 12(3):163–166.

Swinny B. Generalized chronic dermatitis due to tattoo. Ann Allergy 1946; 4:295.

Taylor CR, Anderson RR, Gange W et al. Light and electron microscopic analysis of tattoos treated by Q-switched ruby laser. J Invest Dermatol 1991; 97:131.

Taylor CR, Flotte TJ, Gange RW, Anderson RR. Treatment of nevus of Ota by Q-switched ruby laser. J Am Acad Derm 1994; 30:743–751.

Taylor CR, Gange RW, Dover JS et al. Treatment of tattoos by Q-switched ruby laser: a dose response study. Arch Dermatol 1990; 126:893.

Taylor CR, Anderson RR, Gange RW, Michaud NA, Flotte TJ. Light and electron microscopic analysis of tattoos treated by Q-switched ruby laser. J Invest Dermatol 1991; 97:131–136.

Tazelaar DJ. Herpesensitivity to chromium in a light-blue tattoo. Dermatologica 1970; 141:282.

Thissen M, Westerhof W. Lentigo maligna treated with ruby laser. Acta Derm Venereol 1997; 77:163.

Tong AKF, Tan OT, Boll J et al. Ultrastructural effects of melanin pigment on target specificity using pulsed dye laser (577 nm). J Invest Dermatol 1987; 88:747–752.

Trotter MJ, Tron VA, Hollingdale J, Rivers JK. Localized chrysiasis induced by laser therapy. Arch Dermatol 1995; 131(12): 1411–1414.

Tsao H, Dover JS. Treatment of minocycline-induced hyperpigmentation with the Q-switched ruby laser. Arch Dermatol 1996; 132:1250–1251.

USA Weekend's 14th Annual Special Teen Report on Teens and Parents. USA Weekend 2001; April 29:10–12.

Ueda S, Imayama A. Normal-mode ruby laser for treating congenital nevi. Arch Dermatol 1997; 133:355–359.

Watanabe S, Takahashi H. Treatment of nevus of Ota with the Q-switched ruby laser. N Engl J Med 1994; 331:1745–1750.

Watanabe S, Anderson RR, Brorson S et al. Comparative studies of femtosecond to microsecond laser pulses on selective pigmented cell injury in skin. Photochem Photobiol 1991; 53:757.

Watanabe S, Flotte T, Margolis R et al. The effects of pulse duration on selective pigmented cell injury by dye lasers, J Invest Dermatol 88:523A, 1987.

Watanabe S, Takahashi H. Treatment of nevus of Ota with the Q-switched ruby laser. N Engl J Med 1994; 331(26):1745–1750.

Wheeler ES, Miller TA. Tattoo removal by split thickness tangential excision. West J Med 1988; 124:272–274.

Wilde JL, English JC, Finley EM. Minocycline-induced hyperpigmentation: treatment with the Q-switched Nd:YAG laser. Arch Dermatol 1997; 133:1344–1346.

Yang HY, Lee CW, Ro YS, et al. Q-switched ruby laser in the treatment of nevus of Ota. J Korean Med Sci 1996; 11(2):165–170.

Yules RB, Laub DR, Honey R et al. The effect of Q-switched ruby laser radiation on dermal tattoo pigment in man. Arch Surg 1967; 95:179.

Yun PL, Arndt KA, Anderson RR. Q-Switched laser-induced chrysiasis treated with long-pulsed laser. Arch Dermatol 2002; 138:1012–1014.

Zemtsov A, Wilson L. CO_2 laser treatment causes local tattoo allergic reaction to become generalized. Acta Derm Venereol 1997; 77(6):497.

66

Laser Treatment of Vascular Lesions

Sharon Thornton, Trephina Galloway, and Philip Bailin

Division of Dermatologic Surgery, Department of Dermatology, Cleveland Clinic Foundation, Cleveland, Ohio, U.S.A.

BACKGROUND

Vascular lesions are the most common indication for laser therapy today. While the ruby laser, the neodymium: yttrium-aluminum-garnet (Nd:YAG) laser, the argon laser, and the carbon dioxide laser were developed in the early 1960s, the widespread use of lasers for vascular lesions began in the 1980s with the application of the theory of selective photothermolysis. Selective photothermolysis, described by Anderson and Parrish, is the ability to target and damage a specific chromophore, such as oxyhemoglobin, with minimal damage to the surrounding tissue. By setting the laser pulse duration to a time equal to or shorter than the thermal relaxation time of the target vessel (time for the target vessel to dissipate half of the thermal energy or heat), thermal damage to the surrounding normal tissue is avoided. Oxyhemoglobin is the major chromophore in the cutaneous blood vessels of port-wine stains, hemangiomas, and telengiectases. The major absorption peaks of oxyhemoglobin are 418, 542, and 577 nm. The higher wavelengths are less absorbed by epidermal melanin and allow deeper penetration.

The early argon laser light (488–514 nm), well-absorbed by oxyhemoglobin, effectively treated vascular lesions, however, scarring was a fairly common side effect due to excess thermal damage. The pulsed dye laser, using the theory of selective photothermolysis, revolutionized laser treatment of vascular lesions and dramatically decreased the risk of scarring with treatment.

CLASSIFICATION

There are two recognized types of vascular anomalies: vascular tumors and vascular malformations. Vascular tumors are characterized by cellular proliferation. The most common vascular tumor is the hemangioma. Vascular malformations are thought to be localized defects in angiogenesis. They are subdivided into capillary, venous, lymphatic, and arteriovenous. Vascular tumors will spontaneously regress, whereas vascular malformations never regress. Laser treatment of vascular lesions is possible for vascular tumors such as hemangiomas and vascular malformations of the capillary subtype, including port-wine stains and telengiectases.

Hemangiomas

Hemangiomas are benign proliferations of endothelial tissue. They are the most common tumor to arise in the neonatal period, occurring in 10% to 12% of infants by the first year of life. Hemangiomas occur more often in girls than boys and the more complicated hemangiomas are seen more often in girls.

Hemangiomas are characterized by a rapid growth period during the first year of life, followed by a gradual and spontaneous involution by the teenage years. Hemangiomas can occur anywhere on the skin and mucosal surfaces. The location and depth of the lesion within the skin will determine its clinical appearance. Superficial hemangiomas, located in the superficial dermis, will have a bright red color. Purely superficial lesions account for the majority of hemangiomas, 50% to 60% of cases. Deeper hemangiomas that are located in the deep dermis and subcutis will have a purple/blue appearance. They are not usually noticed in the immediate newborn period. The larger deep hemangiomas can have arterial blood flow during their proliferating phase, and a bruit may be felt on examination. Radiographic studies such as magnetic resonance imaging or ultrasound can help clarify the diagnosis. Deep hemangiomas account for 15% of cases and the other 25% to 35% of hemangiomas are felt to have a mixture of deep and superficial components.

Ulceration is the most frequent complication of hemangiomas, occurring in 10% to 15% of superficial hemangiomas. Ulceration usually causes minor bleeding episodes that are easily controlled with pressure. Certain locations are more likely to have ulceration, including the lip and the perineum. Ulceration can cause pain, increase the risk of infection and result in scarring. For this reason, it is recommended that ulcerated lesions receive early laser treatment.

Large hemangiomas can distort normal tissue and interfere with function. Small hemangiomas in periocular, perioral, and nasal locations can also interfere with normal function, and thus warrant early treatment.

Large cervicofacial hemangiomas are more frequently associated with congenital abnormalities. The Posterior fossa malformation, Hemangioma, Arterial anomalies, Cardiac defects, Eye anomalies, and Sternal defects (PHACES) syndrome describes the abnormalities seen with large cervicofacial hemangiomas. PHACES often does not show characteristics of all anomalies. Specific studies to rule out involvement of each system should be done when a large cervicofacial hemangioma is encountered.

Similarly, hemangiomas in the "beard area" of the lower face can be markers of laryngeal hemangiomatosis, which may cause airway obstruction, and thus these patients should have an otolaryngeal evaluation.

Lumbosacral hemangiomas may be markers of spinal dysraphism and other urogenital malformations, thus adequate imaging to screen for such anomalies should be performed.

Infants with multiple cutaneous hemangiomas should be screened for diffuse neonatal hemangiomatosis, looking for visceral hemangiomas. The liver, gastrointestinal tract, and lungs are the most common internal sites of hemangiomas.

Port-Wine Stains

Port-wine stains are congenital vascular malformations. They occur anywhere on the body and are present in 0.3% of newborns. Port-wine stains begin as pink macules and progressively darken and thicken. Nodules may develop in adulthood. Facial port-wine stains are often distributed along branches of the trigeminal nerve. A midline port-wine stain along the posterior neck or lumbosacral region may signify spinal dysraphism. This is true especially if the port-wine stain is associated with a pit, dimple, or hypertrichosis. There are several syndromes associated with capillary malformations, these include Sturge–Weber syndrome, Klippel–Trenaunay syndrome, and Proteus syndrome.

Telengiectases

Telengiectases are dilated capillaries that appear anywhere on normal skin/mucous membranes at any age. Clinically they appear as small cutaneous vessels that blanch with diascopy. The most common causes of telengiectases are aging/photodamage, rosacea, hyperestrogenemia, and the use of topical steroids. Systemic etiologies of telengiectases are lupus erythematous, scleroderma, dermatomyositis, and cirrhosis of the liver. Telengiectases are also seen in genodermatoses such as xeroderma pigmentosa, Cockayne syndrome, and Bloom syndrome. Medications such as nifedipine and felodipine may also lead to telengiectases in a photodistributed pattern.

PROCEDURE

Preoperative Evaluation

The preoperative assessment should include a detailed history of the cutaneous vascular lesion. Important factors are as follows:

- Location
- Duration
- Changes in appearance, especially color and texture
- Symptoms, especially bleeding or ulceration
- Prior treatments
- Medical illnesses/conditions, including prior isotretinoin use.

A physical examination will allow the physician to determine whether or not the cutaneous vascular lesion is amenable to treatment.

General Principles

Many laser systems may be used to effectively treat cutaneous vascular lesions. Each laser has its own unique treatment consideration, however, some principles of treatment are common to many lasers.

One of the most important aspects of the preoperative assessment is reviewing the procedure and expectations with the patient. Most vascular lesions require a series of laser treatments, usually at 6-week intervals. Laser-specific goggles, plastic eye shields, or eye patches secured for adequate protection of the eyes should be in place before beginning the procedure. If the location of the lesion to be treated is close to the eye, metal corneal shields should be used.

The laser pulse will produce a brief stinging or burning sensation of the skin. Most patients will tolerate the discomfort without anesthesia. However, some patients prefer to use a topical anesthetic (LMX 4®) prior to the procedure. The over-the-counter LMX 4 cream should be applied 1 hour before the procedure and repeated every 20 minutes. Upon arrival to the office, the cream should be removed several minutes prior to treatment to avoid any vasoconstricting effect. General sedation may sometimes be necessary in young children who are unable to lie still for the procedure.

The patient should be instructed to avoid sun exposure and to use sunscreens and sun protection prior to and following the procedure. Patients should avoid anticoagulants and supplements not prescribed by a physician for 2 weeks prior to laser surgery, for example, ibuprofen, aspirin, gingko, ginseng, garlic, and vitamin E. They should avoid alcohol 48 hours before the treatment session.

Treatments are repeated every 6 to 8 weeks as long as improvement continues. Some vascular lesions may nearly resolve with minimal residual telengiectases or pigmentary disturbance. Other lesions, such as hypertrophic port-wine stains, may lighten in color and improve in appearance, but not entirely clear.

Laser science is continually evolving and laser systems and treatment parameters are thus always changing. The laser surgeon must consult latest references to maintain current treatment guidelines.

VASCULAR LASERS

Flashlamp-Pumped Pulsed Dye Laser

The flashlamp-pumped pulsed dye laser is the first laser developed using selective photothermolysis (Table 1). Pulsed dye laser light is generated by a xenon flashlamp exciting a rhodamine dye to generate a yellow light. The original pulsed dye laser emitted a yellow light with

Table 1 Summary of Lasers Used to Treat Vascular Lesions

Laser	Wavelength (nm)	Spectrum of light	Vascular lesion treatment indications
Flashlamp-pumped pulsed dye laser	595	Yellow	Superior for hemangiomas, port-wine stains, redness of rosacea and poikiloderma of civatte. Also effective for facial telengiectases
Variable-pulsed ND:YAG laser	532	Green	Superior for individual telengiectases. Also effective for hemangiomas, port-wine stains, and leg veins
Alexandrite laser	755	Infrared	Leg veins
Diode laser	800	Infrared	Leg veins
Krypton laser	568	Green, yellow	Telengiectases
Copper laser	578	Green, yellow	Telengiectases
Argon-pumped tunable dye laser	488–638	577–585 nm Yellow	Rarely used secondary to risk of scarring

(A) **(B)**

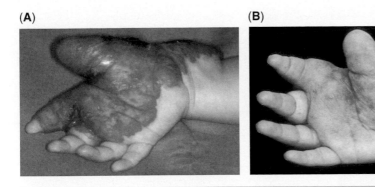

Figure 1 Infant with hemangioma of hand. Before and after treatment with 577-nm flash-lamp-pumped pulsed dye laser. (*See color insert.*)

wavelength of 577 nm, which was later modified to 585 nm to increase the depth of penetration to 1 to 2 mm. The pulse duration of these early lasers was 450 μsec. The laser pulse duration should be a time equal to or shorter than the thermal relaxation time of the target vessel (time for the target vessel to dissipate half of the thermal energy or heat) in order to adequately treat the vascular lesion without damaging the surrounding tissue. The thermal relaxation time of vessels in port-wine stains is longer at 1 to 10 msec for vessels of 50 to 150 μm. This longer relaxation time allows an increased pulse duration to treat large caliber vessels. In addition, a longer wavelength and an increased pulse duration are associated with a lower incidence of postoperative purpura. The newer pulsed dye lasers have pulse durations above 450 μsec.

The 595-nm flashlamp-pumped pulsed dye laser is commonly used for the treatment of cutaneous vascular lesions, including port-wine stains, hemangiomas, telengiectases, and other small vessel cutaneous lesions. The 595-nm pulsed dye laser is generally preferred over the original 585-nm laser because of the lower incidence of post-treatment purpura. Increased pulse durations and higher fluences are useful for the treatment of leg veins.

The laser pulse of the pulsed dye laser feels similar to a rubber band snap to the skin. Most patients require no local anesthesia, however, the preoperative application of topical anesthetic creams may be especially useful in children. The cryogen spray or forced convection cooling devices available with the laser systems provide anesthesia and also serve to protect the epidermal layer of the skin. These epidermal cooling methods help to prevent pigmentary alterations, while allowing penetration of the laser light to the deeper dermal vessels.

Variable-Pulsed 532-nm Nd:YAG Laser

The variable-pulsed 532-nm Nd:YAG laser of the Versapulse (Coherent) laser system is especially useful in treating facial telengiectases. The Versapulse system contains four wavelengths, including the 532-nm Nd:YAG, Q-switched 532-nm, Q-switched 755-nm and Q-switched 1064-nm Nd:YAG. The 532-nm variable-pulsed Nd:YAG laser is generated by passing a 1064-nm laser light through a potassium titanyl phosphate crystal to double the frequency. The 532-nm wavelength lies in the absorption peak of oxyhemoglobin. The cooling device is a glass window that is chilled with water cooled to 4°C passing through it.

Alexandrite and Diode Lasers

Oxyhemoglobin has small absorption peaks in the infrared range of light, therefore, the long-pulsed 755-nm alexandrite

and the 800-nm diode lasers may be used to treat some vascular lesions. They tend to be most effective in treating deeper blue vessels, such as spider veins of the legs.

Krypton Laser

The krypton laser is a quasi-continuous wave laser that emits wavelengths of both 520 to 530 and 568 nm. The quasi-continuous wave is produced by pulses created by a shuttering device. The 568-nm wavelength is used to treat vascular lesions. Treatments are performed with the use of a 1-mm handpiece. The disadvantages of this laser are the small spot size and fixed pulse width, limiting its use to the treatment of telengiectases.

Copper Laser

The copper vapor and copper bromide laser is another quasi-continuous wave laser that emits wavelengths of 511 and 578 nm. This laser is most effective for telengiectases. A common side effect is fine crusting over the treated sites.

Argon-Pumped Tunable Dye Laser

The argon-pumped tunable dye laser uses a fluorescent organic dye as its medium and an argon laser as its power source, emitting a wavelength that can be tuned from 488 to 638 nm. While important in early years of lasers, the argon-pumped tunable dye laser is now rarely used secondary to its risk of scarring.

CLINICAL APPLICATIONS

Hemangiomas

The first-line treatment for hemangiomas is the flashlamp-pumped pulsed dye laser. The pulsed dye laser is effective in the treatment of superficial hemangiomas in the proliferative and involution phases. As the pulsed dye laser is less effective at greater depths, deeper, cavernous liemangiomas are less responsive. The laser treatment of uncomplicated hemangiomas has been shown to be no more effective than

(A) **(B)**

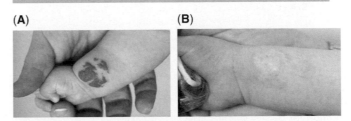

Figure 2 Infant with hemangioma on wrist. Before and after treatment with 577-nm flashlamp-pumped pulsed dye laser.

(A)   **(B)**   **(C)**

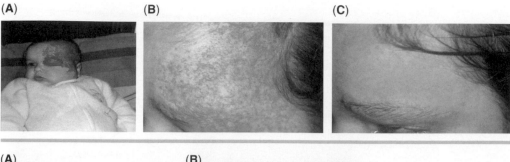

Figure 3 **(A)** Infant with large facial hemangioma. **(B)** Several years later same infant as a child. Resolution of hemangioma with steroid use only. **(C)** Same child after treatment of residual hemangioma with 577-nm flash-lamp-pumped pulsed dye laser. (*See color insert.*)

(A)   **(B)**

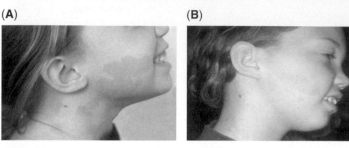

Figure 4 Port-wine stain on child's face. Before and after treatment with 577-nm flashlamp-pumped pulsed dye laser. (*See color insert.*)

(A)   **(B)**

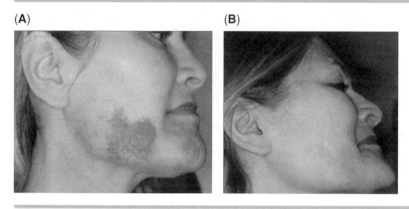

Figure 5 Port-wine stain on face. Before and after treatment with 577-nm flashlamp-pumped pulsed dye laser. (*See color insert.*)

clinical observation. However, hemangiomas that could potentially compromise vital structures and/or impair normal function should be treated early. Also, early laser treatment of ulcerated hemangiomas leads to healing of the ulceration and improvement in the associated pain and discomfort. Usually, multiple treatments are required at 6- to 8-week intervals (Figs. 1–3).

Port-Wine Stains

The treatment of port-wine stains (PWS) with the flashlamp-pumped pulsed dye laser has been studied extensively. Generally, spot sizes of 7 or 10 mm are used and the fluence varies based on the spot size. The smaller spot size requires a greater fluence to achieve the same therapeutic effect. A test spot will determine the subpurpuric fluence. A transitory pink-violaceous color change will occur after the pulse is applied to the skin. If a violaceous or purpuric change occurs and is slow to fade, purpura will be more significant in the postoperative period. Overlapping of pulses by 10% of the spot size will allow uniform treatment of the involved

(A)   **(B)**

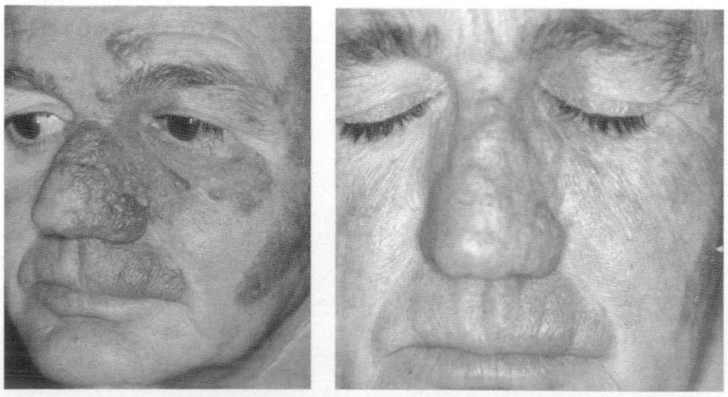

Figure 6 Mature port-wine stain with bleb formation on face. Before and after treatment with 577-nm flashlamp-pumped pulsed dye laser showing reduction in texture changes and color. (*See color insert.*)

(A)   **(B)**

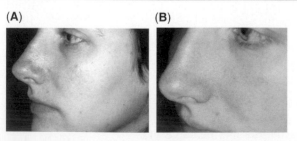

Figure 7 Telengiectases on nasal ala. Before and after treatment with high-energy long-pulsed 532-nm Nd:YAG laser. (*See color insert.*)

(A)　　　　**(B)**

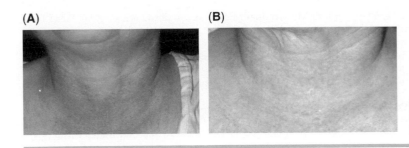

Figure 8 Telengiectases in poikiloderma of civatte before and after treatment with 577-nm flashlamp-pumped pulsed dye laser. (*See color insert.*)

area. Improvement is detectable clinically in approximately 4 to 12 weeks. Characteristics of port-wine stains with poor response to laser treatment include: light pink color, large size, nodules, and thick plaques. Port-wine stains located on the central cheeks and upper lip are also poor responders. Treatments are repeated at 6- to 8-week intervals as long as lightening of the port-wine stains is achieved. Port-wine stains often require eight or more treatment sessions. Combined laser therapy with the 595-nm pulsed dye laser and the variable-pulsed 532-nm Nd:YAG laser may increase efficacy (Figs. 4–6).

Telengiectases

Both the variable-pulsed 532-nm Nd:YAG laser and the 595-nm flashlamp-pumped pulsed dye laser are very effective for the treatment of facial telengiectases. A comparison of the two lasers revealed superior vessel clearance with the pulsed dye laser. However, patients may prefer treatment with the variable-pulsed 532-nm laser due to the lower incidence of purpura. Although uncommon, side effects with this laser may include erythema, swelling, blistering, and hypopigmentation. When treating telengiectases with the variable-pulsed 532-nm laser, transient blanching of the vessel should be seen following the laser pulse. In treating spider telengiectases of the legs, higher fluences and longer pulse durations are required (Figs. 7 and 8).

COMPLICATIONS

Generally, laser treatments of vascular lesions result in minimal complications. However, common side effects include bruising, erythema, and swelling. Bruising usually fades over 7 to 10 days. Swelling and erythema may persist for 2 to 5 days. Often the application of an ice pack for 5 to 15 minutes after the procedure and a few days following the procedure will help to decrease swelling and discomfort. If the treatment site involved the face, patients may also sleep with their head elevated to reduce swelling. Acetaminophen 325 to 500 mg orally may be taken for swelling and discomfort.

Less common side effects are the development of crusts, blisters, ulcerations, hypo- and hyperpigmentation and rarely, permanent scars. If the patient experiences any crusting or blistering in the postoperative period, topical antibiotic ointment or petrolatum jelly should be applied until the areas are healed. Patient should be instructed to avoid disrupting blisters or crusts. Hypo- or hyperpigmentation are more common in patients with Fitzpatrick skin types III to VI. Pigmentary disturbances often gradually resolve over a period of 3 to 6 months following the procedure. Topical bleaching creams may accelerate the fading process in hyperpigmentation.

BIBLIOGRAPHY

Acland KM, Barlow RJ. Lasers for the dermatologist. Br J Dermatol 2000; 143(2):244–255.

Adrian RM, Tanghetti EA. Long pulse 532 nm laser treatment of facial telengiectasia. Dermatol Surg 1998; 24:71–74.

Alster TS, Lupton JR. Lasers in dermatology. Am J Clin Dermatol 2001; 2(5):291–303.

Alster TS, Wilson F. Treatment of port-wine stains with the flashlamp-pumped pulsed dye laser: extended clinical experience in children and adults. Ann Plast Surg 1994; 32:478–484.

Anderson RR, Parrish JA. Selective photothermolysis: precise microsurgery by selective absorption of pulsed radiation. Science 1983; 220:524–527.

Batta K, Goodyear HM, Moss C, et al. A randomized controlled study of early pulsed dye laser treatment of uncomplicated childhood hemangiomas: results of a 1-year analysis. Lancet 2002; 360:521–527.

Cantatore JL, Kriegel DA. Laser surgery: an approach to the pediatric patient. J Am Acad Dermatol 2004; 50(2):165–184.

Dierickx CC, Casparian JM, Venugopalan V, et al. Thermal relaxation of port wine stain vessels probed in vivo: the need for 1–10 millisecond laser pulse treatment. J Invest Dermatol 1995; 105:709–714.

Dohil MA, Baugh WP, Eichenfield LF. Vascular and pigmented birthmarks. Pediatr Clin North Am 2000; 47(4):783–812.

Dover JS, Arndt KA. New approaches to the treatment of vascular lesions. Lasers Surg Med 2000; 26(2):158–163.

Dummer R, Graf P, Greif C, et al. Treatment of vascular lesions using the VersaPulse variable pulse width frequency doubled neodymium: YAG laser. Dermatology 1998; 197:158–161.

Edstrom DW. Flashlamp pulsed dye and argon-pumped dye laser in the treatment of port-wine stains: a clinical and histological comparison. Br J Dermatol 2002; 146:285–289.

Fickarstrand EJ, Svaasand LO, Kopstad G, et al. Photothermally induced vessel-wall necrosis after pulsed dye laser treatment: lack of response in PWS with small sized or deeply located vessels. J Invest Dermatol 1996; 107:671–674.

Fitzpatrick RE, Lowe NJ, Goldman MP, et al. Flashlamp-pumped pulsed dye laser treatment of port-wine stains. J Dermatol Surg Oncol 1994; 20:743–748.

Frieden IJ. Which hemangiomas to treat and how? Arch Dermatol 1997; 133:1593–1595.

Garzoa MC, Frieden IJ. Hemangiomas: when to worry. Pediatr Ann 2000; 29(1):58–67.

Geroaemus RG. Pulsed dye laser treatment of vascular lesions in children. J Dermatol Surg Oncol 1993; 19:303–310.

Hohenleutner S, Badur-Ganter E, Landthaler M, Hohenleutner U. Long-term results in the treatment of childhood hemangioma with the flashlamp-pumped pulsed dye laser: an evaluation of 617 cases. Lasers Surg Med 2001; 28(3):273–277.

Lamb SR, Sheehan-Dare RA. Leg liberation after pulsed dye laser treatment of a vascular malformation. Lasers Surg Med 2003; 32(5):396–398.

Landthaler M, Ulrich H, Hohenleutner S, et al. Role of laser therapy in dermatology—clinical aspects. Dermatology 2004; 208(2):129–134.

Nagore E, Requena C, Sevila A, et al. Thickness of healthy and affected skin of children with port wine stains: potential repercussions on response to pulsed dye laser treatment. Dermatol Surg 2004; 30:1457–1461.

Richards KA, Garden JM. The pulsed dye laser for cutaneous vascular and nonvascular lesions. Semin Cutan Med Surg 2000; 19(4):276–286.

Rothfieisch JE, Klein Kosann M, Levine VJ, et al. Laser treatment of congenital and acquired vascular lesions. Dermatol Clin 2002; 20(1):1–18.

Spicer MS, Goldberg DJ. Lasers in dermatology. J Am Acad Dermatol 1996; 34:1–25.

Tan OT, Murray S, Kurban AK. Action spectrum of vascular specific injury using pulsed irradiation. J Invest Dermatol 1989; 92:868–871.

Travelute Ammirati C, Carniol PJ, Hruza GJ. Laser treatment of facial vascular lesions. Facial Plast Surg 2001; 17(3):193–201.

Waner M. Recent developments in lasers and the treatment of birthmarks. Arch Dis Child 2003; 88(5):372–374.

West TB, Alster TS. Comparison of the long-pulsed dye (590–595 nm) and the KTP (532 nm) lasers in the treatment of facial and leg telengiectasias. Dermatol Surg 1998; 24:221–226.

67

Hair Removal by Photoepilation with Lasers and Intense Pulsed Light Sources

Elizabeth I. McBurney

Department of Dermatology, Louisiana State University, New Orleans, Louisiana, U.S.A.

INTRODUCTION

Technological advances and patient demand have each contributed to the growing popularity of laser/intense pulsed light (IPL) hair removal. The Food and Drug Administration (FDA) reports a growing number of new laser- and light-based hair removal systems being registered each year.

Hair removal with laser or light sources is not new. Prior to the development of the first ruby laser, in 1959, hair removal was attempted using the arc lamp and incandescent lamp epilators. A myriad of patents pertaining to hair removal were filed soon after the first ruby laser was constructed. Goldman reported epilation and the histologic findings of selective damage to pigmented hair follicles in 1967. Despite these earlier observations and reports, lasers intended specifically for hair removal did not become available to physicians and patients until 1995. Since then the goal of permanent hair removal has become a reality with the use of laser photothermal energy.

HAIR PHYSIOLOGY

The hair follicle is divided into three regions: *infundibulum* (epidermal hair follicle opening to the sebaceous gland orifice), *isthmus* (area between the entrance of the sebaceous duct and the arrector pili muscle), and the *inferior or bulbar segment* (extends from the insertion of the arrector pili muscle and the site of the bulge to the base of the follicle to include the hair bulb and matrix). The general anatomy of the hair follicle is shown in Figure 1.

The two primary sites of hair stem cells are within the hair bulb and the bulge. Studies of these germinative centers in scarring alopecia show that the bulge stem cell, not the bulbar region of the hair follicle, is the more important site for follicular regeneration. Consequently, it follows to effect permanent hair removal it is necessary that the bulge stem center must be completely destroyed, in addition to the matrix and hair bulb. The exact follicular target for permanent hair removal—the stem cells of the bulge, the hair bulb or matrix, or the vessels in the dermal papilla—has not been precisely identified.

Human hair grows in a continuous cycle. There are periods of growth (anagen) followed by a relatively brief time in which the bulbar portion of the follicle is almost completely degraded (catagen) and then proceeding into the resting phase (telogen). Each individual anatomic location of the human body has a different anagen/telogen cycle. Table 1 outlines the duration of the anagen cycle for various body sites. The type and cycle of hair growth within a particular anatomic site will vary from location to location and plays a role in determining the sensitivity of an anatomic site to laser treatment and the required frequency of repeat laser/IPL treatments.

Whether hairs are in the anagen or telogen phase when exposed to the laser is vitally important as only anagen hairs are particularly sensitive to insults. Following injury or insult, three reaction patterns of the anagen follicle are seen: premature termination of anagen and movement into telogen, transition from normal anagen to dystrophic anagen, and acute matrix deterioration. It has been suggested that the growth phase of hair at the time of treatment does not affect the ability for permanent hair loss. Permanent hair removal results both from degeneration of follicles and miniaturization of coarse terminal hairs to vellus-like hair follicles, whereas temporary hair removal results mainly from the induction of telogen.

The other component targets for laser hair removal are the chromophores: melanin and melanocytes. Melanin density tends to be highest in the bulb. In contrast, the bulge may contain small amounts of melanin. The melanocytes are located within the hair bulb epithelium around the upper half of the dermal papilla, in the basal layer of the infundibulum, and sparsely within the outer root sheath. Follicular melanocytes produce two types of melanin: eumelanin (brownish black) and pheomelanin (red). The relative composition of the type of melanin pigment and the absolute quantity determine the wide range of hair color. Dark hair contains large amounts of eumelanin. The melanocyte is present throughout the hair cycle, but melanin production is most vigorous during the early anagen phase. Also, the hair follicle bulb lies in close proximity to the bulge during this early growth cycle. As anagen continues, the bulb and the papillae descend deeper into the dermis. Therefore, the seemingly optimal time for laser hair treatment would be during the early anagen phase when the melanin content is the highest and the bulb and the bulge are near to one another (Fig. 2A and B).

DEFINITION OF HAIR REMOVAL

Hair removal is defined differently by physicians, patients, and FDA. It is essential to understand the difference between permanent and complete hair loss. Complete hair loss is defined as a lack of regrowing hairs and may be temporary or permanent. Laser treatment most commonly produces temporary complete hair loss for a few months, and then is followed by partial permanent hair loss. Patients

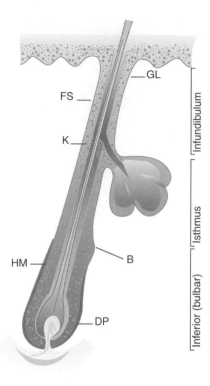

Figure 1 General anatomy of the hair follicle. *Abbreviations*: APM, arrector pili muscle; B, bulge; DP, dermal papilla; HM, hair matrix; HS, hair shaft; SG, sebaceous gland.

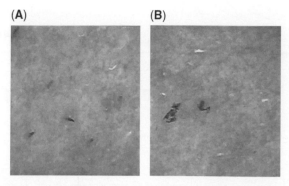

Figure 2 (**A**) Pre-treatment of male beard area with white and dark hairs. (**B**) Post-treatment with 800-nm diode laser, showing destruction of dark hairs and intact white hairs.

would like to obtain complete eradication of all hair with few treatments and no regrowth.

For a hair removal device to meet FDA approval for *temporary* hair reduction, it must show a 30% reduction of hair growth at 3 months after a single treatment. The FDA definition of *permanent* hair reduction is defined as the long-term, stable reduction in the number of hairs regrowing after a treatment regime, which may include several sessions. The number of hairs regrowing must be stable over a time greater than the duration of the complete growth cycle of hair follicles, which varies from 4 to 12 months according to body location. Permanent hair reduction does not necessarily imply the elimination of all hairs in the treatment area.

Table 1 Hair Cycle per Body Site

Body site	Telogen (%)	Anagen (%)	Duration of telogen (mo)	Duration of anagen (mo)
Scalp	10–15	85	3–4	24–72
Eyebrows	85–94	10	3–4	1–2
Upper lip	35	65	1.5	2–5
Moustache	34	66	1.5	2–5
Beard	30	70	2–3	12
Axillae	70	30	3	4
Chest	70	30	2.5	
Back	70	30		
Arms	72–86	20	2–4	1–3
Legs	62–81	20	3–6	4–6
Pubic area	65–81	30	2–3	1–2

Source: From Dierickx (2000); Olsen (1995); Dierickx (2002); Polderman, et al. (2000).

The number of devices for hair removal is expanding so rapidly that the FDA does not maintain an up-to-date list of laser manufacturers whose devices have been cleared solely for permanent hair reduction. To investigate if a specific manufacturer has received FDA clearance one can check the FDA's website at http://www/fda/gpv/cdrh/databases.htm under the 510 (k) database by entering the manufacturer or the device name of the laser. The FDA consumer staff at the Center for Devices and Radiological Health can be contacted at 1–888-INFO-FDA or 301–827–3990 or by fax at 301–443–9535.

LASER PHYSICS AND SKIN OPTICS

Laser hair removal is a multifactorial photothermal process that involves a complex interaction between the laser/IPL light energy and the hair follicle target to achieve destruction of the follicle and sparing of the epidermis.

The principle of selective photothermolysis is the foundation of laser/light-based hair removal systems. According to this principle, selective thermal destruction of a target will occur if sufficient energy is delivered at a wavelength well absorbed by the target within a time period less than or equal to the thermal relaxation time (TRT) of the target. The TRT is the time needed for the target to significantly cool (half of its baseline temperature) and to transfer the heat to the surrounding tissue. Utilizing these concepts, it is possible to selectively destroy hair follicles while minimizing or sparing damage of the surrounding tissue. The target is the endogenous melanin of the hair follicle or an exogenous chromophore applied to the follicle, such as carbon particles or 5-aminolevulinic acid.

An extension of the principle of selective photothermolysis is the thermokinetic selectivity theory which proposes that a longer pulse duration allows intrapulse cooling of smaller targets more rapidly than larger targets for the same chromophore. Longer pulse durations are expected to limit the epidermal thermal damage. For example, if the pulse duration exceeds the TRT of the basal cell layer (about 0.1 msec) this structure's rate of heat transfer will allow it to cool as it is heated during exposure to the laser beam. As a result the larger hair follicle will be selectively injured more than the smaller epidermal target of the same chromophore.

An extension of the traditional hair follicle TRT has evolved into the thermal damage time. Studies indicate that to achieve permanent hair reduction, the ideal pulse duration may be longer than the TRT of the hair follicle. It has been proposed to widen the pulse duration to achieve propagation of the thermal damage throughout the entire volume of the hair and producing permanent damage to the follicular stem cells.

Several laser parameters must be considered to obtain permanent photothermal destruction of the hair follicle: wavelength, pulse duration, spot size, and fluence. Based on the theory of selective photothermolysis, the wavelength of the laser beam must be capable of reaching the target and of being absorbed by the target. Lasers and IPL sources that deliver in the red or near-infrared wavelength region fall in an optical window of the electromagnetic spectrum where selective absorption by melanin is combined with deep penetration into the dermis. Melanin is the primary light absorber between 600 and 1100 nm, but the absorption of the light by melanin decreases with the longer wavelengths. Longer wavelengths in this range are poorly absorbed by water and hemoglobin, although oxyhemoglobin and melanin have similar absorption at the wavelengths at 750 to 850 nm.

The required fluence or energy density to destroy the hair follicle is proportional to the hair shaft diameter. The thinner the hair, the less energy density level is necessary. The fluence of the laser/IPL source should be greater than or equal to the threshold fluence for tissue destruction.

Pulse duration should be longer than the TRT of the epidermis (3–10 msec) and shorter than or equal to the TRT of the hair follicles (40–100 msec) to ensure the full follicular destruction and to spare the epidermal melanosomes from intense heating and vaporization. The pulse width has an important role in determining selective photothermolysis. Short pulses of high energy will cause rapid heating of the target and rapid expansion of the thermal plasma. If the pulse width is too prolonged, there will be unwanted high temperature increases with resultant thermal injury to surrounding nonfollicular tissue and possibly cutaneous scarring and dyspigmentation. To maximize the laser-assisted hair removal it should be appreciated that the actual target is not pigmented, for example, the follicular stem cells that line the outer root sheath. Consequently, it has been proposed that pulses longer than the TRT of the hair shaft would be more efficacious as this would allow propagation of the thermal heat front through the entire volume of the hair and destroy the follicular stem cells.

Spot size diameter may play a role in optimizing laser/IPL hair removal. Larger beam diameters allow for a greater likelihood that the photons will be scattered back into the incident collimated beam and results in a greater photon density being present deeper in the tissue. Larger spot sizes of the beam increase the dermal/epidermal ratio and the relative penetration.

Epidermal cooling is paramount to reduce complications and to enhance the ability to use the highest fluence necessary for maximum response. There are four types of cooling options available for use with laser/IPL equipment. These include: passive cooling with an aqueous gel, active cooling with circulating water in a glass case, active conductive cooling with water encased in a sapphire window, and dynamic active cooling with a cryogenic spray.

CLINICAL EXPERIENCE

The first laser-assisted hair removal device was cleared by the FDA in 1995. Since that time numerous laser/IPL systems have been approved. These systems include ruby (694 nm), alexandrite (755 nm), diode (800–1000 nm), Q-switched and long-pulsed neodymium:YAG (1064 nm), IPL sources (550–1200 nm) with and without radiofrequency (RF), and various combination laser/IPL by a host of manufacturers (Table 2).

It is difficult to compare light systems in terms of long-term or permanent hair removal results because the follow-up periods in some studies are too short, which means that the full growth cycle as well as the recovery time for the hair follicles have not been included. Also confusing is the fact that many studies have included different anatomic sites with different hair growth cycles in the same study. Peer-reviewed studies of laser/IPL hair removal clinical trials often lack adequate hair growth evaluation methods, histologic data, and statistical analysis.

Ruby Laser (694 nm)

The normal-mode ruby laser was the original laser used for melanin-based selective photothermolysis hair removal. The active medium of the ruby laser is a ruby (aluminum oxide) crystal doped with chromium ions and emits light energy at 694 nm in the red portion of the visible light spectrum. The red light of the ruby laser has a very high melanin absorption at 694 nm and is most helpful to remove dark hair in light-skinned patients. There are three ruby lasers approved by the FDA for hair removal: the E2000 (Palomar), the EpiTouch (Sharplan/ESC), and the RubyStar (Aesculap Mediteo). The EpiTouch and the RubyStar lasers can operate in both the long-pulsed and the Q-switched mode.

Grossman et al. introduced the potential of the normal-mode ruby laser for hair removal in 1996. In this study 13 volunteers with brown or black hair were treated with 30 to 60 J/cm^2. Hair growth was assessed by manual terminal hair counts at 1, 3, and 6 months after treatment. At 6 months, four subjects had less than 50% hair regrowth, two of whom showed no change between 3 and 6 months. Significant hair loss was only in the shaved sites treated at the highest fluence. Fluence-dependent selective thermal injury to the follicles was observed histologically.

A long-term follow-up to the 1996 Grossman study was reported in 1998. The efficacy of the normal-mode ruby laser was evaluated at 2 years after a single treatment on the thighs or backs of 13 volunteers. Transient alopecia occurred in all 13 participants after laser exposure. Two years after laser exposure, four patients still had significant hair loss at all laser-treated sites compared with control sites. Laser-induced alopecia correlated histologically with miniaturized, vellus-like hair follicles similar to those found in androgenetic alopecia.

Polderman et al. designed a study to compare the long-pulsed ruby laser system with needle electrolysis and hot wax on three parts (forearm, face, and pubic area)of the body. The 25- and 40-J/cm^2 laser-treated sites showed a statistically significant decrease (38% and 49%, respectively) in the number of hairs at the first visit after the last and third treatment compared to the pretreatment hair counts. Laser therapy gave better results on the forearm than the face or pubic area. No significant decrease was observed in the needle electrolysis and hot wax-treated sites.

A study designed to evaluate the long-term efficacy of the normal-mode ruby laser (Epilaser; 694 nm, 3 msec) was published in 2000 by Campos et al. A wide range of anatomic areas in 51 patient volunteers (Fitzpatrick skin types II–IV) were treated for 2.7 average number of sessions

Table 2 Lasers and Intense Pulsed Light Sources for Hair Removal

Laser or IPL source	Wavelength (nm)	System name (company)	Pulse duration	Fluence (J/cm²)	Spot size	Other features
Long-pulsed ruby	694	E2000 (Palomar)	3100 msec	10–40	10, 20	Cooling, handpiece: 0–10°C; Fiber delivery; Photon recycling
		EpiTouch (Sharplan)	1.2 msec	10–40	3–6	Dual mode: may also be Q-switched
		RubyStar (Aesculap)	2 msec	25–40	7	Dual mode: may also be Q-switched
		Chromos	0.5–1.2 msec	3–20	7, 10	
Long-pulsed Nd:YAG	1064	GentleYAG (Candela)	0.25–300 msec	Up to 600	Up to 18 mm	Dynamic cooling
		Gentle YAG Limited Edition (Candela)	Up to 100 msec	Up to 100	10, 12, 15 mm	
		VARIA (Cool Touch)	0.3–500 msec	Up to 500	3–10 mm	Pulsed cryogen cooling w/pre- and post-cooling
		CoolGuide CV (Cutera)	10–100 msec	10–100		
		CoolGuide Excel (Cutera)	1–300 msec	50–300	10 mm	
		CoolGuide Vantage (Cutera)	0.1–300 msec	Up to 300 J		
		Smart Epil II (Cynosure)	Up to 100 msec	16–200		
		Acclaim 7000 (Cynosure)	0.4–300 msec	300		Air cooled, 110V/220V
		FriendlyLight (FriendlyLight)	0.2–1 msec	Up to 300		
		Lyra i (Laserscope)	20–100 msec	5–900	1–10 mm	
		Gemini (Laserscope)	10–100 msec	up to 990	1–10 mm	
		Lumenis One (Lumenis)	2–20 msec	10–225	2 × 4, 6, 9 mm	Scanner - Athoscan
		Quantel Athos (Med-Surge Technologies)	3–5 msec	Up to 120		30 × 30 mm hi-speed scan, contact cooling
		Profile Console (Sciton)	0.1–200 msec	4–400		Includes chiller
		Profile 1064 Module (Sciton)	0.1–200 msec	Up to 400	30 × 30 mm	Scanner; integrated cooling
		Solo 1.0 + chiller (Sciton)	0.1–200 msec	Up to 400	30 × 30 mm	Scanner, contact cooling
		Profile–ClearScan (Sciton)	0.1–200 msec	Up to 400	30 × 30 mm	Large area scanner (60 × 65 mm).
		Profile-D ClearScan (Sciton)	0.1–200 msec	Up to 400	3, 10 mm	Contact or air cooling
		Mydon (WaveLight)	20–200 msec	15–50		
Long-pulsed Alexandrite	755	GentleLASE (Candela)	3 msec	10–100	Up to 18 mm	Dynamic cooling
		GentleLASE Limited Edition (Candela)	3 msec	10–40	12 mm	
		Apogee 9300 (Cynosure)	5–40 msec	50	7, 10, 12 mm	
		Apogee 5500 (Cynosure)	5–40 msec	50	7, 10, 12 mm	
Diode	800	Arion (WaveLight)	1–50 msec	4–40	3, 10 mm	60 × 65 mm large area scanner
		Lightsheer ET (Lumenis)	5–400 msec	10–100	9 × 9 mm	ChillTip handpiece
		Lightsheer ST (Lumenis)	5–100 msec	10–40	9 × 9 mm	ChillTip handpiece

Type	Wavelength (nm)	Device (Company)	Pulse duration	Fluence/Energy	Spot size	Comments
IPL	810	MeDioStar (Med-Surge Technologies)	4–140 msec	Up to 64	12 mm	Cooled tip, Zimmer cooling.
		Sonata (Orion Lasers)	10–400 msec	Up to 100	10 × 12 mm	SheerCool contact cooling handpieces
		SLP1000 (Palomar)	50–1000 msec	Up to 575		
	550, 580, 615–1200 nm	OmniLight FPL (American Medical BioCare)	Up to 500 msec	Up to 90		
	400–1200	PhotoLight (Cynosure)	5–500 msec	3–30J	46 × 10 mm or 46 × 10 mm	No changing filters or heads. Patented krypton/xenon flashlamp and quad pulsing
	510–1200	Quadra Q4 (DermaMed USA)	60–120 msec	10–20J		Patented xenon flashlamp 19 pre-programmable settings
	480–1200	Quadra 4Q Platinum Series (DermaMed USA)	1–110 min	20		
	550–900	Prolite II (Med-Surge Technologies)	N/A	10–50	10 × 20 mm 20 × 25 mm	
	525–1200	MediLux System (Palomar)	10–100 msec	Up to 30	12 × 28 mm 16 × 46 mm	
	525–1200 nm	EsteLux System (Palomar)	10–100 msec	Up to 28	12 × 28 mm 16 × 46 mm	
	525–1200	NeoLux System (Palomar)	10–20 msec	Up to 25	12 × 28 mm 16 × 46 mm	
	525–1200	StarLux System (Palomar)	1–500 msec	Up to 50	12 × 28 mm 16 × 46 mm	
Combination:						
Optical energy combined w/RF electrical	680–980	Aurora DSR (Syneron)	Up to 200 msec	Optical 5–25		For hair removal and vascular/pigmented lesions
Alexandrite + Nd:YAG	755 and 1064	Apogee Elite (Cynosure)	0.4–300 msec	50	12, 15 mm	SmartCool air cooling
IPL Nd:YAG Diode	515–1200	Lumenis One (Lumenis)	3–100 msec	10–40	15 × 35 mm 2 × 4,6,9	
Diode Combined w/RF Electrical Energy	810	Polaris DS (Syneron)	N/A	Up to 40J/cm^2 RF	8 × 12 mm	No disposal cost, contact cooling
Long-Pulsed Nd:YAG w/IPL	1064 and 600–850	CoolGlide XEO (Cutera)	0.1–300 msec	Optical up to 30J/cm^2 Up to 300J 5–20J (pulsed light)		110V/220V configurations Upgradeable in the field

Abbreviations: IPL, intense pulsed light.
Source: From Moretti (2004); Rogachefsky, et al. (2002).

(range = 1–6). The response rate was assessed in a blinded manner by dermatologists by photographic evaluation. The mean follow-up after the last treatment was 8.37 months. Sixty-three percent of the patients had a sparse regrowth (<25%). Patients treated with higher fluences obtained greater long-term hair reduction.

Chana and Grobbelaar published in 2002 their experience using the pulsed ruby laser (Chromos 694) to remove hair of 402 anatomical sites in 346 consecutive patients. All skin types were treated. Results were recorded in two manners: the percentage reduction in hair density and the hair-free interval. The median reduction in hair density was 55% at a median time of 1 year after the last treatment session. The median hair-free interval was 8 weeks. Darker-colored hair was more effectively removed. Treatment success was not affected by the anatomic site, with the exception of the male face which did not respond well. There was a significant correlation between the number of treatments given and a favorable outcome. Although a greater than 50% reduction in hair density was obtained in half of the 346 patients, complete hair removal was achieved in only 0.7%.

In 2003, Allison et al. reported the results of a 1997–1999 study using the ruby laser (Chromos 694) for hair removal in three treatment sites. The three treatment groups were: top lip, axillae, and legs. Two treatments were given on both sides at each site at monthly intervals and a third treatment was given randomly to one side. Hair counts were made under magnification and using a grid system. The counts were made at monthly intervals for a period of 1 year. Long-term hair reduction was obtained in all patients. The results showed a reduction in hair count of 61% to 75% after a single treatment. Three treatments had an impact for two additional months, but not long term. This ruby laser study showed a persistent two-thirds reduction in hair count over 8 months of follow-up. Extension of the follow-up to 12 months did not show significant regrowth. The investigators postulated that the hair shaft damage is the primary feature in achieving damage to hair growth, not the anagen growth phase.

Q-Switched and Long-Pulsed Neodymium:YAG Lasers

The active medium of the neodymium:YAG laser is a crystal rod of yttrium–aluminum–garnet doped with 1% to 3% neodymium spectrum ions to produce laser light in the near-infrared at 1064 nm. Its beam can be delivered continuous, pulsed, or Q-switched.

On April 3, 1995, the FDA approved the first photoepilation system, the 1064-nm Q-switched Nd:YAG laser (SoftLight; Thermolase Corporation) . This system required pretreatment wax epilation and was followed by a topical carbon-mineral oil suspension. Although this patented process was a rapid method for hair removal, it showed minimal effectiveness for long-term hair reduction. Its ability to delay hair regrowth was limited to no more than a few months and there was full hair regrowth in all anatomic locations after 6 months. This was probably due to its inability to sufficiently heat the follicular unit with its nanosecond pulse duration.

Although the Q-switched Nd:YAG was not a successful permanent hair removal laser because its pulse width was too short to optimally target the hair structure, the long-pulsed Nd:YAG is capable of pulse durations that correspond to the TRT of the hair follicle. This laser system at 1064 nm has decreased melanin absorption which translates into the advantages of reduced epidermal heating and damage, the ability to treat a wider range of Fitzpatrick skin types, and the capacity to use higher fluences. While the decreased melanin absorption is advantageous in terms of decreasing epidermal heating and destruction, it also means that there is less absorption by the primary chromophore of melanin in the hair follicle. This diminished absorption at the target site is overcome by the use of higher fluences and the reduced scatter and deeper penetration of the longer wavelength of this long-pulsed 1064-nm laser. This laser can penetrate from 5 to 7 mm into the dermis, depths more than sufficient to reach the base of the hair bulb.

Alster et al. reported on the safety and effectiveness of the a long-pulsed Nd:YAG laser at 1064 nm (Lyra; LaserScope) in inducing long-term hair reduction in patients with darker skin. Twenty women with Fitzpatrick skin types IV to VI with dark hair on the face, axillae, and legs received three treatments with the 1064-nm laser (40–50 J/cm², 50 msec). Prolonged hair loss was observed 12 months after the last laser treatment (70–90% hair reduction). Axillary hair was more responsive to laser treatment than hair on legs and face. Authors proposed that the difference in sites were due to the skin thickness rather than hair growth cycles of the sites.

A report of 15 Chinese women who had hair removal treatments (13 axillae and two legs) with the diode laser on one side and the long-pulsed Nd:YAG laser on the other was completed by Chan et al. Although regrowth rates were low and similar at 6 weeks for both lasers, most patients had greater than 90% regrowth at week 36. Patients treated with the long-pulsed Nd:YAG experienced significantly a greater degree of immediate pain. The authors concluded that multiple treatment sessions and lasers with a longer pulse width are likely to be important to achieve a better hair reduction.

Galadari showed a 70% reduction of hair regrowth and a 35% reduction at 12 months following three to six treatments in 35 patients with Fitzpatrick skin types IV to VI. The investigator compared these findings to two similar patient groups treated with alexandrite and diode lasers. All three systems were useful in dark skin, but the complication rate was lower in patients treated with long-pulsed Nd:YAG laser.

Tanzi and Alster published a study of 36 adults (Fitzpatrick skin types I–VI) with terminal dark hair treated with long-pulsed Nd:YAG laser (1064 nm, 10 mm spot size, 30–60 J/cm²). The investigators delivered three treatments at 4- to 6-week intervals and performed hair counts and photographic evaluations at baseline, before each session, and at 1, 3, and 6 months after the final treatment. At 6 months after a series of three treatments they reported a mean hair reduction of 41% to 46% on the face and 48% to 53% on the body.

Alexandrite Laser

The 755-nm alexandrite laser offers a longer wavelength than the 694-nm ruby laser and produces a deeper dermal penetration. Melanin absorption is less by the 755-nm wavelength than the 694-nm wavelength. This feature should theoretically minimize side effects related to epidermal pigment change, but it could also diminish the treatment efficacy of hair follicle removal.

McDaniel et al. designed a study to determine the safety and long-term efficacy of the long-pulsed alexandrite laser for hair removal. A total of 31 anatomic areas on 22 patients were evaluated and treated using the 755-nm laser, single pulse technique, fluence of 20 J/cm². They examined the effect of both a 10-mm spot size for 5- and 10-msec pulse durations and a 7-mm spot size for 20-msec pulse duration. Objective-blinded photographic grading was performed by cosmetic surgeons and research assistants at 1, 2, 3, and 6 months after treatment. At 6 months maximum reductions observed were 40% lip, 56% leg, 50% back, and 15% bikini area. Comparison of blinded objective grading at 6 months showed the 10-msec pulse duration treatment sited had significantly better hair reduction rates than for the 5-msec sites ($P = 0.0002$) and moderately better rates than 20-msec sites ($P = 0.04$). There is a significant decrease in the penetration depth using the 7-mm spot size compared with the 10-mm spot size. This would explain the improved reduction with 10 msec (10-mm spot size) over the 20 msec (7-mm spot size).

A study was performed by Nanni and Alster of 36 subjects treated with a long-pulsed alexandrite laser. The laser parameters were an average fluence of 18 J/cm^2, with a 10-mm spot size at either a 5-, 10-, or 20-ms pulse duration. There was a definite delay in hair regrowth compared with control sites at 1 week and 1 and 3 months post-procedurally, but there was no significant hair count reduction at 6-month follow-up. In this published report of 36 patients, two had blonde hair and four had gray hair. Blonde and gray hairs did not respond as well to the alexandrite laser as did brown or black hair, probably because of the reduced melanin content.

Garcia et al. directed a prospective clinical study of 150 patients (Fitzpatrick skin types IV–VI) who were treated with long-pulsed alexandrite laser (12.5-mm handpiece, 40-msec pulse duration, fluence range of 13–24 J/cm^2) in 550 sites. There was an average of three treatment sessions and a 6-month follow-up. Hair reduction or change in quality of existing hairs was documented by hair counts and photography. Approximately 40% reduction in hair count was evident after at least three treatment sessions.

A comparative study of the long-pulsed diode and long-pulsed alexandrite lasers in 20 women with Fitzpatrick skin types I to IV and dark terminal hairs showed significant and equivalent clinical improvement using either laser. Side effects were rare, but more frequently observed after treatment with long-pulsed diode system at the higher fluence of 40 J/cm^2. Histologic changes showed initial follicular injury followed by follicular miniaturization and fewer number of terminal hairs.

Diode Laser

The 800- to 810-nm pulsed diode laser is a versatile, compact hair removal system. Depending on the make and model, the handpiece can be equipped with a cooling tip and the spot size can be as large as 12 × 12 mm. Pulse durations can be adjusted over a wide range (5–400 msec), which when combined with the longer wavelength, will afford some safety for darker-skinned patients. The diode LightSheer (Lumenis) was approved by the FDA for permanent hair reduction in 1999 and has proven to be a safe, efficient hair removal unit (Fig. 3A and B).

Campos et al. reported on the efficacy of the high-power, pulsed diode laser with an actively cooled sapphire tip in the handpiece for eradication of unwanted hair. A total of 38 patients (Fitzpatrick skin types II–VI) were treated in multiple anatomic locations (axillae, arm, back, bikini, buttock, face, shoulder) with fluence ranges from 10 to 40 J/cm^2. One to four treatments were performed. Evaluation of the hair reduction was performed at least 4 months after the last treatment by a blinded assessment of clinical photographs. Sparse hair regrowth was seen at the final evaluation of 59% of the subjects. Higher fluences and multiple treatment sessions achieved greater long-term efficacy. All but two subjects had clinically apparent long-term hair loss. Most had sparse hair regrowth, with a mean follow-up of 8.7 months after the last treatment, at a mean fluence of 33.4 J/cm^2 and a mean of 2.8 treatments.

With a super long-pulsed 810-nm laser, a 34% hair reduction rate in five suntanned subjects (Fitzpatrick skin types II–IV) was achieved at 6 months. The use of variable fluences (23, 45, 57, and 115 J/cm^2) and pulse durations (200, 400, 500, and 1000 msec) did not significantly alter the hair reduction rates. Clinical evaluations rated two treatments superior to one. To achieve the optimal safety in tanned patients the highest fluence (115 J/cm^2) and pulse duration (1000 msec) should be avoided. A follow-up study by the same authors in 10 female patients with Fitzpatrick skin types I to VI showed, at 6 months after the last treatment, an average hair reduction of 25% for two treatments and 22% for one treatment. Optimal hair reduction was achieved at 400 msec, 46 J/cm^2.

The Galadari study of 32 patients showed a 80% reduction in hair growth at 6 months and a 40% diminution in hair growth at 12 months after six treatments with the diode laser in patients with Fitzpatrick skin types IV to VI. This was identical to the alexandrite laser, but the occurrence of side effects was significantly lower.

Intense Pulsed Light

The IPL is not a laser because the light generated is an incoherent, noncollimated, and polychromatic visible-infrared source. The 550- to 1200-nm light pulses are created by a flashlamp, focused by a reflector, and transmitted through a set of filters that determine its spectral characteristics. For hair removal, the filters tailor the spectrum of light to the skin type and hair color of the patient.

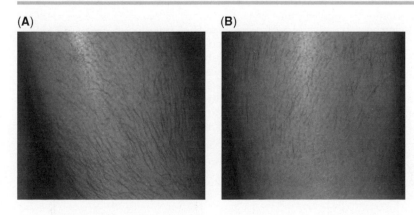

(A) **(B)**

Figure 3 **(A)** Before laser treatment. **(B)** Long-term hair reduction on the lower legs, 6 months after three treatments with the 800-nm diode laser.

A study by Troilius and Troilius evaluated bikini line hair removal with a second-generation IPL source. Ten females with dark hair and skin types II to IV were treated with an IPL device (600 nm) four times with 1-month interval between treatments. Hair counts evaluation was performed using a computer imaging system before treatment and at 4 and 8 months after last treatment. Hair reduction of 74.7% was recorded at 4 months and 80.2% at 8 months.

Sadick et al. published a nonrandomized control trial of 67 subjects with areas of excess body hair (inguinal region, chest, abdomen, face, back, or arms) treated with IPL (EpiLight; ESC Medical Systems). IPL exposure parameters were: filter 590 nm for skin type I, 615 nm for skin type II, 645 nm for skin type III, or 695 nm for skin type IV; fluence 40 to 42 J/cm^2; spot size 10 × 45 mm; pulse duration 2.9 to 3.0 msec with pulse delay of 30 msec. Single or multiple treatments were performed, and follow-up was 6 months or longer. For subjects receiving a single treatment, biopsy samples were taken immediately after treatment and at various intervals up to 20 months.

Mean hair loss after IPL was 49%, 57%, and 54% for a single treatment at follow-up of less than 3 months, 3 to less than 6 months, and 6 months or longer, respectively. For multiple treatments mean hair loss was 47%, 56%, and 64%, respectively. Histologic examination showed morphologic damage confined to the hair follicles and shafts. Terminal–vellus and anagen–telogen ratios, mean hair shaft diameter, and immunohistochemical profiles were not significantly modified by the treatment. The authors concluded that IPL-induced long-term epilation was predominantly due to selective photothermal damage to large, pigmented hair follicles rather than induction of follicular cycle arrest or follicular miniaturization as previously observed with ruby laser hair removal.

Sadick et al. reported on the long-term hair removal efficiency of the IPL (EpiLight) in 34 patients with Fitzpatrick skin types II to V. The mean hair reduction was 76% after a mean of 3.7 treatments and the results were not significantly related to skin type, hair color, anatomic site, or number of treatments.

The long-term effectiveness of IPL (EpiLight) hair removal was addressed in a study published by Gold et al. A 1-year follow-up of 24 of 31 patients who participated in the original 3-month study demonstrated a long-term epilation of 75% one year after a single treatment. The 24 patients had a range of Fitzpatrick skin types of I to VI with hair color of black to light brown. Areas of the body treated included the face, neck, upper limbs, and trunk.

Weiss et al. designed a study of 23 patients with Fitzpatrick skin types I to III (28 sites) to evaluate a single-treatment IPL followed for 3 months. Another 48 patients with Fitzpatrick skin types I to V (56 sites) were randomly enrolled for two IPL treatments 1 month apart and followed for 6 months. Hair reduction was evaluated by hair counts and photography. IPL parameters used were a 2.8- to 3.2-msec pulse duration typically for three pulses with TRT of 20 to 30 msec with a total fluence of 40 to 42 J/cm^2. For the single-treatment protocol a final 63% hair reduction was seen at 12 weeks. For the double-treatment study hair counts were reduced by 33% at 6 months.

A 2004 article from the Netherlands showed that the IPL was effective in achieving 87% long-term hair removal in 70 hirsute females (Fitzpatrick skin types I–V) after a mean of eight treatments and a follow-up mean period of 27.0 months. The number of treatments given was related

to the efficacy of hair removal, but there was no correlation found between hair removal and patient-related and/or technical data.

IPL/Bipolar Radiofrequency Combination

Most dark hair types have benefited from current technologies, but the removal of blonde and white hair has been particularly problematic due to the low concentration of the melanin in the target hair follicle. The photoepilatory effect of a new technological combination of IPL and a bipolar RF device has been explored in patients of diverse skin types and varied hair colors. The theory behind this technology is to decrease optical energy to a level that is safe for all skin types while compensating for the lack of light by utilizing an additive RF energy that is not optical, but is selectively absorbed by the hair structure. The light is absorbed and subsequently heats the hair shaft while the RF directly heats the hair follicle. The combination creates a uniform heat profile across the hair structure and potentially destroys it.

Sadick and Laughlin studied 36 adult women with white and blonde hair on the chin and upper lip regions. They received four treatment sessions with the IPL/RF device over 9 to 12 months with long-term follow-up at month 18 (6 months after last treatment). The level of RF energy was 20 J/cm^3 and the optical fluences varied from 24 to 30 J/cm^2. An average hair removal of 48% was observed at month 18. A slightly higher photoepilatory efficiency was recorded for blonde hair (52%) versus white hair (44%) treatment sites.

Exogenous Chromophore
Photodynamic Therapy

Photodynamic therapy (PDT) consists of the combination of a topical or systemic photosensitizer followed by the exposure to nonionizing radiation. Light of an appropriate wavelength is selectively absorbed by the photosensitizing chemical and may then activate the chemical reactions directly or transfer energy to molecular oxygen to produce a relative intermediary singlet oxygen. The most significant effects of the generated singlet oxygen are lethal alterations of cellular membrane systems through lipid peroxidation and protein damage. As oxygen is consumed during the reaction producing tissue hypoxia, this phenomenon results in tissue damage and a rate-limiting effect since oxygen is required to generate the singlet oxygen.

The concept of PDT has been adopted for hair removal. Topical aminolevulenic acid (ALA) has been used in conjunction with laser light for hair removal. ALA is not itself a photosensitizer, but it can be metabolized in vivo to protoporphyrin IX, a porphyrin intermediate with photosensitizing activity. The optimal wavelength for the in vivo photoactivation of protoporphrin IX has been shown to be 635 nm.

In 1995, Grossman et al. reported on the use of topical 20% ALA solution and laser light for hair removal. In 11 patients the area to be treated was either shaved or waxed, a 20% ALA solution was applied for 3 hours, and then the area was exposed to an argon pumped dye laser at 630 nm with fluences of 100 to 200 J/cm^2. At 3 months there was only a 50% regrowth in areas treated with 20% ALA and 200 J/cm^2 versus 90% regrowth in areas exposed to 100 J/cm^2 and control sites. Fluorescence from the epidemis demonstrated at the photosensitizer was concentrated in the follicular ostium, and an immunofluorescence biopsy showed that the photosensitizer was accumulated in the surrounding follicular epithelium.

This photodynamic technique means that the ability to remove hair is no longer dependent of the hair color but on the concentration of the photosensitizer in the follicular epithelium. The obvious advantage is that all hair colors can be treated. The disadvantages are pain, hyperpigmentation, and the pre-light treatment time necessary for the conversion of ALA to protoporphyrin IX.

The future use of exogenous chromophore to enhance laser/IPL hair removal is an area of active research. A study using nylon microspheres to deliver methylene blue to pilosebaceous units has confirmed this technique in male hairless rates. This method might be used to enhance hair removal, especially blonde or white hair with little or no melanin target.

Laser Selection: Which One to Use?

It is well recognized that the ideal candidate for laser/light hair removal is a fair-skinned individual with dark hair. Any of the available systems will be effective. Studies have shown that patients with darker skin types require longer-wavelength lasers to avoid epidermal damage.

A comparative retrospective investigation was performed in 2004 by Bouzari et al. using the long-pulsed Nd:YAG, alexandrite, and diode lasers for hair removal in 75 patients (Fitzpatrick skin types I–V). A total of 805 consecutive laser hair removal treatments were performed. Patients were evaluated at least 3 months after the last treatment. The mean hair reduction count as performed by a dermatologist and compared to pretreatment photographs showed 42.4%, 65.6%, and 46.9% in Nd:YAG, alexandrite, and diode lasers, respectively. When the number of treatments was taken into consideration, the effectiveness of alexandrite and diode lasers were not significantly different. Both of these lasers were more efficacious than Nd:YAG laser.

In general, thin-haired, lighter-haired patients are a challenge to treat but benefit most from the shorter wavelengths and pulse durations. Longer pulse durations and wavelengths, combined with epidermal cooling, allow safest treatment in darker-skinned patients.

Patient Selection

Prior to initiation of laser hair removal treatment, the physician and patient should have an in-depth consultation. Expectations and goals can be very different for each and need to be outlined and understood. Patients are often seeking complete, permanent hair removal, and this goal is rarely, if ever, achievable with lasers or IPL. The ideal candidate is a patient with fair skin (Fitzpatrick skin types I–III) and relatively dark hair (brown or black). Temporary hair loss (1–3 months) always occurs after laser treatment irrespective of the hair color (except white). Long-term permanent hair reduction is strongly correlated to a patient's hair color (black or brown) and laser/IPL fluence. However, it should be pointed out to the patient that even with lighter colored hair (blonde, red, gray), hair loss can be maintained with regular treatment sessions at approximately 3-month intervals.

A thorough history should be taken with regard to drugs (isotretinoin, photosensitizing medications), herpetic infections in the proposed treatment site, potential of scar formation, exposure to sun or tanning booths, photosensitivity, and seizure disorder triggered by light. Caution should be used in treating patients with immunosuppression. Published studies do not include pregnant females most likely due to the Investigation Review Board restrictions. There are no reported adverse reactions in pregnant patients, so the decision to treat is made by consensus of the patient and physician. It is most likely prudent to err on the conservative side and wait until after the delivery unless there are overriding factors.

If on physical examination the female patient shows evidence of excess androgen production, a gynecologic or endocrine consultation should be considered prior to initiation of hair removal treatment. If there is an underlying hormonal abnormality, and it is not addressed, the efficacy of the hair removal treatment will be compromised.

Special precautions must be taken in particular sites to be treated with the laser or IPL. The axillae and bikini line are more sensitive to blisters and pigmentary changes, especially in darker-skinned patients. Patients should not wax or undergo electrolysis up to 6 weeks before the procedure as the target hair shaft will be removed. Patients may continue to shave up to the day of the procedure.

Laser/IPL hair removal is painful and the patient should be so advised. Topical anesthetic creams are helpful to apply prior to treatment initiation. The epidermal cooling devices also reduce discomfort. Immediately after treatment completion, ice packs and/or cooling aloe vera gel can be quite soothing to the patient and reduce discomfort.

In darker-skinned patients it is always useful to perform a test patch prior to treating a large area. If any epidermal injury, such as immediate whitening, vesiculation, or forced epidermal separation, is observed the starting fluence should be reduced by 20% to 30%. A 2- to 4-week waiting period will allow observation for any complications, particularly dyspigmentation and scarring.

Postoperative Patient Instructions

Careful sun avoidance for 2 weeks and the ongoing diligent regular use of sunscreen is recommended. Use of retinoid products, polyhydroxy-containing potions, cleansing scrubs, or granules are to be avoided for at least 2 to 3 days after the treatment. Oral analgesics are rarely necessary.

COMPLICATIONS

Descriptions of laser/IPL hair removal procedures give the deceiving impression that the technique is simple and has minimal to no complications. In reality the opposite is true. To avoid complications it is crucial that there be careful patient selection, appropriate anatomic site preparation, in-depth patient education regarding expectations, and postoperative care of the treated areas. It is also imperative that the physician or medical personnel performing the procedure be properly trained. Even with the best of training and preparation, side effects can occur, should be anticipated, and dealt with in an expeditious manner to avoid permanent cutaneous damage.

Potential complications can include: edema, erythema (Fig. 4), pain, crusting, vesiculation or blisters, purpura, folliculitis (Fig. 5), infection (bacterial, viral, fungal), dyspigmentation (Figs. 6, 7A and B), scarring, increased hair growth in the treated site, terminalization (conversion of vellus-type hairs to terminal hairs in the laser-treated area), dystrophic hair, whitening or temporary hair color change, and superficial thrombophlebitis. The incidence of adverse effects depends on the patient's Fitzpatrick skin type, the anatomic treatment site, the laser/IPL system and the parameters used during treatment, and the postoperative care. Table 3 describes the complication profile of the major photoepilation hair removal studies.

Nanni and Alster compared the frequency of side effects using three different hair removal laser systems (Q-switched Nd:YAG with pretreatment wax epilation and

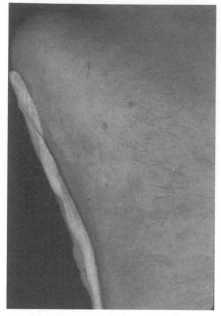

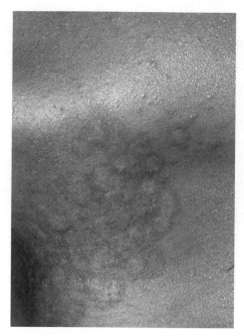

Figure 4   Reactive erythema immediately following laser treatment. (*See color insert.*)

Figure 6   Post-inflammatory hyperpigmentation in patient with Fitzpatrick skin type VI after alexandrite laser treatment. (*See color insert.*)

topical carbon solution, long-pulsed ruby with contact cooling tip, long-pulse alexandrite). Pain at the time of treatment, erythema, edema, hypopigmentation, hyperpigmentation, blistering, crusting, erosions, purpura, and folliculitis were reported. The ruby and the alexandrite lasers induced the majority of the side effects and these occurred in tanned skin or in Fitzpatrick skin types III and higher. The extensor surfaces of the extremities and chin and anterior neck were the anatomic locations with the highest side effect rates. Average duration of postinflammatory

hyperpigmentation was 2 months, whereas hypopigmentation resolved after 3.5 months. Long-term sequelae and scarring were not reported with any of the three lasers systems.

A large multicenter British prospective study by Lanigan was conducted to determine the incidence of side effects in relation to skin types and three different types of lasers (long-pulse ruby, long-pulse alexandrite, and long-pulsed Nd:YAG). There were 480 patients (Fitzpatrick skin types I–VI) who received a total number of 3143 treatments (median 5) on various body sites. The overall incidence of side effects was low, 57 of 480 patients. In addition to the commonly reported adverse effects to laser hair removal there was one case of superficial thrombophlebitis of the submental side of the chin which developed after one of seven treatments with ruby and long-pulsed Nd:YAG lasers and resolved in 7 days. The author reported having one other case of thrombophlebitis as a result of Nd:YAG laser hair removal, but this case was not included in the published study. It is of note to compare the overall incidence of side effects in skin types IV to VI (109 patients) treated with the ruby laser (29.9%) and with the Nd:YAG (9.4%). Lanigan concluded that for darker skin types the long-pulsed Nd:YAG was preferable to the ruby laser.

Jay et al. reported on the safety of the IPL hair removal in 250 patients who underwent 498 treatments. A total of 12 side effects occurred in 11 patients. The three categories of side effects were pigmentary changes, acne-like rashes, and symptoms of tingling or sensitivity without skin changes. All of these complications were brief and transient.

McDaniel et al. reported safety of long-pulsed alexandrite laser hair removal in 22 patients receiving one treatment in 31 various locations (lip, leg, back, bikini region). All patients experienced transient erythema and two patients (9%) with Fitzpatrick skin type III showed transient hyperpigmentation. Four sites (13%) had mild crusting, seven sites (23%) had skin sensitivity, and four sites (13%) developed fine vesiculation. No bruising, purpura, scarring, hypopigmentation, or infections were recorded.

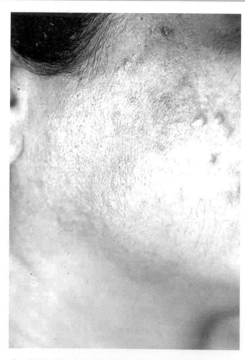

Figure 5   Folliculitis following hair laser removal. (*See color insert.*)

(A)

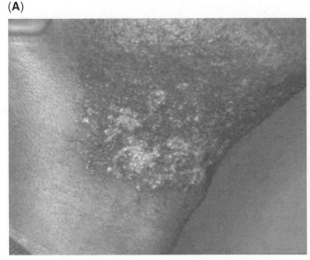

(B)

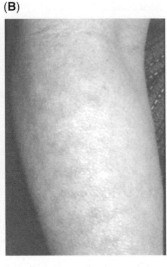

Figure 7 **(A)** Transient post-inflammatory hypopigmentation in a dark-skinned patient following diode laser treatment for pseudo-folliculitis barbae. **(B)** Post-inflammatory hypopigmentation occurring in tanned patient after alexandrite laser hair removal. (*See color insert*.)

Dyspigmentation (hypopigmentation or hyperpigmentation) is extremely more likely following laser hair removal in patients with darker colored skin. Chana and Grobbelaar showed in a study of 346 patients who underwent hair removal at 402 anatomic sites using the ruby laser an overall 9% complication rate. Fitzpatrick skin type I patients remained free of complications while the risk of complications escalated to 24.7% in skin types V and VI.

Pigmentary changes after laser-assisted hair removal in conjunction with cryogen spray cooling have been reported and the injury has been attributed to secondary cryogen damage. Kelly et al. have demonstrated that the pigmentary findings are not related to the cryogen, but rather laser-induced thermal injury. Three recommendations are suggested to reduce or eliminate these types of adverse pigmentary changes: when using a large spot size (15–18 mm) select longer cryogen spurt durations; confirm cryogen coverage before each procedure by firing the beam onto a porous surface; and hold the handpiece perpendicular to the skin surface.

In a study of 38 patients treated with diode laser for hair removal, 11 of the 38 (29%) developed pigmentary changes of hyperpigmentation and/or hypopigmentation, which were well tolerated and cleared spontaneously. Patients with Fitzpatrick skin types of V (3/5, 60%) and VI (2/2, 100%) had an increased incidence of pigmentary changes.

The induction of hair growth by laser/IPL hair removal is an unusual complication. One laser surgeon stated that he saw this in fewer than 5% of his cases. It usually occurred in individuals with skin type IV or V, and the hair usually grew on the lower part of the neck or in the medial malar area. Others have reported similar increase of hair growth in their patients. Most of the patients affected with this complication are Mediterranean women. It is postulated that there may be some type of low-grade biostimulation of the follicle. The hair growth stimulation appears to be more of a problem when short pulses are used rather than long pulses. If the problem arises in a patient, it is suggested to treat with the longest pulses available such as those of the diode laser. It is a rare, but real, complication and the risk of hair growth stimulation should be included in the consent form. There is one ancedotal report of pili bigeminy induced by low fluence hair removal with alexandrite and ruby lasers. Schroeter et al. reported the paradoxical growth of hair after IPL hair removal. This was particularly seen in patients whose treatment intervals were more than 8 weeks. The authors hypothesized that the light helped to stimulate the hair follicle to enter the anagen growth phase more readily and recommended that treatment sessions be spaced 4 to 6 weeks in order to avoid this paradoxical hair growth.

Terminalization or conversion of vellus-type hairs to terminal hair in the laser-treated site was reported in a large comparative study of the long-pulsed Nd:Yag, alexandrite, diode lasers. It occurred in 27% (3/11) of Nd:YAG, 12% (4/29) of alexandrite, and 3% of diode.

There have been reports of whitening of the hair or temporary hair color change from black to blonde after IPL for hair removal. Leukotrichia as a complication of IPL hair removal was reported in 29 patients and the hair color was eventually restored in nine patients. The authors speculated that the heat produced during the procedure was enough to damage the melanocytes permanently, but not enough to destroy the hair germinative cells. In the cases of temporary leukotrichia, the heat produced was insufficient to damage the melanocytes permanently but arrested temporarily the melanogenesis or the melanin transfer to the surrounding keratinocytes. The yellowish discoloration may have had the similar mechanism with melanogenesis reduced or the cause could have been the switching of melanogenesis from eumelanin to pheomelanin.

Following IPL hair removal, hair morphologic changes have been observed. Gross kinking of some hairshafts immediately after IPL treatment (range 0% to 22%; mean ± SD, 10.2 ± 6.5%) has been recorded. Dystrophic hair shapes, including reduced diameter, abnormal tapering, and distorted contours, have been reported after IPL hair removal.

One of the ongoing concerns in patient selection is the safety of performing laser hair removal in patients undergoing isotretinoin treatments. Khatri attempted to answer this dilemma in a small study of seven female patients who had 810-nm diode laser hair removal while concomitantly receiving isotretinoin for acne in dosage of 20 to 80 mg/day. The parameters of the laser were a fluence of 21 to 24 J/cm^2, spot size 12 mm, and a pulse width of 300 msec to remove hair in axillary, bikini, or chin sites. A contact cooling device was used throughout the procedure. The volunteers were evaluated at 1 week and 1 month. There were no incidences of erythema, pigmentary change, swelling, or scarring. One patient developed a bulla 1 week after treatment, which resolved uneventfully. Khatri

Table 3 Complication Profile of Laser/PL Systems Used for Hair Removal

Study	Number of patients	Fitzpatrick skin	Type site Tx	Type of reaction	Number of patients or sites (%)
Long-Pulse Ruby Laser					
Grossman et al. (24)	13	I–III	Back, Thigh	Transient erythemic edenma	6 (100)
				Purpara	6 (100)
				Hyperpigmentation	3 (23)
				Hypopigmentation	2 (15.4)
Poldeman et al. (45)	30	I–III	Forearm	Erythema	3 (10)
			Face	Edema	1 (33)
			Public area	Hyperpigmentation	1 (3.3)
				Hypopigmentation	7 (23.3)
Campos et al. (9)	51	V–IV	Abdomen	Pigmented changes	15 (29.4)
			Arm, Feet	Hyperpigmentation	8 (15.7)
			Shoulders, Axillae	Hypopigmentation	2 (3.9)
			Chest, Thigh, Bikini, Back Face	Both Hyper & Hypopigmentation	5 (9.8)
Chana et al. (11)	346 (402 sites)	I–VI	Face, Neck	Blisters	12 (3)
			Axilla, Chest	Scabs	5 (1.2)
			Abdomen	Hyperpigmentation	14 (3.5)
			Arm, Leg Back	Hypopigmentation	5 (1.2)
Aillson et al. (2)	69	I–III	Lip, Axilla	Reaction of labial herpes	1 (1.4)
			Legs	Superficial burns of anterior aspect of legs	2 (3)
Lanigan et al. (35)	322	I–V	Face, Bikini, Legs, Back, Chest, Abdoman, Upper Lips, Scalp	Blisters	21 (6.5)
				Hyperpigmentation	7 (2)
				Hypopigmentation	4 (1.2)
				Scar	1 (0.3)
Long Pulse Nd:YAG Laser					
Alster et al. (4)	20	IV–VI	Face, Axilla, Leg	Pain	59 (90)[a]
				Vesiculation	1 (1.5)
				Pigmentary alteration	3 (5)
Chan et al. (10)	15	IV–V	Axillae, Legs	Pain	15 (100)
				Erythema	5 (33.3)
				Edema	5 (33.3)
				Folliculitis	5. (33.3)
				Hypopogmentation	1 (7)
Lanigan et al. (35)	224	I–VI	Face, Bikini, Legs, Back, Chest, Abdomen, Upper Limbs, Scalp	Bilsters	11 (5)
				Hyperpigmentation	2 (0.9)
				Hypopigmentation	1 (0.4)
				Thrombophlebitis	3 (1.3)
Tanzi et al. (59)	36	I–VI	Facial, Non-Facial	Pain	108 (100)[b]
				Erythema	103 (65)
				Perifollicular edema	96 (89)
				Hyperpigmentation	1 (1)
Bouzari et al. (7)	11	III–V	Chin, Upper lip, Periauricular Neck	Pain	4 (36)
				Blisters or Erisions	2 (18)
				Hyperpigmentation	1 (9)
				Terminalization	3 (27)
Long-Pulse Alexandrite					
McDaniel et al. (38)	22 (31 sites)	I–III	Lip, Leg, Back Bikini	Erythema	31 (100)
				Crusting	4 (13)
				Vesiculation	4 (13)
				Skin sensitivity	7 (23)
				Hyperpigmentation	2 (9)
Nanni et al. (42)	36 pts	I–V	Lip, Back Legs	Intraoperative pain	31 (85)
				Erythema	35 (97)
				Blisters	1 (< 1)
				Hyperpigmentation	NR (3)
Garcia et al. (20)	150	IV–VI	Upper lip, Chin	Blisters	9 (1.6)
			Beard, Cheeks, Side	Excoriation	1 (.16)
			Burns, Legs, Neck, Axillae, Arms,	Foillculilis	2 (.36)
			Nose, Chest, Ears, Areola,	Hyperpigmentation	3 (.5)
			Forehead, Back, Abdomen,	Hypopigmentation	2 (.36)
			Bikini, Fingers, Thighs, Buttocks		
Lanigan et al. (35)	74	I–V	Face, Bikini, Legs, Back, Chest, Abdomen, Scalp	Blisters	1 (1.4)

(Continued)

Table 3 Complication Profile of Laser/PL Systems Used for Hair Removal (*Continued*)

Study	Number of patients	Fitzpatrick skin	Type site Tx	Type of reaction	Number of patients or sites (%)
Bouzari et al. (7)	29	I–V	Chin, Upper Lip Periauricular Neck	Pain	9 (30)
				Blisters	1 (3)
				Folliculitis	2 (6)
				Hyperpigmentation	2 (6)
				Hypopigmentation	1 (3)
				Terminalization	4 (12)
Diode Laser					
Campos et al. (8)	38	II–VI	Axillae	Erythema	38 (100)
			Arm, Back	Hyperpigmentation	11 (29)
			Bikini, Buttocks Face, Shoulders	Hypopigmentation	3 (8)
Rogachefsky et al. (49)	5 (55 sities)	II–IV	Legs Forearms	Pain	9 (18)
				Erythema	34 (62)
				Persistent erytheme (6 mos)	5 (10)
				Blisters	3 (5)
				Hyperpigmentation	5 (10)
				Hypopigmentation	13 (23)
Chan et al. (10)	15	IV–V	Axillae, Legs	Pain	15 (100)
				Erythema	5 (33.3)
				Edema	5 (33.3)
				Folliculitis	5 (33.3)
				Hypopigmentation	1 (7)
Rogachefsky et al. (48)	10 (108 sites)	I–VI	Neck, Legs	Pain	47 (44)
				Erthema	56 (52)
				Blisters	(5)
				Nikolsky sign	(3)
				Hyperpigmentation[c]	9 (11)
				Hypopigmentation[c]	(57)
Bouzazi et al. (7)	30	II–IV	Chin, Upper lip Periauricular Neck	Pain	11 (35)
				Blisters or erosions	4 (12)
				Hyperpigmentation	4 (12)
				Hypopigmentation	2 (2)
				Terminalization	1 (1)
Intense Pulsed Light					
Gold et al. (21)	24	I–VI	Face, Neck, Upper Limbs, Trunk	Erythema	18 (75)
				Edema	2 (8.3)
				Blisters	4 (16.6)
				Hyperpigmentation	1 (4.2)
Sadick et al. (54)	67	I–IV	Inguinal area Chest, Abdomen, Face, Back, Arms	Transient follicular erythema	67 (100)
				Persistent erythema	1 (1.5)
				Gross kinking of hair shaft	15 (22)
Weisse et al. (63)	71 (84 sites)	I–V	Chin, Back, Bikini, Neck, Lip, Thigh, Shoulder, Abdomen, Submental, Forearm, Ear, Cheek, Preauricular	Erythema	65 (92)
				Urticarial edema	51 (72)
				Crusting	9 (12)
				Vesicle	2 (2.8)
				Hypo/Hyperpigmentation	11 (15.5)
Sadick et al. (55)	34	II–IV	Face, Lip, Back, Mandible, Chest, Abdomen, Chin, Bikini	Crusting	2 (6)
				Hyperpigmentation	3 (9)

[a]Adverse effects calculated from 60 treatment sessions in 20 patients.
[b]Adverse effects calculated from 108 treatment sessions in 36 patients.
[c]6 month follow up on 80 sites in 10 patients.
Abbreviation: NR, not reported.

concluded that his limited study suggested that the diode laser hair removal was safe in patients undergoing isotretinoin treatment. He hypothesized that the laser targeted the melanin in the hair follicles and in theory should not alter the dermal collagen or cause scarring. A commentary written by Goodman following Khatri's article cautioned that short- and long-pulse 1064-nm lasers and IPL devices have been utilized for facial rejuvenation as well as epilation, so it should not be assumed that they will not interact with dermal collagen and have the potential to cause problems of delayed or altered reepithelialization or inhibition of collagenase in patients taking isotretinoin. A judicious, conservative approach would be to wait 6 to 12 months following completion of isotretinoin before initiation of laser/IPL hair removal.

Follicular Scarring Disorders

While laser/IPL hair removal is most often thought of as a cosmetic procedure, it can also have several medical applications for inflammatory scarring disorders, such as folliculitis decalvans, dissecting cellulitis of the scalp, acne keloidalis, and pseudofolliculitis barbae. Removal of the hair follicles may help in the resolution of these conditions. There have been various anecdotal reports of success using lasers and IPL for hair removal in these diseases. Chui et al. presented three patients with various scarring follicular disorders who were treated with the long-pulse ruby laser. The patients tolerated the procedure well and improvement was recorded in all cases. One African-American female developed persistent hypopigmentation. Kauvar reported more than 50% improvement using a diode laser (30–40 J/cm^2 fluence, 20–30 msec pulse duration) to treat pseudofolliculitis barbae in 10 patients with Fitzpatrick skin types I to IV.

BIBLIOGRAPHY

Abell E. Embryology and anatomy of the hair follicle. In: Olsen EA, ed. Disorders of Hair Growth Diagnosis and Treatment. New York: McGraw-Hill, Inc., 1994:1–19.

Allison KP, Kiernan MN, Waters RA, Clement RM. Evaluation of the ruby 694 Chromos for hair removal in various skin sites. Lasers Med Sci 2003; 18:165–170.

Alora MB, Anderson RR. Recent developments in cutaneous lasers. Lasers Surg Med 2000; 26:108–118.

Alster TS, Bryan H, Williams CM. Long-pulsed Nd:YAG laser-assisted hair removal in pigmented skin: a clinical and histological evaluation. Arch Dermatol 2001; 137:885–889.

Anderson RR, Parrish JA. Selective photothermolysis: precise microsurgery by selective absorption of pulsed radiation. Science 1983; 220:524–527.

Anderson RR, Ross EV. Laser–tissue interactions. In: Fitzpatick RE, Goldman MP, eds. Cosmetic Laser Surgery. St. Louis, MO: Mosby, 2000:1–30.

Bouzari N, Tabatabai H, Abbasi Z, Firooz A, Dowlati Y. Laser hair removal: comparison of long-pulsed Nd:Yag, long-pulsed alexandrite, and long-pulsed diode lasers. Dermatol Surg 2004; 30:498–502.

Campos VB, Dierickx CC, Farinelli WA, Lin T, Manuskiatti W, Anderson RR. Ruby laser hair removal: evaluation of long-term efficacy and side effects. Lasers Surg Med 2000; 26:177–185.

Campos VB, Dierickx CC, Farinelli WA, Lin TD, Manuskiatti W. Hair removal with an 800-nm pulsed diode laser. J Am Acad Dermatol 2000; 43:442–447.

Chan HH, Ying S, Ho W, Wong DSY, Lam L. An in vivo study comparing the efficacy and complications of diode laser and long-pulsed Nd:YAG laser in hair removal in Chinese patients. Dermatol Surg 2001; 27:950–954.

Chana JS, Grobbelaar AO. The long-term results of ruby laser depilation in a consecutive series of 346 patients. Plast Reconstr Surg 2002; 110:254–260.

Chui CT, Berger TG, Price VH, Zachary CB. Recalcitrant scarring follicular disorders treated by laser-assisted hair removal: a preliminary report. Dermatol Surg 1999; 25:34–37.

Dierickx CC. Hair removal by lasers and intense pulsed light sources. Dermatol Clin 2002; 20:135–146.

Dierickx CC. Hair removal by lasers and intense pulsed light sources. In: Fitzpatrick RE, Goldman MP, eds. Cosmetic Laser Surgery. St Louis, MO: Mosby, 2000:176–197.

Dierickx CC. Hair removal by light: accomplishments and challenges. In: Arndt KA, Dover JS, eds. Controversies & Conversations in Cutaneous Laser Surgery. American Medical Association Press, 2002:329–331.

Dierickx CC, Campos VB, Lin D, Farinelli W, Anderson RR. Influence of hair growth cycle on efficacy of laser hair removal. Lasers Surg Med 1999; 24(suppl 11):21.

Dierickx CC, Grossman MC, Farinelli WA, Anderson RR. Permanent hair removal by normal-mode ruby laser. Arch Dermatol 1998; 134:837–842.

Dover JS (moderator). Discussion, Part 13. In: Arndt KA, Dover JS, eds. Controversies & Conversations in Cutaneous Laser Surgery. American Medical Association Press, 2002:341–346.

Galadari I. Comparative evaluation of different hair removal lasers in skin types IV, V, and VI. Int J Dermatol 2003; 42:68–70.

Garcia C, Alamoudi H, Nakib M, Zimmo S. Alexandrite laser hair removal is safe for Fitzpatick skin types IV–VI. Dermatol Surg 2000; 26:130–134.

Gold MH, Bell MW, Foster TD, Street S. One-year follow-up using an intense pulsed light source for long-term hair removal. J Cutan Laser Ther 1999; 1:167–171.

Goldberg DJ, Littler CM, Wheeland RG. Topical suspension-assisted Q-switched Nd:YAG laser hair removal. Dermatol Surg 1997; 23:741–745.

Grossman MC, Dierickx C, Farinelli W, Flotte T, Anderson RR. Damage to hair follicles by normal-mode ruby laser pulses. J Am Acad Dermatol 1996; 35:889–894.

Goldman L. Biomedical Aspects of the Laser. New York: Springer, 1967.

Grossman MC, Wimberly J, Dwyer P, et al. PDT for hirsutism. Lasers Surg Med Suppl 1995; 7:44..

Handrick C, Alster TS. Comparison of long-pulsed diode and long-pulsed alexandrite lasers for hair removal: a long-term clinical and histologic study. Dermatol Surg 2001; 27:622–626.

Hirsch RJ, Farinelli WA, Anderson RR. A closer look at dynamic cooling. Lasers Surg Med Suppl 2002; 14:36.

Jay H, Rand D, Delix M, Cabornero R, Asch S. Safety of intense pulsed light hair removal in 250 consecutive new patients. Cosmet Dermatol 2002; 15:15–19.

Kauvar AN. Treatment of pseudofolliculitis with a pulsed infra-red laser. Arch Dermatol 2000; 135:1343–1346.

Kelly AP. Pseudofolliculitis barbae and acne keloidalis nuchae. Dermatol Clin 2003; 21:645–653.

Kelly KM, Svaasand LO, Nelson JS. Further investigation of pigmentary changes after alexandrite laser hair removal in conjunction with cryogen spray cooling. Dermatol Surg 2004; 30:581–582.

Khatri KA. Diode laser hair removal in patients undergoing isotretinoin therapy. Dermatol Surg 2004; 30:1205–1207.

Landthaler M, Hohenleutner U. The Nd:YAG laser in cutaneous surgery. In: Arndt KA, Dover JS, Olbricht SM, eds. Lasers in Cutaneous and Aesthetic Surgery. Philadelphia: Lippincott-Raven, 1997:124–149.

Lanigan SW. Incidence of side effects after laser hair removal. J Am Acad Dermatol 2003; 49:882–886.

Lepselter J, Elman M. Biological and clinical aspects in laser hair removal. J Dermatol Treat 2004; 15:72–83.

Lui H, Bissonnette R. Photodynamic therapy. In: Goldman MP, Fitzpatrick RE, eds. Cutaneous Laser Surgery: The Art and Science of Selective Photothermolysis. St. Louis, MO: Mosby, 1999:437–458.

McDaniel DH, Lord J, Ash K, Newman J, Zukowski M. Laser hair removal: a review and report on the use of the long-pulsed alexandrite laser for hair reduction of the upper lip, leg, back, and bikini region. Dermatol Surg 1999; 25:425–430.

Messenger AG. The control of hair growth and pigmentation. In: Olsen EA, ed. Disorders of Hair Growth Diagnosis and Treatment. New York, McGraw-Hill Inc., 1994:39–58.

Mordon A, Sumian C, Devoisselle JM. Site-specific methylene blue delivery to pilosebaceous structures using highly porous nylon microspheres: an experimental evaluation. Lasers Surg Med 2003; 33:119–125.

Moretti M. Hair Removal Comparison Chart in Aesthetic Buyers Guide. Medical Insight, Inc. 2004; 7:68–70.

Nanni CA, Alster TS. Laser-assisted hair removal: side effects of Q-switched Nd:YAG, long-pulsed ruby, and alexandrite lasers. J Am Acad Dermatol 1999; 41:165–171.

Nanni CA, Alster TS. Long-pulsed alexandrite laser-assisted hair removal at 5, 10, and 20 millisecond pulse durations. Lasers Surg Med 1999; 24:332–337.

Nanni CA, Alster TS. Optimizing treatment parameters for hair removal using a topical carbon-based solution and 1064-nm Q-switched neodymium:YAG laser energy. Arch Dermatol 1997; 133:1546–1549.

Olsen EA. Methods of hair removal. J Am Acad Dermatol 1995; 40:143–155.

Polderman MC, Pavel S, Le Cressie S, et al. Efficacy, tolerability, and safety of a long-pulsed ruby laser system in the removal of unwanted hair. Dermatol Surg 2000; 26:240–243..

Radmanesh M. Temporary hair color change from black to blond after intense pulsed light hair removal therapy. Dermatol Surg 2004; 30:1521.

Rogachefsky AS, Silapunt S, Goldberg DJ. Evaluation of a super long pulsed 810-nm diode hair removal laser in suntanned individuals. J Cutan Laser Ther 2001; 3:57–62.

Radmanesh M, Mostaghimi M, Yousefi I, et al. Leukotrichia developed following application of intense pulsed light for hair removal. Dermatol Surg 2002; 26:572–574.

Rogachefsky AS, Silapunt S, Goldberg D. Evaluation of a new super-long-pulsed 810 nm diode laser for the removal of unwanted hair: the concept of thermal damage time. Dermatol Surg 2002; 28:410–414.

Ross EV, Ladin Z, Kreindel M, Dierickx C. Theoretical considerations in laser hair removal. Dermatol Clin 1999; 17:333–355.

Sadick NS, Laughlin SA. Effective epilation of white and blond hair using combined radiofrequency and optical energy. J Cosmet Laser Ther 2004; 6:27–31.

Sadick NS, Makino Y. Selective electro-thermolysis in aesthetic medicine: a review. Lasers Surg Med 2004; 34:91.

Sadick NS, Shaoul J. Hair removal using a combination of conducted radiofrequency and optical energies—an 18-month follow-up. J Cosmet Laser Ther 2004; 6:21–26.

Sadick NS, Shea CR, Burchette JL, Prieto VG. High intensity flashlamp photoepilation: a clinical, histological, and mechanistic study in human skin. Arch Dermatol 1999; 135:668–676.

Sadick NS, Weiss RA, Shea CR, Nagel H, Nicholson J, Prieto VG. Long-term photoepilation using a broad-spectrum intense pulsed light source. Arch Dermatol 2000; 136:1336–1340.

Schroeter CA, Groenewegen JS, Reineke T, Neumann HA. Hair reduction using intense pulsed light source. Dermatol Surg 2004; 30:168–173.

Szeimies RM, Abels C, Fritsch C et al. Wavelength dependency of photodynamic effects after sensitization with 5-aminolevulinic acid in vitro and in vivo. J Invest Dermatol 1995; 105:672–677.

Tanzi EL, Alster TS. Long-pulsed 1064-nm Nd:YAG laser-assisted hair removal in all skin types. Dermatol Surg 2004; 30:13–17.

Tope WD, Hordinsky MK. A hair's breadth closer?. Arch Dermatol 1998; 134:867–869.

Troilius A, Troilius C. Hair removal with a second generation broad spectrum intense pulsed light source—a long-term follow-up. J Cutan Laser Ther 1999; 1:173–178.

U.S. Food and Drug Administration, http://fda.gov/cdrh/databases.html, 2002.

Weiss RA, Weiss MA, Marwaha S, Harrington AC. Hair removal with a non-coherent filtered flashlamp intense pulsed light source. Lasers Surg Med 1999; 24:128–232.

Weisberg NK, Greenbaum SS. Pigmentary changes after alexandrite laser hair removal. Dermatol Surg 2003; 29:415–419.

Ye JN, Prasad A, Trivedi P, Knapp P, Chu P, Edelstein LM. Pili bigeminy induced by low fluence therapy with hair removal alexandrite and ruby lasers. Dermatol Surg 1999; 25:969.

68

Non-Ablative Facial Rejuvenation

Malcolm S. Ke

Department of Dermatology, University Hospitals of Cleveland, Case Western Reserve University, Orange Village, Ohio, U.S.A.

Mathew M. Avram and Gary P. Lask

Division of Dermatology, University of California, Los Angeles, California, U.S.A.

INTRODUCTION

There are multiple laser, light source, and non-light source-based treatments for photoaging. Photoaging is the characteristic appearance of aging skin after prolonged sun exposure including the appearance of telangiectasias, rhytides, coarse texture, yellow discoloration, and skin laxity. These technologies currently include ablative lasers, non-ablative lasers with epidermal cooling, light sources, light-emitting diodes, radiofrequency devices, and fractional photothermolysis (FP). While each of these technologies improves the appearance of photodamaged skin, their efficacies vary. Importantly, their side effects and patient "downtime" vary considerably as well.

In the past several years, there has been an explosion of interest in non-ablative laser rejuvenation. Non-ablative rejuvenation is the treatment of photoaged skin by thermally targeting dermal collagen in order to stimulate new collagen growth. The epidermis is spared by these treatments. Non-ablative rejuvenation has increased in popularity due to its minimal side effect profile. Additionally, non-ablative lasers do not require the significant, prolonged recovery time associated with other treatment modalities such as laser resurfacing.

There are multiple non-ablative lasers that operate across the visible, near-infrared, and mid-infrared regions of the electromagnetic spectrum. Each modality is designed to stimulate new collagen growth. It is important to note that non-ablative therapies provide subtle, often non-dramatic, improvements in photoaging. It is not a substitute for ablative or more invasive procedures. Currently, the physician and patient must weigh the benefits and risks of therapy carefully with the patient. This chapter will focus on non-ablative laser- and light-based therapies. In order to fully examine this rapidly growing field of treatment, it is first necessary to briefly describe the alternative means of treatment.

Ablative Lasers

For years, ablative laser therapies were the mainstay of treatment of photodamaged skin, providing a more efficient, effective and precise means of treatment than chemical peels, and traditional dermabrasion (for a more detailed treatment of ablative laser modalities, see chapter on "Ablative Laser"). First, the carbon dioxide (CO_2) laser, emitting light at 10,600 nm, was the dominant treatment modality. More recently, the erbium:yttrium-aluminum-garnet (Er:YAG)

lasers (both short- and long-pulsed) have increased in popularity. Emitting infrared light at 2940 nm, near the absorption peak of water, the absorption coefficient of the Er:YAG laser is 16 times that of the CO_2 laser. Both of these lasers effectively ablate epidermal and superficial dermal tissue at controlled, precise depths. Per pass, Er:YAG lasers penetrate less deeply into the dermis than CO_2 lasers thereby producing fewer side effects, at the price of decreased efficacy.

Both lasers produce tissue contraction from thermal denaturation of tissue proteins. This is thought to produce long-term collagen tightening by a process of wound healing and remodeling from adjacent healthy tissue and adnexal structures. Both the CO_2 and Er:YAG lasers are efficacious and have provided significant improvement for patients with photodamaged skin. Currently, no other technology can match their efficacy.

The benefits of ablative lasers, however, must be considered against their side effects. The incidence of adverse events with ablative resurfacing increases with the depth of skin penetration. Additionally, there is significant post-procedure downtime for the patient with ablative resurfacing rendering the patient unavailable for work or social activities. Temporary side effects include: post-procedure edema, oozing, petechiae, erythema, pruritus, contact dermatitis, and pain. More enduring side effects include: milia, permanent hypopigmentation, hyperpigmentation, scarring, and viral, bacterial, or fungal infections. The decision to choose ablative therapy versus non-ablative therapy should be based on a host of factors including: realistic patient expectations, skin type, specific elements of photoaging (wrinkles, telangiectasias, erythema, skin texture, pigmentation), and expected downtime.

Nonetheless, ablative lasers remain the treatments of choice for deeper wrinkles and severe photodamage. Ideal candidates for ablative resurfacing include patients with resting perioral and periocular facial rhytides.

Fractional Photothermolysis

Fractional photothermolysis is neither a purely ablative nor non-ablative technology. Rather, it produces a pattern of multiple columns of thermal damage, referred to as microthermal treatment zones (MTZs), on the skin. These microscopic MTZs can be visualized with magnification. FP can control the pattern density and depth of thermal damage. In this way, different three-dimensional MTZ shapes can be created. This thermal damage extends into the reticular dermis, while producing photocoagulation of the epidermis. Importantly, FP does not affect the tissue surrounding MTZs. Thus, the remaining viable cells support a rapid healing time, with re-epithelialization achieved in one day. With the extrusion and replacement of damaged tissue, a fractionalized resurfacing occurs. In essence, 12% to 18% of the skin is "resurfaced" at one treatment session. The procedure is repeated four to five times at 1- to 4-week intervals. Post-procedure side effects are typically mild and include erythema and edema. Because there is no dermal or epidermal ablation, there is none of the significant recovery time associated with ablative laser therapy.

FP has been studied in the treatment of periorbital rhytides. FP holds the potential to improve rhytides in a superior fashion to non-ablative technologies with more mild side effects than ablative technologies. Further study is awaited to truly assess the efficacy of this technology.

NON-ABLATIVE PHOTOREJUVENATION

While ablative laser remains the most effective means of photorejuvenation, non-ablative technologies have become far more popular among patients and physicians. Their popularity has increased despite the need for multiple treatments and reduced efficacy in treating wrinkles and skin tone. The preference for non-ablative treatments is most likely attributable to patient and physician preferences for treatments with minimal side effects and rapid recovery time. All non-ablative procedures can be performed during a short break from work. Additionally, non-ablative systems offer other benefits over ablative modalities including the selective treatment of telangiectasias, erythema, and superficial pigmentation. Non-ablative rejuvenation technologies include: non-ablative lasers, light sources, and radio-frequency devices.

There are limits to non-ablative treatments. They are most effective for patients with mild to moderate photodamage, skin laxity, and coarseness. As opposed to ablative lasers, epidermal growths such as actinic keratoses, seborrheic keratosis, and lentigines do not respond well to non-ablative therapy. It is important to note that studies assessing the benefits of non-ablative therapy are compromised by non-standardized and non-comparable methods of evaluation. Thus, the true extent of their efficacy remains controversial. Ablative lasers remain the treatment of choice for severe photodamage and deeper wrinkles.

Visible Light and Near-Infrared Lasers

Vascular lasers such as the 585- to 600-nm pulsed dye lasers, the 585- to 595-nm variable-pulsed dye lasers, the 532-nm potassium titanyl phosphate (KTP), and 1064-nm neodymium:yttrium-aluminum-garnet (Nd:YAG) have all been investigated for their efficacy in non-ablative dermal remodeling. It is theorized that selective absorption of laser light by oxyhemoglobin in the dermal vasculature produces thermal damage to vessel walls with subsequent activation of an inflammatory cascade and stimulation of new collagen formation and remodeling. The epidermis is unaffected during treatment since the targeted vascular plexi are located in the dermis. Epidermal cooling also aids in preventing epidermal thermal injury, even at relatively high fluences.

Single-pass, subpurpuric treatments have been shown to produce new collagen. Ideal patients include non-elderly individuals with vascular lesions, coarse skin, skin laxity, and mild rhytides. The 532-nm KTP laser may additionally treat mild dyschromia or lentigines. Adverse effects are typically mild and include purpura, dyspigmentation, erythema, and blistering. As with other forms of laser treatment, care must be taken in darker skin types to prevent hypopigmentation from overly aggressive cryogen cooling. Hyperpigmentation may also occur, especially in individuals with darker skin phototypes.

Other near-infrared lasers such as the 755-nm alexandrite and 810-nm diode have also been shown to be effective in non-ablative resurfacing. The 1064-nm Nd:YAG laser is primarily absorbed by dermal water and oxyhemoglobin. Patients with telangiectasias and mild rhytides may possibly benefit more from using this laser. Individuals with darker skin types will also have less risk of hyperpigmentation with the 1064-nm Nd:YAG laser. However, patients with deeper rhytides alone may choose a longer-wavelength infrared laser to possibly increase penetration and preferentially target deeper dermal tissue. One study noted a greater reduction in redness and pigmentation, and an improvement in rhytides and skin tone with a combination of 1064-nm long-pulsed Nd:YAG and 532-nm KTP lasers than with either modality alone.

Mid-Infrared Lasers

Non-ablative resurfacing systems involve infrared lasers with integrated epidermal cooling mechanisms. These lasers emit wavelengths targeting dermal tissue water, hence creating dermal thermal injury while preserving epidermal integrity. Advantages of these systems over vascular lasers include deeper dermal tissue penetration, greater absorption and dermal thermal injury, and a decreased risk of pigmentation alterations in darker-skinned individuals. These longer wavelengths transmit to the dermis and spare the epidermis as a result of contact cooling. Ideal candidates include those patients with mild to moderate resting rhytides. Acne scarring has also been responsive. The first lasers developed were the 1320-nm Nd:YAG and 1450-nm diode laser.

The 1320-nm Nd:YAG laser (CoolTouch; CoolTouch Inc., Roseville, California, U.S.A.) was first introduced in 1996 and features a thermal feedback device which measures epidermal temperature to allow greater precision in targeting dermal collagen. Based on these readings, the surgeon may change the parameters to attain optimal skin temperature in the 46°C to 48°C range. As with other systems in its class, the 1320-nm Nd:YAG laser also integrates epidermal cooling via a cryogen spray. Neocollagenesis is hypothesized to be induced via host inflammatory cytokines after dermal thermal injury to collagen and vessels (Fig. 1).

The 1450-nm diode laser (SmoothBeam; Candela Corp., Wayland, Massachusetts, U.S.A.) was FDA-approved in 2002 for the treatment of periorbital rhytides. Like the 1320-nm Nd:YAG laser, it targets dermal water. This unit also integrates epidermal cooling via a cryogen spray, but does not contain a thermal feedback device. Specifications include fluences from 8 to 25 J/cm^2, a 250-ms pulse duration, and a 4- to 6-mm spot size. In the treatment of rhytides, efficacy compared with similar laser systems remains to be determined. In the treatment of atrophic facial scars, one study suggested greater efficacy with the 1450-nm diode compared with the 1320-nm Nd:YAG laser.

Side effects of the mid-infrared lasers include temporary pain, swelling, and erythema. At higher fluences, scarring, pigmentary changes, and bulla formation are also

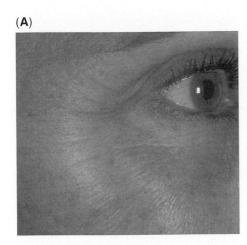

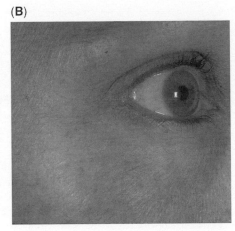

Figure 1 1320-nm Nd:YAG (CoolTouch® photographs) **(A)** baseline; **(B)** 4 weeks post last treatment.

possible. While 1450 nm is not selective for melanin, aggressive cryogen spray can produce temporary pigmentary changes in darker skin phototypes.

Intense Pulsed Light

Broadband intense pulsed-light (IPL) therapy involves polychromatic light delivered by a flashlamp in a continuous spectrum of electromagnetic radiation. This non-laser light emits yellow, red, and infrared light in the range of 500 to 1200 nm, effectively targeting oxyhemoglobin, melanin, and tissue water. Cutoff filters of shorter wavelengths are used in conjunction with IPL to variably narrow the emission range based on the desired target tissue. As part of multiple treatment modalities in photorejuvenation, or as a stand-alone option, IPL can "do a little of everything," partially addressing pigmentation, telangiectasias, erythema, and fine wrinkling (Figs. 2 and 3). Ideal patients display only mild signs of dermatoheliosis. Treatment of specific vascular lesions such as poikiloderma of Civatte can be achieved with cutoff filters focusing on ranges of 550 to 645 nm. Conversely, longer wavelengths are used for dermal remodeling. Advantages over lasers include a wide range of targets to address various elements of photoaging and a larger spot size to efficiently treat large facial and non-facial areas. The flashlamp is housed in the treatment head, thus affording a large spot size. As with other non-ablative systems, postoperative recovery and other inherent risks are minimal. Disadvantages include less dramatic effects on skin toning and usually the necessity of multiple treatments to achieve noticeable results. Adverse effects occur infrequently, but include dyspigmentation, purpura, blistering, and scarring. Transient erythema is common and resolves over several hours. Easy recovery results in high patient satisfaction.

Electrosurgery/Radiofrequency

Introduced in 2002, radiofrequency technology was introduced as a means to "tighten" skin. Based on Ohm's law, where current is proportional to voltage and inversely proportional to resistance, radiofrequency energy is delivered to the target tissue where resistance causes a reduction in current. This loss of energy across tissue resistance is released as heat, thus effectively causing thermal injury. Energy output can be calculated as follows: Energy (Joules) $= I^2$ (Amperes) $\times Z$ (impedance) $\times$ time (seconds).

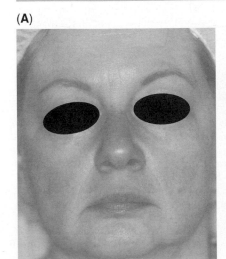

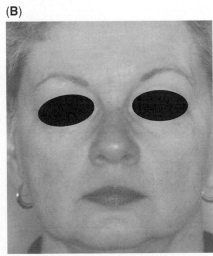

Figure 2 Intense pulsed-light photographs **(A)** baseline; **(B)** 4 weeks post last treatment.

(A)   **(B)**

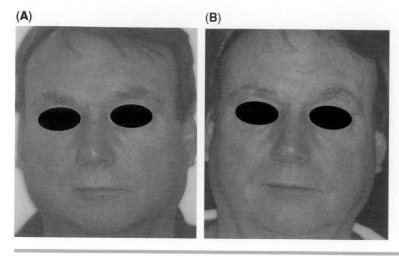

Figure 3 Intense pulsed-light photographs **(A)** baseline; **(B)** 4 weeks post last treatment.

As opposed to the selective targeting and heating of chromophores with lasers, it is believed heat generated from radiofrequency is based on tissue impedance. In theory, this effectively produces heat to shrink collagen and induce neocollagenesis.

There are two systems on the market today: monopolar and bipolar. Like non-ablative laser systems, these radiofrequency systems also contain cryogen-cooled tips to minimize epidermal injury. A monopolar unit (Thermage, Inc., Hayward, California, U.S.A.) uses a capacitive membrane to distribute a 6-MHz alternating-current radiofrequency signal over tissue beneath the membrane surface. This creates a "zone" of effect where impedance converts this current into thermal energy. Up to $220 \, \text{J/cm}^2$ can be delivered with depths of at least 2.5 mm. In addition to initial collagen contraction due to thermal injury, further remodeling and neocollagenesis occurs to further "tighten" dermal tissue over up to six months postoperatively. Bipolar units function by delivering radiofrequency current between two electrodes, thus creating a more selective "zone" of thermal injury. The Polaris system (Syneron Medical Ltd., Yokneam, Israel) delivers energy up to $100 \, \text{J/cm}^2$ and is coupled with a 900-nm diode laser to address the vascular component of photoaging along with a potentially synergistic effect of non-ablative laser therapy and radiofrequency. This unit also contains a 5°C applicator tip for epidermal protection.

Ideal patients are those seeking greater tissue tightening effects than with non-ablative laser systems and want to avoid the complications and recovery associated with ablative laser therapy. The major advantage of radiofrequency devices over non-ablative laser systems is the deeper depth of tissue penetration, creating uniform bulk heating to potentially result in greater "tightening" effects. With depths of at least 2.5 mm, dermal and fascial thermal injury may occur contributing to this effect. The advantage over ablative systems is obvious: favorable dermal effects with minimal downtime since the epidermis is preserved. Best results are seen with patients who desire mild to moderate skin laxity improvement. Patients expecting major, significant improvements are likely to be disappointed. Some patients will experience no improvement. The major complaint is operative pain, usually requiring pre-procedure topical anesthetic creams, nerve blocks, systemic anxiolytics, or opiates. While some have commented that pain thresholds may represent appropriate treatment parameters, common sense dictates that this may vary substantially from patient to patient and thus is an unreliable indicator of appropriate treatment fluences. Common adverse effects include immediate postoperative erythema, edema, and dyspigmentation. Patients may also experience prolonged erythema, edema, paresthesias, scarring, fat atrophy, or first- or second-degree burns, but these major side effects are much less common. These side effects are more common at higher fluences and with multiple-pass treatments.

BIBLIOGRAPHY

Alam M, Dover JS. Nonablative laser and light therapy: an approach to patient and device selection. Skin Therapy Lett 2003; 8:4–7.

Alam M, Hsu TS, Dover JS, Wrone DA, Arndt KA. Nonablative laser and light treatments: histology and tissue effects—a review. Lasers Surg Med 2003; 33:30–39.

Alora MB, Arndt KA. Treatment of a cafe-au-lait macule with the erbium:YAG laser. J Am Acad Dermatol 2001; 45:566–568.

Alster TS. Manual of Cutaneous Laser Techniques. Philadelphia: Lippincott Williams & Wilkins, 2000:259.

Bernstein LJ, Kauvar AN, Grossman MC, Geronemus RG. The short- and long-term side effects of carbon dioxide laser resurfacing. Dermatol Surg 1997; 23: 519–525.

Bitter PH. Noninvasive rejuvenation of photodamaged skin using serial, full-face intense pulsed light treatments. Dermatol Surg 2000; 26:835–842; discussion 843.

Dover JS, Hruza GJ, Arndt KA. Lasers in skin resurfacing. Semin Cutan Med Surg 2000; 19:207–220.

Fisher GH, Geronemus RG. Short-term side effects of fractional photothermolysis. Dermatol Surg 2005; 31:1245–1249.

Fitzpatrick R, Geronemus R, Goldberg D, Kaminer M, Kilmer S, Ruiz-Esparza J. Multicenter study of noninvasive radiofrequency for periorbital tissue tightening. Lasers Surg Med 2003; 33:232–242.

Goldberg D, Tan M, Dale Sarradet M, Gordon M. Nonablative dermal remodeling with a 585-nm, 350-microsec, flashlamp pulsed dye laser: clinical and ultrastructural analysis. Dermatol Surg 2003; 29:161–163; discussion 163–164.

Goldberg DJ, Cutler KB. Nonablative treatment of rhytids with intense pulsed light. Lasers Surg Med 2000; 26:196–200.

Goldberg DJ. Full-face nonablative dermal remodeling with a 1320 nm Nd:YAG laser. Dermatol Surg 2000; 26:915–918.

Goldberg DJ, Sarradet D, Hussain M, Krishtul A, Phelps R. Clinical, histologic, and ultrastructural changes after nonablative treatment with a 595-nm flashlamp-pumped pulsed dye laser: comparison of varying settings. Dermatol Surg 2004; 30:979–982.

Goldberg DJ, Silapunt S. Histologic evaluation of a Q-switched Nd:YAG laser in the nonablative treatment of wrinkles. Dermatol Surg 2001; 27:744–746.

Goldberg DJ. Nonablative resurfacing. Clin Plast Surg 2000; 27:287–292, xi.

Grekin RC, Tope WD, Yarborough JM Jr., et al. Electrosurgical facial resurfacing: a prospective multicenter study of efficacy and safety. Arch Dermatol 2000; 136:1309–1316.

Hale GMQM. Optical constants of water in the 200-nm to 200-m wavelength region. Appl Opt 1973; 12:555–563.

Hohenleutner S, Koellner K, Lorenz S, Landthaler M, Hohenleutner U. Results of nonablative wrinkle reduction with a 1450-nm diode laser: difficulties in the assessment of "subtle changes". Lasers Surg Med 2005; 37:14–18.

Hsu TS, Zelickson B, Dover JS, et al. Multicenter study of the safety and efficacy of a 585 nm pulsed-dye laser for the nonablative treatment of facial rhytides. Dermatol Surg 2005; 31:1–9.

Jacob CI, Dover JS. Birt-Hogg-Dube syndrome: treatment of cutaneous manifestations with laser skin resurfacing. Arch Dermatol 2001; 137:98–99.

Kelly KM, Nelson JS, Lask GP, Geronemus RG, Bernstein LJ. Cryogen spray cooling in combination with nonablative laser treatment of facial rhytides. Arch Dermatol 1999; 135:691–694.

Khatri KA, Ross V, Grevelink JM, Magro CM, Anderson RR. Comparison of erbium:YAG and carbon dioxide lasers in resurfacing of facial rhytides. Arch Dermatol 1999; 135:391–397.

Lask G, Keller G, Lowe N, Gormley D. Laser skin resurfacing with the SilkTouch flashscanner for facial rhytides. Dermatol Surg 1995; 21:1021–1024.

Lee MW. Combination visible and infrared lasers for skin rejuvenation. Semin Cutan Med Surg 2002; 21:288–300.

Leffell DJ. Clinical efficacy of devices for nonablative photorejuvenation. Arch Dermatol 2002; 138:1503–1508.

Lowe NJ, Lask G, Griffin ME, Maxwell A, Lowe P, Quilada F. Skin resurfacing with the ultrapulse carbon dioxide laser.

Observations on 100 patients. Dermatol Surg 1995; 21:1025–1029.

Manstein D, Herron GS, Sink RK, Tanner H, Anderson RR. Fractional photothermolysis: a new concept for cutaneous remodeling using microscopic patterns of thermal injury. Lasers Surg Med 2004; 34:426–438.

Nanni CA, Alster TS. Complications of cutaneous laser surgery. A review. Dermatol Surg 1998; 24:209–219.

Nanni CA, Alster TS. Complications of carbon dioxide laser resurfacing. An evaluation of 500 patients. Dermatol Surg 1998; 24:315–320.

Sadick NS, Weiss R, Kilmer S, Bitter P. Photorejuvenation with intense pulsed light: results of a multi-center study. J Drugs Dermatol 2004; 3:41–49.

Sadick NS, Weiss R. Intense pulsed-light photorejuvenation. Semin Cutan Med Surg 2002; 21:280–287.

Schmults CD, Phelps R, Goldberg DJ. Nonablative facial remodeling: erythema reduction and histologic evidence of new collagen formation using a 300-microsecond 1064-nm Nd:YAG laser. Arch Dermatol 2004; 140:1373–1376.

Sriprachya-Anunt S, Fitzpatrick RE, Goldman MP, Smith SR. Infections complicating pulsed carbon dioxide laser resurfacing for photoaged facial skin. Dermatol Surg 1997; 23:527–535; discussion 535–536.

Tanghetti E, Sherr E. Treatment of telangiectasia using the multipass technique with the extended pulse width, pulsed dye laser (Cynosure V-Star). J Cosmet Laser Ther 2003; 5:71–75.

Tanghetti EA, Sherr EA, Alvarado SL. Multipass treatment of photodamage using the pulse dye laser. Dermatol Surg 2003; 29:686–690; discussion 690–691.

Tanzi EL, Williams CM, Alster TS. Treatment of facial rhytides with a nonablative 1450-nm diode laser: a controlled clinical and histologic study. Dermatol Surg 2003; 29:124–128.

Tanzi EL, Alster TS. Comparison of a 1450-nm diode laser and a 1320-nm Nd:YAG laser in the treatment of atrophic facial scars: a prospective clinical and histologic study. Dermatol Surg 2004; 30:152–157.

Yaghmai D, Garden JM, Bakus AD, Massa MC. Comparison of a 1064 nm laser and a 1320 nm laser for the nonablative treatment of acne scars. Dermatol Surg 2005; 31:903–909.

69

Soft Tissue Augmentation and Fillers

J. Barton Sterling
Spring Lake, New Jersey, U.S.A.

C. William Hanke
Laser and Skin Surgery Center of Indiana, Carmel, Indiana, U.S.A.

INTRODUCTION

Many soft tissue fillers have come and gone in the past decade. The market for fillers is growing. Filler manufactures attempt to show that their filler is safer and longer lasting than their competitor's. Yet no one filler is currently ideal to all practitioners or to all patients.

Most agree that the ideal filler would be long lasting or permanent, inexpensive, has few adverse effects, and consistently produce the desired esthetic effect. Further, to ensure purity and limit the practitioner's medicolegal liability, the product would be approved by the U.S. Food and Drug Administration (FDA).

Fillers have numerous indications. They may be used to correct volume naturally lost as the patient ages. They may be used to enhance the lips, cheek hollows, cheek bones, and chin. They may be used to correct rhytides and blunt facial folds, such as the nasolabial fold. They also may be used to correct depressed scars, such as acne scars.

This chapter will focus on the most commonly used fillers available in the United States: collagen and hyaluronic acid. Poly-L-lactic acid (PLA), calcium hydroxylapatite, and polymethylmethacrylate will also be discussed. Liquid silicone and autologous fat transplantation will not be discussed in this chapter as they are described in subsequent chapters.

COLLAGEN

The most commonly used collagen fillers are CosmoDerm and CosmoPlast (Inamed Aesthetics, Santa Barbara, California, U.S.A.). Both became available in the United States in 2003. These products contain purified collagen derived from cell cultures of human fibrocytes. Cell lines are obtained from the foreskin of newborns. These human collagen products do not require antigen testing and, for this reason, have largely replaced the bovine collagen fillers Zyderm and Zyplast, which require two antigen skin tests and are also manufactured by Inamed Aesthetics.

CosmoDerm is less viscous than CosmoPlast. It is designed to be injected in the upper dermis. A white blanch on the skin surface indicates correct placement (Fig. 1). CosmoDerm works well on superficial rhytides such as crow's feet and upper lip lines. It can be used in the glabella, corners of the mouth, and in undulating acne scars.

CosmoPlast is a more viscous agent and is designed to be injected in the mid dermis. CosmoPlast works best on deep rhytides, folds, and depressions. CosmoPlast is also used to enhance the mucocutaneous junction of the upper lip. A white blanch should not be observed with CosmoPlast, rather a subtle elevation should be seen (Fig. 2). For etched-in lines over deep folds, such as those which typically occur over the nasolabial fold, CosmoDerm can be layered over CosmoPlast.

Both CosmoDerm and CosmoPlast are pre-packaged in 1 cc syringes, containing lidocaine, and are injected through a 30-gauge needle. The fillers must be refrigerated. Correction lasts 2 to 6 months depending on the area injected. In general, correction lasts longer in non-mobile areas such as acne scars and glabellar lines.

Adverse reactions to CosmoDerm and CosmoPlast include bruising, hematoma, reactivation of herpes simplex, and the rare possibility of vascular occlusion. Similar adverse reactions may be seen with Zyderm and Zyplast, which are both more likely to also cause an allergic reaction (Figs. 3–5).

HYALURONIC ACID

Hyaluronic acid is a naturally occurring polysaccharide identical in all animal species and found in all animal tissues. Hyaluronic acid strongly binds water, creating volume. Restylane (Medicis, Scottsdale, Arizona, U.S.A.) and Hylaform (Inamed Aesthetics) are the two FDA-approved hyaluronic acid fillers available in the United States. Captique (Inamed) is another recently available FDA-approved hyaluronic acid. Restylane Fine Lines and Perlane (both Medicis) are hyaluronic acid fillers not yet FDA-approved.

The most widely used hyaluronic acid filler, Restylane, is derived from bacterial fermentation. Restylane is uniquely cross-linked to improve long-term stability and reportedly lasts longer than collagen. Restylane is used to correct deep folds or add volume to the lips (Figs. 6–8). Restylane Touch Fine Lines is less viscous and intended for injection higher in the dermis to fill fine lines similar to the way CosmoDerm is used. Perlane is a more viscous and is intended for injection in the deep dermis to fill large depressions.

Hylaform, unlike Restylane, is derived from rooster combs. Hylaform is less expensive than Restylane and reportedly lasts about as long as collagen. Like CosmoPlast and Restylane, Hylaform is placed in the mid dermis and is used to correct folds or add volume to the lips. Injection is performed using a 30-gauge needle. Similar to Restylane, Hylaform is available in different viscosities. Hylaform Fine Lines is less viscous than Hylaform and is designed for injection in the upper dermis with a 32-gauge needle.

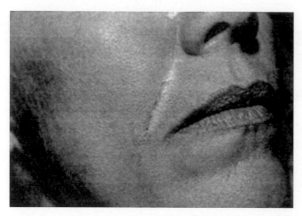

Figure 1 A white blanche indicates that CosmoDerm has been properly placed in the papillary dermis.

(A)   **(B)**

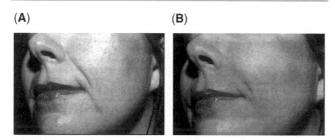

Figure 2 **(A)** A 35-year-old woman has deep nasolabial folds. **(B)** The skin is elevated immediately following CosmoPlast injection. The absence of a white blanche indicates that the implant has been properly placed in the mid dermis.

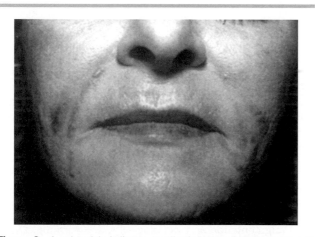

Figure 3 A red nodule indicates an allergic hypersensitivity reaction to bovine collagen.

Hylaform Plus is more viscous and is designed for deep dermal placement using a 27-gauge needle.

Adverse effects of hyaluronic acid injection include significant bruising, swelling of injection sites, and vascular occlusion. Less bruising occurs if patients avoid blood thinners prior to injection. No allergy testing is necessary. Restylane contains trace amounts of gram-positive bacterial proteins and should not be used on patients with known allergies to such substances. Hylaform should not be used in patients allergic to avian products. The hyaluronic acid fillers do not contain lidocaine, so areas to be injected must

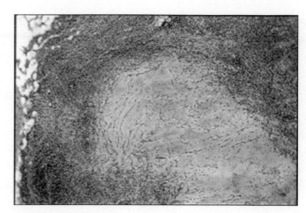

Figure 4 A biopsy from an allergic hypersensitivity reaction reveals granulomatous inflammation.

first be anesthetized. Injection into the lips can be performed with the aid of nerve blocks (Figs. 9 and 10).

POLY-L-LACTIC ACID

Poly-L-lactic acid is a filler recently approved by the FDA for the correction of facial lipoatrophy in patients infected with the human immunodeficiency virus (HIV). Currently, PLA is sold in the United States under the brand name Sculptra (Dermik Laboratories, Berwyn, Pennsylvania, U.S.A.). PLA is the only product approved by the FDA specifically for HIV lipoatrophy. Other alternatives for the treatment of HIV lipoatrophy include liquid silicone and autologous fat transfer. The market for PLA will likely be larger than the HIV-infected population, as physicians use PLA off-label to correct lipoatrophy associated with the normal aging process in non-HIV-infected patients. Correction with PLA is not permanent.

HIV facial lipoatrophy is characterized by sunken cheeks, bitemporal wasting, and deep nasolabial folds. Patients develop a hollow appearing face. This facial appearance is easily recognizable and serves as a social stigma for HIV patients causing psychological stress. HIV facial lipoatrophy commonly occurs in HIV-infected patients who are treated with a combination of antiretroviral medications, especially protease inhibitors and nucleoside

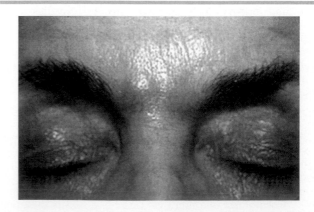

Figure 5 A 45-year-old woman developed a cystic abscess type of allergic hypersensitivity reaction to bovine collagen.

(A) (B)

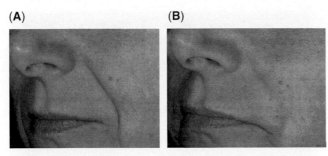

Figure 6 **(A)** A 50-year-old woman has deep nasolabial folds. **(B)** The nasolabial folds have been corrected with Restylane injections.

(A) (B)

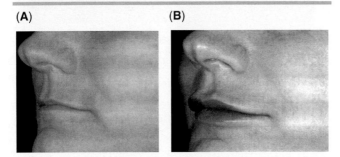

Figure 7 **(A)** A 35-year-old woman has very thin lips. **(B)** The lip volume has been improved following CosmoPlast injections to the vermillion-cutaneous junction and Restylane to the body of the lips.

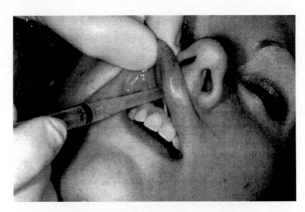

Figure 9 The upper lip can be anesthetized by placing 1 cc lidocaine with epinephrine 1:100,000 in the space between the second and third teeth.

reverse transcriptase inhibitors. Many patients with HIV facial lipoatrophy are eager to correct their appearance.

Poly-L-lactic acid is a synthetic polymer of the α-hydroxy-acid family. PLA in Sculptra is suspended in sodium carboxymethylcellulose and mannitol. PLA presumably creates a tissue response characterized by a foreign body reaction and production of new collagen over the course of weeks to months. PLA is eventually metabolized to lactic acid monomers which are then metabolized to carbon dioxide or incorporated into glucose.

Sculptra is supplied as a freeze-dried product that must be reconstituted with sterile water 2 to 24 hours before injection.

Poly-L-lactic acid is not used to fill individual rhytides but rather to add volume to an entire area, usually the cheeks. One vial of Sculptra is typically necessary for each cheek on every treatment visit. After local anesthesia is injected into the area, the suspension is injected using a one and one-half-inch 26-gauge needle. Needles have a tendency to clog, so multiple 26-gauge needles must be available. Approximately eight puncture sites are needed

for each cheek. Through each puncture site, the suspension is injected in an even fan-like motion, making multiple tunnels in the subcutaneous plane just below the dermis (Figs. 11 and 12).

After finishing the injection, the patient's cheeks are then massaged for 5 minutes to ensure even dispersal of the product. No dressing is needed. To avoid bruising, the patient is instructed to apply ice packs to the treated areas every few hours while awake over the next 24 hours.

Immediately after injection, the patient's cheeks appear fuller, a result of the mechanical effect of the large volume of anesthesia and fluid injected into the skin. Over the next 48 hours, the correction disappears and the patient's appearance returns to baseline. The manufacturer's studies show that the skin will gradually thicken (Fig. 13).

Patients frequently need multiple treatments to achieve the desired correction, making the treatment expensive. Treatments can be spaced up to a minimum of 2 weeks apart. Benefits may last 2 years or more.

The same injection technique can be used to treat facial lipoatrophy associated with the normal aging process in patients not infected with HIV (Fig. 14).

CALCIUM HYDROXYLAPATITE

Radiance (Bioform, Inc., Franksville, WT, U.S.A.) consists of calcium hydroxylapatite microspheres suspended in a polysaccharide gel. Radiance is approved by the FDA for vocal cord augmentation and radiological tissue marking. Use is considered off-label for acne scars, lip augmentation, nasolabial fold and marionette line enhancement, and in HIV facial lipoatrophy.

(A) (B)

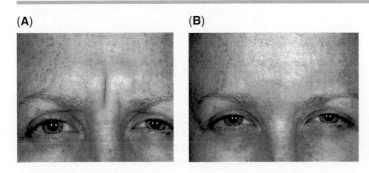

Figure 8 **(A)** A 37-year-old woman has deep glabellar frown lines. **(B)** The frown lines have resolved following Botox and Restylane injections.

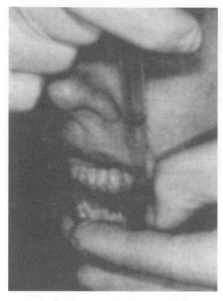

Figure 10   The lower lip can be anesthetized by placing 1 cc lidocaine with epinephrine 1:100,000 between the third and fourth teeth.

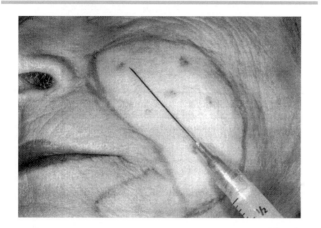

Figure 11   Anesthesia for polylactic acid injections involves placing 1 cc 1% lidocaine with epinephrine 1:100,000 intradermally and subcutaneously into six to seven spots on each cheek.

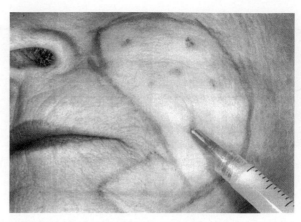

Figure 12   The polylactic acid is mixed using 3 cc sterile water and 2 cc plain 1% lidocaine. The polylactic acid is layered evenly in the upper subcutaneous fat using a 25-gauge 1½-inch needle.

Radiance is injected into the subdermal plane with a 23- to 26-gauge needle using a linear threading technique. The treatment site is molded with the fingers following injection. Results are reported to last 3 to 5 years. Local anesthesia or nerve blocks must be administered prior to injection.

Major drawbacks of calcium hydroxylapatite are reports of calcium deposits, granulomas, and firm nodules. Other adverse reactions include swelling, bruising, and lumpiness. Allergy testing is not required.

POLYMETHYLMETHACRYLATE

Artecoll (Rofil Medical International B.V., Breda, The Netherlands) consists of polymethylmethacrylate microspheres suspended in bovine collagen. This semi-permanent filler is not approved by the FDA for any indication. It was approved in Europe in 1996 and has been used on over 200,000 patients worldwide.

Artecoll is used for the correction of deep folds. Multiple treatments are necessary to achieve the desired correction. Artecoll contains 0.3% lidocaine, but supplemental anesthesia is necessary. After injection of local anesthesia or nerve blocks, Artecoll is injected with a 26-gauge needle

(A)   **(B)**

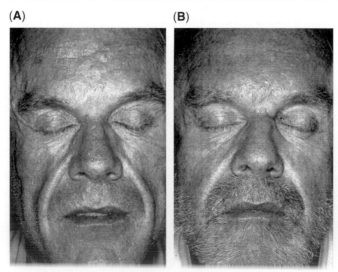

Figure 13   (A) HIV-positive patient has subcutaneous atrophy of the malar areas. (B) Three polylactic acid treatments (one vial per cheek) at 4- to 6-week intervals have added volume to the malar areas.

(A) (B)

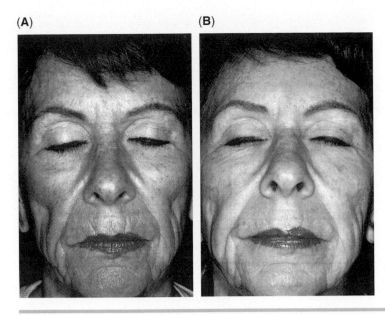

Figure 14 **(A)** A 67-year-old woman (non-HIV) has subcutaneous atrophy on both cheeks. **(B)** The areas of subcutaneous atrophy have been improved following two polylactic acid treatments (one vial per cheek).

with a threading technique. The filler is molded with the fingers following injection. Results can last 2 years or more.

In addition to bruising, adverse reactions include lumpiness and granulomas, which may occur after many years. Skin testing is necessary to screen for bovine collagen hypersensitivity.

BIBLIOGRAPHY

Gogolewski S, Jovanovic M, Perren SM, Dillon JG, Hughes MK. Tissue response and in vivo degradation of selected polyhydroxyacids: polyactides (PLA), poly (3-hydroxybutyrate) (PHB), and poly (3-hydroxybutyrate-co-3-hydroxyvalerate) (PHB/VA). J Biomed Mater Res 1993; 27: 1135–1148.

Hanke CW, Higley HR, Jolivette DM, et al. Abscess formation and local necrosis after treatment with Zyderm and Zyplast collagen implants. J Am Acad Dermatol 1991; 25:319–326.

Jones DH, Carruthers A, Orentreich D, et al. Highly purified 1000-cSt Silicone oil for treatment of human immunodeficiency virus-associated facial lipoatrophy: an open pilot trial. Dermatol Surg 2004; 30:1279–1286.

Lemperle G, Hazan-Gauthier N, Lemperle M. PMMA microspheres (Artecoll) for skin and soft tissue augmentation, part II: clinical investigations. Plast Reconstr Surg 1995; 96:627–634.

Lowe NJ, Maxwell CA, Lowe P, et al. Hyaluronic acid skin fillers: adverse reactions and skin testing. J Am Acad Dermatol 2001; 45:930–933.

Moyle GJ, Lysakova L, Brown, et al. A randomized open-label study of immediate versus delayed polylactic acid injections for the cosmetic management of facial lipoatrophy in persons with HIV infection. HIV Med 2004; 5:82–87.

Narins RS, Brandt F, Leyden J, et al. A randomized, double-blind, multicenter comparison of the efficacy and tolerability of Restylane versus Zyplast for the correction of nasolabial folds. Dermatol Surg 2003; 29:588–595.

Piacquadio D, Jarcho, Goltz R. Hylon B gel (Hylaform) as a soft-tissue augmentation material. J Am Acad Dermatol 1997; 36:545–549.

Reisberger EM, Landthaler M, Wiest L, et al. Foreign body granulomas caused by polymethylmethacrylate microspheres, successful treatment with allopurinol. Arch Dermatol 2003; 139:17–20.

Robinson JK, Hanke CW. Injectable collagen implants: histopathologic identification and longevity of correction. J Dermatol Surg Oncol 1985; 11:124.

Sklar JA, White SM. Radiance FN: a new soft tissue filler. Dermatol Surg 2004; 30:764–768.

Tzikas TL. Evaluation of the Radiance FN soft tissue filler for facial soft tissue augmentation. Arch Facial Plast Surg 2004; 6:234–239.

Valantin M, Aubron-Olivier C, Ghosn J, et al. Polylactic acid implants (New-Fill) to correct facial lipoatrophy in HIV-infected patients: results of the open-label study VEGA. AIDS 2003; 17:2471–2477.

Woerle B, Hanke CW, Sattler G. Poly-L-lactic acid: a temporary filler for soft tissue augmentation. J Drugs Dermatol 2004; 3(4):385–389.

70

Injectable Skin Fillers

Rhoda S. Narins
Dermatology Surgery and Laser Center of New York, White Plains, New York and Department of Dermatology, New York University Medical Center, New York, New York, U.S.A.

Joel L. Cohen
AboutSkin Dermatology and DermSurgery and Department of Dermatology, University of Colorado, Boulder, Colorado, U.S.A.

Kenneth Beer
Palm Beach Esthetic Center, West Palm Beach, Florida and Department of Dermatology, University of Miami, Miami, Florida, U.S.A.

INTRODUCTION

The search for the ideal cutaneous filler has spanned over a century. Presently, interest in soft-tissue augmentation is growing exponentially. As the baby boomer generation enters the market for cosmetic procedures, it is estimated that the number of soft-tissue augmentation procedures performed will rise geometrically. In today's society, cosmetic procedures are more accepted, openly discussed, and are the focus of several prime-time television shows. Within cosmetic dermatology and plastic surgery, the focus of significant time, attention and money is on volume restoration and correction of wrinkles, folds, and scars. There are now more filler options with increased safety profiles than ever before.

Recent advances have expanded our soft-tissue augmentation choices. Several new fillers have recently been approved by the U.S. Food and Drug Administration (FDA) and many more are in the short-term pipeline. These materials amplify our options of treatment modalities for the aging face.

During the normal aging process, there is a loss of connective and subcutaneous tissue, most notably in the face, neck, and hands. Over time, cumulative changes from both dynamic forces and photodamage lead to fine lines, wrinkling, loss of elasticity, and thinning of the dermis. There is a loss and repositioning of fat with hollowing of the cheeks. These changes are responsible for increased visibility of several bony landmarks. Aging also results in atrophy of the lips, descent of the corners of the mouth, and an overall diminished support of the lower third of the face. One of the most prominent stigmata of the aging face is mid-face descent. This descent, combined with the loss of tissue volume, results in prominent nasolabial and melolabial creases. Subcutaneous tissue augmentation with injectable fillers can fill lines, replace lost volume, and re-position structures that have begun to sag. Thus, these materials may be used for a rejuvenating effect to soften the appearance of aging, provide a fuller more youthful face, and recontour lines that form over time.

Fillers frequently work synergistically with surgical procedures (facelifts, laser resurfacing, etc.) to enhance the results of these modalities. Patients who do not want to undergo a surgical or ablative procedure can often obtain excellent results using fillers in conjunction with other low-risk techniques (non-ablative lasers, peels, thread lifts, botulinum toxin, etc.). While the botulinum toxins are unmatched in their ability to rejuvenate the upper third of the face, the lower third of the face is most directly impacted by fillers. The lower third of the face disproportionately bears the brunt of gravitational forces and loss of volume. Fillers can be used to reverse these changes. In addition to rejuvenation, fillers have a significant role in repairing defects such as scars. Scars from acne, surgery, or trauma result predominantly from loss or contraction of tissue. Each of these types of scars can also be greatly improved with fillers.

Each type of filler has different strengths and weaknesses (Table 1). Physicians familiar with multiple fillers have the greatest ability to maximize their patients' benefit with these products—so it behooves the cosmetic dermatologist to know and understand the various properties of the fillers at his or her disposal.

IDEAL FILLER CRITERIA

The ideal filler would be affordable and would provide predictable results for filling lines and scars and restoring volume. Depending on the circumstance, it should persist for months or years without significant degradation. It would be technically easy to use and able to pass through a small gauge needle and injected into the skin with minimal discomfort. This filler would fill superficial lines as well as deep folds and furrows. It would be biocompatible and non-allergenic, allowing injection at the patient's initial visit without the need for a skin test. The ideal filler would have a safety profile that would include being: non-inflammatory, non-toxic, non-carcinogenic, non-teratogenic, stable post-injection, and non-migratory. It would be packaged ready-to-use and shipped and stored at room temperature with a long shelf life. It would be free of transmissible diseases and have minimal post-procedure downtime and morbidity such as swelling, redness, or bruising.

Table 1 Comparison of Filler Characteristics

Filler	Material (source)	Duration in tissue	Primary use	Advantages	Disadvantages
Artecoll®	Collagen (bovine), PMMA (synthetic)	Permanent	Folds, lips	Long-lasting	(permanence a problem?)
Captique®	Hyaluronic acid (bacterial)	3–6 mo	Lips, nasolabial folds, wrinkles	No allergy/skin test	
Cosmoderm®	Collagen (human)	3–5 mo	Wrinkles, fine lines	Not painful	Skin tests required
Cosmoplast	Collagen (human)	3–5 mo	Deep folds/wrinkles, lips	Not painful	Skin tests required
Cymetra®	Micronized dermis	5–7 mo?	Lips, scars, folds	No allergy/skin test (human cadaver)	Short-lasting
Fascian®	Fascia lata	3–6 mo?	Lips, deep defects	No allergy/skin test (human cadaver)	Results not reproducible?
Fat	Fat (autologous)	?	Deep defects	No allergy/skin test	Separate procedure required to harvest fat
Gore-Tex®	ePTFE (synthetic)	Permanent	Deep furrows, lips	Long-lasting, low tissue reactivity	Difficult to remove
Hylaform	Hyaluronic acid (rooster comb)	3–6 mo	Lips, nasolabial folds, wrinkles	No allergy/skin test, less swelling than Restylane	Slightly more pain/ erythema, less longevity than Restylane
Juvederm®	Hyaluronic acid (bacterial)	?	Lips/nasolabial folds/wrinkles	? Longer lasting than other hyaluronic acids	
Sculptra New Fill®	Polylactic acid (synthetic)	Up to 18–24 mo	Lipoatrophy, lifting and filling scars,	No allergy/skin test	Painful upon injection
Radiesse®	Calcium hydroxyapatite	2–5 yr	Deep folds, lips	No allergy/skin test	Painful upon injection
Restylane®	Hyaluronic acid (bacteria)	6–12 mo	Lips, nasolabial folds, medium wrinkles	No skin test required	Painful upon injection
Silicone	Silicone oil (synthetic)	Permanent	Wrinkles, scars	No skin test, inexpensive	Several sessions often required
Zyderm®	Collagen (bovine)	3–5 mo	Wrinkles, fine lines	Not painful	Skin tests required
Zyplast®	Collagen (bovine)	3–5 mo	Deep folds/wrinkles, lips	Not painful	Skin tests required, avoid glabella

Abbreviations: PMMA, polymethylmethacrylate (plexiglas); ePTFE, expanded polytetrafluoroethylene.

To obtain optimal results using fillers for soft-tissue augmentation, the practitioner must be knowledgeable about several important variables including pre-procedure instructions, choice of filler material, proper placement into the desired location, amount of implant deposited, post-procedure instructions, and timing of repeat injections.

Pre-Procedure Instructions

Clarity when conveying pre-procedure instructions to patients is vital to success. Giving patients a brochure or written information sheet pre-treatment is very helpful. Patients should be forewarned that some degree of swelling, bruising or redness of the treated areas may occur and that it may last for several days. This admonition should not only be discussed verbally but should be included in the written consent obtained prior to the procedure. Depending on the amount and type of filler used, it may be prudent to avoid soft-tissue augmentation for approximately 10 to 14 days prior to a significant business or social event (and such as a wedding). Patients should be advised to avoid aspirin, non-steroidal anti-inflammatory drugs (NSAIDs), Vitamin E, and other vitamin as well as herbal supplements for 10 days prior to any injection of soft-tissue augmentation. This will decrease the risk and degree of swelling and bruising. Some dermatologic surgeons routinely give antiviral prophylaxis to patients with a significant history of cold sores (usually beginning 1–2 days prior to the procedure and continuing for two days afterwards—especially for lip augmentation), but there is no evidence to suggest that this is actually necessary.

To increase patient comfort, topical anesthesia may be applied at home 1 hour prior to injection with reapplication using plastic wrap occlusion (provided the treatment area is small) for 15 minutes immediately prior to the injection. It is import ant to remember that some topical anesthetics (such as betacaine and tetracaine) cross-react with sulfa-derivatives, and these should be avoided in patients with sulfa allergies. Due to the prevalence of sulfa allergies, the safest choice for topical anesthetics may be those containing lidocaine without any additional compounds (this includes LMX® by Ferndale Laboratories, Ferndale, Michigan, U.S.A., now available over the counter). In patients without sulfa allergy, a compounded formulation containing beta-caine, lidocaine, and tetracaine (which is referred to by the acronym "BLT") is commonly used and a topical anesthetic mask (S-Caine Peel by Zars) will likely soon be on the market. Most patients will tolerate injections of the more common fillers such as hyaluronic acids or collagen products in the majority of sites (excluding the lips) using only topical anesthesia.

The Choice of Filler

Each filler has individual properties which must be considered when selecting which product is appropriate for a given patient and his or her goals. For example, a permanent, non-organic, high viscosity, thick filler which requires a large bore needle for injection may be acceptable for the treatment of a large atrophic scar but would not be appropriate for the fine, superficial rhytids of the upper lip. A dense hyaluronic acid that might be perfect for correction of nasolabial creases in a middle-aged woman with thick skin, may not be appropriate for treating fine superficial lines in a woman with thin skin who will not tolerate any bumps. Products such as calcium hydroxylapatite

(Radiesse) and poly lactic acid (Sculptra) are not good choices for lip augmentation, but they are viable considerations for the treatment of nasolabial creases. Other factors affecting the choice of filler include budget and time-frame. Some patients cannot afford some of the more expensive products available while others may not want to wait for the delayed volume-enhancement of fillers such as Sculptra and Artefill.

Proper Placement/Location

Selection of the perfect product for a given indication in a particular patient does not guarantee a perfect outcome. Precise placement of any filling substance is critical. This requires anatomic knowledge of the areas being treated as well as an understanding of the intended depth of placement of the material being utilized. For instance, without an understanding of the differences in skin thickness in various areas of the face, placement of fillers may be either too deep or too superficial for the filler to have the intended effect. A filler designed for subcutaneous augmentation should not be placed superficially in the papillary dermis and vice versa. Placement may also be affected by injection technique (linear threading vs. serial puncture, fanning, cross-hatching, and depot injection, etc.) as well as other factors such as needle gauge, needle angle, bevel direction, needle tip depth, and whether the injection was made upon withdrawal, insertion, or both.

Amount of Implant Deposited

One of the most common patient complaints following soft-tissue augmentation is that "it did not work," "did not last," or that a material "did not completely fill" the treatment area. These issues are frequently the result of not injecting enough material to realize the patient's goals. Common etiologies for this are: (i) physicians trying to save the patients' money by using too little volume and (ii) inexperience of the injector with a particular technique or product. Nasolabial folds and other large furrows can be deceiving as to how much volume of a given substance will be required to fill them adequately. This does not necessarily mean complete correction must be achieved at the initial session. On the contrary, gradual correction over several sessions has several advantages over single session correction. The first advantage is that a more precise correction may be obtained. For instance, the lips require some correction for swelling and product absorption that occurs during the injection. Another significant advantage is that staged corrections help guard against overcorrection (a very personal and subjective definition with large inter-patient variation) by requiring the patient to agree "more is needed." As with any cosmetic procedure, the plan for a staged correction should be discussed with the patient prior to the procedure in order to ensure that they are in agreement with this approach. Failure to discuss this type of plan, risks having patients believe that they are being inadequately treated or being treated with inadequate filler. Pre-procedure and post-procedure photography is essential for documentation purposes, and can help show patients the degree of correction achieved—as too often, patients forget what you made go away and simply focus on what is left over.

Timing of Repeat Injections

Different fillers have different tissue residence times, ranging from months to years. There is a great deal of literature to support the duration of correction obtained with collagens, hyaluronans, silicone, and autologous fat but less information about some of the products marketed as semi-permanent (lasting more than a couple of years) such as Radiesse and Sculptra. The dermatologic surgery community is just gaining evidence-based literature about Artefill, a filler which is permanent. With non-permanent fillers, patients obtain incremental benefit from re-evaluation and "touch-up" injections before the implant is completely absorbed. When using a permanent or semi-permanent filler in a patient that has not had fillers in the past, it is prudent to exercise a fair degree of caution. Many experienced dermasurgeons use a non-permanent filler first to give the patient an idea of how they will look. Although one of the authors has never seen a problem with silicone using the micro-droplet technique, others have seen silicone granulomas develop after 15 or 20 years of implantation. Another issue with permanent fillers is what was esthetically pleasing in a 40-year-old face may not be so pretty in a 60-year-old one. The senior author has never found this to be a problem. In addition, esthetic values change over time and one would like to avoid committing ones patients to a particular fashion for life whenever possible (imagine the "Paris Lip" popular in the 1980s in a 60-year-old woman today). Two of the authors recommend use of a non-permanent filler in almost all circumstances—and all of the authors recommend using a non-permanent fillers when possible prior to using a permanent one in order to allow the patient to decide whether soft-tissue augmentation is appropriate for them before they are married to it. Otherwise, make sure to inject the permanent filler over several smaller-volume treatment sessions.

INJECTION TECHNIQUE

Most fillers share a similar treatment protocol: many that are placed superficially or contain lidocaine are injected with only topical anesthesia while those that are injected more deeply (i.e., those that require larger needles such as 27 gauges or larger) are often performed with injectable local anesthesia. Other considerations for deciding upon the use of anesthesia include the region to be treated: lip augmentation is difficult for both patient and dermasurgeon unless nerve blocks or "mini-blocks" (placed focally at the submucosal level) are utilized.

Prior to any injection with soft-tissue augmentation products, makeup should be completely removed. A clean face without makeup is so important not only to allow you to guide your injection sites and help to avoid blood vessels, but also to avoid implantation of a potential foreign body (especially important in lip augmentation as many lipsticks contain various metallic particles). Prior to injection, the treatment area should be cleaned with alcohol. Subsequently, a chlorhexidine or Technicare® prep of the area is recommended. (When injecting the peri-ocular area, however, we recommend specifically Technicare® as chlorhexidine may cause a keratitis.)

During injection in a retrograde fashion, the smallest needle possible should be used to minimize pain as well as vessel trauma. After injection, massaging the implant may help shape it into the desired contour although this should be done gently after hyaluronic acid as more bruising may occur. It is important to change gloves immediately to avoid bacterial contamination of the area if any intra-oral massage is performed. New ice packs are used with each patient in order to avoid the risk of blood-born diseases. Several experienced dermasurgeons warn their patients not to apply makeup to treated areas for at least one day while others apply makeup in the office immediately following treatment. There is minimal evidence-based literature to support either position so the decision is left to the individual injectors. Following injection, patients are instructed to avoid the same list of non-essential medications and vitamin supplements (aspirin, NSAIDs, Vitamin E, Ginko, etc.) for an additional three to four days. Finally, having the patient return in one to two weeks may identify patients who would benefit from "touch-up" treatment as well as to provide the physician with an opportunity to address patients' concerns and questions.

CLASSIFICATION OF FILLERS

Fillers can be classified in many different fashions. These classifications typically separate products into temporary, semi-permanent, and permanent fillers. Other classification systems parse based on animal, non-animal, or autologous source. The authors find a classification based on being biodegradable or non-biodegradable to be the most helpful.

Biodegradable Fillers
Collagen

Over the years, there have been many collagen products used for soft-tissue augmentation. The first collagen product approved for use as a soft-tissue augmentation was Zyderm, a bovine-derived collagen. A cross-linked form of bovine product known as Zyplast and a more dense collagen were also approved and these constituted the soft-tissue augmentation market for a period of several years. More recently, non-animal-based collagen products have emerged. These include cadaveric collagen, non-cadaveric human collagen, and bioengineered autologous collagen.

Bovine Collagen

Zyderm/Zyplast. Zyderm I and II and Zyplast (Inamed, Santa Barbara, California, U.S.A.) have been used successfully as fillers for almost 25 years. Zyderm I appeared first in 1976 and was FDA-approved in 1981. Zyderm I has a collagen concentration of 35 mg/mL. Zyderm II has a collagen concentration of 65 mg/mL. Zyplast has a concentration of 35 mg/mL but has greater duration due to its cross-linking with glutaraldehyde.

These off-white, opaque products are derived from bovine collagen harvested from an isolated U.S.-raised herd. Both come prepackaged in 1 to 2.5 cc syringes for single use. Zyderm is excellent for superficial etched-in lines and Zyplast fills in deeper folds and lines. For both, a double skin test with Zyderm I (which is more immunogenic due to lack of cross-linking) is recommended with treatment delayed until following documentation of two negative skin tests over a six-week period. The first skin test is generally placed 1 cm below the antecubital fossa, and up to 3.5% of patients tested will show a positive reaction (erythema, swelling, or induration) over four weeks. Ninety percent of these positive reactions manifest within 72 hours, while the remaining 10% are seen by four weeks. The second skin test is placed during a four-week follow-up appointment (generally at the left anterior scalp line). Following these two skin tests 1% to 5% of these patients will develop an allergic response at the recommended follow-up two weeks later. After two negative skin tests over six weeks, there is a less than 1% risk of an allergic response with treatment. Augmentation with Zyplast typically lasts three to five months in the nasolabial folds and two or three months in

the lips. The duration of correction with Zyderm 1 or II is slightly less (typically about 3–4 months).

Zyderm I is injected through a 30- to 32-gauge needle into the superficial papillary dermis. The injection technique goal is to raise a bleb as the material flows along superficial lines. It is necessary to overcorrect by approximately 200% with Zyderm as it is diluted with saline. When using this product, it is necessary to explain to patients that the saline is reabsorbed over 24 hours. If placed too superficially, Zyderm can impart a flat yellow look to the skin and care should be taken to avoid this placement. Zyplast is injected using a 30-gauge needle into the mid dermis or deep dermis to fill deeper folds. Each of these fillers should disperse evenly into the tissue and be lightly massaged after injection.

Zyplast can be placed along the vermillion border of the lips for definition of the borders, into the philtrum, or into the body of the lip itself to increase overall volume. When treating the glabella, botulinum toxin chemodernervation is frequently combined with Zyderm injections to enhance and prolong the correction obtained. Cutaneous necrosis, however, has been associated with soft-tissue augmentation of the glabella. This most likely results from deep product placement causing compression of the watershed branches of the supratrochlear vessels or direct intravascular injection of the material. If injection site necrosis is suspected, massage the area with a warm gauze (to encourage temperature-related vasodilation) until a topical 2% nitroglycerine paste can be applied to promote a pharmacological vasodilation of the area. One case of blindness was reported after Zyplast injection into the glabella caused vascular occlusion (likely via retrograde flow reaching the ophthalmic artery). For this reason, low volume Zyderm (which is injected more superficially) rather than Zyplast (which is contraindicated for this location) is recommended for this area. For nasolabial and melolabial "puppet" lines, Zyderm is often layered over Zyplast to get the best correction.

Zyderm and Zyplast offer many advantages for both beginning and advanced cosmetic specialists. They have a long track record of safety, come prepackaged with 30-gauge needles, and are easy to use. In addition, they have the ability to treat etched-in lines as well as folds, and are formulated with 0.4% lidocaine to minimize injection pain.

Their disadvantages include the need for refrigeration, the possibility of allergic reactions (which mandate double skin testing), a relatively short length of duration of improvement (compared with several newer fillers), and the need to use large volumes of product in patients requiring moderate volume correction (rendering treatments very expensive). Over the years, there has been some concern regarding the possibility of bovine collagen inciting "cross-over" auto-antibodies to human collagen with theoretic risk of subsequent induction of collagen vascular disease. Various studies and panels have indicated that this type of induction has not occurred and would be extremely remote. Initially dermasurgeons avoided treatment in patients with a personal or family history of connective tissue autoimmune disease including lupus, scleroderma, rheumatoid arthritis, dermatomyositis, or polymyositis. Presently, however, these patients are treated with collagens. Despite double skin testing, sensitivity reactions (erythema, swelling, induration, or urticaria) occur in less than 1% of patients and these reactions may last one to nine months. For this reason, it is recommended that if a patient has not received treatment for more than one year, a single re-test be done with evaluation at two weeks. Treatment options for sensitivity or allergic reactions to treated areas include topical, intralesional and oral corticosteroids, topical calcineurin inhibitors, pulse dye laser, and non-steroidal anti-inflammatory medications. One case report showed a dramatic and expeditious resolution of collagen sensitivity using cyclosporine.

It is recommended to avoid treating patients who have a history of lidocaine sensitivity, anaphylactoid event, beef allergy and, of course, previous sensitivity to bovine collagen. To reduce the risk of sensitivity to a bovine product, quell any possible concerns of potential risk of transferring some animal-hosted infectious processes and obviate the need for skin testing, Inamed came out in early 2003 with Cosmoderm/Cosmoplast human-derived collagen products.

Human Bio-Engineered Collagen

Cosmoderm/Cosmoplast. Cosmoderm and Cosmoplast (Inamed) contain purified collagen derived from cell cultures of human fibrocytes from a single cell line. They are the only FDA-approved, commercially available dermal fillers that contain non-cadaveric human collagen. These products are analogous to Zyderm and Zyplast in terms of their physical characteristics and indications. The cell line of this human product originates from the foreskin of a newborn, and has been tested for viruses, tumorigenicity, retroviruses as well as known genetic diseases. Cosmoderm and Cosmoplast contain the basic human collagen molecule stripped of antigenic determinates so no skin testing is necessary. They are the first same-day treatment collagen fillers approved in the United States. Thus, soft-tissue augmentation with these two products may occur on the same day as the initial patient consultation.

Cosmoderm and Cosmoplast are opaque and flow through a 30-gauge needle easily. They are both prepackaged in 1-mL syringes and are meant for single use only. Although larger sized syringes are scheduled for production, the current sizes create treatments that are fairly expensive. They are, however, perfect for short-term corrections such as lip enhancement for a special event or photo shoot.

The materials are very similar to the bovine-sourced collagen products. Cosmoplast contains cross-linked collagen fibers while Cosmoderm I has non-cross-linked collagen fibers. Both products have a collagen concentration of 35 mg/mL. Cosmoderm II should soon be approved by the FDA and will have a concentration of 65 mg/mL. Injection of these materials is also similar to Zyderm and Zyplast. Cosmoderm is injected into the superficial papillary dermis, and Cosmoplast is injected into the mid to deep reticular dermis. It is necessary to overcorrect with Cosmoderm as with Zyderm (as their only difference is essentially the human versus bovine source of the collagen) because it is diluted with saline, which is reabsorbed over 24 hours. Care should be used in thin-skinned areas around the eyes and mouth—where bumpy, non-linear placement can be more visible. Cosmoderm is often layered over Cosmoplast for the best results. Superficial placement of Cosmoderm, like Zyderm, is preferred over Cosmoplast for injection in the glabellar area. As all of these collagen products (Cosmoderm/Cosmoplast as well as Zyderm/Zyplast) contain lidocaine, do not inject into patients with rare allergy to amide anesthetics. Other precautions are also similar to those for Zyderm and Zyplast.

The advantage of the Cosmo-products over the previous collagen products, Zyderm and Zyplast, is the ability to use the formulation at the initial consultation visit, as no skin testing is necessary. The disadvantages are the same, including: the need for refrigeration (do not freeze), the cost, the same length of duration as Zyderm and Zyplast (generally between two and five months depending on the site of treatment and the need for large volumes of product patients with deeper lines as with Zyderm and Zyplast. Flu-like symptoms have been reported in 2% to 4% of patients who have received Cosmoderm or Cosmoplast.

Autologous Collagen

Autologen (Collagenesis Inc.). Recently, tissue derived from autologous collagen cultures have been utilized for soft-tissue augmentation. Autologen is collagen harvested from the patient at the time of a surgical procedure. A large piece of harvested tissue is required—usually from abdominoplasty or rhytidectomy. The tissue is frozen and sent for processing, where it can be stored for up to five years or directly processed in a manner where one square inch of harvested skin produces about 3 cc of Autologen product. The processing protocol leaves the telopeptides intact to convey stability and resistance to enzymatic degradation—leading to a durability of the injected product up to 18 months. The syringes of processed material are stable for up to six months. No skin testing is required and patient anxiety over animal or other human-material is alleviated. The material contains no anesthetic, so topical anesthesia is necessary and sometimes local infiltration blocks. The injection sessions are usually spaced at two-week intervals until the desired correction is achieved. The main disadvantages are the need for large tissue harvesting, delay required for tissue processing as well as the high cost of the product.

Isolagen (Isolagen Technologies Inc.). Isolagen is another autologous collagen product, however, harvesting requires only a small piece of tissue, typically a 3-mm punch biopsy harvested from the post-auricular sulcus. The harvested material is sent to the company where it is cultured and grown in vitro for six weeks. The material is then returned to the physician's office in 1 to 1.5 cc aliquots. Injections of the material are accomplished in much the same manner as are traditional collagen injections. Like Autologen, the material does not contain any anesthetic. Injections are usually spaced every two to three weeks until the desired correction is reached. Since the material is autologous, there should not be any risk of allergic or immunologic reaction. Nevertheless, the company still recommends skin testing so that any byproduct allergy could be detected. Finally, since one is injecting viable fibroblasts, collagen matrix and other materials required for replenishment of the dermal support structures, this process offers the opportunity to have a durable correction—but there is little data on the exact duration of the product. When it was available several years ago, the authors of this chapter feel it did not work very well at all and will reserve comments until its efficacy and safety are established.

Cadaveric Collagen

Alloderm (LifeCell Corp.). Alloderm is an acellular dermal allograft derived from cadaveric type IV collagen. As with other donated organs, the product is screened prior to harvesting and, in addition, it undergoes a viral inactivation process after being harvested. It is a decellularized protein framework. Since there are no cells present, there is no risk of immunogenicity and no skin testing is required. It is still recommended, however, to avoid using Alloderm in patients with collagen autoimmune diseases.

The product is made into solid sheets which are inserted into areas of treatment through dissected dermal tunnels. Once these sheets are implanted, they are infiltrated by native fibroblasts which will begin to manufacture collagen and other matrix proteins. Alloderm's most frequent use has been as a skin graft for burn victims. In the cosmetic arena, this product has been used mostly for acne scarring, lip augmentation, and nasal augmentation. The longevity of this product in vivo is unknown, but it reportedly lasts longer than other collagens.

Cymetra (LifeCell Corp.).   Cymetra is the injectable form of Alloderm, and as such is a micronized form of acellular human cadaveric dermis. It is supplied in a prepackaged 5-cc syringe of dried powder. This is reconstituted to 1 cc with saline or lidocaine and is for single use only. The human tissue has been tested, and sterilized. It is a non-immunogenic, soft implant that may last longer than bovine collagen.

Treatment of the nasolabial folds requires, on average, 1.5 to 2 units per side. Prior to injection, the sites are subcised with an 18-gauge 1.5-inch needle. The material is injected with a linear threading technique. If subcision is not utilized, serial puncture technique may be used. Techniques for injecting the lip depend upon the part of the lip being treated. Injection of the vermillion border should be performed with a 22- or 23-gauge needle. The material should be inserted with the bevel up and may be accomplished as the needle is withdrawn. Orientation of the injection should be from the Cupid's bow toward the opposite commissure. This approach should be repeated for the contralateral side while the middle third of the lip is treated by overlapping injections. A total of 0.5 to 1.5 units is used for each lip. To treat the vermilion itself, use the same technique, injecting from one-third of the way across the lip to the other side to deposit roughly twice the amount of Cymetra in the middle-third of the lip. Use about 1.2 units per lip. To treat perioral rhytids, a 26-gauge 3/8-inch needle should be used in a similar manner to deposit material immediately subdermally. A small amount should also be injected parallel to and just above the white roll of the lip in the manner previously described.

The marionette area is treated using a combination of linear threading and serial puncture techniques. The threading technique works best with a 25-gauge, 1.5-inch needle using subdermal subcision from below the fold. Injections should be accomplished while withdrawing the needle. The bevel should be oriented toward the epidermal aspect while the tissue is gently tented upwards. Each marionette line typically requires approximately 0.5 to 1 units of Cymetra on each side.

Treatment of the malar area is accomplished with a 22-gauge 1.5-inch needle: in the subdermal plane, thread the implant three times horizontally and three times vertically for an even crisscross pattern. The area can then be rolled to a homogenous consistency with a common cotton-tipped applicator or massaged bimanually. For all treated areas gentle massage should be performed after injection. Each treated patient should be warned to avoid facial expressions as long as possible (with a minimally acceptable interval of six hours). Several treatments with Cymetra may be necessary for optimal improvement.

Cymetra is advantageous from several perspectives: no skin test is needed so treatment and consultation may occur on the same day. Delivered as a dried powder, it can be stored up to six months. According to information

supplied by the company (Lifecell Corp.) the product must be stored in a refrigerator. It is recommended that this product be avoided in patients with collagen vascular disease and should not be injected into the periorbital or glabellar areas. Several treatments may be necessary for optimal improvement.

Fascian.   Fascian is preserved fascia lata in particulate form. It is made from screened human cadavers and was introduced in 1999. Fascian is a dense material that requires several months to be absorbed by the body. It comes in prepackaged 3-cc luer-lock syringes of dried material. The tissue is screened for various diseases, irradiated, particulated, and vacuum sealed. Fascian particles come in various sizes, < 0.25, < 0.5, and < 2.0 mm. Each of these requires rehydration with between 3 and 5 mL of either saline or lidocaine. Prior to injection, the area to be treated should be anesthetized with either infiltration of local anesthetic or with a regional anesthetic block. Subcision of the treated area is accomplished with a 20-gauge needle. The material is injected subdermally with a 16- to 29-gauge needle, depending on the particle size. Care must be taken in order to avoid intradermal injection of the product which may incite an inflammatory reaction with prominent erythema and lumpiness. Following the injection of this product, collagen formation occurs around the scaffolding injected.

Fascian offers several advantages compared with traditional collagen: it may last slightly longer than either Cosmoderm or Zyderm/Zyplast. In addition, it does not require refrigeration so storage is easier. One disadvantage is that Fascian must be reconstituted and it requires local anesthetic prior to injection. Fascian may contain trace amounts of polymyxin sulfate, bacitracin, or gentamycin and it should not be used in patients who are allergic to any of these substances. Fascian should not be used for superficial lines as intradermal injection can lead to lumpiness or inflammation.

Hyaluronic Acid Gels (Hylans)

Hyaluronic acid (hyaluronan, sodium hyaluronate, HA) is a naturally occurring linear polysaccharide. Unlike collagen, it exhibits no species or tissue specificity; its chemical structure is uniform throughout nature, and thus has no potential for immunogenicity in its pure form. In the skin, it forms the elastoviscous fluid matrix in which collagen fibers, elastic fibers, and other intercellular structures are embedded.

Hyaluronic acid gels (hylans) are swollen with water (95% of weight) and have the unique attribute of *dynamic viscosity*, which decreases with increasing shearing force. Under pressure of injection (high shear rate) the gel can pass through a relatively small gauge needle. Upon removal of the shearing force, viscosity increases, forming a thick gel at the site of tissue implantation, which is unlikely to migrate. Unlike other temporary soft tissue fillers such as collagen, their disappearance from tissue follows *isovolemic degradation*: as individual molecules of HA are degraded, those remaining are able to bind more water, such that the overall volume of the gel remains unchanged. In other words, the concentration of the gel decreases during reabsorption, but volume remains steady until the last molecules of HA are degraded. Clinically, this translates to an implant that maintains $> 95\%$ of its initial space-filling volume until the last of the material is completely resorbed.

Hyaluronic acid products are the most widely used soft-tissue augmentation products at the present time. Among the products presently approved by the FDA are:

Hylaform, Hylaform Plus, Captique, and Restylane. Products which are likely nearing approval in the United States include Juvederm, Perlane, and Restylane Fine Line.

Hylaform

The first hylan preparation widely used for soft-tissue augmentation was hylan B gel (Hylaform Gel®; Biomatrix, Inc., Ridgefield, New Jersey, U.S.A.), which was developed in the mid-1980s. It uses HA derived from the dermis of rooster combs, which is then purified and chemically cross-linked with divinyl sulfone. It has been used in the treatment of soft tissue defects and facial augmentation throughout most of the world (Canada, Europe, Australia, South America, Asia, etc.) for many years, and recently became available in the United States (April 2004). In clinical studies, treatment reactions have included mild erythema, itching, swelling and pain, which usually resolve in less than one week. Hylaform now is available in the United States in two forms: Hylaform and Hylaform Plus. While both have a concentration of 5.5 mg/mL, Hylaform Plus has a particle size that is larger than Hylaform. The larger particle sized product is intended for deeper tissue placement and may be utilized in instances where volume is required whereas Hylaform may be utilized to address more superficial dermal issues. It generally lasts up to three to four months. Studies comparing the duration of Restylane to Hylaform Plus are presently being conducted.

Restylane

Restylane (Q-Med AB, Uppsala, Sweden) is a stabilized, partially cross-linked HA gel. Restylane was the first HA product approved in the United States by the FDA in December 2003. The HA is produced from cultures of *Streptococcus equi* by fermentation in the presence of sugar, which is alcohol-precipitated, filtered, and dried. The HA chains are then chemically stabilized through permanent cross-linking with epoxides. The material is heat sterilized in its final container and has a shelf life of 1.5 years from the date of manufacture. Since its production does not require an animal source, it has been termed a Non-Animal, Stabilized Hyaluronic Acid (NASHA®). Restylane variations available in Europe and Canada include Restylane Fine Line and Perlane. Restylane Fine Line is designed for fine lines and comprised of smaller particles while Perlane is designed for deep rhytids and volume sculpting. Perlane has a larger particle size than Restylane. Restylane Fine Line has a smaller particle size than does Restylane. Perlane has a particle size of 10,000 particles per mL, Restylane has a particle size of 100,000 per mL and Restylane Fine Line has a concentration of 200,000 particles per mL. Since Restylane, Restylane Fine Line and Perlane have the same composition, concentration and manufacturing data, it is anticipated that the latter two products will obtain FDA approval soon. Restylane Sub Q is being designed as a potential replacement for autologous fat and it is presently marketed in Europe and Canada.

In a Swedish study of the clinical safety and efficacy of Restylane, physician evaluation revealed that treatment sites maintained an average of 82% and 69% of correction at 12 and 26 weeks, respectively, while subjects self-reported 75% and 61% improvement at these same time points. An Italian study of Restylane's clinical efficacy and tolerability also showed favorable results, with 78% of patients maintaining moderate to marked improvement after eight months, with nasolabial folds and lips fairing the best.

An American study comparing Restylane® to Zyplast® in the treatment of nasolabial folds reported Restylane® to be superior to Zyplast® in 56.9% of patients, Zyplast® to be superior in 9.5%, and both fillers to be equal in 33.6% after six months.

Injection-related reactions include redness, swelling, darkening of the treatment site and slight pain, most of which resolve spontaneously within several days. In Duranti and Olenius' early efficacy studies, investigators reported such adverse events at an incidence of 13%. Subsequent retrospective reviews of Q-Med Esthetics' adverse events database reported much lower incidences, with only one out of every 650 (0.15%) of an estimated 144,000 patients treated in 1999 reporting temporary redness, swelling, localized granulomatous reactions, bacterial infection, or acneiform lesions. No patients were reported to have systemic symptoms or anaphylaxis, although two cases of injection site necrosis were recorded, both of the glabellar area. Compared to collagen, hylan preparations are slightly more painful on injection (they are more viscous and do not contain lidocaine) and can result in more bruising and swelling at the injection site which may persist for several days to a week.

Although early studies did not demonstrate hypersensitivity or other allergic reactions to hylans, delayed implant site reactions have now been reported to occur in several case series in incidences from 0.4% to 3.7%. In these very rare cases, delayed inflammatory reactions of redness, pruritus, painful swelling, or "nettle-like rash" reactions occurred. None appeared sooner than six to eight weeks after injection; some were reported to last up to 4.5 months without oral treatment. In one instance, patients developed anti-Restylane and anti-Hylaform antibodies. As of mid-2005, Restylane is the most popular filler in the United States.

Captique (Inamed)

Another non-animal-derived HA product is Captique—which was FDA-approved in late 2004. This product is marketed by Inamed and is very similar to Hylaform. Like Hylaform, it has a concentration of 5.5 mg/mL, contains 500 micron particles and is cross-linked by divinyl sulfone. It is also injected with a 30-gauge needle. Captique so closely resembles Hylaform that it is considered to be an extension of it with a new manufacturing source rather than a new product. Captique will likely be a useful product for areas such as lip augmentation which require as minimal edema as possible.

Juvederm

Approved for use in Europe, Juvederm (like Restylane and Captique) is a non-animal-derived HA which is made from bacterial fermentation of Streptococcus and cross-linked by butane-diol-diglycidyl ether. Juvederm, however, is a homogenous gel-based HA. This is in contrast to the other hyalurons which contain particles of different sizes. It is believed that the homogenous nature of the Juvederm gel leads to increased longevity as there is less surface area available for host enzymatic processes to attack and degrade the HA. This however has never been proven, and there are very few published studies to date on this product. In addition, the company feels that the homogenous Juvederm has less friction on injection (i.e., more pliable and viscoelastic) and could be potentially less inflammatory than other HA products. There is also no proof of this theory. Phase

III U.S. trials on Juvederm are nearing completion at the time of the preparation of this manuscript. In Europe, where both Restylane and Juvederm have been used for years, Restylane is twice as popular.

Juvederm is available in five different formulations: Juvederm 18, 24, 24 HV, 30, and 30 HV. Juvederm 18 is composed of 18 mg of cross-linked HA, while both Juvederm 24 and 30 both contain 24 mg of cross-linked non-animal-derived HA. Each formulation is used for different indications, similar to the uses and levels of placement of the Restylane and Hylaform products. Juvederm 18 is used for superficial rhytids, Juvederm 24 for mid dermal defects and Juvederm 30 for deep dermal defects.

These products do not contain anesthetic and thus require either topical anesthetic or injected anesthetic prior to injection for most patient. As with other hyalurons, injection technique is variable with linear threading, serial puncture and cross-hatching being advocated by various skilled injectors.

Treatment with Hylan Fillers

As of the time of this writing, Restylane and Hylaform, Hylaform Plus, and Captique are the only FDA-approved hylans available in the United States, and are only indicated for the treatment of moderate to severe facial wrinkles and folds, such as the nasolabial folds. All other uses are currently considered off-label. They have not been studied in patients who are pregnant, breastfeeding, under 18 years of age, or on immunosuppressive therapy.

The Restylane and Hylaform family of products are designed for use at different dermal depths and understanding what product is appropriate for what area is critical for optimal outcomes with this (or any) soft-tissue augmentation product (Tables 2 and 3). The concentration of HA is identical in all three preparations of each product line (Restylane 20 mg/mL, Hylaform 5.5 mg/ml) as is the chemical composition. Each of these iterations is different in the size of the particle (measured in particles per mL for Restylane products, and in actual size of particle in microns for Hylaform products), as well as the target depth for implantation.

Restylane Fine Lines has the smallest particle size with a size of 200,000 particles per mL. This is the least viscous of the Restylane family. It is injected through a 31-gauge needle and is designed for use in the most superficial dermis. Hylaform Fineline has the smallest particle size of its family of products, 300 microns and is injected through a 32-gauge needle. Placement of both of these products is intended to correct fine lines and superficial, easily distensible defects. Obviously, injection of this low viscosity product in the deep dermis or subcutaneous space will not be efficacious and will lead to sub-optimal correction ("Doc-that filler did not work" syndrome).

Table 3 Comparison of Two Forms of Hylaform

	Hylaform®	Hylaform® Fineline
Material composition	Hylan B polymer (4.5–5.5 mg/mL)	
Syringe fill volume	0.75 mL	0.40 mL
Needle gauge	30 gauges	32 gauges
Gel particle size (median)	500 μm	300 μm
Item code	No. 5340	Not available

Restylane contains particles that are larger with a particle density of 100,000 particles per mL. Hylaform has a gel particle size of 500 microns. These products are both usually injected a 30-gauge needle. They are engineered for injection into the mid dermis. When it is placed too superficially, its large particle size will produce lumps and bumps (especially as the hydrophilic compound absorbs water) and this will result in poor patient satisfaction. Restylane should be utilized for correction of wrinkles that are moderate as well as for facial sculpting (it is remarkable what a small amount of this product can do when placed over the zygomatic arch or against the bone in the tear trough or supraorbital rim).

Perlane is engineered to have a particle concentration of 10,000 particles per mL whereas Hylaform Plus has 700-micron gel particles. These large particle products are injected with a 27-gauge syringe and are designed for deep dermal placement and are ideal for volume correction. Patients that have had successful lip augmentation with Restylane or Hylaform will occasionally benefit from augmentation with Perlane or Hylaform Plus but this should be considered as a treatment for advanced injectors. In the lips, Perlane may last for over a year and it maintains its volume remarkably well.

Obviously, knowledge of each product as well as the techniques and associated anatomy is critical when using soft-tissue augmentation products. A lack of understanding of each of the specific design characteristics of these (or any other injectable products) may lead to poor patient outcomes (just imagine a non-specialist injecting Perlane into the thin skin of the periorbital area).

The Restylane and Hylaform family of products may be used in concert as well as with collagen-based products. This enables the dermatologic surgeon to obtain optimal results from a broad palette. Currently, of the three Restylane products only Restylane itself is FDA-approved for use in the United States (marketed through Medicis Aesthetics, Scottsdale, Arizona, U.S.A., since December 2003), and is officially indicated only for the treatment of moderate to severe facial wrinkles and folds, such as the nasolabial folds. In the Hylaform product line, Hylaform and Hylaform Plus are both FDA-approved for injection into the mid to deep

Table 2 Comparison of Three Forms of Restylane

	Restylane	Restylane Fine Lines	Restylane Perlane
Composition	20 mg/mL stabilized HA	20 mg/mL stabilized HA	20 mg/mL stabilized HA
No. of gel particles/mL	100,000	200,000	10,000
Indications	Wrinkles, lips	Thin superficial lines	Deep folds (e.g., nasolabial), lip augmentation, facial contouring
Target depth	Mid dermis	Upper dermis	Deep dermis/upper subcutis
Degree correction	100%	100%	100%
Syringe volume	0.7, 0.4 mL	0.4 mL	0.7 mL
Needle size	30 gauges	31 gauges	27 gauges

dermis also for correction of moderate to severe facial wrinkles and folds (such as nasolabial folds).

None of the present versions of HA products contains lidocaine although there is no biocompatibility issue with this anesthetic. Future versions (including one product under development by Ortho) will contain lidocaine and this should increase patient comfort with injections of HA. Presently, topical anesthetics (LMX®, compounded "BLT", etc.) can be useful but must be thickly applied for 15 minutes before injection, and the degree of pain reduction provided may not warrant the preparation time involved. Alternatively, small amounts of local anesthetic to function as a "mini block" or as a regional or local nerve block can be used. Some patients can tolerate treatment of nasolabial folds, oral commissures, or the glabellar area without any anesthesia. For injections of the lips, however, peripheral nerve and/or field blocks are usually needed.

Techniques for injection vary and they include the linear threading, cross-hatching, fanning and serial puncture. In addition, one of the authors (KRB) utilizes a technique referred to as the pinch technique whereby the thumb and forefinger are gently pinched to tent up the area being treated as the HA is guided into place between the two fingers.

The linear threading technique is probably the most commonly used: holding the syringe parallel to the length of the wrinkle or fold to be treated, pierce the skin and advance the needle to its fullest extent. Then, while slowly withdrawing the needle, even pressure is applied to inject material into dermis. Fanning and cross-hatching techniques are merely variations on the linear threading technique, most often used when placing a larger amount of filler more deeply. With all of these techniques, pressure should be reduced shortly before the needle leaves the skin to minimize product wastage as well as to avoid creation of superficial dermal blebs. Short, superficial lines and wrinkles can be ablated with a single injection. Larger folds, lines or wrinkles may require several passes with different techniques to obtain a satisfactory correction. For large defects or those that extend into the deep dermis, a filler designed for that indication (such as Perlane or Hylaform Plus) is indicated and using one designed for more superficial placement will be counterproductive for you and expensive for your patients.

Most physicians inject materials with the needle at an angle of 30° or 45°, Some prefer to have the needle parallel to the skin. One key to successful injection of soft-tissue augmentation products is to select one or two methods for a given product and to consistently use it, perfecting ones technique as one gains experience. Although most authors recommend keeping the needle bevel up, this is not mandatory and, in fact, some authors prefer to orient the bevel medially or toward the dermis, depending on the material and location of the injection. Studies have shown that the direction of the bevel does not influence the direction of the flow of the material, which follows the course of least resistance. The authors prefer to inject with the bevel up to see the tip of the needle and more precisely control where it pierces the skin.

Maintaining constant tissue depth during implantation is critical in obtaining consistently good results. The depth of needle placement (and thus filler implantation) should be high dermis for superficial lines, mid dermis for more substantial wrinkles, and deep dermis/subcutaneous border for heavy folds. One way to approximate needle depth is to understand that when one can see the needle contour but not its color, placement is most likely in the mid dermis.

Another very useful device to foster exact tissue placement is the ADG needle distributed with several Inamed products. This needle has an adjustable hub that can be set for a given depth. The exact placement depth can be measured and changed to whatever is needed for optimal product placement. A skilled injector will alter his or her treatment by *visual* response with thinner materials designed for placement in the high dermis (such as Restylane Fine Lines or Cosmoderm) and *tactile* response for materials designed for deeper placement (such as Perlane or Hylaform Plus).

Another useful criterion for correct tissue placement is the resistance to injection. Increased resistance is noted when placing thick products in the deep dermis while a sudden decrease in resistance typically indicates injection into the subcutaneous plane.

For a beginning injector, the most difficult aspect of soft-tissue augmentation is injecting into the correct tissue space. At the early part of the learning curve, it is better to err on the side of injecting too deeply as this will simply not provide ideal correction whereas an injection that is too superficial will produce overcorrection with surface irregularities. Surface irregularities may not be as prominent with the transparent hylan gels but will be markedly noticeable with the opaque materials such as collagen. Superficial placement with semi-permanent fillers such as Sculptra increases the risk of developing subcutaneous papules, and placement of Radiesse in the upper dermis increases the likelihood of developing nodules and granulomas. Thus, precision when injecting material is vital not only to obtaining optimal outcomes but also in avoiding untoward complications.

Following injection of most materials, many practitioners manually massage the treated areas. It is believed that this will smooth out nodular or uneven areas, and ensure the implanted material conforms to the contour of surrounding tissues. Use of an ice pack or other cold compress may minimize swelling (on lips especially), and many patients appreciate the mildly anesthetic effect afforded by this. Post-treatment massage may also help to rectify overcorrection with HAs as they may be manipulated once they are injected. Firm massage of the hylans may help to smooth out any irregularity or asymmetry but be careful because bruising can occur and most bumps will fade away over the first few weeks. This is a very forgiving product. It is better not to overcorrect. It is estimated that as much as a 20% overcorrection can be massaged away while and this increases the opportunity to provide optimal outcomes if correctly utilized. If a significant problem occurs (e.g., too superficial placement of product resulting in a visible nocularity), Vitrase® (hyaluronidase) is an FDA-approved product used commonly in ophthalmologic surgery.

Following treatment, patients may resume normal activities and may apply makeup within a few hours of treatment. The duration of correction depends on character of the defect being treated, tissue stress at the implant site (frequency of muscular activity), implant depth, and injection technique.

Fat

The history of fat transfer dates back to the early part of the twentieth century when fat injections were used to disguise spies going behind enemy lines. Since that time fat has undergone a resurgence for a variety of reasons, the first being the popularity of liposuction among cosmetic surgeons creating an ample supply of fat. In addition, many patients require so much volume that using syringes of

1 mL would simply not be enough and the volume available with fat is more congruous with the needs of these patients.

Fat is an autologous filling substance that is usually available in large quantities, enabling the dermatologic surgeon to fill in large defects, perform mini-face lifts, and rejuvenate the hands. It can be frozen for later use, and often lasts for years in the hollows of the cheeks and after repairing surgical defects. The technique we use (described below) is a modification of that of Dr. Sidney Coleman by several dermatologic surgeons including Dr. Narins and Dr. Donofrio. For completeness, some physicians use the FAMI technique described by Dr. Roger Amar in which fat is injected directly into the muscles supposedly for better blood supply.

Very little equipment is necessary: a sterile tray with several 10-cc syringes, a female–female luer-lock adapter, a test tube rack in which the syringes can be placed upright, various needles (including 30-gauge 0.5-inch, and 18-, 16-, and 22-gauge spinal needles), a Coleman extraction/injection cannula, red syringe caps, and gauze pads. Tumescent lidocaine solution, spinal needles, and syringes or a pressure pump with intravenous tubing are also needed for anesthesia.

The recipient and donor sites are prepped with Betadine, and a small amount of tumescent anesthetic is injected with a 30-gauge 0.5-inch needle using a 3-cc syringe in the "incision" area of the donor site. Tumescent anesthesia is injected radially through this incision site using 10-cc syringes and a spinal needle, or using the Klein pump (very low setting) and intravenous tubing with an 18- or 20-gauge spinal needle.

The incision sites of the recipient areas are then similarly injected and a small amount of tumescent anesthetic is delivered radially into the reinjection area using a 30-gauge 1-inch needle, or, if the area is large, a 22-gauge spinal needle. In this area, very little anesthesia is needed and it should be delivered under barely any pressure with a syringe so that there is no distortion of the tissue. This slight anesthesia of the recipient area makes reinjections much more comfortable for the patient. Tiny needles are necessary to minimize the risk of bleeding, especially here since fat is so vascular. When augmenting the nasolabial fold, the commissures of the mouth, lips, puppet lines, and cheeks, one reinjection site can be used on each side just lateral to the lips. If the chin or area anterior to the jowls is being enhanced, two incision sites are used and the fat injected at multiple levels from both incision sites.

Fat is harvested using syringes rather than a liposuction aspirator since high pressure can injure the fat cells. The skin at the donor site is pierced with a 16-gauge needle. No mark is left from this incision and no suture is necessary. Through this opening, a Coleman extractor attached to a 10-cc syringe can be inserted and used to harvest the fat. Negative pressure is obtained in the syringe by pulling the plunger out and holding it there while the syringe is moved back and forth in the subcutaneous tissue. Fat and fluid fills the syringe that is then placed in the container plunger up so that the fluid can settle to the bottom and fat can rise to the top. This procedure can be repeated with as many syringes and donor sites as are necessary. The negative pressure on the plunger should be small; pull back 0.5 to 1 cc and the fat will come out easily.

The infranatant fluid collects at the bottom of the syringe and is easily be expelled with the plunger. A cap is put on the tip of the syringe and the plunger is removed before centrifuging for one or two minutes. After centrifuging, any oily supranatant fluid is poured off (final amount can be

wicked off with sterile gauze), the plunger is replaced, and the resultant clean yellow fat is ready for transplantation. Fat to be implanted immediately is transferred into 1-cc luer-lock syringes through a female–female adaptor. Any remaining fat is frozen in the 10-cc syringes after capping them. Each syringe is carefully labeled with the patient's name, social security number, and the date before placing it in the freezer at –20°C.

Fresh fat is reinjected through an incision with an 18-guage NoKor needle using a 1-cc luer-lock syringe attached to a Coleman injection cannula. Two or fewer injection sites should be used per area to avoid extrusion of the fat through multiple openings. The cannula is inserted to the furthest point, and a tiny aliquot of fat is injected as the syringe is pulled out. This is done at multiple levels of the skin and subcutaneous tissue. After injection, massage the fat in so that it fills the area smoothly. When injecting, placing a hand around the perimeter of the treatment area can help keep the transplanted fat within the desired site. Some surgeons overcorrect to compensate for fat that is reabsorbed over the first few postoperative days, but we prefer no overcorrection as more can always be added later. When injecting the hands, a single injection site on the back of each wrist should suffice. Five milliliters of fat is injected and massaged to allow an easy spread over the entire hand.

Fat that was previously harvested and frozen is injected into recipient sites using the same technique. It is a good idea to check with the patient the day before the procedure to confirm they are still coming in; the amount of fat necessary for reinjection is then removed from the freezer a few hours prior to the appointment for thawing. The frozen syringes are placed upright in a container and the tray is set up as for fresh fat. The top 0.5 to 1 cc is not used as it is usually just triglycerides and other fatty acids. It is then pushed through a female–female adaptor into 1-cc luer-lock syringes for injection. Some physicians use a sharp 18-guage needle to reinject fat monthly with no local anesthetic. We find less frequent injections suffice when a blunt-tipped instrument is used for injection. We do use local anesthetic as undermining or subcision with the blunt-tipped instrument appears to improve cosmetic results.

The advantage of autologous fat is the ability to harvest, use, and then freeze a large quantity of material. This makes it versatile as it can be used to fill large and small areas over much of the body (face, hands, etc.). As it is the patient's own fat, there is no problem with allergenicity. The disadvantages are the need for a surgical procedure to harvest the fat, the need for frequent touch-ups in areas of heavy movement (nasolabial folds and marionette lines), and the need for a local anesthetic prior to reinjection.

Poly-ʟ-Lactic Acid

Sculptra/New-Fill (Aventis Sanofi/Dermik Aesthetics, U.S.A.). Sculptra, known as New-Fill in Europe, was approved for use in HIV patients with lipoatrophy in the United States in August 2004. It is intended for correction and restoration of HIV-associated facial fat loss. In Europe, it has been approved for general cosmetic use in soft-tissue augmentation of scars and wrinkles.

The product is composed of poly-ʟ-lactic acid (PLA) derived from a vegetable source. PLA has been used in synthetic suture material for more than 40 years. It is non-toxic, synthetic, immunologically inactive, and easily absorbable. No skin testing is required. It is sold in a kit of two vials each containing 150 mg of sterile freeze dried powder stored at room temperature. The product is reconstituted 2 to 72 hours before intended use (the authors prefer at least 8 hours) with 5 cc of sterile water or 4 cc sterile water with 1 cc lidocaine. Recently, it has been suggested by many dermatologic surgeons to reconstitute the product with sterile preserved water. If this preserved sterile water regimen is used and the Sculptra is then refrigerated, it may be viable for about two weeks. Prior to injection, it must be restored to room temperature. Adoption of the technique will enable dermasurgeons to have Sculptra ready for patients that want treatment to begin at the time of consultation, and it is likely that this will increase the usage of this product. In addition, the use of 2% lidocaine instead of 1% has resulted in significant improvement in patient comfort with Sculptra injections.

It is recommended to be injected into the subcutaneous tissue with a 26-gauge needle (but the authors have found less clogging of this particulate product using a 25-gauge needle). In the lower face, the product is tunneled or cross-hatched depositing 0.1 cc aliquots. Above the zygoma and in the temples, depot injections of 0.05 cc are performed.

In the immediate post-injection period, the apparent fill is related to the mechanical action of the volume of liquid injected. The reconstitution fluid is absorbed over five to seven days and the PLA particles (which average 50 μm in size) are said to stimulate collagen growth over weeks to months. Initially, macrophages and proliferating fibroblasts surround the poly-lactide particles. Over time, the product is degraded by a foreign-body giant cell reaction. Degradation is accompanied by an increase in collagen deposition. One to four sessions may be needed for lipoatrophy correction, depending on the severity of the facial fat loss (grade I–IV described as the James Lipoatrophy Severity Scale). The durability of the correction has been reported to last upwards of two years. A local anesthetic is usually used in addition to topical anesthesia. Phase 3 FDA clinical trials comparing Sculptra to Cosmoplast for efficacy and safety in the cosmetic improvement of the nasolabial folds were begun in July 2004.

The advantages of Sculptra/New-Fill PLA are that it does not need to be refrigerated and no skin test is necessary so it can be used immediately. However, it must be reconstituted before injection, a local anesthetic is usually required, and more than one session is often needed for treatment. The original European experience with New Fill as well as the European HIV lipoatrophy studies showed a higher rate of subcutaneous papule formation than has been more recently seen with the two large U.S.-based trials (Blue Pacific and Apex002). Some of these may have been related to superficial injection of this filler which should be injected into the subcutaneous tissue or the more frequent lower-volume dilution (3 cc) than the current volumes of 5 or 6 cc. Other potential issues include: reconstitution duration, ensuring a homogeneous product in syringe, and force used if clog encountered. In addition to at least an eight hour reconstitution time, use of a 5 to 6 total cc dilution, and injection with a 25-gauge needle, the authors recommend agitating each syringe to ensure there is no precipitate prior to injection and immediate withdrawal of the syringe in case of clog.

Radiesse. Radiesse FN (formerly Radiance; Bioform Inc., Franksville, Wisconsin, U.S.A.) is made up of microscopic calcium hydroxyapatite particles suspended in a gel. It has been FDA-approved for several non-cosmetic indications including: dental reconstruction, bone, bladder, neck and vocal cord implants as well as serving as a radiocontrast agent. It is used off-label for cosmetic filling. Radiesse is comprised of calcium hydroxyapatite microspheres suspended in an aqueous polysaccharide gel, similar to Coaptite. The polysaccharide carboxymethylcellulose stays in place long enough for the body's own fibroblasts or osteoblasts to migrate into the implant and resume their native functions. Radiesse FN is thought to act as a scaffolding for bone or for collagen to grow in soft tissue, thereby creating volume. Use of this product for soft-tissue augmentation represents an "off label" indication.

Since Radiesse is completely biocompatible, no skin testing is necessary. Treatment may be given on the day of consultation. It can reportedly last from two to five years, although there are no case-controlled studies to substantiate these claims. When compared with Zyderm I or II, 1 mL of Radiesse will provide significantly more volume of correction. Once assimilated into the dermis, it typically has a natural look and feel. Occasional problems with this product include formation of granulomas and ectopic bone formation. These can typically be managed with intralesional steroid injections.

Anesthesia required for Radiesse injections typically utilizes dental blocks and local infiltration anesthesia. Anecdotal reports indicate a greater degree of discomfort with this product than with hyalurons or collagens although there is no good peer-reviewed data to confirm this notion. Postoperatively, it is common to see swelling for two to three days following the injections.

There is a lack of well-controlled, peer-reviewed clinical data on the use of Radiesse. Despite this, some case reports and anecdotal accounts have described various types of side-effects. Calcium deposits in some instances have risen to the surface of the skin, but apparently are easily excised. Granulomas can sometimes occur. Radiesse is not to be used for superficial lines but is reported to be good for deeper folds and wrinkles. If it is injected too superficially complications can occur, including: lumpiness, extrusion, granulomas, infection, and firmness. Most practitioners feel this product is not to be used for lip enhancement due to various anecdotal reports of "popcorn-like" nodules (perhaps from too superficial placement but also possibly attributable to product being pushed superficially over time from the underlying dynamic musculature). There is a paucity of data on cosmetic use, as the first anecdotal reports on skin placement of this product took place in late 2002. As there are no long-term cosmetic studies on Radiesse, safety and efficacy over time has not been established.

Non-Biodegradable Fillers

In contrast with the fillers previously discussed, these synthetic substances remain in the body permanently. Unfortunately, longer tissue residence time does not always translate to a better result or a more satisfied patient. For a variety of reasons such as long-term complications, changing styles and product migration, permanent fillers may be a poor choice for some patients. One category of patients that are poor candidates for permanent implants are those with no prior experience with soft-tissue augmentation. These patients may find that the contour or texture of the implant does not suit their face. With a non-biodegradable product, the only recourse is to surgically remove them (until the implant arrives that is adjustable using laser or radiofrequency). Since facial contours change with time (aging), placement of any type of permanent implant which does *not* also change will result in an implant that highlights rather than diminishes the signs of an aging face. The senior author, as well as others with a lot of experience using permanent fillers, know that his is an old wives tale and have never seen this to be a problem. In fact, these faces never age as much as untreated face and the patients always look good. They do need more products with advancing years.

Artefill/Artecoll

Artecoll (Artes Medical, San Diego, California, U.S.A.) is a permanent filler consisting of polymethylmethacrylate microspheres (PMMA) (Plexiglas beads) in collagen (microscopic homogenous polymethylmethacrylate beads in 3.5% collagen suspension, mixed with 0.3% lidocaine). At the present it is not approved by the FDA, although it has been approved by the FDA advisory panel so it may enter U.S. markets in the near future. In the United States, the bovine products must meet stringent FDA requirements and the product resulting from this closed American herd is known as Artefill. The European-sourced product is known as Artecoll.

PMMA, commonly called Plexiglas or Lucite, has been used in artificial eye lenses, dentures, and bone cement. The PMMA is polymerized into 30- to 40-μm spheres that are then suspended in the collagen. The collagen is degraded after injection, leaving the PMMA spheres to remain permanently. The company claims that theses spheres cannot migrate as they are encapsulated by the patient's own tissue in two to four months.

Artecoll is injected through a 27-gauge 0.5-inch needle using a threading or tunneling technique at the junction between the dermis and subcutaneous tissue. If it is inadvertently injected high up in the dermis, the skin will blanch and the injection should be stopped immediately—as small nodules can form and prolonged erythema can occur. It is then massaged and molded with the fingers. Two treatment sessions should be used so as not to overcorrect during implantation. Patients should be advised to minimize facial expressions for three days after treatment to reduce the likelihood of muscular contraction pushing the substance more deeply into the subcutaneous tissue. Since Artecoll contains collagen, the product must be refrigerated.

Artecoll is contraindicated in people with thin skin, as it can be palpable or visible after implantation. Patients can experience swelling, redness, and pain over the first few days. Granulomas, some occurring more than 10 years after injection, have been reported. These respond nicely to intralesional injections of 40 mg/cc triamcinolone and often disappear over time by themselves. Similar to injecting Sculptra or really any other filler, if a clog is encountered do not apply more forceful pressure. Pull the needle out of the skin, point the syringe away from yourself and your patient, pull back on the plunger and then push the clog out. Long-lasting redness can occur when the injection is too superficial, and itching can occur and persist for weeks to months.

The FDA panel on fillers has recommended approval for cosmetic use. The FDA has said it will approve this substance when certain manufacturing issues are addressed. We do not yet know if the FDA will require skin testing prior to injection.

Gore-Tex

Gore-Tex (W.L. Gore and Associates, Flagstaff, Arizona, U.S.A.) is a permanent filling substance made of expanded polytetrafluoroethylene (ePTFE) created by the extrusion of Teflon. Nodules of ePTFE are connected by a multidirectional fibril structure to make a polymer. This soft and pliable polymer comes in sheets, patches, and tubes of varying sizes. It has been used in the body since 1971, including abdominal wall and hernia repairs and has been used for skin augmentation since 1991. It is inert and non-allergenic with low tissue reactivity and minimal capsule formation. Its 20- to 30-μm pores allow tissue to grow into and anchor the material, although that also makes it more difficult to remove. Softform is a tubular form of Gore-Tex that comes prepackaged in a trocar to be used in the nasolabial folds and the vermilion border of the lips. After implantation, fibroblastic tissue grows into these tubes within six months and anchors them in place.

After anesthetizing the implantation site, a hollow trocar is used to tunnel subcutaneously through the deepest part of the fold. The implant is then pulled through by dragging back with the trocar, needle or suture and then trimming excess ePTFE. The 3- to 5-mm incision sites are then sutured. Collagen can be layered over this material if more correction is needed.

An advantage of Gore-Tex is that it is stored at room temperature. The disadvantages are many: the implantation is a surgical procedure rather than an injection, the material may become palpable and once implanted, it may migrate. As with any non-biodegradable implant, removal of Gore Tex can be very difficult and involves a surgical procedure that may be complicated by fibrosis. Because of the complications associated with this product, it has not gained widespread acceptance in the cosmetic community.

Silicone

The silicone oil that is used today is Silikon 1000 (Alcon Laboratories, Fort Worth, Texas, U.S.A.) which has a density of 1000 centistokes. The original Dow Corning silicone was 350 centistokes. It is FDA-approved but its use is off-label for wrinkles and scars. It is a purified product as it has been FDA-approved for retinal detachment and has been used for lipoatrophy seen in patients with AIDS. Problems seen in the past were usually due to too much volume injected or adulteration of the fluid with substances such as mineral oil. Silikon 1000 is a sterile, clear, colorless gel that is relatively inert. There are no preservatives or other ingredients. It is distributed in 10-cc vials with 8.5 cc of sterile silicone oil that can be stored at room temperature. Silikon 1000 may be used for off-label use, but as it is a device and not a drug, the physician may not advertise its use in the office, the phonebook, a web site, or the media.

A microdroplet serial injection technique is used to inject silicone oil. Multiple treatments are necessary at intervals of four to six weeks or more, and results may not be apparent for two to three treatments. A 1-cc luer-lock syringe is used and attached to a 27-gauge needle or the RJ Flo 30-gauge, large-bore needle that patients find more comfortable (order 978-532-0666).

Silicone oil is an ideal filling substance in many ways because it is permanent, needs no skin testing as there are no antibodies to liquid silicone, is stored at room temperature, does not support bacterial growth, can be used to treat many areas, is not painful when an anesthetic cream is used before injection and a modified dental block is used for the lips, and does not cause post-injection morbidity. It is relatively inexpensive and has a long shelf life. Granulomas and other side-effects are extremely rare when the proper volume of unadulterated purified silicone is used.

FILLER COMPLICATIONS

In addition to problems such as poor patient selection, inappropriate product placement and injection of an inappropriate product, there are several other potential complications that merit discussion including: infection, sensitivity, necrosis, and embolization.

Infection is one complication that is rare but is a potentially serious risk when injecting soft-tissue augmentation products. Meticulous handling of the material as well as adequate site preparation make the risk of infection very low. However, one should consider the potential for long-term infection with either bacterial, fungal or atypical mycobacterial organisms when injecting patients, especially those that may be colonized by resistant organisms or with impaired immunologic states. Other types of infections that may be seen with any injection include herpes simples virus in those individuals predisposed to outbreaks.

Sensitivity to a given material is another consideration when performing soft-tissue augmentation. Depending on the material used, this risk is quite low. Management of an allergic reaction depends on the nature and severity of the reaction but there is ample literature to suggest that these reactions do occur.

One of the most serious reactions that may occur is *necrosis* of the skin. Typically, this is seen with thicker products which may to either compress blood vessels or, via direct intravascular injection, occlude them. Painless blanching or bruising of the immediate area of injection is the first sign of injection necrosis caused by dermal fillers. Over the next two to three days, the skin usually appears dusky then black. An eschar of necrotic skin soon develops over an ulcer. The area most prone to this appears to be the glabella and use of certain products (such as Zyplast and Cosmoplast) should be considered risky in these areas. It is reasonable to assume that other products with similar physical properties will pose similar risks for the glabellar area.

Embolization of material is another risk when injecting soft-tissue augmentation products. This risk may be minimized although not entirely avoided by withdrawing the hub of the needle prior to insertion of any product. When injecting around the densely vascular periorbital regions, care should be taken to inject slowly and to avoid obvious vessels.

If vascular compromise occurs or there is concern for impending necrosis, one of the authors (JLC) has suggested a protocol that can be used to treat this complication (Dermatologic Surgery, in press). In short if a significant area of blanching occurs while injecting, immediately discontinue the injection and gently massage the treated area. Encourage quick vasodilation to restore blood supply to the area through the immediate application of hot/warm water gauze. This simple and accessible measure can stimulate an immediate mild vasodilation. The application of nitroglycerine paste (which should be kept on hand in the office) can be used for a more significant vasodilation.

CONCLUSION

In conclusion, we are at an exciting time for injectable soft-tissue augmentation products. New injectables are being approved every few months, and the market demand for fillers continues to grow. To ensure success, esthetic physicians must have a keen understanding of the virtues of each product so that we can guide our patients to successful outcomes. Appropriate product selection together with meticulous technique allows us to best meet our patients' expectations.

BIBLIOGRAPHY

Amar RE. Microinfiltration adipocytaire (MIA) au niveau de la face, ou restructuration tissulaire par greffe de tissu adipeux. Ann Chir Plast Esthet 1999; 44:593–608.

Baumann LS, Kerdel F. The treatment of bovine collagen allergy with cyclosporin. Dermatol Surg 1999; 25:247.

Carruthers A, Carruthers J. HIV-associated facial lipoatrophy. Dermatol Surg 2002; 28:979–986.

Coleman SR. Facial recontouring with lipostructure. Clin Plast Surg 1997; 24:347–367.

Cooperman LS, MacKinnon V, Bechler G, Pharriss BB. Injectable collagen: six years' clinical investigation. Aesthetic Plast Surg 1985; 9:145–151.

Duranti F, Salti G, Bovani B, Calandra M, Rosati ML. Injectable hyaluronic acid gel for soft-tissue augmentation. A clinical and histological study. Dermatol Surg 1998; 24:1317–1325 (One of the large clinical studies of Restylane).

Elson ML. Soft tissue augmentation techniques: update on available materials. Cosmet Dermatol 1999; 12(5):13–15.

Elson ML. The role of skin testing in the use of collagen injectable materials. J Dermatol Surg Oncol 1989; 15:301.

Friedman PM, Mafong EA, Kauvar AN, Geronemus RG. Safety data of injectable nonanimal stabilized hyaluronic acid gel for soft tissue augmentation. Dermatol Surg 2002; 28(6):491–494 (A review of the worldwide adverse event database of Q Med Aesthetics for Restylane).

Hanke CW, Coleman WP. Cosmetic Surgery of the Skin. St Louis, MO: Mosby-Year Book, 1997:217.

Jones DH, Carruthers A, Orentreich D, et al. Highly purified 100-est silicone oil for treatment of human immunodeficiency virus-associated facial lipoatrophy: an open pilot trial. Dermatol Surg 2004; 30:1279.

Klein AW. Bonfire of the wrinkles. J Dermtol Surg Oncol 1991; 17:543–544.

Klein AW. In favor of double testing. J Dermatol Surg Oncol 1989; 15:263.

Klein AW, Elson ML. The history of substances for soft tissue augmentation. Dermatol Surg 2000; 26:1096–1105.

Knapp TR, Kaplan EN, Daniels JR. Injectable collagen for soft tissue augmentation. Plast Reconstruct Surg 1977; 60:389–405.

Lemperle G. Artecoll augmentation of wrinkles and acne scars. In: Klein AW, ed. Tissue Augmentation in Clinical Practice: Procedures and Techniques. 2nd ed. New York: Marcel Dekker, 2003.

Lemperle G, Hazan-Gauthier N, Lemperle M. PMMA microspheres (Artecoll) for skin and soft tissue augmentation. Part II. Clinical investigation. Plast Reconstr Surg 1995; 92:331.

Lemperle G, Ott H, Charrier U, Hecker J, Lemperle M. PMMA microspheres (Artecoll) for intradermal implantation. Part I. Animal research. Ann Plast Surg 1991; 26:57.

Lemperle G, Romano JJ, Busso M. Soft tissue augmentation with Artecoll: 10-year history, indications, technique, and potential side effects. Dermatol Surg 2003; 28:573–587.

Lowe NJ, Maxwell A, Lowe P, Duick MG, Shah K. Hyaluronic acid fillers: adverse reactions and skin testing. J Am Acad Dermatol 2001; 45:930–933 (A report of side effects occurring from Restylane at one site).

Lupton JR, Alster TS. Cutaneous hypersensitivity reaction to injectable hyaluronic acid gel. Dermatol Surg 2000; 26(2):135–137 (A case report of a hypersensitivity after a patient's third treatment session using Restylane).

Matti BA, Nicolle FV. Clinical use of Zyplast in correction of age and disease-related contour deficiencies of the face. Aesthetic Plast Surg 1990; 14:227–234.

McClelland M, Egbert B, Hanko V, Berg RA, DeLustro F. Evaluation of Artecoll polymethylmethacrylate implant for soft-tissue augmentation: biocompatibility and chemical characterization. Plast Reconstr Surg 1997; 100:1466.

Micheels P. Human anti-hyaluronic acid antibodies: is it possible? Dermatol Surg 2001; 27(2):185–191 (Clinical study of

Restylane and Hylaform use, including intradermal testing, biopsy and serum antibodies).

Narins RS, Brandt F, Leyden J, Lorenc ZP, Rubin M, Smith S. A randomized, double-blind, multicenter comparison of the efficacy and tolerability of restylane versus zyplast for the correction of nasolabial folds. Dermatol Surg 2003; 29(6):588–595 (A head-to-head comparison of the clinical efficacy and persistence of Restylane versus Zyplast).

Olenius M. The first clinical study using a new biodegradable implant for the treatment of lips, wrinkles, and folds. Aesthetic Plast Surg 1998; 22:97–101 (One of the large clinical studies of Restylane).

Pollack SV. Some new injectable dermal filler materials: Hylaform, Restylane, and Artecoll. J Cutan Med Surg 1999; 3(Suppl 4):27–35 (Great discussion on hylan fillers and specific implantation techniques).

Siegle RJ, McCoy JP, Schade W, et al. Intradermal implantation of bovine collagen. Humoral immune responses associated with clinical reactions. Arch Dermatol 1984; 120:183.

Stegman SJ, Tromovitch TA. Implantation of collagen for depressed scars. J Dermatol Surg Oncol 1980; 6:450–453.

Valantin M, Aubron-Olivier C, Ghosn J, et al. Polylactic acid implants (New-fill) to correct facial lipoatrophy in HIV-infected patients: results of the open-label study. VEGA 2003; 17:2471–2477.

71

Injectable Fluid Silicone

David S. Orentreich
Mt. Sinai School of Medicine, New York, New York, U.S.A.

Norman Orentreich
New York University School of Medicine, New York, New York, U.S.A.

An ideal biocompatible soft-tissue augmentation implant should fulfill certain criteria.

1. Easily obtainable by qualified persons at reasonable cost
2. Capable of fabrication in the form desired
3. Capable of repeated sterilization and prolonged storage at room temperature
4. Easily implanted
5. Self-limiting fibroblastic response
6. Not physically modified by soft tissue
7. Chemically inert
8. Does not invoke inflammation or foreign body reaction
9. Does not produce amaurosis when injected into facial skin
10. Nontoxic
11. Noncarcinogenic
12. Nonteratogenic
13. Produces no state of allergy or hypersensitivity
14. Capable of resisting mechanical strains
15. Physical consistency of treated tissue indistinguishable from normal tissue
16. Long-term persistence of tissue contour restoration
17. Not subject to latent degenerative or calcific changes
18. Persistence in the originally deposited location with minimal or no absorption even with movement of the part

Satisfying these ideal specifications, polydimethylsiloxane fluid of 350 centistokes (cs) is, at present, the safest and most efficacious of all available autogenous and nonautogenous tissue-compatible materials for lifelong dermal and subdermal injection within the human body. Except for number 8 listed above, silicone fluid fulfills these criteria. With rare exception, pure, filtered, sterilized silicone fluid ("injectable-grade") provokes inflammation or foreign-body reaction only to the desirable extent of producing intentional beneficial fibroplasia and hence soft tissue augmentation.

One additional criterion, that of a substance with low abuse potential, is conspicuous by its absence from the foregoing list. Any device, drug, surgical instrument—indeed any tool in the physician's armamentarium—has the potential to be used incorrectly. This does not and should not prevent the training of competent doctors to use tools that enable them to treat disease and correct deformity. This chapter describes the proper use of injectable fluid silicone, but it is in no way a substitute for hands-on training under the careful supervision of a physician experienced in the proper administration of injectable fluid silicone.

DEFINITIONS AND CHEMISTRY

Silicone, a term introduced at the turn of the century by the chemist F. S. Kipping of Nottingham, England, is a generic designation for a family of polymers based on the element silicon. These polymers range from fluids of different viscosities to semisolid (gel) and solid states.

Siloxane is a mnemonic acronym derived from *sil*icon, *ox*ygen, and meth*ane*. Siloxane refers to any one of a class of chemical compounds composed of chains of alternate silicon and oxygen atoms with hydrocarbon groups or hydrogen atoms alone bonded to the silicon. Polyorganosiloxanes $(-R_2SiO-)_x$ are siloxane polymers with organic radicals (R), among which is injectable-grade fluid silicone. Dimethylsiloxane polymers are large molecules of repetitive units $[-(CH_3)_2SiO-]_x$ with viscosities that are a function of the extent of polymerization, which is designated by the subscript x (Table 1; Fig. 1).

The injectable-grade liquid silicone most thoroughly evaluated for use in soft-tissue augmentation is poly dimethylsiloxane with the subscript x having an average value of 130. Although the average value of x for fluid silicone with a viscosity of 350 cs[a] at 25°C is 130, there is *a range of polymer* lengths from the 10s to the 100s. The viscosity of fluid silicone is constant within the range of human body temperature: once injected, silicone fluid does not harden or soften.

Industrial or electrical-grade 350 cs fluid silicone is manufactured by Dow Corning Corporation and is called 200 silicone fluid. It is relatively unpurified and unsuitable for any medical purpose. Dow Corning 200 fluid 350 cs food grade is, however, suitable for human ingestion.

A more purified (nonsterile) grade known as Dow Corning medical-grade 360 liquid silicone (350 cs) was developed in the 1960s. Medical-grade 360 fluid is principally

---

[a] A centistoke is 1/100 of a stoke. A stoke is the cgs (centimeter-gram-second) unit of kinematic viscosity; it is that of a fluid with a viscosity of 1 poise and a density of lg/cm^3. A *poise* is a cgs absolute unit of viscosity that is equal to 1 dyne-second/cm^2. A *dyne* is the unit of force in the cgs system that is equal to the force that gives a free mass of 1 g an acceleration of 1 cm/sec.

Table 1 Relation of Polymer Length to Viscosity of Silicone

Number of dimethyl-siloxane units	Viscosity (cs)	Similar to
2	0.65	Water
10	26.0	
70	100.0	
130	350.0	Mineral oil
160	500.0	
260	1,000.0	
500	12,500.0	Jelly (thick)

used for lubricating disposable hypodermic needles and syringes, coating the inside of containers for medicinals and blood products, and as an emollient in protective skin lotions. This grade was designed to be inserted in the body. It was, however, not initially planned for soft-tissue augmentation, although it was used for this purpose in the United States and other countries. In 1965, Dow Corning Corporation developed a still more highly purified form of the liquid silicone to be used in clinical investigations authorized by the Food and Drug Administration (FDA). This material, which contained fewer heavy metals and other impurities, was 350 cs, sterilized, and labeled MDX 4-4011. The investigational new drug application (NDA) was withdrawn in 1976, for corporate business reasons, even though MDX 4-4011 was found to be safe and effective for injection. Nevertheless, before, during, and after the investigation, material of inferior quality probably did find its way into the hands of physicians and nonprofessionals who injected it into patients.

Due to the ambiguity of the term "medical-grade," the term "injectable-grade" fluid silicone is designated for polydimethylsiloxane fluid of known viscosity (350 cs) that has been filtered and sterilized to remove heavy metals, low-chain-length polymers, and other impurities, to produce a chemically pure product free of paniculate matter suitable for human soft tissue implantation. Injectable-grade fluid silicone is clear, colorless, odorless, tasteless, nonvolatile, and has an oily feel. The fluid is hydrophobic, insoluble in alcohols, and completely soluble in ether and aromatic and chlorinated solvents. Fluid silicone is chemically unaltered by prolonged storage at room temperature or exposure to air, and by most chemicals, sunlight, or microorganisms. Silicone fluid can be contaminated by contact with some rubbers from which it will leach out irritating chemicals, such as agerite alba (monobenzyl ether of hydroquinone). Wide-range thermal stability allows repeated steam autoclaving or dry heat sterilization under standard conditions without significant alteration. Silicone should never be gas-sterilized because of its absorptive properties.

Steam autoclaving may produce a harmless milky color due to accretion of water. It is not necessary to refrigerate silicone; it may be stored at room temperature.

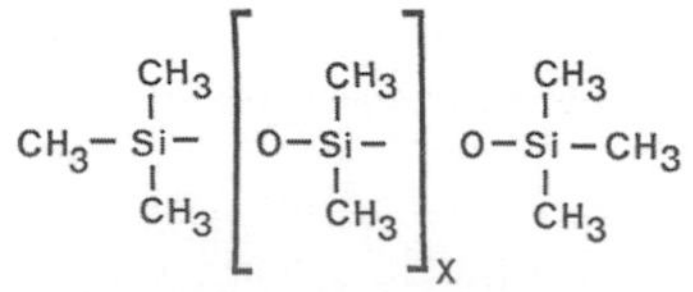

A variety of silicone fluids for soft tissue augmentation have been used since 1952 (Fig. 2). One of the authors (N.O.) participated in the investigational NDA filed in 1965 with the FDA by the Dow Corning Center for Aid to Medical Research, Midland, Michigan.

The basic record to date, apart from the cosmetic improvements and the psychosocial benefits, is one of safety, without serious flaw in approximately 1400 patients under continuous study. Of these patients, half were treated and evaluated by the authors. The beneficial results achieved during the organized study have been substantiated over a 35-year period in patients treated in the years before and after. The results obtained with injectable-grade material and proper (microdroplet) techniques of injection must not, however, be confused with those arising from the use of impure (adulterated) "silicone fluid" and improperly performed injections of large volumes which can result in complications.

BACKGROUND OF CONTROVERSY

Between 1900 and 1935, impure paraffins (mineral oil) were injected for the elevation of facial furrows and depressed contours, augmentation of ocular orbits, correction of saddle-nose deformities, and enlargement of breasts. During the 1940s, paraffins were injected subcutaneously into the scalp for the treatment of male pattern baldness. This procedure took place in Los Angeles, and its rationale was to increase circulation to the hair follicles by loosening an excessively tight scalp. Months and sometimes years later, nodules, plaques, and ulcerations developed at the sites of paraffin deposition. Inflammatory (erysipelas like) responses were also observed, occasionally accompanied by systemic toxicity and fever. Histologic changes in these so-called paraffinomas were in the nature of oil cysts, inflammatory and granulomatous alterations, and eventual extensive fibrosis.

Soft-tissue depositions of animal, vegetable, and mineral oils and various fatty acids, as expected, produce

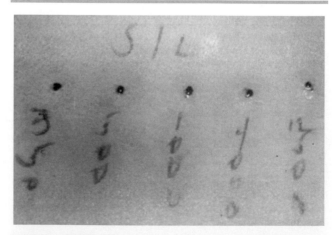

Figure 2 In 1964, 0.2 mL volumes of fluid silicones ranging in viscosity from 350 to 12,000 cs were injected intradermally and subdermally and then each site was tattooed. The response to all viscosities was equal: slight palpable augmentation with no untoward results. All sites were biopsied five years after injection and all showed the persistent presence of silicone.

Figure 1 Linear molecular structure of poly dimethylsiloxane: There are trimethysiloxy units at each end and repetitive dimethylsiloxy units in between. Viscosity is directly related to chain length (Table 1), that is, to the value of x in the above formula.

paraffin-like granulomatous responses. This has been found with camphorated oil, cottonseed oil, sesame oil, fish oil, cod liver oil, beeswax, and a melange of similar substances. The injection of a large volume of liquid paraffin or other oils at one time results in its migration along tissue cleavage planes of least resistance. This adverse effect is compounded in certain places by muscular propulsion of the fluid materials. With the introduction of liquid silicone injections into soft tissues, the already well-recognized physiologic inertness of the pure material often prompted the misguided addition of irritant oils in order to "lock" large volumes of injected silicone into the sites of deposition by induced fibrous encapsulation. Such mixtures were often simply referred to as "silicone." Silicone mixed with 1% sesame oil or 1% oleic acid was used in the California treatments.

Silicone fluids of various viscosities, sometimes containing a variety of additives, were injected directly into skin, subcutaneous tissue, and especially breasts by Japanese, German, and Swiss practitioners who had been using these materials since the 1940s. Clinical reports in the Japanese literature of over 8000 cases claim favorable results, but details of long-term follow-up are not adequately documented. The Japanese experience is further complicated by the fact that one very large clinic practiced injections of a mixture of silicone and 1% "sweet oil" (olive oil). This "Japanese" or "Sakurai" formula was exported to California, where it was used extensively, especially for breast augmentation, in volumes of hundreds to a thousand or more milliliters per breast. This was declared illegal in interstate commerce and further importation of the product into the United States was prohibited by the FDA. In Mexico, a large number of people have received silicone/foreign material injections in different parts of the body.

Variations in the composition of "silicone" preparations and in the manner of injection, especially in augmentation of disallowed sites (mainly breasts), have led to misunderstandings about harmful results (Figs. 3 and 4A). For example, according to the Dow Corning Center for Aid to Medical Research, foreign-body reactions attributed to silicone were cases in which either the "Japanese" formula or another impure preparation had been used rather than pure injectable-grade silicone. This was established by extensive

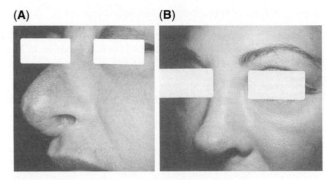

Figure 4 **(A)** Granulomatous nasal deformity about two years after the macrovolume injection of adulterated silicone intended to correct a poor result of rhinoplasty. **(B)** Marked improvement in the appearance of the nose following surgical revision for redundancy of skin (Dr. R. Webster) and two dermabrasions (Dr. N. Orentreich). This patient subsequently received injectable-grade silicone by the microvolume technique to facial rhytes without untoward results (Dr. N. Orentreich).

follow-up of all traceable cases. The injection of massive quantities of even pure silicone into breasts together with the trauma produced by a large needle most likely caused compression of fat with release of fatty acids, fat atrophy, and granulomatous or inflammatory reactions. Additional complications encountered after injection of materials into breasts, such as lymphedema, peau d'orange (Fig. 3), infection, and ulceration, could be related to factors other than inherent nonreactivity of tissues to fluid silicone. Foremost are mechanical compression of tissue and blockage of lymphatic channels. Nevertheless, apart from complications following injections into breasts or into other glandular tissues (the glandular nature being another aspect of unsuitability), to date there is no clear-cut evidence of serious, untoward sequelae from properly performed subcutaneous injections of injectable-grade silicone into other sites. We have injected atrophic cutaneous defects in skin overlying breasts with beneficial results and long-term safety.

Additives to silicone fluids, henceforth referred to as "adulterants," are but one factor beclouding the medical use of injectable-grade silicone. Putatively safe and effective materials touted for the augmentation of soft-tissue came to be administered in massive doses by unqualified individuals or charlatans who injected "secret formulas." The consequences were disastrous. Well-publicized fiascoes were misrepresented as resulting from the use of "silicone." In fact, some of the injected concoctions contained no polydimethylsiloxane at all.

The following letter to the editor of *Plastic and Reconstructive Surgery*, written in 1970 by S. Braley, the Director of the Dow Corning Center for Aid to Medical Research, indicates the degree to which the situation regarding silicone use had deteriorated:

> Sir:
> It is well known that some physicians have augmented soft tissue by the injection of silicone fluids to which adulterants have been added. The patient is generally told that the injected fluid is "silicone." Should any foreign-body reactions occur, they are attributed by the patient (and often by the original or subsequent physician) to the silicone. This is in spite of the fact that the adulterant is added for the express purpose of causing foreign-body reactions not obtainable from pure silicone fluid.

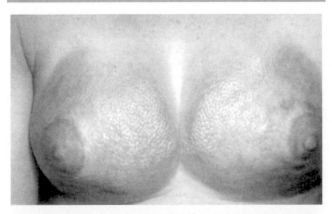

Figure 3 Lymphatic blockade in breasts after the injection of considerable amounts of "silicone." Information is lacking about adulterating additives and amount injected. Note the erythema and peau d'orange surface. An intradermal and subdermal skin test on this patient's abdomen with 0.1 mL of injectable-grade silicone fluid was observed for five years. There was no untoward response at the test sites.

We have now encountered 3 extreme cases of this.... Each of these 3 cases happened to be breast injections; the patients showed severe reactions to what they had been told were silicone injections. In each case, removal of all or portions of the breasts was necessary after extended efforts to reduce the pain, swelling, and nodules.

Portions of the excised tissue were sent to us for analysis. The analysis technique used for the detection of the silicone fluids in tissue is based upon the fact that the silicon-carbon bond is not found in nature. If, upon infrared analysis of an extract of the tissue, the presence of such bonds is seen, this is considered unequivocable evidence of the presence of a silicone. The test is accurate to about 0.1 percent and we use it extensively for tissue analysis. We cannot determine the source of silicone fluid, *nor can we determine if it was an adulterated silicone* [Emphasis added].

When 3 samples under discussion were tested in this manner, they showed *a complete absence of any silicone* [Emphasis added]; rather, the infrared curve obtained was from a linear hydrocarbon, most likely paraffin....

A glaring misstatement of silicone's effects was reported in the *New York Daily News*, February 4, 1983. An article entitled "Silicone Kills Eight" reported that transvestites seeking a womanly figure had injected themselves with an industrial silicone mixed with *laxatives*, which left 8 of them dead and another 30 deformed. A fourth-year engineering student had sold the material to the transvestites, one of whom died of cardiac arrest after an injection of two pints of the mixture into his buttocks.

In 35 years of administering injectable-grade polydimethylsiloxane fluid into approximately 100,000 patients in the authors' practice, there has never been one single allergic reaction. All patients who claimed to have had a reaction to "silicone" administered elsewhere, those who by physical examination had evidence of reaction to an injected implant material of undetermined composition, and those who desired proof and reassurance of safety, received a skin test with injectable-grade silicone. None of these patients has ever developed an untoward reaction at the test site before, during, or after treatment.

Except possibly for very rare, temporary, inflammatory, idiosyncratic reactions to injectable-grade silicone, major problems reported to have resulted from injections of liquid silicone are explainable by qualitative and quantitative factors of misuse and by injections into unsuitable locations, such as the glandular breast. Qualitative factors of misuse include intentional or accidental contamination of the fluid silicone. The main quantitative consideration is the injection of excessive amounts of fluid in a particular site at once or cumulatively.

CRITICAL ANALYSIS OF PUBLISHED PURPORTED "SILICONE" REACTIONS

Reviewing the literature on purported silicone reactions reveals several fundamental weaknesses. Proof is often lacking that the complications presented are due to dimethylpolysiloxane. Such proof would involve establishing the source of all the silicone used in each patient, its purity, the exact technique and frequency of injections, the amount injected each time, the exact location of each injection, the preparation of the skin prior to the injection, the use of any massage over the area after injection, and whether the "reaction" was associated with any concurrent systemic or local infection.

There is a fundamental weakness in any document based on a critique of complications occurring in patients treated by other physicians. Condemning an unknown agent as the cause of a serious complication solely on the basis of another physician's operative report or the label on a bottle is subject to errors of communication.

Common pitfalls in "silicone" reporting include:

1. Authors who report "complications," especially when observed in patients treated by another physician, and do not themselves independently establish the source and, more importantly, the purity of all silicone used in each patient.
2. Reports of adverse reactions to "silicone" in patients who received known (documented) adulterated material.
3. Absent or incomplete documentation of the method of skin preparation prior to silicone injection; technique of injection; location; frequency (interval between sessions); and volume of fluid injected.
4. No pathologic examination of tissues involved by the "reaction."
5. Analysis for silicone was not performed on pathologic tissues.
6. No analysis for "adulterants" in pathologic specimens.
7. No indication of whether the "reaction" was associated with any concurrent infection, systemic or local, such as adjacent furuncle or acute sinusitis.

Dr. Blocksma reported two patients, one with swelling and one with redness at the site of injection. In each case, the "reaction" developed several years after silicone injections and was associated with an adjacent furuncle in one and an acute sinusitis in the other. He suggested that tissues infiltrated with silicone fluid may have a decreased resistance to infection from adjacent lesions or via a bacteremia. While this sounds logical, and may be applicable to large-volume injections, we have not observed a decreased resistance to infection in tissue treated with injectable-grade silicone by the microdroplet injection technique.

In one report, the presence of concomitant infection was cited but overlooked as a possible pathogenic agent. In this case, "inflammatory episodes" occurred on the right cheek of a woman seven years after she received her last injection of 12 mL of silicone given in 0.5 to 2 mL increments over a four-year period. Apparently, the silicone was used to correct facial atrophy incurred after an episode of either Weber-Christian disease (relapsing febrile nodular nonsuppurative panniculitis) or atypical mycobacteria (Runyon group 3) infection. The atypical mycobacteria were "noted" from the facial lesions one year prior to commencement of silicone injections. The patient was treated with *p*-aminosalicylic acid and isoniazid for several months. Primary skin disease due to *Mycobacterium avium-intracellulare* (Runyon group 3 mycobacteria) has been reported in rare instances. A chronic, slowly progressive skin condition of many years' duration has been described. Where feasible, surgical treatment is advised since the organism seems to be poorly susceptible to chemotherapeutic agents. Silicone injections into the infected cheek area may have been coincidental with a recrudescence of the mycobacterial infection.

A 33-year-old Asian woman, who 12 years earlier had undergone bilateral breast augmentation in Thailand with injections of an undocumented substance, developed an *M. avium-intracellulare* infection. Mycobacterial cultures of material obtained from bronchial washings, incision, and drainage of the right breast, and pilar lymph node biopsy were all positive. Although the title of the report was "*M. avium* infection in a silicone-injected breast," there was no analysis of the liquid evacuated from the involved breast for silicone, adulterants, or paraffin. These two reports suggest that *M. avium-intracellulare*, either by needle introduction or via a bacteremia, may be capable of infecting tissue into which a fluid implant material was injected.

Another pitfall is that the "complications" were caused by overinjection of an excessive volume at a single sitting.

In 1977, Wilkie reported his 10-year experience with injections of silicone into 92 patients, of whom 13 developed "granulomas." Eight of the 13 "granulomas" occurred within the first 12 months. From the data and observations reported, several conclusions can be drawn. The purity of silicone used was in question. The intradermal injection technique he used in some patients could explain the chronic pink discoloration of the overlying skin. The fanning technique used may have made precise placement and microdroplet injection difficult and resulted in pooling along needle tracts. The volumes injected per site were probably excessive (up to 1.0 mL). Injection intervals of two weeks are usually too short. The swellings shown in the photographs of the reported patients are compatible with classic overcorrection almost certainly due to overinjection of silicone. Pathologic findings were consistent with a tissue response to an undetermined foreign material.

In one case, approximately 4 mL was injected into the frown lines over a 10-week period. This amount is approximately 13 times that routinely used to treat frown lines over a comparable period of time (0.1 mL per session for three sessions spaced at monthly intervals for a total of 0.3 mL).

Poor results may be caused by injecting sites too frequently, e.g., intervals of one to two weeks. An untoward reaction may be caused by injection of contraindicated sites, such as the eyelids and breasts, or reactions attributed to "silicone" may most likely have been caused by subsequent treatment with agents such as intralesional triamcinolone acetonide, which by themselves may have been responsible for the reported "complication."

In reviewing the literature of purported reactions to "silicone," we found that no cases were substantiated by appropriate fundamental intradermal skin testing to the material actually used on the patient for augmentation and by a control skin test of injectable-grade silicone. In the authors' experience, when patients with alleged "silicone" reactions are seen, they have never had a positive skin test reaction to injectable-grade silicone.

Failure to distinguish fact from fiction in the "silicone" literature creates confusion regarding silicone's safety and efficacy and leads to the drawing of unjustified conclusions.

CURRENT STATUS OF INJECTABLE FLUID SILICONE FOR SOFT-TISSUE AUGMENTATION

Silicone microdroplet injection therapy is of recognized therapeutic value. Dating back 35 years, this treatment has wide support in the clinical and medical literature. Subcutaneous injections of filling material (e.g., silicone) are specifically included in the *Physicians' Current Procedural Terminology* (Nos. 11950–11954), a comprehensive listing of medical and surgical procedures prepared by the American Medical Association in 1985.

Only one commercial manufacturer (Dow Corning Corporation) completed an FDA application for approval to market liquid injectable silicone as a medical device for soft tissue augmentation. The FDA did not have an opportunity to act on this application since the corporation withdrew it in 1976. At that time Dow Corning Corporation issued a statement that the study showed the product to be safe and effective. Because of the need for the material for use in severe facial defects, especially in children, the FDA allowed the study to be continued and the material to be supplied by Dow Corning Corporation to physicians for this purpose. On October 25, 1979 the FDA Bureau of Devices gave written investigational drug evaluation approval to the University of California, San Francisco (UCSF), Department of Ophthalmology, Dr. Walter Stern, to evaluate the use of 1000 cs silicone fluid for replacement of the vitreous of the eye as a part of the treatment for vitrectomy. In the early 1980s, the University of California, Los Angeles, Department of Ophthalmology, Dr. Steven Ryan, joined the original sponsor (UCSF) and the investigation became a joint study. However, liquid silicone has been approved by the FDA for many years for other purposes [e.g., as a lubricant for disposable syringes and needles and for human ingestion in Pharmaceuticals and foodstuffs (simethicone)].

The Food, Drug and Cosmetic Act permits physicians to use for therapeutic purposes medical devices made to a physician's order (custom devices) and intended to meet the special needs of his or her practice. In the circumstances of medical practice, the use of liquid silicone complies with these provisions of the Food, Drug and Cosmetic Act.

TISSUE RESPONSE TO DEPOSITIONS OF SMALL VOLUMES

Soft-tissue reaction to depositions of small volumes of fluid silicone (equal to or less than 0.1 mL) is slight when they are properly injected in single treatments. Injectable-grade silicone elicits less physiologic reactivity than almost any other foreign material, though in a strict and desirable sense it is not absolutely biologically inert.

The combination of puncture with a needle and deposition of silicone results in early migration of polymorphonuclear leukocytes to the area, followed in several days by a moderate infiltrate composed mainly of small round cells. The infiltrate largely dissipates in about six months. Slight phagocytic activity is evident even later by the presence of macrophages in limited numbers and banal giant cells, which do not proliferate or agglomerate into gross granulomatous nodules.

At first, small globules of fluid silicone deposited at the dermal-subcutaneous interface displace connective tissue bundles and thus are surrounded by pseudocapsules of preexistent collagen. Later, a microscopically observable thin-walled collagen capsule forms around tiny globules of silicone. Deposition of initially large or cumulatively large volumes produces many "honeycomb" cysts lined by opaque and thicker capsules.

The eventual tissue response to silicone is fibroblastic, resulting in increased collagen deposition localized to the immediate surrounding area. The production of collagen by fibroblasts coupled with the mass displacement of dermal connective tissue by the silicone microdroplets corrects the contour defect. This fibrosis is self-limited and does not become extensive even with deposition of large volumes, provided that lymphatics and blood vessels have not been compressed. The limited, rather constant, and predictable degree of fibroplasia is especially beneficial for optimal

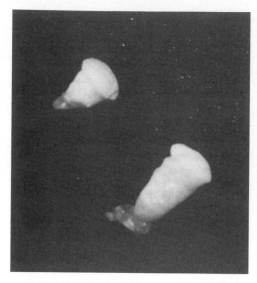

Figure 5 A site on the medial aspect of an arm was injected with 0.2 mL of injectable-grade silicone. One year later, this site and an untreated adjacent site were punch excised. Collagen augmentation in the treated site (specimen on the right) is obvious.

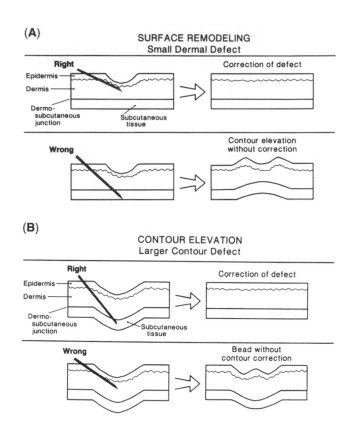

Figure 6 (**A**) Surface remodeling applies to augmentation by relatively superficial (i.e., intradermal) injection of fluid silicone. Top shows correct and bottom shows incorrect technique. (**B**) Contour elevation applies to subdermal injections of fluid silicone that alter facial contours. Top shows correct and bottom shows incorrect technique.

augmentation by the introduction of microdroplets of silicone fluid (about 0.005–0.01 mL) utilizing the technique of serial punctures (Fig. 5). Antibodies to silicone have never been demonstrated and true adjuvant disease has never been provoked.

INDICATIONS AND RELATIVE VOLUME REQUIREMENTS

When using the microdroplet serial (multiple) puncture technique, each needle puncture and injection deposits between 0.005 and 0.01 mL of injectable-grade fluid silicone (a "microdroplet"). As a basis for comparison, the average treatment session for a middle-aged woman with facial rhytes requires between 0.50 and 0.75 mL of silicone fluid. Injection of this volume entails between 50 and 150 individual needle punctures and would suffice to treat the neck, labial commissure grooves, nasolabial lines, malar grooves, crow's feet, frown lines, and forehead lines. Treatment sessions are usually repeated at intervals of one month or longer until the desired degree of augmentation is achieved. The number of sessions will, of course, depend on the degree of dermal atrophy and the individual's fibroplastic response.

Depositing silicone at different depths in the skin may produce either desirable or undesirable effects (Fig. 6). Excess intradermal injection of silicone into skin of normal thickness will usually produce a "beading" effect, especially when the skin overlies bone (i.e., forehead); visible beading is to be avoided. However, certain scars and rhytes lack dermal thickness; in these circumstances, controlled intradermal injection is preferable and produces the precise desired augmentation (microelevation). If silicone were injected at the deeper dermal-subcutaneous interface under these same defects, a less optimal correction would usually result. We apply the term *surface remodeling* to augmentation by the relatively superficial (i.e., intradermal) injection of fluid silicone with the express purpose of obtaining a smoother skin surface (Fig. 6A). Examples of surface remodeling are augmentation of depressed (broad and atrophic) acne scars and chickenpox scars.

Conversely, with depressions and rhytes, where skin of normal thickness overlies subcutaneous tissue of less than desirable depth, it is preferable to deposit the silicone just below the dermis. (Intradermal injection in these cases may produce undesirable beading.) This type of augmentation is called *contour elevation*: subdermal injections of fluid silicone that alter facial contours but minimally change surface skin topography (Fig. 6B). Examples of contour elevation are augmentation of nasolabial folds, malar grooves, and zygomatic arch.

Scars

Fluid silicone may be injected to lift depressed scars that result from various causes (Fig. 7), provided they are not bound down by strong fibrous adhesions. The silicone fluid is incapable of freeing up the strong adhesions surrounding and underlying bound-down defects. Attempted elevation of an unyielding, bound-down scar, such as the "ice pick" scars of acne vulgaris, will force silicone fluid into surrounding skin and produce a "doughnut effect," making the depression still more pronounced. "Ice pick" scars are best treated by other modalities (i.e., punch excision with or without full-thickness autologous skin grafting). The broad distensible atrophic scars that are the aftermath of acne, neurotic and psychopathic excoriations, adventitious trauma, varicella, microbial infection, scarring dermatoses, conventional surgery, and skin grafting can effectively be raised to skin-surface level. For a depression less than 1 cm^2, a small total volume (less than 0.5 mL) of silicone injected in two or three repeated treatments usually suffices.

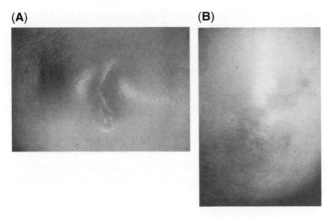

(A) **(B)**

Figure 7 **(A)** Persistent atrophy of the scalp following local injection of a suspension of an adrenocorticosteroid for treatment of alopecia areata. **(B)** Elevation of the depression to normal surface level after three injections of 0.2 mL injectable-grade silicone at monthly intervals.

Depressed scars stand out because scar edges cast shadows by blocking incident visible light. Raising the scars out of the shadows results in major cosmetic improvement. Surface characteristics of scar tissue, such as hyper- or hypopigmentation, telangiectasia, and adnexal pore size, are usually unaffected by silicone augmentation. Some bound-down chicken pox scars respond poorly to silicone. In certain discolored pox scars, the skin's contour may be improved; however, the color match may not be optimal, and further correction may require other therapeutic modalities.

Rhytes

For age-associated furrows or sunken contours of the face, small to moderate volumes injected beneath the depressions (up to a few milliliters per region divided in repeated treatments) suffice for acceptable cosmetic correction (Fig. 8). For furrows on the forehead and depressions in skin closely stretched over bony or cartilaginous prominences, each deposition is optimally 0.005 to 0.01 mL. Small volumes are effective for the vertical and oblique "frown lines" in the glabellar region (Fig. 9) and for deep wrinkles elsewhere on the face. The amount injected in the glabellae needs to be controlled to avoid a general fullness that may develop in

the area. Nasolabial folds can be lifted by repeated injections of silicone using a total volume of a few milliliters (Fig. 10). Care must be taken not to inject laterally into cheek tissue that is already relatively full. Doing so would cause further protrusion and accentuate the nasolabial folds. Lateral tissue bulge, should it inadvertently be incurred, may be reduced by subcutaneous injection of triamcinolone acetonide, 2.5 to 5 mg/mL, evenly dispersed (e.g., 0.05–0.1 mL aliquots) at 0.5 to 1.0 cm intervals.

Sunken facial contours on the upper cheeks, such as the malar groove, can be effectively augmented. Suitable augmentation of facial eminences (brow, malar including zygomatic arch, and angle of the mandible) can also be achieved. Volumes should be kept small for depressed planes on the lower portion of the face to avoid accentuation of the jowls. Cutaneous pores are not visibly altered by injection of small amounts of underlying fluid silicone.

A few patients develop "beading" at augmentation sites even after all precautions have been followed. In such cases, the effect is often temporary; the papulation subsides in ensuing months or may be reduced with locally injected suspensions of triamcinolone acetonide (2.5–5 mg/mL).

Eyes

Some cosmetic improvement may be achieved in periorbital crow's feet wrinkles. Great care and caution must be taken to inject very small quantities of fluid silicone. Use of the silicone tattooing technique may be appropriate for these superficial wrinkles.

Many adults' eyelid skin has developed fine lines characteristic of actinic and chronologic aging. Except in special circumstances, eyelid skin is too thin and swells (augments) too easily to be a suitable site for silicone-induced soft tissue augmentation. Eyelid deformities were reported in patients who received unknown quantities of adulterated material. Eyelid rhytes are usually better treated with blepharoplasty and resurfacing techniques such as chemical peel or dermabrasion rather than soft tissue replacement. On the other hand, atrophy of eyelid skin (traumatic scarring and linear scleroderma) has been successfully corrected with microdroplet (0.005 mL) injections of silicone fluid.

Dark "circles" under the eyes are a common cosmetic complaint. They can first appear in patients in their early 20s and generally intensify with age. Several factors contribute to their development. The fat pads of the lower eyelids

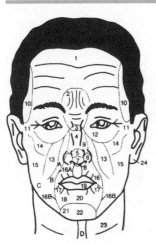

RHYTES:
1 Forehead furrows
2 Glabella "frown lines" (verticle and oblique)
3 Radix (horizontal) furrows
4 Dorsum of nose
5 Tip of nose
6 Ala
7 Columella
8 Columella - labial junction
9 Lateral nasal wall
10 Temple

11 Periorbital ("crow's feet") creases
12 Infra-orbital groove (dark "circle" under the eye)
13 Malar groove
14 Malar eminence (including zygomatic arch)
15 Cheek
16A Upper nasolabial (cheek-lip) groove
16B Lower nasolabial (cheek-lip) groove
17 Labial commisure groove

18 Lips (perioral radial creases)
19 Vermilion
20 Chin-lower lip groove
21 Chin-cheek groove
22 Chin
23 Neck
24 Earlobe
REDUNDANCIES:
A Nasolabial ridge
B Cheek pouch
C Jowls
D Dew-lap

Figure 8 Facial topography.

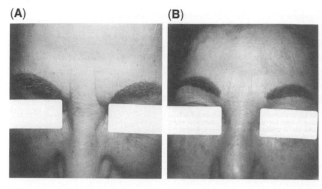

Figure 9 (A) Pronounced glabellar "frown lines" before treatment. (B) Improvement in appearance after a course of six injection treatments of injectable-grade silicone.

enlarge and cause pouches with aging. In addition, hypertrophy of the orbicularis oculi muscle may occur. A bulging lower eyelid casts a shadow (dark "circle") on the lower eyelid or infraorbital groove (Fig. 8) by blocking incident visible light. Correction usually requires lower lid blepharoplasty with the removal of the enlarged fat pads, hypertrophied muscle, and excess skin.

Also with aging, a rift develops in the dermal support tissue between the lower eyelid and the upper cheek. This separation leads to a broad, thin-skinned, semicircular depression below the eye. This depressed area adjacent to pouching of the lower lid results in a deeply shadowed infraorbital groove, especially when the face is lit from above. Gentle digital pressure on the upper cheek to ease the soft upper-cheek tissue back into the depression will illustrate what silicone augmentation can accomplish.

Other factors contributing to dark circles under the eyes are a semicircular pattern of hyperpigmentation caused by chronic ultraviolet light exposure or melasma; a reddish-blue tint (hue) imparted to the inherently thin skin by the underlying orbicularis oculi muscle and network of blood vessels; the dense concentration of large sebaceous glands; and shadowing produced by lower eyelid fullness due to fluid retention.

The infraorbital groove may be augmented by careful injection of small volumes of silicone fluid, such as 0.005 mL per puncture for a total of 0.025 mL per side. The injection

is best made with an acute skin-to-needle angle to avoid needle contact with the infraorbital.

Hands

Wrinkled and thinned skin covering the dorsal surface of the hands due to aging and actinic changes may be improved in appearance, texture, and fullness by injections of silicone fluid (Fig. 11). Silicone injections can correct contour deformity due to loss of muscle in the interosseous spaces. Prominent veins may also be camouflaged. Response has been observed with minute amounts and small cumulative volumes. Special care is taken to avoid intravascular injection.

Contouring

Relatively large cumulative volumes may be required for extensive, deeply depressed contours of the face or other parts. Such depressions, especially in the face, may be associated with alveolar bone resorption following rejected dental implants or other dental problems. They may also result from surgery or trauma, especially in the nasal, orbital, or zygomatic regions or from various conditions of congenital, hereditary, and unknown causes that are responsible for atrophy, dystrophy, or underdevelopment of tissue.

Facial Contouring

Restoration of facial contour has been especially successful in hemifacial atrophy (Romberg's disease, linear scleroderma, or coup de sabre) (Fig. 12). Augmentation should proceed gradually over many visits, and the serial puncture microdroplet injection technique should be used to reduce the possibility of "drift" of silicone fluid and "overcorrection," since the cumulative volume injected may be considerable. The total volume required usually varies between 10 and 50 mL, but as much as 69 mL was reported in a 17-year-old girl. The quantity recommended per treatment of the affected side ranges from 0.5 to 2 mL, delivered in multiple small divided volumes. Migration of fluid has not been a problem when proper procedures are followed.

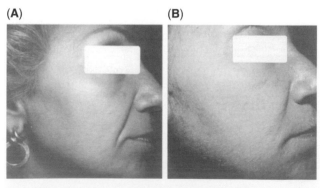

Figure 10 (A) Nasolabial grooves before treatment. (B) Improvement in appearance after 21 injection treatments with injectable-grade silicone over 30 months.

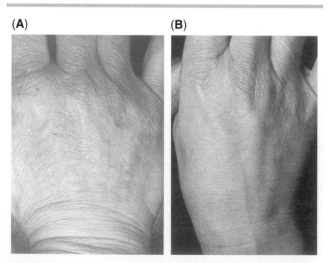

Figure 11 (A) Dorsal aspect of a hand immediately after initial treatment. Note temporary urticarial wheals due to trauma of needle punctures. (B) Improvement in appearance of the hand after six sessions of injections with injectable-grade fluid silicone.

Hemifacial atrophy that is already evident in infancy often portends a severe defect. With later onset the defect tends to be less severe. Rarely is the atrophy bilateral. The treatment of hemifacial atrophy that develops during childhood need not be delayed until the process has run its course since it is difficult to predict the progress. Improvement of appearance and reapproximation of facial symmetry in children and adults has usually been far more successful with fluid silicone than with other reconstructive measures, such as the use of autografts of various tissues and attempts at augmentation with other alloplastic materials.

Still larger volumes of fluid silicone may be required for restoration of facial contour in progressive lipodystrophy because of bilateral involvement. Progressive lipodystrophy may result in loss of subcutaneous fat from the neck, upper portion of the trunk, and arms, but it is generally judicious not to inject large volumes of silicone into the loose subcutaneous fat of the anterior aspect of the neck and to evaluate treatment carefully for marked defects on arms and trunk that are easily concealed by clothing.

Injections of fluid silicone have also been effective in augmenting flattened hemifacial contour in cases of the first and second branchial arch syndrome. Variable characteristics of this syndrome include underdevelopment of bone and muscle, the external and middle ear, and the parotid gland of the affected side of the face. Other features are macrostomia and branchial cleft sinus. The volume of fluid required for augmentation is of the same order as that required for hemifacial atrophy. Mandibular hypoplasia and maxillary retrusion are also correctable. Defects created by parotid gland removal also respond well to silicone-induced soft tissue augmentation, as does posttraumatic facial atrophy, and muscle wasting from paralytic disease.

Body Contouring

Trunk deformities amenable to correction by silicone are pectus excavatum of minor degree, subclavicular depression caused by congenital absence of the pectoralis major muscle, depression in the abdominal wall caused by partial absence or secondary (neurotrophic) atrophy of the rectus abdominus muscle, and indentations secondary to trauma, surgery, atrophodermas, necrobiosis lipoidica, and localized scleroderma. Good results may be difficult to achieve in cases of localized scleroderma in which pigmentation and cutaneous atrophy are very pronounced. Depressions left after lipoma removal or liposuction are correctable by silicone injections. Localized atrophy associated with insulin or other intramuscular (parenteral) injections is also readily repaired.

In patients who have had poliomyelitis, gradual and progressive silicone augmentation of the skin of an atrophied limb has been achieved to dimensions nearly those of the unaffected extremity. Although the required cumulative volume for such a purpose is considerable, each treatment should be limited to 3 to 10 mL, given in multiple injections in a uniform grid pattern for even distribution of silicone to induce a smoothly contoured augmentation. This microdroplet injection technique is designed to prevent migration of the fluid.

Podiatry

With advancing years, loss of protective subcutaneous fat over the sole or toes contributes directly to localized pain and the most common of foot problems: clavi (corns) and calluses. Poorly fitting shoes that apply pressure to bony prominences also contribute.

Injections of silicone in the foot have been used to provide a subdermal cushion between digital and plantar bony prominences and intractably painful corns, calluses (Fig. 13), and scar tissue. Silicone implantation is useful for the treatment of healed, chronically recurring neuropathic ulcers and for local areas of pain in the absence of keratotic formation. Reducing friction and pressure is the mechanism by which silicone improves these clinical conditions.

Seven hundred and forty patients received fluid silicone injections (Dow Corning Medical Fluid 360, 350 cs viscosity) in one or both feet over a period of 19 years (1964–1983). Patients with diabetes, rheumatoid and psoriatic arthritis, scleroderma, pernicious anemia, and neurofibromatosis were treated with benefit. Some feet assessed as having mild peripheral arterial impairment were injected; those with known significant lower extremity vascular insufficiency were not.

Sites were anesthetized by a cryogenic freeze-spray used in conjunction with a local anesthetic. Local migration of the fluid, a possible side effect following large volume subdermal injection, was considerably reduced by use of only fractional amounts. Digital sites received 0.03 to 0.1 mL per injection and 0.1 to 0.4 mL total, with plantar areas receiving 0.05 to 0.2 mL per injection and 0.5 to 1.5 mL total volume for a single site.

Typical locations injected included the hallux, the dorsal aspect of the lesser toes, distal aspect of the toes, sole, weight-bearing surfaces of the metatarsal heads, the heel, or the interdigital web space (soft corns). Patients were seen

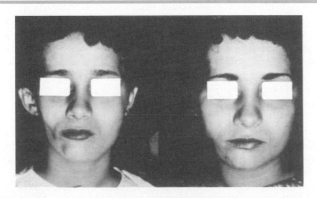

Figure 12 A young woman with severe hemifacial atrophy (*left*). Improved appearance following multiple injection treatments (*right*).

(A)　　　　**(B)**

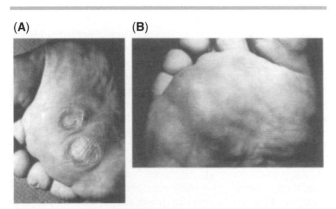

Figure 13 **(A)** Plantar keratoses of 15 years' duration in rheumatoid arthritic patient. **(B)** No need for care for six years following fluid silicone implantation. *Source*: Courtesy of S.W. Balkin, Los Angeles, CA; Balkin SW. The fluid silicone prosthesis. Clin Podiatry 1984; 1:145–164.

at one- to four-week intervals, with all involved sites treated during a single session and an immediate return to regular activity. Dispersal of weight or pressure transmitted at bony prominences in such cases was followed by relief from pain and tenderness and reduction or complete resolution of keratoses.

Pressure keratoses on the diabetic or neuropathic foot present a special challenge since they almost invariably precede ulceration. To date, Dr. Balkin has evaluated 104 patients (19 diabetics) to time of death without any known evidence of skin breakdown or vascular-related complications at an injected site (personal communication). In these high-risk patients, surgery on weight-bearing bone can often be averted with fluid silicone augmentation.

Following fluid silicone implants into the foot, two types of side effects have been reported, either localized asymptomatic fluid migration or skin discoloration with or without migration. Each response has been attributed to overinjection in some early cases. When the micro volume serial puncture technique is used, observable fluid drift or discoloration is rare. Complications, such as infection, ulceration, tumor formation, rejection of fluid, or increase in symptoms, have not been observed in these 740 patients treated over a 19-year period. Histologic examination of long-term biopsy and necropsy specimens has revealed no adverse tissue response.

The procedure should be contemplated when there is considerable disability and as an alternative to orthopedic surgery. In cases of corns that failed to resolve following the injections, surgical excision of the involved skin and bony prominences corrected the problem. Uneventful healing of the silicone-injected tissue took place. Our own experience corroborates these results. We have successfully treated painful clavi and scars following plantar wart removal by surgery or radiation.

Decubitus Ulcers

Any skin area exposed to chronic continuous pressure can eventually break down and ulcerate due to diminished vascularity. Patients prone to these conditions include the chronically bedridden or wheelchair bound, and those with amputation stumps who wear a prosthesis. As with podiatry patients, fluid silicone injections may produce a significant degree of improvement. Treatment for decubitus ulcers is best started when the earliest skin signs of chronic pressure become visible over a bony prominence.

PREPARATION OF PATIENTS

As with any cosmetic surgical procedure, a review with the patient of indications and expected results, techniques of injection, expected sequelae and possible adverse side effects, and limitations of the procedure is essential before treatment is started. It is made clear that silicone replaces lost tissue and does not resurface damaged skin or redrape redundant areas. The patient is told that the needle punctures alone may induce some pain or discomfort and temporary localized bruising, redness, and swelling. After the swelling subsides, in several hours or days, progress in augmentation may be most adequately gauged or predicted at subsequent stages of treatment. There is usually an interval between sessions from one month or more to allow time for new collagen to develop. Silicone augmentation is designed to be performed in stages; the number of sessions required will be proportional to the amount of augmentation necessary to correct the defect. Benefit may not be

obvious until after three to six visits, depending on the site and nature of the defect under treatment. Patients are advised as to the permanent nature of silicone implantation and are told that silicone-induced natural collagen will last as long as their original collagen. It corrects previous loss of collagen but cannot prevent future loss of collagen caused by further aging, facial expression mannerisms, or scarring. Therefore, maintenance injections at 6 to 12 month intervals may be helpful. Silicone injection therapy is completely compatible with, and may be administered before or after, such procedures as rhytidectomy, dermabrasion, chemical peel, liposuction, or grafting. Patients are assured that there has never been an allergic reaction to injectable-grade silicone and that migration does not occur when the microdroplet serial puncture technique is used. In selecting and accepting patients for treatments their motivations, preconceived expectations, uncertainties, and general psychological makeup should be taken into account. Photographs taken before treatment are desirable. Patients are made aware of pretreatment facial redundancies and bulges due to dermatochalasis and subcutaneous localized lipomatous accumulations, such as cheek pouches, jowls, and dewlaps (Fig. 8). We do not recommend administering silicone to patients who refuse pretreatment photographs.

As a test procedure to judge the probable outcome of soft-tissue augmentation or whether a scar will yield to elevation, infiltration with a lidocaine solution may be performed. This procedure is especially useful when you are assessing the suitability of silicone augmentation for correction of nasal deformities. If success is judged to be likely, silicone may then be injected after the trial treatment with the advantage of local anesthesia. Sedation before injection is rarely required for adults, but may be needed for children undergoing treatment for a deformity such as hemifacial atrophy.

Alternative augmentation procedures should be discussed with the patient prior to use of silicone injections.

INSTRUMENTATION

The injectable-grade fluid silicone is stored in glass bottles with either glass or Teflon-coated bottle caps. The silicone fluid should not come in contact with rubber, dust, lint, fingerprints, etc., as these may provoke foreign body reactions.

Syringes used for the injection of injectable-grade silicone should be of the long tuberculin type to allow accurate control of amounts injected and to provide mechanical power for the propulsion of viscous fluids. For fine work, especially for the serial puncture technique, a 0.25-mL syringe is preferable. The conventional 0.25-mL tuberculin-type syringe made of glass is not much shorter than the 1-mL tuberculin syringe; therefore, it provides even better propulsive power and even more precision in the control of amounts injected. Unfortunately, the thin stem of the glass plunger is fragile, and there is no Luer-Lok attachment for the needle. Other 0.25-mL syringes with metal plungers, Luer-Loks, and glass barrels fracture under the hydraulic pressure needed to inject through a 30-gauge needle.

A modified 0.25-mL syringe for injection of viscous fluid (U.S. patent 4,664,655) has a narrow-bore stainless steel barrel and a long stainless steel rod plunger that provides more precision in the control of amounts injected (Fig. 14). The tip of the plunger has a Teflon coating to ensure a tight seal and to facilitate movement. With this syringe, a 0.005 to 0.01 mL microdroplet of silicone liquid can be delivered easily and reproducibly. This allows for 25 to 50 individual

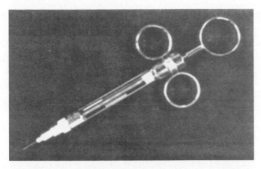

Figure 14 Stainless steel syringe (U.S. patent 4,664,655) for high-viscosity fluid delivery with a capacity of 0.025 mL and equipped with three rings and a Luer-Lok bearing a 30-gauge metal hub needle.

serial punctures before the syringe requires refilling. A further aid to mechanical efficiency is a three-ring grip at the handle end of the syringe. Two rings are attached to the barrel, into which the index and middle fingers are inserted, and a third ring at the end of the plunger is provided for the thumb. At the other end of the syringe, a Luer-Lok attachment prevents dislodgement of the needle during injection. Syringes of this type have been modified to accept cartridges containing small amounts of injectable-grade fluid silicone that remains uncontaminated (U.S. patent 4,664,655). Fluid silicone of 350 cs is injected through metal disposable hypodermic 30-gauge needles. The needle the authors use for almost all silicone injections is manufactured by MPL and called Solo Pak. It is a 30-gauge hypodermic needle with metal hub and specially designed extra large flanges to ensure a firm grip when inserted and locked into the Luer-Lok tip of the silicone syringe. The needle shaft length is 0.5 in. (12 mm); it has a tribeveled point and a polymerized silicone coating (MPL, Inc., Chicago, Illinois, U.S.A.; Catalog No. P63230 Metal Hub Special). It is impossible to draw up fluid silicone of 350 cs into a syringe through a 30-gauge hypodermic needle. The syringe may be repeatedly filled from a multiple-dose bottle fitted with a large-bore needle (U.S. patent 4,664,655).

TECHNIQUES OF INJECTION

As with other transdermal injections, there is minimal risk of infection with injectable-grade silicone microdroplet injection; aseptic precautions are followed as with any injection procedure. The skin should first be thoroughly cleansed to remove cosmetic material or any other residue. Makeup, dirt, etc., can be inadvertently tattooed into the skin and may cause foreign-body reactions that are mistakenly attributed to the silicone. For evaluation and marking of facial defects, the patient is placed in a sitting position and the lighting adjusted to allow the best visualization of the cosmetic defects. The areas to be augmented are marked with a cotton-tipped applicator dipped into an antimicrobial dye. Povidone-iodine 10% solution serves the dual role of topical antiseptic microbicide and visible dye. No sequelae have been observed from the injection of silicone fluid through skin marked with povidone-iodine solution. Rarely, a patient may be allergic to povidone-iodine solution, and another dye can be substituted (metaphen or merthiolate). Depending on personal preference, the patient can be injected in a supported sitting position or first repositioned

to recumbency (Fig. 15). Occasionally, it is advantageous to inject the patient in other positions that accentuate the defect's appearance.

Three principal methods have been advocated for the injection of liquid silicone: the fanning technique, whereby the subcutaneous course of injection parallels the skin surface; the microdroplet serial puncture technique, whereby a fine needle is directed at an angle to the skin surface and the subdermal depositions of silicone are closely spaced from the outside; and the tattooing technique, whereby the needle is stabbed rapidly into and out of the skin with constant digital pressure upon the plunger and silicone expulsion. The characteristics of the cosmetic defect (its shape, depth, and size) may suggest the use of one or the other method or a combination.

Partial local anesthesia may be optimal for the fanning technique, produced by injection of a small amount of anesthetic, raising a wheal at the site where the needle for silicone injection will then be introduced. Larger infiltrations of anesthetic solution will distort contour, making it difficult to assess the required amount and distribution of silicone. Block anesthesia may be performed, in which case no change in the contour of the tissue defect will result. The injection needle is first inserted subcutaneously and then directed parallel to the skin surface until it is fully inserted, after which the first small amount of silicone is introduced. The needle is slowly withdrawn and, at intervals of several millimeters, more small depositions are made until the tip of the needle is near its original point of entry. As a precaution, aspiration should be performed to test for entry into a blood vessel. The needle is then redirected along a new line, then another and another in a radial pattern from its first point of insertion until a fan of injections has been made. For a linear depression, the same technique is practiced along a single subcutaneous tract. After years of comparison the authors do not recommend the fanning technique and advise that it be used with utmost caution because of its tendency to produce pooling of the injected silicone in the injection tract.

With the microdroplet serial puncture technique, some local anesthesia may be obtained by spraying ethyl chloride or freon refrigerant onto the skin just prior to injection. Mucous membranes (lips) may be anesthetized using topical anesthetics. For those patients who have a low tolerance for the discomfort of silicone injections, the use of

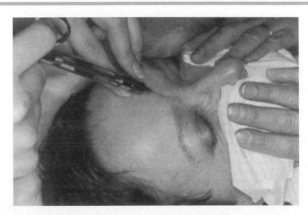

Figure 15 Technique of injecting an area on the face. Patient applies pressure to recently injected sites to prevent or minimize bruising.

nitrous oxide inhalation anesthesia may be helpful. Generally, however, adults require no anesthesia. The needle is inserted into the skin at intervals 5 to 10 mm apart at the appropriate angle for optimal penetration and deposition. The angle of insertion may vary: more oblique (toward 90°) for greater depth or more acute (approaching parallel to the skin) for superficial deposition, deposition in thin skin, and to avoid underlying bony, vital, and vascular structures. With the syringe illustrated in Figure 14, a 30-gauge needle is always used. A minute amount of fluid silicone (0.005–0.01 mL), depending on the extent and depth of the depression, is deposited subcutaneously upon each insertion of the needle. When using a 30-gauge needle and the microdroplet serial puncture technique, it is not necessary or practical to aspirate prior to injection. When injected into a blood vessel, the silicone microdroplets act as an anticoagulant and are well tolerated.

When injecting silicone with a three-ring syringe, it is important to puncture the skin by exerting downward force only with the two fingers that are placed in the two side rings. When the needle has achieved the desired tissue depth, force is then applied to the plunger ring to expel a dose of silicone (usually 0.005–0.01 mL). If pressure is applied to all three rings during needle insertion, a small amount of silicone may be deposited in the upper levels of the skin. This may produce a beading effect after collagen deposition occurs. Superficial deposition of minute amounts of silicone is performed intentionally to correct certain (dermal) defects and when one is using the tattooing technique.

Pinching and elevating the area to be injected between thumb and index finger of the free hand has been recommended by some to stabilize loose skin; however, this also distorts the tissue and may make precise injection difficult. We find that gently placing the free hand adjacent to the area being treated usually provides adequate stabilization with minimal distortion of the area.

When injecting certain areas of the face, there is a likelihood of needle tip contact with facial bones. This is common where the skin overlies bony prominences, such as the point of the chin, infraorbital rims, and forehead.

Contact of the needle tip with a bony surface is neither painful nor harmful; however, blunting and damage to the needle tip which takes the form of a tiny burr usually results. This damage, is immediately obvious to the physician as an increased resistance to insertion and removal of the needle. The patient also experiences more pain with injection, greater trauma to the tissues, and possibly an increased incidence of edema and ecchymosis. Gentle digital stroking of the needle tip reveals the burr. To minimize pain and tissue trauma, the needle should be replaced.

Due to the high pressure that develops within this syringe, the needle occasionally dislodges from its tight Luer-Lok attachment. This may be detected as a decreased resistance to digital force applied to the plunger and by leaking of silicone fluid around the needle hub. When a loose fit is suspected, the needle is promptly tightened using its plastic cover.

For fine work, especially on the face, the deposition of many tiny silicone droplets produced by the microdroplet serial puncture technique has an advantage over the bulkier deposition of silicone by the fanning technique. A given volume of silicone dispersed into small droplets provides a larger total surface area for contact with the patient's tissues than would the same volume divided into fewer but larger globules. Since fibroplasia and augmentation occur at the surface of silicone droplets, the amount of

new collagen formed will be directly proportional to the surface area of the injected silicone implant. Therefore, a soft-tissue augmentation will be greater for a given volume of silicone fluid dispersed into microdroplets than if it is divided into fewer larger globules.

The serial puncture technique has been used to best advantage when small to moderate total volumes of silicone are required, as for facial contours, furrows, and small depressed scars. The deposition of such tiny amounts of silicone results in limited fibroplastic responses that are best for continuous and precise augmentation of soft-tissue to desired degrees. Microdroplet injection also effectively eliminates migration by stimulating a collagen capsule that traps the silicone at the site of implantation.

Intervals between sessions are usually one month in the early phases of treatment in the same area(s) of the face. This interval allows time for new collagen to develop in response to the silicone injections and is necessary to achieve the desired effect without overcorrection. Treatments given less than one month apart are permissible if different areas are treated. Intervals longer than one month pose no problem for the physician or patient. As soft-tissue augmentation progresses and the defects improve, intervals of one to three months or more are appropriate. Follow-up sessions once or twice a year may be desirable as the degenerative effects of aging, actinic damage, and facial expression mannerisms continue to take their toll.

With the microdroplet serial puncture technique a smaller proportion of fluid in the syringe is deposited than with the fanning technique, due to some leakage from the syringe and needle tracks onto the surface of the skin. The leakage appears in the form of blood and silicone at points of puncture. The loss is minor and inconsequential, and is minimized by the pressure applied right after injection primarily to prevent ecchymosis. There is no need to seal puncture sites with collodion or suture. A more important advantage of the microdroplet serial puncture technique is that it minimizes the risk of embolism and drift of fluid.

The silicone tattooing technique is done by rapidly stabbing the 30-gauge needle through the epidermis repeatedly at 2 to 3 mm intervals into the dermal or superficial subcutaneous layers while constant pressure is maintained on the syringe plunger. Silicone is thus expelled during both insertion and withdrawal of the needle. However, due to the speed of injection and short time the needle is in the skin, minute quantities of silicone (less than 0.005 mL) are actually deposited. This technique requires a high degree of manual dexterity and is best practiced after one has achieved facility with the microdroplet serial puncture technique. It is suitable for treatment of fine lines, such as crow's feet, some forehead creases, and neck folds. Beading is more likely to occur with this technique.

Do not massage, snap a tongue depressor against the skin, or apply a hand-held vibrating machine to ensure dispersement of silicone after injection: (i) The injection of microdroplets at each puncture site obviates the need for imprecise dispersion by massage; (ii) it is unlikely that massage can adequately disperse silicone injected intradermally or subdermally into facial skin; and (iii) massage may unnecessarily traumatize delicate facial tissues.

In contradistinction to bovine collagen injections, the intentional production of a slight overcorrection immediately after injection is to be avoided. Since silicone is a permanent implant, it is important that proper technique be used to *avoid overcorrection*. The defect should be undercorrected, with gradual augmentation induced over several sessions

ADVERSE REACTIONS AND PRECAUTIONS

Pain

Some pain is expected from the injection of the needle but is not related to the silicone. Discomfort may be minimized by using the finest needles feasible and by local or inhalation anesthetics. Replace burred needles, as discussed previously.

Edema

Edema is related to the trauma caused by the needle and usually resolves within several hours to days. Judgment of cosmetic improvement should be made after this time because edema produces temporary correction of defects. A transitory urticarial papular reaction (wheal and flare) is occasionally seen at the sites of needle puncture within minutes of injection (dermographism) (Fig. 11A).

Ecchymosis

If ecchymosis occurs, it is usually mild and related to needle puncture, needle gauge, thinness or looseness of the skin, and the surface anticoagulant property of silicone. Bruising may be more prominent in areas with a dense vascular network. It may be advisable for patients to avoid use of aspirin for seven days prior to treatment. The application of firm pressure reduces the incidence and extent of ecchymosis and prevents loss of fluid silicone through the needle track puncture site (Fig. 15). Resolution of ecchymosis may be hastened by applying cold compresses for the first 24 hours and warm compresses thereafter. Patients are informed they can apply makeup immediately after the treatment.

Erythema

Slight to moderate transient erythema may appear immediately after injection. The triple response of Lewis (wheal and flare) reaction may be more pronounced in patients with dermographism and a tendency toward contact or pressure urticaria. It usually persists for a few hours and may be masked by makeup. Persistent erythema of an injected area may result if the injection of silicone has been made too superficially (i.e., intradermally or with adulterated "silicone"). Persistent erythema may be diminished by topical application of anti-inflammatory adrenocorticosteroid preparations.

Dyschromia

The intradermal injection of silicone has also been reported on rare occasion to cause temporary brownish-yellow pigmentation of the skin. This is probably caused by injection of adulterated "silicone." A bluish tinge may result from superficial deposition of fluid silicone in thin (translucent) skin, such as striae, atrophic scars, and some chickenpox scars. Hemifacial atrophy is frequently associated with cutaneous hyperpigmentation on the lower portion of the forehead and along the canine fossa (a maxillary depression). This occurs apart from, and should not be attributed to, silicone treatment. Pigmentary changes may be a natural sequela of other dystrophic conditions, postinflammatory states, and surgery (i.e., cosmetic surgery and dermabrasion). It is important to have careful documentation of preexisting pigmentation in the form of written records and photographs. As important is making the patient aware of the rare pigmentary changes associated with treatment.

Texture and Sensation

The texture of soft tissue containing evenly dispersed, minute droplets of fluid silicone is very natural. The patient does not experience any unnatural sensation or sensitivity to touch in such locations. Larger amounts of silicone, as may be required to correct hemifacial atrophy, may impart a slight rubbery consistency on palpation. This change is usually acceptable to patients and often reverts to a natural texture given sufficient time. Injection of fluid silicone in greatly excessive amounts or, purportedly, too superficially in the dermis has been known to cause stretching of the skin and blockage of lymphatics. Brawny fullness or a peau d'orange texture may result (Fig. 3).

Excessive Elevation

Only small amounts of silicone should be injected into any one site at any one treatment. Augmentation should proceed gradually over the course of months. Overcorrection at a particular silicone implantation site may occur if an excessive quantity is injected at one time or cumulatively over several sessions. Multiple injections at intervals as short as one week make it more difficult to control augmentation and may produce overcorrection; these have erroneously been reported as "granulomas." When a patient is unable to return for the next treatment session for six months or longer, two to three sessions, at intervals of one week, may be carefully and safely performed. Overcorrection may result in excessive edema and discoloration of the skin over the injected site. These effects may be corrected with intralesional injections of antiinflammatory corticosteroid, usually triamcinolone acetonide 2.5 to 5 mg/mL, with approximately 0.1 mL injected per cubic centimeter of elevated tissue.

Where skin overlies bone tightly, as on the forehead, or overlies cartilage, as on the nose, very small amounts of silicone are injected to avoid excessive elevation or "beading" (Fig. 16). This may be prevented by the injection of minute amounts (0.005 mL) to sufficient depth.

When rapid augmentation has been done in order to produce instant gratification and large volumes injected, a variety of dispersal techniques have been used including massage, vibration, and snapping a tongue blade against the skin. Massage right after injection has been purported to help dispersal of the fluid and to prevent beading. There are significant differences of opinion in this matter. The authors' belief is that the volume and level of controlled injections should be the only factors that influence deposition and dispersal and that massage and vibration are uncontrollable methods.

Beading and overcorrection are amenable to intralesional injections of triamcinolone acetonide (Fig. 16B), microelectrodesiccation, and, if necessary, dermabrasion or tangential shave-excision surgery. Although experience is limited, the use of suction-assisted lipectomy to treat excessively augmented tissues injected with unknown fluid implant materials, adulterated silicone, or even injectable-grade silicone may be worthwhile in selected cases.

Embolism

Care must be taken to avoid intravascular injection of fluid silicone. This precaution applies to injection of any materials that is immiscible in blood or of a particle size that may cause embolism. It applies even to soluble preparations such as local anesthetic agents containing epinephrine, which may cause vasospasm ("functional embolism").

Subcutaneous and submucosal blood vessels of the face connect with the ophthalmic and meningeal vessels. Forceful injection into the superficial dermal arterial branches of the face and scalp could cause retrograde

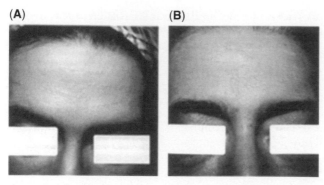

Figure 16 **(A)** Beading following injections of injectable-grade silicone into forehead wrinkles. **(B)** The condition responded in time to intralesional injections of adrenocorticosteroid.

movement into the retinal arteries. Symptoms and signs of embolism by these routes are acute pain at the site of injection and in the ipsilateral eye and orbit, dilatation of the pupil, impairment of vision, paresis of extraocular muscles, cephalagia, mottling of facial skin, reflex nausea, hypotension, and back pain.

Fortunately, the authors have never had any personal experience or heard any reports of ophthalmic symptoms after injectable-grade silicone injection in the face using the microdroplet serial puncture technique. Nor are we aware of any published or unpublished reports of such. This may be a result of silicone's fluid nature and its anticoagulant properties. Unlike silicone, injectable bovine collagen has been associated with at least one case of amaurosis, probably as a result of its particulate nature, propensity to polymerize once injected, and hemostatic properties. Tragic fiascoes from massive, instantaneous injections of "silicone" (e.g., hundreds of milliliters into a breast) have resulted in emboli to other organs and have caused rare fatalities.

Granulomatous Reactions

Granulomatous inflammatory reactions to injected "silicone" have been called "siliconomas," a misnomer since silicone itself cannot become a tumor ("-oma"). Nor do cells that phagocytize silicone (macrophages) multiply in a tumorous fashion. Reports of granulomatous reactions to "silicone" fall into several categories: cases of overinjection, injection into contraindicated sites, injection of adulterated materials, and injection of substances of unknown chemical composition.

In most cases of overinjection, the tissue reaction to silicone may be typical but its degree is exaggerated because of the excessive volume of silicone injected (overinjection). Milojevic reported a patient who developed a "granuloma" in the zygomatic region on both sides four weeks after the injection of 4 mL of "fluid silicone." A second patient showed signs of "granuloma" five weeks after the injection of 6 mL silicone into the nasolabial folds. The histologic description of these "granulomas" was consistent with an appropriate tissue response to silicone fluid. In comparison, all four areas (right and left zygomatic region and nasolabial folds) should be treated in a single patient with a total of 0.25 to 0.50 mL, divided into 25 to 50 microdroplet serial punctures. Additional sessions would usually take place at a minimum of one-month intervals. Overinjection was also the primary factor for the development of "granulomas" reported by Wilkie, as reviewed previously.

On rare occasion, an excessive inflammatory reaction has been seen, especially to adulterated silicone, in the glabella, nasolabial folds, angle of mouth, cheek pouch, or jawline. Histologically, there is an acute to subacute inflammatory response with granulomatous elements. Since the face has a ubiquitous and dense population of pilosebaceous adnexae, inflammatory reactions are often associated with a granulomatous infiltrate (as is often seen in acne vulgaris) secondary to dermally entrapped pilosebaceous material. When injected at the aforementioned facial sites, silicone, especially if adulterated, can produce a recurrent inflammatory acute, subacute, or chronic reaction. This reaction is rarely, if ever, seen when injectable-grade fluid silicone is used properly.

When inflammatory reactions do occur, as in acne-prone individuals, surgery is rarely needed to correct the problem and should not be used as primary treatment. Intralesional corticosteroids are most effective and will usually suffice. Oral steroids and antibiotics are also effective. Sometimes all three are appropriate.

Intralesional corticosteroids are injected with a 30-gauge needle directly into the body of the indurated area. A 0.25 to 1 mL glass tuberculin syringe offers the best hydraulics for injection of steroid suspensions into dense tissue. Triamcinolone acetonide 5 to 10 mg/mL should be used every two to four weeks. If recurrences are frequent, the longer-lasting steroid triamcinolone hexacetonide can be substituted for or mixed with the triamcinolone acetonide. Injections of triamcinolone hexacetonide need not exceed more than 5 mg/mL administered in aliquots of 0.1 mL per 1 cm² tissue.

Idiosyncratic Reactions

These rare, local, isolated, idiosyncratic reactions of an inflammatory nature are characterized by an isolated area of swelling with slight erythema. They occur with an approximate incidence of 1:10,000 patients treated in our practice. These reactions usually appear months after injection and usually involve one, or rarely two, of the many areas treated. Patients invariably have a negative intradermal skin test to injectable-grade fluid silicone. The reactions respond within days to intralesional corticosteroid injections and oral antibiotics. Further silicone augmentation can be performed without difficulty. When a biopsy is performed, the histopathologic specimen shows a nonspecific chronic inflammatory reaction. One explanation may be the proximity of the idiosyncratic reaction to a nidus of inflammation or infection (e.g., a tooth abscess or acne lesion).

Drift

There is a great deal of confusion in the literature and in the minds of physicians and patients about the concept of silicone "drift." The term "drift" has been applied to different phenomena, which accounts in part for some of the confusion.

The transport of silicone droplets to sites distant from injection may occur as a result of inadvertent intravascular injection (embolism). When the microdroplet serial puncture injection technique is used, intravascular introduction is inconsequential and, in our experience, unassociated with untoward sequelae.

Dispersion by low-grade phagocytic activity and reticuloendothelial cell migration is harmless and analogous to that occurring with the pigment in a tattoo. Most tattoos fade slightly with age as some of the pigment is carried off by tissue macrophages. Some of the tattoo pigment may be found in regional lymph nodes as a result of this benign migration.

Drifting of silicone liquid (or any other injectable implant, for that matter) will occur when large volumes (several to 1000 mL) are injected into a single site, such as the breast or leg. Distant migration of silicone gel from ruptured breast implants has also been reported. These large volumes, which cannot be contained by the receiving tissues, are propelled in a cephalad or caudad direction by muscle action and external pressure along tissue planes of least resistance.

A "migratory silicone granuloma" of the left upper portion of the chest and left upper arm was reported in a 38-year-old woman about four months after rupture of a silicone-gel–containing breast implant. The large volume of gel released accounted in part for its migration and the exaggerated degree of tissue response.

Silicone has erroneously been held responsible when areas of redundant facial tissue develop coincidentally to silicone injections administered over time. These areas usually correspond to typical bulges seen with chronologic and actinic aging, such as the nasolabial ridges, cheek pouches (just lateral to labial commissure groove), the lower jawline jowls, and dewlaps. In some instances these bulges existed prior to silicone treatment but were not noticed by the patient and physician. Increased attention to cosmetic appearance leads to closer scrutiny of the face by both patient and doctor. General dissatisfaction with an aged appearance causes the patient and occasionally the physician to blame the problem falsely on silicone "drift." Examination of pretreatment photographs will usually dispel this misconception. Furthermore, since silicone liquid does not halt the aging process, most patients will in all probability develop typical "natural" facial redundancies years after receiving silicone injections, as their skin continues to age.

Finally, gravitational or dependent drift of silicone has been putatively reported to occur months to years after injection. This type of "drift" is difficult to reconcile with the laws of physics because the specific gravity of silicone is less than that of water. Silicone liquid floats on water. Since the specific gravity of human soft tissue is even greater than that of water, silicone fluid would migrate or drift, if indeed it did, upward in a cephalad direction. The authors have never observed the presence of silicone liquid in the scalp months or even years after it was injected into caudal areas, nor are we aware of any such published reports.

Rather than being produced by gravitational attraction, the "drift" of silicone liquid to areas adjacent to the puncture (introduction) site may be caused by the unintentional dispersal of silicone liquid along tissue planes of least resistance at the time of injection. Propelled by the high pressure generated in the syringe, the silicone cannot be contained by tissue in the immediate vicinity of the needle tip. Like an ameba sending out pseudopods, a relatively too large silicone globule will extend beyond the point of injection. For example, when one is injecting circumoral oral lines on the upper lip, the needle usually points toward the oral cavity. If these lines are overinjected, the "pseudopods" of silicone will most likely find room for themselves in the direction the needle points (toward the vermilion), thereby giving the false impression of "drift" months later when soft tissue augmentation takes place. The microdroplet injection technique effectively eliminates "migration" by stimulating a collagen capsule that holds the silicone at the site of implantation.

RELATIVE AND ABSOLUTE CONTRAINDICATIONS
Breasts
Injection of fluid silicone into grandular breast tissue is absolutely contraindicated. The great majority of severe complications attributed to fluid "silicone" involved improper injection of breasts and the probable use in most cases of large volumes of adulterated material (Fig. 3). Aside from the unlikelihood of improving the appearance of certain types of breasts (i.e., the sagging variety with stretched ligamentous attachments), interference with clinical, mammographic, or other known methods to detect neoplastic masses is a serious sequela. Nevertheless, in human beings, there is no known causal relation between the injection of silicone into the breasts and breast cancer. Additional complications that developed after breast injections have been discussed previously. Subcutaneous mastectomy followed by the insertion of a mammary prosthesis has been successful for selected women who had adulterated silicone or some other poorly tolerated foreign material injected into their breasts.

Eyelids
Except in very special circumstances, such as atrophic traumatic scars and linear scleroderma (coup de sabre), eyelid tissue is usually unsuitable for augmentation because of its thinness, overdistensibility, and tendency for discoloration. This does not include the lower eyelid groove.

Vascular Abnormalities
As a precaution against embolism, fluid silicone should not be injected where arteriovenous communications may have resulted from surgery or trauma. Injections are best avoided in areas of lymphostasis.

Bound-Down Scars
Depressed scars that are tightly bound down by fibrotic adhesions (nondistensible), especially the "ice pick" scars of acne vulgaris, resist elevation. Overzealous attempts to inject beneath such scars may result in collarette elevation of surrounding skin ("doughnut effect"), thus exaggerating the depressions. This is also a problem in some chickenpox scars.

Fibrocystic Lesions
Cavities of cysts should not be filled with silicone, but the depressed scars that remain after spontaneous or surgical resolution of epidermal or inflammatory cysts may be elevated by injection of silicone.

Genitalia
Foreign fluid materials have been injected into the penis to correct impotence and premature ejaculation, for augmentation, and in cases of sexual deviance. These injections have frequently been performed by nonprofessionals. The foreign body reaction that develops following injections of vegetable oil, mineral oil, or adulterated silicone has been termed sclerosing lipogranuloma. "Paraffinoma" of the penis has also been reported. Clinical findings are characterized by the presence of hard, lobular subcutaneous masses in the penis. Penile or scrotal edema and draining sinus tracts are sometimes present. In addition, some men complained of impotence, painful erection, and inability to copulate because of size deformity.

All reported cases of sclerosing lipogranuloma involved injections of foreign or adulterated fluids. It is prudent at this time to consider the genitalia an untested site for the administration of injectable-grade silicone. The judicious use of injectable-grade silicone to repair selected cutaneous defects of the genitalia may be appropriate.

Expectation of Perfect Transformation

Facial wrinkles and deep furrows correspond to underlying fibromuscular attachments of skin to fascia. Elevation by properly injected silicone generally produces some cosmetic improvement, but attempts to obliterate linear depressions completely may be unwise, if feasible at all, and are not warranted for the creases that are natural during young adulthood. Such practice may result in a fullness of tissue that is not aesthetic.

Soft-tissue augmentation with liquid silicone does not substitute for rhytidectomy and liposuction, which *redrapes* redundant skin and removes excess fat; dermabrasion or chemical peel, which *resurfaces* by abrading away wrinkled, scarred, or actinically damaged skin; and full-thickness punch autografting, which *replaces* defective skin, such as "ice pick" scars.

Treatment During Pregnancy

To the best of our knowledge, there have been no adverse reports concerning the subcutaneous injection of silicone in pregnant women. Polydimethylsiloxane of various viscosities is reportedly devoid of adverse reproductive, teratogenic, and mutagenic effects in the mice, rats, and rabbits studied. The authors have never encountered any adverse effects on pregnancy from injectable-grade silicone injections; however, definitive studies have not been done.

Actively Inflamed or Infected Sites

Injection into sites of active inflammation (i.e., bovine collagen reactions and allergic contact dermatitis) or active infection (i.e., acneiform lesions, ulcers, and herpes lesions) is best deferred until the underlying process has been controlled.

Silicone "Allergy"

Although never encountered in the authors' practice or review of the literature, should a patient develop an allergic reaction (proven by intradermal skin testing) to silicone or silicone type implants, he or she is not a candidate for silicone implantation.

ANIMAL TOXICITY, EFFECTS OF DEPOSITION OF LARGE VOLUMES, AND LACK OF CARCINOGENICITY

More than 1000 laboratory animals, mostly rodents, have been studied for the effects of fluid silicone depositions. Studies have been carried out on mice, rats, guinea pigs, rabbits, dogs, monkeys, baboons, and apes. Massive subcutaneous injections of polydimethylsiloxane in rodents, on the order of 50 to 300 mL in mice and guinea pigs and even larger volumes in rats, have not resulted in systemic toxicity. The sheer weight and bulk of the material decreased the mobility of some test animals.

The sequence of local tissue response to large subcutaneous depositions of fluid silicone in rodents is essentially the same as with small volumes. Large amounts of silicone result in proportionately thicker fibrous capsules of opaque character. Granulomatosis does not occur from injectable-grade silicone. Antibodies to silicone could not be demonstrated in guinea pigs, even when intentionally sought with the additive effect of complete Freund's adjuvant.

Relative to body weight and size, much larger quantities of fluid silicone have been tested for effects in laboratory animals than have been injected in human beings for cosmesis. In patients closely studied during the past 35 years, no consistent or significant alterations have been found in complete blood cell counts and differentials, blood chemical levels (glucose, urea nitrogen, uric acid, cholesterol, total protein, albumin, bilirubin, alkaline phosphatase, glutamic oxalacetic transaminase, lactic acid dehydrogenase, calcium, phosphorus), and urinalysis.

Little dissipation of injectable-grade silicone from sites that were properly injected has been found. Minute quantities of the material may be phagocytized and transported via the reticuloendothelial system but with no known harmful effects.

Polydimethylsiloxane of various viscosities was reportedly devoid of adverse reproductive, teratologic, and mutagenic effects in the mice, rats, and rabbits studied.

Injectable-grade fluid silicone has never been found to be carcinogenic. More than 1000 experimental animals have been tested for the possibility of carcinogenesis, and among lower mammals the period of observation has been for the major portion of their life-spans. No development of carcinoma or sarcoma directly attributable to silicone has been verified in human beings. This has been the authors' 35-year experience in approximately 100,000 patients treated. Spontaneous development of malignant neoplasms in a control population is crucial to determine if a given substance has carcinogenic potential. Thus, a claimed relationship between malignancy and silicone fluid deposition in two mice (out of 36 injected) was not confirmed by additional studies with controls and by later revised interpretation of the original histologic slides as benign mammary adenomas, a common neoplasm in mice. The claim of carcinogenicity from silicone was subsequently retracted by the original author.

Malignancies were reported in Bethesda black rats following the implantation of silicone rubber. This strain of rats is particularly susceptible to the spontaneous development of neoplasms and to the development of malignancies following implantation of various materials other than silicone.

Silicone fluid should never be injected directly into human breast tissue, as we have emphasized. However, in thousands of recipients of large volumes of the material in the past, no induction of carcinoma in mammary tissue attributable to silicone fluid has been demonstrated to date. With so large a population, the usual incidence of spontaneous development of carcinoma (unrelated to silicone) must be expected, and yet no excess incidence has occurred. Special concern remains for those patients in whom massive quantities of silicone may have caused blockage of lymphatics, because lymphatic blockage for other reasons is well known to have been followed in rare instances by the development of angiosarcoma in the lymphedematous tissue (i.e., the Stewart-Treves syndrome). To our knowledge, this has not been reported.

Prolonged living with solid silicone materials embedded internally has not been carcinogenic in over a million patients with synthetic devices, such as shunts for drainage of hydrocephalus; heart valves; coverings for pacemakers; joint, breast, and penile implants; arterial prostheses; and ocular bands installed for repair of detached retinas. Material for suturing is often silicone-coated. Of the many other medical uses of liquid silicone, its wide use as an internal lubricant in disposable syringes and cartridges attests to its safety. Each time an injection is given with a silicone-lubricated needle or syringe, a small quantity of silicone fluid is also administered. The average diabetic taking daily injections of insulin with disposable syringes (which are internally lubricated with silicone) receives about 5 mL of liquid silicone each year.

METABOLISM, EXCRETION, AND DETECTION
Metabolism and Excretion
The slight tissue reactivity to small volume depositions of injectable-grade fluid silicone was discussed previously, as was dispersal from the site of injection. Traces of the material may be found in urine and stool. In these respects fluid silicone is not entirely inert in the subcutaneous tissue of the host, although local reaction is less than with other synthetic materials used for augmentation.

Fluid silicone is not known to be altered in vivo. Its consistency is unchanged at environmental temperatures compatible with mammalian life. Fluid silicone does not support the growth of microorganisms, nor is it altered by them. Infections that followed improper injections of "silicone," as discussed above, were probably consequences of contaminated materials; unsuitability of glandular and ductal tissue of the breast for fluid augmentation; built-up pressure in tissue with vasoconstriction, lymphostasis, and local hypoxia; or a combination of such factors.

Detection
Fluid silicone is not stainable or usually retained during routine preparation of tissue for microscopic examination. It has been claimed, especially in examination of frozen preparations or thick sections stained with hematoxylin and eosin, that "silicone" may be discernible as thin refractile sheets or membranes lying in spaces surrounded by histiocytes. However, this is neither a specific nor a sensitive method of identification. Electron microscopy cannot be used to identify positively fluid silicone in tissues. The location of silicone in tissue may be suspected from rounded extracellular spaces and vacuoles within cells. However, an indistinguishable picture may be left by various nonsilicone oily substances.

Specific physical or chemical detection of silicone requires fairly sophisticated equipment because of the inert character of the material in vitro.

Methods of detection include the following.

1. Infrared spectroscopy is an accurate physical method of detecting the silicon-carbon and silicon-oxygen bonds. Since the silicon-carbon bond is synthetically produced and does not occur spontaneously in nature, a positive test implies that one or more silicones is present. The test does not reveal the nature of the remainder of the silicone molecules; the source, quantity or purity of the material present; or the presence or absence of adulterants.
2. Thin-layer chromatography is useful to detect paraffin (mineral oil) and other adulterants.
3. A laser-Raman microprobe has been used to identify microscopic inclusions of silicone polymer (rubber) in standard sections of axillary lymph node from a patient with a silicone elastomer finger-joint prosthesis.
4. Silicone shows no anisotropic optical behavior; it is nonpolarizing and not birefringent. Reports of bright shining crystals and fluorescent granules seen when pathologic specimens are viewed with polarizing light probably indicate the presence of adulterants.
5. X-ray spectroscopy of biopsy tissue can only demonstrate the presence of elements, including silicon.

Other analytic techniques that can only detect Si (silicon) include atomic emission spectrography, atomic absorption spectrometry, and energy-dispersive x-ray analysis.

COMPATIBILITY WITH OTHER SURGICAL/COSMETIC PROCEDURES
To test if there is an adverse influence of fluid silicone on wound healing, fresh cutaneous autografts in rats were injected peripherally with silicone. Vascularization proceeded normally with no interruption in the take of the grafts. Preservation of skin in a fluid silicone medium for up to four days at 4°C was followed by successful graft vascularization.

Proper human tissue augmentation with injectable-grade silicone does not interfere with local surgical procedures and wound healing. Dermabrasion has been successfully performed even in areas where excessive amounts of silicone have been deposited (Fig. 4). Confined areas of soft-tissue augmentation with silicone may be excised, when indicated, with no impairment of wound healing.

Additional improvement of the appearance of the face has been achieved by silicone augmentation in patients treated before or afterward by dermabrasion, chemical peel, rhytidectomy, blepharoplasty, or "facials." The procedures differ in rationale, mechanisms, and effects. Proper injection of silicone provides controlled augmentation and lifting of furrows and depressed distensible scars.

Sites properly augmented by fluid silicone do not require special care. There have been no adverse interactions following exposure to the sun. Makeup may be applied in the usual manner.

Thousands of patients with facial acne scarring have had concomitant or subsequent correction of depressed scars by silicone-induced collagen augmentation, and of "ice pick" scars by full-thickness punch autografting, without any negative influence of one technique upon the other.

COMPARISON WITH OTHER AUGMENTING IMPLANTS
Injectable-grade liquid silicone has several advantages over other injectable augmentation prostheses. With silicone there is no hypersensitivity and, therefore, no pretesting is necessary. The product contains no lidocaine or other adulterants. There are no contraindications to its use in atopic patients or patients with a personal or family history of autoimmune diseases, such as rheumatoid arthritis, lupus erythematosus, scleroderma, polyarteritis nodosa, and polyarthralgia rheumatica. There is no fear of amaurosis when the microdroplet serial puncture technique is used, and the long-term effects (35 years) and proven safety are well established. Silicone is not biodegradable or reabsorbed, so that the physician and patient can depend upon persistence of the desired soft tissue augmentation.

Fibrin collected from the blood of the patient is processed (Fibrel) and then injected under a depressed site. The site may be undermined by the needle used for injection before the fibrin is injected. Since fibrin gets completely absorbed by the body, lasting improvement may be related to the undermining and trauma of implantation and not the fibrin. Fibrel requires venipuncture, plasma preparation, and pretreatment intradermal skin testing. In preliminary studies approximately 2% of patients have positive skin tests and cannot be treated.

For more than 100 years, collagens from various sources (most recently bovine skin) have been used in attempts to replace lost collagen. Although chemically processed to reduce allergenicity, these collagens can cause allergic reactions. Before a person can receive collagen injections, he or she must have a test injection. As many as 3% to 5% react to this test. Of those who are treated, between 1% and 5% develop an adverse reaction during treatment. Inflammation at the injected sites may be precipitated by sun, alcohol, aspirin, beef, heat, cold, and menses. Since foreign collagens are degraded and absorbed, improvement gradually fades and retreatment is needed within 6 to 24 months. Collagen is a coagulant and can, therefore, cause thrombosis when injected into a blood vessel. Since the eyes and face share a common blood supply, injection of collagen into the face carries the risk of causing permanent loss of vision. One such case has already been reported.

A relatively new technique of withdrawing small amounts of adipose tissue from the abdominal or other areas and injecting them into atrophic skin is currently being used. Whether this technique will produce comparable cosmetic improvement or be long-lasting remains to be seen. The relatively large size of the adipose "grafts" and the impracticality of injecting them through a 30-gauge needle (18-gauge needles are necessary) make this technique unsuitable for many finer deformities for which silicone is suited. Fat transplantation is especially useful for subcutaneous augmentation.

BIBLIOGRAPHY

Abraham JL, Etz ES. Molecular microanalysis of pathological specimens in situ with a Laser-Raman microprobe. Science 1979; 206:716–718.

Achauer BM. A serious complication following medical-grade silicone injection of the face. Plast Reconstr Surg 1983; 71:251–254.

Andrews JM. Cellular behavior to injected silicone fluid: a preliminary report. Plast Reconstr Surg 1966; 38:581–583.

Arduino LJ. Sclerosing lipogranuloma of male genitalia. J Urol 1959; 82:155–161.

Aronsohn RB. Reconstruction observations on the use of silicone in the face. Arch Otolaryngol 1965; 82:191–194.

Aronsohn RB. A 22-year experience with the use of silicone injections. Am J Cosmet Surg 1984; 1:21–28.

Arthaud JB. Silicone-induced penile sclerosing lipogranuloma. J Urol 1973; 110:210.

Ashley FL, Braley S, McNall EG. The current status of silicone injection therapy. Surg Clin North Am 1971; 51:501–509.

Ashley FL, Braley S, Rees TD, Goulian D, Ballantyne DL. The present status of silicone fluid in soft-tissue augmentation. Plast Reconstr Surg 1967; 39:411–420.

Ashley FL, Rees TD, Ballantyne DL, et al. An injection technique for the treatment of facial hemiatrophy. Plast Reconstr Surg 1965; 35:640–648.

Ashley FL, Thompson DP, Henderson T. Augmentation of surface contour by subcutaneous injections of silicone fluid. A current report. Plast Reconstr Surg 1973; 51:8–13.

Balkin SW. Silicone injection for plantar keratoses. Preliminary report. J Am Podiatr Assoc 1966; 56:1–11.

Balkin SW. Plantar keratoses: Treatment by injectable liquid silicone. Report of an eight-year experience. Clin Orthop 1972; 87:235–247.

Balkin SW. Treatment of corns by injectable silicone. Arch Dermatol 1975; 111:1143–1145.

Balkin SW. Silicone augmentation for plantar calluses. J Am Podiatr Assoc 1976; 66:148–154.

Balkin SW. Treatment of painful scars on soles and digits with injections of fluid silicone. J Dermatol Surg Oncol 1977; 3:612–614.

Balkin SW. The fluid silicone prosthesis. Clin Podiatry 1984; 1: 145–164.

Ballantyne DL, Rees TD, Seidman I. Silicone fluid: response to massive subcutaneous injections of dimethylpolysiloxane fluid in animals. Plast Reconstr Surg 1965; 36:330–338.

Ben-Hur N, Ballantyne DL, Rees TD, Seidman I. Local and systemic effects of dimethylpolysilox-ane fluid in mice. Plast Reconstr Surg 1967; 39:423–426.

Ben-Hur N, Neuman Z. Malignant tumor formation following subcutaneous injections of silicone fluid in white mice. Isr Med J 1963; 22:15–20.

Ben-Hur N, Neuman Z. Siliconoma—another cutaneous response to dimethylpolysiloxane. Experimental study in mice. Plast Reconstr Surg 1965; 36:629–631.

Berger RA. Dermatologic experience with liquid silicones. NY State J Med 1966; 66:2523–2526.

Berger RA. Use of silicone injections in facial defects. Arch Otolaryngol 1975; 101:525–527.

Berman WE. Synthetic materials in facial contours. Trans Am Acad Ophthalmol Otolaryngol 1964; 68:876–880.

Blocksma R. Experience with dimethylpolysiloxane fluid in soft-tissue augmentation. Plast Reconstr Surg 1971; 48:564–567.

Blocksma R. The voice of polite dissent: complications following silicone injections for augmentation of the contours of the face. Plast Reconstr Surg 1978; 62:109.

Blocksma R, Braley S. Implantation materials. In: Grabb WC, Smith JW, eds. Plastic Surgery. 2nd ed. Boston: Little, Brown, 1973:131–156.

Braley S. The silicones as tools in biological engineering. Med Electron Biol Eng 1965; 3:127–136.

Braley S. The chemistry and properties of the medical-grade silicones. J Macromol Sci-Chem A4 1970; 3:529–544.

Braley S. Silicone fluids with added adulterants—letter to the editor. Plast Reconstr Surg 1970; 45:288.

Braley S. The status of injectable silicone fluid for soft-tissue augmentation. Plast Reconstr Surg 1971; 47:343–344.

Brooks N. A foreign body granuloma produced by an injectable collagen implant at a test site. J Dermatol Surg Oncol 1982; 8:111–114.

Brown AF, Joergenson EJ. Genito mammary paraffin oil granulomas in the male. Ann West Med Surg 1947; 1:301–305.

Bulcao de Moraes H. Liquid silicone in the dorsum of the hand. Ann Plast Surg 1981; 6:500–502.

Capozzi A, Du Bou R, Pennisi VR. Distant migration of silicone gel from a ruptured breast implant. Case report. Plast Reconstr Surg 1978; 62:302–303.

Chaplin CH. Loss of both breasts from injections of silicone (with additive). Plast Reconstr Surg 1969; 44:447–449.

Chastre J, Basset F, Viau F, et al. Acute pneumonitis after subcutaneous injections of silicone in transsexual men. N Engl J Med 1983; 308:764–767.

Christ JE, Askew JB Jr. Silicone granuloma of the penis. Plast Reconstr Surg 1982; 69:337–339.

Clauser SB, Fanta cm, Finkel AJ, Perlman JM, eds. Physicians' Current Procedural Terminology. 4th ed. Chicago: American Medical Association, 1985.

Datta NS, Kern FB. Silicone granuloma of the penis. J Urol 1973; 109:840–842.

De Cholnoky T. Augmentation mammoplasty: survey of complications in 10,941 patients by 265 surgeons. Plast Reconstr Surg 1970; 45:573–577.

Delage C, Shane JJ, Johnson FB. Mammary silicone granuloma: migration of silicone fluid to abdominal wall and inguinal region. Arch Dermatol 1973; 108:104–107.

Dingman R. Silicon injections. In: Epstein E, ed. Skin Surgery. 3rd ed. Springfield, IL: Charles C Thomas, 1970:578–584.

Durst S, Johnson BS, Amplatz K. The effect of silicone coatings on thrombogenicity. Am J Roentgenol 1974; 120:904–906.

Edgerton MT, Wells JH. Indications for and pitfalls of soft-tissue augmentation with liquid silicone. Plast Reconstr Surg 1976; 58:157–165.

Ellenbogen R, Ellenbogen R, Rubin L. Injectable fluid silicone therapy: human morbidity and mortality. JAMA 1975; 234:308–309.

Freeman BS, Bigelow EL, Braley SA. Experiments with injectable plastic. Use of silicone and silastic rubber in animals and its clinical use in deformities of the head and neck. Am J Surg 1966; 112:534–536.

Frisch EE. Technology of silicones in biomedical applications. In: Rubin LR, ed. Biomaterials in Reconstructive Surgery. St. Louis: CV Mosby, 1983:73–90.

Goin JM. Silicone for facial furrows (letter). JAMA 1974; 229:1581.

Gonzalez Ulloa M, Stevens E, Loewe P, Vargas de la Cruz J, Noble G. Preliminary report on the subcutaneous perfusion of dimethyl polisiloxane to increase volume and alter regional contour. Br J Plast Surg 1967; 20:424–431.

Grasso P, Goldberg L, Fairweather FA. Injections of silicones in mice. Letter to the editor. Lancet 1964; 2:96.

Harris HI. Survey of breast implants from the point of view of carcinogenesis. Plast Reconstr Surg 1961; 28:81–83.

Hawthorne GA, Ballantyne DL, Rees TD, Seidman I. Hematological effects of dimethylpolysilox- ane fluid in rats. J Reticuloendothel Soc 1970; 7:587–593.

Huang TT, Blackwell SJ, Lewis SR. Migration of silicone gel after the "squeeze technique" to rupture a contracted breast capsule. Case report. Plast Reconstr Surg 1978; 61:277–280.

Hueper WC. Cancer induction by polyurethan and polysilicone plastics. J Natl Cancer Inst 1964; 33:1005–1027.

Jaques LB, Fidlar E, Feldsted ET, MacDonald AG. Silicones and blood coagulation. Can Med Assoc J 1946; 55:26–31.

Kagan HD. Sakurai injectable silicone formula. A preliminary report. Arch Otolaryngol 1963; 78:663–668.

Karfik V, Smahel J. Subcutaneous silicone granuloma. Ada Chir Plast 1968; 10:328–332.

Kennedy GL Jr, Keplinger mL, Calandra JC. Reproductive, teratologic, and mutagenic studies withsome polydimethylsiloxanes. J Toxicol Environ Health 1976; 1:909–920.

Kipping FS, Blackburn JC, Short JF. Organic derivatives of silicon. Part XLIV. J Chem Soc 1931; 133:1290–1298.

Klein AW, Rish DC. Substances for soft-tissue augmentation: collagen and silicone. J Dermatol Surg Oncol 1985; 11:337–339.

Klein JA, Cole G, Barr RJ, Bartlow G, Fulwider C. Paraffinomas of the scalp. Arch Dermatol 1985; 121:382–385.

Kopf EH. Injectable silicones. Rocky Mt Med J 1966; 63:34–36.

Kopf EH, Vinnik CA, Bongiovi JJ, Dombrowski DJ. Complications of silicone injections. Rocky Mt Med J 1976; 73:77–80.

Kozeny GA, Barbato AL, Bansal VK, Vertuno LL, Hano JE. Hypercalcemia associated with silicone-induced granulomas. N Engl J Med 1984; 311:1103–1105.

Kuiper D. Silicone granulomatous disease of the breast simulating cancer. Michigan Med 1973; 72:215–218.

Le Van P. The causes and prevention of poor cosmetic results from injection of fluid silicone. J Dermatol Surg Oncol 1978; 4: 328–332.

Lever WF, Schaumberg-Lever G, eds. Histopathology of the Skin. 6th ed. Philadelphia: JB Lippincott, 1983:222.

Lewis CM. Inflammatory carcinoma of the breast following silicone injections. Case report. Plast Reconstr Surg 1980; 66:134–136.

Lighterman I. Silicone granuloma of the penis. Case reports. Plast Reconstr Surg 1976; 57:517–519.

Mason J, Apisarnthanarax P. Migratory silicone granuloma. Arch Dermatol 1981; 117:366–367.

May JA, Pickering PP. Paraffinoma of the penis. Calif Med 1956; 85:42–44.

May SB, Balkin SW. Plantar callus and diabetic ulceration treated by injectable liquid silicone. Arch Dermatol 1973; 108: 287–288.

McCurdy H, Solomons ET. Forensic examination of toxicological specimens for dimethylpolysiloxane (silicone oil). J Anal Toxicol 1977; 1:221–223.

McDowell F. Complications with silicones—what grade of silicone? How do we know it was silicone?. Plast Reconstr Surg 1978; 61:892–895.

Milojevic B. Complications after silicone injection therapy in aesthetic plastic surgery. Aesth Plast Surg 1982; 6: 203–206.

Montgomery H, ed. Dermatopathology. New York: Harper & Row, 1967:403–415.

Mullison EG. Silicones and their uses in plastic surgery. Arch Otolaryngol 1965; 81:264.

Mullison EG. Current status of silicones in plastic surgery. Arch Otolaryngol 1966; 83:59–63.

Mullison EG. Silicones in head and neck surgery. Arch Otolaryngol 1966; 84:91–95.

Nedelman CI. Oral and cutaneous tissue reactions to injected fluid silicone. J Biomed Mater Res 1968; 2:131–143.

Newcomer VD, Graham JH, Schaffert RR, Kaplan L. Sclerosing lipogranuloma resulting from exogenous lipids. Arch Dermatol 1956; 73:361–372.

Noll W, ed. Chemistry and Technology of Silicones. New York: Academic Press, 1968.

Nosanchuk JS. Silicone granuloma in breast. Arch Surg 1968; 97:583–585.

Nosanchuk JS. Injected dimethylpolysiloxane fluid. A study of the antibody and histologic response. Plast Reconstr Surg 1968; 42:562–566.

Ohmori S, Hirayama T. Is it possible to produce adjuvant's disease in human beings by the injection of silicone?. Jpn J Plast Reconstr Surg 1966; 13:132–166.

Orentreich DS, Orentreich N. Acne scar revision update. Dermatol Clin. In press.

Orentreich N. Preventive and therapeutic measures for aging skin. Proc Sci Sec Toilet Goods Assoc 1964; 41:37–43.

Orentreich N. Dermabrasion. J Am Med Womens Assoc 1969; 24:331–336.

Orentreich N. Soft-tissue augmentation with medical-grade fluid silicone. In: Rubin LR, ed. Biomaterials in Reconstructive Surgery. St. Louis: CV Mosby, 1983:859–872.

Orentreich N, Durr NP. Rehabilitation of acne scarring. Dermatol Clin 1983; l:405–413.

Orentreich N, Durr NP. The four R's of' skin rehabilitation. In: Graham JAG, Kligman AM, eds. The Psychology of Cosmetic Treatments. New York: Praeger, 1985:227–237.

Orentreich N, Selmanowitz VJ. Cosmetic improvement of factitial defects. Med Trial Tech Q 1970; XVII:172–180.

Ortiz-Monasterio F, Trigos I. Management of patients with complications from injections of foreign materials into the breasts. Plast Reconstr Surg 1972; 50:42–47.

Parsons RW, Thering HR. Management of the silicone-injected breast. Plast Reconstr Surg 1977; 60:534–538.

Pearl RM, Laub DR, Kaplan EN. Complications following silicone injections for augmentation of the contours of the face. Plast Reconstr Surg 1978; 61:888–891.

Perry RP, Jaques DP, Lesar MS, et al. Mycobacterium avium infection in a silicone-injected breast. Case report. Plast Reconstr Surg 1985; 75:104–106.

Piechotta FU. Silicone fluid, attractive and dangerous: Collective review and summary of experience. Aesth Plast Surg 1979; 3:347–355.

Pucevich MV, Rosenberg EW, Bale GF, Terzakis JA. Widespread foreign-body granulomas and elevated serum angiotensin-converting enzyme. Arch Dermatol 1983; 119:229–234.

Rees TD. Silicone injection therapy. In: Rees TD, Wood-Smith D, eds. Cosmetic Facial Surgery. Philadelphia: WB Saunders, 1973:232–267.

Rees TD. Local and systemic response to injectable silicone fluid. In: Rubin LR, ed. Biomaterials in Reconstructive Surgery. St. Louis: CV Mosby, 1983:529–543.

Rees TD, Ashley FL. Treatment of facial atrophy with liquid silicone. Am J Surg 1966; 111:531–535.

Rees TD, Ashley FL. A new treatment for facial hemiatrophy in children by injections of dimethylpolysiloxane fluid. J Pediatr Surg 1967; 2:347–353.

Rees TD, Ashley FL, Delgado JP. Silicone fluid injections for facial atrophy. A ten-year study. Plast Reconstr Surg 1973; 52:118–127.

Rees TD, Ballantyne DL, Coburn RJ. Liquid silicone therapy—a decade's experience. In: McMahon FG, ed. Drug Induced Clinical Toxicity. MT. Kisco, NY: Futura Publishing, 1974:169–181.

Rees TD, Ballantyne DL, Hawthorne GA. Silicone fluid research. A follow-up summary. Plast Reconstr Surg 1970; 46:50–56.

Rees TD, Ballantyne DL Jr, Hawthorne GA, Seidman I. The effects of dimethylpolysiloxane fluid on rat skin autografts. Plast Reconstr Surg 1968; 41:153–156.

Rees TD, Ballantyne DL, Seidman I. Eyelid deformities caused by the injection of silicone fluid. Br J Plast Surg 1971; 24:125–128.

Rees TD, Ballantyne DL, Seidman I, Hawthorne GA. Visceral response to subcutaneous and intraperitoneal injections of silicone in mice. Plast Reconstr Surg 1967; 39:402–410.

Rees TD, Coburn RJ. Silicone treatment of partial lipodystrophy. JAMA 1974; 230:868–870.

Rees TD, Platt J, Ballantyne DL. An investigation of cutaneous response to dimethylpolysiloxane (silicone liquid) in animals and humans: a preliminary report. Plast Reconstr Surg 1965; 35:131–139.

Rich JD, Shesol BF, Gottlieb VG. Supraclavicular migration of breast-injected silicone: case report. Milit Med 1982; 147:404–405.

Scales JT. Discussion on metals and synthetic materials in relation to tissues: tissue reactions to synthetic materials. Proc R Soc Med 1953; 46:647.

Selmanowitz VJ, Orentreich N. Cosmetic treatment of factitial defects. Cuds 1970; 6:549–552.

Selmanowitz VJ, Orentreich N. Cutaneous corticosteroid injection and amaurosis. Arch Dermatol 1974; 110:729–734.

Selmanowitz VJ, Orentreich N. Medical-grade fluid silicone: a monographic review. J Dermatol Surg Oncol 1977; 3:597–611.

Smetana HF, Bernhard W. Sclerosing lipogranuloma. Arch Pathol 1950; 50:296–325.

Solomons ET, Jones JK. The determination of polydimethylsiloxane (silicone oil) in biological materials: a case report. J Forensic Sci 1975; 20:191–199.

Sperber PA. Chemexfoliation and silicone infiltration in the treatment of aging skin and dermal defects. J Am Geriatr Soc 1964; 12:594–601.

Stough DB. Medical silicone in dermofacial defects. Cutis 1970; 6:1243–1245.

Stough DB. Silicone treatment of plantar keratoses. Cutis 1971; 8:575–576.

Symmers WS. Silicone mastitis in "topless" waitresses and some other varieties of foreign-body mastitis. Br Med J 1968; 3:19–22.

Travis WD, Balogh K, Abraham JL. Silicone granulomas: report of three cases and review of the literature. Human Pathol 1985; 16:19–27.

Urbach F, Wine SS, Johnson WC, Davies RE. Generalized paraffinoma (sclerosing lipogranuloma). Arch Dermatol 1971; 103:277–285.

Vinnik CA. The hazards of silicone injections (editorial). JAMA 1976; 236:959.

Walsh FB, Hoyt WF, eds. Clinical Neuro-Ophthalmology. 3rd ed. Vol. 3. Baltimore: Williams & Wilkins, 1969:2501–2510.

Webster RC, Fuleihan MD, Gaunt JM, Hamdan US, Smith RC. Injectable silicone for small augmentations: twenty-year experience in humans. Am J Cosmet Surg 1984; 1:1–10.

Webster RC, Fuleihan NS, Hamdan US, Gaunt JM, Smith RC. Injectable silicone for small augmentations: recommendations for controlled release to medical profession. Am J Cosmet Surg 1984; 1:11–21.

Webster RC, Kattner MD, Smith RC. Injectable collagen for augmentation of facial areas. Arch Otolaryngol 1984; 110:652–656.

Wilkie TF. Late development of granuloma after liquid silicone injections. Plast Reconstr Surg 1977; 60:179–188.

Winer LH, Sternberg TH, Lehman R, Ashley FL. Tissue reactions to injected silicone liquids. A report of three cases. Arch Dermatol 1964; 90:588–593.

Wustrack KO, Zarem HA. Surgical management of silicone mastitis. Plast Reconstr Surg 1979; 63:224–229.

Wynn SK. Combining cosmetic rhinoplasty with nasolabial silicone injection. Wise Med J 1966; 65:179.

Zalar JA Jr, Knode RE, Mir JA. Lipogranuloma of the penis. J Urol 1969; 102:75–77.

Zandi I. Use of suction to treat soft tissue injected with liquid silicone. Plast Reconstr Surg 1985; 76:307–309.

72

Botulinum Toxin Type A: Cosmetic Applications in the Face and Neck

Alastair Carruthers
Department of Dermatology, University of British Columbia, Vancouver,
British Columbia, Canada

Jean Carruthers
Department of Ophthalmology, University of British Columbia, Vancouver,
British Columbia, Canada

INTRODUCTION

Botulinum toxin type A (BTX-A) was introduced for cosmetic use in the early 1990s, and has since become extremely popular with patients seeking safe, effective, and minimally invasive treatment to address the appearance of premature aging caused by facial lines. The outstanding results yielded by BTX-A treatment in tandem with the simplicity of the treatment process itself have combined to place BTX-A injections among the most commonly performed cosmetic procedures today. The exponential growth of this modality shows no signs of abating.

As clinical experience with this powerful neurotoxin grows, the techniques for its application are becoming more sophisticated. Clinicians wishing to offer BTX-A treatment can now draw on significant accumulated experience and a wealth of literature to provide patients with highly satisfying cosmetic outcomes. This chapter will provide an overview of the cosmetic use of BTX-A in the face and neck, including discussion of patient selection, specific injection techniques, maximizing results, and postoperative considerations, as well as complications and adverse events.

BACKGROUND

Development of BTX-A

BTX-A was isolated in pure crystalline form in 1946, and its mechanism of action was identified in the 1950s. In the 1960s, Dr. Alan Scott of the Smith-Kettlewell Eye Research Foundation began to study the effects of BTX-A on strabismus in primates. Dr. Scott's work over the next 20 years would ultimately lead to the use of BTX-A in human treatment. BTX-A received FDA approval for strabismus and blepharospasm in 1989 and for cervical dystonia in 2000.

We began using BTX-A in 1982, and in 1987 we observed that patients receiving BTX-A injections for blepharospasm showed improvement in the appearance of glabellar lines. In 1992, we published the first report describing cosmetic use of BTX-A; other reports describing a reduction in facial lines in facial dystonia patients began to appear around this time. In 2002, BTX-A (BOTOX Cosmetic) received FDA approval for the treatment of glabellar lines.

Botulinum Neurotoxins

Clostridium botulinum produces seven distinct serotypes of botulinum neurotoxin (BTX A–G). Each BTX serotype differs slightly in both mechanism of action and clinical effect, but all block neuromuscular transmission by binding to receptor sites on motor nerve terminals and inhibiting acetylcholine release. Intramuscular injection of therapeutic doses of BTXs causes temporary chemodenervation of the injected muscle and a localized reduction in muscle activity. Administration of appropriate doses in patients without underlying neuromuscular dysfunction produces no systemic clinical effects.

BTX Formulations

Two commercial BTX formulations are currently available in North America: BOTOX®, BOTOX Cosmetic™, and Vistabel (BTX-A) and MYOBLOC™ (BTX-B; Elan Pharmaceuticals, San Diego, California, U.S.A.). A third product, Dysport® (BTX-A; Ipsen Limited, Maidenhead, Berkshire, U.K.), has been available in Europe for several years, is under review by the FDA and will be marketed in North America under the name Reloxin by Allergan, Inc. (Irvin, California). At the present time, BOTOX Cosmetic™ is the only botulinum toxin approved for cosmetic use in North America. It is important to stress that BOTOX, MYOBLOC, and Dysport are unique products with many differences, not only in biological and clinical effect, but with respect to *C. botulinum* strain, potency, manufacturing process, and therapeutic dose. Our clinical experience lies primarily with BOTOX. Unless otherwise noted, all references in this chapter to BTX-A will refer to the BOTOX, BOTOX Cosmetic, or Vistabel formulations. This is especially true of dose information.

Storage and Reconstitution

BOTOX Cosmetic™ is supplied in vials containing 100 mouse units of vacuum-dried *C. botulinum* type A neurotoxin complex. The product should be stored in a freezer at or below –5°C or in a refrigerator between 2 and 8°C. Diluent volume is determined by the desired concentration of the injection solution. In general, our preference is to use low volumes of concentrated toxin (100 U/mL), as this allows precise delivery of BTX-A while minimizing diffusion. We have shown that higher volumes of less concentrated toxin (5–10 U/mL) will produce more diffuse effects, which may be desirable in some applications. Other investigators have reported similar findings . Positive results have been described using dilutions as high as 10 U/mL to treat the periorbital area (crow's feet) and the brow area.

Instructions provided by the manufacturer suggest that BTX-A be reconstituted with sterile, non-preserved 0.9% saline solution and that the reconstituted product be discarded after 4 hours. Clinical experience, however, indicates that reconstitution with preserved saline may reduce pain on injection and does not affect the stability of the product, and that BTX-A retains efficacy for up to 6 weeks following reconstitution. BTX-A should not be frozen once reconstituted.

PREOPERATIVE CONSIDERATIONS
Patient Selection and Education
Successful outcomes following cosmetic use of BTX-A depend in large part on appropriate patient selection. BTX-A is most effective in reducing negative facial signals caused by underlying muscle pull in patients aged 20 to 45 years. In patients with age-related loss of dermal elasticity, substantial facial lentigines, telangiectasia, and telangiectatic matting with fine rhytides and diminished skin texture, BTX-A treatment alone may not yield a satisfactory response . Many of these individuals will retain the overall appearance of age and fatigue that led them to seek treatment.

The clinician should ensure that the patient has a realistic understanding of the anticipated benefits of treatment, the time course of the clinical effect, and the necessity of periodic re-treatment to maintain the desired effect. Patients who undergo BTX-A treatment with unrealistic or exaggerated expectations are likely to be disappointed with the outcome, regardless of whether the procedure was clinically successful. The patient's motivations and expectations can be clarified by taking a history of prior cosmetic interventions and the patient's satisfaction with the results. During the initial consultation, safety concerns should be addressed and the patient should be informed about what to expect following treatment.

Documentation
In addition to ensuring that expectations are realistic, the clinician should carefully document the facial anatomy using pre- and postoperative photography. Special attention should be paid to atypical facial features. Digital photography is particularly valuable because it enables the capture of video clips as well as still images, providing a more complete and accurate record to demonstrate the dynamic effects of BTX-A treatment.

Contraindications
Contraindications include a known hypersensitivity to any of the product contents; inflammation or infection at the injection site; and underlying neuromuscular disorders including myasthenia gravis, Eaton–Lambert syndrome, myopathies, or amyotrophic lateral sclerosis. Caution should be exercised in disorders that produce a depletion of acetylcholine, and in patients receiving aminoglycosides or other drugs that interfere with neuromuscular transmission. No studies concerning the safety of BTX-A in pregnant or nursing women have been published.

INJECTION TECHNIQUES
General Technique
Photography of the target region when muscles are at rest and during maximal contraction will reveal the individual patient characteristics that are key to successful treatment. With the patient seated upright, natural muscle movement and corresponding facial lines can be precisely delineated by marking the area to be injected.

The desired dose is drawn into the syringe. We use the Becton-Dickinson Ultra-Fine II short-needle 0.3-mL insulin syringe. With an integrated 30-gauge, silicon-coated needle, this syringe minimizes pain on injection and reduces drug waste compared to syringes with a needle hub. B-D has now introduced a similar syringe with an even finer 31-gauge needle. The needle remains sharp for approximately six cutaneous punctures and should then be discarded. We use a bottle opener to carefully remove the rubber stopper from the vial prior to drawing up the solution, a measure that will prevent the needle from becoming prematurely dull through perforating the hard rubber of the stopper. Reconstituting with preserved saline (containing 0.9% benzyl alcohol), infusing slowly with a 30- or 31-gauge needle, and injecting small volumes of relatively concentrated solution will help to minimize pain associated with injections. Distracting the patient by gently rubbing the skin adjacent to the injection site can help to reduce the initial pain of injection, and we have demonstrated a benefit to the use of lidocaine 4% topical anesthetic cream prior to BTX-A injection for crow's feet. Vibration anesthesia has also been reported to be effective in reducing pain on injection. Standard skin preparation and sterility procedures should be followed.

The Upper Face
The first reports of cosmetic use for BTX-A were in the upper face, and to date, treatment of the upper face has provided the greatest wealth of clinical experience. The lines and wrinkles common in the aging face include glabellar frown lines, horizontal forehead lines, and crow's feet. In older patients these presentations are caused by loss of dermal elasticity associated with age, though they may be accelerated or exacerbated by factors such as smoking and photodamage. In younger patients, hyperactivity of the facial muscles yields significant lines, giving the patient an appearance of age and fatigue. It is in these younger patients that BTX-A will provide the greatest benefits through its dramatic effect in relaxing the underlying musculature.

Glabellar Frown Lines
BTX-A treatment for glabellar frown lines typically produces a clinical effect of three to four months duration, although the effects may persist for six to eight months in some patients. In determining appropriate doses and injection sites, the clinician must consider individual anatomical characteristics, including the type and degree of brow arch and asymmetry, whether the brow is ptotic or crosses the orbital rim, and the amount of muscle mass in the brow. In males, doses of 60 or 80 U BTX-A may be required to produce a satisfactory reduction in glabellar lines, due to the greater muscle mass in the typical male brow. In female patients, good clinical effect can often be achieved with doses of 30 or 40 U. Our method for reconstituting BTX-A when treating males is to reduce the diluent volume by half, thereby doubling the dose of BTX-A while reducing the injected volume. We use an initial dose of 30 and 60 U for

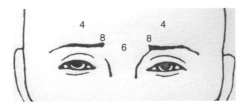

Figure 1 Injection sites and doses for the treatment of glabellar frown lines.

women and men, respectively, diluted to 1 or 2 U per 0.01 mL. If the desired response is not achieved, we titrate up to a dose of 40 and 80 U in women and men, respectively.

The patient should be seated, with the chin down and the head slightly lower than the clinician's. We insert the needle just above the eyebrow, directly above the caruncle at the inner canthus. Eyebrow position will differ from one patient to the next, but the injection site is always above the bony supraorbital ridge. Bleeding may occur during the procedure, as the supratrochlear vessels are located immediately medial to the injection site; therefore, it is important to choose an injection site where pressure can be applied safely following treatment.

We inject 4 to 6 U and then slowly withdraw the needle, with the tip kept superficially beneath the skin. We reposition the needle and inject a further 4 to 5 U superiorly and superficially to at least 1 cm above the previous injection site in the orbicularis oculi. We then repeat the procedure on the opposite side of the brow to maintain a balanced appearance. We inject another 5 to 10 U into the procerus in the midline, at a point below a line joining the brows and above the intersection of the "X" formed by joining the medial eyebrow to the contralateral inner canthus (Fig. 1). In patients with horizontal brows (the majority), we inject an additional 4 to 5 U into a point 1 cm above the supraorbital rim in the midpupillary line.

We instruct patients to remain vertical and to frown as much as possible while the toxin is binding in the two to three hours immediately following treatment. We also warn patients not to rub, press, or otherwise manipulate the treated area. A follow-up appointment is scheduled for two to three weeks following treatment. At this time, we assess the clinical effect and perform "touch-up" injections if necessary.

Horizontal Forehead Lines

BTX-A treatment of horizontal forehead lines has a clinical effect of four to six months duration in most patients. A conservative, cautious approach is needed to achieve satisfactory outcomes when treating horizontal forehead lines. Inducing paresis in the frontalis without a corresponding weakening of the depressors will produce unopposed action of the depressors, lowering the brow and yielding an angry countenance (Fig. 2). The clinician must endeavor to leave some function in the frontalis intact. Ensuring that injection sites are positioned above the brow will avoid ptosis or a lack of expressiveness. In patients with a narrow brow (defined as less than 12 cm between the temporal fusion lines at mid-brow level) fewer injections (four sites, compared to five) and lower doses should be used than in patients with a broader brow.

We have found that the greatest improvement in horizontal forehead lines and a satisfactory duration of clinical effect can be achieved with a total of 48 U injected in the procerus, frontalis, lateral orbicularis oculi, and depressor muscles (Fig. 3). It should be noted, however, that adverse effects are dose-related.

Brow Shaping

BTX-A can be used to alter the shape of the brows, producing a more pleasing appearance through brow elevation or correction of brow asymmetry. A thorough knowledge of the underlying musculature and of the action of BTX-A in the glabellar complex is required to achieve these effects. As we know, the positive cosmetic effect of BTX-A lies in its neuroparalytic action, blocking neuromuscular transmission and producing weakness of the treated muscles. However, we now recognize that BTX-A produces its effects both by reduction in resting tone in treated muscles and by increasing tone in adjacent muscles. As described in the following section, the brow lift we see following BTX-A treatment of the glabella is due to partial weakening of the glabellar complex/lower frontalis producing an increase in resting tone in the untreated part of frontalis.

Brow Elevation

Elevation of the brow following BTX-A treatment of glabellar lines has been described by several authors, and we have reported the beneficial result of lateral and mid-pupil elevation following administration of 30 and 40 U BTX-A in the glabellar region. We initially believed that this elevation resulted from the action of the BTX-A on the medial (corrugator supercilii, procerus, and the medial portion of the orbicularis oculi) and lateral (the lateral portion of the orbicularis oculi) brow depressors, but further study revealed that a total of 10 U BTX-A injected in the glabella produced mild, medial brow ptosis that persisted for two months. Furthermore, doses of 20 to 40 U yielded an initial lateral eyebrow elevation, followed by central and medial

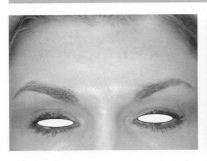
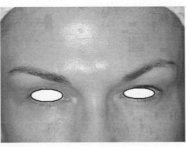

Figure 2 Poor technique in the treatment of horizontal forehead lines can yield a lowered brow and an angry expression.

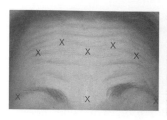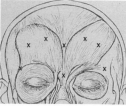

Figure 3 Musculature and injection sites for the treatment of horizontal forehead lines.

eyebrow elevation that peaked at 12 weeks but was still significantly present at 16 weeks. BTX-A typically reaches peak effect in skeletal muscle at four weeks, and this marks the first time we have observed peak effect at 12 weeks. The primary effect is lateral, in an area not injected; this leads us to believe that the brow elevation results from partial inactivation of the frontalis, rather than from the action of the toxin on the brow depressors. The subsequent elevation of the central and medial brow may be caused by a gradual lift following the adjustment of resting tone in the frontalis muscle, meaning that the eyebrow elevation is the result of increased tone in the untreated portion of frontalis, which in turn is due to the reduction in tone in the treated portion of frontalis.

These observations lead us to conclude that adjustment in the amount of treated frontalis is the main determinant of eyebrow position and shape. Reducing the dose of BTX-A delivered to the frontalis muscle will decrease the brow elevation and, if carried to an extreme, may result in brow ptosis. Injecting frontalis more medially or laterally will likewise alter the shape of the eyebrows. Patient response to changes in dose and treatment site will vary significantly. We strongly advise keeping accurate and detailed records describing exact injection patterns. This will allow adjustment in future treatments if the desired eyebrow shape is not achieved with the first treatment.

Eyebrow Asymmetry

BTX-A injections can be used to correct asymmetry of the eyebrows. Typically, the toxin is used to elevate the lower eyebrow to the same level as the higher. This can be achieved both by reducing depressor activity and by increasing tone in relevant parts of frontalis, as described above. In some patients, however, a portion of one eyebrow may be significantly elevated; in such cases it is appropriate to lower that while raising the other eyebrow in order to achieve a symmetrical appearance (Fig. 4).

Some practitioners use a technique in the glabella area employing deep injections into corrugator above the inner canthus to preferentially affect the depressor muscles and produce greater brow elevation, while using more superficial injection of the inferomedial portion of frontalis, yielding reduced elevation of the central brow. We do not recommend this technique, for two reasons. First, BTX-A diffuses extremely well and our experience indicates that differences of a few millimeters in injection site do not dramatically change the treatment effect. Second, as discussed above, we believe that the BTX-A brow lift is due to the treated portion of frontalis causing an increased tone in the untreated portion of frontalis. It could therefore be argued that the above technique may have an effect completely opposite to the desired result. There is currently insufficient evidence to support either position.

Though eyebrow asymmetry is very common and is not noticeable in the majority of individuals, minor asymmetry following surgical brow lift can be extremely distressing for both clinician and patient, and BTX-A treatment offers an easy way to correct this. Again, we stress the importance of careful patient assessment, both at rest and dynamically in tandem with detailed recording of injection sites and dose to achieve a satisfying response.

Crow's Feet

Even in patients with severely photodamaged skin, BTX-A can dramatically reduce the appearance of crow's feet rhytides by relaxing, rather than paralyzing, the lateral orbicularis oculi (Fig. 5). Clinical effects from the initial treatment session typically persist for approximately 4 months, but the duration of treatment effect may increase on subsequent treatments.

Crow's feet are treated by injecting lateral to the lateral orbital rim, and equal doses of toxin (approximately 4–7 U/site; 12–20 U/side) are delivered at two to three injection sites. There is a lack of consensus regarding optimal dosage in the lateral orbital region. A recent dose-ranging study found no significant difference in efficacy between 6 and 18 U/side. Other reported total dose ranges include 5 to 15 U and 4 to 5 U per eye over two or three injection sites. Our preference is to use 12 to 15 U/side, distributed equally over two to four sites. We recommend minimizing the number of injections and injecting as superficially as possible to minimize bruising.

To identify the injection sites for crow's feet, ask the patient to smile maximally. Determine the center of the crow's feet; the first injection site is in the center of the area of maximal wrinkling, approximately 1 to 2 cm lateral to the lateral orbital rim. The second and third injection sites are approximately 1 to 1.5 cm above and below the first

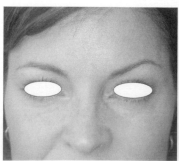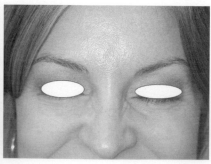

Figure 4 BTX-A injection can be used to good effect in the correction of eyebrow asymmetry.

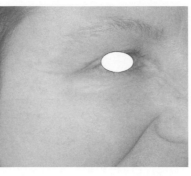

Figure 5 Relaxing the muscles responsible for the formation of crow's feet rhytides can produce dramatic effects.

injection site, respectively (Fig. 6). Distribution of crow's feet will differ from one patient to the next. Some patients will present with equal distribution above and below the lateral canthus; in others, crow's feet appear primarily below the lateral canthus (Fig. 7). In the latter case, the injection sites may be in a line that angles from anteroinferior to superoposterior. In all patients, regardless of the distribution, the most anterior injection should be placed lateral to a line drawn vertically from the lateral canthus. To avoid having the toxin affect the ipsilateral zygomaticus complex, causing ptosis of the upper lip, ensure that the patient is not smiling while the toxin is injected.

The Mid- and Lower Face

As the cosmetic use of BTX-A continues to expand, recent years have seen a dramatic increase in its use in the mid- and lower face. As with the upper face, recognition of differences in individual patient characteristics is key to achieving good outcomes. Severe impairment of muscular function and expression can result from poor technique in the mid- and lower face, and for this reason the use of electromyographic guidance is recommended in some patients. These procedures should only be performed by physicians with a thorough understanding of both facial vasculature and dynamic and resting facial anatomy.

Perioral Rhytides

Vertical perioral rhytides radiating outward from the vermilion border are the result of overactivity of the orbicularis oris, and these lines can be effectively treated by weakening the orbicularis oris. Care must be taken to avoid causing

a paresis that could interfere with speech and suction. Small doses of BTX-A (1–2 U per lip quadrant) are usually sufficient, and in this application BTX-A is often used in combination with a soft-tissue augmenting agent. The dilution is increased and a total dose of 6 U is applied to eight injection sites (0.75 U in 0.03 mL per injection), carefully measuring the sites to balance on either side of the columella or the lateral nasal ala (Fig. 8).

Hypertrophic Orbicularis

In patients of Asian heritage and in some others, the perceived size of the palpebral aperture may be transiently diminished when smiling. We have shown that injecting 2 U into the lower pretarsal orbicularis will relax the palpebral aperture, both at rest and while smiling. Mean palpebral aperture increases of 1.8 mm (at rest) and 2.9 mm (at full smile) have been reported after subdermal injections of 2 U, delivered 3 mm inferior to the lower pretarsal orbicularis, and three, 4-U injections placed 1.5 cm from the lateral canthus, with 1 cm between injection sites (Fig. 9).

Nasalis

The appearance of "bunny lines," radial rhytides that fan obliquely across the radix of the nose, can be significantly diminished by injecting BTX-A anterior to the nasofacial groove on the lateral wall of the nose. It is important to inject well above the angular vein, and to avoid injecting the nasofacial groove, as this can affect the levator labii superioris and levator labii superioris aleque nasi. To assist in diffusing the toxin, the clinician should gently massage the area

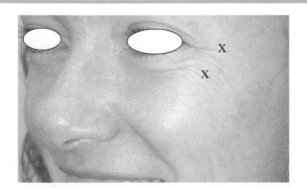

Figure 6 Injection sites for crow's feet are identified by asking the patient to smile maximally.

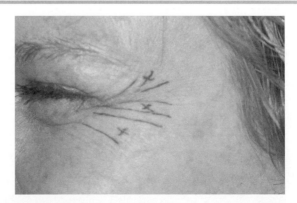

Figure 7 Distribution of crow's feet relative to the lateral canthus varies by individual patient.

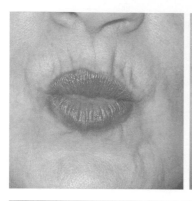
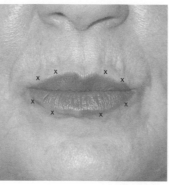

Figure 8 Injection sites and dose distribution for the treatment of perioral rhytides.

following injection. Patients with repeated nasal flare resulting from involuntary dilation of the nostrils can also benefit from injection of the nasalis. In these patients, the nasalis fibers, which drape over the lateral nasal ala, are injected.

Nasolabial Folds

In patients with a naturally short upper lip, application of 1 U BTX-A to each lip elevator complex in the nasofacial groove will elongate the muscles of the upper lip, but will also collapse the upper aspect of the nasoiabiai fold and flatten the mid-face, an effect that many patients may not desire. The cosmetic result of weakening the lip levator, zygomaticus, and risorius muscles should be carefully explained to the patient, in addition to the long duration of clinical effect (approximately six months) associated with this treatment.

Depressor Anguli Oris

The depressor anguli oris is a cosmetically important muscle that extends inferiorly from the modiolus and attaches at the inferior margin of the mandible on the lateral aspect of the chin. Contraction of the depressor anguli oris causes a downward turn to the corner of the mouth, creating a negative appearance. The depressor anguli oris overlies the depressor labii inferioris, and to avoid the asymmetrical paresis that may result from direct injection, we use 3 to 5 U at the posterior margin of the mandible, close to the anterior margin of the masseter. The result is significant weakening, but not paralysis, of the muscle (Fig. 10).

As discussed in the section on brow elevation, BTX-A does not act on muscles in isolation. The effect of BTX-A on one muscle often produces a positive or negative effect on another muscle. Another example of the complementary effect of BTX-A can be seen in treating patients with "mouth frown," a permanent downward angulation of the lateral

corners of the mouth caused by the action of the depressor anguli oris and the upward motion of the mentalis. Treating mouth frown simply by injecting the depressor anguli oris or mentalis alone may produce the desired effect in some patients, but carries the possibility of suboptimal results and unacceptable side effects in many individuals.

We therefore inject both the depressor anguli oris and mentalis simultaneously. In females we achieve a subtle weakening effect by using a total dose of 12 U:3 U injected into each depressor anguli oris, and 3 U into each side of the mentalis. Careful counseling is required to ensure that patients understand the risk of adverse effects and the desired outcome, and pre- and post-procedure photographic documentation must be undertaken. This procedure is not recommended in patients naive to BTX-A treatment.

Melomental Folds

Cosmetic improvement of melomental folds, deep skin folds extending from the depressed corner of the mouth to the lateral mentum, has traditionally been achieved using soft-tissue augmentation. The clinical effect of filling agents can be improved in these folds by injecting BTX-A into the depressor anguli oris. This will extend the duration of soft-tissue augmentation and will minimize contortion and repeated molding that may occur with filling agents when used as monotherapy.

Mental Crease

The mental crease can be weakened by injecting the mentalis anterior to the point of the chin. The aim of treatment, as in the perioral area, is to relax, rather than paralyze, the muscle. To achieve this effect, we inject 3 to 5 U into each side of the midline under the point of the chin, just anterior to the bony mentum, instead of injecting centrally. Toxin should not be applied at the level of the mental crease, as

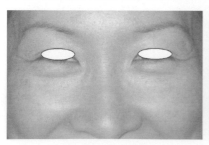
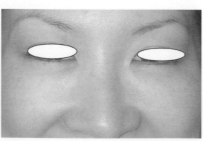

Figure 9 BTX-A can be used to increase the size of the palpebral aperture in patients of Asian heritage.

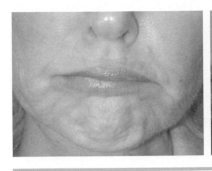
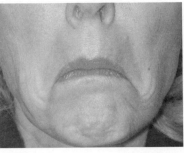

Figure 10 Treatment of the depressor anguli oris can produce a more positive resting facial expression in patients with a downward turn to the mouth.

this will weaken the lower lip depressors and orbicularis oris, causing serious adverse effects that may persist for 6 months or more, depending on the dose.

"Peau d'Orange" Chin

Loss of subcutaneous fat and dermal collagen produces a "peau d'orange" appearance in the chin that becomes evident when the mentalis and depressor labii muscles are used in speech requiring co-contraction of the orbicularis oris (Fig. 11). Again, while the traditional approach involved the use of filling agents and laser resurfacing, the appearance of "peau d'orange" chin can be significantly improved by combination treatment with soft-tissue augmentation and BTX-A in the mentalis, or, in patients who do not require filling agents, by BTX-A injection alone.

The Neck

The appearance of necklace lines and platysmal bands, common signs of aging in the neck, can be effectively reduced by injection of BTX-A.

Necklace Lines

The easiest way to treat necklace lines—horizontal lines of skin indentation caused by subcutaneous muscular aponeurotic system attachments—is to apply 1 to 2 U at several sites along the lines, injecting into the deep intradermal plane. It is important to employ deep dermal injections while avoiding both venous perforators, which may bleed, and the underlying muscles of deglutition, which are cholinergic and may be adversely affected by BTX-A (Fig. 12). We use a total dose of no more than 20 U per treatment session. Bruising can be minimized by massaging the injected area following treatment.

Platysmal Bands

Platysmal bands, traditionally treated with rhytidectomy surgery, respond well to BTX-A injection in carefully selected patients. Appropriate patient selection is paramount,

as the appearance of platysmal bands may be exacerbated in individuals with jowl formation and bone resorption. Good candidates for this procedure include patients with obvious platysmal bands, minimal fat descent, and good cervical skin elasticity. As with necklace lines, care must be taken to avoid injecting the muscles responsible for deglutition and neck flexion. To avoid the possibility of profound dysphagia, we recommend using a total dose of no more than 30 to 40 U per treatment session.

Facial Asymmetry

BTX-A can be applied to correct facial asymmetry resulting from underlying muscular activity or consequent to surgery. In patients with hemifacial spasm, repeated tonic and clonic facial movements will distort the facial midline toward the hyperfunctional side. Using BTX-A to weaken the zygomaticus, risorius, and masseter on the hyperfunctional side of the face will return the facial midline to a central position. In patients with hypofunctional asymmetry following VII paresis, BTX-A applied on the normofunctional side of the face at doses of 1 to 2 U in the zygomaticus, risorius, and orbicularis and 5 to 10 U in the masseter will restore facial symmetry. Intraoral injection of 10 to 15 U BTX-A into the internal pterygoid can be used to correct asymmetry of jaw movement.

Facial asymmetry may also result from surgical causes. For example, surgical or traumatic cutting of the orbicularis oris or risorius muscle can produce unopposed action of the corresponding muscles in the normally innervated side, resulting in decentration of the mouth. Injecting the overdynamic risorius immediately lateral to the lateral corner of the mouth and in the mid-pupillary line will correct the off-center position of the mouth when the face is at rest. Individuals with either acquired or congenital weakness of the depressor anguli oris will exhibit an inability to depress the corner of one side of the mouth; a balanced appearance and improved function can be achieved in these patients by injecting BTX-A in the corresponding muscle.

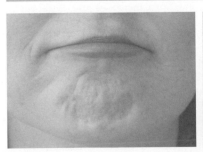
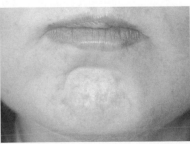

Figure 11 "Peau d'orange" chin can be treated by BTX-A injection of the mentalis.

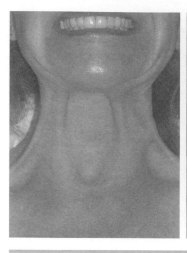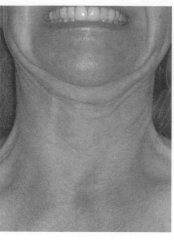

Figure 12   In the treatment of necklace lines, deep dermal injections are required.

Masseteric Hypertrophy

Where shaping of the jaw is desired, BTX-A provides a simple, non-surgical means to achieve the desired cosmetic effect with the advantage of brief recovery time. Though the literature on this intervention is primarily derived from small series, one larger trial indicates that a gradual reduction in masseter thickness can be achieved by using a total dose of 25 to 30 U distributed evenly across five to six sites on the mandibular angle. The duration of clinical effect was between six and seven months; side effects lasted one to four weeks and included difficulty chewing, muscle pain, and speech difficulties. The average reduction in masseter thickness in this study was 1.5–2.9 mm.

ADJUNCTIVE THERAPY

BTX-A is highly effective as monotherapy in the treatment of rhytides caused by underlying muscular activity. In patients with non-dynamic rhytides, however, it is not effective alone. Lentigines, telangiectasias, and pore-sized elements of the aging face have traditionally been treated with surgery, soft-tissue augmentation, laser resurfacing, and broadband light (BBL) therapy. BTX-A represents a highly effective adjunct to these interventions, yielding impressive results. Some of the most dramatic and successful applications of BTX-A result from its use in combination with other agents and modalities.

Surgery

Application of BTX-A prior to surgery can enable greater surgical correction by relaxing and reducing the action of the facial muscles, facilitating tissue manipulation. Following surgery, BTX-A has been reported to limit the reappearance of facial lines by reducing the activity of underlying musculature. A number of authors have reported successful outcomes with BTX-A in the surgical context. Use of BTX-A to weaken the brow depressor complex 1 week prior to brow lift surgery has been reported to produce greater elevation of the brow, and greater duration of clinical effect following brow lift surgery has been reported with post-surgical application of BTX-A. Cosmetic outcomes for surgical brow lifts may vary based on postoperative healing, and therefore stabilization of brow musculature is important to achieving a predictable final brow position.

In patients undergoing periorbital rhytidectomy, BTX-A treatment improves and increases the longevity of the surgical results. Relaxing the muscles responsible for crow's feet with BTX-A prior to surgery enables greater accuracy in estimating the amount of skin to be resected during surgery and better placement of the incision. Similarly, the application of BTX-A during lower eyelid ectropion and "roundeye" repair relaxes the lateral fibers of the orbicularis, reducing the muscular pull on the medial side of the temporal incision and the possibility of post-surgical dehiscence.

Soft-Tissue Augmentation

In patients undergoing soft-tissue augmentation, BTX-A is a valuable adjunct that increases the effect and duration of results by eliminating or reducing the muscular activity responsible for the formation of rhytides and increasing the longevity of the augmenting material.

A prospective, randomized study of 38 patients with moderate-to-severe glabellar rhytides demonstrated that combination therapy with BTX-A plus non-animal stabilized hyaluronic acid (NASHA) produced a better response both at rest and on maximum frown than monotherapy with NASHA (Restylane™). The combination also significantly increased the duration of response compared to either intervention alone. The median time to return of pre-injection furrow status occurred at 18 weeks in the NASHA or BTX-A monotherapy groups, compared with 32 weeks in the BTX-A plus NASHA group.

Used in combination with filling agents, BTX-A may decrease the amount of augmenting agent required. We inject BTX-A first, wait two to four weeks for BTX-A to soften the muscle contractions, and then inject the filling agent to correct the remaining lines.

Laser Resurfacing

In laser resurfacing procedures, adjunctive use of BTX-A improves clinical outcomes and increases the duration of cosmetic effect. BTX-A prevents muscle movement during resurfacing and the recurrence of dynamic lines following resurfacing, while the laser treatment stimulates production of collagen and targets static facial lines. Regular postoperative BTX-A injections administered at 6- to 12-month intervals prolong the effects of resurfacing, especially for the improvement of forehead, glabellar, and canthal rhytides. Additionally, a greater duration of effect in forehead, glabellar, and canthal rhytides has been reported in patients treated with postoperative BTX-A injections in conjunction with CO_2 laser resurfacing compared to patients treated with laser resurfacing alone. Combination BTX-A injection and laser therapy has been shown to yield greater treatment success in patients with crow's feet compared with ablative resurfacing alone.

Broadband Light Therapy

Broadband light therapy is a non-invasive treatment modality with brief recovery time and little epidermal damage. Our investigation of BTX-A and BBL combination therapy suggests that the two interventions may act together to improve facial signs of aging, and may represent a promising approach to the treatment of patients with extensive photodamage and facial aging. A prospective, randomized study of BTX-A and BBL therapy in 30 patients with moderate to severe crow's feet found that the BTX-A plus BBL group demonstrated better response at rest and on maximum smile compared to BBL alone. Patients receiving combination therapy also had an improved response to treatment of associated lentigines, telangiectasia, pore size, and facial skin texture compared to BBL alone, and a 15% global aesthetic improvement compared to BBL alone.

POSTOPERATIVE CARE

Instructing the patient in appropriate postoperative care will help to ensure the best cosmetic outcome and minimize undesired effects. We instruct patients not to lie down in the hours immediately following injection, and not to rub, press, or otherwise manipulate the injected area. The toxin binds in the first two to three hours following treatment, and we instruct patients to exercise the facial muscles as much as possible during this time by performing a range of facial expressions. We schedule a follow-up appointment two to three weeks following treatment. At this time, we assess treatment response and patient satisfaction, and perform touch-up injections as required. While unlikely, the possibility of an immunological response to the toxin requires caution in re-injecting new patients. For this reason, we do not perform touch-up injections sooner than two weeks following the initial treatment session.

ADVERSE EFFECTS AND COMPLICATIONS

Reports of adverse effects associated with BTX-A treatment are few and anecdotal, and are often related to poor injection technique. There have been no reported long-term adverse effects or health hazards for any cosmetic indication of BTX-A. When adverse effects do occur, they are usually mild and transient. They include swelling or bruising at the injection site, mild headache, and flu-like symptoms. We have observed that smaller doses are less likely to cause problems than larger doses, and therefore we recommend a conservative approach in most patients.

Upper Face Complications

Brow Ptosis

Brow ptosis occurs when the injected toxin affects the frontalis during glabellar or brow treatment, and is the result of poor injection technique. Using a higher concentration of BTX-A will facilitate accuracy of placement and greater duration of effect, and will minimize side effects. Toxin spread produces a radius of denervation of about 1 to 1.5 cm (diameter, 2–3 cm) at each injection site. Using lower concentrations of BTX-A will encourage the spread of toxin. Patients are instructed to remain upright, to avoid

manipulating the injected area for 2 hours, and to exercise the treated muscles as much as possible during the first four hours following treatment.

Brow ptosis produces an extremely negative appearance and can persist for up to three months. It can be avoided through careful patient selection (in particular, do not inject frontalis in individuals with significant brow ptosis) and pre-injection of the brow depressors if necessary (i.e., in patients with low-set brows or mild brow ptosis, and those over the age of 50 years). We always inject the depressors when treating frontalis, even in younger patients.

Diminished expressiveness may result from injection of the frontalis lateral to the mid-pupillary line. To avoid this, we inject above the lowest fold produced when the patient elevates the frontalis, and limit the treatment of forehead lines to the portion 3 cm or more above the brow. Brow ptosis is more likely to result if the glabella and the whole forehead are injected in a single session. Mild brow ptosis can be disguised with Apraclonidine (Iopidine® 0.5%), alpha-adrenergic agonist ophthalmic eye drops that stimulate Muller's muscle, though it is important to note that allergic contact conjunctivitis can occur with the prolonged use of apraclonidine.

Cocked Eyebrow

When injecting the lateral fibers of the frontalis muscle, poor injection technique can cause the untreated portion of the frontalis pull upward on the brow, producing a quizzical or "cockeyed" appearance (Fig. 13). This can be corrected by applying a small amount of toxin in the lateral frontalis fibers exerting the upward pull. When injecting to correct this unwanted outcome, a conservative approach is recommended. Overcompensating with too high a dose can yield a hooded brow that partially covers the eye. Keeping the glabellar treatments more medial will help ensure that the increased tone in frontalis produces a smooth arch to the brow.

Upper Eyelid Ptosis

As with brow ptosis, upper eyelid ptosis is the result of poor injection technique. It is caused by diffusion of toxin through the orbital septum, affecting the upper eyelid levator muscle, and it is most often seen following BTX-A treatment of the glabellar region. Ptosis may be evident at 48 hours post-treatment, or may appear as late as 14 days after injection; duration is from 2 to 12 weeks. Upper eyelid ptosis can be avoided by using small injection volumes, ensuring that injection sites are no closer than 1 cm above the central bony orbital rim. and not injecting at or under

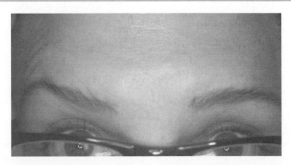

Figure 13 A quizzical or "cockeyed" expression may result from incorrect technique in the lateral fibers of the frontalis muscle.

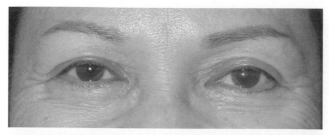
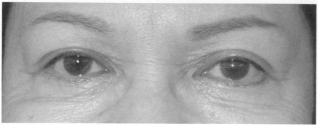

Figure 14 In older patients, injection of the infraorbital orbicularis may produce an effect opposite to that desired.

the mid-brow. To raise the eyelid by 1 to 2 mm and compensate for the loss of the levator palpebrae superioris, one or two drops of apraclonidine may be administered daily until the ptosis resolves.

Periorbital Complications
Bruising, diplopia, ectropion, or a drooping lateral lower eyelid and an asymmetrical smile are among the complications reported following treatment of the periorbital area. Ensure that toxin is injected laterally at least 1 cm outside the bony orbit or 1.5 cm lateral to the lateral canthus and avoid choosing injection sites close to the inferior margin of the zygoma. Superficial injections administered in a wheal or series of continuous blebs can reduce ecchymoses. Placing each injection at the advancing border of the previous injection will assist in avoiding blood vessels.

While BTX-A delivered to the infraorbital orbicularis can produce significant benefit in younger individuals, it may produce the opposite effect in older patients (Fig. 14). Patients who have previously undergone major surgery beneath the eye and individuals with a significant amount of scleral show pre-treatment, increased lid laxity, or a large amount of redundant skin under the eye are poor candidates for infraorbital orbicularis injection. Patients with clinically significant dry eyes may find their symptoms worse following treatment, due to weakening of the infraorbital orbicularis oculi. We advise asking patients about dry eye symptoms prior to treatment. A Schirmer's test may be performed to ascertain the presence of clinically significant dryness.

Lower Face and Cervical Complications
Use of excessive doses of toxin can yield significant complications in the lower face, negatively affecting muscular function and impairing facial expression . Using low doses and ensuring that the toxin is not delivered too deeply will reduce the incidence of complications such as drooling and facial asymmetry, and injecting symmetrically will aid in producing uniform muscle movement following treatment. When injecting the depressor anguli oris, avoid injecting too close to the mouth and do not inject the mental fold. Poor technique in the depressor anguli oris can yield a

flaccid cheek, oral incompetence, or an asymmetrical smile. Overzealous use of large doses (> 100 U) of toxin in the platysma may weaken the neck flexors and cause dysphagia.

Immune Response
BTX-A contains proteins capable of producing neutralizing antibodies and eliciting an immune response, causing patients to cease responding to treatment. Secondary lack of effectiveness due to the development of immunologic resistance is extremely rare in patients receiving BTX-A for cosmetic treatment. Data are sparse, and the factors affecting this phenomenon are not well understood, though the total protein concentration and number of units injected are important in determining potential immunogenicity, and it has been suggested that frequent, high-dose injections of BTX-A may be associated with a greater incidence of antibody formation. Current lots of BOTOX contain lower protein concentrations and therefore have reduced potential for antigenicity compared with early formulations of the product.

CONCLUSION
With careful patient selection and education, a thorough understanding of facial anatomy and musculature, and appropriate injection technique, the skilled clinician can employ BTX-A to great effect in cosmetic treatment of the face and neck. BTX-A injections are effective as monotherapy in treating premature signs of aging caused by underlying muscular activity and, when used in combination with filling agents, laser resurfacing procedures, and surgery, BTX-A can enhance and extend the benefits of these more traditional cosmetic interventions. Driven by safety, efficacy, and ease of treatment, this remarkable toxin has assumed a unique and important role in cosmetic treatment. As new and innovative applications for BTX-A are developed and refined, its use will expand and become increasingly sophisticated.

BIBLIOGRAPHY
Ahn MS, Catten M, Maas CS. Temporal brow lift using botulinum toxin A. Plast Reconstruct Surg 2000; 105:1129–1135.

Alam M, Dover JS, Arndt KA. Pain associated with injection of botulinum A exotoxin reconstituted using isotonic sodium chloride with and without preservative: a double-blind, randomized controlled trial. Arch Dermatol 2002; 138:510–514.

Blitzer A, Brin MF, Keen MS, et al. Botulinum toxin for the treatment of hyper-functional lines of the face. Arch Otolaryngol Head Neck Surg 1993; 9:1018–1022.

Borodic GE. Botulinum A toxin for (expressionistic) ptosis overcorrection after frontalis sling. Ophthal Plast Reconstr Surg 1992; S:137–142.

Carruthers A, Carruthers J. A single-center, double-blind, randomized study to evaluate the efficacy of 4% lidocaine cream vs. vehicle cream during botulinum toxin type A (BTX-A) treatments. Dermatol Surg 2005; 31(2):1655–1659.

Carruthers A, Carruthers J. Botulinum toxin type A: history and current cosmetic use in the upper face. Semin Cutan Med Surg 2001; 20:71–84.

Carruthers J, Carruthers A. Botox use in the mid and lower face and neck. Semin Cutan Med Surg 2001; 20:85–92.

Carruthers A, Carruthers J. Botulinum toxin type A for treating glabellar lines in men: a dose-ranging study. Presented at the 20th World Congress of Dermatology, Paris, France, July 1–5, 2002.

Carruthers J, Carruthers A. The effect of full-face broadband light treatments alone and in combination with bilateral crow's feet Botulinum toxin type A chemodenervation. Dermatol Surg 2004; 30:355–366.

Carruthers A, Carruthers J. Glabella BTX-A injection and eyebrow height: a further photographic analysis. Presented at the Annual Meeting of the American Academy of Dermatology, San Francisco, CA, March 21–26, 2003.

Carruthers J, Carruthers A. A prospective, randomized, parallel group study analyzing the effect of BTX-A (Botox) and nonanimal sourced hyaluronic acid (NASHA, Restylane) in combination compared with NASHA (Restylane) alone in severe glabellar rhytides in adult female subjects: treatment of severe glabellar rhytides with a hyaluronic acid derivative compared with the derivative and BTX-A. Dermatol Surg 2003; 29:802–809.

Carruthers JDA, Carruthers JA. Treatment of glabellar frown lines with C. botulinum-A exotoxin. J Dermatol Surg Oncol 1992; 18:17–21.

Carruthers A, Carruthers J, Cohen J. Dose dependence, duration of response and efficacy and safety of botulinum toxin type A for the treatment of horizontal forehead rhytids. Presented at the American Academy of Dermatology 2002 Winter Meeting, New Orleans, LA, February 22–27, 2002.

Carruthers A, Carruthers J, Said S. Dose-ranging study of botulinum toxin type A in the treatment of glabellar lines. Presented at the 20th World Congress of Dermatology, Paris, France, July 1–5, 2002.

Carruthers J, Carruthers A, Zelichowska A. The power of combined therapies: Botox and ablative facial laser resurfacing. Am J Cos Surg 2000; 17:129–131.

Dyer WK, Yung RT. Botulinum toxin-assisted brow lift. Facial Plast Surg 2000; 8:343.

Fagien S, Brandt FS. Primary and adjunctive use of botulinum toxin type A (Botox) in facial aesthetic surgery: beyond the glabella. Clin Plast Surg 2001; 28:127–148.

Flynn TC, Carruthers JA, Carruthers JA. Botulinum-A toxin treatment of the lower eyelid improves infraorbital rhytides and widens the eye. Dermatol Surg 2001; 27:703–708.

Flynn TC, Carruthers A, et al. Surgical pearl: the use of the Ultra-Fine II short needle 0.3-cc insulin syringe for botulinum toxin injections. J Am Acad Dermatol 2002; 46:931–933.

Garcia A, Fulton JE Jr. Cosmetic denervation of the muscles of facial expression with botulinum toxin: a dose–response study. Dermatol Surg 1996; 22:39–43.

Guerrissi JO. Intraoperative injection of botulinum toxin A into orbicularis oculi muscle for the treatment of crow's feet. Plast Reconstr Surg 2000; 105:2219–2228.

Hexsel DM, de Almeida AT, Rutowitsch M, et al. Multicenter, double-blind study of the efficacy of injections with botulinum toxin type A reconstituted up to six consecutive weeks before application. Dermatol Surg 2003; 29:523–529.

Hsu TSJ, Dover JS, Arndt KA. Effect of volume and concentration on the diffusion of botulinum exotoxin A. Arch Dermatol 2004; 140:1351–1354.

Huang W, Rogachefsky AS, Foster JA. Brow lift with botulinum toxin. Dermatol Surg 2000; 26:55–60.

Huang W, Foster JA, Rogachefsky AS. Pharmacology of botulinum toxin. J Am Acad Dermatol 2000; 43:249–259.

Huilgol SC, Carruthers A, Carruthers JDA. Raising eyebrows with botulinum toxin. Dermatol Surg 2000; 25:373–376.

Kane MA. Nonsurgical treatment of platysmal bands with injection of botulinum toxin A. Plast Reconstr Surg 1999; 103:656–663.

Keen M, Kopelman JE, Aviv, et al. Botulinum toxin: a novel method to remove periorbital wrinkles. Facial Plast Surg 1994; 10:141–146.

Klein AW. Dilution and storage of botulinum toxin. Dermatol Surg 1998; 24:1179–1180.

Klein AW. Complications, adverse reactions, and insights with the use of botulinum toxin. Dermatol Surg 2003; 29:549–556.

Lowe N, Lask G, Yamauchi P, Moore D, Patnaik R. Botulinum toxin type A (BTX-A) and ablative laser resurfacing (Erbium:YAG): a comparison of efficacy and safety of combination therapy vs. ablative laser resurfacing alone for the treatment of crow's feet. Presented at the American Academy of Dermatology 2002 Summer Meeting, New York, NY, July 31–August 4, 2002.

Lowe NJ, Lask G, Yamauchi P, et al. Bilateral, double-blind, randomized comparison of 3 doses of botulinum toxin type A and placebo in patients with crow's feet. J Am Acad Dermatol 2002; 47:834–840.

Park MY, Ahn KY, Jung DS. Application of botulinum toxin A for treatment of facial contouring in the lower face. Dermatol Surg 2003; 29:477–483.

Pribitkin EA, Greco TM, Goode RL, Keane WM. Patient selection in the treatment of glabellar wrinkles with botulinum type A injection. Arch Otolaryngol Head Neck Surg 1997; 123:321–326.

Product monograph. BOTOX Cosmetic (botulinum toxin type A for injection) Purified Neurotoxin Complex. Markham, Ontario: Allergan Inc., 2001; revised July 2004.

Schantz FJ. Botulinum toxin: the story of its development for the treatment of human disease. Persp Biol Med 1997; 40:317–327.

Smith KC, Comite SL, Balasubramanian S, Carver A, Liu JF. Vibration anesthesia: a noninvasive method of reducing discomfort prior to dermatologic procedures. Dermatol Online J 2004; 10:1.

To EW, Ahuja AT, Ho WS, et al. A prospective study of the effect of botulinum toxin A on masseteric muscle hypertrophy with ultrasonographic and electromyographic measurement. Br J Plast Surg 2001; 54:197–200.

von Lindern JJ, Niederhagen B, Appel T, Berge S, Reich RH. Type A botulinum toxin for the treatment of hypertrophy of the masseter and temporal muscle: an alternative treatment. Plast Reconstr Surg 2001; 107:327–332.

West TB, Alster TS. Effect of botulinum toxin type A on movement-associated rhytides following CO_2 laser resurfacing. Dermatol Surg 1999; 25:259–261.

73

Dermabrasion

Henry H. Roenigk, Jr.

Arizona Advanced Dermatology, Scottsdale, Arizona, U.S.A.

INTRODUCTION

"Dermabrasion is dead. CO_2 laser resurfacing is the best method for removing acne scars and wrinkles. Microdermabrasion is a new technique with no downtime and can clear up acne scars and improve wrinkles. Dermabrasion has too many complications and is operator or technique dependent. CO_2 laser resurfacing is much easier to learn than dermabrasion. There is too much bleeding and risk of scarring with dermabrasion." The lists of claims and counterclaims about a time-honored technique as dermabrasion go on. The truth is that dermabrasion still remains a vital technique in the hands of a properly trained and experienced dermatologic and plastic surgeons. The complications from dermabrasion are no different or more frequent than any other resurfacing technique.

Jacob reviewed the different types of acne scarring and attempted to fit the treatment to the type of scar. They recommend punch excision, subcision, and laser resurfacing. Dermabrasion is not even considered but in the discussion they say "dermabrasion was once the main treatment modality for skin resurfacing but complications, technique dependent with steep leaning curves make it less attractive than laser resurfacing." They quote uncontrolled laser studies on acne scars. Controlled studies of wrinkles treating one side with dermabrasion and the other with CO_2 laser show equal clinical results with slower healing time with CO_2 laser resurfacing. Whang have combined chemical peel, excision, punch grafting, CO_2 laser and dermabrasion with excellent results. What a clever idea for a dermatologic surgeon to use many different techniques.

HISTORY

Kromayer described his cylindrical knives for punching scars, tattoos, pigmentation, abscesses, hair, nevi, and other defects in 1905. Later he described rasps or burrs with either clockwise or counterclockwise rotation for scar removal to which he attached motor-driven instruments from the dental clinic. He adapted his punches and rasps to perform "scarless operations," which were described in his book *Cosmetic Treatment of Skin Complaints*. Kromayer showed that healing of wounds occurs beneath a scab without obvious cicatrization if the injury does not penetrate the reticular dermis. Freezing the skin with carbon dioxide snow and ether spray provided rigidity as well as anesthesia suitable for dermabrading.

Kurten, who was a dermatologist, reawakened interest in wire brush motor-driven dermabraders using refrigeration for anesthesia in 1953. He reported improvement in acne scars, seborrheic and actinic keratosis, tattoos, wrinkles, keloids, traumatic scars, adenoma sebaceum, nevi, and lichenoid plaques. Orentriech who worked with Kurten, popularized dermabrasion and refined much of today's equipment. Burke's textbook *Wire Brush Surgery in the Treatment of Certain Cosmetic Defects and Diseases of the Skin*, published in 1956 and revised in 1979 gave creditability to dermabrasion as an accepted procedure. There have been minor modifications in techniques since then. The author and others have used dermabrasion to treat nonacne-related lesions such as trichoepithelioma, epithelioma adenoids cysticum, and others.

Dermabrasion reached its peak in popularity in the 1950s. There was criticism of the procedure in the 1960s and early 1970s but with the renewed interest in dermatologic surgery in the 1970s and 1980s, dermabrasion became more popular. Dermabrasion has lost some popularity since the technique is old and not taught much in residency or fellowship.

INDICATIONS

Dermabrasion was developed as a method of treating acne scars. It has been used to treat a variety of problems including hypertrophic scars, traumatic scars, actinically damaged and wrinkled skin, and correction of pigmentary abnormalities. Among the cosmetic indications for dermabrasion are acne scars, fine wrinkling, scar revision, melasma, perioral rhylides, and tattoo removals (laser is probably treatment of choice for tattoos).

There are many other therapeutic reasons for selecting dermabrasion: epidermal nevus, epithelioma adenoids cysticum, rhinophyma, nevus angiomatosus, syringoma, adenoma sebaceum, keloids, scar of discoid lupus erythematosus, actinic keratosis and solar elastosis, seborrheic keratosis, basal cell carcinoma, and Darier's disease. Hanke provided a list of 50 conditions that have been treated with dermabrasion (Table 1).

The correction of old and new scars by dermabrasion is very effective. Superficial sharply demarcated scars can often be completely removed while soft saucer like depressions can be improved but not eliminated. Emphasize to the patient that improvement is expected, but do not promise to eliminate all scars. Dermabrasion will soften sharp edges and improve the crater-like appearance of these scars caused by shadows in the depression. Deep ice-pick-type scars will require scar revision by punch excision and suturing, punch elevation or punch grafting at the same time as dermabrasion is done. Dermabrasion can also be used for cysts or to marsupialize epithelialized sinuses when chronically infected. In another chapter, Yarborough shows that

Table 1 Various Entities Treated with Dermabrasion

Postacne scars	Adenoma sebaceum
Traumatic scars	Neurotic excoriations
Smallpox or chickenpox scars	Multiple trichoepitheliomas
Rhinophyma	Darier's disease
Professionally applied tattoos	Fox–Fordyce disease
Amateur-type tattoos (India ink)	Lichenified dermatoses
Blast tattoos (gunpowder)	Porokeratosis of Mibelli
Multiple pigmented nevi	Lichen amyloidosis
Actinically damaged akin	Verrucous nevus
Age- and sun-related wrinkle lines	Molluseum contagiosum
Active acne	Keratoacanthoma
Freckles	Xanthalasma
Pseudofolliculitis barbae	Hemangioma
Telagiectasia	Leg ulcer
Acne rosacea	Scleromyxedema
Chioasma	Striae distensae
Vitiligo	Early operative scars
Congenial pigmented nevi	Hair transplantation
Syringocystadenoma papilliferum	(elevated recipient sites)
Nevus flammeus	Linear epidermal nevus
Keloids	Syringoma
Dermatitis papilaris capilliti	Angiofibromas of tuberous sclerosis
Lupus erythematosus	Chronic radiation dermatitis
Basal cell carcinoma	Xeroderma pigmentosum
(superficial type)	Lentigines

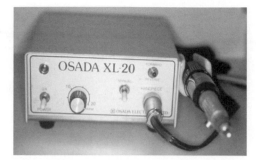

Figure 1 Osada XL 20 dermabrasion with foot pedal control.

scars from excisional surgery or trauma can be dermabraded six to eight weeks after sutures are removed to camouflage these wounds by forming a more natural epidermal surface. Older wound do not respond as well unless they are re-excised, followed by dermabrasion. Dermabrasion has become a tool for treatment of photoaging skin, although most prefer lasers because of the tissue contraction that helps wrinkles.

Rhinophyma can be greatly improved with dermabrasion when combined with electrofulguration or CO_2 laser resurfacing for the contraction of tissue. Actinically damaged skin and aging skin is a growing indication for dermabrasion. Today, CO_2 laser, erbium laser, and noninvasive lasers may be better. In a study of half-face dermabrasion of actinically damaged skin, Burke showed that precancerous lesions were substantially reduced and their future development was retarded over a 5-year period. This work has been corroborated by Coleman et al., more recently. Aside from the benefit of the prophylactic effect on the development of new keratosis and the resolution of old ones, improvement in facial wrinkling is seen in dermabrasion patients.

EQUIPMENT

Proper outpatient operating room facilities must be available to perform dermabrasion. Most dermatologists perform dermabrasion in an office surgical unit separate from general offices or an ambulatory surgical center. Hospitalization with general anesthesia is not necessary and adds to the expense and risk of the procedure but should be offered to the patients. There should be a versatile operating table capable of placing the patient in several different positions. Adequate lighting and proper emergency equipment should be available. The patient's past medical history and current medications should be noted. The operator and assistant should wear surgical gowns and gloves. A plastic face

shield and mask is worn for protection from blood and tissue particles that spray.

Hand engines are the most popular dermabraders because they are small, hand-held engines that are quiet and easy to maneuver. The Bell Hand Engine and Osada models (Fig. 1) can reach rotational speeds of 18,000 to 35,000 rpm in both directions, depending on the model. A rheostat adjusts the speed, which can also be controlled with a foot pedal. The combination of rotational speed of the machine, abrading attachment, and pressure applied by the operator allows rapid planning, which is not as convenient as hand engines.

Nitrogen-driven machines, such as the Stryker unit, are well built, provide excellent torque, and reach 50,000 rpm easily. The handpiece is larger than the hand engine. It is necessary, however, to store and replace large tanks of nitrogen.

The abrading end pieces for dermabrasion are diamond fraise, wire brush (Fig. 2), or serrated wheel. Diamond fraises are stainless-steel wheels on which diamond chips of different grades of coarseness (regular, coarse, or extra coarse) are bonded. Most experienced surgeons use the coarse or extra coarse fraises. The cylinder type comes in various widths and diameters, while other shapes such as pear, are helpful in specific locations.

The wire brush is a stainless-steel wheel with wires arranged at an angle. The wires of the brush cut deep and

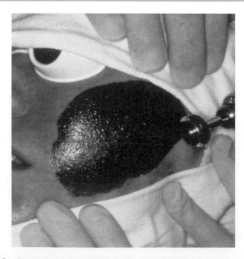

Figure 2 Dermabrasion operative site. Gentian violet to mark areas for dermabrasion, towels, and wire fraise on dermabrader. (*See color insert.*)

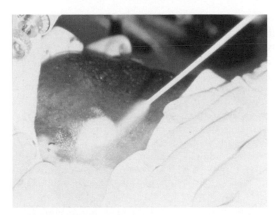

Figure 3 Cryoanesthesia to skin with Frigiderm spray.

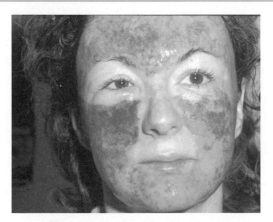

Figure 4 Immediately postoperative after full-face dermabrasion. (*See color insert.*)

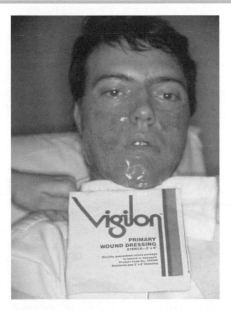

Figure 5 Immediately postoperative with the Vigilon dressing applied to areas of dermabrasion.

rapidly in frozen skin. Most experienced surgeons prefer the wire brush, but for the novice these are much harder to control and can gouge easily. The wire brush should be used for the deep scars and the diamond fraise to feather the edges

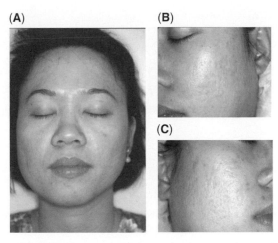

Figure 6 (**A–C**) Preoperative pitted scars of moderate severity on entire face. (*See color insert.*)

or plane more smoothly than an area treated with the wire brush. The CO_2 laser may be used after epidermis is removed to get more contraction of collagen of scars.

PATIENT SELECTION AND PREOPERATIVE ASSESSMENT

The preoperative consultation is extremely important. You must tell the patient clearly what to expect from the procedure, as well as get a feel for what he or she really understands. List alternative procedures such as chemical peel, collagen, collagen implants, microdermabrasion, and CO_2 laser. The use of photographs, video, or PowerPoint® presentation to demonstrate the procedure, as well as before and after pictures including that of complications, are helpful in the consultation. This discussion should be documented in the chart. Pamphlets and handout brochures are good.

Patients who seek cosmetic surgery to improve their appearance for a variety of personal reasons have particular personalities. The surgeon must have a basic understanding of psychology and specifically the psychopathology of the

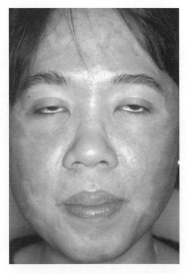

Figure 7 Ten days postdermabrasion with edema and erythema. (*See color insert.*)

(A)   (B)

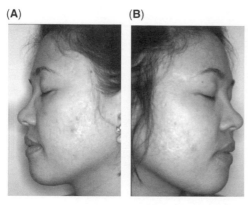

Figure 8 (**A–B**) Six weeks after dermabrasion with return of normal colored skin and marked improvement in scars. (*See color insert.*)

cosmetic surgery patient. Therapeutic dermabrasion may relieve some of the pressure to achieve perfect results. Avoid promoting dermabrasion and list the other options available and the complications that can occur. There are adjunctive procedures that are often combined with dermabrasion and these should be carefully covered in the consultation. The physician must decide who is a good candidate and if a reasonable improvement can be expected. Avoid the patient who has a minimal scar and cannot tolerate what seems like a slight blemish. Also, avoid patients critical of care given by previous physicians. The patient's criticism may be valid, but you too may be unable to live up to the patient's expectations.

Preoperative work-up includes a medical history, specifically other medication (especially aspirin) and diseases such as hepatitis, HIV infection, and recurrent herpes simplex. Evaluate atypical scars or keloids from previous surgery that may be predictive of poor results. Laboratory evaluation includes complete blood cell count, serum chemistry values, and bleeding time, although frequently these test are not necessary. Other tests include evaluation of hepatitis B antigen and antibody and HIV antibody titers. These are done to protect the surgeon and staff.

Outstanding reviews by Roenigk, Yarborough, and Alt of techniques using the wire brush and diamond fraise require little elaboration. It must be emphasized that dermabrasion is a hands-on technique that requires adequate preceptorship training under the auspices of someone experienced in this art. Most authors agree that a wire brush requires considerably more skill and runs higher potential risk for injury as it is able to cut much deeper and more quickly than is the diamond fraise. Wire brushes do produce superior results in deeper scars.

Many patients requesting dermabrasion have been previously treated with 13 isotretinoin (Accutane®) systematically. This potent acne therapy causes sebaceous gland atrophy, a cause for concern in the healing process. Initial reports suggested that dermabrasion patients were unaffected by previous treatment with isotretinoin then later reports suggested that patients who were dermabraded after isotretinoin exhibited atypical scarring. Subsequently, other surgeons have compiled patients that have been treated with isotretinoin and dermabraded without difficulty. This controversy has not been settled but has significant medical and legal implications. There is still no definite answer to the question of isotretinoin treatment and postdermabrasion scarring but it can occur unpredictably after use of isotretinoin. It is prudent for physicians to suggest that isotretinoin patients be fully informed of the potential risks and wait a period of at least six months to a year before undergoing dermabrasion.

Another preoperative consideration is the HIV. Dermabrasion results in the aerosolization of blood and tissue products and potentially, live infective viral particles. Wentzell indicated that aerosolized particles produced during dermabrasion were of sufficient size to allow access to, and retention by, mucosal and pulmonary surfaces. The studies suggested that commonly used personal protection devices, such as operating masks, goggles, and scatter shields, do not prevent the inhalation of these particles. Risks clearly exist to the physician, his assistants, and other personnel, as well as to the HIV-infected patient. A thorough history, HIV titers and all protective equipment must be used when doing dermabrasions and there must be the realization that with all of these measures, there still remains a degree of risk. Therefore, doing dermabrasion in HIV

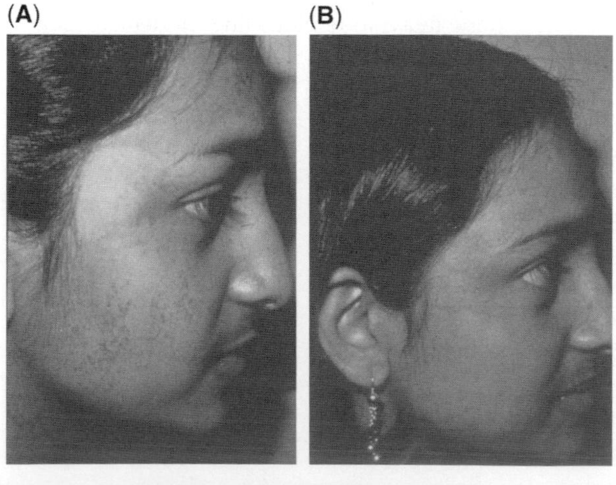

(A)   (B)

Figure 9 Dark-skinned patient with facial epidermal nevus. Test spot dermabrasion in right temple, then entire cheek treated. There is good repigmentation. (*See color insert.*)

(A)   (B)

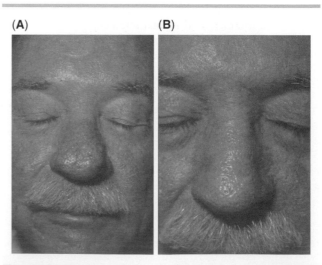

Figure 10 Rhinophyma before and after dermabrasion combined with CO_2 laser. (*See color insert.*)

(A) **(B)**

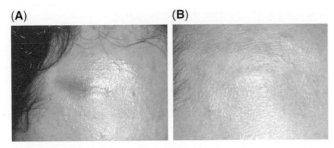

Figure 11 Surgical excision with dermabrasion six weeks after the wound healed. Nice cosmetic improvement of scar.

patients is not recommended. Other alternative procedures can be used. Similar precautions regarding hepatitis are recommended.

Surgical scars respond so well to dermabrasion that patients who are receiving excisional surgery are told preoperatively that dermabrasion in six weeks may be a viable option as a "touch-up." Dermabrasion can also be done at the time of the surgical scar if its location can be improved cosmetically by dermabrasion. The results of waiting six weeks of doing simultaneously with the surgery show equal results.

ANESTHESIA

Preoperative medication should relax the patient and reduce pain since most dermabrasion is done with local anesthesia. Intramuscularly meperidine hydrocloride (50–100 mg) and intravenous diazepam (10–20 mg) provide sedation, although other agents may be used. These can also be given during the procedure by keeping an intravenous line open. The blood pressure, pulse, and heart rate should be monitored continuously. A pulse oximeter is necessary for all patients under heavy sedation. Ibuprofen or corticosteroids may help reduce edema and bleeding. Preoperative topical retinoic acid may reduce the incidence of milia postoperatively and enhance wound healing.

For small areas, it is preferable to use a local anesthesia field block. Nerve blocks with lidocaine may be used on the central face, based on the distribution of facial sensory nerves. Approximately, 3 ml of lidocaine is injected bilaterally at the supraorbital notch, supratrochlear region, infraorbital foramen, and mental foramen.

Tumescent anesthesia may be useful in dermabrasion and can eliminate nerve blocks and cryoanesthesia. This takes more time to deliver to the entire face. It also distorts the scars that are to be dermabraded.

Prechilling of the skin with ice packs enhances the anesthestic effect of hydrocarbon sprays used for topical cryoanesthesia. The skin is sprayed by the assistant in a circular motion for 10 to 20 seconds until it becomes frigid and developed a white frost (Fig. 3). Freezing too aggressively will result in deep cryonecrosis in the dermis, especially over the mandibular bone. The area to be sprayed is usually not greater than 2 to 3 cm. Towels not gauze should be used to protect the adjacent skin.

The choice of spray anesthesia is important. Ethyl chloride is the oldest agent and is not used much because it is explosive and inflammable, has general anesthetic properties and requires a blower for rapid evaporation. Frigiderm (Freon) and Fluro-Ethyl are Freon 114 and Freon 114 plus ethyl chloride, respectively. They generally freeze the skin surface to −42°C in 25 seconds. Freon and Fluro-Ethyl are the preferred agents for cryoanesthesia.

General anesthesia is used more frequently by nondermatologic surgeons. Except for special circumstances, this only adds to the risk, cost and time to do this procedure. The vast majority of dermabrasions are done in office surgical suites.

TECHNIQUES

Dermabrasion requires at least one assistant to help with freezing and to hold the skin taut. Both the operator and assistant should wear gowns, rubber gloves, and plastic face shields. The assistant should wear cotton gloves over rubber gloves to protect the fingers. Cotton towels are preferred over gauze, which easily gets caught in the wire brush. The area should be painted with Gentian violet to serve as a guide (Figs. 2 and 3). Gentian violet deep in the scars also indicates whether the abrasion has gone to the sufficient depth to obliterate them. Disposable eye patches are the best cover for the eyes. The patient lies supine on the table.

Dermabrasion of the face is usually done in sections: four on each cheek, two on the chin, two on the nose, two on the upper lip, and three on the forehead. Spraying and abrading one area at a time, the surgeon starts at the outermost and dependent areas and moves toward the central and upper areas of the face (Fig. 4). The operator moves the brush or fraise over the frozen skin with firm, steady, back-and-forth strokes, and even pressure. In areas with deeper scars, more pressure may be applied. Dermabrasion is done in anatomic units, so it is usually done to the natural folds of the face (nasolabial fold, hairline, or submandibular). This is done to avoid obvious lines of demarcation that can occur with spot dermabrasion. CO_2 laser resurfacing of the lower eyelids and lip, if necessary, is preferred over dermabrasion. Localized dermabrasion of a small area of scarring is also risky because texture and pigment changes may be readily apparent. Although the trunk is usually not dermabraded, lesions on arms and legs may respond well.

(A) **(B)** **(C)**

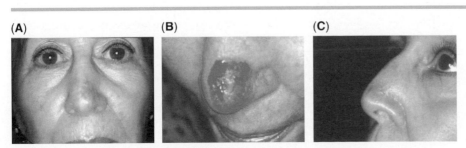

Figure 12 Skin graft on nose following Mohs surgery for basal cell carcinoma. Immediately after and six weeks after dermabrasion of graft and edges.

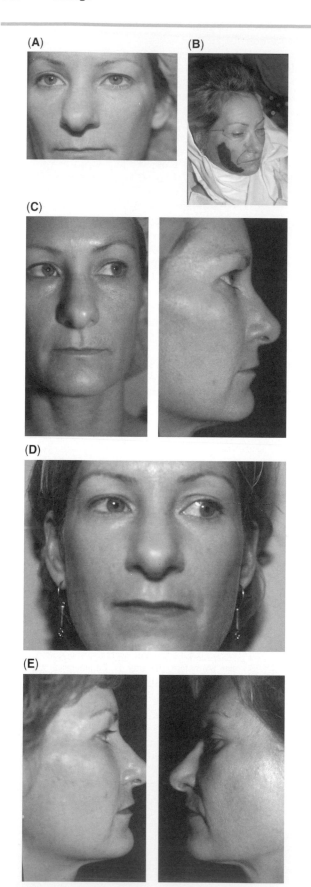

Figure 13 Mild acne scar on cheek and wrinkle under eyes and upper lip (A–B). CO$_2$ laser under eyes and upper lip. Dermabrasion of cheek six weeks postoperative (C–E).

POSTOPERATIVE CARE AND DRESSING

The author has tried many types of dressings in more than 30 years of performing dermabrasion. For the past 15 years, the dressing choice has been Vigilon or second skin (Spenco).

Vigilon appears to fulfill more criteria for the ideal wound dressing than any of the other wound dressings. It is composed of 4% polyethylene oxide and 96% water in a colloidal suspension on a polyethylene mesh support. Prior to application, a polyethylene film is removed from the side of the dressing that will cover the wound. Vigilon, unlike other occlusive dressings permits a moist environment while allowing for absorption of wound exudates (Fig. 5). It is also nonadherent. The Vigilon is changed daily for about five days and then the wound is left open with lubrication applied.

Biological dressings, in patients undergoing full-face dermabrasion, act by preventing dehydration to allow rapid epithelial migration. Healing time or re-epithelialization is reduced by as much as 50%. Vigilon (second skin) may be the best dressing to use the following dermabrasion. Re-epithelialization will occur in five to seven days without crusting compared to 10 to 12 days when crusts are allowed to form.

Op-site was the first in a series of thin, transparent, semipermeable, synthetic polyurethane membranes to be used as a wound dressing. Several others have been introduced, including Bioclusive (Johnson & Johnson), Tegaderm (3M), and Ensure (Deserat). Each is a thin, elastic film, transparent and permeable to air and water vapor without being porous. They do not adhere to the wound, but stick to intact skin and conform to the curves of the face. The membrane protects nerve endings like a second skin, giving immediate pain relief. They keep the wound moist and prevent eschar formation thus providing optimal conditional for re-epithelialization.

The patient is given written instruction for postoperative care. Pain medication such as acetaminophen with codeine is helpful. Systemic antibiotics (dicloxacillin or Keflex 500 mg two times a day) and a short course of prednisone starting at 40 mg/day and tapering in one week are useful in reducing infection and postoperative edema. Antiviral drugs such as acyclovir or valacyclovir are essential prior to and 10 days after postoperative.

The patient is seen in 24 hours for dressing change. The Vigilon dressing is then changed on a daily basis at home or in the office depending on the patient's choice. Office dressing changes are better and you can detect any problems early. The patient should be evaluated regularly at 7, 14, and 30 days—more often if necessary.

Avoidance of sun is important after dermabrasion. Sun exposure may easily burn the new skin and will predispose to postinflammatory hyperpigmentation.

CLINICAL RESULTS FROM DERMABRASION

Dermabrasion is most frequently done for acne scars (Figs. 4–6). You can expect improvement but frequently touch up dermabrasion is needed. Even patients with oriental skin color or darker skin colors (Figs. 7A and B) will respond and heal with normal repigmentation.

Other therapeutics indications are rhinophyma (Figs. 8A and B), surgical scars (Fig. 9A and B), and skin grafts (Fig. 10C). Photoaging skin and wrinkles are more often treated by CO$_2$ laser because of the collagen contraction but dermabrasion in the past has been effective (Fig. 11C). Deep acne scar may

(A)

(B)

(C)

(D)

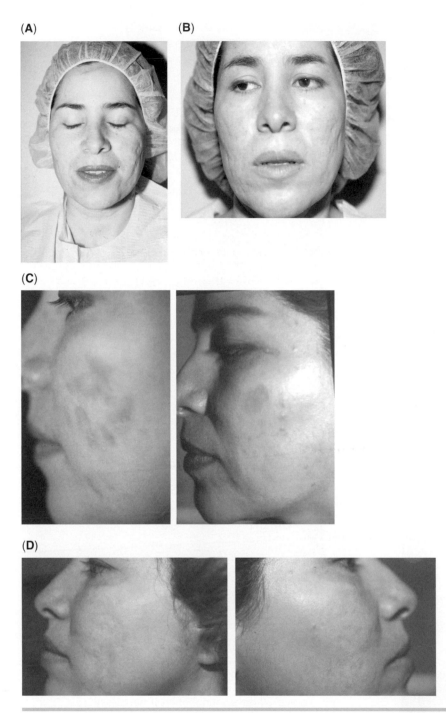

Figure 14 Deep acne scars requiring both dermabrasion **(A)** before, **(B)** after 1st Dermabrasion and follow-up touch up with CO_2 laser. **(C)** 2 weeks after CO_2 laser, **(D)** 3 months after Dermabrasion and CO_2 laser.

require repeat dermabrasion (touch up) and/or CO_2 laser to get tissue contraction of edges of scar (Figs. 12 and 13D).

COMPLICATIONS AND CONTRAINDICATIONS

Among the most common complications are keloids (Fig. 14)-hyperpigmentation, hypopigmentation (Fig. 15), hypertrophic scars, gouging of skin, herpes simplex, milia, persistent erythema, and telangiectasia (Fig. 16).

Erythema is expected in the postoperative period, but it may persist for weeks or months with some telangiectasia. Milia formation is very common and can easily be

corrected by abrasive soaps or simple extraction. Pinpoint electrodesiccation can also be used. The use of topical retinoic acid prior to and after dermabrasion may be reduced with the incidence of milia.

Hypertrophic scars or keloids may occur in a small number of patients (Fig. 14). A personal or family history of keloid formation is a relative contraindication. African-American patients tend to form keloids more frequently. The use of refrigerants, especially on the mandible may be partially responsible. Atypical keloids develop in atypical locations such as the buccal skin after dermabrasion of patients still on or having recently taken isotretinoin.

(A)

(B)

(C)

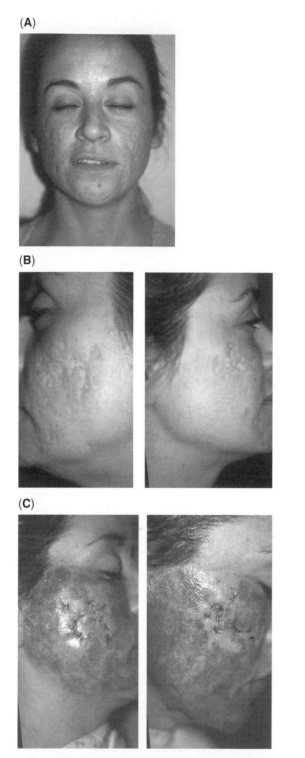

(D)

(E)

(F)

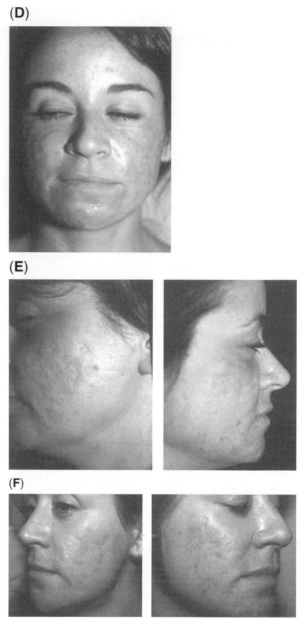

Figure 15 (Continued)

Figure 15 Deep acne scars which need deep dermabrasion, punch excision, and CO_2 laser. (**A–B**) pre-operative, (**C**) after dermabrasion and punch excision, (**D–E**) 2 month postoperative, (**F**) after CO_2 laser.

Patients now wait six months to one year after stopping isotretinoin before the procedure. Treatment of these scars with intralesional triamcinolone is helpful. Early treatment with flashed pumped dye vascular laser may stop the development of keloids if used early.

Patients with a history of recurrent herpes simplex should be approached with caution. The surgeon should avoid

dermabrasion in the trigger areas of previous herpes simplex. All patients regardless of history of herpes simplex are treated with an anti-viral agent. Oral acyclovir 400 mg three times a day or valacyclovir 1.0 mg two times a day for three days before and until the skin has re-epithelialized, should be given prophylactically. If disseminated herpes simplex develops, hospitalization and intravenous acyclovir are indicated.

Hypopigmentation and hyperpigmentation are common but usually temporary. Pigmentary problems are more common in dark-skinned patients (skin types IV–VI). It is most noticeable at the edges of the dermabrasion or in spot dermabrasion. Postinflammatory hyperpigmentation usually fades in several months and topical hydroquinone 4% may be helpful.

Acne will occasionally recur after dermabrasion, although most patients with minimally active disease will

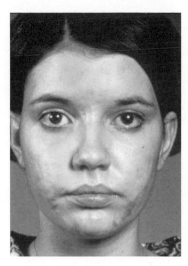

Figure 16 Complication—keloids on chin. (*See color insert.*)

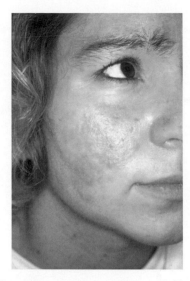

Figure 18 Complication—persistent erythema and telangiectasia. (*See color insert.*)

actually improve. Infection with *Staphylococcus* and *Pseudomonas* occurs occasionally and needs prompt topical and systemic therapy. *Candida albican* infection can occur and culture prompt treatment with Diflucan® is essential.

Dermabrasion is usually contraindicated in patients with chronic radiodermatitis, pyoderma, herpes simplex, psychosis, severe psychoneurosis, alcoholism, xeroderma pigmentosum, verrucae planae, or burn scars.

ADJUNCTIVE PROCEDURES WITH DERMABRASION

Subcision of depressed scars using a Nokar™ (B-D) needle will release fibrous bonds. Larger deeper scars that do not respond well to dermabrasion alone may be treated in other ways. Punch excision with a circular punch can be sutured closed. Occasionally, the depressed scar can be removed with 4 to –5 mm punch and elevated flush to the surface

of the surrounding skin and held in place with steristrips. In addition, punch excision of the scar with a full-thickness punch graft replacement taken from the postauricular area will fill these defects. Dermabrasion is usually done six weeks after these procedures have corrected the deeper

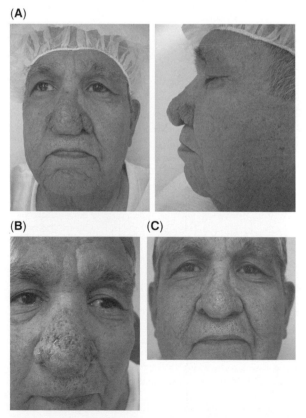

Figure 19 Severe rhinophyma treated with dermabrasion and CO_2 laser at the same time. (**A**) Preoperative; (**B**) immediately postoperative; (**C**) 2 months postoperative.

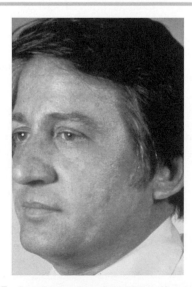

Figure 17 Complication—hypopigmentation. (*See color insert.*)

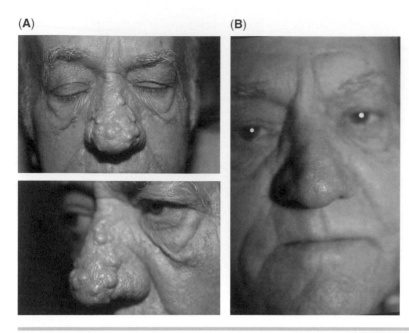

Figure 20 Severe rhinophyma and multiple cysts of nose treated by combination dermabrasion and CO_2 laser at the same time. (**A**) preoperative; (**B**) postoperative.

scars to smooth the skin surface. We now do both procedures at the same time with similar results.

Bovine collagen (zyderm I or II or Zyplast™) or hyaluronic acid (Restylane™) used to augment soft depressions remaining after dermabrasion. Dermabrasion should probably be done just to eliminate as many scars as possible. Collagen implant or autologous fat implants can be used to fill out the remaining scars. Zyderm will last only four to six months. Restylane last longer than Zyplast—up to six months. Fat implants may be more permanent. Fat implants have been used in recent years to correct the soft shallow larger scars not corrected by dermabrasion. Dermabrasion can safely be done on patients who have previously received collagen or silicone injections.

COMBINING RESURFACING

Resurfacing of the face to remove acne scars, wrinkles, actinic keratosis, and photodamaged skin is not a new technique. The recent boom in resurfacing lasers leads one to believe that lasers invented the technique of resurfacing and rejuvenation the face. Many techniques have been available for almost 100 years, but certainly, in the past decade the whole field has shown new promise. Sometimes the technique or device (i.e., laser) is brought to the public's attention with publicity on television, in newspapers, women's magazines before adequate clinical trials can be completed, and long-term results and potential complications can be evaluated.

The Er:YAG laser was developed in an attempt to reduce healing time and minimize erythema while still trying to achieve the results of CO_2 laser resurfacing. There are also lasers which combine the CO_2 laser with the Er:YAG laser, as well as lasers with two different Er:YAG delivery systems. There have been some comparative studies with clinical and histologic evaluation to try to evaluate the benefit:risk ratio of all lasers.

We can incorporate new technology where it has an advantage over previous techniques (i.e., CO_2 laser for contraction of collagen), but we should retain chemical peels, dermabrasion, and soft-tissue augmentation in combination where indicated. The next several cases will illustrate the points of combination resurfacing with emphasis on dermabrasion.

COMBINATION RESURFACING CASES

Dermabrasion plus CO_2 laser combined with dermabrasion is usually performed first followed by CO_2 laser for touch up and contraction (Figs. 12 and 13). Dermabrasion can be combined with CO_2 laser in different locations to achieve different goals (Fig. 11). Dermabrasion and CO_2 laser can be used at the same time for severe cases of rhinophyma (Figs. 17 and 18C). Severe photoaging skin may require full-face CO_2 laser plus dermabrasion (Figs. 19B and C, 20, and 21).

COMPARSION WITH OTHER MODALITIES

All resurfacing techniques result in upper to mid-dermal wound. Dermabrasion relies on mechanical "cold steel" injury, acid peels result in a "caustic" injury, and lasers result in a thermal injury. Studies in the porcine model comparing carbon dioxide laser, trichloracetic acid, and dermabrasion by Fitzpatrick and Campbell have shown that histological and ultrastructural changes seen following these procedures are comparable. A study by Giese revealed that when dermabrasion was compared with chemosurgical peels, significant alterations were seen in the elastic fibers in histological and mechanical properties. Holmkvist reported that half-face perioral dermabrasion contrasted with half-face CO_2 laser resurfacing yielded identical clinical results but that dermabrasion healed in approximately half the time with significantly less postoperative erythema and morbidity. Most surgeons practicing resurfacing agree that extended postoperative erythema and delayed hypopigmentation are more common with phenol or CO_2 laser than dermabrasion. A review by Baker points out that dermabrasion equipment is inexpensive, portable, and widely available, requires no specialized accessory equipment, and poses no fire hazard in the operating room. Dermabrasion should not become a lost art. It has many advantages over other resurfacing techniques.

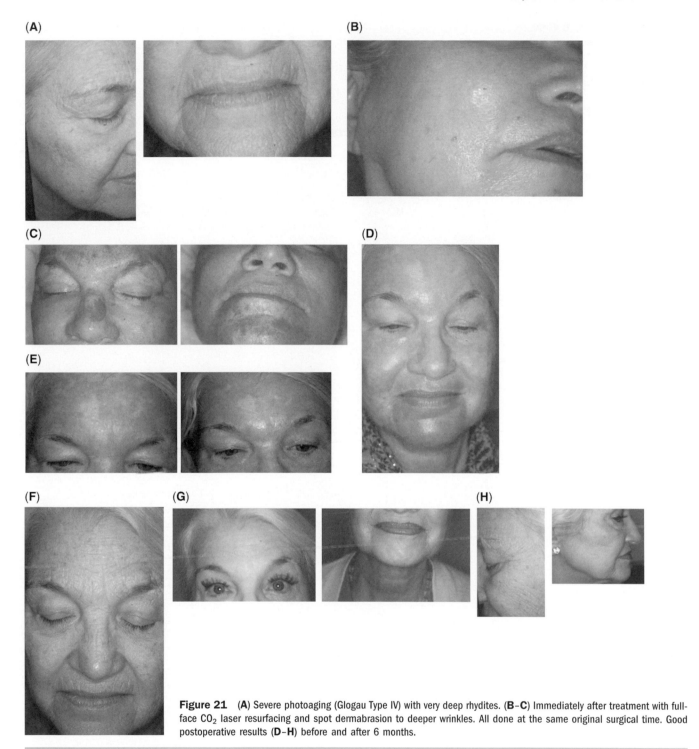

Figure 21 (**A**) Severe photoaging (Glogau Type IV) with very deep rhydites. (**B–C**) Immediately after treatment with full-face CO_2 laser resurfacing and spot dermabrasion to deeper wrinkles. All done at the same original surgical time. Good postoperative results (**D–H**) before and after 6 months.

BIBLIOGRAPHY

Alt T. Facial dermabrasion: advantages of the diamond fraise technique. J Derm Surg Oncology 1987; 13:618.

Baker TM. Dermabrasion as a complement to aesthetic surgery. Clin Plast Surg 1998; 25:81–88.

Burke J, Marascalco J, Clark W. Half-face planning of precancerous skin after five years. Arch Dermatol 1963; 88:140.

Burks J. Dermabrasion and Chemical Peeling, in the Treatment of Certain Defects and Disease of the Skin. Springfield, IL: Charles C. Thomas, 1979.

Burks JW. Wire Brush Surgery. Springfield, IL: Charles C. Thomas, 1956.

Campbell JP, et al. The ultrasound comparison of mechanical dermabrasion and carbon dioxide laser resurfacing in the Minipig model. Arch Otalaryngeal Head Neck Surg 1998; 124:758–760.

Coleman WP, Yarborough JM, Mandy SH. Dermabrasion for prophylaxis and treatment of actinic keratosis. J Dermatol Oncol 1996; 22:17–21.

Fitzpatrick RE, et al. Pulsed carbon dioxide laser trichloracetic acid, Baker–Gordon phenol and dermabrasion: a comparative clinical and histologic study of cutaneous resurfacing in a porcine model. Arch Dermatol 1996; 132:469–471.

Giese SY, McKinney P, Roth SI, Zukowski M. The effect of chemosurgical peels and dermabrasion on dermal elastic tissue. Plast Reconstr Surg 1997; 100:489–498.

Hanke CW, O'Brian JJ, Solow EB. Laboratory evaluation of skin refrigerants used in Dermabrasion. J Dermatol Surg Oncol 1985; 11:45–49.

Holmkvist KA. Treatment of perioral rhytids: a comparison of dermabrasion and superpulsed carbon dioxide laser treatment. Presented to The American Society for Dermatologic Surgery, May 1998.

Jacob CF, Dover JS, Kaminer MS. Acne scarring: a classification system and review of treatment option. J Am Acad Dermatol 2001; 45:109–117.

Kurtain A. Corrective surgical planning of skin. Arch Dermatol Syphilol 1953; 68:389–397.

Kromayer E. Die Heilung der Akne durch in Neves Norbenlases Operationsverfahren Das Stanzen. Illustr Monatsschr Aerztl Polytech 1905; 27:101.

Roenigk HH Jr, et al. Acne retinoids and Dermabrasion. J Dermatol Oncol 1988: 11;396–396.

Roenigk HH Jr. Dermabrasion and aging skin. J Gertiatr Dermatol 1994: 2(1):24–29.

Roenigk HH Jr. Dermabrasion for miscellaneous cutaneous lesions (exclusive of scarring from acne). J Dermatol Surg Oncol 1977; 3:322–328.

Roenigk HH Jr. Dermabrasion for rejuvenation and scar revision. In Surgical Dermatology.

Roenigk HH Jr. Dermabrasion: state of the art. J Dermatol Surg Oncol 1985; 11(3):306–314.

Roenigk R, Roenigk H. London: Martin Dunitz, 1992:509–519.

Rubenstein R, Roenigk HH Jr. Atypical keloids after dermabrasion of patients taking Isotretinoin. J Am Acad Dermatol 1986; 15(LpLl):280–285.

Wentzell MJ, Robinson JK. Physical properties of aerosols produced by dermabrasion. Arch Dermatol 1989; 125: 1637–1643.

Whang KK, Lee M. The principle of a three staged operation in the surgery of acne scars. J Am Acad Dermatol 1999; 40: 95–97.

Yarborough JM. Dermabrasion by wire brush. J Dermatol Surg Oncol 1987; 10:13–610.

Yarborough JM. Dermabrasive surgery state of the art. In: Millikan, ed. Clinics in Dermatology, Advances in Surgery. Vol 5. Philadelphia: Lippincott, 1987:75.

74

Chemical Peel

William P. Coleman III
Tulane University School of Medicine, New Orleans, Louisiana, U.S.A.

Harold J. Brody
Emery University School of Medicine, Atlanta, Georgia, U.S.A.

Randall K. Roenigk
Mayo Clinic, Rochester, Minnesota, U.S.A.

Henry H. Roenigk, Jr.
Arizona Advanced Dermatology, Scottsdale, Arizona, U.S.A.

INTRODUCTION

Chemical exfoliation has been used by physicians for as long as 3500 years, beginning when the Egyptians applied a variety of irritants in an attempt to improve the appearance of skin. Over the last century, dermatologists have attempted to study chemical peeling in a scientific manner while refining techniques.

The primary indications for chemical peeling are

- actinic damage,
- pigmentary dyschromias,
- wrinkles,
- superficial scarring.

Chemical wounding of the skin is often classified as superficial, medium, or deep. Superficial peels wound through the epidermis. Medium peels penetrate through the papillary dermis, while deep peels extend into the mid-reticular dermis.

The decision about what type of peel to perform should be based on the type of skin pathology present in the patient. Deeper skin problems require deeper peels. The depth of the peel also determines the length of the healing phase and the chance of complications.

SUPERFICIAL PEELS

A variety of peeling agents are capable of producing a superficial peel. The most commonly used ones are listed in Table 1. Jessner's solution (Table 2) is commonly employed as an epidermal wounding agent. Applying additional coats of Jessner's solution produces deeper penetration. This provides a convenient clinical mechanism for modulating the peel depth.

Alpha-hydroxy acids are nontoxic organic chemicals derived from food products, featuring one or more carboxyl groups with a hydroxyl group on the adjacent skeleton carbon atom. Major alpha-hydroxy acids are listed in Table 3. In low concentrations (10–20%) these acids diminish comeocyte cohesion. In higher concentrations (over 50%) they cause epidermolysis. Of these, the most useful for chemical peeling is glycolic acid.

Glycolic acid is derived from sugar cane, although it can be more conveniently manufactured by a chemical process. It is available in a variety of concentrations and can be diluted with water. Many commercial formulations of glycolic acid are available for peeling. Some contain buffers to raise the pH and diminish the potency.

Glycolic acid 50% to 70% is best employed as a superficial wounding agent. If allowed to penetrate into the dermis, it can cause unpredictable healing and may scar the skin. Glycolic acid is only applied for short periods of time to limit penetration. Physical signs such as vesiculation or intense erythema can be used as end points. Once the desired effect is achieved, the acid must be diluted with water or an alkaline agent to stop the epidermal destruction. Failure to thoroughly dilute the acid may lead to dermal penetration and crusting or scars. The length of time the acid is left undiluted is a convenient indicator for controlling the peel intensity. Usually, glycolic peels are performed monthly to gradually improve the appearance of the skin. Repeated peels continue to provide more improvement, although numerous glycolic acid peels will not provide the same improvement as one medium-depth peel.

Salicylic acid can also be used as a superficial peeling agent. An example of a potent formulation can be found in Table 4. Salicylic acid is contraindicated in the presence of malignancy. It may also cause salicylate sensitivity when used in high concentrations or over large surface areas.

There have also been reports of hearing impairment. Salicylic acid has recently become available in pre-prepared commercial formulations.

MEDIUM PEELS

Trichloroacetic acid

Trichloroacetic acid (TCA) has been used as a destructive agent for the treatment of warts, keratoses, photoaging, and as a cauterant for over 100 years. Ayres first delineated the use of TCA as therapy for aging skin; however, its use in dermatology has been documented in British literature from 1926. There are now many cosmetic and therapeutic indications for TCA chemexfoliation that correspond with the

Table 1 Commonly Used Superficial Peeling Agents

Jessner's solution
Glycolic acid
Salicylic acid
Trichloroacetic acid 10–30%

Table 3 Alpha-Hydroxy Acids

Benzylic acid	Malic acid
Citric acid	Mandelic acid
Gluconic acid	Taxtaxic acid
Lactic acid	Glycolic acid

heightened interest in facial chemical peeling. Various application techniques and combinations with other procedures are now used (Table 5).

TCA can be used as a superficial or medium-depth peeling agent. In concentrations of 10% to 30%, TCA destroys the epidermis resulting in a superficial peel. Higher concentrations of TCA (35% or greater) will chemically destroy both the epidermis and the upper dermis, causing a slough of devitalized skin within five to seven days. In patients with extensive photodamage and actinic keratoses, atypical keratinocytes are replaced by normal cells derived from the adnexa. Dermal collagen begins regeneration within two to three weeks. The remodeling of collagen fibers, including homogenization of the superficial dermal collagen and increased elastic staining, continues for up to six months. The degree of this effect is based principally on the concentration of TCA. These histologic changes are essentially permanent.

Treatment of actinic keratoses and photodamage are the principal indications for TCA peels (Table 6). Other common methods of epidermal destruction such as cryotherapy are effective, but in some cases the number of actinic keratoses is so extensive that more complete treatment is warranted. TCA chemical peel compares favorably with 5 fluorouracil and imiquimod creams for correction of extensive actinic damage because of the need for prolonged application and the severe dermatitic reaction that results with application of the creams. It is not uncommon that patients using 5 fluorouracil or imiquimod cream will not complete a therapeutic trial. In contrast, a TCA chemical peel is applied by the physician and is normally performed only once.

The cosmetic benefit obtained after a TCA chemical peel for photoaging is due to the decrease in mild-to-moderate wrinkling of facial skin by new collagen formed in actinically damaged, solar elastotic dermis. TCA improves fine cross-hatched facial rhytides and mild perioral wrinkles as well. However, the deepest rhytides that are caused by muscles of facial expression or excessively lax skin will not respond well to chemical peel with TCA at safe concentrations.

Indications

Indications for TCA chemical peel also include solar-induced pigmentary disorders, especially lentigo simplex. Other pigmentary problems such as postinflammatory hyperpigmentation or melasma may respond, but the results are highly variable and the condition may be worsened in patients with type 3 or 4 skin. A test patch is suggested in these cases, and patients should be cautioned

about variable results. These patients also require prolonged use of hydroquinone to control postinflammatory hyperpigmentation. Many patients ask about TCA chemical peel for acne scarring. Most patients are better served by dermabrasion. Another common request is for treatment of dilated pilosebaceous pores that rarely respond to TCA peels.

Formulation of Trichloroacetic Acid

Chemical peeling with TCA is a versatile, elegant procedure. The concentration is chosen by the physician operator and reliably correlates with the depth of dermal damage. However, more than one method has been used to formulate TCA solutions, causing confusion in the literature. The standard pharmaceutical method for calculating and labeling the strength of any solution in which a solid is dissolved in a liquid is the weight in volume method (w/v). TCA crystals should meet the standards of United States Pharmacopeia. Standard concentrations of TCA are usually referred to as weight of the TCA crystals in grams to the volume of the water diluent (w/v). Twenty percent to 35% TCA (w/v) formulations are most commonly used for TCA peels. Higher concentrations of TCA cause unacceptable scarring on facial skin and in animal models. Gynecologists routinely use 70% TCA w/v to treat vaginal and cervical condyloma. However, the moist mucosal surface effectively reduces the concentration, so submucosal damage is less and scar does not result. Recently, there has been interest in using high concentrations of TCA (70–90%) for ice pick scars. The concentrated TCA is applied focally with a sharp stick like a toothpick into the depth of the scar to obliterate it. Unpredictable scarring commonly occurs, however, if TCA greater than 40% w/v is applied widely to the face.

TCA is not light sensitive and may be stored refrigerated or nonrefrigerated in clear or amber glass or TCA-resistant plastic containers for at least 23 weeks, providing the solution is not contaminated. At least one manufacturer has analyzed the potency of solutions 20% through 100% w/v through two years.

Communication between the physician and pharmacist is important to avoid complications, and communication between practitioners should be standardized. To avoid ambiguities, all TCA solutions should be fully labeled according to the preparation method used. Ideally, all TCA preparations should be labeled % w/v.

Procedure

In many ways, the preoperative consultation is more important than the procedure itself. Accurate medical and psychological evaluation requires years of experience. It is

Table 2 Jessner's Solution

Lactic acid USP 14% w/v
Salicylic acid USP 14% w/v
Resorcinol USP 14% w/v
In ethyl alcohol, USP

Abbreviation: USP, United States Pharmacopeia; w/v, weight in volume.

Table 4 Salicyclic Acid Peel Formulation

Salicylic acid powder, USP 2 oz
Methyl salicylate 16 gtt
Croton oil 4–8 drops
Aquaphor qs 4 oz

Abbreviation: USP, United States Pharmacopeia.

Table 5 Some Variations of Chemical Peel with TCA

Superficial peel with 20% TCA w/v (single or repeated)
Intermediate peel with 30–40% TCA w/v
Tape Occlusion (more superficial peel)
TCA plus tretinoin cream (pre- and postoperatively)
TCA plus 5-FU
TCA plus Jessner's solution (medium depth)
TCA plus solid CO_2 ice (medium depth)
TCA plus glycolic acid (medium depth)
TCA plus dermabrasion (chemabrasion)
TCA plus phenol (combination peel)
Focal treatment with 50–80% TCA w/v

Abbreviations: TCA, trichloroacetic acid; w/v, weight in volume.

vitally important to choose the appropriate patients. The preoperative consultation is a learned art, as the clinician must not only determine a patient's candidacy for chemical peel on the basis of physical findings but also judge their motivation and the ability to emotionally to handle the temporary postoperative disfigurement. Some medically appropriate candidates for chemical peel may have little interest in this procedure because it is cosmetic. Conversely, some patients may have normal skin but because of their concern about cosmetic appearance are willing to try anything including chemical peel, for the perceived benefit. Medium-depth (mid-dermal) TCA chemical peeling results in a superficial wound that takes months to heal completely. The residual erythema that typically lasts two to three months after a moderate or deep TCA chemical peel can be anxiety provoking or depressing for an ill-prepared patient who expects rapid results quickly. In some cases, a superficial TCA peel or a less aggressive alpha-hydroxy acid peel might be more appropriate.

The physician should also emphasize the importance of avoiding the sun for three to six months postoperatively. In temperate climates, patients may prefer to have a chemical peel in the fall or winter, when they are less likely to be outside. If the potential outcome is questionable, a small test patch can be performed on facial skin in a relatively hidden site (although this is routinely unnecessary).

Patients may be pre-prepared with daily use of tretinoin (0.05% or 0.10% Retin-A® cream) for two weeks. This is used for mild debridement of the stratum corneum including hypertrophic actinic keratoses. It may also mildly degrease the skin, as it decreases the activity of facial sebaceous glands. The patient should not apply makeup, moisturizer, hair conditioners, mousse, or hairspray for 24

Table 6 Some Indications for TCA Peels

TCA commonly used and effective
   Actinic keratoses
   Lentigo simplex
   Photoaging—solar elastosis
   Rhytides (superficial to medium depth)
TCA occasionally used and variably effective
   Acne scars (superficial or distensible)
   Alopecia areata
   Dilated pilosebaceous pores
   Melasma
   Neurotic excoriations
   Postinflammatory hyperpigmentation
   Rosacea

Abbreviations: TCA, trichloroacetic acid; w/v, weight in volume.

hours preoperatively. Oils on the skin prevent transepidermal penetration of TCA.

A tray is prepared with the following materials: bottles containing appropriate concentrations of TCA, cotton-tipped applicators, square cotton gauze pads, and a small glass cup to hold quantities of the TCA. A readily accessible container of water should be available as a rinse in the event of an accidental eye splash.

The face is scrubbed with acetone until the sebaceous oils have been thoroughly removed. Remember that acetone is flammable, so electrosurgery or laser should not be performed while preparing the skin with acetone. When this step is complete, the skin feels like fine sandpaper. The small scales on the face turn white because the oil has been removed. The eyes may be protected with an antibiotic ointment, gauze pads, and hypoallergemic tape or goggles; however, simply closing the eyes is usually sufficient and allows application of the TCA closer to the lid margins. Oral or intramuscularly administered sedatives may be used in anxious patients. Local anesthetic is not required. Topical anesthetics such as ELMX® or EMLA® may be applied, occluded or not, for 30 minutes at this point to reduce the pain of TCA penetration. Studies have shown up to a 70% reduction in discomfort using this approach. However, the topical anesthetic cream residue must be removed by acetone or soap prior to application of the TCA.

A cotton-tipped applicator or gauze sponge is moistened with TCA and rolled against the wall of the glass cup to remove excess fluid. The TCA is applied to a small area by firmly rubbing in a circular or linear fashion. Once the skin has been treated, it slowly changes color, becoming whitish-gray as a result of chemical coagulation of the epidermis (Fig. 1). This color change is called a "frost." The frost appears more rapidly with high concentrations of TCA and may not appear at all with low concentrations, especially if the skin has not been adequately degreased. Once the pad or the cotton-tipped applicator is soiled, it should be discarded.

The acid stings moderately when applied, and correlates with the concentration of TCA. The pain crescendos, normally peaking approximately half way through the procedure. Dry cool or ice compresses are helpful to soothe the discomfort, as is a patient hand-held fan. Some practitioners

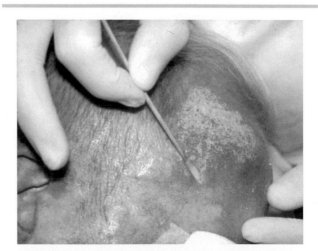

Figure 1 Forty percent trichloroacetic acid w/v applied with cotton-tipped applicator. Note "frost," fine scale on untreated area due to acetone scrub, eye protection.

like to perform chemical peel in a specific pattern by peeling anatomic units of the face in the same order for all patients. Some anatomic facial subunits require different concentrations of TCA (i.e., forehead, cheeks, chin—35% w/v; eyelids 25% w/v). As a matter of habit, for example, one might start with the highest concentration to be used on the forehead, followed by the cheeks, chin, nose, ears, lips, and eyelids (lowest concentration). The moistened cotton-tipped applicator is kept away from the eyes at all times. When the eyelids are being treated, particular care is used to avoid seepage of excess TCA onto the sclera. If the patient complains of eye discomfort, immediate lavage with water will dilute the acid and protect the eye from injury.

Postoperative Care

After the peel is complete (determined by an even frost over the face), cool water compresses or ice packs can be used to sooth the burning. Application of water has no effect on the penetration of the peel as it does with glycolic acid. Postoperative care includes a thin coat of a petrolatum-based ointment such as Aquaphor®. This causes immediate relief from the burning sensation. Some dermatologists employ a hydrogel dressing such as Vigilon® postoperatively. A face mask is fashioned from multilayered gauze placed over the hydrogel dressing and left intact for one day. The patient is instructed to sleep with the head elevated and to avoid excessive activity. Ice packs help reduce swelling and diminish any remaining burning. Most patients go home and sleep or relax until the follow-up appointment the next day. One day postoperatively, patients may be quite swollen depending on the concentration of TCA used (Fig. 2).

Patients are instructed to wash the peeled areas with a mild soap two to four times daily and reapply the emollient ointment. Another visit at two to three days postoperatively allows the physician to monitor healing and respond to problems. These visits also provide an opportunity to reinforce

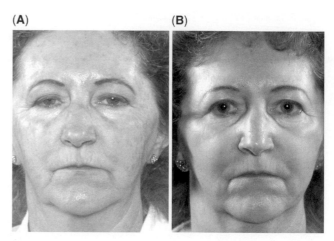

Figure 3   **(A)** Prior to peel using 40%, 30%, 18% trichloroacetic acid w/v in different anatomic subunits. **(B)** Seven months postoperative. (*See color insert.*)

postoperative instructions and reassure patients that healing is progressing normally.

Re-epithelialization is normally complete within one week, at which point emollient applications can stop, with the substitution of lubricating lotions and sunscreens. TCA peels of lower concentrations may re-epithelialize more rapidly (those in the 10–20% w/v range may not completely slough the epidermis). Diffuse erythema may last up to several months for deeper TCA peels, but cosmetics may be used after one week. Some examples of patients treated for photoaging, actinic keratoses, and lentigo simplex are demonstrated in Figures 3–6.

Combination TCA peels have become quite popular among dermatologists over the last 20 years. Pretreatment with a superficial wounding agent prior to application of the TCA allows deeper penetration with lower concentrations of TCA. The most popular of these combinations is the Jessner's plus TCA peel. Jessner's solution is applied first to increase penetration of the TCA. A similar approach is the Glycolic plus TCA peel, which relies on Glycolic acid for the first step. The CO_2 ice plus TCA peel is based on the application of CO_2 ice prior to the TCA to augment penetration. All three of these approaches provide a reliable dermal peel when 35% TCA is used. The CO_2 ice plus TCA peel penetrates deeper into the dermis than the other two approaches and allows the surgeon to "sculpt" deeper scars or wrinkles by rubbing harder with the CO_2 ice.

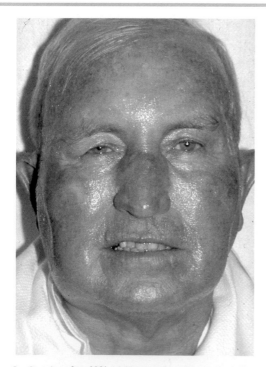

Figure 2   One day after 40% trichloroacetic acid w/v peel. Note edema. Skin has yet to exfoliate.

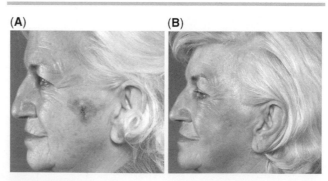

Figure 4   **(A)** Note lentigo prior to 40% trichloroacetic acid w/v peel. **(B)** Five months postoperative. (*See color insert.*)

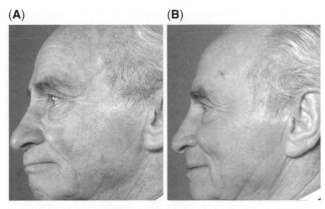

Figure 5 (**A**) Solar elastosis, actinic keratoses, lentigines prior to 40% trichloroacetic acid w/v peel. (**B**) Six weeks postoperative. (*See color insert.*)

Histologic Effects of Trichloroacetic Acid on the Skin

The depth of wounds created by various concentrations and application techniques of TCA and phenol has been evaluated by several researchers using human and animal models. The therapeutic effects of TCA are destruction of the epidermis and dermis with subsequent re-epithelialization from epidermal appendages, and new collagen formation (Figs. 7 and 8). The depth of the wounds caused by various dilutions of TCA is directly correlated to therapeutic efficacy.

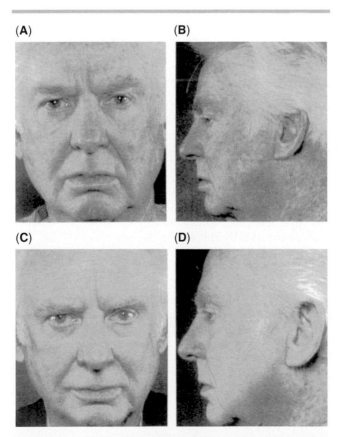

Figure 6 (**A**) Prior to 40% trichloroacetic acid (TCA) w/v to forehead, cheeks, chin, nose, ears; 30% TCA w/v to upper and lower lips; 18% TCA w/v to upper and lower eyelids. Front view. (**B**) Side view. (**C**) Six months postoperative. Front view. (**D**) Side view.

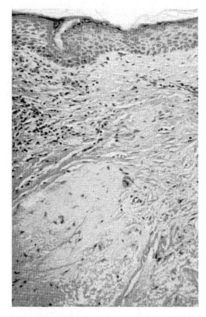

Figure 7 Histology (hematoxylin and eosin ×40) three months after 40% trichloroacetic acid w/v in a human. Note frbroblasts forming new collagen in papillary dermis. Also note persistent nodule of solar elastosis in reticular dermis, deeper than peel penetrated.

Immediate Histologic Effects of Trichloroacetic Acid

The depth of tissue necrosis increases with the concentration of TCA (Table 7). The concentration of a TCA solution used for actinic keratoses should be at least 30% to 40% w/v because this is what is required for complete removal of the epidermis and superficial dermis, allowing re-epithelialization by appendage keratinocytes. The appropriate concentration of TCA used for facial rejuvenation depends on the desired effect. A solution of 18% TCA w/v results in mild epidermal exfoliation. This is well tolerated, but the degree of rejuvenation is relatively short term and superficial. Serial applications (weekly or biweekly) of 18% TCA w/v may directly or indirectly induce remodeling of the papillary dermis because of the repeated caustic damage to temporarily thinned epidermis.

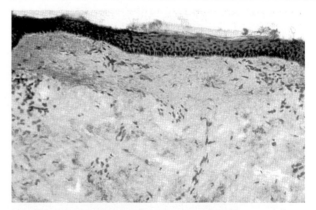

Figure 8 Histology (hematoxylin and eosin ×40) one year after 40% trichloroacetic acid w/v in a human. Note band of mature new collagen that overlies blue stain scar damage.

Table 7 Depth of Necrosis (mm) in a Porcine Model at Various Concentrations of TCA

Depth of necrosis (mm)

TCA concentration (w/v) difference	Unoccluded technique	Occluded technique	
18%	0.044	0	–
30%	0.2555	0.075	0.180
40%	0.500	0.178	0.322

Abbreviation: TCA, trichloroacetic acid; w/v, weight in volume.
Source: From (1989).

Solutions of 30% and 40% TCA w/v cause not only replacement of the epidermis but also longer lasting dermal changes. Histologically, 0.3 to 0.5 mm of dermal necrosis results (Fig. 9). There is an associated reduction in fine- and medium-depth facial wrinkles. There are no reports of the clinical use of 80% TCA on humans for facial rejuvenation procedures. Because of dermal necrosis noted in experimental studies (0.8–0.9 mm depth), scarring would likely result (as was noted clinically in animal studies) and would be cosmetically unacceptable.

Tape occlusion after chemical peeling has in the past been thought to increase the depth of penetration of TCA. Increased penetration and a deeper peel after skin occlusion with tape may occur with phenol (Baker's formula). In several studies, it has however been confirmed that occlusion of TCA with tape reliably decreases the depth of dermal necrosis (Fig. 10). In a porcine model, at all TCA concentrations tested, the occluded technique produced significantly less necrosis than the unoccluded technique. Hypothetically, less dermal necrosis in the occluded specimen could be the result of interstitial humidification (Fig. 11). Occlusion accomplishes this by the prevention of transepidermal water loss, which leads to increased interstitial water content in the epidermis and dermis. Therefore, the effective concentration of TCA is decreased or more rapidly diluted.

There is histologic benefit to pretreating the skin with tretinoin cream for two weeks and acetone immediately preoperatively. Although both degrease the skin, they also thin and dedifferentiate the epidermis, including the stratum corneum, which may contain hypertrophic actinic keratoses. The depth of damage in the skin correlates directly with the concentration of TCA and is constant. Thinning the epidermis causes relatively deeper dermal necrosis at a given concentration (Fig. 12). The effect on the epidermis is relatively short lived. The longer-lasting dermal effect is usually preferable. Higher concentrations of TCA might be used in place of preparing the skin with tretinoin and acetone but may cause unpredictable results, risking a scar. Re-epithelialization time is shortened by the use of preoperative tretinoin.

Long-Term Histologic Effects of Trichloroacetic Acid

In long-term histologic studies of TCA on porcine skin, test sites have been treated with 20%, 35%, 50%, and 80% TCA and with either tape-occluded or tape-unoccluded techniques, in addition to serially applied 20% TCA on six occasions over nine weeks. Biopsy specimens have been obtained over a 28-week period. Specimens stained with hematoxylin and eosin and sel Giemsa microscopically showed epidermal changes that include thinning and orthokeratosis of the stratum corneum at four weeks after treatment with TCA. This change is transient. At eight and 28 weeks, the stratum corneum is similar to its baseline status. The change in the epidermal thickness is variable, depending on the concentration of TCA, the time of the biopsy, and the application technique (Table 8).

At 24 hours and four weeks, collagen is distinctly basophilic, representing the zone of necrosis. Collagen is altered at eight and 28 weeks, as the staining tends to be much paler in the superficial dermis, and the level of dermal necrosis much less distinct. The bundles are haphazardly organized, smaller, fragmented, and have less well-defined borders.

The number of fibroblasts is increased in the superficial dermis at four, eight, and 28 weeks in skin treated with 30% TCA w/v or higher concentrations. These fibroblasts appear histologically to be metabolically active and are characterized by abundant basophilic cytoplasm. Solutions with high concentrations of TCA induce a greater number of fibroblasts than solutions with low concentrations. At 28 weeks, the number of fibroblasts remains greater than that at baseline.

Elastic fibers are histologically unchanged in skin treated with 18% TCA w/v and the serial application technique. However, skin treated with higher concentrations has a decrease in the quantity of elastin (stained with sel Giemsa) at four and eight weeks. At 28 weeks, the amount of elastin is increased. The depth of these alterations in elastin corresponds roughly to the depth of basophilic necrosis. The morphology of new elastic fibers at 28 weeks shows no characteristic pattern and range from short, thin fragments to long, branching, and thick fibers.

The long-term (28 weeks) histologic effects vary depending on the concentration used and the application technique. Serial applications of 18% TCA w/v have very little long-term effect. However, further clinical investigation of the serial application of 18% TCA w/v is warranted because there are some short-term histologic changes. Specimens treated with 35%, 50%, and 80% TCA have definite

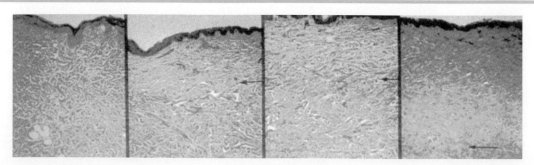

Figure 9 Histology (hematoxylin and eosin ×40) of porcine skin 24 hours after application of trichloroacetic acid. Arrows indicate depth of necrosis. Open technique. Left to right 20%, 25%, 50%, 80% TCA (w/v formulation).

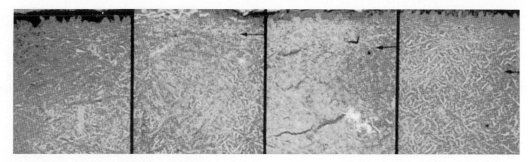

Figure 10 Histology (hematoxylin and eosin ×40) of porcine skin 24 hours after application of trichloroacetic acid (TCA) by closed technique (tape occlusion). Arrows indicate depth of necrosis. Left to right 20% (no necrosis noticeable), 35%, 50%, 80% TCA (Mayo formulation). Depth of necrosis less at all concentrations compared with Figure 9.

alterations, which persist. Generally, the degree of histologic alteration increases in proportion with the increase in TCA concentration. The histologic effects were most intense with 80% TCA. Scar and pigmentary alteration (decreased pigment) are evident in porcine skin treated with solutions of 80% TCA but not in skin treated with 35% and 50% TCA. When the long-term histologic effects of tape-occluded and tape-unoccluded techniques were compared, the tape-occluded specimens have significantly less long-term histologic alteration than the tape-unoccluded specimen.

Complications

The complications of TCA chemical peel, when performed by a skilled operator, are rare and tend to be minor or easily corrected (Table 7). Superficial bacterial pustulation and eczematization may rarely occur as early complications and are managed with appropriate antibacterial therapy. Routine postoperative care includes topical petroleum jelly applied after cleansing with mild soap. Latent herpes simplexvirus may reactivate, so patients with this history should be treated prophylactically with oral antiviral agents (prior to and five days after).

Milia frequently form early in the postexfoliation period but are easily treated with incision and drainage or mild abrasive scrubs and otherwise resolve spontaneously. Hyperpigmentation and hypopigmentation are the most common long-term problems (Figs. 13 and 14). Generally, hyperpigmentation is more likely to occur after superficial peels whereas hypopigmentation may occur after deep peels. These problems are more visually obvious in patients with darker complexions.

Scars may occur on skin less richly endowed with cutaneous adnexa such as the dorsal aspects of the hand. Scar formation may also occur in certain sites due in part to greater skin movement during normal activity, such as the lip and neck, associated with interdigitation of muscle fibers with the skin. We normally perform nonfacial chemical peels with lower concentrations of TCA or using other agents (such as alpha-hydroxy acids) that typically cause only epidermolysis. Hypertrophic scars may form on the face, but keloids are rare.

Other complications include accentuation of telangiectasias, apparent enlargement of pores, darkening of pigmented nevi, persistent erythema, and increased sensitivity to wind, sunlight, and temperature variation.

Advantages of Trichloroacetic Acid for Chemical Peel

The goal of facial chemical peeling is to achieve the appropriate result for the patient. Various solutions used for facial chemical peel have been employed, as each clinician tries to achieve "better" results; but these formulations should be studied scientifically to establish their safety and efficacy. The use of TCA for facial chemical peeling has been tested and used for decades as a safe, effective, elegant, regularly reproducible method for treating common problems associated with photoaged skin (Table 9).

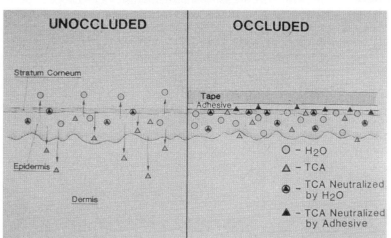

Figure 11 Theoretically, occlusion increases interstitial water causing a relative decrease in trichloroacetic acid concentration causing less necrosis.

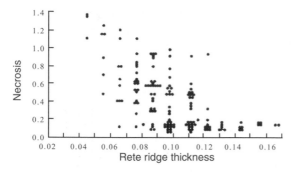

Figure 12 Thicker epidermis causes less dermal necrosis at a given concentration. Supports pretreatment with tretinoin and acetone to thin or equalize the epidermis (specifically the stratum corneum).

DEEP PEELS

The chemical peel that penetrates into the mid-reticular dermis to correct most severe actinic damage utilizes a formula containing phenol, or carbolic acid. Liquefied phenol consists of an 88% solution of phenol in water.

The traditional chemical peel with 55% phenol as described in 1961 by Baker and Gordon is still currently in use. This measured formula is the modification made by lay peelers in Los Angeles and Miami that evolved from the use of phenol to treat gunpowder burns in World War I (Table 10). This specific formula has been studied histologically and clinically. Full-strength 88% phenol for many years was thought to cause immediate coagulation of epidermal keratin proteins and to self-block further penetration of phenol. The specific formula dilutes the concentration to approximately 50% to 55%. Liquid hexachlorophene soap in alcohol (Septisol-Delasco, Council Bluffs, Iowa, U.S.A.) as a surfactant reduces surface tension to promote a more even peel. Croton oil, the fixed oil from the seed of the plant Croton tiglium, is an epidermolytic vesicant in a 2.1% concentration in the formula that may increase inflammation. The freshly prepared emulsion is not miscible and must be stirred constantly in a clear glass cup immediately prior to patient application. Baker and Gordon originally described the application of waterproof tape following the peel to increase penetration, presumably through a mechanism of maceration. The modification of this peel by McCollough and Beeson promotes more aggressive defatting of the skin and aggressive removal of the epidermal barrier with acetone prior to a heavier application of the formula. This elimination of the taping and tape removal discomfort with optional sedation is advantageous. However, in spite of claims of similar results and possibly less risk of scarring, histologic evidence supports the increased wound depth of phenol from taping.

Table 8 Potential Complications of Chemical Peels

Accentuation of telangiectasia, nevi, and pores
Bacterial infection
Hyperpigmentation (usually superficial peels, dark skin)
Hypopigmentation (usually deep peels)
Milia
Persistent erythema
Reactivation of herpes simplex
Scars
Sensitivity to sun, wind, temperature change

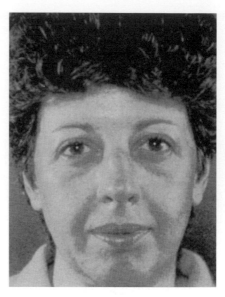

Figure 13 Postinflammatory hyperpigmentation at three months after 30% trichloroacetic acid w/v peel.

Hetter's landmark work published in 2000 describes a series of formulas designed to be applied to moderately photoaged skin. The formulas are thoroughly investigated histologically based on photoaging and application to different cosmetic units. They eliminate the heavier application and taping that could be used to regulate penetration of the Baker/Gordon formula. The work is based on the premise that croton oil is the active ingredient in the formula and phenol is the carrier. Higher concentrations of croton oil make it possible to use a weaker strength of phenol in the formula, reducing systemic effects of phenol toxicity. Addition of 0.2% croton oil increases phenol peel depth by 20%. The phenol concentration is not the important variable. Hetter's 1.2% croton oil concentration formula is a strength for moderately photodamaged perioral skin as opposed to

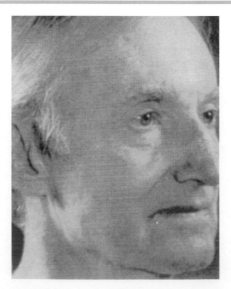

Figure 14 Postinflammatory hypopigmentation at one year after 40% trichloroacetic acid w/v peel.

Table 9 Advantages of TCA peels

Few medical contraindications
Elegant (adjust depth of necrosis by concentration of TCA)
No allergic reactions
No systemic toxicity
Scarring rare at standard concentrations
Wound healing time shorter than with 5-fluorouracil cream (better compliance)
More practical than repeated cryotherapy for patients with extensive actinic keratoses

Abbreviation: TCA, trichloroacetic acid.

Table 11 Hetter's Heavy Peel Perioral for Moderately Wrinkled Skin

Phenol, 4 cms (33%)
Water, 6 cms
Septisol liquid soap, 16 drops
Croton oil, 3 drops (1.1% Croton oil)

the 2.1% croton oil concentration of the traditional Baker/ Gordon formula, originally used for severely photo-damaged skin (Table 11).

All techniques have merit, and unoccluded Baker/ Gordon formula produces an excellent peel as long as the wound depth is deep enough to efface defects. It is easier to selectively tape very severe, thick, actinically damaged skin, and rest assured that the deepest peel possible is produced over these areas. The Hetter formula is ideal for less photodamaged perioral skin. The phenol formulas for the other facial cosmetic units are less necessary with TCA peeling being safe and available.

Procedure

Much of the time, deep peeling solutions will be applied to only one cosmetic unit and TCA formulas will be applied to the remainder of the face. No cardiac or renal precautions or sedation are needed for this small application. In full face applications, at least half the volume of phenol in the formula is discarded with multiple cotton-tipped applicators. The actual amount of phenol applied to the skin is probably a little more than 1 mL. Thus, the amount applied to one cosmetic unit is equivalent to that applied to a nail bed for a phenol nail matrixectomy. Oral hydration may be given in the form of 8 to 16 Oz of water prior to the peel if they have not been drinking much fluid on the day of the procedure.

With full face application, the use of regional supraorbital, infraorbital, mental, superior alveolar, and preauricular block anesthesia can electively be employed by using the long-acting local anesthetics bupivacaine or etidocaine. Mild tumescence of the cheeks with 0.1% lidocaine may be helpful for adequate anesthesia in some patients. If blocks are not employed, the intravenous combination of fentanyl citrate, an analgesic, and midazolam, a sedative, can be administered and titrated to the needs of the patient.

Intravenous fluids are still used to flush the phenol through the kidneys. Immediately prior to the administration of intravenous fluids with or without sedation, the patient is placed in a sitting position, and a line of small dots is placed slightly inferior to the mandible. The peel is extended to this point to minimize possible permanent color change, which would fall into the shadow cast by the mandible. Because phenol is partially detoxified in the liver and excreted by the kidney and because phenol may induce cardiac arrhythmias in large doses, the good health of these

Table 10 Heaviest (Baker–Gordon) Perioral for Very Wrinkled Skin

Phenol, USP, 88%, 3 cms (55%)
Tap water, 2 cms
Septisol liquid soap, 8 drops
Croton oil, 3 drops [2.1 % Croton oil if 1 gutta = 27 drops/ cms]

organs should be established prior to full face peeling. A preoperative history and physical examination to rule out cardiac and hepatorenal disease is performed, and a recent electrocardiogram, complete blood count, hepatorenal profile, and electrolyte values are obtained. Hydration with 500 cm^3 of lactated Ringer's solution prior to the procedure and 1000 cm^3 during and after the peel will prevent phenol toxicity to these organ systems and ensure an increased output of alkaline urine.

The face should be washed thoroughly with soap and water the night before and the morning of the procedure. No makeup should be employed on the morning of the peel. The fine facial hair is shaved first to avoid the discomfort of depilating these hairs during tape removal after surgery. A thorough three-minute acetone scrub or a combination of acetone followed by alcohol to degrease the skin is utilized immediately prior to the application of wounding agent. The gentle abrasion of the skin with acetone on gauze until a sandpaper-like sound is heard when the sponge is rubbed across the skin may result in more wounding agent absorption but less need for a taped mask, assuming that more Baker/Gordon solution is applied. We do not abrade to this aggressive end point, since it may result in irregular penetration of wounding agent. We prefer to occlude that only what we judge clinically needs to be taped as the most severely photodamaged.

The application of phenol should be accomplished with moist but not very wet cotton-tipped applicators. Whether continued application and rubbing produce increased penetration has been discussed and argued between different cosmetic surgical specialties. There is no question that phenol formulas penetrate immediately through the papillary dermis. The continued penetration for an extra 10th of a millimeter more or less is achieved by continued rubbing and optional taping of the cosmetic unit. Continued rubbing and the subsequent application of a greater quantity of phenol with a very moist cotton-tipped applicator past a white color until a gray-white color is seen are necessary for elimination of severe rhytides. A single application with one cotton-tipped applicator to the individual deepest rhytides may precede the application to the rest of the cosmetic unit. If the rhytides are not very deep and only of a moderate photoaging variety, the Hetter formula is a consideration. Optionally, a single application of the Baker/Gordon formula with one cotton-tipped applicator that has been "wrung out" against the lip of the peel container with no continued rubbing is adequate. This might be termed a "light" versus a "heavy" application of phenol since the gray-white end point is not achieved here. In relatively normal skin, the light application less likely to be a reality because it is the sun damage that retards wounding agent penetration (Fig. 15).

The face is divided into six cosmetic units: forehead, left cheek, right cheek, perioral, nose, and periorbital areas. Peel solution is usually applied in this order—moving from the least sensitive to the most sensitive areas. The solution should be feathered into all hair-bearing areas including the scalp and eyebrows. An electric fan to vent the phenol

(A)   **(B)**

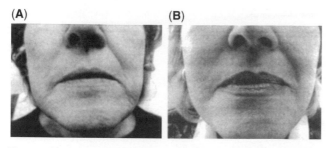

Figure 15 **(A)** Severe perioral photoaging in a Fitzpatrick II female. **(B)** Two months after deep peeling with unoccluded Baker/Gordon formula.

fumes accompanied by good central ventilation in a room with outdoor air access is important for the comfort of the staff. To minimize renal and cardiac toxicity, 10 to 15 minutes are allowed between cosmetic units, so it requires 60 to 90 minutes for an entire face. One or two fresh single cotton-tipped applicators are used for each application of solution. These many applicators are discarded during the procedure and are soaked with substantial amounts of wasted phenol. In reality, the amount of phenol in contact with the skin is less than half of the total 3 cms in the formula. This small total amount along with slow application and hydration accounts for the excellent safety record of this procedure over the last 40 years. If there are many folds and rhytides indicating more surface area, the cosmetic units may be subdivided, and application may be slower. The extent of cutaneous absorption of phenol depends more upon the total area of skin exposed than upon the concentration of solution employed. An immediate burning sensation is present for 15 to 20 seconds and quickly subsides. Pain returns in 20 minutes to persist for six to 10 hours. The use of EMLA (eutectic mixture of local anesthetic: lidocaine 2.5% and prilocaine 2.5%—AstraZeneca LP, Wilmington, Delaware, U.S.A.) or L-M-X Cream (lidocaine cream 5%, Femdale Labs, Ferndale, Michigan, U.S.A.) once immediately after application on the frost to reduce this pain in peels without tape may have some measure of success in pain relief. Throbbing and burning still persist but may be more tolerable. Rebound stinging may occur if the patient overuses the topical anesthetic at home multiple times.

Baker's solution is usually needed for the crow's feet area, but full-strength phenol or a more moderate Hetter formula may be used for the upper and/or lower eyelid unit as determined by actinic damage. From the superior border of the tarsal plate to the upper eyelash ciliary margin, 35% TCA may be adequate.

Zinc oxide tape may be applied to selected segments as the peel progresses, although one can wait until the entire face is covered with phenol/croton oil solution. Tape must adhere properly, or skip areas may result. The eyebrows, eyelids, and earlobes should be peeled but not taped. Microfoam tape (3M) can be used to occlude the perioral area because the tape is elastic and will both stretch and contract with lip movement. Stuzin has found that immediate application of petrolatum applied only once immediately following the Baker/Gordon peel may obviate the need for the mask and serve as a vapor barrier to prevent phenol evaporation and increase maceration and penetration. However, they concede that deeply lined faces that appear weather-beaten still require use of the tape.

Postoperative Care

Although the pain subsides within six to eight hours, the edema is severe, and the eyelids are frequently swollen shut. The patient should sleep with the aid of oral hypnotics and analgesics if necessary in a sitting or semireclining position to reduce this edema. The mask is removed in 48 hours when the exudate has lifted the tape and drainage is beginning under the chin. Wet to dry soaking gently three to five times daily with tap water while standing in the shower or dilute antiseptic skin cleansers can be used to dry the exudative edema, followed by an occlusive moisturizer of petrolatum-based ointment. The original thymol iodide powder forming an overlying dry crust, or second "mask," that was used by lay peelers and in Baker's original description should seldom be used today. Its use may be associated with an increased healing time or increased degree of hypopigmentation or depigmentation.

Biosynthetic occlusive dressings have been successfully implemented to prevent desiccation and speed epithelialization in dermabrasion. They may be used after tape removal in deep peeling, but are less necessary because of the protective desiccated epidermis that remains in place for several days if occlusion is not used. Daily cream-based sunscreens and tretinoin are reinstituted as soon as tolerated within one to four weeks of re-epithelialization. Complete avoidance of sunlight is imperative during the healing period. Petechiae may result from strenuous physical exercise within a month after peeling. Milia are a common occurrence and may be extracted with a no. 11 scalpel blade or may resolve spontaneously.

After deep peeling, the erythema is so intense and the skin so tender that special attention should be paid to assist the patient with cosmetics. Cosmetics with a green foundation that are cream based will mask the intense red erythema for the immediate weeks after peeling and may be applied as soon as the crusts have disappeared. Men do not handle erythema even from medium-depth peels very well, and they generally are not good candidates for deep peeling with phenol-based formulas. Dermabrasion or laser resurfacing may be better alternatives.

A suggested interval of at least one to three months is recommended between any procedure that involves undermining or a flap closure. This includes rhytidectomy, brow lift or blepharoplasty. This time interval is supported by histologic study since collagen remodeling is not complete in medium-depth or deep peeling until 60 to 90 days later. Regional perioral and periorbital peels can be done at the completion of a face-lift if a blepharoplasty or perioral surgery is not performed. Deep plane face-lifting may be at less risk from simultaneous peeling. A transconjunctival blepharoplasty performed by laser or by scalpel does not involve undermining or closure of the skin. Therefore, chemical peeling of any variety may be performed concurrently with less risk.

The usual complications that occur with any dermal resurfacing can occur with deep peeling. Pigmentary changes, scarring, infection, prolonged erythema, and textural changes are the most feared complications. Mild hypopigmentation is expected and depth related. Photodamaged faces are uniformly darker than the rest of the body prior to peeling, and loss of pigment is predictable and not generally a problem. Acne, milia, and contact dermatitis from improper use of ointments are manageable. Complications previously occurring chiefly from the hospitalization of deep peeling patients are less common today in the era of outpatient medicine. These include toxic shock syndrome, laryngeal edema, and cardiac arrhythmias.

Many patients today that are peeled with phenol/croton oil formulas have been using combinations of tretinoin and alpha-hydroxy acids prior to the procedure. They may have had superficial peels prior to phenol application. These factors should be considered additional risks for increased penetration of the deep peel. Exact time interval precautions to restrict exfoliation prior to phenol peeling are uncertain because the extent of epidermal insult is very variable with the many skin care programs and superficial peels in use today.

It is increasingly unnecessary to perform a full face phenol/croton oil peel if each cosmetic unit has been properly evaluated. However, the reliability and predictability of the deep peel reflect evidence of its 40-year safety record. A tried and true technique such as deep peeling has a solid position alongside lasers and dermabrasion as another complimentary resurfacing modality. Clinical comparison between the ultrapulsed CO_2 laser and Baker's solution reveals that the laser improves severe photodamage by approximately 50%. Evaporation of all the intracellular and intercellular water in the skin by the laser is the limiting factor in laser penetration. After evaporation occurs, it may be necessary to use complimentary lasers or dermabrasion immediately following ultrapulsed CO_2 laser to further penetrate to the mid-reticular dermis to eliminate deepest rhytides. The Baker/Gordon phenol peel, however, can eliminate the vast majority of rhytides in one treatment. No procedures for this indication are immune to residual hypopigmentation, and depth-dependent pigment loss is expected for all of the resurfacing modalities.

BIBLIOGRAPHY

Alt TH. Occluded Baker/Gordon chemical peel: review and update. J Dermatol Surg Oncol 1989; 15:980–993.

Ayres S III. Superficial chemosurgery in treating aging skin. Arch Dermatol 1962; 85:385–393.

Baker TJ. The ablation of rhytides by chemical means. A preliminary report. J Fl Med Assoc 1961; 48:451.

Beeson WH, McCollough EG. Chemical face peeling without taping. J Dermatol Surg Oncol 1985; 11:985–990.

Brodland DG, Cullimore KC, Roenigk RK, et al. Depths of chemexfoliation induced by various concentrations and application techniques of trichloroacetic acid in a porcine model. J Dermatol Surg Oncol 1989; 15:967–971.

Brodland DG, Roenigk RK. Trichloroacetic acid chemexfoliation (chemical peel) for extensive premalignant actinic damage of the face and scalp. Mayo Clin Proc 1988; 63:887–896.

Brody HJ. Chemical Peeling. St. Louis, MO: Mosby-Yearbook, Inc, 1992.

Brody HJ. Deep Peeling. In: Chemical Peeling and Resurfacing. 2nd. London, U.K.: Mosby-Harcourt, 1997:137–160.

Brody HJ, Hailey CW. Medium-depth chemical peeling of the skin: a variation of superficial chemosurgery. J Dermatol Surg Oncol 1986; 12:1268–1275.

Coleman WP III, Futrell JM. The glycolic acid trichloroacetic acid peel. J Dermatol Surg Oncol 1994; 20:76–80.

Heria O, Nemeth AJ, Taylor JR. Tretinoin accelerates healing after trichloroacetic acid chemical peel. Arch Dermatol 1991; 127:678–682.

Hetter GP. An examination of the phenol-croton oil peel: parts I-IV. Plast Reconstr Surg 2000; 105:227, 240, 752, 1061.

Lober CW. Chemexfoliation—indications and cautions. J Am Acad Dermatol 1987; 17:109–112.

Matarasso SL, Glogau RG. Chemical face peels. Dermatol Clin 1991; 9:131–150.

Matarasso SL, Salman SM, Glougau RC, et al. The role of chemical peeling in the treatment of photo damaged skin. J Dermatol Surg Oncol 1990; 16:945–954.

Monash S. The uses of diluted trichloroacetic acid in dermatology. Urol Cutan Rev 1945; 49:119.

Monheit GD. The Jessner's TCA peel: a medium depth chemical peel. J Dermatol Surg Oncol 1989; 15:945–950.

Morrow DM. Chemical peeling of the eyelids and periorbital area. J Dermatol Surg Oncol 1992; 18:102–110.

Roberts HL. The chloroacetic acids: a biochemical study. Br J Dermatol 1926; 38:323, 375.

Spinowitz AL, Rumsfield J. Stability-time profile of trichloroacetic acid at various concentrations and storage conditions. J Dermatol Surg Oncol 1989; 15:874–875.

Spira M, Gerow FJ, Hardy SB. Complications of chemical face peeling. Plast Recon Surg 1974; 54:397.

Stegman SJ. A comparative histologic study of the effects of three peeling agents and dermabrasion on normal and sun damaged skin. Aesth Plast Surg 1982; 6:123.

Stegman SJ. A study of dermabrasion and chemical peels in an animal model. J Dermatol Surg Oncol 1980; 6:490.

Stuzin JM, Baker TJ, Gordon HL. Chemical peel: a change in the routine. Ann Plast Surg 1989; 23:166–169.

Taylor MB. Letter to the editor–EMLA for effective pain relief following chemical peeling. Dermatol Surg 1995; 21:738–739.

Van Scott EJ, Yu RJ. Hyperkeratinization, comeocyte cohesion and alpha hydroxy acids. J Am Acad Dermatol 1984; 11:867.

Wang B, Carey WD. Chemical peeling as adjuvant therapy for facial neurotic excoriations. J Am Acad Dermatol 1994; 30(4):669–670.

Zelickson AS, Mottaz JH, Weiss JS, et al. Topical tretinoin in photo aging: an ultrastructural study. J Cut Aging Cosm Dermatol 1988; 1:41.

75

Hair Restoration

Dow B. Stough

*Department of Dermatology, University of Arkansas for Medical Sciences,
Little Rock, Arkansas, U.S.A.*

THE FOLLICULAR UNIT

The advent of follicular unit transplantation is credited to Bob Limmer in San Antonio, who, in the late 1980s, began using microscopes for creation of small one- to five-hair grafts inserted into needle slits. Limmer removed all excess non–hair-bearing tissue, which allowed for the natural hair groupings to be transplanted into 18-gauge needle sites. While improvements are still being made, most follicular unit transplants today are quite similar to Limmer's original technique. Around 1995, William Rassman documented the natural growth patterns of hair as seen through a hair densitometer. He stated that, "hairs grow in groups, most frequently in pairs, sometimes in groups of three, and more rarely in groups of four and five; understanding this architecture is critical, the incorporation of the patient's growing hair groups is to be exploited in the design of the restoration." In 1997, Robert Bernstein and Bill Rassman described their technique under the moniker "follicular unit transplantation," thus contributing the term "follicular unit" to the nomenclature.

Follicular unit "purists" insist that the term applies only to grafts containing hair in its natural groupings. In Caucasians, follicular unit grafts are often created utilizing microscopes for tissue dissection; in dark-haired races, this is not a necessity. While hair density following transplantation may occasionally be less than optimal, some surgeons feel strongly that the capacity for a (pure) follicular unit transplant to produce a natural result, coupled with the demonstrated advantages of stereomicroscopic subsection of donor tissue (related to low hair transection rates), make follicular unit transplantation a superior method of hair restoration. The latest development in the field involves the ability to produce a single session result utilizing only follicular unit grafts. David Seager, Victor Hasson, Jerry Wong and others have pioneered this work.

MEDICAL TREATMENT

Currently, there are only two medically proven treatments for hair loss; one being minoxidil and the other finasteride. Minoxidil exerts its effects on the cells of the hair follicle, although its precise mechanism of action in androgenetic alopecia and female-pattern alopecia is not known. Minoxidil is approved by the food and drug administration to regrow or stop hair loss. With continued use of the product, a patient would expect to produce longer, larger-caliber hairs. Common side effects of topical minoxidil include unwanted facial hair growth (especially disconcerting for women) and skin irritation or localized skin allergy to a component of the minoxidil solution. Rarely patients may complain of headache or chest pain.

The only oral medication indicated for use in the treatment of androgenetic alopecia is finasteride in a 1-mg/day dose (Propecia®). Finasteride is a specific inhibitor of Type II 5α-reductase, which is responsible for converting testosterone to dihydrotestosterone. Dihydrotestosterone causes for miniaturization of hair follicles seen with androgenetic alopecia.

The longest controlled clinical trial of a hair-loss treatment ever reported examined the effects of finasteride vs. placebo in men with androgenetic alopecia. Men who took finasteride had a considerable difference in hair counts after five years compared to men who took a placebo (Fig. A., *see color insert*; Fig. 1). This study showed that, following five years of treatment, the men on finasteride had an average of 277 more hairs in a 1 inch. diameter circle than those who received a placebo. The net benefit of treatment with finasteride compared to those men treated with placebo also increased each year. At the end of the five-year study, a panel rated 90% of men treated with finasteride as having no visible hair loss compared to baseline vs. 25% of men on placebo only.

Possible side effects include changes in sexual function that manifest in men as decreased libido, ejaculatory dysfunction, or erectile dysfunction. It should be noted that the incidence of these side effects is only slightly higher than the placebo, and less than 2% overall. All patients who discontinued finasteride had a resolution of the side effect, as did 58% of men who continued taking finasteride. Gynecomastia is also a side effect infrequently reported with finasteride administration. Finasteride is not indicated for use in women due to the potential for birth defects in the form of feminization of a male fetus.

The advantages of medical therapy are well established. Both minoxidil and finasteride are likely to slow or halt male-pattern hair loss in a given individual. For this reason, medical therapy should be considered in all patients with mild to moderate androgenetic alopecia. For patients who desire hair restoration surgery, medical therapy can stabilize their hair loss; therefore, necessitating less donor harvesting and also allowing the patient to maintain a more natural appearance

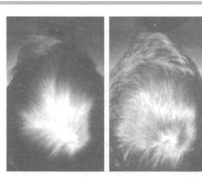

Figure 1 Before and after five years of treatment with Propecia® in patient with androgenetic alopecia. *Source*: Courtesy of Merck & Co., Inc.

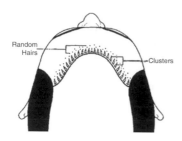

Figure 3 Microirregularities of frontal hairline: Clusters, gaps, and random single hairs are the most commonly used designs for the transition zone allowing the hairline to have a soft appearance and avoiding an abrupt hairline. *Source*: Rose, Parsley. Science of hair design. In: Hair Transplantation. Procedures in Cosmetic Dermatology. Haber, Stough (ed.). Elsevier, 2006.

in smaller sessions, or those in individuals with exceptionally dense hair, the asymmetric approach is utilized. After one session using this approach, the resulting scar will always be asymmetric and occupy a greater portion of the right or left side of the donor area. The strip width is kept narrow (ranging from 8 mm to 1.1 cm). In session two, the opposite side of the parietal scalp will become the initial point of harvesting. Some overlap of the initial scar, which will be located in the inferior portion, is expected. Using this approach, the patient is always left with a single scar because the original scar is removed. The resulting scar is minimal because the width of the donor strip has been significantly shortened by increasing the overall length of the strip. By decreasing the width and increasing the length, the resulting scar is minimal. In the past, many surgeons began by making a symmetrical incision occupying the entire occipital region with no harvesting into the parietal areas. When the prime occipital donor area becomes depleted, the surgeon was forced to take relatively small strips in the parietal areas. Such harvesting techniques are quite inefficient and proper preoperative planning will negate this need (Figs. C–E; *see color insert*).

With this technique, several precautions are necessary. The physician must first gauge the number of follicular units to be harvested. (This is covered elsewhere in the text). Then the physician must choose the strip width and length. The desired width of the strip in the mid occipital area may not be advisable in the posterior auricular zones and the parietal areas of the scalp. In these areas, a smaller width must be taken. It is important to keep the previous scar in the inferior portion of strip after session one.

When keeping the donor width between 8.0 mm and 1.1 cm, this approach will consistently yield a donor scar between 1 and 3 mm width. When donor width is repeatedly harvested in the central occiput between 1 to 1.1 cm, the resultant tension and stretch on the occipital area will frequently yield unacceptably wide donor scars.

Prior to surgery, 10 cc of 0.5% lidocaine with 1:200,000 epinephrine (adrenaline) is administered to the donor area, followed by 10 cc of naropin after excising the area.

The goal of donor strip removal is to minimize transection of hair follicles, during both the harvesting phase and the dissection phase. Using an elliptical incision with a double blade, one scores the surface of the scalp, being careful not to extend beyond 1 mm in depth. The double-blade knife can be used as a template to insure uniform width of the donor strip.

For donor strip dissection, four skin hooks are placed into a 2 mm depth incision. Tension is exerted away from the incision, and the blade being held parallel to the patient's hair follicle. The strip is then pulled apart, with minimal to no assistance, from the surgical scalpel blade. The strip of tissue is tapered into an elliptical pattern and cut from the base using scissors. Hemostasis is obtained with light cautery or, rarely, ligation with sutures. The preferred method of wound closure is with surgical staples (Fig. F; *see color insert*).

Graft Dissection

Once the donor tissue is harvested, the strip is immediately placed in a Petri dish containing chilled isotonic saline, where it is kept until dissection. Technicians subsection the elliptical donor tissue into slivers, each approximately 2 mm in width (Fig. 4). Considerable skill and experience is required to avoid transection during slivering (Fig. G; *see color insert*). Each sliver is further dissected into follicular unit grafts with a surgical razor blade or number 10 surgical blade using backlighting and microscopic magnification (Fig. 5). Grafts are observed and separated into one, two, three, or greater hairs per follicular unit (Fig. 6). These follicular unit grafts are placed back into chilled isotonic saline. It is imperative these grafts stay cool and moist in order for them to maintain viability. The benefits of hair in a complete nontransected state are controversial. There is evidence that transected hairs will grow, but these hairs have demonstrated a decreased diameter of growth.

Anesthesia

The recipient scalp is anesthetized in preparation for creating the incisions for graft placement. The author routinely performs a bilateral supraorbital nerve block, which produces anesthesia of the midfrontal portion of the scalp. The nerve blocks are achieved by infiltrating initially with buffered 0.5% lidocaine, followed by 0.2% ropivacaine Hcl.

Fifteen to thirty minutes before making the incisions, the area is injected with a saline and epinephrine mixture at a concentration of 1:80,000, approximately 10 ml of this mixture is used.

THE RECIPIENT SITE

Success in densely packing follicular units is dependent upon small recipient sites. This necessitates using a rectangular blade varying from 0.7 to 1.0 mm in size.

The density of placement varies from case to case due to existing recipient site hair, tissue characteristics, vascularity, and graft size. Angulation is defined as the angle of insertion

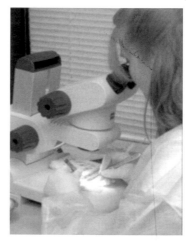

Figure 4 Dissection of silvers is best accomplished with the aid of a stereomicroscope.

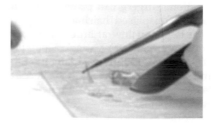

Figure 5 A single hair follicular unit graft produced under the stereomicroscope.

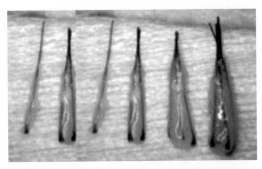

Figure 6 *left to right*: 1, 2, 3, and 4 hair follicular unit graft. *Source*: Parsley B. Terminology in hair transplant surgery. In: Hair Transplantation. Procedures in Cosmetic Dermatology. Haber, Stough (eds). Elsevier, 2006.

of the needle into the recipient scalp. A sharp angle of insertion, i.e., less than 20°, is favorable in the anterior hairline. Larger angles (20°–45°) can be used more posteriorly. Dense packing techniques require skillful graft creation and placement, which can only be achieved by experienced technicians (Fig. H; *see color insert*). One surgeon inserting all the grafts would be inefficient and offers no benefit to the patient. Thus, a rotating team of well-trained technicians is standard practice.

Insertion Phase

In the separated needle stick and graft placement technique, the surgeon has complete control of graft positioning. The surgeon dictates the spacing and angle by recipient site creation. The technicians then insert all the grafts. A modified approach is one in which the physician makes the site and the technician places the grafts. The technicians then simultaneously make additional sites as needed. This is a hybrid of the two methods and can routinely achieve over 30-grafts/cm² in recipient site density. Many surgeons routinely transplant over 2000 grafts per session.

Nuances

The most important factors for successful follicular unit transplantation are: the need for binocular stereoscopic microscope dissection, skillful atraumatic graft planting, and, above all, the need to keep the grafts completely moist. The latter is by far the most important factor influencing the success of follicular unit transplantation. Partial drying of grafts is the most common reason practitioners are unable to achieve adequate growth from follicular unit transplantation, despite otherwise immaculate technique. The authors advocate total immersion of grafts in saline and believe that drying of grafts even for brief periods (less than one minute) is detrimental to survival. Binocular stereoscopic microscopic dissection has become the standard for slivering an intact donor strip. Other methods without magnification can be used, but the transection rates are higher. Growth yield may be affected.

Postoperative

Immediately after hair restoration surgery, the surgeon should supply the patient with instructions on wound care and permissible activities. All grafts should be kept moist for at least 48 hours. The patients usually will need approximately three days of recovery before the redness and scabbing of the scalp resolve. Postoperative explanations are crucial and compliance is important to the ultimate outcome.

Ergonomics

There are practical difficulties, pertaining to staff, associated with large megasessions. In addition to the extra recruitment and training, there is the added problem of maintaining staff for the prolonged hours required during large graft sessions. Planting for many hours on a daily basis can and does lead to physical ailments, such as repetitive strain syndrome. To combat this, close attention must be paid to ergonomics. For instance, it is important that planters position their elbows or forearms on a firm, supportive surface while using wrist and finger movements. If the planters have to support the entire weight of their arms throughout their planting, they will often develop muscle fatigue in their neck, shoulders, and forearms. The staff should also rotate duties; that is, after a certain interval of planting they should do some other type of work, such as cutting grafts or administrative work, prior to returning to graft placement. They must have frequent relaxation breaks; and they must do regular stretching exercises at least every hour during their planting and cutting of grafts.

SUMMARY

One must remember that alopecia progression may impart a desire for further hair restoration procedures. Some of the most common observations that warrant subsequent treatments are recessions along the parietal and temporal scalp, which result in the isolation of transplanted hair. Careful planning and appropriate candidate selection produce results that withstand the test of time.

Follicular unit hair transplantation surgery, when performed with regard to future hair loss and the patient's own hair characteristics, offers patients an alternative that appears natural. It is important to note that many patients transplanted in the 1990s and 2000s have results that mimic nature so closely that their spouses, and even hair stylists are unaware a hair transplant procedure has been performed. The standard of hair restoration for the 2000s is to achieve this degree of naturalness in one or two sessions (Figs. 7–10; and I–L; *see color insert*).

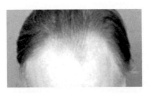

Figure 7 54-year-old Caucasian male prior to transplantation. (*See color insert*.)

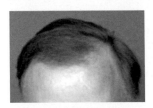

Figure 8 Patient in Fig. 12 after 1958 grafts. Note the softness of the feathering zone and the macro and microirregularities. Abrupt hairlines occur with follicular unit grafts if meticulous attention is not given to developing random irregularities into the frontal hairline. (*See color insert*.)

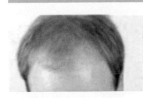

Figure 9 A 31-year-old Caucasian male prior to transplantation. (*See color insert*.)

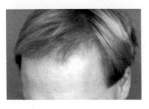

Figure 10 Patient in Fig. 14 after 2100 grafts; a soft irregular feathering zone of 1.5 centimeters was created along the anterior border. (*See color insert*.)

BIBLIOGRAPHY

General

Baden HP. Diseases of the Hair and Nails. London: Year Book Medical Publishers. 1987.

Brandy DA. A technique for hair-grafting in between existing follicles in patients with early pattern baldness. Dermatol Surg 2000; 26:801–805.

Camacho FM, Randall VA, Price VH. Hair and Its Disorders–Biology, Pathology and Management London: Martin Dunitz: 2000.

Cash TF. The psychosocial consequences of androgenetic alopecia: a review of the research literature. Br J Dermatol 1999; 141:398–405.

Cather JC, Lane D, Heaphy MR Jr., et al. Finasteride–an update and review. Dermatol Surg 1999; 64:167–171.

Commo S, Gaillard O, Bernard BA. The human hair follicle contains two distinct k19 positive compartments in the outer root sheath: a unifying hypothesis for stem cell reservoir? Differentiation 2000; 66:157–164.

Dawber R, Van Neste D. Hair and Scalp Disorders–Common Presenting Signs, Differential Diagnosis and Treatment. Philadelphia: Martin Dunitz. 1995.

Diani AR, Mulholland MJ, Shull KL, et al. Hair growth effects of oral administration of finasteride, a steroid 5α-reductase inhibitor, alone and in combination with topical minoxidil in the balding stumptail macaque. J Clin Endocrinol Metab 1992; 74:345–350.

Dzubow LM. A redefinition of male pattern baldness and its treatment. Yale University/Glaxo Dermatology Lectureship Series In Dermatology. 1995.

Guess HA, Gormley GJ, Stoner E, et al. The effect of finasteride on prostate specific antigen: review of data. J Urol 1996; 155:3–9.

Headington JT. Telogen effluvium: new concepts and review. Arch Dermatol 1993; 129:356–363.

Kaplan SA, Holtgrewe HL, Bruskewitz R, et al. Comparison of the efficacy and safety of finasteride in older versus younger men with benign prostatic hyperplasia. Urology 2001; 57:1073–1077.

Kaufman KD, et al. Finasteride in the treatment of men with androgenetic alopecia. J Am Acad Dermatol 1998; 39(4 Pt 1):578–589.

Limmer BL. Elliptical donor stereoscopically assisted micrografting as an approach to further refinement in hair transplantation. J Dermatol Surg Oncol 1994; 20:789–793.

Ludwig E. Classification of the types of androgenetic alopecia (common baldness) occurring in the female sex. Br J Dermatol 1977; 97:247–254.

Matzkin H, Barak M, Braf Z. Effect of finasteride on free and total serum prostate-specific antigen in men with benign prostatic hyperplasia. Br J Urol 1996; 78:405–408.

Norwood OT. Male pattern baldness: classification and incidence. South Med J 1975; 68:1359–1365.

Olsen EA, ed. Disorders of Hair Growth: diagnosis and treatment. New York: McGraw-Hill. 1993:257–283.

Orentreich DS. The history of hair restoration surgery. In: Stough DB, Haber, B (eds). Hair Restoration, Surgical and Medical. St Louis: Mosby. 1996:50–62.

Overstreet JW, Fuh VL, Gould, et al. Chronic treatment with finasteride daily does not affect spermatogenesis or semen production in young men. J Urol 1999; 162:1295–1300.

Price VH. Treatment of hair loss. N Engl J Med. 1999; 341:964–973.

Price VH, Menefee E. Quantitative estimation of hair growth I. Androgenetic alopecia in women: effect of minoxidil. J Invest Dermatol 1990; 5(6):683–687.

Price VH, Menefee E, Strauss PC. Changes in hair weight and hair count in men with androgenetic alopecia after application of 5% and 2% topical minoxidil, placebo, or no treatment. J Am Acad Dermatol 1999; 41(5 Pt 1):717–721.

Price VH, et al. Lack of efficacy of finasteride in postmenopausal women with androgenetic alopecia. J Am Acad Dermatol 2000; 43(5 Pt 1):768–776.

Roenigk RK, Roenigk HH Jr. Roenigk & Roenigk's Dermatologic Surgery, Principles and Practice. 2nd ed. New York: Marcel Dekker; 1996:1211–1212.

Rook A, Dawber R. Diseases of the Hair and Scalp. 2nd ed. Oxford: Blackwell Scientific Publications; 1991.

Staughton RCD. The Color Atlas of Hair and Scalp Disorders. London: Richard C.D. Staughton and Wolfe Publishing. 1988.

Stough D, Haber R. Hair Replacement–Surgical and Medical. Philadelphia: Mosby; 1996.

Rassman WR. Technique–small graft hair transplantation. In: Stough D, Haber R (eds). Hair Replacement–Surgical and Medical. St Louis: Mosby; 1996.

Stough D, Whitworth J. Methodology of follicular unit hair transplantation. Hair restoration and laser hair removal. Dermatol Clin 1999; 17(2):297–306.

Unger WP. Hair Transplantation. 3rd ed. New York: Marcel Dekker, 1995.

Unger WP. The history of hair transplantation. Hair Transplant Forum Intl 2000; 10:97–108.

Van Neste D, Fuh V, Sanchez-Pedreno P, et al. Finasteride increases anagen hair in men with androgenetic alopecia. Br J Dermatol 2000; 143:804–810.

Whiting DA. Chronic telogen effluvium: increased scalp hair shedding in middle-aged women. J Am Acad Dermatol 1996; 35:899–906.

Whiting DA. Diagnostic and predictive value of horizontal sections of scalp specimens in male pattern androgenetic alopecia. J Am Acad Dermatol 1993; 29:554.

Whiting DA, Howsden FL. Color Atlas of Differential Diagnosis of Hair Loss. London: Canfield Publishing; 1996.

Whitworth JM, Stough DB, et al. A comparison of graft implantation techniques for hair transplantation. Semin Cutan Med Surg 1999; 18(2):177–183.

Repair

Leavitt ML. Corrective hair restoration. In: Stough DB, Haber RS (eds). Hair Replacement–Surgical and Medical. St Louis: Mosby. 1996; 306–313.

Shiell R. Management of widened donor scars. Hair Transplant Forum International. 2002; 12:116.

Avram M. Management of widened donor scars. Hair Transplant Forum Intl 2002; 12:116.

Epstein E. Management of widened donor scars. Hair Transplant Forum Intl 2002; 12:116.

Kabaker S. Management of widened donor scars. Hair Transplant Forum Intl 2002; 12:116.

Puig C. Management of widened donor scars. Hair Transplant Forum Intl 2002; 12:116.

Mangubat T. Management of widened donor scars. Hair Transplant Forum Intl 2002; 12:116.

Swinehart J. Hair repair surgery. Derm Surg 1999; 25:523–529.

History

Okuda S. Clinical and experimental studies of transplantation of living hairs. Jpn J Dermatol 1929; 46:135–138.

Tamura H. Pubic hair transplantation. Jpn J Dermatol 1943; 53:76.

Unger WP. The history of hair transplantation. Dermatol Surg 2000; 26:181–189.

Orentreich N. Autografts in alopecias and other selected dermatological conditions. Ann NY Acad Sci 1959; 83:463.

Limmer BL. Elliptical donor harvesting. In: Stough DB and Haber RS (eds). Hair Restoration–Surgical and Medical. St Louis: Mosby; 1996.

Bernstein RM, Rassman WR. Follicular transplantation: patient evaluation and surgical planning. Dermatol Surg 1997; 23:771–784.

Bernstein RM, Rassman WR. The aesthetics of follicular transplantation. Dermatol Surg 1997; 23:785–799.

Unger WP. Commentary on: Follicular Transplantation by Bernstein and Rassman. Dermatol Surg 1997; 23:801–805.

Reed W. Rethinking some cornerstones of hair transplantation. Hair Transplant Forum Intl 1999; 9:133,138–139.

76

Treatment of Veins and Varicosities

Robert A. Weiss

Department of Dermatology, Johns Hopkins University School of Medicine, and MD Laser Skin and Vein Institute, Baltimore, Maryland, U.S.A.

INTRODUCTION

Minimally invasive methods for treatment of varicose and spider veins have advanced dramatically over the last few years. This revolution has provided dermatologic surgeons with a completely new array of techniques. These include endovenous vein occlusion methods using simple access to the vein lumen and sealing the vein with radiofrequency (RF) or various wavelengths of laser, each different in its benefits dependant upon the absorption characteristics. Other new methods include the use of agitation of sclerosing solution with air to create microbubble foam for larger veins and tributary veins of the saphenous system. Another new development is the use of glycerine as a sclerosing agent for telangiectasias to minimize matting and pigmentation. This chapter will discuss primary concepts and the use of these methods to treat both large and small varicose veins as well as accompanying telangiectasias.

PATHOPHYSIOLOGY

Vein size is not the most important indication of the association with symptoms. Surprisingly, isolated small reticular veins and telangiectasia often cause severe symptoms that are worsened by prolonged standing or sitting and may be relieved by wearing support hose or by elevation of the legs. Vessels causing symptoms may be as small as 1 mm in diameter or less. Women typically curb their activities and modify their lifestyles to avoid situations in which their legs are exposed. This is in addition to experiencing symptoms of pain, burning, and fatigue. Treatment, typically by sclerotherapy, not only offers the possibility of remarkably good cosmetic results, but also has been reported to yield an 85% reduction in symptoms. Successful treatment requires the correct technique, the correct diagnosis, and the correct treatment plan for the type and size of vein to be treated.

OVERVIEW AND TREATMENT PLAN

Treatment of varicose and telangiectatic veins follows a logical approach. Saphenous trunks leading to varicose veins are first eliminated by endovenous ablation techniques such as RF occlusion or endovenous laser, then branch varicosities are treated by ambulatory phlebectomy (AP) or foam sclerotherapy; finally related reticular veins and telangiectasias can be treated. It is important to understand that overall treatment proceeds from largest to smallest vessels. Success rates of sclerotherapy are generally high with 80% to 90% of vessels responding to a one to two treatments.

The anatomy of the venous system is akin to an upside-down tree. The trunk is in the thigh and the branches extend distally below. The main trunk veins are the great saphenous vein (GSV) in the medial thigh and the short saphenous vein (SSV) in the posterior calf. These are referred to as truncal veins in the literature and the primary varicose tributaries seen on the skin as branch varicosities. If valves fail in the saphenous system, this leads to pressure below and the formation of varicosities, reticular veins, and telangiectasias. It is important to be able to recognize high venous pressure originating from the saphenous system and it is imperative to treat these veins with an endovenous occlusion technique first. Most often medial leg varicosities or posterior calf varicosities are related to the saphenous system.

AP allows treatment of virtually all large truncal varicose veins; compression sclerotherapy can be used to treat large varicose veins, and reticular varicose veins. Once venous pressure is addressed, telangiectasias may either be treated with sclerotherapy or with intense pulsed light devices. In patients with isolated telangiectasia without pressure problems, sclerotherapy or laser/light therapy may be instituted primarily. In cases where an incompetent valve occurs at the main valve of the GSV at the junction of the femoral vein, the new endovenous occlusion techniques may be required. All these approaches may be performed in the office setting.

No matter how small and how localized the telangiectasia, every patient must initially be evaluated by detailed history and physical examination, with noninvasive diagnostic vascular tests performed as necessary. Once any reflux in the saphenous system has been identified and treated by endovenous techniques, then treatment of the smaller branch veins may begin.

Telangiectasia can also develop due to reflux from reticular veins, thin-walled blue superficial venules that are part of an extensive network of the lateral subdermic venous system; a system that is separate from the saphenous system. A typical network is shown in Figure 1. Reticular veins associated with telangiectasia are commonly called "feeder" veins. Both handheld Doppler and Duplex ultrasound has been used to demonstrate transmission of venous pressure from small reticular veins into telangiectasia.

High-pressure reflux through failed valves is at the root of nearly all telangiectatic webs, although there are some exceptions due to A–V malformations or shunts. This has been estimated to occur approximately 1 in 20 times, although it may be a high estimate. Typically, localized

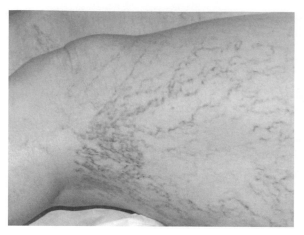

Figure 1 Typical telangiectatic web-reticular vein complex of the lateral subdermic venous system. This is not associated with saphenous reflux and requires no further work-up unless poor response to treatment is observed.

valve failure will produce arborizing networks of dilated cutaneous venules that are direct tributaries of underlying larger veins. Arborization occurs through a recruitment phenomenon in which high pressure causes dilatation of a venule, failure of its valves, and transmission of the high pressure across the failed valves into an adjacent vein. Treatment of an arborizing system must be directed at the entire system, because if the point source of reflux is not ablated, the web will rapidly recur.

Given the success rate of sclerotherapy and endovenous techniques, it is recommended that laser and light therapy be utilized only in certain situations. When a needle-phobic patient has only isolated telangiectasias, laser may be appropriate. Additionally, telangiectasias, which are too small to be injected or vessels, which remain after feeding vessels are treated or suspected arteriolar spider malformations should be considered for laser and light treatment. The most often utilized laser in our office is the 1064 nm Nd:YAG, utilized most often for telangiectasia unassociated with pressure arising from the saphenous system.

ENDOVENOUS TECHNIQUES

Endovenous Radiofrequency. The first procedure that was developed to replace stripping was the use of a specially designed bipolar RF catheter. RF energy can be delivered through a specially designed endovenous electrode to accomplish controlled heating of the vessel wall, causing vein shrinkage or occlusion by contraction of venous wall collagen. The mechanism by which RF current heats tissue is resistive (or ohmic) heating of a narrow rim (less than 1 mm) of tissue that is in direct contact with the electrode. Deeper tissue planes may be slowly heated by conduction from the small volume region of heating. This is part of the process, whereby heat is dissipated by conduction into surrounding tissue. By carefully regulating the degree of heating with microprocessor control, subtle gradations of either controlled collagen contraction or total thermocoagulation of the vein wall can be achieved.

When the RF catheter is pulled through the vein while feedback controlled with a thermocouple, the dermatologic surgeon can heat the section of vein wall to a specified temperature. This is a relatively safe process because the temperature increase remains localized around the active electrode provided that close, stable contact between the active electrode and the vessel wall is maintained. By limiting temperature to 85° to 90°C, boiling, vaporization, and carbonization of the tissues is avoided. With worldwide clinical experience on over 60,000 procedures since 1999, this technique has been a valuable addition to treating large varicose veins resulting from saphenous reflux.

Dermatologic surgeons are experts in the use of tumescent anesthesia for liposuction and were the first to apply tumescence to endovenous techniques as well as AP. Tumescent anesthesia or the placement of large volumes of dilute anesthesia in a perivascular position serves several purposes: (i) to protect perivascular tissues from the thermal effects of intravascular energy from RF or laser, (ii) to decrease the diameter of the treated vein to allow for better contact of the RF electrodes with the vein wall, (iii) to reduce vein diameter to have less risk of vein explosion from too much heating of blood during the endovenous laser procedures reducing bruising and pain, and (iv) provide more effective and safer anesthesia for patients.

Using tumescent anesthesia, saphenous veins can be sealed with endovenous techniques as a virtually painless procedure with little downtime and immediate ambulation. Having performed endovenous techniques over six years treating over 1000 saphenous veins using tumescent anesthesia, there are greatly reduced risks of side effects. The incidence of deep venous thrombosis (DVT) as measured by Duplex ultrasound follow-up at 3 to 14 days is 0%. Other side effects are also reduced. No skin injury has been observed using the tumescent anesthesia technique and the incidence of nerve injury presenting as focal anesthesia is virtually zero.

Endovenous Lasers

Shortly after the development of RF Closure™, endoluminal lasers were also demonstrated to be able to close truncal veins through thermal damage to endothelium with subsequent thrombosis and resorption of the damage vein. Endovenous laser treatment allows delivery of laser energy directly into the blood-filled vessel lumen, which heats the blood in order to produce adjacent endothelial and vein wall damage with subsequent fibrosis. The target for lasers with 810, 940, and 980 nm wavelengths is intravascular red blood cell absorption of laser energy. There must be some blood in the vein for these wavelengths to heat and this heat gets transmitted to the surrounding vein wall. Steam bubbles have been shown to occur within blood in the lumen as the primary mechanism for laser effects. Direct thermal effects on the vein wall without the presence of blood probably do not occur. The extent of thermal injury to tissue is strongly dependent on the amount and duration of heat the tissue is exposed to, which for these lasers are dependent on multiple factors include blood in the lumen, rate of pullback, and amount of tumescent anesthesia placed around the vein.

Patients treated with an 810 nm diode laser have shown an increase in posttreatment purpura and tenderness. Functional normality of leg movement is typically not seen for two to seven days as opposed to the one-day "down-time" with RF or 1320 nm endovenous treatment of the GSV. Recent studies suggest that pulsed 810 nm diode laser treatment with it's increased risk for perforation of the vein as opposed to continuous treatment, which does not have intermittent vein perforations, may be responsible for the increase symptoms with 810 nm laser versus RF treatment.

In an attempt to bypass the problems associated with laser wavelength absorption of hemoglobin a 1320 nm endoluminal laser was developed. At this wavelength, tissue water is the target and the presence or absence of red blood cells within the vessels is unimportant. The CoolTouch CTEV™ treatment is an endovenous ablation method using a special laser fiber coupled to the intraluminal use of an infrared 1320 nm wavelength with an automatic pullback device preset to pullback at 1 mm/sec (Fig. 2). This 1.32-micron wavelength is unique among endovenous ablation lasers in that this wavelength is absorbed only by water and not by hemoglobin. This makes it significantly different to the other (hemoglobin targeting) wavelengths used for endovenous laser treatments.

When using a wavelength strongly absorbed by hemoglobin, such as 810 nm, there is a lot of intraluminal blood heating with transmission of heat to the surrounding tissue through long heating times. Temperatures in animal models have been reported as high as 1200°C. When ex vivo vein treatment is performed without blood, the 810 nm wavelength simply chars the inside of the vein.

Our overall success with the different techniques is confirmed using duplex ultrasound to measure elimination of saphenous reflux. With the endoluminal RF techniques the success rates are 90% (five-year follow-up), with endoluminal 810 nm the long-term success is 80% (three-year follow-up), and with 1320 nm the success rate is 95% (two-year follow-up). Postoperative symptoms are markedly reduced with RF and 1320 nm (less than 5%), while postoperative pain and bruising are fairly high for 810 nm involving over 50% of patients.

AMBULATORY PHLEBECTOMY

AP is a surgical procedure attributed to Swiss dermatologist, Robert Muller. He first performed the technique in an office setting in Neuchâtel, Switzerland in the late 1950s as an alternative to hospital-based surgery and sclerotherapy. Acceptance of this technique was very slow. It became popular in the 1990s when reduced time to resolution and longer lasting resolution was realized. Importantly, new instruments became more widely available.

The decision to treat by AP versus sclerotherapy usually is determined by anatomic location, patient preference and estimated thickness of vein wall. Phlebectomy leads to good results except when significant reflux at the sapheno-femoral and sapheno-popliteal junctions is present. When reflux is present in the saphenous veins, then the endovenous techniques are used as in the section above.

AP also avoids possible complications of sclerotherapy for larger subcutaneous varicose veins including intra-arterial injection, superficial thrombophlebitis, skin necrosis, and months of hyperpigmentation. The recurrence rate of large varicose veins is also reduced, but only when the major source of reflux (if present) at the sapheno-femoral or sapheno-popliteal junctions is eliminated as well.

Instrumentation requirements are relatively simple. The Muller hook, available in four sizes, with a blunt tip, resembles a crochet hook, which elevates the vein from below. Oesch's hook, available in three sizes, is characterized by a massive squared off grip, and is designed with a small barb at the tip to pierce the vein from the lateral aspect and elevate. Ramelet's hook, available in two sizes, is a smaller, fine, sharp, hook, elevating the vein from above by lifting from adventitia.

Local anesthesia using a tumescent anesthesia technique requires a higher concentration than tumescent anesthesia for liposuction. Typically, 0.2% Lidocaine with 1:500,000 epinephrine in normal saline is prepared. Cutaneous incisions performed with number 11 scalpel blade or 18-gauge needle should be vertical along the thigh and lower leg and follow the skin lines at the knee or the ankle. The distance between the incisions varies from 2 to 15 cm, but is typically 3 to 4 cm. Once the AP hook is inserted into the puncture site, the targeted vein is gently dissected by undermining with the shaft of the phlebectomy hook. As the vein loop is exposed and pulled through the small incision, mosquito forceps are then used to clamp the vein loop. Traction is maintained by pulling as far as the vein slides easily. Too much tension will result in breakage.

Novices are warned to avoid the popliteal fossa, dorsum of the foot, peripatellar or pretibial region, and recurrent varicose veins after phlebitis or sclerotherapy. Hemostasis is achieved with intra- and postoperative local compression and by Trendelburg positioning of at least 10°. Venous ligation is not necessary as stretching of the vein causes rapid hemostasis most likely due to more exposed endothelial sites for platelet aggregation. Avoiding ligation eliminates all the additional complications of foreign material left just below the skin.

A typical session lasts 30 to 60 minutes with the major portion of a varicose vein extending from thigh to mid-calf. Occasionally, incision sites in the mid-thigh may stretch

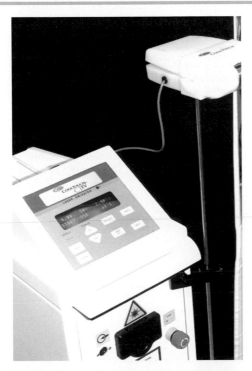

Figure 2 The 1320 nm endovenous treatment system with automatic pullback to insure uniform and predictable treatment results.

with removal of large truncal veins and may require one 5–0 suture. Postoperative pain seldom occurs due to long action of the tumescent anesthesia but some patients have reported a slight burning at the site of incisions during the first post-surgical night. Analgesia is easily achieved by acetaminophen. Immediate ambulation reduces risks of DVT to a negligible rate.

An elastic graduated compression stocking is also worn to obtain high resting pressure. The patient walks for 10 minutes in the office and the dressing is observed for any signs of bleeding. If the dressing remains dry, the patient may drive home without assistance as long as local anesthesia has not compromised motor function.

Surgical puncture sites are usually totally invisible after 3 to 6 months, but may persist much longer in younger patients with tighter skin. Hematomas rapidly disappear and pigmentation usually fades within two to three weeks. Long-term results are excellent as long as the source of venous reflux has been correctly eliminated.

FIRST SCLEROTHERAPY TREATMENT "TEST"

The first treatment session is usually limited to a small number of sites in order to observe the patient for any allergic reactions, ability to tolerate the burning or cramping of a hypertonic solution, judge the effectiveness of a particular concentration and class of sclerosing agent, and to observe the ability to comply with compression. It also serves to familiarize the patient with the treatment, treating physician, clinic surroundings and the sensation of the fine needle. This allows more extensive treatment on the second visit, with the patient being familiar with the technique and surroundings. The test site also complies with the suggestion in the package insert of sodium tetradecyl sulfate (STS) (Sotradecol™, Bioniche Pharma, Belleville, Ontario, Canada).

When the patient returns in four to eight weeks, the "test" site or limited treatment area is compared with pre-treatment photographs. Any side effects such as matting and pigmentation can be explained to the patient. Reasonable time intervals for clearance of treated vessels can be reinforced. At each session, all sites treated are noted in anatomic diagrams in the chart.

SCLEROTHERAPY TREATMENT OF RETICULAR VEINS

Reticular veins usually feed a group of telangiectasias on the lateral thigh from a varicose lateral subdermic venous system. During the treatment session, treatment would begin with reticular veins from which reflux is suspected to arise and would proceed along the course of the reticular vein, with injections every 3 to 4 cm along the feeder.

Our typical treatment regimen is to foam or agitate STS at 0.1% to 0.2% using a ratio of one part sclerosant to four parts air. This foam mixture is injected into reticular veins that are directly connected to visible telangiectasias (Fig. 3). It is not advisable to treat every reticular vein of the thigh; only those reticular veins visibly connected to a telangiectatic web should be targeted.

As sclerosing solution/foam flows away from the point of injection, it is clearly seen for a distance of several centimeters before it is diluted by blood and becomes less potent.

When injecting a reticular vein, the sclerosing foam is sometimes seen flowing into the telangiectasia. When this

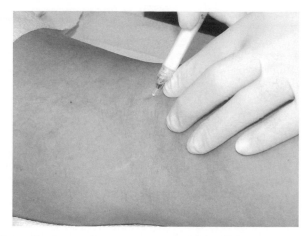

Figure 3 Foam mixture of sodium tetradecyl sulfate 0.1% comprised of liquid sclerosant agitated with air at a ratio of one part liquid to four parts air. Here the foam is seen injected into reticular veins.

is observed, the telangiectasias do not need to be injected directly. Similarly, sclerosing solution injected into a telangiectasia may be seen flowing into the feeder vein, but reticular veins usually still need to be injected directly, because it is difficult to deliver an effective volume and concentration of sclerosant foam to the reticular vein indirectly.

The technique used for injection of small reticular "feeder" veins is the direct cannulation technique used for the injection of larger, deeper reticular veins, and varicose veins.

The patient is recumbent in a position that allows convenient access to the reticular veins to be treated. A 3 cc syringe with a 27 or 30 gauge is used, and the needle is bent to an angle of 10° to 30° to facilitate cannulation (rather than transfixion) of the vein (Fig. 4). The syringe is held in the dominant hand, which rests on the patient's leg, and the needle is advanced at a shallow angle through the skin and into the reticular vein. When the physician feels the typical "pop-through" sensation of piercing the vein, the plunger is pulled back gently until blood return is seen in the transparent plastic hub. Typically one injects up to 2 cc of foamed sclerosant and then massages the solution toward

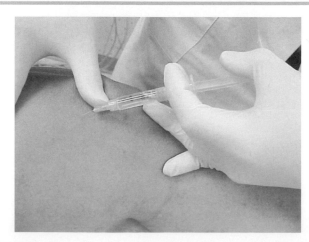

Figure 4 The position of the syringe with needle bend in the hands of the injecting physician for injecting reticular veins.

any associated telangiectasias. Injection must stop immediately if any signs of leakage occur or if a bleb or bruising is noted. As the needle is withdrawn, pressure is applied immediately either with cotton ball then tape or compression bandaging.

The cannulation of a reticular vein can be quite difficult at times, because reticular veins can go into spasm, and may virtually disappear during an attempt at cannulation. It is best to avoid applying alcohol to the skin just prior to treatment as the evaporative cooling may cause venospasm of the reticular vein. Any resistance to injection means the needle tip is not inside the vein. When this happens, the injection should be terminated immediately and the needle withdrawn. Failed cannulation will rapidly produce a bruise at the site of injection.

With use of STS, it is recommended to use latex free syringes. In high enough concentration STS (0.5% and above) will dissolve the rubber from the plunger thereby releasing rubber and rubber products into solution. There is a relatively high and increasing incidence of latex allergy in the general population. Theoretically the risk of a severe allergic reaction may be increased with latex containing syringes. We have not yet seen allergic reactions to STS in over 500,000 injections since switching to latex free syringes in 1994.

SCLEROTHERAPY TREATMENT OF TELANGIECTASIA

The patient is recumbent in a position that allows convenient access to the telangiectasias to be treated. If available, a motorized table with height adjustment will facilitate easy access to all regions of the leg. Use of double

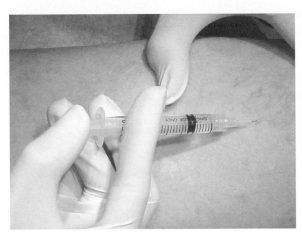

Figure 6 Position of hand during injection of telangiectasias.

polarized lighting (InVu Vantage, Syris Scientific, Grey, ME) has also proven to be helpful (Fig. 5). The neck and back position of the treating physician must be optimal to avoid injury over the long term to the physician. Indirect lighting is best as harsh halogen surgical lights bleach out reticular veins and some telangiectasias.

A syringe of sclerosant is prepared with a 30-gauge needle that has been bent to an angle of 10° to 30° with the bevel up. The needle is placed flat on the skin so that the needle is parallel to the skin surface. The usual position is indicated in Figure 4. The nondominant hand plays an important role in stabilization of the syringe. The injecting hand rests on the patient's leg with the fourth and fifth finger providing stabilization in a fixed position to facilitate controlled penetration of the vessel. The nondominant hand is used to stretch the skin around the needle and may offer additional support for the syringe. The firmly supported needle is then moved slowly 1 to 2 mm forward, piercing the top of the tiny vein just sufficiently to allow infusion of solution with the most minimal pressure on the plunger.

The technique requires a gentle, precise touch, but with practice the beveled tip of the 30-gauge (0.3 mm diameter) needle may be used to cannulate vessels as small as 0.1 mm. The bevel of the needle usually can be seen within the lumen of the telangiectasias with use of 1.75 to 2× magnification. Needles smaller than 30 gauge or longer than $\frac{1}{2}$ inch are difficult to use because they tend to veer off course when advanced through the skin. Depending on the patient's skin type, needles can become dull rather quickly, and should be replaced whenever resistance to skin puncture is noted. This typically occurs within 3 to 10 punctures.

Concentrations of sclerosants used for telangiectasias are less than those used for reticular veins. Typically the solutions are not foamed. We now prefer to use 72% glycerine for the telangiectasias of a telangiectatic web-reticular vein complex (Table 1). When sclerosing solutions are injected into telangiectasia, blood is usually flushed out of the vessel ahead of the solution, thus the sclerosant usually is not diluted at all. For this reason, the initial treatment of telangiectatic webs begins with the minimal effective concentration of sclerosant. At the next visit, the same concentration is used if sclerosis is effective, and a higher concentration is used if sclerosis is ineffective.

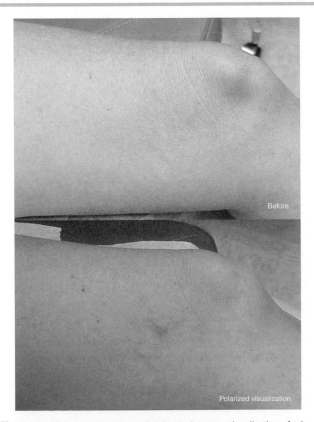

Figure 5 Use of cross polarized lighting to increase visualization of telangiectasias. (*See color insert.*)

Table 1   Sclerosant Concentrations

Varicose branch	0.5%	1.0%	Yes	Sodium tetradecyl sulfate (STS)
Reticular 3–5 mm	0.2%	0.5%	Yes	STS
Reticular 1–3 mm	0.1%	0.25%	Yes	STS
Telangiectasias 0.2–1 mm	0.2%	0.5%	No	Polidocanol (Laureth-9)
Telangiectasias 0.2–1 mm	0.1%	0.2%	No	STS
Telangiectasias 0.2–1 mm	72% in water	Same	No	Glycerine 72%
Telangiectasias 0.2–1 mm	10% hypertonic saline and 25% dextrose	Same	No	Sclerodex™

Abbreviation: STS, sodium tetradecyl sulphate.

The injection of telangiectasias is performed very slowly, with minimal pressure on the syringe. A few drops of sclerosant are sufficient to fill the vein and maintain contact with the vessel wall for 10 to 15 seconds. The amount infused is approximately 0.1 to 0.2 cc per site, and this often is sufficient to produce blanching in a radius of 2 cm from the site of injection. Rapid flushing of the vessels with larger volumes of sclerosant or with higher pressures leads to problems with extravasation, tissue necrosis, and ulceration, as well as an increased incidence of telangiectatic matting and of hyperpigmentation.

For glycerine injection, the telangiectasia are filled with solution and the injection is stopped. Glycerine has the least risk of causing subsequent matting or pigmentation. When detergent sclerosants are used, small volumes and small areas of short-duration blanching are still important to minimize side effects such as telangiectatic matting. Sometimes, there is no blanching at the site of injection, but the sclerosing solution flows easily through the telangiectasia or can even be seen flowing through adjacent telangiectasias or reticular veins several centimeters away from the injection site. In this case the injection is stopped after no more than 0.5 cc of sclerosant has been injected. Immediately after injection, the treated area is gently massaged in the desired direction of further spread of sclerosant. We strongly recommend against the use of hypertonic saline as it is painful and highly ulcerogenic.

To minimize skin necrosis, extravasation must be avoided, although the risks are minimized with glycerine or very low doses of liquid 0.1% STS. If there is resistance to the flow of sclerosant, or if a "bleb" begins to form at the injection site, the injection must be stopped immediately. Extravasation of low concentrations of polidocanol does not cause tissue necrosis, but significant extravasation of higher concentration (greater than 0.1%) STS or of hypertonic saline will cause necrosis and ulceration. A randomized study in animals found the incidence of ulceration to be greater when attempts were made to dilute the extravasated sclerosant by the injection of normal saline into the area. Vigorous massage of any blebs is recommended to minimize the chance of necrosis. Application of 2% nitroglycerine paste, if bone white blanching is observed, is applied to cause immediate vasodilatation and minimize risks of small areas of necrosis.

COMPRESSION

Compression will speed vessel clearance and reduce staining from any vessel that protrudes above the surface of the skin. After treatment of telangiectasias, compression is provided by ready-to-wear gradient compression hose (15–20 mm Hg) placed over cotton balls secured with tape at the sites of injection. If larger reticular veins (greater than 3 mm) are treated at the same session then compression consists of Class I 20–30 mm Hg compression. Some authorities recommend that continuous compression be applied for as long as the patient will tolerate it (usually one to three days). Then the stockings are removed and the cotton balls discarded; the patient bathes and reapplies the stockings, wearing them for the next two weeks except when bathing and sleeping. We have the patient remove both stockings and cotton balls at bedtime of the day of treatment. Compression hose are then worn daily for two weeks except when bathing and sleeping. Patients are encouraged to walk, and the only restrictions on activity are those such as heavy weightlifting that result in sustained forceful muscular contraction and venous pressure elevation.

TREATMENT INTERVALS

Physician and patient preferences play a large role in determining treatment intervals. New areas may be treated at any time, but retreatment of the same areas should be deferred for 6 to 12 weeks, because the immediate posttreatment appearance of telangiectasias is either bruising, matting, or pigmentation and this will ultimately clear after two to four weeks. Patients often are anxious to speed their course of treatment, but allowing a longer time between treatment sessions may minimize the number of sessions needed. We strongly recommend waiting as long as four to eight weeks between treatments.

After the initial series of treatments, a "rest" period of four to six months will allow time for pigmentation and matting to clear, and for any remaining reticular veins to establish "new" routes of reflux or drainage. Approximately 80% of patients will clear to their satisfaction during the first course of treatment. Any remaining telangiectatic webs or new telangiectasias are then reassessed to determine the best approach for another round of treatment.

POOR RESPONSE TO TREATMENT

When patients have had a poor response to the initial series of treatments, the original diagnosis must always be called into question. Unsuspected sources of reflux can include truncal varices, incompetent perforating veins, and unrecognized reticular vessels. If no untreated source of reflux can be identified, the patient must be carefully questioned about proper compliance with compression. Many patients abandon compression immediately after sclerotherapy, and this can lead to treatment failures. The concentration and volume of sclerosant used should also be reexamined. It is not uncommon to find that the concentrations selected were ineffective for the size and type of vessel being treated.

SUMMARY

When based upon a correct diagnosis and an appropriate treatment plan, treatment of varicose and spider veins is highly effective. Formulating an effective treatment plan requires a detailed knowledge of venous anatomy and all the techniques used in phlebology. This is accompanied by a thorough understanding of the principles and patterns of reflux, and intimate familiarity with a range of volumes and concentrations of sclerosing solutions as well as endovenous techniques and AP.

Treatment of varicose and telangiectatic veins follows a logical approach, which proceeds largest and most proximal to smallest and most distal vessels. Saphenous trunks leading to varicose veins are first eliminated by endovenous ablation techniques such as RF occlusion or endovenous laser, then branch varicosities are treated by AP or foam sclerotherapy; finally related reticular veins and telangiectasias are treated. Isolated telangiectasias can be treated by percutaneous lasers. The results obtained depend greatly on the experience of the clinician, but with care and with attention to detail, clearing rates of 90% can be achieved in most patients. Sufficient time must be allowed between treatments to allow gradual clearing so that excessive number of treatments is avoided.

BIBLIOGRAPHY

Bihari I, Muranyi A, Bihari P. Laser-doppler examination shows high flow in some common telangiectasias of the lower limb. Dermatol Surg 2005; 31(4):388–390.

Cheng L, Lee D. Review of latex allergy. J Am Board Fam Pract 1999; 12(4):285–292.

Duffy DM. Small vessel sclerotherapy: an overview. Adv Dermatol 1988; 3:221–242.

Georgiev M. Postsclerotherapy hyperpigmentations. Chromated glycerin as a screen for patients at risk (a retrospective study). J Dermatol Surg Oncol 1993; 19:649–652.

Goldman MP, Amiry S. Closure of the greater saphenous vein with endoluminal radiofrequency thermal heating of the vein wall in combination with ambulatory phlebectomy: 50 patients with more than 6-month follow-up. Dermatol Surg 2002; 28(1):29–31.

Goldman MP, Weiss RA, Bergan JJ. Diagnosis and treatment of varicose veins - a review [review]. J Am Acad Dermatol 1994; 31(3 Pt 1):393–413.

Haines DE. The biophysics of radiofrequency catheter ablation in the heart: the importance of temperature monitoring. Pacing Clin Electrophysiol 1993; 16(3 Pt 2):586–591.

Haines DE, Verow AF. Observations on electrode-tissue interface temperature and effect on electrical impedance during radiofrequency ablation of ventricular myocardium. Circulation 1990; 82(3):1034–1038.

Martin DE, Goldman MP. A comparison of sclerosing agents: clinical and histologic effects of intravascular sodium tetradecyl sulfate and chromated glycerin in the dorsal rabbit ear vein. J Dermatol Surg Oncol 1990; 16:18–22.

Muller R. [Ambulatory phlebectomy]. Ther Umsch 1992; 49: 447–450.

Muller R. Traitement des varices par la phlebectomie ambulatoire. Bull Soc Franc Phlebologie 1966; 19:277–279.

Proebstle TM, Sandhofer M, Kargl A, Gul D, Rother W, Knop J, et al. Thermal damage of the inner vein wall during endovenous laser treatment: key role of energy absorption by intravascular blood. Dermatol Surg 2002; 28(7):596–600.

Ramelet AA. La phlebectomie ambulatoire selon Mueller: technique, avantages, desavantages. J Mal Vasc 1991; 16: 119–122.

Ramelet AA. Le Traitement Des Telangiectasies: Indications De La Phlebectomie Selon Muller. Phlébologie 1995; 47(4):377–381.

Ramelet AA. Muller phlebectomy. A new phlebectomy hook. J Dermatol Surg Oncol 1991; 17:814–816.

Sadick NS. Sclerotherapy of varicose and telangiectatic leg veins. Minimal sclerosant concentration of hypertonic saline and its relationship to vessel diameter [see comments]. J Dermatol Surg Oncol 1991; 17(1):65–70.

Smith SR, Goldman MP. Tumescent anesthesia in ambulatory phlebectomy. Dermatol Surg 1998; 24(4):453–456.

Somjen GM, Ziegenbein R, Johnston AH, Royle JP. Anatomical examination of leg telangiectases with duplex scanning [see comments]. J Dermatol Surg Oncol 1993; 19(10):940–945.

Weiss RA. Comparison of endovenous radiofrequency versus 810 nm diode laser occlusion of large veins in an animal model. Dermatol Surg 2002; 28(1):56–61.

Weiss MA, Weiss RA. Efficacy and side effects of 0.1% sodium tetradecyl sulfate in compression scleortherapy of telangiectasias: comparison to 1% polidocanol and hypertonic saline [abstr]. J Dermatol Surg Oncol 1991; 17:90–91.

Weiss RA, Weiss MA. Controlled radiofrequency endovenous occlusion using a unique radiofrequency catheter under duplex guidance to eliminate saphenous varicose vein reflux: a 2-year follow-up. Dermatol Surg 2002; 28(1):38–42.

Weiss RA, Weiss MA. Doppler ultrasound findings in reticular veins of the thigh subdermic lateral venous system and implications for sclerotherapy. J Dermatol Surg Oncol 1993; 19(10):947–951.

Weiss RA, Weiss MA. Incidence of side effects in the treatment of telangiectasias by compression sclerotherapy: hypertonic saline vs. polidocanol. J Dermatol Surg Oncol 1990; 16:800–804.

Weiss RA, Weiss MA. Resolution of pain associated with varicose and telangiectatic leg veins after compression sclerotherapy. J Dermatol Surg Oncol 1990; 16:333–336.

Weiss RA, Feied CF, Weiss MA. In: Vein Diagnosis and Treatment: A Comprehensive Approach. New York: McGraw-Hill, 2001.

Weiss RA, Goldman MP. Advances in sclerotherapy. Dermatol Clin 1995; 13(2):431–445.

Weiss RA, Heagle CR, Raymond-Martimbeau P. The Bulletin of the North American Society of Phlebology. Insurance Advisory Committee Report. J Dermatol Surg Oncol 1992; 18:609–616.

Zimmet SE. The prevention of cutaneous necrosis following extravasation of hypertonic saline and sodium tetradecyl sulfate. J Dermatol Surg Oncol 1993; 19:641–646.

77

Liposuction and Fat Transfer

Rhoda S. Narins

Dermatology Surgery and Laser Center of New York, White Plains, New York and Department of Dermatology, New York University Medical Center, New York, New York, U.S.A.

Paul H. Bowman

The Bowman Institute for Dermatologic Surgery, Tampa, Florida, U.S.A.

INTRODUCTION

For centuries, physicians and surgeons have sought after ways to alter body contour. The modern phase of fat removal for contour change began in the late 1970s when Fischer and Fischer reported on their use of a sharp, hollow aspiration tube to extract subcutaneous fat, the forerunner of liposuction. Illouz modified the technique by designing a blunt cannula, and preoperatively injecting hypotonic saline into the tissues to be removed (wet technique). These changes greatly decreased perioperative bleeding, and allowed preservation of adipose septae in which vessels, lymph channels, and nerves survived.

The next significant advance was in 1986 to 1987, when Klein introduced the tumescent technique of anesthesia, directly infiltrating the target fatty tissue with large volumes of dilute anesthetic solution consisting of lidocaine, epinephrine, and sodium bicarbonate in physiologic saline, enabling the procedure to be performed using local anesthesia alone. This change has revolutionized how liposuction surgery is performed by further decreasing blood loss, avoiding complications associated with general anesthesia, minimizing postoperative pain and shortening recovery time. In addition, performing the procedure with an awake, interactive patient who can move into different positions decreases the incidence of complications such as diaphragmatic and abdominal perforation, thrombophlebitis and subsequent pulmonary embolus, and also enables the surgeon to remove tissue more precisely with uniformity for superior results.

Further advances in cannula design, anesthetic solution administration, extraction technique, and postoperative care continue to improve the procedure of tumescent liposuction. Due to Occupational Safety and Health Administration (OSHA) standards, disposable tubing and canisters and viral filters have been developed. Smaller incision areas, direct crisscross approaches to the removal of fat, using larger cannulas in deep areas and tiny cannulas in superficial areas to avoid rippling have contributed to the evolution of "liposculpture." Power and ultrasonic liposculpture have evolved as adjunctive techniques.

Liposuction surgery can be useful in many different body sites. The lateral cheeks, jowls, and upper neck are common areas for liposuction that respond beautifully in both men and women. The most common body areas in younger women are lateral thighs, with or without the hips and buttocks, and in older women the abdomen. In addition, the waist, back, breast, inner and anterior thigh, arms, calf, and ankle fat can be treated. Circumferential liposuction is excellent for the abdominal area in patients where the waist, lower back, and hips are treated at the same time as the abdomen for a more youthful, hourglass shape. The most common body areas in men are the flanks and the abdomen. Gynecomastia and pseudogynecomastia can be treated in males. Disorders such as lipomas, buffalo humps, lipodystrophy, and axillary hyperhidrosis can also be treated.

Fat accumulation in different anatomic sites occurs for a variety of reasons. Some are considered evolutionary caloric storehouses, others facial and genetic configurations, and still others hormonally controlled. Removing such tissues safely and with excellent cosmetic results is easily attainable by appropriately trained liposuction surgeons. Guidelines for liposuction surgery have been written by the American Academy of Dermatology and the American Society for Dermatologic Surgery.

PATIENT SELECTION AND RISK MANAGEMENT

Appropriate patient selection and adequate preoperative evaluation and planning are paramount to achieving optimal cosmetic results and avoiding complications. The preoperative consultation is perhaps the most important part of the procedure, because identifying patients that ought to do well versus those that won't goes a long way toward achieving "good" outcomes and avoiding complications and dissatisfied patients. A good consent form and operative flow sheet are also extremely important when dealing with risk management. Liposuction is appropriate for any individual, with an indication for the procedure, who can tolerate the pre-, intra-, and postoperative stresses and risks, and who accepts realistic limitations.

Preoperative photographs are mandatory, and patients refusing these should be categorically denied any intervention. Pre- and postoperative photographs of other patients with "good" results can be reviewed with the patient, to ensure they have realistic expectations. The necessity for possible "touch-up" procedures should also be mentioned, the charge for such being each surgeon's decision. Inquiring about past experiences with liposuction and other cosmetic procedures is also a good idea—what was their experience like? Were there any complications?

Were they pleased with the results? Patients must be told that this is not a procedure to correct obesity, striae, spider veins, skin turgor, or cellulite. This is a contouring procedure. Deformities and unusual prominence of anatomic bony structures must be evaluated and discussed with the patient.

A complete medical history, including a history of bleeding, medication, allergies, etc., should also be taken to identify any contraindications or risks. All medical problems must be evaluated individually. Any patient taking significant systemic medications should consider evaluation by his or her family physician prior to the procedure.

Once it has been determined that the patient is a good candidate for liposuction surgery by evaluation of his or her objectives and the realistic goals that can be achieved from the examination of fat and skin turgor, then possible complications and other risks are discussed with the patient. If the patient decides to proceed with the procedure, a photograph is taken; blood pressure, urine, and blood tests, including a CBC, SMAC, PT, PTT, Hep-C surface antibodies, Hep-B surface antigen, and HIV tests, are obtained. Preoperative directions are discussed, including avoidance of all salicylates and nonsteroidal anti-inflammatories two weeks prior to surgery. Forms are given to the patient with extensive preoperative and postoperative instructions. Patients undergoing tumescent liposuction procedures require no general anesthesia, but may receive some type of intramuscular (IM) and/or oral (PO) sedation, along with local tumescent anesthesia. The surgeon should evaluate the patient's desire for such sedation, as well as any evidence of anxiety on the day of consultation to make this decision.

Most patients are extremely realistic about the results that they can achieve. If they are already nearly perfect, you can give them a perfect contour, but most patients, especially those who are older and who have had children and whose skin is somewhat loose, will find that liposuction surgery gives extremely gratifying results with very little scarring or morbidity but will not make them look like 18 again. Most patients are happy to look better in clothing and have a nicer contour.

EQUIPMENT
Cannulas

Many different cannulas are now available, and it is important to choose the appropriate size and style for different applications. Multiple cannulas are used on every patient, and are chosen by the anatomic location to be addressed, the amount of fat in the area, the fibrousness of the tissue, the depth of the fat to be removed, and the experience of the surgeon. Cannula shafts vary by length, curvature, and diameter, with the "size" decreasing as the diameter increases (such as needle gauge sizes). The original Illouz cannulas were blunt and went up to size 10, which looks enormous by today's standards. Large cannulas (even up to size four) are still used occasionally when there is a great amount of deep adipose tissue to be removed. Larger cannulas are meant to stay deep in the fatty tissue, away from the overlying dermis, so as not to get rippling on the surface of the skin. Tiny microcannulas have now been developed for use in superficial tissues, allowing very precise removal of small amounts of fat (liposculpture).

The number, shape, size, and placement of apertures along the cannula most directly determine the cannula's effect on tissue. An "aggressive" cannula is one with many large (compared to the diameter of the shaft) holes placed close to the tip, as it will most effectively remove fat with the fewest number of passes. They are also more likely to cause bleeding and tissue trauma. Examples are the Cobra, Pinto, and Accelerator cannulas. Less aggressive cannulas, with fewer, smaller apertures located further from the tip are more forgiving, requiring more passes to remove the same amount of fat, and are best for less experienced liposuction surgeons. These include the Klein, Fournier, standard, and spatula cannulas. These safer cannulas also tend to avoid apertures on the dorsal surface of the shaft, in order to avoid possible trauma to the overlying dermis. As one gain more experience, more aggressive tips can be used to remove fat more quickly.

The size and type of grasping handle on the proximal end of the cannula—round or angled, large or small, smooth or textured—is a matter of individual preference and comfort. The handle also usually provides some means of identifying the orientation of the cannula tip, so the surgeon does not unknowingly turn the ventral surface upward and damage the dermis with resultant scarring. Not all manufacturers use the same handle/tubing diameters, so if varied combinations are desired, graded attachments may be required to allow adaptation of varying manufacturers' diameters. Single handles with interchangeable tips are also available, some of which are adaptable for fat transplantation.

Aspiration Pump and Tubing

A variety of manufacturers in several countries now produce aspiration pumps that develop negative air pressures approaching 30 in. (1 atm) negative pressure. This reference point is sought by the instrument makers, but adequate suction for some areas may be obtained with readings as low as 15 to 18 in. Today's canisters are either disposable as a unit or come with removable/disposable bags. The tubing is also disposable, and a viral filter is used and changed according to direction. Dr. Pierre Fournier has developed a syringe technique and can aspirate thousands of cubic centimeters by hand without using a pump at all.

Pulse Oximeter

A pulse oximeter is a useful adjunct to measure the oxygen saturation as toxicity to lidocaine is related to decreased oxygen saturation. Another advantage of working with conscious patients is that the surgeon can simply ask them to take a deep breath if oxygen saturation decreases.

ANESTHESIA

Presently, the available anesthesia techniques for liposuction are the rarely used "dry" technique using general anesthesia without preinfiltration of any vasoconstrictive solution, the "wet" technique using general anesthesia and preinfiltration with a low volume of vasoconstrictive solution, which is fairly commonly used, especially by plastic surgeons, the addition of tumescent anesthetic solution to general or intravenous (IV) anesthesia, again a technique used mostly by plastic surgeons who understand the benefits of high-volume tumescent anesthesia, and the true tumescent technique of local anesthesia alone, with no general anesthesia and the preinfiltration of a high volume of low-dosage lidocaine/epinephrine anesthetic solution.

The advantages of the true tumescent technique include (i) the decreased incidence of bleeding and subsequent transfusions, (ii) no need for IV fluids because the large volume of anesthetic solution itself provides volume replacement, (iii) effective and long-lasting anesthetic effect, such that often no other pain medication is required in small treatment areas, and (iv) increased safety to the patient because the risks of general anesthesia are avoided. Because the surgery can be performed with the patient awake, able to report discomfort, and move into different positions during the procedure, other advantages include (i) decreased likelihood of perforation into the thoracic or abdominal cavities, (ii) decreased likelihood of deep venous thrombosis and subsequent pulmonary embolus, (iii) more precise and complete treatment of difficult to reach anatomic sites, and (iv) faster recovery postoperatively. The tumescent technique, described herein, is used mostly by dermatologic surgeons and has essentially revolutionized the liposuction process to become the current state of the art for this procedure.

The hallmark of the tumescent technique of local anesthesia is the concentration of lidocaine, which is usually 0.05%, 0.075%, or 0.1%, and the concentration of epinephrine, which is usually 1/1,000,000. The formulas for these are given in Table 1. For smaller volumes, a 250 mL bag of saline can be prepared rather than the 1000 mL bag by dividing the recipe appropriately. The total safe concentration of lidocaine is based on the published figure of 55 mg/kg. Thus, if a patient weighs 150 lb, (divided by 2.2, to equal 68 kg), multiply 68 kg by 55 mg/kg to arrive at a safe limit of 3740 mg of lidocaine. A 1000 cc bag of 0.1% lidocaine anesthetic solution has 1000 mg of lidocaine and a 1000 cc bag of 0.05% lidocaine anesthetic solution has 500 mg of lidocaine. This 68 kg patient can, therefore, use approximately 3 3/4 bags of 0.1% solution or seven bags of 0.05% solution to stay under the safe limit of 3740 mg of lidocaine. If greater amounts of fluid are necessary for the surgery (a large number of treatment areas), then the 0.05% solution can be used. Indeed, any mixture of solutions that totals 3740 mg of lidocaine is acceptable in a patient who weighs 150 lb. The preceding calculations and formulas can easily be extrapolated to determine the "safe" amount and concentration that can be utilized in any given patient. In very sensitive areas like the abdomen, buttock, inner thighs, and knees, one should try to use the 0.1% solution. If many areas are being treated and one needs to conserve anesthesia, then use the 0.5% lidocaine in the less sensitive areas such as the lateral thigh, arms, neck, etc.

In the tumescent technique, the anesthesia is delivered in a three-step procedure, wherein the incision sites (through which the cannulas are inserted) are first injected with a small amount of local anesthetic using a syringe and a 30-gauge needle. The second stage is the delivery of a small amount of the anesthetic solution through a spinal needle radially through these incision sites, fanning out to achieve a preliminary anesthesia. This preliminary anesthetic can be pushed in with a pressure cuff around a bag of saline or by the use of an infiltration pump on a low setting. For large areas, many of us have progressed from

60 cc syringes attached to a three-way stopcock to the Klein infiltrator to using a pressure cuff around the bag of anesthesia to an electric infiltration pump. Although each gives the desired results, the easiest to use is the electric pump. These machines were first developed in the 1990s and make the administration of anesthesia much more simple. Finally, the anesthetic solution is delivered through an infiltration cannula with multiple openings ("showerhead" cannula). During this final step, the infiltration pump is increased to higher settings and the tissue is infiltrated ("tumesced") until firm (*L. tumidus*, swollen). The solution is injected along deep and intermediate levels in order to attain full effect. After the target tissue has been tumesced, it is necessary to wait 30 minutes or so for the full vasoconstricting effect of the epinephrine solution to occur.

In addition to the infiltrated anesthetic solution, some patients may require additional analgesics, anxiolytics, or sedatives. While nonanxious patients and those having small areas (such as the neck, knees, lipomas, etc.) treated may require nothing at all, others usually do very well with PO diazepam, IM meperidine, promethazine, and/or midazolam. Various combinations of these agents are used by dermatologic liposuction surgeons, while surgeons in other specialties may use other methods (general anesthesia, epidural, or IV sedation, especially when the procedure is performed in a hospital, or with a nurse anesthetist or anesthesiologist present).

PREOPERATIVE PROCEDURE

Having bathed with an antiseptic antimicrobial skin cleanser for seven days preoperatively, the patient reports to the office wearing loose-fitting clothing that can be easily removed. The patient washes his or her hair that morning and is given postoperative support garments by the nurse.

It is important to weigh the patient before the procedure. If the patient gains weight after the surgery, it will be distributed over the body and not accumulate in the surgical area. However, some fat will accumulate there and may appear to make the surgical results less significant. As previously stressed, it is also extremely important to take preoperative photographs of the patient (usually front, back, and side views) to compare to postoperative visits. Preoperative photographs can also be referred to during the liposuction procedure.

Once the patient is weighed and photographed, the areas to be treated are marked using an indelible marking pen. Several systems of marking have evolved, and each surgeon will adopt what is most comfortable for them. Some mark bony prominences and preexisting soft-tissue depressions (to avoid making them more prominent), while others delineate only the areas of fat to be removed. Some like to use multiple colors (green for treatment areas and red for "avoid"). It is a good idea to observe the areas to be treated with the patient in multiple positions (standing, sitting, etc.) when marking the sites, to maximize the likelihood of achieving the desired clinical result. Incision sites should also be planned and marked for each area to be treated. Once the areas have been marked and mapped, the surgeon must not deviate from that after the patient is supine or prone. These markings should also be reviewed with the patient.

All of the patient's questions are answered, and the consent sheet is then signed. At this time the patient receives any preoperative medications. The patient should go to the restroom at this point, otherwise he or she may have to interrupt the procedure because of the large amounts of fluid injected.

Table 1 Formula for Tumescent Anesthetic Solution

Ingredient	Amount (cc)
Normal saline (0.9%)	1000
Epinephrine 1/1000	1
Bicarbonate 8.4%	12.5
Triamcinolone acetonide 10 mg/cc	1
Lidocaine 1%	50 (to make 0.05% solution)
OR	
Lidocaine 2%	50 (to make 0.1% solution)

TECHNIQUE

The patient is positioned on a power operative table draped with a sterile sheet. All areas to be treated are prepped with a bactericidal solution such as Hibiclens (some surgeons prewarm the prep solution and/or the anesthetic tumescent solution in a microwave or water bath so the patient won't become chilled). Body parts that will not be involved in the procedure are covered with blankets, and the exposed treatment areas are lined with sterile towels, in order to insulate the patient and reduce heat loss. After a small amount of local anesthetic at each of the premarked incision sites, small stab incisions are made with a number 11 blade. These incisions ("adits") are generally 2 to 4 mm in length, depending on the size of the cannulas to be used. Some surgeons prefer few incisions, while others use a grid work with multiple, tiny incisions both to deliver the anesthetic solution and to remove the fat. The tumescent anesthetic solution is then instilled through the incision sites in a three-stage process as previously described.

After waiting 15 to 30 minutes beyond complete tumescence to allow the epinephrine to effect maximal vasoconstriction, (easily noted by blanching on the surface of the skin) liposuction can begin. If fat is to be harvested and stored, it is often extracted by hand at this point: sterile 10 cc syringes attached to cannula extractors are used to harvest fat by hand, using manual back-pressure on the syringe's plunger. As a syringe is filled, pressure is released from the plunger so the syringe can be changed to an empty one without removing the cannula from the patient. Once an appropriate number of syringes are filled, they are set aside for storage and the electric aspirator tubing is connected to continue liposuction.

Deeper areas are treated first, using larger cannulas, to effect the "first pass" through the target area. Areas are covered with a radial "crisscross" fashion. With the noncannula-grasping hand (Fournier's "thinking, educated hand"), the surgeon guides the cannula to those areas from which adipose tissue is to be systematically removed within a prearranged pattern using a series of piston-like movements at varying depths to accomplish the liposculpturing process. Limits are determined by the preoperative markings, the surgeon's estimate of how much fat should be removed from a particular area, and visual observation of the quality of aspirant and assessment of the amount of blood loss occurring. With the tumescent technique the amount of blood loss is minimal. Liposuction should be performed in crisscross channels, using larger cannulas more deeply to begin with and smaller cannulas more superficially for liposculpturing. The immediate effect of liposuction is to debulk the subcutaneous fat from the area, while the fibrous tissue that forms afterwards serves to retract the skin. A windshield wiper-like sweeping movement is never allowed in any part of the body except the submental area (and even its use there is the subject of controversy). Preservation of some neurovascular septae is imperative to preclude cavity formation with the attendant risks of hematoma, seroma, infection, and significant postoperative deformity.

After the initial first pass over the treatment area, the surgeon can begin to focus on individual sites. In defatted areas, residual palpable masses of fat may be noted. Smaller cannula with either more aggressive or flatter aspirating tips may be directed into these residual islands. Peripheral mesh undermining may then be performed using solid rods or smaller cannula with or without suction. One must also be cautious to avoid localized overtreatment, causing a depression.

In general, postoperative surface irregularities are more frequent along the horizontal than the vertical axis of the body. The path of cannula movement should, therefore, be predominantly along vertical axes, utilizing the crisscross technique.

Prior to the use of tumescent anesthesia, the safe amount of fat to remove was generally considered to be less than 2000 cc. However, with the use of large amounts of anesthetic fluid volume used, many surgeons routinely remove between 2000 and 4500 cc, with 2500 cc being the average removed at any one time. The American Society for Dermatologic Surgery 2004 Guidelines of Care for Liposuction cite the maximum safe volume to be removed in any setting as less than or equal to 5000 cc total aspirate.

Many surgeons no longer suture the incision sites. During the procedure a significant amount of fluid drains, so if you do decide to suture with either a subcutaneous or skin suture, do not do so until all liposuction is finished so that drainage can occur. Especially in anatomic lines such as the suprapubic line, groin, etc., incision lines can be left open and will heal with virtually no scarring.

ULTRASONIC AND POWERED LIPOSUCTION

Ultrasonic and powered liposuction techniques were introduced as ways to more easily remove fat from fibrous areas, such as female backs, male flanks, and areas that are fibrotic from being treated previously. Ultrasonic liposuction was promoted by Zocchi in the early 1990s and became quite popular in the United States. It is based on the premise that ultrasonic energy disrupts the lipocytes and liquefies the fat, making it easier for the surgeon to remove. Unfortunately, most of the initial "benefits" reported with the technique (decreased bleeding and pain) were not from the use of ultrasound, but rather from the tumescent technique of local anesthesia that was required for the ultrasound to work. Later, complications such as seromas, burns, and sloughing were reported and limited the popularity of ultrasonic liposuction. It is still a useful adjunct to conventional liposuction for treating scars or fibrous areas such as male gynecomastia, but has a definite learning curve. Many surgeons feel that other benefits have never been adequately documented such as the reduction of cellulite, the retraction of skin, and the reported lack of harm to septae that carry nerves, blood vessels and lymphatics. Some surgeons use a hollow ultrasonic cannula to remove the fat while aspirating, while others use a solid probe to liquefy the fat and then manually express it or aspirate it with conventional liposuction. The problem with using a probe is that there is no feedback to the surgeon about what is going on under the skin, plus the procedure is very time consuming, necessitating two steps. Limiting the ultrasonic portion to just a minute or two, then witching to conventional liposuction once decreased resistance is felt, as well as keeping the ultrasonic cannula in a deep plane (1 cm away from the surface) seems avoid most of the burns and other complications and emulate the same safety profile as conventional tumescent liposuction.

Powered liposuction was developed as another way to minimize surgical effort in moving through large or fibrous areas, while avoiding the negative effects seen with ultrasonic liposuction. In the mid-1990s, manufacturers began to experiment with various designs incorporating moving blades inside the conventional blunt cannula. Although they promised to be effective, they did not become widely popular due to concern of increased bleeding. Later, powered blunt cannulas that moved in a to-and-fro "reciprocating" motion were developed. These would vibrate through a distance of several millimeters, thousands of times per minute. Because they did not create the thermal energy associated with ultrasonic liposuction, burns and sloughing were not a problem. Studies have shown benefits to using powered liposuction, though, like ultrasonic liposuction, there is a learning curve.

POSTOPERATIVE CARE

At the completion of the procedure, the patient is washed with warm water and dried with towels. Compression is then applied to the treatment area(s) to assist with drainage and minimize postoperative seromas and hematomas. Originally, tape and tight dressings were used. Now most surgeons use compression garments of some type, or a combination of both. Many different garments are available from a number of manufacturers; most are machine-washable and can be re-used for the entire recovery period. The patient wears these garments 24 hours a day for five to seven days and then, depending on the area, 12 to 24 hours a day for the next one to three weeks. The patient can shower the next day but should be advised that the areas will drain for 24 to 48 hours. Sanitary napkins can be used over the incision sites, and towels can be used to sit on. Towels over a large plastic bag should be used in the car when going home after surgery to collect the fluid and prevent staining. Depends diapers can also be useful.

Many patients take it easy for a day, but depending upon the number of areas treated and how they feel, they can usually return to work within two to three days. They can return to non-jarring non-contact exercise as soon as they feel up to it (stationary bicycle, walking) but should avoid heavier activity (aerobics, tennis, or jogging) for three weeks. Patients often feel better when they wear the garments, which support the treatment area(s) and minimize soreness. The tumescent technique causes much less bruising than other types of liposuction: Ecchymoses generally disappear within two to three weeks, if they occur at all.

Most surgeons prescribe prophylactic broad-spectrum antibiotics (cephalexin, etc.) and some also use IM corticosteroids preoperatively. Antibiotics are begun two days preoperatively and continued for one week. It is also prudent to call the patient within 24 hours of surgery to make sure they are doing well. Patients should drink plenty of fluids (Gatorade, etc.), minimize their caloric intake, especially their intake of fat, and begin an exercise program as soon as they feel up to it.

COMPLICATIONS

When true tumescent liposuction surgery is performed according to guidelines, serious complications are rare. The usual postoperative sequelae include dysesthesias in the area for a limited period of time, ecchymoses, and soreness. Postoperative complications ranging from infection to development of hematomas or seromas, waviness, dimpling, cicatrical retraction, fat embolism, death, etc., are rarely seen. Several deaths have been reported with general and IV anesthesia. A death from fat embolism was reported, but the "tumescent" liposuction surgery had been combined with open abdominal lipectomy.

FOLLOW-UP VISITS

If there are no problems, the patient is seen at two to three days, seven days, one month, three months, and six months postoperatively. At the end of the third and sixth month visits, photographs are taken so that the patient can follow his or her own improvement. It is amazing that patients who have lived with deformities for most of their lives cannot remember those three months later. It is important that when photographs are taken, patients should also be weighed so that the surgeon can compare it with the weight before the procedure.

CONSIDERATIONS
Head and Neck

Submental adipose tissue may be removed with small diameter, spatula-type cannulas usually through a single small incision placed within the submental fold. Often this incision can hardly be seen a few days postoperatively. If a patient has a larger deposit of fat on the neck, three incisions can be used: a submental incision and one behind each ear to crisscross the area. Usually when the neck is treated, the jowls are included. In this area, extra small cannulas are used very gently so as not to injure the marginal mandibular nerve. The skin pulls back nicely in this area. Removal of even a small deposit from the neck can take 10 years off a person's appearance.

The neck is one area where it is permissible to turn the cannula so that the openings face upwards toward the skin in order to remove as much fat as possible and maximize the number of tracts and encourage skin retraction after the procedure. Usually, the volume aspirated from this area is quite small; ranging from 10 to 100 cc, yet the improvement may be astonishingly great. This is an easy procedure for the patient, and with tumescent anesthesia, there is often no bruising at all. The patient can go out two or three days later without any problem.

When wrapping the neck, one good option is to tape the area for two days and then have the patient wear a chin guard. The initial pieces of tape are separated by 1 in. in the center of the neck so that there is less chance of getting vertical folds. These folds, if they occur, are temporary. Occasionally, the skin is so thin that it is advisable to add a neck lift. In patients who want a simpler procedure and understand its limitations, liposuction with a submental excision can be performed. The submental incision is made easier because the undermining has already been performed by the preceding liposuction. An occasional patient may need to have the platysmal bands addressed.

Facial liposuction should be reserved for experienced liposuction surgeons. The results in this area can be disappointing and unattractive if the procedure is not performed with great care.

Upper Extremities

Many women accumulate fat in the upper arms as a result of heredity and/or obesity, and request liposuction for this area. The best results are obtained when liposuction is performed before the skin gets so loose that it results in unsightly, loosely hanging skin. In the usual patient with moderate to good skin turgor, an excellent result can be achieved through a single incision above the elbow.

Torso

The "buffalo hump" or dowager deformity responds strikingly. One or two tiny incisions allowing the operator to crisscross the cannula easily removes the loose and soft fat from this area.

Adipose pseudogynecomastia responds beautifully to liposuction, but is more challenging to treat. The approach incision can be in the axillae. This is another area (in addition to the neck) where the cannula may need to be turned upside-down so that as much breast tissue as possible can be removed. Care should be taken to avoid scarring. This maneuver is performed in the infra-areolar and periareolar areas only. This procedure allows a patient to have vast improvement in the gynecomastic area without scarring and without loss of time from work. This is another area in which maximizing the number of tracts that will later fibrose will help to retract the skin. Many patients with pseudogynecomastia have true gynecomastic tissue in a subareolar location. An aggressive cannula can remove more of this tissue. Histologic examination of the aspirated subareolar tissue would be appropriate. Sometimes this tissue has to be removed surgically through the liposuction incision.

Flanks

Flanks are the most common area in which men lay down fat. This responds beautifully to liposuction surgery. Many patients are in wonderful shape and still have this unsightly protrusion, which can hang over their waistbands. Fibrosis and retraction occur in this area and significant contour improvement results.

Back

The back is often treated along with the flanks in men and the waist and hips in women. This area tends to be more fibrous and, therefore, more aggressive cannulas should be used. The waist and back areas can often be approached from the same incision used for the flanks, abdomen, or hips. At other times more direct approaches are necessary. The location and number of incisions used to approach the area is a matter of personal preference, but remember that incisions into the taut tissue of the back may leave more of a scar than those hidden a slight distance away, in the looser skin of the waist or flanks.

Abdomen

This is one of the most common areas for liposuction. The fat is soft and easy to remove and is found mainly in two locations: the rounded infraumbilical and periumbilical protuberance that extends laterally, and the more doughy protuberance extending from the costal margin downwards to meet the major abdominal fat deposit. Fat below and lateral to the umbilicus responds very well. The fat cells in the upper abdomen are arranged in large fibrous clumps that can be difficult to aspirate and should be aspirated from two tiny incisions directly adjacent to them so as not to break the fibrous banding that often occurs at the waist.

Usually the fat in the abdomen of women is anterior to the muscle, and thus is easily amenable to surgery. It is amazing how even an abdominal apron will pull back after liposuction surgery. Occasionally, there are women whose skin is so loose due to pregnancies that in addition to doing liposuction, a superpubic excision of skin can be performed to give a nicer result. A very small number of people really do not benefit from liposuction and would be better off with an open lipectomy and repair of the rectus abdominus muscle. The "beer belly" fat occurs in many men and lies behind the muscle, and, as such, one cannot remove it. This concern generally responds to diet and exercise.

It is important to rule out the possibility of an umbilical or ventral hernia before performing surgery. In addition, the area around the umbilicus is especially sensitive; after tumescent anesthesia, injecting an extra 10 cc of undiluted 1% lidocaine with epinephrine around the umbilicus and down the central line to the pubic area is very helpful in maximizing the patient's comfort during the procedure.

Multiple techniques have been used in the abdomen, including a grid pattern with 20 to 40 tiny incisions and injection of the tumescent solution and liposuction into each of these radially. We prefer to use three to five incisions for the lower abdomen and two for the upper abdomen. For the lower abdomen, the incisions can be well hidden on either side of the superpubic fold, above the umbilicus, and in each of the two lines extending out from the umbilicus. For the upper abdomen, tiny incisions placed just laterally to each fat pad work well. If the hip is being treated as well, a lateral abdominal incision will allow access to both areas, and the umbilical incisions can be skipped. The incisions always have to be geared to the patient and the areas that are being corrected.

Lateral Thighs ("Saddle Bags") and Buttocks

Along with the abdomen and neck, lateral thighs are the most common areas for which women request liposuction. Often the hip is also involved in a "violin deformity." Both the hip and lateral thigh can be treated through a single incision between them. Moving the cannula vertically upward removes the fat in the hip area and vertically downward removes fat from the lateral thigh. Crisscrossing the lateral thigh area from a second incision in the infragluteal region completes the procedure. Both of these incisions will suffice for the buttocks as well. Generally the lateral thigh has good skin turgor and responds very well. Although the fibrous septae around cellulite globules are sometimes broken, it is better to tell the patients that there will probably be no change in the appearance of "cellulite" in the treated area. Adipose deposits in the lateral thigh can even occur in thin women and is usually inherited.

Circumferential Thigh Reduction

Circumferential thigh reduction is performed from multiple incisions above the knee going around the entire thigh. Very large extremities can be reduced, but usually serial reductions are necessary.

Pubic Area

Both men and women may have undesirable deposits of fat in the pubic area. Although patients do not frequently complain, when queried they may state bulges are displeasing to them (especially when sitting). This fat is easily aspirated from any of the abdominal incisions, but some mons veneris softness should remain. Patients of both sexes should be forewarned of transient genital swelling and ecchymoses, which can be alarming.

Knees

Knees are not too difficult and can often be treated through one incision per knee. Small cannulas should be used, and one has to be careful not to do too much work just above the knee anteriorly. Often the upper medial part of the calf is treated as well to give a better contour.

Calves and Ankles

With the advent of the smaller Klein cannulas, liposuction surgery for calves and ankles has become easier. With the smaller cannulas multiple tiny incisions can be made with fat carefully sculpted from these areas. This is another area (like the face) where the surgeon must be experienced.

Lipomas

The removal of even massive lipomas can be accomplished through very small incisions. However, the fibrous stroma within the lipoma may be very difficult to remove. This is a much more difficult procedure in general, especially if the lipoma extends into the muscle, than removal of adipose tissue. After the mass of the lipoma has been removed, an excision must be performed through the tiny incision area. The tissue will have to be teased out with counterpressure from the operator's fingers. This area must be taped with a pressure dressing and heals beautifully.

FAT TRANSPLANTATION

Fat transfer, or microlipoinjection of autologous fat, is a safe, effective method for correcting contour defects that result from aging, trauma, surgery, and various atrophic diseases. While attempts to transplant fat over the last century have met with variable success, the technique of microlipoinjection has taken on new life with the advent of liposuction surgery. Dr. Yves-Gerard Illouz first reported reinjecting viable fat that had been obtained during liposuction surgery to correct body contour defects, presenting his findings in 1986. Today, fat is harvested by hand using the syringe technique (described above) and injected immediately (fresh fat) or frozen for later use.

There are many areas where fat transfer is useful. These include the nasolabial folds, oral commissures, lips, chin, cheeks, temples, earlobes, and depressed scars. Transplanted fat seems to last longest in those areas with the least movement. Autologous fat has also been useful in nonfacial areas such as body-contour defects (such as trochanteric depressions), depressions caused by liposuction or trauma, scars, hand rejuvenation, and breast enlargement.

In most people, adequate donor fat can be found in the abdomen, buttocks, hips, lateral thighs, knees, or flanks. In some patients (with little body fat), tissue must be harvested from multiple sites. Pinski and Roenigk reported that adipose tissue from the thigh lasted longer than that from the buttock or abdomen. Katz prefers the buttock for donor fat, while Scarborough and colleagues prefer fat from the medial knee. Most physicians feel that harvesting fat by syringe is preferable to harvesting via liposuction procedures, as it avoids damaging the fat with high negative suction pressure.

The technique is straightforward: After choosing a suitable donor site, the area is marked with an indelible marking pen and prepped with sterile technique. A small amount of tumescent anesthesia is initially injected with a 30-gauge, $\frac{1}{2}$ in. needle using a 3 cc syringe. Larger syringes or a spinal needle attached to IV tubing and an infiltration pump is then used to complete anesthesia of the donor site. Anesthesia of the recipient site is similar, though very little anesthesia is needed, and it should be delivered with a syringe under minimal pressure to avoid distortion of the tissue. To harvest the fat, a small incision is made at the donor site using a 16-gauge needle, through which a Coleman extractor or spinal needle attached to a 10 cc syringe is introduced. Negative pressure is produced in the syringe by pulling the plunger out and holding it there while the syringe is moved back and forth in the subcutaneous tissue. Fat and fluid fills the syringe that is then placed in the container plunger up so that the fluid can settle to the bottom and the fat can rise to the top. This procedure can be repeated with as many syringes and donor sites as needed. The negative pressure on the syringe should be small; pull back $\frac{1}{2}$ to 1 cc and the fat will come out easily. The fluid infranatant collects at the bottom of the syringe and is easily expelled by a push of the plunger. A cap is placed on the tip of the syringe and the plunger is removed before centrifuging for one to two minutes. The lock on the tip is removed, any remaining infranatant drains off, the oily supranatant is poured off and any remaining supranatant wicked off with sterile gauze. The plunger is replaced and the fat can then be used for transplantation. The fat appears yellow and clean. The fat that will be used at the time of harvesting is transferred into 1 cc luer lock syringes through a female-female adaptor. The rest of the fat is frozen in the large syringes after being labeled with the patient's name and date.

The technique for reinjecting the fat is similar to injecting other fillers, although only one or two injection sites should be used per area in order to minimize extrusion of the injected fat through multiple openings. A 1 cc syringe attached to an 18-gauge needle or Coleman injection cannula is inserted through the incision to its furthest point, then a tiny aliquot of fat is injected as the syringe is withdrawn. This is repeated at multiple levels of the skin and subcutaneous tissue until the procedure is complete. When injecting, the surgeon should keep the other hand on the outside of the recipient area to monitor the deposition of the fat. Afterwards, the area can be gently massaged so the fat fills the area in smoothly. Some surgeons "over correct" the area, because some of the injected fat may disappear within the first few days. When using frozen fat, be sure to check with the patient the day before to confirm they are coming in for treatment. The appropriate number of syringes can then be removed from the freezer a few hours prior to the appointment and placed upright so any fluid can collect in the dependent part of the syringe and be expelled.

Postoperatively, the recipient site is iced, and antibiotic ointment and pressure dressings are applied to both the recipient site and donor sites. As with tumescent -liposuction (above), most surgeons use oral antibiotics for several days and ask the patient to avoid aspirin, non-steroidal anti-inflammatory drugs (NSAIDs), etc., to minimize the chance of infection and bleeding. Problems are very rare but include infection, hematomas, and swelling. Of note, cases of blindness have resulted from fat injection into the glabella, due to fat embolism. Otherwise, it is a very safe procedure and complications are rare.

TRAINING IN LIPOSUCTION SURGERY

For dermatologists embarking on a career of liposuction surgery, many pathways are open to them. Basic courses are being given by the American Society of Dermatologic Surgery, the International Society of Dermatologic Surgery, the American Academy of Liposuction Surgery under the auspices of the American Academy of Cosmetic Surgery, and members of the Tumescent Liposuction Council who gives courses under the American Society for Dermatologic Surgery. The American Academy of Dermatology has guidelines for liposuction surgery, and the Tumescent Liposuction Council puts out a newsletter several times a year with valuable tips and up-to-date instruction sheets. Acquaintance with a variety of experiences from different surgeons with varying approaches and philosophies is urged and encouraged.

Because the tumescent technique has been proven to be safe and effective, this field will continue to expand.

BIBLIOGRAPHY

Baker JL Jr. A practical guide to ultrasound-assisted lipoplasty. Clin Plast Surg 1999; 26(3):363–368.

Coleman WP III. The history of dermatologic liposuction. Dermatol Clin 1990; 8:381.

Coleman WP III. The history of liposuction and fat transplantation in America. Dermatol Clin 1999; 17(4):723–727.

Committee on Guidelines of Care. Guidelines of care for liposuction. J Am Acad Dermatol 2004.

Courtiss EH, Chouair RJ, Donelan MB. Large-volume suction lipectomy: an analysis of 108 patients. Plast Reconstr Surg 1992; 89:1068.

Dillerud E. Suction lipoplasty: a report on complications, undesired results, and patient satisfaction based on 3511 procedures. Plast Reconstr Surg 1991; 88:239.

Field L, Narins R. Liposuction surgery. In: Epstein E, Epstein E Jr., eds. Skin Surgery. 6th ed. Philadelphia: W.B. Saunders, 1987:370–378.

Field LM. Liposuction surgery, a review. J Dermatol Surg Oncol 1984; 10:530.

Field LM. The dermatologic surgeon and lipsculpturing. In: Fournier PF, ed. Liposculpture: The Syringe Technique. Paris: Arnette Blackwell, 1991:265–266.

Fournier P. Body Sculpturing Through Syringe Lipo-Extractions and Autologous Fat Re-Injection. Solana Beach, CA: Samuel Rolf International, 1988.

Fournier PF. Liposculpture: The Syringe Technique. Paris: Arnette Blackwell, 1991:163.

Glogau RG. Microlipoinjection. Arch Dermatol 1988; 124:1340.

Grazer FM, Meister FL. Complications of the tumescent formula for liposuction. Plast Reconstr Surg 1997; 100:1893–1896.

Illouz YG. History and current concepts of lipoplasty. Clin Plast Surg 1996; 23(4):721–730.

Illouz YG. The fat cell "graft": a new technique to fill depressions. Plast Reconstr Surg 1986; 78:122.

Klein JA. Anesthesia for liposuction in dermatologic surgery. J Dermatol Surg Oncol 1988; 14:1124–1132.

Klein JA. The two standards of care for tumescent liposuction. Dermatol Surg 1997; 23:1194–1195.

Klein JA. The tumescent technique: anesthesia and modified liposuction technique. Dermatol Clin 1990; 8:425.

Klein JA. Tumescent liposuction: totally by local anesthesia. In: Lask GP, Moy RI, eds. Principles and Practice of Dermatological Surgery. New York: McGraw-Hill, 1993.

Lauber JS, Abrams H, Coleman WP. Application of the tumescent technique to hand augmentation. J Dermatol Surg Oncol 1990; 16:369–373.

Mateo JM, Vanquero Perez MM. Systematic procedure for ultrasonically assisted lipoplasty. Aesthetic Plast Surg 2000; 24:259–269.

Teimourin B. Blindness following fat injections (letter). Plast Reconstr Surg 1988; 82(2):361.

Troilius C. Ultrasound-assisted lipoplasty: is it really safe? Aesthetic Plast Surg 1999; 23:307–311.

Zocchi M. Clinical aspects of ultrasonic liposculpture. Perspect Plast Surg 1993; 7(2):153–174.

Zocchi M. Ultrasonic liposculpturing. Aesthetic Plast Surg 1992; 16:287–298.

78

Fat Transplantation

Kevin S. Pinski
American Institute-Dermatology, Chicago, Illinois, U.S.A.

Henry H. Roenigk, Jr.
Arizona Advanced Dermatology, Scottsdale, Arizona, U.S.A.

INTRODUCTION

Aging of the face is influenced by loss of skin elasticity and by atrophy of subcutaneous fat. This results in loss of volume and fullness, which does not allow the skin to drape comfortably over the decreased facial framework, thus creating the illusion of facial sagging and wrinkling. Therefore, the answer to facial rejuvenation is not only skin resurfacing and/or tightening but also volume filling of the atrophied areas. In many cases, microlipoinjection may be the most sensible procedure to reverse some of the signs of aging.

Soft-tissue augmentation with adipose tissue has been utilized for many years. Historically, constituents of this tissue have been implanted anywhere from the periosteum through the dermis. However, the more traditional approach has involved the placement of adipose tissue into the subcutis to correct cosmetic defects.

HISTORY

Fat transplantation surgery began almost a century ago, when, in 1893 Neuber reported on his technique of free-fat transplantation. He used 1 cm pieces of free fat from the upper arm to reconstruct depressed facial defects. In 1911, Bruning reported the technique of fat injection. He placed small pieces of fat into a syringe and, by injecting this adipose tissue, corrected postrhinoplasty deformities.

Free fat transplants were largely neglected in the mid-20th century because most surgeons preferred to use pedicle flaps. These preserved the blood supply to the fat, thus making the outcome more predictable. In addition, artificial injectable substances such as paraffin and silicone became available and were used to fill defects in the skin at that time. In 1950, Peer reported a series of experiments with autologous human fat transplants in which over 50% of the fat remained as a viable transplant one year following grafting.

The current phase of fat transplantation began in 1976 when Fisher and Fisher performed fat extraction with the cellusuctiotome. Two years later, Illouz introduced simplified instrumentation for the technique known today as liposuction. This new procedure provided the cosmetic surgeon with an abundant supply of viable adipose tissue that could be used to augment soft-tissue deformities.

Coincident with the appearance of liposuction surgery, there was a resurgence of interest in fat grafting as a natural mode of soft-tissue augmentation. Pierre Fournier pioneered a syringe-extraction fat-grafting technique called "microlipoinjection." Illouz reported a similar approach. Microlipoinjection is currently performed as an outpatient surgical procedure for soft-tissue augmentation of the aging face and for minor contour defects.

PREOPERATIVE CONSIDERATIONS/CONSULTATION

Aging of the face is most notable by fat wasting and deepening of wrinkles, all of which can be augmented with fat transplantation. Other areas such as acne scars, buccal fat wasting, facial asymmetries, and senile earlobes can also be improved with microlipoinjections. In addition, senile lipoatrophy of the hands and atrophy secondary to linear morphea or lupus panniculitis can be treated in a similar fashion.

Before beginning the procedure, the surgeon and the patient must sit together to discuss their goals andconcerns. It is important for the surgeon to take a few moments to examine the face thoroughly for general proportions, asymmetries, and predicted volumes necessary to accomplish the desired results. The patient should be given a hand mirror to follow along.

It is imperative that the surgeon determine whether the cosmetic defect is of a superficial–dermal or deeper–subcutaneous nature. Subcutaneous defects are best augmented with fat transplants, whereas these are inappropriate for dermal defects. Superficial dermal defects, however, can be treated with lipocytic dermal augmentation (autologous collagen). Combined superficial and deep defects are best corrected with a layered approach.

It is also necessary to examine the patient's potential donor sites preoperatively. Occasionally, it may be difficult to obtain a sufficient amount of fat from a very slender patient to perform even one procedure. In this situation, it may be prudent to suggest an alternative approach.

As previously mentioned, the nature of the cosmetic defect is an important consideration in regard to fat-graft longevity. Graft longevity varies with the nature of the cosmetic defect being treated and with the location of the recipient site. The less mobile the recipient site, the greater the degree of graft longevity.

During the preoperative consultation, the patient should be informed that touch-up procedures would be required. It has been observed that long-term results are markedly improved when these transplants are repeated two to three times every three to six months after the initial procedure. Each subsequent transplant has a cumulative effect, with higher percentages of fat surviving after each

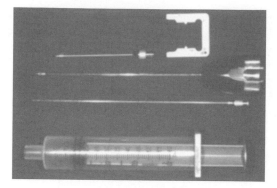

Figure 1 Fat transplantation set-up.

successive procedure. This has also been reported by others and documented by magnetic resonance imaging.

One final consideration is whether one should utilize freshly harvested fat for each procedure. From a longevity standpoint, one should certainly use fresh material each time. In order for the fat transplant to survive as a true graft, it should be as unadulterated as possible. However, from a convenience standpoint, it is much easier to freeze any fatty tissue left after the initial procedure for subsequent touch-ups. It has been recently demonstrated that frozen adipocytes are still viable upon thawing. Thus, frozen tissue should be adequate for microlipoinjections. It has been effectively and safely utilized after one to two years of storage.

EQUIPMENT

A simple setup is used, which includes 500 ml tumescent solution (Fig. 1). This is infiltrated using a Medex pressure cuff (Tiemann Surgical Supply, Inc.) that pushes the anesthetic solution through intravenous tubing to a connected Klein infiltrating cannula. The remainder of the tray consists of 3 ml and 60 ml syringes, a Johnnie-Lok device (The Tulip Co.), a 1 ml syringe, a 30-gauge needle, a 16-gauge needle, a #11 blade, a surgical marking pen, sterile gauze, a 15 cm 2.7 mm blunt-tipped uniport Toomey cannula (Bryon Supply Co.), a fat transfer adaptor (Byron Supply Co.), a Coleman 16-gauge injection cannula (Byron Supply Co.), a sterile basin or tray, and 100 mL sterile saline solution (Figs. 2 and 3).

In addition, if harvesting fat during a liposuction procedure, one may wish to use Lipivage™ (Genesis Biosystems, Inc.). This is a closed sterile collection device, which can gently harvest adipocytes at low vacuum levels. There is no need for centrifugation, washing, or separating fat from fluid. Most importantly, a closed system is continuously maintained (Fig. 4).

TECHNIQUE LIPOEXTRACTION

Microlipoinjection involves extracting and reimplanting adipose tissue by a closed technique. Generally, the quantity of

Lidocaine	1%	50cc
Epinephrine	1:1000	1cc
Ringer's Lacatate		950cc

Figure 2 Tumescent anesthesia formula.

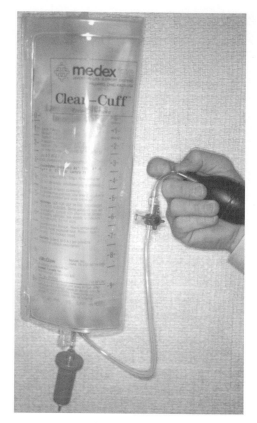

Figure 3 Medex pressure cuff.

fat needed for correcting facial defects is small: 10 to 20 mL. It is imperative that the surgeon respect the extracted tissue and minimize hydraulic and chemical trauma. It is for this reason that we prefer to harvest via a syringe.

The majority of fat transplantation procedures are performed under local anesthesia. If necessary, nerve blocks and/or Valium 5 mg orally can be administered. Great care must be taken to avoid causing pain as well as diminishing postoperative swelling and ecchymosis. If these occur, the patient may be discouraged from following up with subsequent procedures, thus diminishing one's chance for good long-term results.

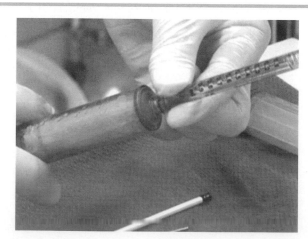

Figure 4 Lipivage™ device for harvesting fat during a liposuction procedure.

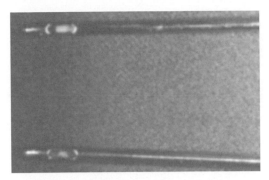

Figure 5 Blunt-tipped uniport harvesting cannulae.

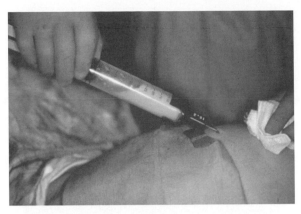

Figure 6 Harvesting of adipose tissue with 60 cc syringe.

Before beginning, the donor area is marked with the patient in a standing position, as if to perform a standard liposuction, with attention paid to irregularities and asymmetries. We prefer to utilize the upper outer quadrant of the buttocks whenever possible. The fat is easy to obtain here and if a resultant harvesting deformity occurs, it is usually very unobtrusive. It is important to plan to remove adequate tissue for storage for subsequent touch-ups. Typically, less than 100 mL is sufficient.

Utilizing the tumescent anesthesia, an intradermal wheal is raised at the incision site of the chosen donor area. A 2 to 3 mm incision is made in the skin with a #11 blade. Tumescent anesthesia is then instilled using a 15 cm Klein infiltrating needle. The donor area should be tumesced in a very slow and nonpainful fashion, proceeding from the subcutaneous-fascial plane and progressing superficially.

Before harvesting, the surgeon must wait a minimum of 15 minutes for the maximum effect of the tumescent anesthesia. During this time, one should consider anesthetic options for the recipient areas. If EMLA or a regional nerve block is to be employed, they can be safely administered at this time.

Lipoextraction begins by suctioning with a blunt-tipped 15 cm, 2.7 mm uniport cannula attached to a 60 mL syringe (Fig. 5). This is preferred over a 14-gauge needle, multiple port cannulas, or Cobra tip cannulas, which tend to retrieve more fibrous tissue and are more traumatic to the fat. It is important to respect this part of the procedure because a rough and hasty lipoextraction will result in destruction of fat cells, which will have little chance of survival. Keep in mind that this is harvesting of viable adipocytes for transfer and not destructive removal of fat by liposuction.

The syringe is primed for harvesting by submerging the distal end of the attached cannula into the basin filled with saline. All air should be expelled from the syringe and 5 to 10 mL saline should be aspirated. The cannula is then inserted into the fat through the incision site and the plunger of the syringe is pulled out to create negative pressure. This relative vacuum is sufficient to extract the fat as the cannula is maneuvered back and forth within the adipose layer (Fig. 6).

The cannula and syringe are moved back and forth five or six times in the same tunnel, after which the procedure is repeated in a radial fashion until sufficient fat has been aspirated. During the extraction the plunger is kept in the same position. A "Johnnie Lok" device aids in maintaining the negative pressure of the syringe (Fig. 7). During the entire procedure, the skin is constantly palpated by the surgeon's free hand.

TREATMENT OF THE COLLECTED FAT

When the extraction is complete, the filled syringe is capped, placed vertically (plunger up), and allowed to decant. It should be allowed to stand for 10 to 15 minutes. This will cause the tumescent fluid to accumulate near the tip of the syringe (Fig. 8). By removing the syringe cap, this fluid is discarded, leaving only "pure fat," which is then transferred into 3 mL syringes (Fig. 9).

We feel that washing the collected fat is an unnecessary step. Simply letting the syringe of adipose material stand for 10 to 15 minutes allows the tumescent anesthesia to wash the adipocytes. One is left with pure bloodless fat.

Some claim that centrifugation of collected fat provides a more concentrated graft, while other studies have documented decreased viability after such processing. In an effort to treat harvested adipocytes as gently as possible, we choose not to centrifuge.

KEIMPLANTATION

Lipoinjection is typically performed with a 1 or 3 mL syringe and a 16-gauge Coleman injection cannula (Fig. 10). Fat injected through a lumen smaller than 18-gauge is damaged, as measured by nuclear, cellular, and globular morphology. This has been confirmed by checking the biochemical integrity of the adipocyte as measured by glucose metabolism, fatty acid synthesis, and insulin stimulation. zA 16-gauge cannula seems to be the optimal size for transferring fat, for both ease of injection and minimizing trauma to the transplanted adipocytes. In addition, it does not scar the skin and its blunt tip reduces the risk of vascular laceration.

A small intradermal wheal is raised at each injection site with 1% Xylocaine. A 16-gauge needle is used to pierce

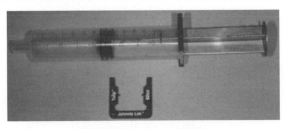

Figure 7 Johnnie-Lok device.

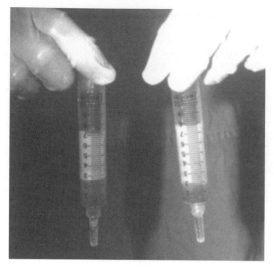

Figure 8 Tumescent anesthesia collects as infranatant by gravitational pooling.

a hole in the skin to make the entry site for the transplant cannula. The cannula is then guided into the anesthetized recipient sites, parallel to the surface of the skin, sliding just along the subcutaneous-fascial plane, until it reaches its most distal point. As the cannula is slowly withdrawn, the fat is injected in a retrograde fashion in microdroplet amounts. Multiple passes are made at various levels, extending from the subcutaneous-fascial plane up to the dermal subcutaneous junction in a fan-shaped pattern.

The injection of fat in different areas and levels ensures sufficient peripheral circulation around each graft to allow its incorporation in the surrounding tissue. A column of injected fat seems to survive better than a large bolus. Therefore, the endpoint of microlipoinjection should be correction of the cosmetic defect. Overcorrection is not necessary and should be avoided. Control of fat deposition is maintained by applying manual pressure bilaterally along the edges of the defect. Once the injection is complete, the fat should be gently molded into a desired position. This technique is the mainstay of autologous fat injections used by others and us.

Intact adipocytes can be placed in many different tissues, provided that vascularization of the graft is obtained. Fat is harvested as previously outlined, it is centrifuged to condense the fat, and then small parcel grafts are injected into multiple tissue planes other than just the subcutis. This technique has been popularized by Dr. Sydney Coleman and reported extensively in the literature as Lipostructure®. Reported results of correction and longevity have

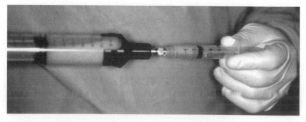

Figure 9 Transferring adipose tissue from 60 cc syringe to 3 cc syringes.

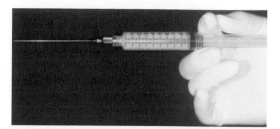

Figure 10 Fat injection using 16-gauge Coleman injection cannula.

been gratifying. It is important to understand that the short-term morbidity from such extensive multiple injections is substantial, with edema potentially lasting for months.

An additional approach is the F.A.M.I. technique, developed by Roger Amar, a French plastic surgeon. It is based on two premises. First is that the volume lost during aging is not only fat, but involves atrophy of muscle and bone. The second premise is that transplanted fat survives best next to muscle. The F.A.M.I. procedure involves injection of autologous fat in or near the muscles of facial expression. Because it parallels the blood supply, trauma is supposedly minimized and fat survival is optimized. Unfortunately, this is a very technique-dependent procedure involving the usage of specific injection cannulae. Because of intramuscular placement of fat injections, nerve blocks and sedation are typically required. In addition, patients generally experience marked edema with minimal bruising for five to seven days postoperatively.

If required, superficial defects can be corrected with the injection of nonviable, fat-derived tissue into the dermis via small (i.e., 25-gauge) needles. This technique was termed Dermal Lipocytic Augmentation by Pinski and Coleman. Once the fat has been harvested, it is passed into 3 cc syringes and mixed with sterile distilled water for injection. This hypotonic mixture is then passed back and forth through an adapter with a decreasing aperture in a forceful manner. This leads to a homogeneous emulsion, which following centrifugation and separation can be easily injected via a 25-gauge needle into the dermis in a fashion similar to Zyderm®. This material differs from others used in the techniques above in that no viable tissue is retained and therefore "grafting" will not take place. It has been shown that the injected material stimulates host fibrosis. When combined with traditional fat transplantation, it enables correction of both superficial and deep defects.

INDICATIONS

Multiple cosmetic defects are amendable to augmentation with adipose tissue. The best response is seen with less-mobile recipient sites and areas that have significant atrophy (i.e. morphea, facial hemiatrophy, etc.). Strategic positioning of injection sites is shown in Figure 11.

Some ideal indications for lipoinjection are as follows:

1. Glabellar furrows: Typically, less than 2 cc of fat are required here. These furrows should be injected away from the eye to avoid intrusion of fat into the periorbital area. Marks left by the 16-gauge needle, if any, are not noticeable in the medial aspects of the eyebrows.
2. Nasolabial furrows/melomental creases/oral commissures: All three areas can be approached through the same entry point lateral to the commissures of the

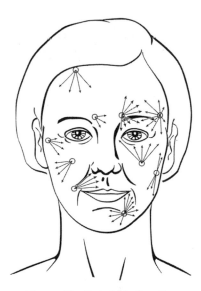

Figure 11 Typical injection sites.

mouth (Fig. 12). Patients should be cautioned about excessive facial manipulation and exertion for the first 12 to 24 hours postoperatively.

3. Lips: The same lateral entry points may be used. This will give the lips a fuller appearance and consequently diminish wrinkles. Perpendicular rhytides or "smoker's lines" will not be eradicated. This can also be used to evert the lips by injecting 1 to 3 cc of fat between the inner mucosa and muscular layers.

4. Cheeks: Whenever fat is injected into the face, it should be directed away from orifices if possible. Cheekbones can be augmented with lipoinjection. Hollow cheeks (Figs. 13 and 14) and infraorbital grooves are good indications (Fig. 15). Atrophic acne scars are amenable as well, but the scars should have associated atrophy of the subcutis (Fig. 16). If the scars are pitted or purely dermal defects, the chance of correction is very unlikely.

5. Morphea/Lupus profundus: Both of these conditions respond quite well to lipoinjections (Fig. 17). However, the disease process should be inactive prior to beginning cosmetic correction. A biopsy may aid in documenting this.

6. Facial hemiatrophy: Congenital defects such as facial hemiatrophy can be successfully treated (Fig. 18).

However, as more fat is injected into one area, be careful to inject at different levels to insure maximal vascularity to each graft. The patient should be aware that several injections may be needed, usually two to three months apart.

7. Hands: Fat transplantation plays an integral role in hand rejuvenation. Transplanted fat provides thickness to an atrophic subcutaneous compartment, decreasing the prominence of blood vessels and tendons, thus giving the hands an overall younger appearance. The cannula is inserted at the dorsal wrist crease and threaded along the tendon sheath distally to each metacarpophalangeal joint. The fat should be massaged distally to avoid plump hands with skinny fingers (Fig. 19).

COMPLICATIONS

To date this has been a relatively safe and effective procedure. Temporary swelling and minor bruising at the recipient site and mild tenderness at the donor site may occur. In rare cases, temporary lumpiness or cyst formation may occur (Fig. 20). In addition, we have had two hematomas develop over the years. There has been one report of unilateral blindness following transplantation of autologous fat to the glabella. Care must be exercised when injecting any particulate substance near the eye. Because of the large size of these particles, however, intravascular penetration of fat is rare.

SUMMARY

Our current procedure for fat transplantation has been a progressive evolution since 1989. When we first began, adipose tissue was harvested by a suction apparatus and a sterile-filter trap (Robbins Instrument Co.). Large volumes were injected into each recipient site because of high reabsorption rates. Most cases involved 30% to 50% over-correction in an effort to compensate. However, this led to significant inflammation and swelling, which forced patients to heal for a period of days to weeks.

In the mid-1990s, being somewhat disenchanted with long-term results, we started to transplant smaller volumes of adipose tissue. We were also influenced by others who reported better graft viability with smaller injected volumes. This, combined with less traumatic harvesting, has led to more acceptable long-term results. The ideal fat graft appears to be tubular, less than 3 mm in diameter, and placed at various levels to ensure adequate vascularity.

(A)

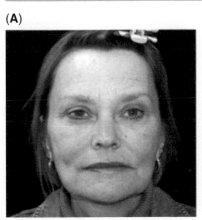

(B)

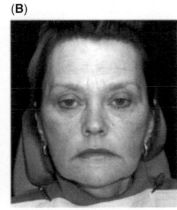

Figure 12 **(A)** Before fat transplantation for senile lipoatrophy. **(B)** Four weeks after fat transplants to cheeks and nasolabial furrows.

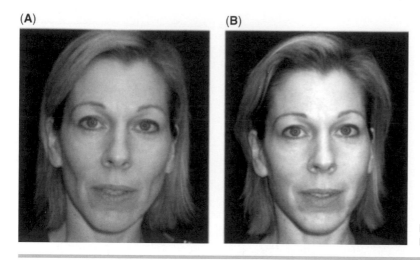

Figure 13 (A) Before fat transplantation for senile lipoatrophy. **(B)** Four weeks after fat transplants to cheeks.

The other major change through the decade is the freezing of adipose tissue for subsequent touch-up procedures. We believe that utilizing freshly harvested tissue each time would be ideal. However, as a matter of convenience, freezing excess tissue is more practical. In addition, a recent report has shown viability of adipocytes after freezing and thawing.

When one is storing human tissue for subsequent transplantation, extreme care must be taken to ensure proper identification. Each syringe and storage bag should be labeled with the patient's name, Social Security number, and date of harvesting.

This is checked carefully by the physician prior to each reinjection.

Touch-up procedures are repeated two to three times every three to six months. This is scientifically justified by work done by Horl et al. with magnetic resonance imaging of fat transplants. They identified 49% volume loss at three months and 55% loss at six months, with negligible decrease in volume between 9 and 12 months.

The current hypothesis regarding fat-graft transfer supports the cell survival theory. The volume of fat, when surgically removed from the donor site, becomes ischemic. After transfer into the recipient site, some cells may die,

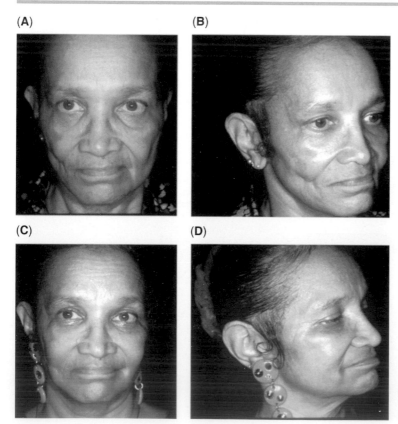

Figure 14 (A,B) Before fat transplantation for senile lipoatrophy. **(C,D)** Three months after fat transplants to cheeks and nasolabial furrows.

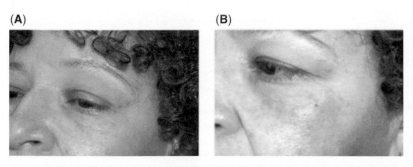

Figure 15 (**A**) Before fat transplantation to infraorbital groove. (**B**) Immediately after fat transplantation.

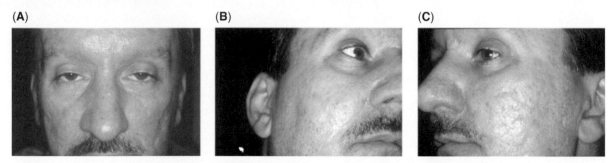

Figure 16 (**A**) Prior to fat transplantation for atrophic acne scarring. (**B,C**) One year after fat transplantation.

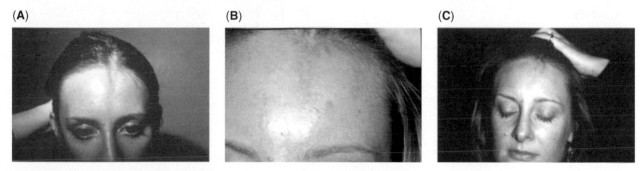

Figure 17 (**A**) Prior to fat transplantation for linear morphea (Coup de Sabre) of the scalp. (**B**) Six months after fat transplantation. (**C**) Four years after two episodes of fat transplantation.

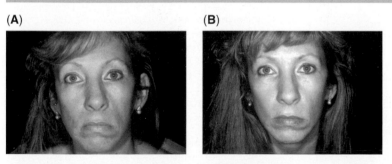

Figure 18 (**A**) Facial hemiatrophy. (**B**) Three months after fat transplantation of 4 cc adipose tissue.

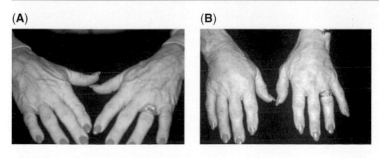

Figure 19 (**A**) Senile Lipoatrophy of the hands. (**B**) Six months after fat transplantation of 8 cc to each hand.

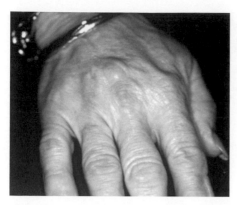

Figure 20   Triglyceride cyst formation after fat transplantation.

some survive as adipocytes, and others dedifferentiate into preadipocyte cells. The preadipocyte cells, after recovery from the transfer process, can accumulate fat and mature into an adipocyte. Ultimately, the fat graft regains its blood supply from the periphery and those cells that have survived will remain and function. Those that die will be cleared and replaced by the normal process of fibrosis.

BIBLIOGRAPHY

Amar RE. Fat Autograft Muscle Injection, AACS Annual Meeting, Feb 2002.

Amar RE. Microinfiltration adipocytaire (MIA) au niveau de la face, ou restructuration tissulaire par greffe de tissu adipeux. Ann Chir Plast Esthet 1999; 44(6):593–608.

Billings E Jr., May JW Jr. Historical review and present status of free graft auto transplantation in plastic and reconstructive surgery. Plast Reconstr Surg 1989; 83:368.

Brandow K, Newman J. Facial raultilayered micro lipoaugmentation. Int J Aesthet Restor Surg 1996; 4:95–110.

Bruning P. (cited by Brockaert TJ) Contribution a 1'etude des greffes adipeusses. Bull Acad R Med Belg 1919; 28:440.

Campbell G-L, Laudenslager N, Newman J. The effect of mechanical stress on adipocyte morphology and metabolism. Am J Cosmet Surg 1987; 4:85–87.

Carpaneda C, Ribeiro MT. Study of the histological alterations and viability of the adipose graft in humans. Aesthetic Plast Surg 1993; 17:43–47.

Chajchir A, Benzaquen I, Moretti E. Comparative experimental study of autologous adipose tissue processed by different techniques. Aesthetic Plast Surg 1993; 17:113–115.

Coleman SR. Long-term survival of fat transplants: controlled demonstrations. Aesthetic Plast Surg 1995; 19:421–425.

Coleman SR. Facial recontouring with lipostructure. Clin Plast Surg 1997; 24:347–367.

Coleman WP, Lawrence N, Sherman RN, Reed RJ, Pinski KS. Autologous collagen? Lipocytic dermal augmentation a histopathologic study. J Dermatol Surg Oncol 1993; 19:1032–1040.

Eppley BL, Smith PG, Salove AM, et al. Experimental effects of graft revascularization and consistency on cervicofacial fat transplant survival. J Oral Maxillofac Surg 1990; 48:54–62.

Fischer A, Fischer GM. Revised technique for cellulite fat. Reduction in riding breeches deformity. Bull Int Acad Cosmet Surg 1977; 2:40.

Fournier PF. Collagen Autologue: Liposculpture ma Technique. Paris: Arnette, 1989:227–229.

Fournier PF. Facial recontouring with fat grafting. Dermatol Clin 1990; 8:523–537.

Glogau RG, Matarasso SL, Markey AC. Microlipoinjection: autologous fat grafting. In: Lask G, Moy R, eds. Principles and Techniques of Cutaneous Surgery. New York: McGraw-Hill, 1996:437–444.

Horl HW, Feller AM, Biemer E. Technique for liposuction fat reimplantation and long-term volume evaluation by magnetic resonance imaging. Ann Plast Surg 1991; 26:248–257.

Hudson DA, Lambert EV, Bloch CE. Site selection for autotransplantation: some observations. Aesthetic Plast Surg 1990; 14:195.

Illouz Y-G. Communications at the Societe Francaise de Chirurgie Esthetique, June 1978, 1979.

Illouz Y-G. L'Avenir de la reutilization de la graisse aprds liposuction. Rev Chir Esthet Lang Franc 1985:10.

Illouz Y-G. The fat cell "graft", a new technique to fill depressions. Plast Reconstr Surg 1986; 78:122–123.

Jones JK. Am Acad Cosra Surg Mtg 1977.

Klein JA. The tumescent technique for liposuction surgery. Am J Cosmet Surg 1987; 4:263–267.

Lewis CM. The current status of autologous fat grafting. Aesthetic Plast Surg 1993; 17:109–112.

Matsudo PKR, Toledo LS. Experience of injected fat grafting. Aesthetic Plast Surg 1988; 12:35.

Neuber F. Fat grafting. Cuir Kongr Verh Otsum Ges Chir 1893; 20:56.

Newman J, Levin J. Facial lipo-transplant surgery. Am J Cosmet Surg 1987; 4:131–140.

Nguyen A, Pasyk KA, Bouvier TN, et al. Comparative study of survival of autologous adipose tissue taken and transplanted by different techniques. Plast Reconstr Surg 1990; 85:378–387.

Peer LA. Loss of weight and volume in human fat grafts. Plast Reconstr Surg 1950; 5:217.

Pinski KS, Roenigk HH. Autologous fat transplantation: a long-term follow-up. J Dermatol Surg Oncol 1992; 18:179–184.

Polsy RI. Adipocyte survival. The Third Annual Scientific Meeting of the American Academy of Cosmetic Surgery and the American Society of Liposuction Surgery, Los Angeles, Feb 1987.

Sattler G, Sommer B. Liporecycling: immediate and delayed. Am J Cosmet Surg 1997; 14:311–316.

Temourian B. Blindness following fat injections, correspondence and brief communications. Plast Reconstr Surg 1988; 80:361.

Van Akkerveeken PF, Van de Kraan W, Muller JWT. The fate of the free fat graft. A prospective clinical study using CT scanning. Spine 1986; 11:501.

Van RL, Bayliss CE, Roncari DA. Cytological and enzymological characterization of adult human adipocyte precursors in culture. J Clin Invest 1976; 58:699.

Van RL, Roncari DAK. Isolation of fat cell precursors from adult rat adipose tissue. Cell Tissue Res 1977; 181:197.

Weisz GM, Gal A. Long-term survival of a fat free graft in the spinal canal. A 40 month postlaminectomy case report. Clin Orthop 1986; 205:204.

79

Blepharoplasty and Brow Lifting

Robert C. Langdon
Shoreline Dermatology, Guilford, Connecticut, U.S.A.

INTRODUCTION

The peri-orbital area is an important esthetic unit because it is highly visible. During face-to-face conversation, the eyes are the part of the face most viewed by an interlocutor. Aging changes in the eyelids, temples, glabella, and forehead frequently prompt patients to seek cosmetic improvement. As is true for the face in general, aging of the peri-orbit and upper face occurs by three primary mechanisms: photo-aging (affecting the skin), gravitational aging (causing ptosis of all soft tissue), and volumetric aging (atrophy of soft tissues and, with advanced age, of bone). All three aging mechanisms synergize with overuse of facial muscles of expression to produce characteristic wrinkles such as frown lines in the glabella, horizontal forehead wrinkles and, "crow's feet" wrinkles.

Because many of the aging changes in the peri-orbital and upper face regions are interrelated, evaluation of prospective patients for cosmetic surgery in this area should be comprehensive. In particular, redundant upper eyelid skin (dermatochalasis) is generally partly or largely the result of brow ptosis. Deep horizontal forehead creases result from overuse of the frontalis muscle to elevate the ptotic brow. Ptosis of temporal skin accompanies brow ptosis and contributes to deep "crow's feet" wrinkles. Although patients may complain mainly about "droopy eyelids," the constellation of the aforementioned signs would indicate that the underlying problem is brow ptosis.

The endoscopic forehead-lift can potentially improve all stigmata of a ptotic brow and even one of its causes (glabellar muscle activity). The endoscopic procedure described herein includes brow and temple elevation (enabled by the appropriate release of soft tissues) as well as myotomies and neurotomies of glabellar frown muscles and their motor nerve supply. With endoscopic visualization the surgery can be performed using minimal incisions, thus avoiding the adverse sequelae of the traditional coronal incision, including a visible scar, alopecia, and sensory nerve injury. A biodegradable fixation device, the Endotine™, assures stable and symmetric elevation of the undermined and mobilized soft-tissue layers, which firmly reattach to underlying immobile tissues at a more cephalad level. Correction of brow ptosis partially improves upper eyelid dermatochalasis, but in many cases a subsequent blepharoplasty is required for full correction. Weakening or eliminating glabellar muscle activity improves the stability of brow elevation because these muscles are brow depressors. Brow elevation also lessens the patient's need to constantly contract the frontalis muscle in order to improve the visual field. Thus, deep forehead rhytids will improve secondary to lessened frontalis activity.

Direct improvement of upper eyelid dermatochalasis is achieved by blepharoplasty. The surgery is well suited to use of the carbon dioxide (CO_2) laser, which, in focused mode, will incise soft tissues while simultaneously providing hemostasis. Hemostasis is critical to the safety of any surgery in the well-vascularized eyelid area. In addition to redundant skin, excessive or herniated orbital fat can be removed during upper eyelid blepharoplasty. If both forehead-lift and upper blepharoplasty are contemplated in a given patient, the forehead-lift should be performed first. This is because the amount of correction of brow ptosis may be difficult to predict. Brow position should be stable prior to blepharoplasty so that the latter procedure can be used to precisely remove residual excess skin of the upper lid.

In the lower eyelid, orbital fat may be prominent because of actual herniation of orbital fat pads and/or atrophy of adjacent soft tissues (volumetric aging of the anterior face). Ptosis of the malar fat pad, a gravitational change, can also contribute to prominence of lower lid orbital fat. The primary goal of lower lid blepharoplasty is to remove excessive orbital fat.

The lower eyelid is a free margin and is vulnerable to caudal traction, which can result in scleral show or even ectropion. The transconjunctival approach to lower blepharoplasty is less likely to result in altered postoperative lid position because with this method the orbital septum is not violated (see Anatomy). The orbital septum can contract on healing, resulting in excessive caudal traction on the lower lid. Thus, the transcutaneous approach, in which the septum is traversed, should be avoided. Any excessive skin is safely reduced by a subsequent laser resurfacing or conservative pinch excision of skin only. As is the case for upper blepharoplasty, transconjunctival lower blepharoplasty is advantageously performed with the CO_2 laser because of the hemostatic properties of this instrument.

This chapter is intended as an introduction to these procedures. In-depth discussion of anatomy, surgical techniques, and avoidance and management of complications is available from many sources.

ANATOMY

Thorough familiarity with the anatomy of the forehead, temporal fossa, orbit and peri-orbital tissues is essential for the safe performance of forehead-lift and blepharoplasty. Knowledge of the location of fascial and muscle layers as well as motor and sensory nerve branches is required.

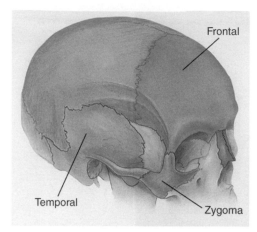

Figure 1 Bones of the skull. The bones of the forehead and temporal fossa include the frontal, zygoma, and temporal bones.

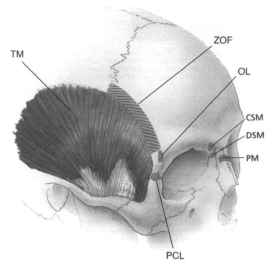

Figure 2 Soft-tissue anchor points of forehead and temporal fossa. The temporalis muscle fills the temporal fossa. Anchor points between periosteum and superficial musculoaponeurotic system include the zone of fixation, orbital ligament and pre-canthal ligament, all of which must be released during a forehead-lift to allow adequate elevation of the lateral brow. Also shown are the bony origins of the glabellar muscles: corrugator supercilii, depressor supercilii, and procerus. *Abbreviations*: ZOF, zone of fixation; OL, orbital ligament; CSM, corrugator supercilii; DSM, depressor supercilii; PM, procerus; PCL, pre-canthal ligament.

Forehead and Temporal Fossa

The bones of the skull compose the substructure of the forehead and temporal fossa (Fig. 1). The frontal bone underlies the entire forehead. The bones of the lateral skull form a depression in the temple (the temporal fossa), which accommodates the temporalis muscle. The supero-medial edge of this fossa is called the temporal crest. This edge is palpable as a bony ridge between the forehead and temple. The temporalis muscle attaches to the floor of the temporal fossa and extends caudally beneath the zygomatic arch (composed of processes of the temporal and zygoma bones) toward its insertion into the coronoid process of the mandible. The orbital rim is composed largely of the aforementioned bones and on its supero-medial surface contains (in most patients) the supraorbital notch, the skull foramen through which the supraorbital nerve (SON) emanates.

An important soft-tissue structure, which also defines the juncture between the forehead and temporal fossa, is the zone of fixation (Fig. 2). This structure, also referred to as the temporal crest ligament, is a curvilinear band of dense connective tissue that attaches the superficial musculoaponeurotic system (SMAS) elements to underlying frontal bone. This band is approximately 6-mm wide and runs just medial to the bony ridge of the temporal crest. The zone of fixation approaches the superior orbital rim, at which is a discrete ligamentous attachment between the frontal bone of the orbital rim and the overlying SMAS and dermis (the orbital ligament).

Another connective tissue attachment between bone and SMAS is the pre-canthal ligament (PCL), an adherence between the lateral orbital rim (just lateral to the lateral canthus) and the overlying superficial temporal fascia (Fig. 2).

In the temporal fossa the temporalis muscle is covered by the deep temporal fascia. This fascia is relatively thick and striated in appearance, and lies on the surface of the muscle. Immediately superficial to the deep fascia is the superficial temporal fascia (also called tempero-parietal fascia), the local representative of SMAS (see below).

Superficial Musculoaponeurotic System

The SMAS is composed of the superficial muscles of expression (whose purpose is to move the skin of the face in order to express emotion) and their associated fascia and connective tissue attachments to dermis. In the scalp cephalad to the forehead, the SMAS is composed of a dense fascial layer, the galea aponeurotica. In the forehead, the galea splits into superficial and deep layers to envelop the frontalis muscle (Fig.3). In the lower forehead the deep galea (DG) splits yet again to envelop the galea fat pad. The fascia underlying the fat pad splits once more to form the glide plane space.

These various DG layers fuse together at the superior orbital rim and attach to the underlying frontal bone of the orbital rim (Fig. 3). Within the orbit the fused DG layers form the orbital septum. More superficially, the frontalis muscle interdigitates with orbicularis oculi just cephalad to the orbital rim. These muscles, together with various galea layers, compose the SMAS of the forehead and upper eyelid.

Motor Nerves of Forehead and Temporal Fossa

Motor nerve supply to the forehead, glabella, and eyelid is provided by the temporal and zygomatic branches of the facial nerve (Fig. 4). Rami of the temporal branches are the structures at greatest risk of injury during surgery in the temporal fossa. The temporal branch rami innervate the frontalis muscle and the supero-lateral part of the orbicularis oculi. The temporal branch also supplies motor input to the corrugator supercilii. These rami run within the superficial temporal fascia (the SMAS of the temple) and are vulnerable during sub-SMAS undermining in the temple.

The zygomatic branch of the facial nerve innervates the lower orbicularis oculi and provides varying amounts of input to the glabellar musculature (8). This branch is generally not at risk of injury during the endoscopic forehead-lift as described in this chapter.

Sensory Nerves of Forehead

The SON emanates from the supraorbital foramen, which in 90% of cases is a notch in the superior orbital rim just medial

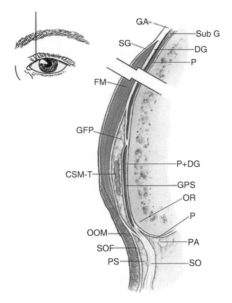

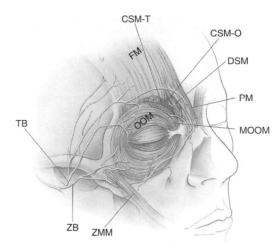

Figure 3 Relationships of SMAS components in the forehead and superior orbit. A saggital cross-section of the frontal bone and overlying soft tissues of the forehead and upper orbit is depicted at the level of the medial limbus. In the upper forehead the local SMAS element is the GA, which overlies the sub-galea fascial plane. Caudally, the GA divides into the SG and DG to envelop the FM. In the lower forehead (beneath the FM) the DG divides once more to envelop the GFP, through which passes the transverse head of the CSM-T. Deep to the GFP the DG divides a final time into two layers that can glide over each other, creating the GPS; beneath the GPS the deepest layer of DG is fused to periosteum of the frontal bone. At the orbital rim the OS is formed by the fusion of most of the layers of the DG, except for a superficial layer of DG that becomes the suborbicularis fascia, the undersurface of the orbicularis oculi muscle. Pre-septal fat also known as retro-orbicularis oculi fat, and PA lie superficial and deep to the OS, respectively. *Abbreviations*: SMAS, superficial musculoaponeurotic system; GA, galea aponeurotica; Sub G, sub-galea fascial plane; SG, superficial galea; DG, deep galea; CSM-T, corrugator supercilii muscle; FM, frontalis muscle; GFP, galea fat pad; GPS, glide plane space; OR, orbital rim; OS, orbital septum; SOF, suborbicularis fascia; OOM, orbicularis oculi muscle; ROOF, retro-orbicularis oculi fat; PA, pre-aponeurotic fat.

Figure 4 Motor nerve supply to the forehead and periocular area. The temporal branch of the facial nerve supplies the ipsilateral frontalis, corrugator and superior orbicularis oculi muscles. The zygomatic branch supplies the inferior orbicularis oculi and the glabellar muscles via an infra-orbital approach. *Abbreviations*: DSM, depressor supercilii; PM, procerus; OOM, orbicularis oculi muscle.

The supratrochlear nerve emerges from the supero-medial orbital rim and traverses the glabellar musculature to innervate the skin of the glabella and central forehead. In the glabella, the nerve branches usually run within the fibers of the depressor supercilii muscle.

Eyelids and Orbit
The orbital septum is an important fascia layer that partitions the eyelid into superficial and deep compartments.

to the midpoint of the rim. The nerve consists of two major divisions: superficial and deep. The superficial division has several branches that pass through the frontalis muscle to innervate the skin of the ipsilateral forehead. The deep division consists of one or more branches that travel at a deep level, just superficial to periosteum (Fig. 5). The deep division traverses laterally across the lower forehead at brow level and then cephalad just medial to the zone of attachment. This division finally innervates fronto-parietal scalp cephalad to the distribution of the superficial division. It is important to note the course of the deep division because it can be injured if the periosteum is violated during subperiosteal undermining during the endoscopic forehead-lift.

In approximately 10% of patients the deep division of the SON separates "earlier" from the main trunk of the nerve and emanates from its own bony foramen in the lower forehead. This separate foramen is usually 1 to 2-cm supero-lateral to the supraorbital foramen. To avoid injury to a potentially separate deep division of the SON, subperiosteal undermining over the lowermost frontal bone should be done under direct endoscopic visualization.

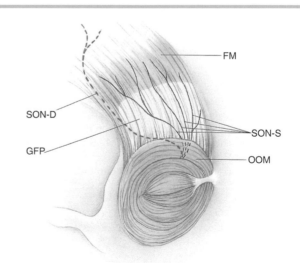

Figure 5 Supraorbital nerve. The supraorbital nerve has a superficial and a deep division. The superficial branches pass through the frontalis muscle to provide sensory innervation to the ipsilateral forehead skin. The deep division traverses laterally and in a cephalad direction, just medial to the zone of fixation, at a deep level just superficial to the periosteum. The deep division innervates the superior fronto-parietal region of the scalp. Also shown are the orbicularis oculi muscle and the position of the galea fat pad. *Abbreviations*: SON-D, supraorbital nerve-division; SON-S, supraorbital nerve-superficial; FM, frontalis muscle; GFP, galea fat pad; OOM, orbicularis oculi muscle.

The septum attaches circumferentially to the bony orbital rim and is a continuation of the DG from the forehead (Fig. 3). In both upper and lower lids, the deep layer of the eyelid margin is composed largely of the tarsal plate, a somewhat rigid cartilaginous structure. The orbital septum in each lid approaches the tarsal plate but fuses with another fascial layer (lid retractors) that itself attaches directly to the tarsal plate (Fig. 6). Each lid retractor is a musculo-fascial system whose function is to open the eye by retracting the eyelid. (The eye is closed via contraction of the sphincteric orbicularis oculi.) The lid retractor of the upper lid is the levator aponeurosis (elevated by the levator palpebrae muscle). The lower lid retractor is the capsulopalpebral fascia, which is attached to the inferior rectus extraocular muscle. (As the globe "looks downward" via contraction of the inferior rectus, the lower lid is retracted by the capsulopalpebral fascia.) Posterior to the orbital septum and anterior to the lid retractor layers lie the superficial components of the orbital fat pads (referred to as pre-aponeurotic fat).

One of the primary goals of cosmetic blepharoplasty is to remove excessive superficial orbital fat. The surgical approach to pre-aponeurotic fat must be precise in order to avoid injury to neighboring structures. In the upper lid, excessive skin (dermatochalasis) is almost always removed along with the intimately attached underlying orbicularis oculi muscle. If orbital fat is to also be removed, the orbital septum must be incised. The septum should be incised at a high (cephalad) level in order to avoid injuring the underlying levator aponeurosis, which merges with the septum near the upper edge of the tarsal plate. A division of the orbital septum should be performed cephalad to the level halfway between the upper edge of the tarsal plate and the superior orbital rim.

In the lower lid, the orbital septum should not be violated in order to minimize the risk of healing with contraction. If the orbital septum contracts, it may produce caudad pull on the lower lid, resulting in possible scleral show or even ectropion. The most direct access to the anterior orbital fat of the lower lid is through the conjunctiva of the inner lid and subjacent capsulopalpebral fascia (transconjunctival route). This approach avoids the orbital septum entirely.

PATIENT EVALUATION

During the initial consultation every patient should look into a mirror and describe the physical features that they would like to have improved. Although the primary problem may be brow ptosis, the patient may complain mainly of excessive upper eyelid skin. The need for brow elevation should be pointed out to the patient and the expected improvement in dermatochalasis by elevation of the lateral brow can be demonstrated by lifting the brow with one's finger. In many patients, the degree of brow elevation achieved by an endoscopic forehead-lift will not be adequate to fully correct the upper lid dermatochalasis. The additional benefits of the forehead-lift include significant improvement in glabellar and forehead rhytids. A patient who would like to achieve lateral brow elevation and wrinkle reduction is a suitable candidate for forehead-lift with subsequent blepharoplasty to eliminate residual dermatochalasis. Patients whose concerns are primarily dermatochalasis and herniated orbital fat may be better suited to blepharoplasty first, but they should understand that this procedure will not improve wrinkles and brow position.

Prior to blepharoplasty, careful history and evaluation of the eye, the orbit and peri-orbit are mandatory. Casual observation of the patient will elicit important physical and functional information. Deep forehead and glabellar wrinkles suggest brow ptosis. Upper lid ptosis, the result of weakness or stretching of the levator system, is suggested by asymmetry of lid position. The normal upper lid margin is halfway between the pupil and the upper limbus (the edge of the iris), a span that is typically 4 mm. The lower lid margin should cover the lower limbus (there should be no "scleral show").

Extraocular muscle function, accommodation, and pupillary light reflex should be assessed. Normal levator and lower lid retractor function can be tested by observing lid excursion accompanying upward and downward gaze, respectively. Lower lid tone should be evaluated with the distraction and snap back tests, in which the lower lid is distracted away from the globe and then released. Distraction distance should be 7 mm or less and the lid should snap back into position in less than one second. The presence of lower lid laxity or of frank ectropion or entropion should prompt referral for lid-tightening surgery, because blepharoplasty may exacerbate the problem. Correction of lid ptosis requires oculoplastic repair of the levator.

The patient should be asked to close the eyes, a maneuver accomplished by contraction of the orbicularis oculi (dependent on facial nerve integrity). Visual acuity should be documented by recent optometric testing or by in-office Snellen chart reading.

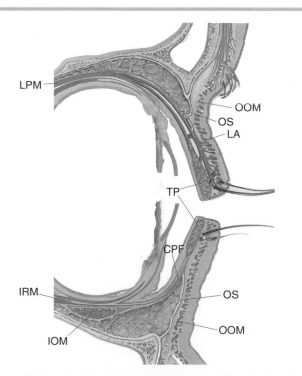

Figure 6 Cross-section of the eyelid and orbit at mid-pupillary level. A saggital cross-section shows in each lid, moving from superficial to deep, the orbicularis oculi muscle, the orbital septum, the pre-aponeurotic fat (not labeled), musculo-fascial system and the lid retractor layer. The retractor layer of the upper lid is the levator aponeurosis, which is retracted by the levator palpebrae muscle. The retractor layer of the lower lid is the capsulopalpebral fascia, which is retracted by the inferior rectus muscle. Also shown are the tarsal plate and the inferior oblique muscle. Abbreviations: OOM, orbicularis oculi muscle; OS, orbital septum; LPM, levator palpebrae muscle; CPF, capsulopalpebral fascia; IRM, inferior rectus muscle; TP, tarsal plate; IOM, inferior oblique muscle.

A history of dry eye as well as tolerance for contact lens use should be assessed. Contact lens intolerance may be a sign of marginal dry eye. Previous refractive surgery may predispose patients to dry eye symptoms.

A history of or predisposition to dry eye is a major concern because all blepharoplasties result in temporary worsening of dry eye. Removal of excessive eyelid tissue may result in chronic increased exposure to evaporation of the tear film. An ophthalmologic consultation is recommended prior to surgery. Tear production can be quantitated by the Schirmer test. After topical anesthesia (proparacaine HCl) a strip of number 41 filter paper is placed in the inferior cul-de-sac and the degree of wetting of the paper is measured after five minutes. Normal tear production will produce wetting of 10 mm or more. The quality of the tear film is another parameter that can be tested by the ophthalmologist.

Grave's disease is a multisystem autoimmune disorder with endocrine, ophthalmic, and cutaneous abnormalities. The most common manifestation, hyperthyroidism, may occur by itself or in combination with ophthalmopathy and/or dermopathy. The eye signs of Grave's disease are largely infiltrative and proliferative. In the retrobulbar area, extraocular muscles are enlarged because of fibroblast overactivity and production of excessive glycosaminoglycans. The engorged muscle cone causes proptosis (exophthalmos), which can result in a widening eye fissure. Unstable or progressive proptosis is a contraindication to cosmetic blepharoplasty and demands investigation. Because eye disease may be independent of thyroid pathology, thyroid studies may be normal. Patients who have been successfully treated for Grave's disease and who have limited and stable proptosis of greater than one year's duration may be considered for cosmetic blepharoplasty.

Preoperative laboratory evaluation should include complete blood count (with platelets), prothrombin time and International Normalized Ratio (INR). Strict adherence to preoperative avoidance of anticoagulant medications is essential. Aspirin must be discontinued at least 14 days prior to blepharoplasty.

TECHNIQUE: UPPER LID BLEPHAROPLASTY USING THE CO_2 LASER

The goal of upper lid blepharoplasty is to remove excess skin and orbital fat. Excess skin (dermatochalasis) causes the lid to appear heavy and redundant. Bulging orbital fat also contributes to upper lid fullness. In many cases, only the medial fat pad is excessive; in patients with heavier upper lids the central fat pad may also require reduction.

The most important step to assure an esthetically pleasing upper lid blepharoplasty is to properly mark the skin to be removed. The excised skin should be in the shape of a curvilinear ellipse that removes the bulk of the skin excess (Fig. 7). The first line drawn is the lower side of the excision. This line is placed in the natural crease of the upper lid (8–10 mm above the eyelid margin) and will define the postoperative eyelid crease. The line extends medially nearly to the level of the caruncle. The line (i.e., the lid crease) is higher in the mid portion of the lid than at either end of the lid; it is lower near the medial canthus that it is near the lateral canthus. The line extends lateral to the lateral canthus for varying distances (sometimes beyond the inner orbital rim) depending on the amount of "lateral hooding" (skin excess lateral to the canthus). Lateral to the canthus the line should extend into a "crow's foot" wrinkle slanted in a cephalad direction.

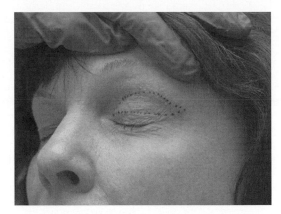

Figure 7 Markings for upper lid blepharoplasty.

The next line drawn is the upper side of the excision. The placement of this line will determine how much skin is excised. This marking must be done with great care. Inadequate skin removal will result in less than optimal improvement. Excessive skin removal could result in a postoperative lagophthalmos (inability to close the eye fully). During marking, the patient should be relaxed, with the eyes closed. A general guideline that will not result in excessive skin removal is to place the upper line at a level no higher than 12 mm below the lower edge of the eyebrow, at the midpoint of the lid (Fig. 8). To assess the amount of skin redundancy, curved tip forceps can be used to gently approximate the skin between the lower line and the proposed upper line; the patient's closed eyelid should not be opened (Fig. 9). This pinch test is performed at several sites along the planned excision to verify that skin removal will not be excessive.

Sedation and Anesthesia

Both upper and lower blepharoplasty as well as endoscopic forehead-lift can be safely performed using local anesthesia and low-dose intramuscular (IM) sedation. After upper lid markings are completed, sedation should be administered. For most patients midazolam 5-mg IM, along with hydroxyzine HCl 25-mg IM, provides adequate sedation. Monitoring oxygen saturation with pulse oximetry is mandatory.

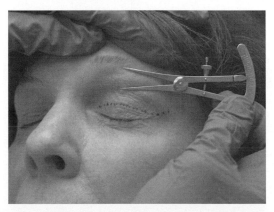

Figure 8 Measuring skin to be removed. The upper dotted line is placed at a level 12 mm below the eyebrow at the mid-pupillary level. The lower line is within the natural lid crease.

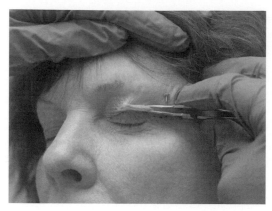

Figure 9 Pinch test to assess skin to be removed from upper lid.

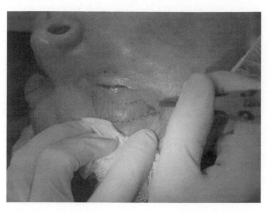

Figure 11 The initial skin incision with the focused CO_2 laser. (*See color insert.*)

Patients older than 65 years or with a history of reactive airway or obstructive pulmonary disease may be overly sensitive to respiratory depression and should receive an initial dose of 2.5-mg midazolam. Blood pressure should be monitored throughout the procedure.

The eye surface is anesthetized with proparacaine HCl ophthalmic drops. Then, an ophthalmic lubricant (e.g., Lacrilube®) is placed in the inferior fornix and spread over the corneal surface. Next, sterile stainless steel Cox scleral shields are placed on the scleral surfaces. After the shields are placed, local anesthesia solution (2%lidocaine HCl with epinephrine 1:100,000 buffered with 1/10 volume, 8.4% sodium bicarbonate) is instilled into upper eyelid skin. A total volume of 3 cc is typically injected using a 30-gauge needle (Fig. 10). The needle is placed intradermally at three points within the planned skin/muscle excision (any bruise from the needle will, therefore, be excised). Boluses of anesthetic can be spread laterally or medially by finger pressure. One should wait at least 15 minutes before surgical incision begins.

The focused continuous wave (CW) CO_2 laser is used to make the initial skin incision (Fig. 11), using a spot size of 0.2 mm or less and power settings of 5 W. The incision follows the outline drawn previously and is made just through the skin and into underlying muscle. Next, the skin/muscle flap is excised, from lateral to medial, with the laser set to 7 W (Fig. 12). Lateral to the lateral canthus the division is kept relatively superficial, leaving most of the orbicularis muscle

intact. There are frequently larger blood vessels deeper in the muscle in this area, which are thus avoided. Medial to the lateral canthus, the division is done at a deeper level, immediately on the surface of the orbital septum, thus removing the entire thickness of muscle along with the attached skin. A curved, burnished bone plate is used as a backdrop during final excision near the medial canthus (Fig. 13). Defocused laser energy is used to coagulate any bleeding vessels as well as the exposed orbicularis muscle in the lateral area of the excision (in order to minimize postoperative "crow's feet" wrinkles).

If orbital fat is to be removed, the focused laser energy is then used to incise the orbital septum. Gentle finger pressure on the globe will cause the orbital fat to exude, increasing its exposure. The septum should be excised at a level cephalad to the point halfway between the upper edge of the tarsal plate and the superior orbital rim (in order to avoid injury to the underlying levator aponeurosis as discussed under Anatomy). After an initial buttonhole incision is made, a saline-soaked cotton-tipped applicator can be inserted beneath the septum to be incised, to serve as a backdrop for the laser.

Fragments of orbital fat are then similarly excised using slightly defocused laser energy to provide coagulation (Fig. 14). To remove medial fat, the incision through the septum is extended in an infero-nasal direction. The medial fat is whiter in color than central fat and is removed as described above. Any bleeding vessels should be coagulated

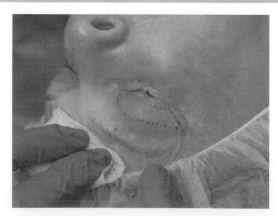

Figure 10 Upper lid after injection of local anesthetic solution (surgeon's view).

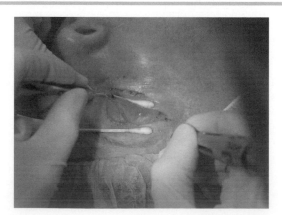

Figure 12 Excising the skin/muscle flap with the focused CO_2 laser. (*See color insert.*)

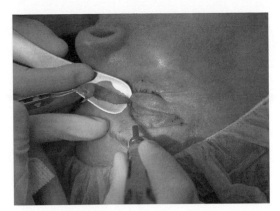

Figure 13   A burnished bone plate is used as a backdrop for the laser near the medial canthus. (*See color insert.*)

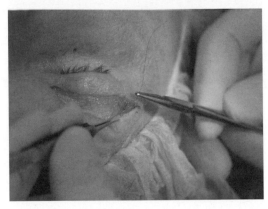

Figure 15   Suture "bites" are taken 2 mm from the laser-incised wound edge. (*See color insert.*)

with defocused laser energy or bipolar electrocautery. Bipolar energy should be used with great care to avoid contact with any conductive material (such as stainless steel scleral shields). Assessment of the completeness of fat removal is accomplished by applying gentle pressure on the globe and observing any residual fat herniation.

Upon completion of one lid, a cotton ball soaked in local anesthetic is applied to the wound; while, blepharoplasty is performed on the contralateral lid. After a final check for hemostasis, the scleral shields are removed and the wound edges are sutured. Because of laser-induced thermal damage to the incised skin edges, while suturing, a bite of no less than 2 mm should be made on either side of the wound (Fig. 15). If smaller bites are taken, the sutures may dehisce a few days later. After the most lateral wound edges are carefully approximated, the remaining sutures are placed using the "rule of halves" to assure that sutures are evenly distributed (Fig. 16). Frequently, the lids are pulled slightly open after the blepharoplasty wound is sutured because the volume of local anesthetic has not yet been absorbed.

Ice packs are applied to each lid surface and the patient is kept for observation for at least one hour. For the remainder of the day, the patient should apply ice packs for periods of 15 minutes every half hour. During sleep, head elevation (at least one extra pillow) helps to minimize edema on the following morning. The patient is seen the next day and returns at seven days for suture removal. After sutures are removed, Steri-Strips™ can be placed over the incision.

Complications

The most feared complication is postoperative hemorrhage. Minor oozing of blood tinged local anesthetic solution is expected during the first few hours. Superficial bleeding (anterior to the orbital septum) may cause bruising or hematoma. Active bleeding mandates a return to surgery to locate and coagulate the responsible vessel.

More serious is the bleeding posterior to the orbital septum. A retrobulbar hematoma may threaten the optic nerve or retinal artery via compression of their blood supply, and may lead to blindness. Retrobulbar hemorrhage is a medical emergency. The patient's caregiver should be instructed to call urgently if significant unilateral bruising, pain, or vision loss develops, and the patient should be seen promptly. Severe bruising accompanied by proptosis, pain, or vision loss may indicate retrobulbar hemorrhage. Ophthalmologic consultation should be immediately procured. Retrobulbar hemorrhage is managed by surgical lysis of the lateral canthal tendon (lateral canthotomy) and medical treatment to lower intraocular pressure.

Blepharoplasty is fraught with many more potential complications, including damage to extraocular muscles, the levator aponeurosis, lacrimal gland, and cornea;

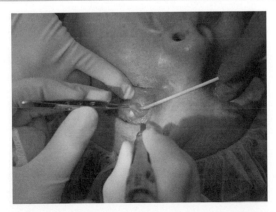

Figure 14   Fragments of orbital fat are excised using defocused laser energy. (*See color insert.*)

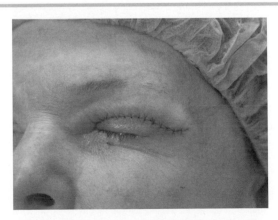

Figure 16   Final sutures in place. (*See color insert.*)

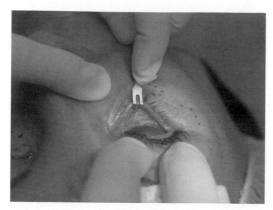

Figure 17 The transconjunctival incision is made approximately 5 mm from the lower lid margin and is directed toward the orbital rim. (*See color insert.*)

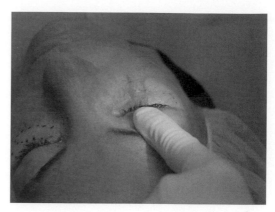

Figure 19 Completeness of fat removal is assessed by applying gentle pressure to the globe and observing for bulging of fat pads. (*See color insert.*)

lagophthalmos and eyelid malposition; dry eye; and under- or over-resection of orbital fat. These complications and their management are discussed in detail in books on blepharoplasty.

TECHNIQUE: TRANSCONJUNCTIVAL LOWER LID BLEPHAROPLASTY USING THE CO₂ LASER

Preoperative markings are optional and can include outlining the three orbital fat pads. If fat is more prominent on one side, the involved fat pad can be highlighted as a reminder that more fat should be removed from that side.

Sedation and placement of scleral shields are performed as described above. A block of the infraorbital nerve is performed. As an assistant retracts the lower lid, local anesthetic is injected into the lower lid via the conjunctiva. A 1 in. 30-gauge needle is directed toward the lower orbital rim and is advanced to the rim. Anesthetic is injected, as the needle is withdrawn, into the orbital fat, retractor layer, and conjunctiva. The central lid receives 1.5 cc. The medial and lower lid each receive 0.75 cc (3 cc total). Surgery is delayed for 15 minutes to allow for vasoconstriction.

As an assistant retracts the lower lid, gentle pressure on the globe is applied using a bone plate. The focused CO₂ laser at 5 W power is then used to incise through the conjunctiva over most of the horizontal length of the lid.

This incision should be made at a level approximately 5 mm caudal to the lid margin, and is directed toward the underlying orbital rim (Fig. 17). A second pass is then made using 7 W of power in order to incise more deeply through the lid retractor layer (capsulopalpebral fascia). The incision is deepened while pressure is applied to the globe, causing orbital fat to extrude (Fig. 18). Fat fragments are excised using slightly defocused laser energy as described above.

Incisions are deepened over each fat pad (while pressure is applied to the globe) and fat fragments are excised. As in the upper lid, the medial fat is whitish in color and lies near larger blood vessels. Hemostasis is achieved as described above. The inferior oblique muscle is often identified between the medial and central fat pads. Injury to the muscle is avoided by incising only orbital fat that extrudes during pressure on the globe. The lateral fat pad is generally more difficult to access via the transconjunctival route but will present more readily if pressure on the globe is applied more medially (closer to the nose). An assistant can also "push" the lateral fat into the operative field using a cotton-tipped applicator. Completeness of fat removal should be repeatedly assessed, with all instruments withdrawn, by applying gentle pressure to the globe (Fig. 19). This simulation of gravity will cause residual fat to bulge. The final distribution of fat removed from each fat pad should be recorded (Fig. 20).

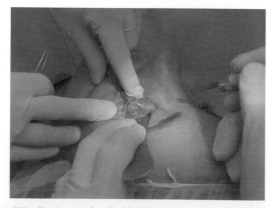

Figure 18 The transconjunctival incision is deepened while gentle pressure is applied to the globe, causing the central orbital fat to extrude. (*See color insert.*)

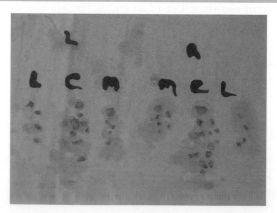

Figure 20 The amount of excised fat from each fat pad (lateral, central, and medial) is assessed. (*See color insert.*)

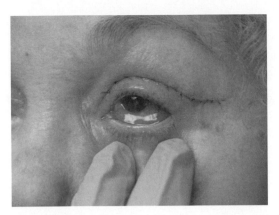

Figure 21 Edema of the bulbar conjunctiva produces a gelatinous appearance (chemosis).

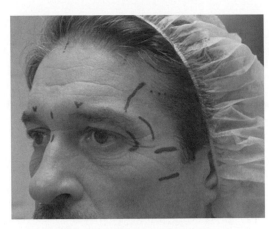

Figure 22 Preoperative markings for endoscopic forehead-lift. At the glabella, the midline and supraorbital notches are marked. Solid lines demarcate the inner and outer lateral orbital rim, the superior and inferior edges of the zygomatic arch, and the palpable temporal crest. Dotted lines indicate the sites of the midline, para-medial, and temple incisions.

After a final check for hemostasis, the scleral shields are removed. The incised conjunctival edges should be in apposition to each other. No sutures are needed. Ice packs are applied and postoperative care is given as described above for upper blepharoplasty.

Complications

Many of the complications associated with upper blepharoplasty are also encountered in lower transconjunctival blepharoplasty (see previous discussion). One complication unique to the lower lid procedure is chemosis: edema of the bulbar conjunctiva (Fig. 21). This edema results from inflammation associated with healing of the palpebral conjunctival incision. The swelling results in a gelatinous appearance and can be treated with corticosteroid eye drops (e.g., dexamethasone) or with nonsteroidal anti-inflammatory drops (e.g., ketorolac tromethamine). Chemosis generally improves within a few days of initiating treatment.

TECHNIQUE: ENDOSCOPIC FOREHEAD-LIFT

The purpose of endoscopic forehead-lift is to provide long-lasting elevation to the ptotic soft tissues of the forehead and temple. Attachments of more superficial soft-tissue layers to underlying structures must be released in order to allow cephalad movement. After advancement, the mobilized layers will reattach to the fixed underlying layers, providing long-term elevation. Use of an endoscope enables the procedure to be accomplished through minimal incisions and increases safety because many anatomic features can be visually identified. The described technique includes avulsion of glabellar muscles and neurotomies of terminal motor nerve supply to some of these muscles.

After preoperative photographs are obtained, the patient is marked (Fig. 22). Five incisions to be used for entry of the endoscope are marked with dotted lines within the frontal and parental scalp. In the forehead, three sagittally oriented 1.5-cm incisions are marked just behind the frontal hairline. These include a midline site and two paramedian sites (each 5 cm from the midline). Two oblique 3-cm incisions are marked within the temporal hair, 2 to 3 cm behind the hairline. The temporal incisions are lateral to the temporal crest and lie over the superior part of the temporalis muscle.

The palpable temporal crest is marked with a solid line, as are the superior and inferior edges of the zygomatic arch and the inner and outer lateral orbital rim. The palpable supraorbital notches, which are generally about 2.7 cm from the midline, are also marked with a "V."

Sedation for this procedure is given as for blepharoplasty. Local anesthesia consists of nerve blocks and tumescent infiltration. The supraorbital and supratrochlear nerves are blocked using 0.5% bupivacaine with epinephrine 1:200,000. The zygomaticotemporal and zygomaticofacial nerves are similarly blocked. Tumescent anesthetic solution is prepared as outlined in Table 1. This solution is instilled subcutaneously, using a 27-gauge needle on a 10-cc syringe, at the incision sites and in the temple (30–40 cc per side). In the temple, the area inferior to the incision, anterior to the ear, and superior to the zygomatic arch is infiltrated. The needle is pushed to bone in the lateral orbital rim to provide deep anesthesia to this area. Tumescent solution (approximately 10 cc) is also injected across the brow and glabella (within the superficial musculature).

Table 1 Composition of Tumescent Anesthetic Solution for Endoscopic Forehead Lift

Ingredient	Stock concentration	Volume	Amount	Final concentration
Sodium Chloride (normal saline)	0.9%	500 mL		
Lidocaine HCl	2%	50 mL	1000 mg	0.18%
Epinephrine	1 mg/mL (1:1000)	2 mL	2 mg	3.6 mg/L (1:278,500)
Sodium Bicarbonate	8.4% (1 mEq/mL)	5 mL	5 mEq	9 mEq/L

Note: The indicated volumes of stock solutions of lidocaine HCl, epinephrine, and sodium bicarbonate are added to a 500-mL bag of normal saline.

Next, incisions are made. The three forehead incisions are taken down to bone. In the temple, the incisions are made just through the dermis. Then iris scissors are used to bluntly dissect (by spreading the scissor tips) through subcutaneous tissue and through each of the three layers of superficial temporal fascia until the deep temporal fascia is reached. The deep fascia is striated in appearance and is immobile; all superficial tissue will move along with the skin when tested by finger motion. It is important to verify that the dissection has reached the level of the deep temporal fascia, which is generally 8 to 10 mm deep to the skin surface.

Undermining in the forehead is done at the subperiosteal level. A periosteal elevator is introduced through each of the three forehead incisions. Movements of the instrument directly on bone are verified by a slightly "gritty" sound and feel. The release is done blindly and is relatively easy cephalad to the level approximately 2 cm above the brow, below which the periosteum is much more firmly attached to bone. The area of blind subperiosteal release should extend from 2-cm cephalad to the incisions to 2-cm cephalad to brow level and lateral to the zone of fixation, where the periosteum is also much more adherent to bone. In the lowermost forehead, the undermining should be done under endoscopic visualization in order to avoid injuring a potentially separate deep division of the SON (present in 10% of cases).

From the temple incisions, the periosteal elevator is introduced and is used to undermine on the surface of the deep temporal fascia. This release should extend from 1-cm cephalad to the incision to the superior edge of the ear and anterior along the superior border of the zygomatic arch. Anterior of the midpoint of the zygomatic arch, and along the lateral orbital rim, within approximately 2 cm of these structures, the release becomes more difficult because the superficial and deep temporal fasciae fuse. This region of fusion includes the course of the temporal branch rami of the facial nerve; undermining in this area should be done with endoscopic guidance to ensure that the nerve is protected (see below).

From the temple incision, the periosteal elevator is used to bluntly release the upper half of the zone of fixation, always from lateral to medial (and requiring significant force). Continuity is, thus, established between the temple dissection (just superficial to deep temporal fascia) and the forehead dissection (subperiosteal). Only the upper half of the zone is released blindly.

The endoscope is used to guide all further dissections. The endoscope is introduced through the paramedial forehead incision. Release of the lower zone of fixation is accomplished using small Metzenbaum scissors introduced through the temple incision (Fig. 23). The zone is released, caudad down to the level of the orbital rim. The frontal periosteum is released down to and just over the superior orbital rim. The supraorbital neurovascular bundle is identified (Fig. 24). More laterally, the lower and anterior temple is undermined. This division must be kept at the level of deep temporal fascia. The adherent superficial temporal fascia is separated from the deep fascia using a scissor-tip spreading technique. The medial zygomaticotemporal vein (sentinel vein) is encountered in the infero-medial temple and becomes visible upon development of the space between the deep and superficial temporal fasciae (Fig. 25). This vein serves as a landmark for the "danger zone" in which the temporal branch rami are running within the superficial temporal fascia.

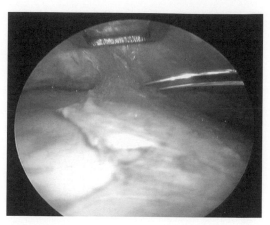

Figure 23 Endoscopic view of the lower zone of fixation. Scissors are used to release the connective tissue. (*See color insert.*)

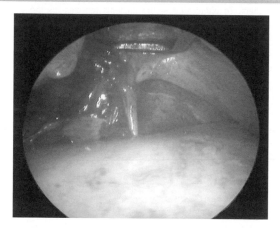

Figure 24 Endoscopic view of the supraorbital neurovascular bundle. In the foreground is the lower frontal bone. The periosteum (upper part of image) has been raised and incised just caudal to the orbital rim. (*See color insert.*)

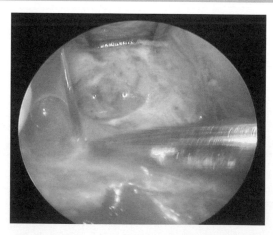

Figure 25 Endoscopic view of the lower temple dissection. The medial zygomaticotemporal vein (sentinel vein) is visible on the left side of the image. (*See color insert.*)

Over the superior zygoma and lateral orbital rim, the dissection is done at the supraperiosteal level. Lateral to the lateral canthus the PCL connects the periosteum of the lateral orbital rim to the overlying SMAS. This ligament should be partly or totally severed to enhance suspension

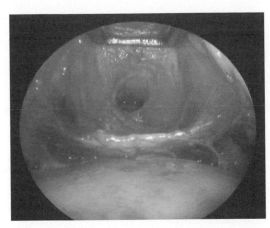

Figure 26 Endoscopic view of the glabella. The lower frontal bone is in the foreground. The left and right procerus muscles are visible below the steel dissector and have been separated by the previous passage of a probe between them. To either side of the procerus muscles lay the depressor supercilii muscles (through which run the supratrochlear veins). Closer to the foreground and obliquely oriented are the corrugator supercilii muscles. (*See color insert.*)

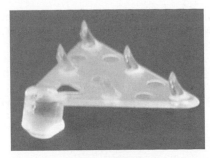

Figure 27 The biodegradable Endotine™ anchoring device. The cylindrical component is inserted into a hole that is drilled into the skull table. Five sharp tines engage the suspended soft tissues.

of the superficial temporal fascia. More medially, across (and just caudal to) the superior orbital rim, the periosteum should be released in the area between the orbital ligament and the supraorbital neurovascular bundle. This release is accomplished with sharp-tipped scissors. Next, the overlying DG layer (see Fig. 3) is similarly released.

After all soft-tissue releases are effected, attention is directed toward the glabella. The periosteum is incised at the level of the orbital rim and a periosteal elevator is pushed into the glabellar space. The space is opened by moving the instrument to the root of the nose and then back-and-forth. Through the endoscope the glabellar muscles are identified (Fig. 26). Myotomies of the procerus and depressor supercilii are performed; the muscle tissue is avulsed by spreading the sharp tips of scissors. Branches of the supratrochlear nerve are visible within the avulsed fibers of the depressor supercilii.

In the suprabrow region, a myotomy is performed at the juncture of corrugator supercilii and orbicularis oculi. Just lateral to the level of the supraorbital neurovascular bundle, and superior to the brow, sharp-tipped scissors are used to puncture, and then spread, the periosteum (the periosteum is not cut because the deep division of the SON may run just superficial to this layer). The scissor tips are used to cut the more superficial muscle tissue, up to the level of the dermis. Just medial to the supraorbital neurovascular bundle, a similar incision through periosteum is performed to effect a neurotomy of the terminal motor nerve branch to the corrugator, which runs in this area.

(A) **(B)** **(C)**

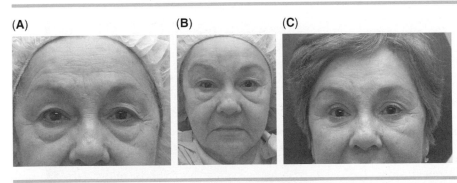

Figure 28 This 69-year-old female patient is shown before surgery (**A**), after endoscopic forehead-lift (**B**) and after subsequent upper and lower transconjunctival laser blepharoplasty (**C**). In (**B**), note improvement in upper lid dermatochalasis and reduced glabellar and forehead rhytids.

(A) **(B)**

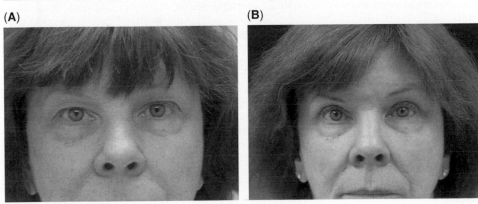

Figure 29 This 61-year-old female patient is shown before (**A**) and after (**B**) upper lid laser blepharoplasty.

(A)

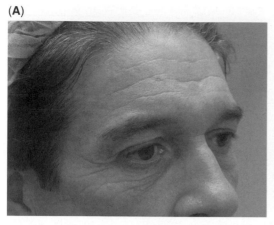

(B)

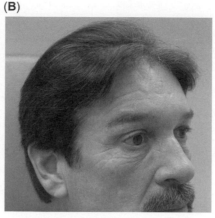

Figure 30 This 59-year-old male patient is shown before (**A**) and after (**B**) endoscopic forehead-lift. Note improved brow position and upper lid dermatochalasis, and lessened glabellar and forehead rhytids.

(A)

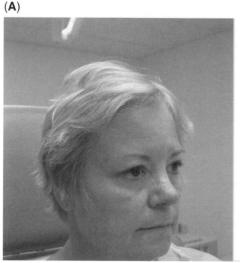

(B)

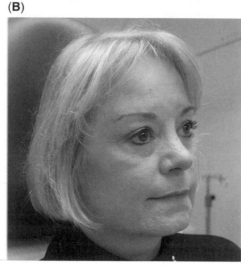

Figure 31 This 53-year-old female patient is shown before (**A**) and after (**B**) endoscopic forehead-lift. Note improved brow position and upper lid dermatochalasis, and lessened glabellar and forehead rhytids.

Finally, multiple incisions throughout the soft tissues deep to the lateral brow are performed. Beneath the brow, all soft tissue up to the dermis is cut with the scissor tips, in the region between the supraorbital neurovascular bundle and the lateral brow. These incisions accomplish myotomies of orbicularis oculi and neurotomies of motor nerve supply to frown muscles (see Fig. 4).

A small Jackson-Pratt drain is placed subperiosteally at brow level. The drain passes through a small stab wound just behind (lateral to) the temporal hairline and extends across the forehead to the contralateral temple. The drain is held in place with an anchoring suture and a vacuum bulb is attached.

The Endotine anchoring device is used to suspend the lateral brow. This biodegradable device (Fig. 27) is placed in a drill hole in the skull table just lateral to the lower end of each paramedial upper forehead incision. The forehead tissues are elevated *en bloc* and anchored by pushing down on the multiple tines of the device, which pierce the periosteum to provide anchorage. Within two weeks the periosteum re-adheres firmly to bone. At the temple incisions, sutures (2-0 Vicryl, Ethicon, Somerville, New Jersey, U.S.) are used to suspend the superficial temple tissue. The suture is placed through superior temporal fascia of the undermined temple flap and through deep temporal fascia cephalad to the incision site. Tying this suture elevates the temple flap.

All five incisions are closed with buried sutures (Vicryl). At the three central incisions, the suture includes all soft-tissue layers, including periosteum (in order to prevent a postoperative depression). Final skin closure is with 5-0 Prolene (Ethicon, Somerville, New Jersey, U.S.).

A head-wrap style dressing provides mild compression and incorporates the vacuum bulb of the drain. The patient returns one day later, at which time the drain is pulled out. Surface sutures are removed after seven days.

Complications

Although undermining is performed in relatively avascular planes, some bruising is typical after endoscopic forehead-lift. Bruising is mainly the result of muscle avulsion and myotomies and appears primarily in the infraorbital area. Bruising can be significantly reduced by the placement of a drain postoperatively.

Transient neuropraxia of the temporal branch of the facial nerve is not uncommon. Compression or irritation of the temporal branch rami during undermining in the temple may result in a unilateral paresis of the frontalis muscle. The use of a fixation device such as the Endotine minimizes brow ptosis and assures that tissue layers readhere at the appropriate suspended level. Neuropraxia typically resolves within a few weeks.

Sensory nerve deficits are much less common with the endoscopic method compared to traditional coronal forehead-lift. With careful technique, there is generally no transection of sensory nerve branches. Hyperesthesia over the distribution of the deep division of the SON (superior fronto-parietal scalp) may result from nerve irritation caused by the tines of the Endotine. These symptoms may persist for several weeks and will diminish as the device dissolves.

CLINICAL RESULTS

Patients who have undergone laser blepharoplasty of the upper lids are demonstrated in Figures 28 and 29. A patient who underwent laser blepharoplasty of the lower lids is seen in Figure 28. Patients who received endoscopic forehead-lift are seen in Figures 28,30 and 31.

BIBLIOGRAPHY

Isse NG. Endoscopic facial rejuvenation. Clin Plast Surg 1997; 24:213–231.

Knize DM. The Forehead and Temporal Fossa: Anatomy and Technique. Philadelphia: Lippincott Williams and Wilkins, 2001.

Knize DM. Muscles that act on glabellar skin: a closer look. Plast Reconstr Surg 2000; 105:350–361.

Krejci-Papa NC, Langdon RC. Skin aging in three dimensions. In: Krutmann J, Gilchrest BA, eds. Skin Aging. Berlin: Springer-Verlag. (In press).

Langdon RC, Herbich GJ. The mid-face suspension lift. In: Moy R, ed. Procedures in Cosmetic Dermatology Series: Face-lift. Edinburgh: Elsevier. (In press).

Langdon RC, Sattler G, Hanke CW. Minimum incision face lift. In: Robinson J, et al., eds. Surgery of the Skin. Edinburgh: Elsevier, 2005.

Spinelli HM. Atlas of Aesthetic Eyelid and Periocular Surgery. Philadelphia: Saunders, 2004.

Wolfort FG, Kanter WR. Aesthetic Blepharoplasty. Boston: Little, Brown, 1995.

80

Facelift Surgery

Hayes B. Gladstone
Stanford University, Stanford, California, U.S.A.

Greg S. Morganroth
*University of California, San Francisco, California and Stanford University, Stanford,
California, U.S.A.*

INTRODUCTION

Perhaps the most dramatic intervention in esthetic surgery is the face-lift. It has become a symbol for what is good and bad in cosmetic surgery. If it is performed in the appropriate patient, and with meticulous technique and appropriate vectors, it can produce a very satisfying, natural-appearing rejuvenation. Yet, it is not a forgiving procedure. If the superficial musculoaponeurotic system (SMAS) and skin are pulled too tight and in a horizontal manner, the patient will have a wind tunnel, saran wrap appearance, which neither produces a youthful look nor a happy patient.

Historically, rhytidectomies have been reserved for those in their sixth and seventh decades. Similar to most other cosmetic procedures, the large majority of face-lifts have been performed in females. Yet, with increased longevity of life, an emphasis on physical well being and activity in the baby boomer generation, as well as increased competitiveness in the workplace, lifting procedures are now more common in those in their 40s and 50s and in men. Because these patients have less facial laxity, and are very concerned about minimizing downtime, there have been adaptations to the standard face-lift to maximize results with a shorter recovery. The length of the incision, and whether to involve the neck needs to be tailored to each individual. While always significant, understanding the extent of anatomical changes and patient desires has taken on a new degree of importance. No longer does one face-lift fit all. Dermatologic surgery with its emphasis on minimally invasive surgical procedures has played an important role in this change. Dermasurgeons have substantially contributed to developing the short scar face-lift, incorporating liposuction into the procedure and performing this method under local anesthesia using the tumescent technique.

While it is not clear which specialty first performed the face-lift, Marie Noel, a Parisian cosmetic dermatologist popularized the procedure in the early 20th century (Fig. 1). Her book La Chirurgie Esthetique Son Role Sociale, published in 1926, described her face-lift technique, which she had been practicing for the past decade. Her version included only a short preauricular skin incision. While this method was minimally invasive and produced some improvement along the jaw line, it was not long lasting. Over the next several decades, the incision was lengthened into the temporal hairline, and in the postauricular region including the hairline. These modifications developed by plastic surgeons under general anesthesia produced more dramatic results, but again did not last long. Sagging would return within one to two years. Because of these short-lived changes, the face-lift fell into disrepute.

In the 1970s, revival of the rhytidectomy was due to the description and role of the superficial muscular aponeurotic system by Mitz and Peyronie. Skoog, a plastic surgeon, incorporated it into his lifts and made other modifications, which produced long-lasting results. Webster, a facial plastic surgeon, added further refinements and made important contributions in describing plication and imbrication of the SMAS. The face-lift enjoyed a new popularity, particularly among movie stars and the jet set. It was longer lasting, and usually effected a dramatic change, one that was very noticeable and in many patients produced the telltale wind tunnel look.

In the 1980s, dermatologic surgeons such as Chrisman and Fields described using less invasive techniques including liposuction to produce face-lift-like results. The development of tumescent anesthesia by Klein enabled less invasive procedures under local. Because of the perceived limitations of the supra SMAS face-lift in terms of results, longevity, and lack of mid-face-lifting, in the early 1990s, Hamra and Kamer among others developed the deep plane face-lift. This approach addressed some of the issues, but also was a technically more demanding procedure with greater down time, and a higher potential for facial nerve injury. The subperiosteal face-lift promised long-term results with a less risk of complications; yet the reported down time was still significant. In the mid to late part of the decade, the face-lift approaches swung toward less invasive methods. The composite approach incorporated aspects of both the deep plane and the traditional rhytidectomy. The endoscopic face-lift utilized small incisions, but did not appear to have dramatic results or to be long lived.

In dermatologic surgery, practitioners were focused on improving the neck and jowls through minimally invasive liposuction. Cooke described his "weekend" face-lift. Saylan, at the end of the century, adapted Noel's face-lift by incorporating SMAS plication with a short anterior incision. He popularized the S-lift, which improved the lower third of the face with minimal recovery time. Saylan and Fulton followed by Alster and Hopping demonstrated that this lift could be combined with careful laser resurfacing to optimize lower face rejuvenation. While this approach has

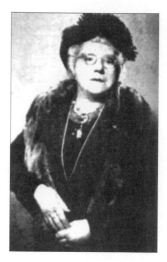

Figure 1 Suzanne Noel.

some significant limitations such as not addressing the neck and providing only a very moderate lift and a questionable longevity, it galvanized the surgeons in all of the esthetic specialties to reexamine the face-lift. This short scar approach also satisfied the public's demand for instant results and minimal down time from daily activities.

Concurrent with the emphasis on a shorter excision was the reexamination of the importance of facial volume, and loss as one ages. Practitioners from dermatologic surgery, facial plastics, and plastic surgery all contributed to using pan facial fat transfer to restore facial volume and fill the deflated skin envelope. In regard to lifting procedures, both Hamra and Little elaborated on the three dimensional aspects of facial volume.

Baker combined these concepts with a lateral SMA-Sectomy and a shortened scar, which provided tightening without flattening the face. Another major modification of the face-lift has been "vector verticalization." Tonnard and Verpaele described a plication technique using multiple purse strings oriented in a near 90° angle to the jaw line.

The authors have combined all of the above minimally invasive techniques while adding further modifications. With this approach, the 21st century patient can have near full face-lift-like results, but without undergoing general anesthesia and having an extended recovery time. In addition, the extent of incision, liposuction, and plication is tailored to the individual's needs.

RELEVANT FACIAL ANATOMY

The lower face is bounded superiorly by an imaginary horizontal line from the earlobe, traversing across the cheek to the base of the columella and extending across the contralateral cheek and earlobe. The inferior border of the lower face is demarcated by the mandibular line. The superior portion of the neck extends from the mandibular line to the thyroid notch. In the lower face, the soft tissue envelope includes skin, subcutaneous fat, SMAS, and muscle. In the upper neck, the layers are similar, though the platysma is continuous with the SMAS. A subplatysmal fat pad is located in the midline. Other structures include the submandibular glands that are located in the fascial plane at the anterior aspect of the mandible bilaterally, and the hyoid

bone, which is located in the anterior neck deep to the strap musculature.

The sensory innervation of the lower face is provided by the third branch of the trigeminal nerve. In the postauricular region, C2 and C3 contribute to the greater auricular nerve, which innervates the lower portion of the auricle. The facial nerve provides the major motor innervation of the face and neck. The temporal branch innervates the frontalis muscle and courses most superficially at the malar arch. The marginal mandibular branch innervates the lip depressor muscles. It runs slightly inferior to the mandible before traveling more superficially as it reaches the lip commissures. While the zygomatic and buccal branches are susceptible to injury, there are many anastomoses between them, so that functional impairment if traumatized is usually minimal and transient. In the neck, the platysma is innervated by the cervical branch of the facial nerve. The spinal accessory nerve is found in the posterior triangle, but runs across the body of the sternocleidomastoid, and is susceptible to injury. The blood supply of the lower face consists of branches of the facial arteries. There is an analogous venous system, which has many perforators. Branches from the external carotid supply the majority of the neck.

The two major anatomic structures that influence the appearance of the lower face are the SMAS and the platysma. The SMAS is fascia that invests the facial mimetic musculature, and is intimately related to the skin by ligamentous attachments. It connects with the galea superiorly and inferiorly with the platysma (Fig. 2).

The platysma is the shield-like thin muscle that originates from the pectoralis fascia, extends to the neck, ultimately interdigitating with the SMAS, and attaching to the risorius muscle. In most individuals, the platysma decussates—intertwines at the midline. Yet, in a significant minority—39% in one study—the platysma divides at the midline. Combined with concomitant hypertrophy from years of lower facial expression, platysmal banding results in a gobbler-like appearance (Fig. 3).

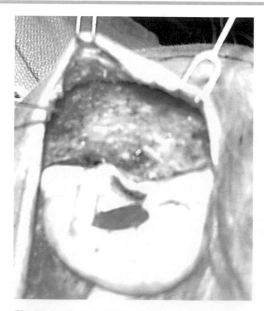

Figure 2 The superficial musculoaponeurotic system.

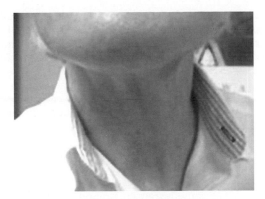

Figure 3 Example of platysmal bands.

FACIAL ESTHETICS AND GOALS OF THE RHYTIDECTOMY

The foundation of western facial analysis is based on the golden proportion. It initially was addressed by the Egyptians, defined by the Greeks, and expanded and popularized for the face by Leonardo da Vinci. This proportion addresses the relationship between the division of a single line into two unequal parts. The ratio of the shorter line to the longer line is the same as that of the longer line to the whole. Mathematically, this is represented by a ratio of 1:1.618. The Greeks felt that this proportion was naturally pleasing. Da Vinci applied this both to the horizontal and vertical proportions of the face. Optimally, the facial height: width ratio is 4:3. Ideal facial width can be divided into five equal parts. Each division is equal to one eye width. Vertically, the face is divided into thirds. Though the eyes are included in discussions about the upper face, anatomically, the upper third of the face is defined superiorly by the hairline, and by the inferior extent of the eyebrow. The mid-face extends from this level to the base of the nasal tip. The lower third is bounded by the base of the nose and the chin. Each third is equal in length.

How the face relates to the neck is an important anatomic esthetic consideration. This relationship can be measured in several ways. The classic method is to determine the angle between the vertical neck and the submandibular plane. This cervicomental angle should be less than 120°. Ellenbogen referred to the angle bound by the submentum and the sternocleidomastoid muscle because it was easier to visually assess. The SM–SCM angle should be 90 degrees to provide a youthful look (Fig. 4).

Many factors contribute to the structural changes of the aging face. For many years, it was felt that gravity played the dominant role in the aged face. While it certainly is a contributor, photodamage, loss and redistribution of fat, muscle atrophy and hypertrophy, bony reabsorption, and genetics produce sagging and jowling. Solar elastosis and collagen damage in the skin create rhytides and a superficial flaccidity. Loss of fat in the periorbital region, malar region, and lower cheeks causes a hollowness and volumetric decrease that contributes to sagging. Fat accumulation in the upper neck blunts the cervicomental angle. Muscle atrophy, particularly in the temporal region, leads to volumetric changes, decreasing anchoring points, and consequently increases the sagging of the more superficial tissues. Hypertrophy as well as separation of the platysma produces bands that disrupt the cervicomental angle and the smooth neck contour. Over time, the face's bony foundation, which provides buttresses for the soft tissues, reabsorbs. This reabsorption is particularly apparent in the lower face. This phenomenon leads to more volume depletion, hollowing, and sagging of the more superficial tissues.

To optimally correct these deficits in order to restore a youthful appearance, a comprehensive approach should be taken. Recently, much attention has been devoted to volume correction. An infant's face has been used as an example of what to strive for; however, in examining an individual in their third decade, there is "angular roundness" to their face and neck (Fig. 5). It retains the softness of youth, but also the hard edge of adulthood. A properly executed rhytidectomy with fairly steep vector angles and concomitant neck liposuction with prudent sculpting in the lower face along with platysmaplasty will restore this angular roundness. A chin implant can dramatically enhance this quality. Adjuvant procedures such as fat transfer or synthetic filler substances will supplement the volume and recreate symmetry, while laser resurfacing and chemical peels can generate a smooth, homogenous surface.

(A) **(B)**

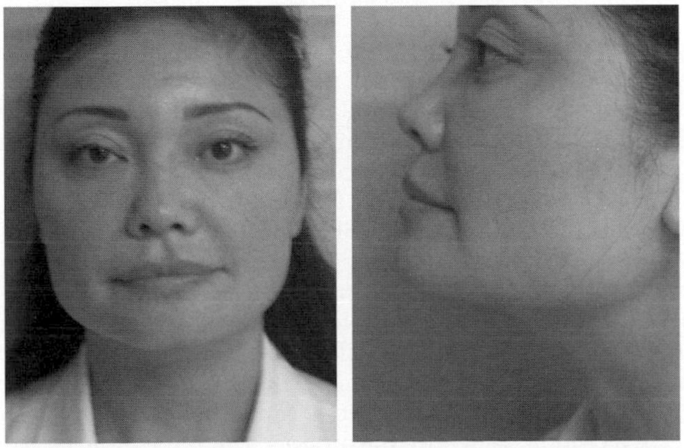

Figure 4 (A, B) Frontal and profile of angle. A youthful submental-sternocleidomastoid angle.

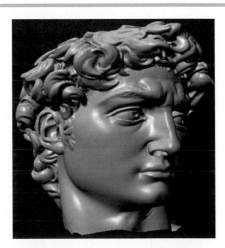

Figure 5 Angular roundness of the lower face, which is considered a youthful quality.

Patient Criteria

In the past, rhytidectomies have been reserved for those patients in their sixth decade or older, who generally have severe skin laxity. The vast majority of these patients have been women. Yet, face-lifts can and should be customized to the needs of the individual. Because the current philosophy that facial rejuvenation should be performed gradually over decades in order to maintain a natural appearance, an individual in their early 40s may be appropriate for a short scar face-lift. As long as the patient can tolerate the procedure and has no underlying medical condition that would contraindicate the procedure, age really is not a major factor particularly since this procedure can be performed under local anesthesia. The age ceiling is determined by the health and vibrancy of the individual.

The determining physiologic criteria are the lower face and neck soft tissue laxity. The degree of laxity is a combination of genetic, Fitzpatrick Skin Type, and sun exposure/protection factors. A fair-skinned 40-year-old native Californian who has not protected herself from the sun may be an excellent candidate for a short scar face-lift.

With the baby boomer generation, there is an increasing number of men undergoing lifting procedures. The criteria of jowling and neck flaccidity are no different in men. However, as will be discussed below, the anesthesia, incision, and occasionally the postoperative care may be modified.

Patient Consult

The initial patient consult should take place in a quiet, well-appointed room. This room should have patient education handouts on face-lifts. It should also have a book with before and after photos, patient testimonials, the surgeon's credentials/affiliations, and any relevant publications authored by the surgeon. Some practitioners prefer a computer to display their preoperative and postoperative images.

While a cosmetic consultant is not absolutely necessary, this individual can improve patient care and service. This consultant initially interviews the patient to obtain an understanding of the patients cosmetic concerns and needs. Often a patient may want a face-lift because a friend had one, but this may not be the most appropriate intervention. The cosmetic consultant can describe the various procedures and answer some of the patients' questions. Essentially, the cosmetic consultant forges a bond with the patient and is an integral member of the cosmetic surgery team. The cosmetic consultant will then summarize the patients concerns to the physician that he/she can focus on the issues that are important to the patient.

The cosmetic consult is streamlined, but comprehensive. During this consultation, the practitioner should not only address the patient's physical concerns, but also her/his motivations, expectations, and any body-image issues. Obviously, the patient should not desire facial rejuvenation in order to please someone else. Nor will the face-lift make the individual appear as they were in their third decade. Nor will a face-lift alone dramatically change the person's lifestyle or status. Initially, it can be difficult to diagnose the body dysmorphic syndrome, and some practitioners employ a questionnaire. The authors use their judgment and experience rather than a formal process, which can also be problematic, and decrease trust between the patient and physician.

If a rhytidectomy is indicated, the procedure including preoperative preparation and the postoperative course should be summarized. Expected results should be discussed.

Some practitioners use a computer program to simulate a postoperative result; however, the authors feel that this computer simulation may not be an accurate portrayal and may confuse the patient. The risks of the procedure should also be discussed. The patient's history is reviewed. Bleeding disorders or wound healing abnormalities such as a history of keloids would be a contraindication for this procedure. Immunosuppression is a relative indication. Because the authors perform the face-lift under local anesthesia, the risks are less for most patients.

If the patient genuinely wants to address lower face laxity, this integrated process of the cosmetic consultant and esthetic surgeon should result in the scheduling of the surgery. While some surgeons prefer to discuss the fee, the authors prefer to leave this to the cosmetic consultant in order to preserve the doctor–patient relationship and focus on the actual procedure. Therefore, after the physician leaves the room, the consultant will discuss the fee, answer any additional questions, provide the patient contacts of previous face-lift patients, and schedule the preoperative appointment. The cosmetic consultant becomes the liaison between the doctor and the patient for the remainder of this relationship. Though this procedure is performed under local anesthesia, it is prudent to obtain an electrocardiogram, a CBC/Platelets, PT/PTT, HIV, Hepatitis screen and CETs for all patients as well as a physical examination by the primary care provider. During the preoperative appointment, the consent should be signed (Fig. 6), which will generate more questions, the procedure and postoperative instructions reviewed, and antibiotics and pain medications prescribed. The initial postoperative appointment should also be scheduled.

Decision-Making

When deciding which procedure(s) is/are most appropriate, it is important to classify the patient's aging pathology. A series of questions should be addressed, and then an algorithm should be followed. Does the patient have rhytides, sagging, or both? Where is the laxity? The neck? In the jowls? Lower cheeks or malar region? Does the patient have prominent nasolabial folds and marionette lines? Does the patient have a receding chin? Does the patient have platysmal banding? Does the patient have cheek hollowing?

Subjectively, what are the patients concerns? If it is just with wrinkling, then only a lifting procedure will not be satisfactory. A resurfacing procedure alone or in combination with a lift would be more appropriate. If the patient's concern is primarily with prominent nasolabial folds, it should be explained that a face-lift will only modestly modify them, and a filler will need to be injected in the future. If the patient is concerned about her neck only, then only a neck lift is necessary. If there is fat, but the skin is taut, neck liposuction will be effective. Similarly, a patient with lower face laxity and a tight neck may only require an anterior face-lift. Yet, in the authors' experience, it is rare that a patient will benefit from only an anterior face-lift. Including even a limited postauricular incision will improve the jaw line. If the patient wants reasonable results, but less downtime, then a shorter scar face-lift needs to be considered. If the patient is concerned about her lowered "cheek bones," then a suture-based mid-face-lift will be indicated in addition to the traditional face-lift. While the procedures for each patient needs to be customized to fit their objective and subjective criteria, generally the authors will perform neck and judicious lower face liposuction, a platysmaplasty, and then tailor the length of the face lift incision to the patient's needs.

AUTHORIZATION AND INFORMED CONSENT

_____
(Patient's Name)

1. I request and authorize M. Eugene Tardy, Jr., M.D. (the "Doctor") to perform an operation upon me (or my _____) entitled (description of procedure): _____
_____
_____

2. The nature and effects of the operation, the risks, ramifications, complications involved, as well as alternative methods of treatment, have been fully explained to me by the Doctor and I understand them.

3. I authorize the Doctor to perform any other procedure which he may deem desirable in attempting to improve the condition stated in paragraph 1 or any unhealthy or unforeseen condition that may be encountered during the operation.

4. I consent to the administration of anesthetics by the Doctor or under the direction of the physician responsible for this service. If an anesthesiologist assists in my surgery, I understand that the anesthesiologist will take full charge of the administration and maintenance of the anesthesia, and that this is an independent function of the surgery.

5. I have been thoroughly and completley advised that the object of the operation I have requested is primarily an improvement in appearance. Since I understand that the practice of medicine and surgery is not an exact science and therefore that no reputable surgeon can guarantee results, I acknowledge that imperfections might ensue and that the operative result may not live up to my expectations. I certify that no guarantees have been made by anyone regarding the operation(s) I have requested and authorized.

6. I understand that the two sides of the human body are not the same and can never be made the same.

7. I have been advised that part of this surgery is/maybe performed through external skin incisions which will leave permanent scars whose extent and location have been described to me. I have been advised that all scars may require up to a year or more to mature.

8. For the purpose of advancing medical education, I consent to the admittance of authorized observers to the operating room.

9. I give permission to M. Eugene Tardy, Jr., M.D. to take still or motion clinical photographs with the understanding that such photographs remain the property of the doctor. If, in the judgment of the Doctor, medical research, education or science will be benefitted by their use, such photographs, and related information may be published and republished in professional journals or medical books, or used for such publication or use. I shall not be identified by name.

10. I understand that if Dr. Tardy judges at any time that my surgery should be postponed or cancelled for any reason, he may do so.

11. I hereby authorize that the information furnished by Dr. Tardy by me during my diagnostic evaluation is correct.

12. I agree to follow the instructions given to me by Dr. Tardy to the best of my ability before, during and after my surgical procedure.

I certify that I have read the above authorization, that the explanations referred to therein were made to my satisfaction, and that I fully understand such explanations and the above authorization.

Signed _____
     (Patient or person authorized to consent for patient)

Witness _____ Date _____

Figure 6 Example of a consent form for an anterior lift.

ANESTHESIA

Traditionally, rhytidectomies have been performed under general anesthesia. More recently, they have been performed using "twilight" sedation with Propofol. Both of these modalities are effective, however, in the vast majority of patients are not necessary. The only patient who would require these two techniques is one who is adamant about not being awake for the procedure. If the advantages of using tumescent anesthesia have been clearly explained—no nausea; less drowsiness and quicker recovery time; and less bleeding and risk for postoperative complications—the patient should recognize the superiority of this anesthesia technique.

The classic Klein tumescent solution is 0.1% lidocaine with 1/1000,000 epinephrine. This mixture is adequate for a cervicofacial rhytidectomy. Yet, both authors will routinely increase the epinephrine concentration to 1/500,000 because of the vascularity in the head and neck. In men who have a

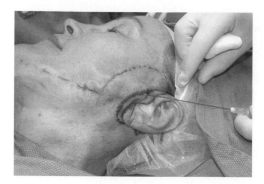

Figure 7 Tumescing the face and neck.

tendency to bleed more (most likely secondary to increased vascularity due to follicles), a concentration of 1/500,000 is prudent. One author (GM) uses 0.3% lidocaine given the extensive dissection of this procedure. Because approximately 250 cc of tumescent fluid will be infiltrated, patient toxicity is not an issue. While some patients may not want oral sedation, most will want to be relaxed and have a degree of amnesia regarding the surgery. One author (HBG) routinely gives 0.50 to 0.75 mg Xanax; 1 hydrocodone tablet; and 25 mg Phenergan. The other author (GSM) gives IM Demerol and 25 mg phenergan and 1–2 mg oral Ativan.

The tumescent solution can be infiltrated with either a 20 g spinal gauge needle or a cannula (Fig. 8). After injecting blebs of 1% lidocaine with 1/100,000 epinephrine, infiltration is begun in the neck. The patient should be warned that she may feel a fullness in the neck. While it has never occurred in the authors' experience, the patient should also be instructed to tell the surgeon if she has any difficulty breathing. The anesthetic is delivered in a fan-like motion so that it is uniform. When infiltrating at the level of the mandible, and superior to it, it is necessary to be careful not to traumatize the marginal mandibular nerve. The cheeks, temples, and pre- and postauricular regions are anesthetized. Tumescent anesthesia not only provides excellent hemostasis, but also hydrodissects the tissue. This tissue separation is important in the postauricular/neck region where the skin is bound down particularly in men with severe actinic damage. By facilitating dissection in this

region, there is less likelihood of injuring the great auricular nerve, which has been the most frequently traumatized in conventional cervicofacial rhytidectomies. While the tumescent technique provides excellent anesthesia, a small amount of 1% lidocaine with 1/100,000 epinephrine is injected along the incision lines.

TECHNIQUES

Essentially, the different techniques are variations on the same theme of creating a natural lift that addresses the major aging pathology and concerns of the patient. The placement and extent of the incision depend on which region needs to be modified. An anterior lift will only address the lower face and, possibly, the midface. If there is significant neck laxity, then a postauricular incision, undermining, and plication sutures are necessary.

Anterior Lifts
The S-Lift
Photography

Preoperative photographs should always be taken. They need to be standardized in terms of lighting, focal length (usually 1:3), height, and angle (frontal, oblique, profile). The lighting must be consistent, and should be softened with bounce cards in order to better demonstrate the facial topography. The patient must not wear makeup in either the pre- or postoperative photos. While a studio is optimal, with the advent of digital photography, and instant evaluation of the image quality, it is not necessary.

Marking

Following consent and photographs, the patient is marked in an upright position. The jaw line, thyroid cartilage, base of neck, and submental crease are initially marked using either gentian violet, a surgical marking pen, or a Sharpie indelible marker. These markings are important for the liposuction portion of the procedure. The preauricular skin is pinched to determine laxity. The incision line begins at the root of the helix and extends interiorly along the auricular border on to the tragus (pretragal for women), then extending to the base of the earlobe. Depending on the laxity of skin, second identical undulating line is drawn on the preauricular area. They are connected superiorly and at the inferior pole. In most patients, the lines are separated by 1 cm of skin. These connected lines resemble an "S" (Fig. 8).

Finally, the extent of undermining needs to be marked. While Saylan described a very short 4 cm flap, the authors prefer a longer 6 to 7 cm flap. This flap is still significantly lateral to the nasolabial folds (NLFs). Several points are marked 6 cm from the tragus, and a gentle arc is drawn representing the extent of the flap.

Anesthesia

The patient is placed in a supine position. A neck roll will help extend the neck and provide better exposure. The tumescent anesthesia is prepared as described as above. It can be infiltrated with a syringe or a Klein pump. A 20 gauge spinal needle or an infiltrating cannula may be used. If using a Klein pump, it should be set at 3 to 4. The infiltration in this region is gradual. The submentum is first infiltrated followed by the other areas of the neck and the jaw line. The preauricular region and cheek can also be

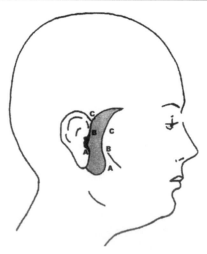

Figure 8 Marking for the S-lift.

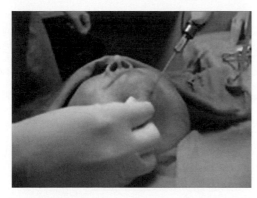

Figure 9 Liposuction of the neck, which is an integral part of the facelift under local anesthesia.

accessed from this area, Yet, the tumescent anesthesia should also be infiltrated from the incision site and medially underneath the flap in the subcutaneous plane. This infiltration will hydrodissect the flap.

Liposuction

Liposuction of the neck is approached both from a stab incision in the submental crease and from postauricular sulcus. A smaller cannula such as a 16 or 14 are initially used, which serves to break apart the connective tissue and dissect the fat. Then a 12 gauge and occasionally a 3 mm cannula may be used. Great care should be exercised when using larger cannulas. When approaching the jaw line or sweeping above it, it is prudent to use a smaller cannula such as a 14 gauge cannula. Combined with grasping the overlying skin, this technique will minimize the risk of trauma to the marginal mandibular nerve (Fig. 9). The liposuction should be performed in a crisscross fashion, which results in uniform fat removal. In many individuals, less than 50 cc of fat will be removed; however, the liposuction promotes contraction of the skin and possibly the platysma by mechanically wounding them.

Incision

Using a #15 blade, the lateral outline of the S is incised in a superior to inferior fashion, followed by incision of the lateral line. Thus, 1 cm of skin is pre-excised in the shape of an S. This skin pre-excision facilitates the initial flap development.

Undermining

For the S-lift, undermining can be started with the 12 gauge or 3 mm cannula without suction. It can create tunnels, which will facilitate raising the flap. The flap is initially developed with sharp dissection using a #15 blade in order to obtain the correct plane. The SMAS should not be in the flap. The flap is generally thin without compromising its vascular supply. Following sharp dissection, the flap is developed with either a "baby" Metzenbaum, Mayo, or Gorney scissors. Each has its advantages, and the choice is surgeon dependent. When raising the flap, the scissors tips should be "up," which aids in crating a thin flap and minimizes injury to the parotid gland. The scissors' orientation should alternate between horizontal and vertical. The latter facilitates the creation of tunnels and the flap.

Hemostasis is very important. Inadequate control of bleeding will surely lead to a postoperative hematoma, which could compromise the flap. Fortunately, the tumescent anesthesia produces excellent hemostasis. Yet, there will be some bleeding particularly at the flap's medial aspect. The authors prefer to cauterize "as they go," which ensures excellent visibility.

Plication

Addressing the SMAS is a key component in any rhytidectomy. It may be plicated or imbricated. While trimming, the SMAS does eliminate its laxity; studies have shown that it does not carry an esthetic or functional advantage over plication sutures. In addition, there is a higher risk of nerve injury for imbrication. The authors prefer plication because the superior suspension of the SMAS also lends a roundness to the lateral cheeks.

Plication sutures can be absorbable or nonabsorbable. One author (HBG) uses 3-0 prolene and the other author prefers (3-0 Vicryl). The nonabsorbable potentially could cause more tissue reaction, but is permanent. In the past, plication sutures were oriented horizontally. This led to a wind tunnel and pulling effect. It was not effective, because it did not reverse the aging process, which causes the skin to sag. The proper orientation should be more vertical—between 60° to 90°; though some procedures may place the more superior sutures at 90°. These suspension sutures are buried, and the lateral anchor suture grasps the fascia. Because SMAS plication is such an important aspect of the face-lift, the authors believe that there should be many sutures. In an anterior face-lift, this may range from 8 to 10 depending on the facial size.

Trimming/Closure

While an S-lift pre-excises the skin, this does not mean that there will not be additional skin to trim. Closure must be without tension. As with Mohs Surgery closures, the skin should be closed in layers. Layered closure will decrease the risk of a widened scar—the aspect that the patient will notice most. Buried 4-0 absorbable should be used for the deep layer. When closing this layer, the skin flap is sutured to the preauricular skin in a superior fashion. This suturing reinforces the vertical vector. The skin is approximated with either 6-0 fast-absorbing gut or nylon sutures (Fig. 10).

G-Lift

The G-lift evolved from the S-lift, because many patients had neck bands and laxity in addition to their jowling, but did not want the down time of a full face-lift. In addition,

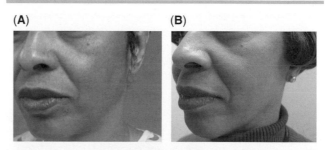

(A)   **(B)**

Figure 10 (A and B) Pre and post photos for the S-lift. The postoperative photo is at two years. The S-lift improves mild jowling and improves the contour of the lower face.

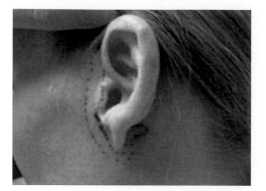

Figure 11 Marking the G-lift, which includes a postauricular incision, which travels 1.5 cm postauricularly into the scalp.

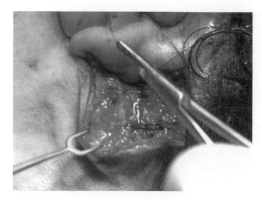

Figure 13 Plication of the lateral platysma.

many patients desired an anterior scar that was hidden—without the temporal extension. The G-lift addresses these concerns, and is indicated for those patients with jowling, and mild-to-moderate neck laxity.

Markings/Incision

As with the S-lift, the skin is pre-excised. The incision begins at the superior helix without any medial extension. It travels inferior around the lobule and then hugging the postauricular sulcus to the level of the superior aspect of the external auditory canal. At this point, it travels posteriorly for 1.5 cm. While some surgeons prefer to incise the skin along the posterior auricle, because this technique will more effectively camouflage the ear, it may lead to retraction or tethering of the auricle. The excised skin should resemble an upper case "G" (Fig. 11).

The Neck

The neck is marked in a similar fashion to the S-lift. In many patients, there will also be platysmal bands. These are marked.

Liposuction is performed as with all other versions of the rhytidectomy. However, because platysmal plication is also performed, a small submental ellipse is excised, and the liposuction is vigorously performed through this portal as well as from the postauricular sulcus. The latter can be performed more easily following the skin pre-excision.

The combination of tumescent anesthesia and the liposuction will remove most of the fat from the platysma. The two bands will need to be further dissected from the overlying skin with a metzenbaum scissors. Hemostasis

should be performed with an insulated cautery tip. One author (HBG) prefers the Colorado needle. Because of this anterior access, the neck is widely undermined. While there a many methods to address the platysma including trimming it and using a corset suturing technique, the authors will use simple interrupted sutures to recreate approximate the bands. These sutures begin inferiorly at the level of the thyroid cartilage, and end just inferior to the submental incision. Either 4-0 prolene or an absorbable suture may be used (Fig. 12). Depending on the size of the neck, there are usually 4 to 6 plication sutures.

In addressing the posterior neck, it is important to develop a thin flap because of the risk of injury to the greater auricular nerve and the marginal mandibular branch of the facial nerve. Initial undermining with a cannula sans suction will aid in raising the flap, since the postauricular skin is bound down, particularly in those patients with extensive actinic damage. Undermining with Mayo/Gorney scissors will facilitate a continuous plane to the midline.

Because of the contour of the neck, the plication sutures should be placed in a 60° vertical vector (Fig. 13). There will be usually two to three, because of the short posterior excision. Generally, the skin will need to be trimmed, and there may be a dog-ear. While a tensionless closure is the goal, there may be some tension in the postauricular region. In closing the skin, the buried sutures should be anchored to the stable skin by taking large deep bites. The

(A)   **(B)**

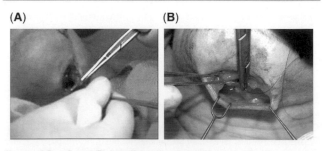

Figure 12 (**A** and **B**) Identifying the platysmal band. Plicating the platysma with interrupted sutures.

(A)   **(B)**

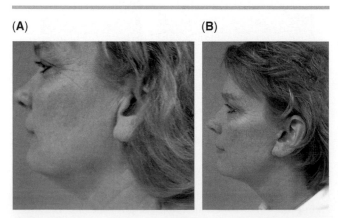

Figure 14 (**A** and **B**) Pre- and post-G-lift. In this lift, the posterior incision extends approximately 1.5 to 2 cm into the scalp. This lift will provide some improvement to the neck compared to the S-lift.

postauricular epidermis is approximated with 5-0 fast-absorbing gut (Fig. 14).

The Facial Lipo-Lift and Extended Facial Lipo-Lift

The Facial Lipo-Lift and its extension (GSM) is a multistep procedure that owes its foundation from the rhytidectomies performed by Webster, Alt, Asken, Moy, and others. It involves more aggressive and extensive liposuctioning as well as an emphasis on the vertical vector of sints plication. The procedure is indicated for patients with facial ptosis, excess jowl and neck fat, mild platysmal banding, and good neck skin elasticity.

Technique

The zone of neck liposuction is defined by the anterior border of the sternocleidomastoid muscle and the inferior border of the neck above the sternal notch. The facial liposuction zones are dependent on facial adipose deposits and may include lower cheek above the mandible, jowl, and, rarely, the nasolabial folds. Platysmal bands, if present, are outlined, and the submental incision planned just anterior to the submental crease. The anterior face-lift incision is drawn starting at the medial-third of the sideburn parallel to the top of the helix and extends inferiorly along the preauricular crease, along the edge of the tragus, around the earlobe, and in the postauricular crease to the junction of the middle- and top-third of the ear. Unlike the common practice of placing the incision onto the posterior surface of the conchal bowl in anticipation of scar stretch back, this incision is placed in the postauricular crease to allow the posterior flap to be anchored to the mastoid fascia to prevent any scar movement. The incision is then extended posterolaterally into the scalp approximately 2 cm. The anterior flap zone of undermining zone is created in a semicircular manner approximately 5 to 7 cm medially, 4 cm inferior to the earlobe, and 3 cm in the postauricular region (Fig. 15).

The face-lift incision and submental incision are infiltrated with 1% lidocaine with 1:100,000 epinephrine. A #11 blade is used to create 2 mm punctures in the submental crease, sideburn incision, postauricular horizontal incision, and inferior earlobe crease for subcutaneous infiltration of

250 to 350 cc of 0.3% tumescent lidocaine solution with 1:500,000.

The face and neck liposuction is performed via the submental, infra-auricular, and melolabial fold stab incisions with 3 mm spatula and 16 g Klein Finesse cannulae. The extent of liposuction is determined by the individual patient's adipose deposits. The suction is turned off, and a 2 mm spatula cannula is used via the sideburn and postauricular incision punctures to undermine the anterior and posterior skin flaps and connect them to the subcutaneous plane of the neck liposuction.

The submental puncture is extended approximately 1 cm bilaterally. A Gorney scissors is used to undermine the anterior neck skin, and a strip of adipose tissue is scissor excised to reveal the edges of the platysmal bands. Five to seven interrupted 4.0 Prolene sutures are used to plicate the muscle bands to the level of the hyoid bone. If indicated, a subperiosteal chin-jowl or jowl implant is placed through the same submental incision. The incision is closed in a layered linear closure with 4.0 Vicryl and 5.0 nylon sutures.

The patient is positioned with the left face down. Using a #15 blade, the incision is created along the natural curve of the ear, edge of the tragus, within earlobe crease, and within the postauricular crease (not over conchal bowl cartilage).

The anterior flap is undermined in the subcutaneous plane with a Gorney scissors with vertical and horizontal spreading until the anterior pocket matches the preoperative markings in extent and shape. Elevation of the flap is facilitated by a combination of transillumination, direct fiberoptic illumination, and countertraction by surgical staff. The posterior flap is undermined in the subcutaneous plane to allow free tissue movement for the creation of the standing cone of redundant tissue in the superior region of the postauricular crease. Meticulous hemostasis is obtained with electrocoagulation, and surgical drains are not required.

The SMAS plication is performed with 3.0 Polydioxanone (PDS) buried, interrupted sutures and begins in the preauricular region. Five to seven sutures are placed for the direct vertical plication parallel to the preauricular incision. The postauricular plication is completed with two sutures posterosuperior to the earlobe 4.0 prolene sutures are also placed inbetween the PDS sutures for added security. Every suture that is placed sequentially creates an increasingly upward vector. Following plication, additional undermining is required to release retracted skin over at the edge of the undermining zone.

The anterior and posterior skin is retracted superolaterally in a vertical manner. For the anterior flap, the lateral and superior retraction is balanced to prevent distortion of the lateral canthus. 4.0 Prolene sutures are used to anchor the skin flap at the superior aspect of the preauricular incision and central tragus. While the face-lift flap is retracted superiorly, a 1 to 1.5 cm incision is made in the flap overlying the earlobe to allow the earlobe to project anterior to the pre- and postauricular flaps. The postauricular skin is then stretched in a vertical manner to create a standing cone of redundant skin in the superior aspect of the postauricular crease. A 4.0 Prolene suture is placed to anchor the flap to the superior aspect of the postauricular crease. The excess skin is then excised to create a smooth flap edge corresponding to the original incision pathway and shape of the ear.

The anterior incision is closed with numerous 4.0 Vicryl-buried sutures for complete skin edge apposition. The postauricular incision is closed with multiple 3.0 Vicryl sutures that are first passed through the mastoid fascia in the postauricular crease to lock the flap edge deep in the postauricular crease to the residual ear skin. Each of

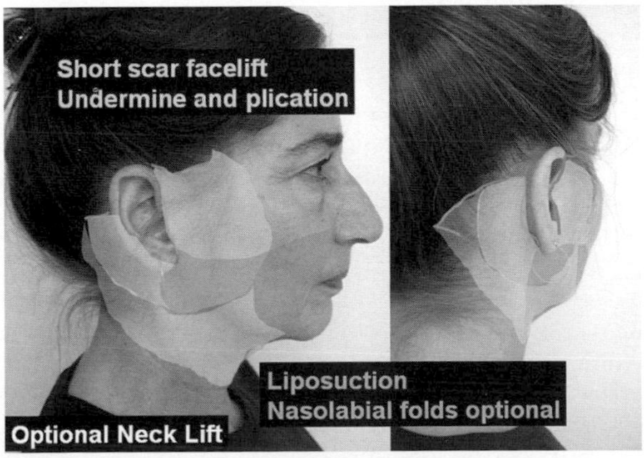

Figure 15 The facial lipo-lift combines a short scar face incision (red line) and vertical vector lift (orange) with facial and neck liposuction (blue) with or without a neck lift (white) under local anesthesia. *Source*: Courtesy of Greg S. Morganroth, MD.

the anterior and posterior periauricular sutures is placed with the flap bite approximated 5 mm inferior to the anchor bite of fascia or cartilage. The pre- and postauricular Vicryl anchor sutures allow for complete closure of the earlobe portion of the incision without any visible tension on the lobe and will prevent downward displacement of the earlobe (pixie ear deformity) with relaxation of the skin. The skin edges are already approximated by the numerous buried sutures; however, additional 5.0 nylon running and interrupted sutures are placed for additional support.

The Extended Facial Lipo-Lift

The extended version of the Facial Lipo-Lift differs by its longer postauricular incision extending 5 cm or more into the occipital scalp to allow for full neck undermining, lateral platysmal plication, and excision of neck skin similar to a Webster face-lift. This extended anterior–posterior technique provides rejuvenation for patients with the most severe neck ptosis, wrinkling, and elastosis that will not adequately respond to liposuction alone and would be considered candidates for a traditional face-lift under sedation.

The Extended Facial Lipo-Lift procedure differs from the facial lipo-lift in the following manner: The postauricular flap undermining zone is much larger and extends from the postauricular scalp incision inferiorly to the midline of the neck. Undermining of the postauricular flap takes place in the adipose plane just below the hair follicles in the plane created by the 2 mm spatula during the suction-free undermining phase of the procedure. A combination of vertical and horizontal spreading assists in remaining superficial through the fibrous fascia over the sternocleidomastoid to avoid injuring the great auricular and lesser occipital nerves.

The postauricular plication in this procedure involves a vertical elevation that is not possible in a solo neck lift, where a more lateral vector is employed. The multiple buried 3.0 PDS plication sutures anchor the edge of the SMAS and platysma anterior to the sternocleidomastoid muscle to the immobile mastoid fascia 4.0 prolene sutures are also placed inbetween the PDS sutures for added security. The postauricular zone tends to bleed more often than the anterior flap. Jackson-Pratt drains are commonly placed for men and rarely placed for women.

After fixing the anterior flap, the postauricular skin is retracted in a superolateral vector. The postauricular incision is closed with 3.0 Vicryl sutures that are first passed through the mastoid fascia in the postauricular crease to lock the flap edge deep in the postauricular crease to the residual ear skin. Each of the posterior sutures is placed with the flap bite approximated 5 mm inferior to the anchor bite of mastoid fascia. These anchor sutures prevent stretchback of the incision and allow for tension-free closure of the earlobe portion of the incision (Fig. 16).

POSTOPERATIVE CARE

All incisions are dressed with Polysporin antibiotic ointment, nonstick bandages, and 4 × 4 gauze. Kerlex and coban may be used to complete the pressure dressing. Alternatively, neck liposuction compression garments may be placed over the gauze as well as a cervical collar to prevent flexion and formation of abnormal, skin folds.

The patient returns the next day for a wound check and may return daily for one or more days depending upon the amount of swelling, pain, need to assess proper wound care in certain patients, and to check drains, if present. For one author (HBG), the neck liposuction garment is placed on Post Operative Day (POD)#1 in order to avoid soiling from immediate postoperative drainage. The garment is worn for at least one week. The author (GSM) continues the compression garment, and cervical collar for three days. If nonabsorbable sutures have been placed, they are removed at seven days for the anterior flap and submental incision and the then the postauricular flap sutures are removed at 10 days.

Most patients experience only moderate postoperative discomfort lasting for a few days. For extended facial lipo-lifts, they may experience postauricular discomfort during the first two months postoperatively. The bruising and edema in these lifting procedures typically resolves over 5 to 10 days, and most patients return to work after one week. For shorter scar face-lifts, they can return to work after a long weekend. Numbness, mild edema, and evolving fibrosis will be present in variable amounts for up to 8 to 10 weeks. Frequent gentle, daily massage is useful to accelerate healing. A significant number of patients experience temporary swelling and discomfort that requires hand-holding during the first few weeks. All patients are seen every three to four weeks until all swelling resolves. They may be seen at three months and six months depending on their recovery. The patients are reassured from the preoperative consult and through the postoperative course of the one year duration for healing.

MULTIPLE PROCEDURES

A major advance in face-lift surgery has not only been the use of local anesthesia, but the ability to perform multiple simultaneous facial cosmetic procedures without general anesthesia. The most common adjunct procedure is the medium-strength chemical peel or single-pass laser resurfacing. Because a rhytidectomy does not truly address rhytides, these two procedures are complementary. The combination of lifting and refining the skin texture can lead to stunning results. Radiofrequency or nonablative lasers may have an additive effect, particularly for anterior-only lifts. Other adjunct procedures include a suture mid-face-lift, which can be performed through the rhytidectomy incision, and may flatten the nasolabial folds, and lift the malar fat pads.

As discussed above, a chin implant can be performed through the submental incision for the platysmal plication.

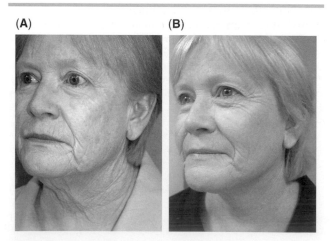

(A)   **(B)**

Figure 16 **(A and B)** Pre- and post-solo rhytidectomy under local anesthesia.

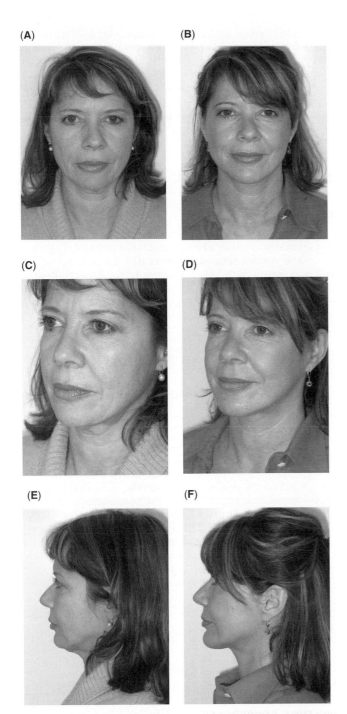

(A) **(B)**

(C) **(D)**

(E) **(F)**

Figure 17 (A–C) Preprocedure. **(D–F):** Post multiple procedures performed under local anesthesia: facial lipo-lift, chin-jowl implant, upper blepharoplasty, periorbital and perioral laser resurfacing, and facial TCA peel. *Source*: Courtesy of Greg S. Morganroth, MD.

increases in blood pressure during a rhytidectomy could potentially increase the risk for periorbital bleeding (Fig. 17).

COMPLICATIONS

The most common complication is the hematoma. It occurs from 1% to 10% of all face-lift patients. Hematomas occur more commonly in males than females. While there is not enough data to determine if short-scar face-lifts result in less hematomas than the traditional rhytidectomy, one study did show an overall low complication rate of short-scar face-lifts using a tumescent solution for anesthesia.

While they have occurred weeks after surgery, hematomas most commonly occur in the first 24 hours. They present as expanding masses, and the patient complains of increased pressure or pain. Because they can be a nidus for infection, and cause puckering of the skin and asymmetry, hematomas need to be evacuated. If small and discrete, they can be aspirated. This may involve daily aspirations and pressure bandages for up to a week. For significant hematomas, sutures may need to be removed, the blood/clot evacuated, the area cauterized, and a drain placed. A less-invasive method is to use a liposuction cannula to eliminate the hematoma. The best way to prevent a hematoma is a thorough preoperative evaluation and instruction regarding aspirin as well as meticulous intraop hemostasis.

The other common complication is nerve injury. In supra-SMAS rhytidectomies, nerve injury is approximately 2%. The most common injury is to great auricular nerve. This nerve, which receives contributions from C2 and C3, crosses the sternocleidomastoid, and becomes very superficial. It innervates the lower portion of the ear including the earlobe. If it is injured, then there will be numbness of the earlobe, which makes putting on earrings problematic. The spinal accessory nerve also crosses the SCM, but is most superficial in the posterior triangle of the neck. Although it is uncommon, it can be injured in a full face-lift while undermining the neck. Injury to this nerve, which innervates the trapezius, leads to a painful drooping of the shoulder.

While its sequelae are the most feared, injury to the facial motor nerves is uncommon. The temporal branch is the most commonly injured branch. It is very superficial as it crosses over the malar arch. Injury to this nerve will result in the inability to raise the ipsilateral eyebrow. The patient will complain of a heavy eyelid that may impair vision. Correction of this clinical complication is a direct brow-lift. The marginal mandibular branch may also be injured. As it courses under the mandible, it can be traumatized by aggressive liposuction. This branch becomes very superficial as it approaches the lateral commissure of the lip. Injury to the marginal mandibular will lead to lip depressor function loss. This may affect speech and eating. Over time, it may evolve into a drool that can lead to perleche. Although it is difficult to determine if a nerve has been severed, because of the local anesthesia, if possible, the nerve should be immediately reanastomosed. These nerve injuries can be avoided, understanding the anatomical relationships, by remaining in the correct plane, and raising a thin flap. Tumescent anesthesia, which facilitates hydrodissection and hemostasis, plays an important role in the prevention of nerve injuries.

Other significant complications include skin slough and frank necrosis, widened and hypertrophic scars (Fig. 18), infection, seromas, contour irregularities, premature sagging, and contact dermatitis. As with any skin

A chin implant, particularly the extended implant can dramatically enhance the jaw line definition and provide a sharper cervicomental angle. Because most short scar face-lifts require less than three hours, separate procedures such as blepharoplasties and brow-lifts can also be performed under local anesthesia. Although some may prefer to perform the eyelid procedures before the face-lift because they require finer manual skills, from a patient standpoint, it is advantageous to perform these procedures after the face-lift since the surgical manipulation movement, and possible transient

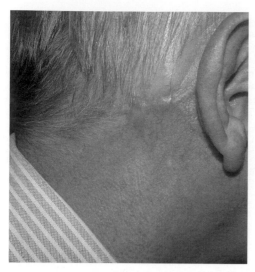

Figure 18 Hypertrophic scar along the postauricular incision line. The risk of this complication can be reduced by reducing the tension on the flap through undermining, accurate trimming, and taking large anchoring bites when placing the buried sutures.

wound, tensionless closure is desirable. Increased tension decreases vascular viability and enhances the opportunity for infection and skin slough. If the trimming has been performed correctly, then there should be no tension for the anterior portion of the face-lift. Because of the difference in skin elasticity and the vectors, there may be some tension in the posterior flap. Layered closure and taking deep anchoring bites of the stable tissue will decrease the risk. The buried sutures will reduce the risk for widened scars.

Given the head and neck's blood supply and the sterile conditions, the risk for infection is low. As mentioned, this can be increased if there is significant wound tension. Immunocompromised individuals also have a higher risk for infection. Although there is not good data, the authors place the patient on broad-spectrum antibiotics before the surgery and postoperatively.

Seromas are rare, though they will be surely increased if the parotid gland is injured. These may take several weeks to resolve, and a drain will be needed. Contour irregularities can occur with inadequate undermining or plications sutures placed in the incorrect plane. Initially, there may be neck contour irregularities from the liposuction. Overtime, many of these abnormalities will smooth out particularly with massage. Occassionally, using a liposuction cannula through a stab incision may correct the contour. Premature sagging is usually the result of plication suture failure. It is important to grasp a significant portion of the SMAS as well as the fascia, and tying several secure knots; so the suture does not slip. Contact dermatitis occurs unpredictably. Although it will not compromise the result, it cause patient anxiety, and will slow the healing process. Removing the offending agent whether it is the tape or antibiotic ointment, and applying a weak topical steroid will resolve the dermatitis.

SUMMARY

Rhytidectomies have evolved over the past century to take into account the SMAS for longevity and methods to decrease recovery time for the patient. This procedure and its variants are indicated for patients with moderate to severe lower face laxity, effacement of the cervicomental angle, and redundant neck skin. While several specialties most notably plastic and facial plastic surgery have contributed to the rhytidectomy, dermatologic surgeons have demonstrated that it can be performed safely and effectively under local anesthesia using the tumescent technique, and that the rhytidectomy should be combined with at least neck liposuction and in many patients judicious lower-face liposuction.

BIBLIOGRAPHY

Alster TS, Doshi SN, Hopping SB. Combination surgical lifting with ablative laser skin resurfacing: a retrospective analysis. Dermatol Surg. 2004; 30:1191.

Asken S. Cervicofacial rhytidectomy. In: Cosmetic Surgery of the Skin. William Coleman III, ed. Mosby: St. Louis, 1997:428–452.

Baker DC. Minimal incision rhytidectomy (short scar face lift) with lateral SMASectomy: evolution and application. Aesthetic Surg 2001; 21:14.

Baker DC, Conley J. Avoiding facial nerve injuries in rhytidectomy: anatomic variations and pitfalls. Plast Reconstr Surg 1979; 64:781.

Barton FE. Rhytidectomy and the nasolabial fold. Plast Reconstr Surg 1992; 90:601.

Bisaccia E, Khan AJ, Scarborough DA. Anterior face-lift fpr correction of middle face aging utlilizing a minimally invasive tehcnique. Dermatol Surg 2004; 30:769.

Chrisman BB, Field LM. Facelift surgery update: suction-assisted rhytidectomy and other improvements. J Dermatol Surg Oncol 1984; 10:544.

De la Plaza R, Valentine E, Arroyo JM. Supraperiosteal lifting of the upper two thirds of the face. Br J Plast Surg 1991; 44:325.

Duffy MJ, Friedland JA. The superficial plane rhytidectomy revisited. Plast Recosntr Surg 1994; 93:1392.

Furnas DW. The retaining ligaments of the cheek. Plast Reconstr Surg 1989; 83:11.

Gonzalez-Ulloa M. The history of rhytidectomy. Aesthic Plast Surg 1980; 4:1.

Hamra ST. Composite rhytidectomy. Plast Reconstr Surg 1992; 90:1.

Hamra ST. The deep plane rhytidectomy. Plast Reconstr Surg 1990; 86:53.

Hinderer UT. Vertical preperiosteal rejuvenation of the frame of the eyelids and midface. Plast Recosntr Surg 1999; 104:1482.

Hoefflin SM. The extended supra platysmal plane (ESP) face lift. Plast Reocnstr Surg 1998; 101:494.

Ivy EJ, Lorenc ZP, Adston SJ. Is there a difference? A prospective study comparing lateral and standard SMAS face lifts with extended SMAS and composite rhytidectomies. Plast Reconstr Surg 1996; 98:1135.

Jones BM, Grover R. Avoiding hematoma in cervicofacial rhytidectomy:a personal 8 year quest. Reviewing 910 patients. Plast Reconstr Surg 2004; 113:381.

Jones BM, Grover R. Reducing complications in cervicofacial rhytidectomy by tumescent infiltration: a comparative trial evaluating 678 consecutive facelifts. Plast Reconstr Surg 2004; 113:398.

Jost G, Lamouche G. SMAS in rhytidectomy. Aesth Plast Surg 1982; 6:69.

Kamer FM, Mingrone MD. Deep plane rhytidectomy: a personal evolution. Facial Plast Surg Clin North Am 2005; 13:115.

Klein JA. Tumescent technique chronicles. Local anesthesia, liposuction, and beyond. Dermatol surg 1995; 21:449.

Lemmon ML, Hamra ST. Skoog Rhytidectomy. A five year experience with 577 patients. Plast Reconstr Surg 1980; 65:283.

Little JW. Hiding the posterior scar in rhytidectomy. The omega incision. Plast Reoncstr Surg 1999; 104:259.

Marchac D, Brady JA, Chiou P. Facelifts with hidden scars: The vertical U incision. Plast Reconstr Surg 2002; 109:2539.

Massiha M. Short scar facelift with extended SMAS plaatysma dissection and lifting and limited skin undermining. Plast Reconstr Surg 2003; 112:663.

Mitz V, Peyronie M. The superficial musculo-aponeurotic system (SMAS) in the parotid and cheek area. Plast Reconstr Surg 1976; 58:80.

Noel S. La Chirurgie Esthtetique: Son role sociale. Paris: Masson, 1926.

Owlsey JQ. Face lifting: problems, solutions, and an outcome study. Plast Reconstr Surg. 2000; 105:302.

Owsley JQ. Lifting the malar fat pad for correction of prominent nasolabial folds. Plast Reconstr Surg. 1993; 91:463.

Panfilove DE. MIDI facelift and tricuspidal SMAS flap. Aesth Plast Surg 2003; 27:27.

Ramirez OM. The subperiosteal rhytidectomy: the third generation facelift. Ann Plast Surg 1992; 28:218.

Roberts TL III, Pozner JN, Ritter E. The RSVP facelift: a highly vascular flap permitting safe simultaneous, comprehensive facial rejuvenation in one operative setting. Aesth Plast Surg 2000; 24:313.

Scarborough D, Bisaccia E. The Webster-type face and neck lift:an extensive cervic-facial rhytidectomy employing a minimally invasive technique. Dermatol Surg 201; 27:747.

Skoog T. Plastic Surgery: New Methods and Refinements. Philadelphia: Saunders, 1974.

Stuzin JM, Baker TJ, Baker TM. Refinements in facelifting: Enhanced facial contouring using Vicryl mesh incorporated into SMAS fixation. Plast Reconstr Surg 2000; 105:290.

Tonnard P, Verpaele A, Monstrey S, et al. Minimal access cranial suspension lift: a modified S-lift. Plast Reconstr Surg 2002; 109:2074.

Webster RC, Smith RC, Papsidero MJ, et al. Comparison of SMAS plication with SMAS imbrication in facelifting. Laryngoscope 1982; 92:901.

Webster RC, Smith RC, Smith KF. Part I: Extent of undermining of skin flaps. Head Neck Surg 1983; 5:525.

Whetzel TP, Stevenson TR. The contribution of the SMAS to the blood supply in the lateral face lift flap. Plast Reconstr Surg 1997; 100:1011.

81

Endoscopic Facial Plastic and Reconstructive Surgery

Oren Friedman
Department of Otorhinolaryngology, Mayo Clinic, Rochester, Minnesota, U.S.A.

Tom Wang
Department of Otolaryngology, Oregon Health Science Center, Portland, Oregon, U.S.A.

INTRODUCTION

The pursuit of a permanent youthful look is an endeavor that is not unique to our time, but rather spans world history from ancient Egypt to the present. Ancient Egyptians portrayed ideal facial aesthetics in their sculptures and carvings, and utilized facial makeup to enhance the appearance of the face and hide facial blemishes. Greek artists, followed by artists of the Renaissance period, continued to portray esthetic facial ideals through their works. Since these early times, the concepts of facial aesthetic ideals continue to evolve (Fig. 1).

Over the past century, surgical procedures to enhance one's external appearance have emerged from secrecy to become the fastest growing medical specialty. During this same time period, technological advances have propelled the development of minimally invasive surgical techniques. Endoscopic surgery for facial rejuvenation has become increasingly popular as surgeons and patients seek techniques with reduced morbidity and recovery time, while providing excellent results.

Minimally invasive facial rejuvenation allows for small incisions which are placed at a distance from the intended operative site, thereby eliminating visible scars. While brow-lift and midface-lift procedures have been the most common facial plastic procedures performed under endoscopic guidance, a number of other endoscopic procedures have also been described. Endoscopic rhinoplasty, endoscopic face-lift, endoscopic facial fracture repair, endoscopic facial reanimation, and endoscopic dacryocystorhinostomy have gained increasing popularity among many surgeons.

ENDOSCOPIC INSTRUMENTATION

Advances in endoscopic surgery have emerged as a direct result of highly specialized surgical instrumentation. The rod lens endoscope is made of a series of rod-shaped glass lenses. The lenses lie in a small diameter sheath. Within the rod lens endoscope there is also an objective lens, optical illumination fibers, an image reversal system, and an image collecting eyepiece. The rod lens endoscope produces a wide viewing angle, large depth of field, and outstanding image illumination and resolution. The most commonly used endoscopes for facial plastic procedures measure 4 or 5 mm in diameter, with 0° and 30° angles (Fig. 2). These endoscope specifications allow for ideal lighting, maneuverability, and visualization in the limited spaces of the face.

Halide or xenon light provide excellent sources for endoscopic illumination. Xenon light is whiter than halogen light and is thought to produce more natural and neutral lighting on the video monitors, with limited color distortion. A fiberoptic cable connects the light source to the endoscope.

A camera may be built into the endoscope itself, or it may be attached to the endoscope through a coupler. The video camera allows for the procedure to be viewed on a monitor rather than through the eyepiece of the endoscope, which enhances magnification, increases the mobility of the surgeon, improves teaching of trainees, and allows all in the operating room to better assist the surgeon. The video monitor should be of medical quality with high resolution, a reasonable screen size, and compatibility with the specific camera and endoscopic system. It is useful to have a system that allows for recording of still images as well as moving images, useful for educational and documentation purposes.

A variety of outstanding instruments are offered by a number of different companies. Instruments with different degrees of curvature, head shapes, and sharpness are available, including periosteal elevators, scissors, hooks, and forceps. Insulated instruments allow for electrocautery (Fig. 3).

ENDOSCOPIC BROW-LIFT

In an attempt to rejuvenate the periorbital area in the most natural and esthetically pleasing way, consideration must be given to all of the elements that constitute the region surrounding the eye. The position and orientation of the eyebrows are essential determinants of facial esthetics. Brow ptosis gives the face a tired, crowded, angry, and unattractive appearance, and may also accentuate upper eyelid skin redundancy. As the brow descends below the supraorbital rim, it pushes skin over the upper eyelid, worsening the cosmetic appearance of preexisting baggy eyelids. Successful management of brow malposition necessitates an understanding of the ideal brow position, and a detailed understanding of the anatomy of the forehead.

Esthetic Ideals of the Periorbital Area

The ideal brow anatomy in the male differs from that in the female. The classical brow position in women describes the medial brow as having its medial origin at the level of a vertical line drawn to the nasal alar-facial junction. The lateral extent of the brow should reach a point on a line drawn

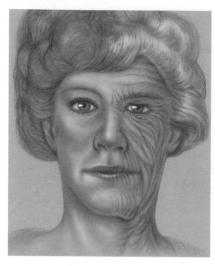

Figure 1 The aging face with youthful aesthetic ideals depicted to contrast facial aging.

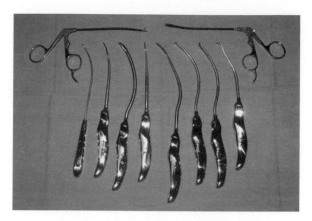

Figure 3 Endoscopic instruments for brow-lift, neck-lift, and face-lift surgery.

from the nasal alar-facial junction through the lateral canthus of the eye. The medial and lateral ends should lie on the same horizontal plane (Fig. 4). The medial end should have a clubhead appearance and the lateral end should gradually taper to a point. The brow should arch superiorly, well above the supraorbital rim, with the highest point classically described as lying at the lateral limbus, and more recently described as lying at the lateral canthus. In men, there should be less of an arch to the brow position, and more of a horizontal contour along the supraorbital ridge. The distance between the midpupillary line and the inferior brow border should be approximately 2.5 cm. The distance from the superior border of the brow to the anterior hairline (in the absence of alopecia) should be 5 cm. In addition to brow ptosis, the aging brow may reveal dynamic wrinkles or even wrinkles at rest. These furrows in the glabella and forehead are caused by the repeated pull on the skin by the facial mimetic muscles combined with the effects of gravity. The distance between the two eyebrows should be the same as the distance between the alar-facial junctions on either side of the nose, which is equivalent to the distance between the left and right medial canthus.

Sensory and Motor Innervation

Sensation of the brow and anterior scalp region is provided by the ophthalmic division of the trigeminal nerve. The ophthalmic division divides into the supraorbital and supratrochlear nerves. The supratrochlear innervates the conjunctiva, upper eyelids, and inferomedial aspect of the forehead, while the supraorbital nerve innervates the upper lid skin, forehead, and anterior scalp (Fig. 5). The supratrochlear nerve lies 1.5 to 1.7 cm from the midline, while the supraorbital nerve lies 1 cm lateral to the supratrochlear nerve. The zygomaticotemporal and zygomaticofacial nerves, branches of the maxillary division of the trigeminal nerve, supply the lateral orbit, lateral eyelids, and the skin of the temporal region.

The temporal, or frontal, division of the facial nerve supplies the muscles of the forehead and the orbicularis oculi muscle. This division of the facial nerve courses from the parotid gland, anterior to the superficial temporal artery, toward its final destination where it pierces the undersurface of the frontalis muscle 1.5 cm above the lateral canthus. The frontal branch of the facial nerve lies deep to the superficial musculoaponeurotic system (SMAS) fascia and its continuation in the temporal region, the temporoparietal fascia (Fig. 6). Below the zygoma, the nerve lies fairly deep to the SMAS, whereas above the zygoma the nerve lies on the deep surface of the temporoparietal fascia. As the nerve crosses over the zygomatic arch, it lies between the perios-

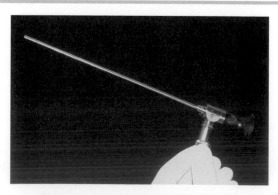

Figure 2 Endoscope used for facial surgery.

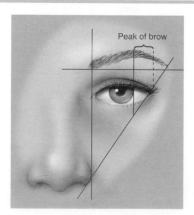

Peak of brow

Figure 4 Ideal peak brow position is located between the lateral canthus and lateral limbus.

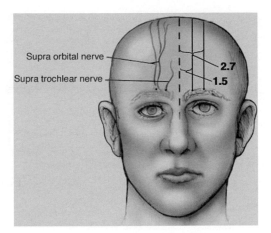

Figure 5 The ophthalmic division of the trigeminal nerve provides sensation to the forehead and scalp by way of the supraorbital and supratrochlear nerves.

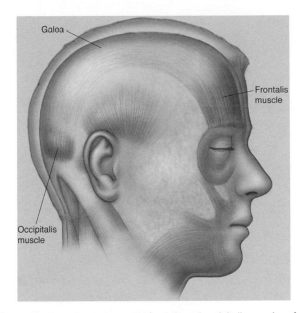

Figure 7 The galea connects the frontalis and occipitalis muscles of the scalp.

teum of the zygoma and the SMAS. Dissection in the region of the zygomatic arch requires caution to avoid injury to the nerve, and should be carried out either subcutaneously or subperiosteally. The course of the nerve may be approximated by a line drawn from a point 0.5 cm anterior to the tragus to a point 1.5 cm lateral to the lateral brow. The nerve enters the orbicularis oculi muscle and frontalis muscle along the deep surface of the muscles.

Fascial Layers of the Forehead and Temporal Region

The central forehead and scalp consist of five layers, the skin, subcutaneous tissue, galea aponeurosis, loose areolar tissue, and periosteum. The galea is a tendinous, inelastic sheet of tissue, which connects the frontalis muscle of the forehead with the occipitalis muscle (Fig. 7). The frontalis muscle originates from the galea and inserts into the forehead skin. At the superior orbital rim, the galea becomes tightly adherent to the periosteum. Laterally, the galea continues as the temporoparietal fascia which lies in the

immediate subcutaneous plane in the temporal region. The temporoparietal fascia is continuous with the SMAS layer of the face and the platysma layer of the neck (Fig. 8). Deep to the temporoparietal fascia lies the deep temporal fascia, which envelops the temporalis muscle. The deep temporal fascia, temporoparietal fascia, and the calvarial periosteum are contiguous at the temporal line of the skull, an area known as the conjoint tendon. The temporal fat pad, just superior to the zygomatic arch, is ensheathed by the temporal fascia inferior to the level of the supraorbital ridge. At that point, the temporal fascia splits to become the intermediate temporal fascia and the deep temporal fascia, separated by the fat pad. The intermediate fascia layer attaches to the superior aspect of the zygoma laterally, while the deep layer attaches medially (Fig. 9).

MUSCULATURE

There are four muscles in the forehead: frontalis, procerus, corrugator supercilii, and orbicularis oculi (Fig. 10). The frontalis is a paired subcutaneous muscle which inserts into the dermis of the eyebrow at the level of the supraorbital rim. Laterally, the frontalis terminates at the conjoint tendon. The frontalis muscle has no bony insertions, and its only action is brow elevation. It is the only brow elevator, while the other three forehead muscles depress the brows. Horizontal forehead rhytids correspond to the long-term effects of frontalis activation.

The frontalis muscle's dermal insertion at the brow extends inferonasally to form the procerus muscle, which originates from the caudal aspect of the nasal bones. Activity of the procerus muscle produces inferior brow displacement, and is responsible for horizontal glabellar wrinkles (Fig. 11).

The corrugator muscle originates from the nasal process of the frontal bone, near the superomedial orbital rim, and inserts into the dermis at the middle third of the eyebrow after blending with the frontalis and orbicularis muscles. Its action produces inferior and medial forehead

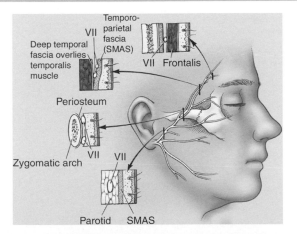

Figure 6 The frontal branch of the facial nerve has a variable depth along its course to the frontalis and orbicularis muscles. *Abbreviation*: SMAS, superficial musculoaponeurotic system.

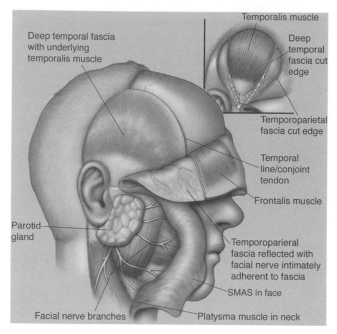

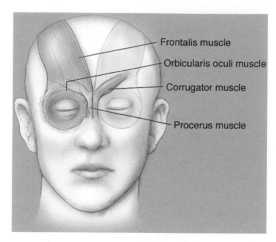

Figure 8 Temporoparietal fascia of forehead, superficial musculo-aponeurotic system layer of face, and platysma layer in the neck form a continuous fascial layer. The deep temporal fascia surrounds the temporalis muscle.

Figure 10 Forehead musculature. There are four muscles in the forehead, three of which are brow depressors and only one of which is a brow elevator (frontalis).

and brow movement, and results in vertical glabellar wrinkle (Fig. 12).

The orbicularis oculi muscle acts as a sphincter around the eye. The actions of the orbicularis muscle contribute to lateral brow depression, counteracting the effects of the frontalis muscle's elevator function.

Blood Supply

The internal and external carotid artery systems supply the blood to the forehead. The internal carotid artery, via the ophthalmic artery, branches to form the frontal, supraorbital, and

supratrochlear arteries. The external carotid artery system supplies the largest area of the scalp via the superficial temporal artery. Thus, there is a rich anastomotic complex of vessels providing adequate nutrients to the forehead, allowing for safety in esthetic surgery of the forehead.

ENDOSCOPIC BROW-LIFT TECHNIQUE

Until recently, the coronal approach to the forehead and brow was the gold standard. In recent years, with the development of endoscopic techniques, the endoscopic brow-lift has become increasingly popular. The long and potentially visible incisions of the coronal and trichophytic brow-lift, the high rate of alopecia, the widening of the scar, and the potential for pruritus and numbness prompted the demand for endoscopic techniques by the patient. The following is a

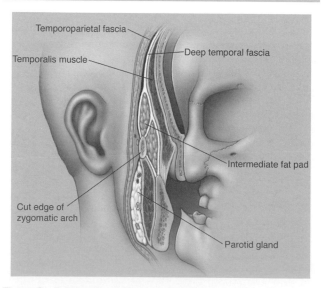

Figure 9 Relationship of zygoma to facial nerve temporoparietal fascia, deep temporal fascia, temporalis muscle, fat pads, and parotid gland.

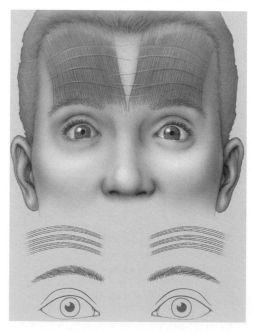

Figure 11 Activity of frontalis muscle is responsible for horizontal forehead wrinkles.

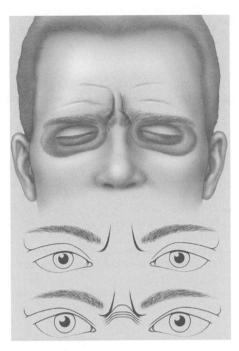

Figure 12 The corrugator muscle (vertical glabellar wrinkles) and the procerus muscle (horizontal glabellar wrinkles) are responsible for glabellar wrinkling.

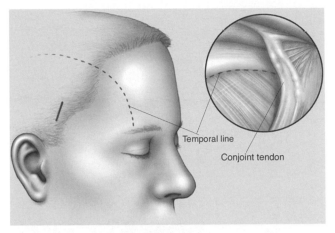

Figure 13 Incision used for endoscopic brow-lift and endoscopic mid-face-lift. (*Inset*) Conjoint tendon/temporal line marked with dotted line. Medial to this mark, subperiosteal dissection is performed while lateral to the mark, subtemporoparietal fascia dissection required.

standard technique; however, a number of subtle differences may exist among different surgeons.

Prior to administering sedation in the holding area, the patient is assessed in the sitting position. Brow positioning is determined, as is the degree of desired brow elevation. Skin markings may be performed in the holding area or in the operating room. Incision markings are 1 to 1.5 cm in length and 1.5 cm posterior to the anterior hairline. They are located in the midline and in the paramedian areas corresponding to the sites of desired vectors of pull (Fig. 13). Generally, the paramedian incision should be placed at the desired peak of the lateral brow, which typically corresponds to the lateral canthus. Incisions are carried down through all layers of the scalp to the skull with a number 15 scalpel blade. Temporal incisions are made 1 cm posterior to the temporal hairline, 3 cm superior to the helical root, in the region anterior to the superficial temporal vessels. These incisions are carried down to the level of the superficial layer of the deep temporal fascia. Elevation of the temporal region is achieved directly on the superficial layer of the deep temporal fascia, deep to the temporoparietal fascia, to avoid injury to the frontal branch of the facial nerve. Identification of the sentinel vein, located approximately 1 cm lateral to the lateral canthus and 1.3 cm cephalic to this point, is then achieved. Bipolar cautery of the sentinel vein is achieved at the deepest plane possible to avoid frontal nerve injury. The temporal line at the medial-most extent of the temporalis fascia is elevated off the frontal bone by entering a subperiosteal plane through the conjoint tendon (Fig. 14). The skull is exposed through the central and paramedian incisions. These access incisions allow for subperiosteal elevation of the forehead soft tissues to a point just inferior to the supraorbital rim. This subperiosteal elevation is performed under endoscopic visualization with a 30° endoscope to help preserve the supraorbital and supratrochlear neurovascular bundle. If necessary, the corrugator and procerus muscles may be

addressed at this time with transaction, resection, or denervation (Fig. 15). Once the supraorbital neurovascular pedicle is identified and preserved, periosteal relaxation incisions are made below the level of the brow with cautery to allow for optimal brow elevation. This is achieved along the entire width of the brow on either side of the forehead. Additional relaxing incisions may be made in a vertical direction at the glabella to help widen the interbrow distance and flatten the vertical glabellar rhytids. After adequate relaxing incisions are made in the periosteum, brow elevation is secured by fixation of the galea to the skull through the paramedian incisions. Lateral traction is supplied by fixation of the temporoparietal fascia to the deep temporal fascia through the lateral temporal incisions. Our preferred method for fixation of the forehead and brow to the skull utilizes a bone bridge and suture technique (2-0 Ethibond), although a variety of different fixation techniques and devices are available (Fig. 16). All incisions are closed in a single layer of 5-0 Vicryl Rapide suture.

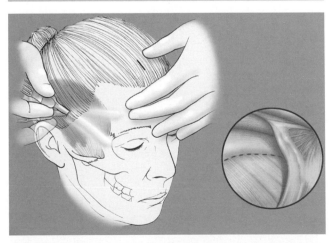

Figure 14 Dissection through temporal line allows for a transition from the subtemporoparietal fascia plane of dissection to a subperiosteal medial dissection. The subperiosteal plane allows access for brow-lift and midface-lift.

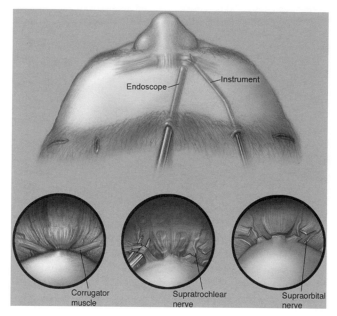

Figure 15 Subperiosteal dissection through the midline and paramedian incision exposes the corrugator and procerus muscles, and allows for preservation of the supratrochlear and supraorbital nerves and vessels.

The advantages of endoscopic forehead and brow-lifts are multiple. The incisions are well hidden, and may even be used in bald patients, as they heal inconspicuously. There is minimal alopecia and hairline alteration. There is less numbness in the forehead and scalp. Recovery time is less than with the open approach. Glabellar furrows are easily addressed through the endoscopic route.

The disadvantages of this procedure lie primarily in the learning curve required for facility with endoscopic equipment. In addition, specialized, expensive instrumentation is required for this procedure. As the endoscopic brow-lift procedure has only been used in recent years, the best method for fixation of the brow is still debated. The longevity of the endoscopic brow-lift has not yet been definitively established. Similar to the open coronal and pretrichial brow-lifts, the long distance between the brow and fixation point makes for less accurate and possibly less effective brow elevation.

ENDOSCOPIC MIDFACE-LIFT

Midface Anatomy

The presence of a high and prominent cheek bone conveys a youthful midfacial appearance. In addition to the underlying bony malar eminence, the malar mound is formed by a variety of soft-tissue components. The orbicularis oculi muscle extends beyond the eyelids to lie over the bony malar eminence. Both the superficial and deep surfaces of the malar orbicularis oculi muscle are associated with a fat pad. Superficial to the orbicularis is the subcutaneous malar fat pad. Deep to the orbicularis lies the suborbicularis oculi fat, also known as the SOOF. The SOOF layer of fat is in close contact with the periosteum of the inferior orbital rim as well as with the insertions of the zygomaticus muscles. The inferior and lateral orbital rims should be padded with malar fat and SOOF. In youth, the orbicularis maintains a sling around the orbital rim, but with the loss of orbicularis tone associated with aging, descent of the malar soft-tissue complex prevails (Fig. 17). As a result, there is a deepening of the nasolabial crease and exposure of the inferior and lateral orbital rims. Descent of the subcutaneous malar fat pads, and the suborbicularis oculi fat, results in a flattened malar eminence and prominent orbital rims which are esthetically displeasing. As midface aging progresses, the corners of the mouth sag to create a sad look in the perioral region. The mandibulolabial lines (marionette lines) deepen, and jowling occurs along the mandibular line. This combination of midfacial changes gives the face an aged appearance.

Midface-Lift Technique

Extended face-lifts may help to restore some youthfulness to the midface, but they are involved cases, requiring a great deal of operative and healing time. Standard face-lift techniques have been unable to correct the aging midface. Aging of the midface may occur independently of lower face and neck aging, thus extended face-lift and neck-lift procedures may be unnecessary. Minimally invasive techniques, which specifically address the midface, have become a great tool in facial esthetic surgery. They allow us to overcome the shortcomings of standard face-lift procedures, which neglected the midfacial structures, and also allow for a more defined area of enhancement with low morbidity and rapid recovery. Midface suspension may be performed by extension of endoscopic forehead-lifting procedures or through a subciliary approach to lower eyelid blepharoplasty.

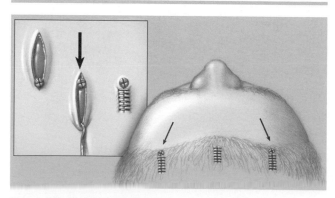

Figure 16 Staples and screws may be used for fixation of the brow in an elevated position.

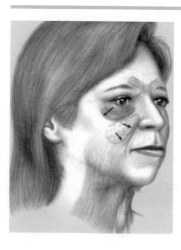

Figure 17 Descent of molar soft tissue and orbicularis muscle is responsible for midfacial aging.

With these techniques, midface tissues are repositioned superiorly to offset the effects of gravity and time.

The standard lateral temporal incision utilized for the endoscopic brow-lift also provides access to the midface. The skin incision is carried down to the superficial layer of deep temporal fascia, leaving the temporoparietal fascia attached to the skin and subcutaneous tissue. A lighted retractor or endoscope is then used to elevate in the subtemporoparietal fascia plane anteriorly toward the conjoint tendon, and inferiorly along the temporal line to the superior orbital rim (Fig. 14). Multiple vessels will be seen during the course of this dissection, and they act as indicators of the proximity to the frontal branch of the facial nerve. These vessels are cauterized with the bipolar cautery at the deepest plane possible so as to remain at a distance from the frontal branch. The frontal branch of the facial nerve is located within the temporoparietal fascia, superficial to the plane of dissection. The conjoint tendon is released with blunt and sharp dissection, allowing access to the subperiosteal plane and subsequent identification of the zygomaticofrontal suture line. Dissection continues in the subperiosteal plane from the zygomaticofrontal suture inferiorly along the lateral and inferior orbital rims, then to the malar eminence and the face of the maxilla (Fig. 18). A 1-cm gingivobuccal incision is made beginning at the canine and extending laterally. This facilitates dissection along the face of the maxilla and identification of the infraorbital nerve. Additionally, the zygomaticotemporal and zygomaticofacial nerves may be identified emanating from the corresponding suture lines. Dissection continues to the pyriform aperture and nasal bones in order to allow the greatest degree of mobility to the midface structures. A heavy absorbable suture is then used to secure the periosteum of the midface to the superficial layer of the deep temporal fascia. The suture may either be placed endoscopically or transorally through the gingivobuccal incision. The needle is then passed subperiosteally, along the face of the maxilla and zygoma, to the lateral temporal incision, and secured to the deep temporal fascia. A second suture may be used to further secure the midfacial tissues superiorly. The skin and gingivobuccal incisions are then closed.

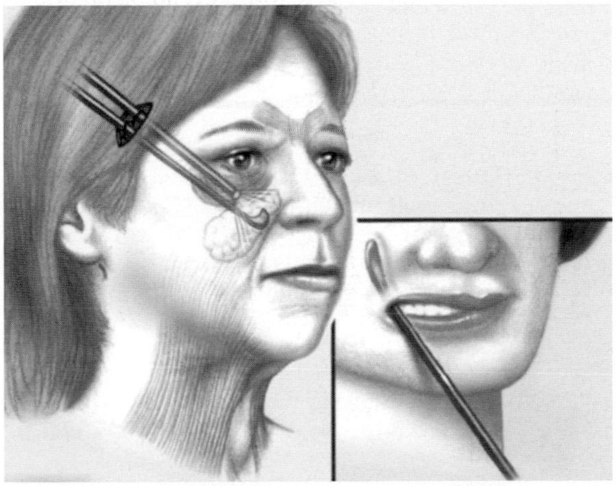

ENDOSCOPIC FACE-LIFT AND NECK-LIFT

In youth, the perioral area has minimal nasolabial folds and maximal fullness to the lips. With age comes prominence of the nasolabial folds, vertical rhytids around the mouth, and loss of exposed red lip. In youth, a well-defined mandibular line separates the face from the neck, creating two distinct esthetic units. As one ages, definition along the mandibular line is diminished due to loss of mandibular bone height, excess fat in the neck, platysmal dehiscence, and ptosis of skin and fat along the jaw line. This deformity of aging appears as a tissue bulge that hangs lateral and inferior to the mandibular body. Traditionally, the characteristics of aging of the lower face and neck have been managed with standard face-lift and neck-lift techniques. In recent years, techniques of endoscopic face and neck-lifting have been described.

In addition to the previously described brow-lift and midface-lift incisions in the lateral temporal region, access incisions for the lower face and neck are made behind the earlobe in the region of the mastoid bone, and in the submental crease. About 1 to 2-cm incisions allow for the introduction of an endoscope into the face and neck cavities (Fig. 19). Subcutaneous dissection is performed along the cheek, mandibular line, and neck, utilizing endoscopic scissors or dissectors. The dissection should free all of the skin from the underlying tissues to the midline of the neck (superficial to the platysma) and to the nasolabial fold. The endoscope is useful to insure that all fibrous bands that connect the skin to the deeper tissues are released, as well as to visualize any bleeding sites that require cautery for hemostasis. Under endoscopic visualization, the SMAS layer may be plicated and suspended vertically with sutures to the deep temporal fascia through the lateral temporal brow-lift incisions. Similarly, the platysma may be plicated at its lateral boundary and vertically suspended to the mastoid periosteum. The midline platysmal dehiscence may be addressed with placation and subcutaneous fat excision through the submental incision. The excess skin, which results from plication of the underlying tissues, may itself

Figure 18 Endoscopic access to midface tissues achieved through the lateral temporal access route and the intraoral route where dissection along the face of the maxilla occurs.

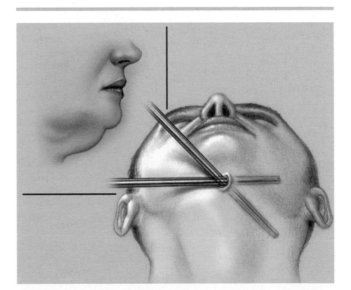

Figure 19 Endoscope introduced into submental incision to gain access to the neck for removal of fat and elevation of skin for neck-lift and face-lift procedures.

be plicated and hidden behind the ear. The midface is elevated through the lateral temporal brow-lift incision by grasping tissue in the nasolabial fold and suture suspending it to the deep temporal fascia, as described in the endoscopic midface-lift section. Endoscopic assistance in face and neck-lift procedures is limited to those cases in which a minor lift is desired. If significant face-lifting is achieved, the amount of excess skin may be too great to allow for postauricular plication. In such cases, excess skin must be excised with external incisions.

ENDOSCOPIC ASSISTANCE IN SEPTORHINOPLASTY

Rhinoplasty is generally performed through invisible intra-nasal incisions, or through external incisions. External approaches to rhinoplasty have been employed to aid with visualization and access to different areas of the nose. It is felt by many surgeons that the external rhinoplasty approach allows for more accurate management of nasal deformities because there is less reliance on palpation of deformities and more reliance on inspection of the deformities and their surgical corrections under direct vision. The application of endoscopic techniques to septorhinoplasty allows for outstanding visualization and may eliminate the need for an external incision.

Nasal septal deformities that are difficult to visualize and to correct surgically with traditional anterior rhinoscopy with a nasal speculum may be more easily visualized and surgically corrected with endoscopic guidance. Nasal endoscopy allows for the visualization of high dorsal and posterior septal deformities which may not have been addressed with traditional septoplasty techniques. The septum is approached in the standard fashion with a hemitransfixion incision, followed by elevation of the muco-perichondrial flaps under indirect endoscopic visualization. A 0° endoscope allows for visualization of the entire bony and cartilaginous septum under the mucosal flap. The Cottle or Freer (with or without suction) elevator may be used to transect and resect fragments of septal deviations. A thorough and safe septoplasty may be performed endoscopically due to the significantly improved visualization provided by the endoscopic view.

During the standard endonasal approach to rhino-plasty, the skin and soft-tissue envelopes are elevated off the nasal dorsum to allow for a direct view of, and access to, the dorsum. Because the view of the upper nasal dorsum (at the root of the nose) is somewhat limited, palpation of the nasal dorsum is essential in rhinoplasty. In order to improve visualization of the dorsum and to allow for more accurate dorsal alterations, the 0° endoscope may be introduced under the skin soft-tissue flap. The nasal hump, both cartilaginous and bony, may be rasped or resected under excellent endoscopic view. Once all alterations to the dorsum have been completed, the nasal endoscope may be reintroduced for final inspection to insure that all cartilaginous and bony fragments have been removed and that the dorsal surface is smooth. Thus, the endoscope may be used to prevent one of the most common causes for revision rhinoplasty—dorsal irregularities.

Endoscopic assistance in rhinoplasty is not intended to replace the standard rhinoplasty techniques which afford outstanding surgical control with minimal incisions. Rather, with increasing experience, endoscopic assistance may improve surgical results and limit the need for revision rhinoplasty. Small dorsal irregularities may easily be seen, and septal deformities may be more precisely addressed utilizing the endoscope for assistance.

CONCLUSION

Facial rejuvenation surgery has grown in popularity alongside our aging population. The increased demand for facial rejuvenation along with major technological advances in recent years has prompted the development of low morbidity procedures. Endoscopic facial plastic and reconstructive surgery has been established as a standard approach with outstanding success including lower morbidity and more rapid recovery when compared with open techniques.

BIBLIOGRAPHY

Aiache AE. Evolution of the endoscopic facelift. Facial Plast Surg Clin North Am 1997; 5(2):167–177.

Anderson RD, Lo MW. Endoscopic malar/midface suspension procedure. Plast Reconstr Surg 1998; 102:2196–2208.

Bergin DJ. Anatomy of the eyelids, lacrimal system, and orbit. In: McCord CD, Tanenbaum M, Nunery WR, eds. Oculoplastic Surgery. New York: Raven Press, 1995:51.

Byrd HS. The extended browlift. Clin Plast Surg 1997; 24:233.

Cook TA, Brownrigg AJ, Wang TD, et al. The versatile midforehead browlift. Arch Otolaryngol Head Neck Surg 1989; 115:163.

Giles WC, Gross CW, Abram AC, Greene WM, Avner TG. Endoscopic septoplasty. Laryngoscope 1994; 104:1507–1509.

Hochberg J, Miura Y, De Moura Paulo, Faria-Correa MA. Endoscopically assisted nasal surgery. Facial Plast Surg Clin North Am 1997; 5(2):203–210.

Howard BK, Leach J. Aesthetic Surgery of the Upper Third of the Face. A Self Instructional Package. Washington DC: American Academy of Otolaryngology Head and Neck Surgery Foundation, Inc.

Isse NG. Endoscopic facial rejuvenation: case reports. Aesthetic Plast Surg 1994; 18:21.

Isse NG. Endoscopic facial rejuvenation. Clin Plast Surg 1997; 24(2):213–231.

McKinney P, Massie RD, Zukowski ML. Criteria for the forehead lift. Aesthetic Plast Surg 1991; 15:141.

Millman B, Core GB. Endoscopic instrumentation and equipment for facial aesthetic surgery. Facial Plast Surg Clin North Am 1997; 5(2):85–94.

Mitz V. Endoscopic control during rhinoplasty. Aesthetic Plast Surg 1994; 18:153–156.

Quatela VC, Graham D, Sabini P. Rejuvenation of the brow and midface. In: Papel, Frodel, Holt, et al., eds. Facial Plastic and Reconstructive Surgery. 2nd ed. New York: Thieme, 2002:171.

Ramirez OM. Cervicoplasty: nonexcisional anterior approach. Plast Reconstr Surg 1997; 99(6):1576–1585.

Ramirez OM. Why I prefer the endoscopic forehead lift. Plast Reconstr Surg 1997; 100:1033.

Sykes JM. Applied anatomy of the forehead and brow. Facial Plast Surg Clin North Am 1997; 5(2):99–112.

82

Postsurgical Cosmetics

Zoe Diana Draelos

*Department of Dermatology, Wake Forest University School of Medicine,
Winston-Salem, North Carolina, U.S.A.*

INTRODUCTION

The postsurgical patient emerges with a new self-image whether the surgery was therapeutic or cosmetic. The patient may view the therapeutic surgery as deforming and experience a period of depression during which the patient withdraws from social situations with family and friends. Even when an elective cosmetic procedure is performed, there is a brief time during which uncertainty about the positive outcome of the surgery may cause emotional problems for the patient. The physician should anticipate these postsurgical difficulties and provide counseling.

Appropriate counseling should include expected time to healing and wound care instructions. The patient should thoroughly understand what changes are expected in the surgical site and are part of the normal healing process. Warning signs indicating problems and requiring medical evaluation should also be discussed.

Another often overlooked area of postsurgical counseling is helping patients maximize their appearance during and after the healing process. This counseling should include recommendations for appropriate skin care routines and the use of cosmetics. The patient should understand how to select appropriate cleansers, moisturizers, and sunscreens. Camouflage techniques should also be discussed, whether they are employed on a temporary or a permanent basis. Postsurgical cosmetics and skin care products are important for both the physical and the emotional well-being of the patient following surgery.

SKIN CHANGES IN THE POSTSURGICAL PATIENT

In the postsurgical patient, skin no longer functions as a barrier to the external environment. Therefore, all applied substances have much greater access to the dermal vasculature. This increases the probability of experiencing adverse reactions to topical products, including irritation (stinging, burning, itching, tingling), sensitization, and urticaria. Products must be carefully selected to meet the strictest standards to hypoallergenicity in the postsurgical patient. Unusual erythema, vesiculation, or urticaria in and around the postsurgical site suggests adverse reactions to topically applied material.

POSTOPERATIVE WOUND CARE AND COLORED COSMETICS

Cosmetics should not be applied to wounds that are healing by either first or second intention immediately following surgery. This generally is not a problem since cosmetics will not adhere to skin until the serous drainage from the wound has stopped. Premature application of colored cosmetics can create a foreign body reaction from the iron oxide or other pigments contained in the formulation.

Facial foundations are the most commonly used colored cosmetic in the postsurgical period. These cosmetics are pigmented lotions or creams that are applied to the face to hide blemishes and create an even skin tone. They are especially useful in the postsurgical patient to mask erythema and bruising. Facial foundations are composed of titanium dioxide, a covering agent, and iron oxide pigments. Both of these substances represent powders that could act as foreign bodies and impede wound healing by initiating an inflammatory response or providing an impetus for milia formation. Therefore, facial foundations and all other cosmetics should be avoided until re-epithelialization has occurred or the sutures have been removed.

TOPICAL THERAPEUTICS

Topical therapeutic agents may be used during the postsurgical period to enhance wound healing. Commonly employed topical products include antibiotic preparations and corticosteroids. The absence of an intact stratum corneum requires careful selection of postsurgical topical agents.

Topical antibiotics with the least sensitizing potential should be selected. Therefore, neomycin, a cause of allergic contact dermatitis, and polymixin B, a mast cell degranulater, should be avoided. Less sensitizing antibiotics such as polysporin, bacitracin, erythromycin, and mupirocin should be recommended for topical use. Patients who experience delayed wound healing should be patch-tested for topical antibiotic sensitivity.

Topical corticosteroids may also be used to decrease inflammation during the postsurgical period. Ointment preparations are preferred over gels, creams, and emollients as they have a petrolatum base and are less likely to contain cutaneous irritants, such as propylene glycol. Anhydrous, or water-free, preparations do not require high preservative concentrations, thus eliminating another potential source of irritancy or sensitization. Statistically, corticosteroids preserved with parabens have the least sensitizing potential, while products preserved with Kathons sensitize patients most often.

SKIN CARE PRODUCT SELECTION

Physicians should provide patients with a grooming routine during the postoperative period designed to optimize wound healing. Cleanser, moisturizer, and sunscreen products should be selected for each patient's individual requirements.

Cleansers

Cleansers used during the postoperative period should be nonirritating to minimize damage to newly formed epithelium. Immediately postoperative, lukewarm water may be the only cleanser required. As serum crusting begins, a synthetic detergent soap (e.g., Dove, Unilever; Cetaphil, Galderma; Oil of Olay, Procter & Gamble) gently cleanses without overdrying the skin. Synthetic detergent soaps are generally labeled as "beauty bars."

A newer variation on the beauty bar soap is the body wash. These emulsion cleansers combined water- and oil-soluble partitions into one continuous liquid phase. The water-soluble components dissolve sebum and skin debris, while the-oil soluble components, such as soybean oil, dimethicone, or petrolatum, leave behind a thin moisturizing film on the skin surface. Petrolatum-rich body washes (e.g., Olay Complete Bodywash for Dry Skin, Procter & Gamble) are useful in patients with large body surface areas devoid of an intact barrier, such as following dermabrasion, laser resurfacing, or chemical peeling.

Lipid-free cleansing lotions (e.g., Cetaphil, Galderma; CeraVe, Coria), used with or without water, can also gently cleanse a wound. They do not possess substantial antibacterial properties, however. In surgical sites where bacterial contamination may be a problem, deodorant soaps containing triclosan (e.g., Dial, Dial Corporation) may be appropriate. Antibacterial beauty bar soaps are available (e.g., Lever 2000, Unilever) and may be helpful in sensitive complected patients who are at risk of a wound infection.

Moisturizers

Moisturizer use is important for the postsurgical patient since the barrier to transepidermal water loss is absent. This allows free water evaporation from the skin, creating a tight sensation accompanied by pruritus. Furthermore, desiccation impedes wound healing, which proceeds most rapidly in a moist environment.

Immediately after surgery, pure white petroleum jelly may be the best moisturizer. It is an excellent occlusive, thus trapping moisture within the skin. It is used as a negative control for dermatologic patch testing because its irritation and sensitization potentials are low. Furthermore, it is extremely economical. Drawbacks to petroleum jelly are its greasy appearance, odor, and ability to stain natural fiber fabrics.

Once re-epithelialization has begun, oil-in-water formulations (Eucerin Cream, Biersdorf; Acid Mantle Cream, Doak) may be substituted and are more cosmetically elegant. Creams should be selected over lotions since they are better moisturizers and, are less likely to contain irritants. Products should be chosen for their paucity of ingredients. Therefore, creams with fragrances, herbal or biological additives, and specialty ingredients should be avoided until complete healing has occurred.

There are several new moisturizer ingredients that may be of importance for the postsurgical patient. One of the more interesting substances that may facilitate healing is synthetic ceramide 3 (Nouriva Cream, Ferndale Laboratories). Ceramide 3 is a synthetic analog of one of the ceramides found in the intercellular lipids necessary for barrier restoration. Ceramide 3 acts as an occlusive moisturizer, but may also cut down in the stratum corneum healing time making it useful in the postoperative period.

Another important ingredient functioning to enhance the water holding capacity of injured resurfaced skin is glycerin. Twice daily application of a high-concentration glycerin moisturizer (Norwegian Formula Hand Cream, Neutrogena) can create a glycerin reservoir and prevent tissue desiccation. Creation of a glycerin reservoir provides excellent skin hydration, especially in patients who have prolonged scabbing and crusting following a resurfacing procedure.

Lastly, patients may not find petrolatum very cosmetically acceptable, but need a highly occlusive moisturizer due to loss of the skin barrier. Facial moisturizers containing acrylate, a film-forming polymer, can provide an artificial barrier without the greasy feeling of petrolatum (Cetaphil Cream, Galderma). Acrylate moisturizers can be used in the resurfacing patient one week following the procedure.

A variety of specialty ingredients have entered the postsurgical moisturizer market. Two worthy of note are niacinamide and gluconolactone. Niacinamide is the amide derivative of niacin, which is a component of NADPH. NADPH is part of the energy production machinery of the cell. Niacinamide (Olay Total Effects, Procter & Gamble) functions as a vitamin exfoliant speeding turnover and maintaining a smooth skin surface immediately after healing has occurred. This nonirritating therapeutic moisturizer additive may be useful following resurfacing procedures after early re-epithelialization has occurred. For patients who require more aggressive exfoliation, gluconolactone-containing moisturizers may be useful. Gluconolactone is a polyhydroxy acid capable of inducing exfoliation on the skin surface without irritation following resurfacing. It can also function as a humectant enhancing the water-binding capacity of the skin. It is a larger molecular weight hydroxy acid minimizing dermal penetration and the stinging and burning that can accompany exfoliation following resurfacing. However, gluconolactone should not be applied to the skin surface until healing has been completed.

Sunscreens

Sun exposure to the surgical site should be avoided after surgery, as the skin has lost its ability to adequately protect against photodamage. Postinflammatory hyperpigmentation may also result. Many patients will continue their daily activities, which may include casual sun exposure. All chemical sunscreening agents (cinnamate derivatives, benzophenones, etc.) are potential causes of both irritant and allergic contact dermatitis.

The physician may suggest use of an inorganic or particulate sunscreen, such as zinc oxide or titanium dioxide. These are broad-spectrum UVA and UVB screens that both reflect and scatter radiation. They are inert and thus cause neither irritant nor allergic contact dermatitis. Zinc oxide is the preferable sunscreen active for daily wear because the silicone-coated particles do not cause wound inflammation and do not whiten the skin (Olay Complete Daily Facial Moisturizer SPF 15, Procter & Gamble). Titanium dioxide is the preferred sunscreen ingredient for beachwear or under high humidity conditions because the larger particle size stays in place better (Neutrogena SPF 15 for Sensitive Skin, Neutrogena).

COSMETIC SELECTION

Cosmetics available for camouflage purposes in the postsurgical patient include foundations, cover creams, and color correctors.

Foundations

Facial foundations are designed to add color, cover blemishes, and blend uneven facial color. Postsurgical patients commonly have residual erythema for two weeks to six months following the procedure depending on the type of surgery, speed of healing, and skin color of the patient. Facial foundations are an excellent method of camouflaging postsurgical erythema.

Facial foundations used for blending erythema do not require the coverage necessary for surgical camouflaging. These facial foundations can be powders that are stroked across the skin, such as Maybelline Purestay Powder Foundation, Cover Girl Simply Powder, L'Oreal Air Wear Breathable Long-Wearing Powder Foundation, or Cover Girl Ultimate Finish Liquid Powder Makeup (higher coverage). If more complete coverage is required, a surgical cover cream is preferred.

Cover Creams

Cover creams are also facial foundations, but they are designed to provide opaque cover, thus completely obscuring the underlying skin. They are formulated as creams, sticks, and compressed powders. Cream and stick formulations may be waterproof, while the compressed powders are not water resistant. The most widely marketed cover cream is Dermablend. This product is available at department stores where a trained consultant can assist the patient in proper color selection and demonstrate application techniques. Surgical cover creams require skill and practice to achieve a good cosmetic result.

Color Correctors

Color correctors are liquid or cream facial foundations in specialty colors designed to aid in blending of unwanted skin tones. They contain additional pigments to produce colors of green, of purple, orange, peach, pink, etc. Their use will be more fully discussed later.

BASIC CAMOUFLAGE TECHNIQUES

Postsurgical cutaneous defects can be divided into pigmentation abnormalities and contour abnormalities. Surgery may also destroy appendageal structures resulting in the absence of cutaneous texture and landmarks.

Pigmentation Abnormalities

Pigmentation abnormalities can be corrected by the use of facial foundations, cover creams, and color correctors. Facial foundations can be used if the pigmentation problem is minor erythema, hypopigmentation, or hyperpigmentation. If bruising, depigmentation, or dark hyperpigmentation is present then a cover cream such as Dermablend should be selected.

Cover creams, also known as surgical camouflaging cosmetics, require special application and removal techniques. They are completely opaque and can cover any underlying pigmentation problem. In order to obtain high coverage, long wearability, and waterproof qualities, proper application is essential.

Prior to application of the cosmetic, a proper color match should be determined. The stock cosmetic color closest to the patient's natural skin color should be selected and a small amount should be scooped from the jar onto the back of the patient's hand. The back of the hand is an excellent surface for warming the stiff cosmetic and blending the appropriate color. Additional makeup colors can

be blended with a cosmetic spatula until the desired color is obtained. All hues present in the patient's skin should be represented, but it is better not to blend more than three colors.

Once the final color has been obtained, it is dabbed (not rubbed) over the face. Application should begin over the central face with blending into the hairline, over each tragus, and down beneath the jawline. No lines of demarcation should be present where cosmetic application has stopped. It is important to dab the cosmetic, since rubbing may remove foundation applied earlier. Foundation does not adhere to facial scars as well, since appendageal structures are decreased or absent.

The cover cream must now be set with a translucent powder. The powder is pressed into the foundation to impart a matte finish and waterproof characteristics. The foundation may require some touch-up, but surgical facial foundations are designed to wear eight hours, and most colored cosmetics applied on top of the surgical foundation wear better than when applied directly to the skin.

An alternative to an opaque surgical cover cream is the use of color correctors. Color correctors are applied under a facial foundation to avoid the use of surgical cosmetics. They are based on the principle of complementary colors. For example, red pigmentation defects can be camouflaged by applying a green color corrector foundation. The blending of red skin with green foundation yields a brown tone, which can be readily covered by a more conventional facial foundation. Yellow skin tones can be blended with a complementary colored purple foundation to also yield brown tones. Bluish bruising can be camouflaged with a peach- or orange-colored corrector.

Contour Abnormalities

Contour abnormalities represent areas of hypertrophy or atrophy within the surgical scar. Contour defects cannot be masked with foundations, cover creams, or color correctors and may accentuate contour abnormalities with a shiny finish.

High- and low-skin areas are camouflaged by shading. Contour camouflaging is based on the principle that dark areas recede while light areas project. Thus, a depressed scar will appear darker than the surrounding skin simply due to the shadows created. Conversely, a hypertrophied scar will appear lighter than the surrounding skin due to the lack of shadows. A lighter cosmetic, either a facial foundation or a blush, can be applied to depressed scars while a darker cosmetic, either a facial foundation or blush, can be applied to hypertrophied scars. Achieving a good cosmetic result requires some artistic skill and practice. Fortunately, poor results can be easily removed. Patients left with chronic contour abnormalities may wish to seek the services of a paramedical camouflage artist who can assist them in cosmetic selection, color blending, and cosmetic application.

Recreating Cutaneous Texture and Landmarks

Many procedures, such as Mohs micrographic surgery, flaps, or grafts, destroy appendageal structures, thus creating skin of different texture once healing has occurred. Furthermore, surgery requiring removal of significant amounts of normal tissue may remove folds and contours on the face that create important landmarks, such as the nasal groove, nasolabial fold, chin crease, etc. Camouflage techniques are also available to restore these cutaneous textures and landmarks.

Scarred skin may be devoid of hair. If the male beard is missing in a key area on the face, cover creams alone will not be able to adequately reproduce the color or texture of beard stipple. Beard stipple can be added by dipping a coarse sponge into black theatrical powder and then pressing the sponge into the surgical foundation.

If there are areas where it is critical to more accurately reproduce hair, such as the eyebrow area, a prosthesis can be constructed. Crepe wool, yak hair, and human hair are three materials from which missing eyebrows can be created. Crepe wool is a wool-like material that is inexpensive and available in a wide variety of colors. Yak hair and human hair give more realistic results but are more expensive and require greater application skill. The fibers can be glued with spirit gum on a daily basis to the affected area, or a permanent prosthesis can be constructed, if necessary.

Skin folds, wrinkles, bags, jowls, or pouches are actually painted on the face. Powdered or cream colors in various shades of gray, red, and brown are used to artistically create these landmarks and minimize the appearance of the facial deformity. More detailed discussion of the techniques used can be obtained from texts on stage makeup.

SPECIFIC CAMOUFLAGE TECHNIQUES

Specific camouflage techniques are used following dermabrasion and face peels, cryosurgery and electrosurgery, laser surgery, and incisional surgery.

Dermabrasion and Face Peels

Dermabrasion and face peel patients have temporary erythema, which can be easily camouflaged with a superior facial foundation (Workout Makeup, Clinique). The oily foundations will help smooth skin scale and decrease transepidermal water loss. The foundation should not be applied, however, until re-epithelialization has occurred. Once the reddish skin hues have faded to pink, the patients may resume their normal foundation. For individuals with long-standing vibrant red skin tones, especially following a vigorous dermabrasion, a green color corrector may be used under the foundation to aid in camouflage.

CRYOSURGERY AND ELECTROSURGERY

Cryosurgery and electrosurgery usually induce localized wounding that is allowed to heal by second intention. Once a serum crust has formed, a dab of cover cream can be applied to the area and blended with the patient's usual facial foundation. If erythema is persistent following re-epithelialization, a green color corrector may be used under the foundation.

Laser Surgery

Bruising may be a sequlae following facial treatment with some lasers. Purplish-red bruising is best camouflaged with a green color corrector under foundation, while bluish bruising is best camouflaged with an orange color corrector under foundation. As the bruise resolves and the yellowish-brown hemosiderin pigments become apparent, a purple color corrector may be used.

Incisional Surgery

Incisional surgery creates scars that are generally permanent. If extensive Mohs micrographic surgery is performed or if a graft or flap is required, contour and pigmentation abnormalities may occur. These patients generally do best with surgical facial foundations such as Dermablend. If the scarring is severe, the patient should receive professional instruction in application of the product. Lightening of depressions and darkening of hypertrophic areas may be needed to minimize contour abnormalities. Cutaneous textures and landmarks can be recreated, as previously discussed.

SUMMARY

It is important for the dermatologist to make the postsurgical patients comfortable with their new image following surgery. This entails counseling the patient on postoperative wound care, the appropriate use of skin care products, cosmetic selection, and camouflage techniques, if appropriate. The dermatologist who has knowledge in these areas can improve both the patient satisfaction and, ultimately, the final result.

BIBLIOGRAPHY

Allsworth J. Skin Camouflage. Cheltenham, U.K.: Stanley Throes Ltd, 1985.

Cash TF, Cash DW. Women's use of cosmetics. Int J Cosmet Sci 1982; 4:1.

Draelos ZK. Atlas of Cosmetic Dermatology. Edinburgh: Churchill Livingstone, 2000.

Draelos ZK. Cosmetic camouflaging techniques. Cutis 1993; 52(6):362–364.

Rayner V. Clinical Cosmetology. Albany: Milady Publishing, 1993.